The ASAM Essentials of
Addiction
Medicine

THIRD EDITION

The **ASAM Essentials** of
Addiction Medicine

THIRD EDITION

Abigail J. Herron, DO
Vice President for Behavioral Health
Director of Psychiatry and Addiction Medicine
The Institute for Family Health
New York, New York

Tim K. Brennan, MD, MPH
Director, Fellowship in Addiction Medicine Program
Icahn School of Medicine at Mount Sinai
Vice President, Medical and Academic Affairs
American College of Academic Addiction Medicine
New York, New York

A summary text of *The ASAM Principles of Addiction Medicine,*
6th Edition, **edited by Shannon C. Miller, David A. Fiellin,**
Richard N. Rosenthal, and Richard Saitz

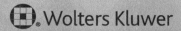

. Wolters Kluwer

Philadelphia · Baltimore · New York · London
Buenos Aires · Hong Kong · Sydney · Tokyo

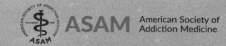

ASAM American Society of
Addiction Medicine

Acquisitions Editor: Chris Teja
Development Editor: Ariel S. Winter
Editorial Coordinator: Ashley Pfeiffer
Editorial Assistant: Brian Convery
Marketing Manager: Rachel Mante Leung
Production Project Manager: David Saltzberg
Design Coordinator: Terry Mallon
Manufacturing Coordinator: Beth Welsh
Prepress Vendor: Absolute Service, Inc.

Third Edition

9 8 7 6

Printed in the United States of America

Library of Congress Cataloging-in-Publication Data

Names: Herron, Abigail J., 1977- editor. | Brennan, Timothy, editor. |
    American Society of Addiction Medicine, issuing body.
Title: The ASAM essentials of addiction medicine / [edited by] Abigail J.
    Herron, Tim K. Brennan.
Other titles: Principles of addiction medicine (Cavacuiti) | Abridgement of
    (work): ASAM principles of addiction medicine.
Description: Third edition. | Philadelphia : Wolters Kluwer
Health/Lippincott
    Williams & Wilkins, [2020] | Abridgement of: The ASAM principles of
    addiction medicine / senior editor, Shannon C. Miller ; associate
editors,
    David A. Fiellin, Richard N. Rosenthal, and Richard Saitz. Sixth edition.
    [2019]. | Includes bibliographical references.
Identifiers: LCCN 2018058204 | ISBN 9781975107956 (paperback)
Subjects: | MESH: Substance-Related Disorders—therapy | Behavior, Addictive
    | Substance-Related Disorders—diagnosis | Handbook
Classification: LCC RC564 | NLM WM 34 | DDC 362.29—dc23 LC record available
at https://lccn.loc.gov/2018058204

shop.lww.com

Editors of *The ASAM Principles of Addiction Medicine, Sixth Edition*

SENIOR EDITOR

Shannon C. Miller, MD, DFAPA, DFASAM
Director, Addiction Services
VA Medical Center
Faculty, Neuroscience Graduate Program
Professor of Clinical Psychiatry, Affiliated
University of Cincinnati College of Medicine
Cincinnati, Ohio
Past Founding Co-Editor, Journal of Addiction
Medicine (2006–2016), American Society of
    Addiction Medicine
Lieutenant Colonel, United States Air Force, Retired

ASSOCIATE EDITORS

David A. Fiellin, MD, FASAM
Professor of Medicine, Emergency Medicine and
    Public Health
Director, Program in Addiction Medicine
Yale School of Medicine
New Haven, Connecticut

Richard N. Rosenthal, MA, MD, DFAPA, DFAAAP, FASAM
Professor of Psychiatry
Director of Addiction Psychiatry
Department of Psychiatry
Stony Brook University Medical Center
Stony Brook, New York

Richard Saitz, MD, MPH, FACP, FASAM
Chairman, Department of Community Health
    Sciences (CHS)
Professor of Community Health Sciences & Medicine
Boston University Schools of Public Health and
    Medicine
Clinical Addiction Research and Education (CARE)
    Unit
Section of General Internal Medicine
Boston Medical Center
Boston, Massachusetts

SECTION EDITORS

Peter Banys, MD, MSc
Clinical Professor of Psychiatry
University of California at San Francisco (UCSF)
San Francisco, California
Technical Expert, Addiction Treatment
WHO and European Union EPOS
Manila, Philippines

William C. Becker, MD
Associate Professor of Medicine (General Internal
    Medicine)
Yale University School of Medicine
New Haven, Connecticut
Co-Director, Opioid Reassessment Clinic
VA Connecticut Healthcare System
West Haven, Connecticut

J. Wesley Boyd, MD, PhD
Associate Professor of Psychiatry and Faculty, Center
    for Bioethics
Harvard Medical School
Boston, Massachusetts
Staff Psychiatrist
Cambridge Health Alliance
Cambridge, Massachusetts

Tim K. Brennan, MD, MPH
Director, Fellowship in Addiction Medicine Program
Icahn School of Medicine at Mount Sinai
Vice President, Medical and Academic Affairs
American College of Academic Addiction Medicine
New York, New York

Martin D. Cheatle, PhD
Associate Professor, Department of Psychiatry
Perelman School of Medicine
University of Pennsylvania
Director, Pain and Chemical Dependency Program
Center for Studies of Addiction
Perelman School of Medicine
University of Pennsylvania
Philadelphia, Pennsylvania

Wilson M. Compton, MD, MPE
Deputy Director
National Institute on Drug Abuse
National Institutes of Health
U.S. Department of Health and Human Services
Bethesda, Maryland

John A. Dani, PhD
David J. Mahoney Professor of Neuroscience
Perelman School of Medicine
University of Pennsylvania
Chair, Department of Neuroscience
Director, Mahoney Institute for Neuroscience
Perelman School of Medicine
Philadelphia, Pennsylvania

Lori J. Ducharme, PhD
Program Director for Health Services Research
National Institute on Alcohol Abuse and Alcoholism
Bethesda, Maryland

Robert L. DuPont, MD
President, Institute for Behavior and Health, Inc.
Rockville, Maryland
Clinical Professor of Psychiatry
Georgetown University School of Medicine
Washington, District of Columbia

Rollin M. Gallagher, MD, MPH
Clinical Professor of Psychiatry and Anesthesiology
Director for Pain Policy Research and Primary Care
Perelman School of Medicine
University of Pennsylvania
Philadelphia, Pennsylvania

R. Jeffrey Goldsmith, MD
Professor of Clinical Psychiatry
Department of Psychiatry and Clinical Neuroscience
University of Cincinnati College of Medicine
Staff Psychiatrist
Mental Health Care Line
Cincinnati VA Medical Center
Cincinnati, Ohio

Adam Joseph Gordon, MD, MPH, FACP, DFASAM, CMRO
Elbert F. and Marie Christensen Endowed Research
   Professorship
Professor of Medicine and Psychiatry
University of Utah School of Medicine
Section Chief, Addiction Medicine
Salt Lake City VA Health Care System
Salt Lake City, Utah

David A. Gorelick, MD, PhD, DLFAPA
Professor of Psychiatry
University of Maryland School of Medicine
Baltimore, Maryland

Jon E. Grant, MD, JD, MPH
Professor
Department of Psychiatry & Behavioral Neuroscience
Pritzker School of Medicine
University of Chicago
Chicago, Illinois

John R. Knight Jr., MD
Associate Professor of Pediatrics
Harvard Medical School
Director, Center for Adolescent Substance Abuse Research
Division of Developmental Medicine
Boston Children's Hospital
Boston, Massachusetts

Thomas R. Kosten, MD
Waggoner Chair and Professor of Psychiatry,
   Neuroscience, Pharmacology, Immunology &
   Pathology
Director, Dan Duncan Institute for Clinical and
   Translational Research
Baylor College of Medicine, Michael E. DeBakey
   VAMC
Houston, Texas

Kevin Kunz, MD, MPH, DFASAM
Executive Vice President
The Addiction Medicine Foundation
Chevy Chase, Maryland

Patrick G. O'Connor, MD, MPH
Dan Adams and Amanda Adams Professor of General
   Medicine
Chief, Section of General Internal Medicine
Department of Internal Medicine
Yale School of Medicine
New Haven, Connecticut

Theodore V. Parran Jr., MD, FACP, FASAM
Isabel and Carter Wang Professor and Chair in
   Medical Education
CWRU School of Medicine
Co-Medical Director, Rosary Hall
St. Vincent Charity Medical Center
Cleveland, Ohio

Richard K. Ries, MD, FASAM, FAPA
Professor of Psychiatry
Director Addictions Division
Department of Psychiatry and Behavioral Sciences
University of Washington School of Medicine
Seattle, Washington

Richard N. Rosenthal, MA, MD, DFAPA, DFAAAP, FASAM
Professor of Psychiatry
Director of Addiction Psychiatry
Department of Psychiatry
Stony Brook University Medical Center
Stony Brook, New York

Seddon R. Savage, MD, MS, DFASAM
Adjunct Associate Professor of Anesthesiology
Geisel School of Medicine at Dartmouth
Hanover, New Hampshire

Andrew J. Saxon, MD
Professor
Psychiatry and Behavioral Sciences
University of Washington School of Medicine
Director, Center of Excellence in Substance Addiction
    Treatment and Education
Mental Health Service
VA Puget Sound Health Care System
Seattle, Washington

Corinne L. Shea, MA
Director of Programs and Communications
Institute for Behavior and Health, Inc.
Rockville, Maryland

Daryl Shorter, MD
Director of Residency Education
Assistant Professor
Menninger Department of Psychiatry and
    Behavioral Sciences
Staff Psychiatrist
Michael E. DeBakey VA Medical Center
Houston, Texas

Deborah R. Simkin, MD
Adjunct Assistant Professor
Emory School of Medicine
Atlanta, Georgia

Jeanette M. Tetrault, MD, FACP, FASAM
Associate Professor of Medicine
Yale School of Medicine
Program Director
Addiction Medicine Fellowship
Yale Hospital
New Haven, Connecticut

Bonnie B. Wilford, MS
Executive Vice President
Coalition on Physician Education in Substance Use
    Disorders (COPE)
Easton, Maryland

Christine Yuodelis-Flores, MD, FAPA, FASAM
Associate Professor
Department of Psychiatry and Behavioral Sciences
University of Washington
Harborview Medical Center
Seattle, Washington

Joan E. Zweben, PhD
Clinical Professor
Psychiatry
University of California, San Francisco
Staff Psychologist
Substance Abuse
Veterans Affairs Medical Center
San Francisco, California

Contributors to *The ASAM Essentials of Addiction Medicine, Third Edition*

Catreena Al Marj, MD
Post-Doctoral Fellow
University of Utah
Salt Lake City, Utah

Laith Al-Rabadi, MD
Assistant Professor
Internal Medicine-Renal Division
University of Utah
Salt Lake City, Utah

Daniel P. Alford, MD, MPH, FACP, DFASAM
Professor of Medicine
Section of General Internal
    Medicine
Boston University School of
    Medicine
Director, Clinical Addiction
    Research and Education
    (CARE) Unit
Section of General Internal
    Medicine
Boston Medical Center
Boston, Massachusetts

Jeffrey Allgaier, MD, FACEP
Medical Director
Ideal Option, PLLC
Dunbarton, Washington

Christopher A. Arger, PhD
Clinical Psychologist
Iora Health
Mesa, Arizona

Ashraf Attalla, MD
Associate Professor of Psychiatry
Emory University School of
    Medicine
Atlanta, Georgia
Program Director
Youth Services at Ridgeview
    Institute
Smyrna, Georgia

Sanford Auerbach, MD
Associate Professor
Departments of Neurology,
    Psychiatry and Behavioral
    Neurosciences
Boston University School of
    Medicine
Director
Sleep Disorders Center
Boston Medical Center
Boston, Massachusetts

Robert L. Balster, PhD
Butler Professor of Pharmacology
    and Toxicology, Research
    Professor of Psychology and
    Psychiatry
Virginia Commonwealth
    University
Richmond, Virginia

Kristen L. Barry, PhD
Research Professor Emeritus
Department of Psychiatry
University of Michigan
Ann Arbor, Michigan

Andrea G. Barthwell, MD, DFASAM
Clinical Professor
School of Social Welfare
State University of New York,
    Stony Brook
Stony Brook, New York

Michael H. Baumann, PhD
Chief
Designer Drug Research Unit
    (DDRU)
IRP, NIDA, NIH, DHHS
Baltimore, Maryland

Nicolas Bertholet, MD, MSc
Private Docent, Senior Lecturer
Faculty of Biology and Medicine
Lausanne University
Deputy Physician
Department of Community
    Medicine and Health, Alcohol
    Treatment Center
Lausanne University Hospital
Lausanne, Switzerland

Roger L. Bertholf, PhD
Professor
Clinical Pathology and Laboratory
    Medicine
Weill Medical College of Cornell
    University
New York, New York
Medical Director of Clinical
    Chemistry
Department of Pathology and
    Genomic Medicine
Houston Methodist Hospital
Houston, Texas

James Besante, MD
Resident Physician
Mount Auburn Internal Medicine
Residency Program
Cambridge, Massachusetts

Thomas J.R. Beveridge, MSc, PhD
Assistant Professor
Physiology and Pharmacology
Wake Forest School of Medicine
Winston Salem, North Carolina
Medical Director
Medical Affairs, Oncology
Ipsen Biopharmaceuticals
Cambridge, Massachusetts

Jennifer Bielenberg, PsyD
Psychology Postdoctoral
  Fellow, Substance Use and
  Co-Occurring Disorders
Mental Health Service
San Francisco VA Medical Center
San Francisco, California

Joyce N. Bittinger, PhD
University of Washington
Seattle, Washington

Erika Litvin Bloom, PhD
Assistant Professor (Research)
Department of Psychiatry
  and Human Behavior and
  Department of Medicine
Alpert Medical School of Brown
  University
Psychologist
Division of General Internal
  Medicine
Rhode Island Hospital
Providence, Rhode Island

Frederic C. Blow, PhD
Professor
Department of Psychiatry
Adjunct Professor
Department of Psychology
University of Michigan
Director
University of Michigan Addiction
  Center
Substance Abuse Section
Michigan Medicine
Ann Arbor, Michigan

Jacob T. Borodovsky, BA
PhD Candidate
Center for Technology and
  Behavioral Health & The
  Dartmouth Institute for Health
  Policy and Clinical Practice
Dartmouth Geisel School of
  Medicine
Lebanon, New Hampshire

Gilbert J. Botvin, PhD
Professor Emeritus
Department of Healthcare Policy
  and Research
Weill Cornell Medical College
New York, New York

Andria M. Botzet, MA, LAMFT
Family Therapist
Department of Psychiatry
University of Minnesota
Minneapolis, Minnesota

J. Wesley Boyd, MD, PhD
Associate Professor of Psychiatry
  and Faculty, Center for
  Bioethics
Harvard Medical School
Boston, Massachusetts
Staff Psychiatrist
Cambridge Health Alliance
Cambridge, Massachusetts

Katharine A. Bradley, MD, MPH
Senior Investigator
Kaiser Permanente Washington
  Health Research
Kaiser Permanente Washington
Affiliate Professor
Medicine and Health Services
University of Washington
Seattle, Washington

Alyssa M. Braxton, MD
Addiction Fellow
Department of Psychiatry
Medical University of South
  Carolina
Charleston, South Carolina

Robert M. Bray, PhD
Chief Scientist (Retired)
Division of Behavioral Health and
  Criminal Justice
Research Triangle Institute
Research Triangle Park, North
  Carolina

Tim K. Brennan, MD, MPH
Director, Fellowship in Addiction
  Medicine Program
Icahn School of Medicine at
  Mount Sinai
Vice President, Medical and
  Academic Affairs
American College of Academic
  Addiction Medicine
New York, New York

Traci L. Brooks, MD
Instructor in Pediatrics
Department of Pediatrics
Harvard Medical School
Boston, Massachusetts
Medical Director, School-Based
  Health Centers
Cambridge Health Alliance
Cambridge, Massachusetts

**Lawrence S. Brown Jr., MD,
MPH, DFASAM**
Clinical Associate Professor of
  Medicine, Healthcare Policy and
  Research
Department of Medicine
Weill Medical College of Cornell
  University
New York, New York
Chief Executive Officer
START Treatment & Recovery
  Centers
Brooklyn, New York

Richard A. Brown, PhD
Research Professor
School of Nursing
University of Texas at Austin
Austin, Texas

Deepa Camenga, MD, MHS
Assistant Professor
Emergency Medicine
Yale School of Medicine
Attending Physician
Pediatrics
Yale New Haven Hospital
New Haven, Connecticut

James W. Campbell, MD, MS
Professor of Family Medicine
Case Western Reserve University
Chair
Geriatrics
MetroHealth Medical Center
Cleveland, Ohio

Faye Chao, MD
Assistant Professor
Department of Psychiatry
Icahn School of Medicine at
  Mount Sinai
New York, New York
Attending Psychiatrist
Department of Psychiatry
James J. Peters VA Medical Center
Bronx, New York

Martin D. Cheatle, PhD
Associate Professor, Department
  of Psychiatry
Perelman School of Medicine
University of Pennsylvania
Director, Pain and Chemical
  Dependency Program
Center for Studies of Addiction
Perelman School of Medicine
University of Pennsylvania
Philadelphia, Pennsylvania

Benjamin M. Clemens, MSW
Associate Vice President
Behavioral Health
The Institute for Family Health
New York, New York

Jeffrey S. Cluver, MD
Associate Professor of Psychiatry
  & Behavioral Sciences
Deputy Chair & Vice Chair for
  Education & Training
Medical University of South
  Carolina
Charleston, South Carolina

Andrea Cole, PhD, MSW
Behavioral Health Research
  Coordinator
Behavioral Health
Institute for Family Health
New York, New York

John J. Coleman, MA, MS, PhD
President
Prescription Drug Research Center
Chicago, Illinois

Wilson M. Compton, MD, MPE
Deputy Director
National Institute on Drug Abuse
National Institutes of Health
U.S. Department of Health and
  Human Services
Bethesda, Maryland

David J. Copenhaver, MD, MPH
Associate Professor
Director of Cancer Pain
Anesthesiology and Pain Medicine
University of California at Davis
UC Davis Medical Center
Sacramento, California

Gail D'Onofrio, MD, MS
Professor and Chair
Department of Emergency
  Medicine
Yale University School of Medicine
Physician-in-Chief
Emergency Department
Yale-New Haven Hospital
New Haven, Connecticut

Dennis C. Daley, PhD
Professor of Psychiatry
Department of Psychiatry
University of Pittsburgh School of
  Medicine
Senior Clinical Director, Substance
  Use Services
Behavioral Health Integration
  Division
UPMC Health Plan
Pittsburgh, Pennsylvania

John A. Dani, PhD
David J. Mahoney Professor of
  Neuroscience
Perelman School of Medicine
University of Pennsylvania
Chair, Department of Neuroscience
Director, Mahoney Institute for
  Neuroscience
Perelman School of Medicine
Philadelphia, Pennsylvania

**Itai Danovitch, MD, MBA,
DFASAM, FAPA**
Associate Clinical Professor
Department of Psychiatry and
  Behavioral Neurosciences
Chairman
Department of Psychiatry and
  Behavioral Neurosciences
Cedars-Sinai Medical Center
Los Angeles, California

Danielle R. Davis, MA
Predoctoral Fellow
Departments of Psychology &
  Psychiatry
University of Vermont
Burlington, Vermont

George De Leon, PhD
Clinical Professor
Psychiatry
NYU School of Medicine
New York, New York

Adam R. Demner, MD
Assistant Professor
Department of Psychiatry
New York University School of
  Medicine
Unit Chief
Chemical Dependency Outpatient
  Program
Bellevue Hospital Center
New York, New York

Laura Diamond, LMHC, EdM, MA
Inpatient Counseling Supervisor
Department of Psychiatry
Addiction Institute at Mount Sinai
  West
New York, New York

Patricia Jean Dickmann, MD
Assistant Professor
Department of Psychiatry
University of Minnesota Medical
  School
Medical Director, Addiction
  Recovery Service
Mental Health
Minneapolis VA Health Care
  System
Minneapolis, Minnesota

Coreen Domingo, DrPH
Assistant Professor
Department of Psychiatry
Baylor College of Medicine
Houston, Texas

Edward F. Domino, MS, MD
Active Emeritus
Department of Pharmacology
The University of Michigan Medical
  School
University of Michigan
Ann Arbor, Michigan

Dennis M. Donovan, PhD
Professor Emeritus
Department of Psychiatry &
  Behavioral Sciences
University of Washington
Seattle, Washington

Antoine Douaihy, MD
Professor of Psychiatry & Medicine
Psychiatry
University of Pittsburgh School of
  Medicine
UPMC Western Psychiatric
  Hospital
Pittsburgh, Pennsylvania

Robert L. DuPont, MD
President, Institute for Behavior
  and Health, Inc.
Rockville, Maryland
Clinical Professor of Psychiatry
Georgetown University School of
  Medicine
Washington, District of Columbia

Jon O. Ebbert, MD
Professor of Medicine
Mayo Clinic
Rochester, Minnesota

Xiaoduo Fan, MD, MPH, MS
Associate Professor
Department of Psychiatry
University of Massachusetts
   Medical School
Director
Psychotic Disorders Program
UMass Memorial Health Care
Worcester, Massachusetts

**James L. Ferguson, DO,
D-FASAM, C-MRO**
Medical Director
Recovery Management Services
FS Solutions
Chalfont, Pennsylvania

Sergi Ferré, MD, PhD
Senior Researcher
Integrative Neurobiology
National Institute on Drug Abuse,
   IRP, NIH
Baltimore, Maryland

James W. Finch, MD, DFASAM
Director of Physician Education
Governor's Institute on Substance
   Abuse
Raleigh, North Carolina
Medical Director
Changes By Choice
Durham, North Carolina

**Deborah S. Finnell, DNS, RN,
CARN-AP, FAAN**
Professor
Johns Hopkins School of Nursing
Baltimore, Maryland

Marc Fishman, MD
Medical Director
Psychiatry and Behavioral Sciences
Johns Hopkins University School
   of Medicine
Maryland Treatment Centers
Baltimore Maryland

Scott M. Fishman, MD
Fullerton Endowed Chair of Pain
   Medicine
Department of Anesthesiology &
   Pain Medicine
University of California Davis
   School of Medicine
Chief of Pain Medicine
UC Davis Health
Sacramento, California

James H. Ford II, PhD
Assistant Professor
School of Pharmacy
University of Wisconsin–Madison
Madison, Wisconsin

P. Joseph Frawley, MD
Co-medical Director
Department of Internal Medicine
Santa Barbara Cottage Hospital
Santa Barbara, California

**Peter D. Friedmann, MD, MPH,
DFASAM, FACP**
Associate Dean for Research &
   Professor of Medicine
Professor of Quantitative Health
   Sciences
University of Massachusetts
   Medical School (UMMS)
Chief Research Officer & Endowed
   Chair for Clinical Research
Office of Research
Baystate Health
Springfield, Massachusetts

Angela M. Galka, MPH
Research Program Administrator
Psychiatry
University of Michigan
Ann Arbor, Michigan

Mark S. Gold, MD
Adjunct Professor
Psychiatry
Washington University School of
   Medicine in St. Louis
St. Louis, Missouri

Bruce A. Goldberger, PhD
Professor
Department of Pathology,
   Immunology and Laboratory
   Medicine
University of Florida College of
   Medicine
Gainesville, Florida

R. Jeffrey Goldsmith, MD
Professor of Clinical Psychiatry
Department of Psychiatry and
   Clinical Neuroscience
University of Cincinnati College of
   Medicine
Staff Psychiatrist
Mental Health Care Line
Cincinnati VA Medical Center
Cincinnati, Ohio

**David A. Gorelick, MD, PhD,
DLFAPA**
Professor of Psychiatry
University of Maryland School of
   Medicine
Baltimore, Maryland

Brian Grahan, MD, PhD
Assistant Professor
Medicine
University of Minnesota
Physician
Addiction Medicine
Hennepin Healthcare
Minneapolis, Minnesota

Jon E. Grant, MD, JD, MPH
Professor
Department of Psychiatry &
   Behavioral Neuroscience
Pritzker School of Medicine
University of Chicago
Chicago, Illinois

Walter Green, MD
Emergency Medicine Physician
Department of Emergency
   Medicine
Yale University School of
   Medicine
New Haven, Connecticut

William M. Greene, MD
Associate Professor
Psychiatry
University of Florida College of
   Medicine
Medical Director, Dual Disorders
   Unit
Psychiatry
UF Health Shands Psychiatric
   Hospital
Gainesville, Florida

Kenneth W. Griffin, PhD, MPH
Professor
Department of Healthcare Policy
    & Research
Weill Medical College of Cornell
    University
New York, New York

Roland R. Griffiths, PhD
Professor
Departments of Psychiatry and
    Neuroscience
Johns Hopkins University School
    of Medicine
Baltimore, Maryland

Kathleen A. Gross, MD
Clinical Research Coordinator
Center for Clinical Research
Homer Stryker M.D. School of
    Medicine
Western Michigan University
Kalamazoo, Michigan

Joel W. Grube, PhD
Senior Research Scientist
Prevention Research Center
Pacific Institute for Research and
    Evaluation
Berkeley, California

Paul J. Gruenewald, PhD
Senior Research Scientist
Prevention Research Center
Pacific Institute for Research and
    Evaluation
Berkeley, California

**Carolina L. Haass-Koffler,
PharmD**
Assistant Professor
Psychiatry and Human Behavior
    and Behavioral and Social
    Sciences
Brown University
Providence, Rhode Island

**Paul S. Haber, MD, FRACP,
FAChAM**
Professor and Head
Discipline of Addiction Medicine
University of Sydney
Sydney, Australia
Clinical Director
Drug Health Services
Royal Prince Alfred Hospital
Camperdown, NSW, Australia

Timothy M. Hall, MD, PhD
Assistant Clinical Professor
Department of Family Medicine
David Geffen School of Medicine
    at UCLA
Los Angeles, California

Manassa Hany, MD
Assistant Professor
Department of Psychiatry
Icahn School of Medicine at
    Mount Sinai
Medical Director
Addiction Institute at Mount Sinai
    St. Luke's
New York, New York

Sion Kim Harris, PhD, CPH
Associate Professor
Department of Pediatrics
Harvard Medical School
Research Associate
Department of Medicine Division
    of Adolescent/Young Adult
    Medicine
Boston Children's Hospital
Boston, Massachusetts

Karen J. Hartwell, MD
Assistant Professor
Department of Psychiatry and
    Behavioral Sciences
Medical University of South
    Carolina
Medical Director
Substance Treatment and Recovery
    Program
Ralph H. Johnson VA Medical
    Center
Charleston, South Carolina

Colette L. Haward, MD
Attending Psychiatrist
The Department of Psychiatry
The Institute for Family Health
New York, New York

Kathryn Hawk, MD, MHS
Assistant Professor
Emergency Medicine
Yale University
Attending Physician
Emergency Medicine
Yale New Haven Hospital
New Haven, Connecticut

J. Taylor Hays, MD
Professor of Medicine
Nicotine Dependence Center
Mayo Clinic College of Medicine
    and Science
Consultant
Department of Medicine
Mayo Clinic
Rochester, Minnesota

Sarah H. Heil, PhD
Professor
Psychiatry and Psychological
    Sciences
University of Vermont
Burlington, Vermont

Abigail J. Herron, DO
Vice President for Behavioral Health
Director of Psychiatry and
    Addiction Medicine
The Institute for Family Health
New York, New York

Stephen T. Higgins, PhD
Director
Vermont Center on Behavior &
    Health
University of Vermont
Burlington, Vermont

Kenneth Hoffman, MD, MPH
Adjunct Assistant Professor
Department of Psychiatry
Uniformed Services University
Bethesda, Maryland
Medical Director
Steven A. Cohen Military Family
    Clinic
Easterseals
Silver Spring, Maryland

Kim A. Hoffman, PhD
Senior Research Associate
School of Public Health and
    Preventive Medicine
Oregon Health and Science
    University
Portland, Oregon

The Hon. Peggy Fulton Hora, JD
Judge of the Superior Court of
    California (Retired)
Walnut Creek, California

Mark Hrymoc, MD
Assistant Clinical Professor
Department of Psychiatry
UCLA
Medical Staff
Department of Psychiatry
Cedars-Sinai Medical Center
Los Angeles, California

Keith Humphreys
Esther Ting Memorial Professor
Psychiatry
Stanford University
Stanford, California
Senior Career Research Scientist
Health Services Research and
    Development
VA Palo Alto Health Care System
Palo Alto, California

Richard D. Hurt, MD
Emeritus Professor of Medicine
    and Emeritus Director of the
    Nicotine Dependence Center
Mayo Clinic
Rochester, Minnesota

Ryan T. Hurt, MD, PhD
Professor of Medicine
General Internal Medicine
Mayo Clinic
Rochester, Minnesota

Steven L. Jaffe, MD
Professor Emeritus
Psychiatry
Emory University School of
    Medicine
Atlanta, Georgia

Julie K. Johnson, PhD
Postdoctoral Researcher
Mental Health
Johns Hopkins Bloomberg School
    of Public Health
Baltimore, Maryland

**Kimberly Johnson, MSEd, MBA,
PhD**
Associate Professor
Mental Health Law and Policy
College of Behavioral and
    Community Sciences
University of South Florida
Tampa, Florida

**Christopher M. Jones, PharmD,
MPH**
Senior Advisor and Director of
    Strategy and Innovation
National Center for Injury
    Prevention and Control
US Centers for Disease Control
    and Prevention
Atlanta, Georgia

Hendrée E. Jones, PhD
Professor/Executive Director
UNC Horizons
Department of Obstetrics and
    Gynecology
University of North Carolina
Carrboro, North Carolina

Laura M. Juliano, PhD
Professor
Department of Psychology
American University
Washington, District of Columbia

Christopher W. Kahler, PhD
Professor
Center for Alcohol and Addiction
    Studies
Department of Behavioral and
    Social Sciences
Brown University School of Public
    Health
Providence, Rhode Island

David Kan, MD, DFASAM
Clinical Faculty
Department of Psychiatry
University of California, San
    Francisco
San Francisco, California

Lori D. Karan, MD, DFASAM, FACP
Professor
Internal Medicine and Preventive
    Medicine
Substance Treatment and Recovery
Loma Linda University School of
    Medicine
VA Loma Linda Healthcare System
Loma Linda, California

Jag H. Khalsa, MS, PhD
Special Volunteer at NIDA/NIH
Chief, Medical Consequences
    of Drug Abuse and Infections
    (Retired)
Division of Pharmacotherapies
    and Medical Consequences
National Institute on Drug Abuse,
    NIH
Bethesda, Maryland

Jason R. Kilmer, PhD
Associate Professor
Psychiatry & Behavioral Sciences,
    School of Medicine
Assistant Director of Health &
    Wellness for Alcohol & Other
    Drug Education
Health & Wellness, Division of
    Student Life
University of Washington
Seattle, Washington

Simeon D. Kimmel, MD
Fellow
Department of Medicine
Boston University School of
    Medicine
Fellow, Infectious Diseases and
    Addiction Medicine
Department of Medicine
Boston Medical Center
Boston, Massachusetts

Drew D. Kiraly, MD, PhD
Assistant Professor
Psychiatry & Neuroscience
Icahn School of Medicine at
    Mount Sinai
Attending Physician
Psychiatry
The Mount Sinai Hospital
New York, New York

Barbara M. Kirrane, MD, MPH
Medical Toxicology Consultant
Department of Emergency Medicine
Saint Barnabas Medical Center
Livingston, New Jersey

John R. Knight Jr., MD
Associate Professor of Pediatrics
Harvard Medical School
Director, Center for Adolescent
    Substance Abuse Research
Division of Developmental Medicine
Boston Children's Hospital
Boston, Massachusetts

George F. Koob
Director
National Institute on Alcohol
    Abuse and Alcoholism
Bethesda, Maryland

Thomas R. Kosten, MD
Waggoner Chair and Professor
    of Psychiatry, Neuroscience,
    Pharmacology, Immunology &
    Pathology
Director, Dan Duncan Institute
    for Clinical and Translational
    Research
Baylor College of Medicine,
    Michael E. DeBakey VAMC
Houston, Texas

Kevin Kunz, MD, MPH, DFASAM
Executive Vice President
The Addiction Medicine Foundation
Chevy Chase, Maryland

Maritza E. Lagos, MD, DABAM
Associate Professor
Department of Psychiatry
Homer Stryker M.D. School of
    Medicine
Western Michigan University
Attending Physician
Department of Psychiatry
Ascension Borgess Hospital
Kalamazoo, Michigan

Mary E. Larimer, PhD
Professor, Director
Department of Psychiatry &
    Behavioral Sciences
University of Washington School
    of Medicine
Seattle, Washington

Celine Larkin, PhD
Postdoctoral Research Fellow,
    Department of Emergency
    Medicine
University of Massachusetts
    Medical School
Worcester, Massachusetts

Sonya Lazarevic, MD
Evolution Medicine PC
New York, New York

David Y.W. Lee, PhD
Associate Professor
Neuroscience
Harvard Medical School
Boston, Massachusetts
Director
Bio-Organic & Natural Products Lab
McLean Hospital
Belmont, Massachusetts

David Lehman, MD, MS
Associate Attending
Psychiatry Department
Mount Sinai West
Unit Chief Inpatient Detox & Rehab
Psychiatry Department
Mount Sinai Health System
New York, New York

**Janet H. Lenard, EdD, LCSW,
CCS, CAC II**
Department of the Army Clinical
    Program Manager (Retired)
Army Substance Abuse Program
Installation Management
    Headquarters Command
Fort Sam Houston
Houston, Texas

Adam M. Leventhal, PhD
Professor
Department of Preventive Medicine
University of Southern California
Los Angeles, California

Annie Levesque, MD, MSc
Assistant Professor
Psychiatry
Icahn School of Medicine at
    Mount Sinai
Medical Director, Opioid
    Treatment Program
Addiction Institute at Mount
    Sinai West
New York, New York

Frances R. Levin, MD
Chief, Division on Substance Use
    Disorders (NYSPI)
Kennedy-Leavy Professor of
    Psychiatry
Department of Psychiatry
Columbia Universtiy Medical
    Center/New York State
    Psychiatric Institute
Associate Attending Psychiatrist
Department of Psychiatry
New York-Presbyterian
New York, New York

Aron H. Lichtman, PhD
Professor of Pharmacology and
    Toxicology and Medicinal
    Chemistry
Associate Dean of Research and
    Graduate Studies, School of
    Pharmacy
Virginia Commonwealth
    University
Richmond, Virginia

Ty W. Lostutter, PhD
Assistant Professor
Center for the Study of Health &
    Risk Behaviors
Department of Psychiatry &
    Behavioral Sciences
University of Washington
Director, Psychology Internship
    Program
Department of Psychiatry &
    Behavioral Sciences
University of Washington's School
    of Medicine
Seattle, Washington

**Karsten Lunze, MD, MPH, DrPH,
FACPM, FAAP**
Assistant Professor
Boston University School of
    Medicine
Director of Global Health
Department of Medicine, General
    Internal Medicine
Boston Medical Center
Boston, Massachusetts

Joseph Lurio, MD, FAAFP
Associate Professor
Family Medicine and Community
    Health
Icahn School of Medicine at
    Mount Sinai
Director
Addiction Medicine Fellowship
Institute for Family Health
New York, New York

Robert Malcolm, MD
Professor of Psychiatry
Family Medicine and Pediatrics
Associate Dean for SME
Medical University of South
    Carolina
Charleston, South Carolina

Yonina C. Mar, MBBS, MSc
Addiction Medicine Fellow
Icahn School of Medicine at
Mount Sinai
Addiction Institute at Mount Sinai
West
New York, New York

Marianne T. Marcus, EdD, RN, FAAN
Professor Emerita
Emeritus Faculty
Cizik School of Nursing
University of Texas Health Science
Center
Houston, Texas

G. Alan Marlatt, PhD†
Professor of Psychology
University of Washington
Seattle, Washington

Lisa A. Marsch, PhD
Director, Center for Technology
and Behavioral Health
Andrew G. Wallace Professor
Geisel School of Medicine at
Dartmouth
Dartmouth College
Lebanon, New Hampshire

Ashwin Jacob Mathai, MD
Clinical Assistant Professor
Psychiatry
SUNY Downstate Medical School
Integrated Addiction Psychiatrist
Behavioral Health
Kings County Hospital
Brooklyn, New York

Andrea L. Maxwell, MD
Associate Training Director,
Psychiatry Residency Training
Program
Department of Psychiatry and
Behavioral Sciences
Medical University of South Carolina
Addiction Psychiatrist
Mental Health Service
Ralph H. Johnson VA Medical
Center
Charleston, South Carolina

Elinore F. McCance-Katz, MD, PhD
Professor of Psychiatry and
Human Behavior
Alpert Medical School
Brown University
Chief Medical Officer
Rhode Island Department of
Behavioral Healthcare
Developmental Disabilities and
Hospitals
Providence, Rhode Island

Thomas W. McCarry, LMHC, NCC
Director of Substance Abuse
Prevention
The Institute for Family Health
New Paltz, New York

Barbara S. McCrady, PhD
Distinguished Professor
Department of Psychology and
Center on Alcoholism, Sub-
stance Abuse, and Addictions
University of New Mexico
Albuquerque, New Mexico

David D. McFadden, MD
Assistant Professor of Medicine,
College of Medicine
General Internal Medicine
Mayo Clinic
Rochester, Minnesota

Mark McGovern, PhD
Professor
Psychiatry and Behavioral
Sciences; Medicine
Stanford University School of
Medicine
Clinical Psychologist
Psychiatry
Stanford Health Care/Stanford
Hospital
Palo Alto, California

A. Thomas McLellan, PhD
Professor Emeritus
Perelman School of Medicine
University of Pennsylvania
Philadelphia, Pennsylvania

David Mee-Lee, MD
President
DML Training and Consulting
Davis, California

Lisa J. Merlo, PhD, MPE
Associate Professor
Department of Psychiatry
University of Florida
Gainesville, Florida

Shannon C. Miller, MD, DFAPA, DFASAM
Director, Addiction Services
VA Medical Center
Faculty, Neuroscience Graduate
Program
Professor of Clinical Psychiatry,
Affiliated
University of Cincinnati College of
Medicine
Cincinnati, Ohio
Past Founding Co-Editor, Journal
of Addiction
Medicine (2006–2016), American
Society of Addiction Medicine
Lieutenant Colonel, United States
Air Force, Retired

Samar Ali Mirzaei, MD
Psychiatry Resident
Psychiatry
Rutgers New Jersey Medical School
Newark, New Jersey

Margaret R. Moon, MD, MPH
Associate Professor of Pediatrics
Johns Hopkins University, School
of Medicine
Chief Medical Officer, The Johns
Hopkins Children's Center
Core Faculty, The Johns Hopkins
Berman Institute of Bioethics
Baltimore, Maryland

Kenneth L. Morford, MD
Addiction Medicine Fellow
Department of Internal Medicine
Yale University School of Medicine
New Haven, Connecticut

Kelly S. Mulé, PhD
Assistant Director
CARES
Department of Psychiatry and
Behavioral Health
Mount Sinai St. Luke's
New York, New York

---

†Deceased.

Hugh Myrick, MD
Acting Chief Mental Health
    Officer VISN 7
ACOS, Mental Health Service Line
Ralph H. Johnson VAMC
Associate Professor of Psychiatry
Director, Addiction Sciences
    Division
Director, Military Sciences Division
Medical University of South Carolina
Charleston, South Carolina

Edgar P. Nace, MD
Clinical Professor
Department of Psychiatry
University of Texas Southwestern
    Medical School
Dallas, Texas

Eric J. Nestler, MD, PhD
Director, Friedman Brain Institute
Neuroscience
Icahn School of Medicine at
    Mount Sinai
New York, New York

Dmitry Ostrovsky, MD
Resident
Department of Psychiatry
Mount Sinai St. Luke's and Mount
    Sinai West
New York, New York

James A.D. Otis, MD, PhD
Associate Professor of Neurology
Director, Headache and Pain
    Management Group
Department of Neurology
Boston University School of
    Medicine
Boston Medical Center
Boston, Massachusetts

Simy K. Parikh, MD
Fellow
Department of Neurology
Thomas Jefferson University
Philadelphia, Pennsylvania

Kimberly D.L. Parks, MD
Assistant Professor
Menninger Department of
    Psychiatry and Behavioral
    Sciences
Baylor College of Medicine
Attending Psychiatrist
Department of Psychiatry
Ben Taub General Hospital
Houston, Texas

**Theodore V. Parran Jr., MD,
FACP, FASAM**
Isabel and Carter Wang Professor
    and Chair in Medical Education
CWRU School of Medicine
Co-Medical Director, Rosary Hall
St. Vincent Charity Medical Center
Cleveland, Ohio

Mallie J. Paschall, PhD
Senior Research Scientist
Prevention Research Center
Pacific Institute for Research and
    Evaluation
Berkeley, California

David L. Pennington, PhD
Associate Professor
Department of Psychiatry; UCSF
    Weill Institute for Neurosci-
    ences
University of California, San
    Francisco
Clinical Research Psychologist
Research/Mental Health Service
San Francisco Veterans Affairs
    Health Care System
San Francisco, California

India Perez-Urbano, BA
MD Candidate
School of Medicine
University of California, San
    Francisco
San Francisco, California

Michael Perloff, MD, PhD
Assistant Professor of Neurology
Interventional Pain Management
Boston University School of
    Medicine
Boston, Massachusetts

Steven Pfau, MD
Associate Professor of Medicine
Department of Medicine
    (Cardiology)
Yale University School of Medicine
New Haven, Connecticut

Karran A. Phillips, MD, MSc
Senior Clinician and Clinical
    Director
National Institute on Drug Abuse
National Institutes of Health
Baltimore, Maryland

Marc N. Potenza, MD, PhD
Professor
Departments of Psychiatry, Child
    Study and Neuroscience
Yale University School of Medicine
Connecticut Mental Health Center
New Haven, Connecticut

James O. Prochaska, PhD
Professor and Director
Cancer Prevention Research Center
Psychology
Health Sciences College
University of Rhode Island
Kingston, Rhode Island

Janice M. Prochaska, PhD
Adjunct Professor
Human Development and Family
    Studies
University of Rhode Island
Kingston, Rhode Island

**Yelena Gorfinkel Pyatkevich,
MD**
Instructor of Neurology
Department of Neurology
Boston University School of
    Medicine
Neurology Attending
Department of Neurology
Boston Medical Center
Boston, Massachusetts

Gary M. Reisfield, MD
Associate Professor
Department of Psychiatry
University of Florida College of
    Medicine
Gainesville, Florida

**Launette Marie Rieb, MD, MSc,
CCFP, FCFP, CCSAM, dip. ABAM**
Clinical Associate Professor
Department of Family Practice
University of British Columbia
Addiction Medicine Consultant
Department of Family and Com-
    munity Medicine
St. Paul's Hospital
Vancouver, Canada

Richard K. Ries, MD, FASAM, FAPA
Professor of Psychiatry
Director Addictions Division
Department of Psychiatry and
    Behavioral Sciences
University of Washington School
    of Medicine
Seattle, Washington

Felipe Bolivar Rincon, MD
Post Graduate Year 3
Internal Medicine
Icahn School of Medicine at
    Mount Sinai
Resident
Internal Medicine
Mount Sinai St. Luke's–West
New York, New York

Richard N. Rosenthal, MA, MD, DFAPA, DFAAAP, FASAM
Professor of Psychiatry
Director of Addiction Psychiatry
Department of Psychiatry
Stony Brook University Medical
    Center
Stony Brook, New York

Stephen Ross, MD
Associate Professor
Department of Psychiatry
NYU Langone Medical Center
Director, Addictive Disorders
    and Experimental Therapeutics
    Research Laboratory
Department of Psychiatry
NYU Langone Medical Center
Bellevue Hospital Center
New York, New York

Stanley Sacks, PhD
Senior Research Scientist Emeritus
National Development and
    Research Institutes, Inc.
New York, New York

Radha Sadacharan, MD, MPH
Clinical Instructor
Family Medicine
Brown University
Pawtucket, Rhode Island
Attending Physician
Family Medicine
The Miriam Hospital
Providence, Rhode Island

Richard Saitz, MD, MPH, FACP, FASAM
Chairman, Department
    of Community Health
    Sciences (CHS)
Professor of Community Health
    Sciences & Medicine
Boston University Schools of
    Public Health and Medicine
Clinical Addiction Research and
    Education (CARE) Unit
Section of General Internal
    Medicine
Boston Medical Center
Boston, Massachusetts

Robert F. Saltz, PhD
Senior Scientist
Prevention Research Center
Pacific Institute for Research and
    Evaluation
Berkeley, California

Jeffrey H. Samet, MD, MA, MPH
Professor of Medicine
Section Chief
General Internal Medicine
Boston University School of
    Medicine
Boston Medical Center
Boston, Massachusetts

Ammar El Sara, MD
Addiction Psychiatry Fellow
Mount Sinai Health System
Department of Psychiatry
New York, New York

Christine L. Savage, PhD, RN, FAAN
Professor, Emerita
Johns Hopkins School of Nursing
Baltimore, Maryland

Andrew J. Saxon, MD
Professor
Psychiatry and Behavioral Sciences
University of Washington School
    of Medicine
Director, Center of Excellence in
    Substance Addiction Treatment
    and Education
Mental Health Service
VA Puget Sound Health Care System
Seattle, Washington

Emmanuelle A.D. Schindler, MD, PhD
Assistant Professor
Department of Neurology
Yale School of Medicine
New Haven, Connecticut
Staff Neurologist
Neurology Service
VA Connecticut Healthcare System
West Haven, Connecticut

Simone H. Schriger, BA
PhD Student
Psychology
University of Pennsylvania
Philadelphia, Pennsylvania

Frank J. Schwebel, MS
Graduate Student
Department of Psychology
University of Washington
Psychology Intern
Department of Psychiatry and
    Behavioral Sciences
University of Washington School
    of Medicine
Seattle, Washington

Samit Shah, MD, PhD
Instructor
Section of Cardiovascular Medicine
Department of Internal Medicine
Yale University School of Medicine
Clinical Fellow
Section of Cardiovascular
    Medicine
Yale New Haven Hospital
New Haven, Connecticut

Harshit Sharma, MBBS
Research Scholar
Center for Psychiatric Neuroscience
Zucker Hillside Hospital
Glen Oaks, New York

Steven Shoptaw, PhD
Professor
Family Medicine
University of California, Los Angeles
Los Angeles, California

Gerald D. Shulman, MA, MAC, FACATA
President
Shulman & Associates, Training &
    Consulting in Behavioral Health
Jacksonville, Florida

Jason J. Sico, MD, MHS, FAAN, FAHA, FACP, FANA
Associate Professor
Neurology (Vascular and Headache Medicine) and Internal Medicine (General Medicine)
Yale School of Medicine
New Haven, Connecticut
Director of Stroke Care
Director of Research and Clinical Care Headache Center of Excellence (HCoE)
Neurology
VA Connecticut Healthcare System
West Haven, Connecticut

Deborah R. Simkin, MD
Adjunct Assistant Professor
Emory School of Medicine
Atlanta, Georgia

Prameet Singh, MD
Associate Professor
Department of Psychiatry
Icahn School of Medicine at Mount Sinai
Interim Chair
Department of Psychiatry
Mount Sinai St. Luke's and West
New York, New York

David Smelson, PsyD
Director
Center of Excellence in Addiction
University of Massachusetts Medical School
Worcester, Massachusetts
Translational Research
Edith Nourse Rogers Memorial Veterans Hospital
Bedford, Massachusetts

Tricia H. Smith, PhD
Biology Department
Virginia Commonwealth University
Richmond, Virginia

David Son, DO, MPH
Addiction Medicine Fellow
Addiction Institute at Mount Sinai West
New York, New York

Sharon Stancliff, MD, FASAM
Medical Director (Former)
Harm Reduction Coalition
New York, New York

Jack B. Stein, PhD
Director, Office of Science Policy and Communications
National Institute on Drug Abuse, National Institutes of Health
Bethesda, Maryland

Randy Stinchfield, PhD
Emeritus
Psychiatry
University of Minnesota Medical School
Minneapolis, Minnesota

Susan A. Storti, PhD, RN, NEA-BC, CARN-AP
The Substance Use and Mental Health Leadership Council of RI
Warwick, Rhode Island

Carol A. Sulis, MD
Associate Professor
Department of Medicine
Boston University School of Medicine
Hospital Epidemiologist; Attending Physician
Department of Medicine, Division of Infectious Diseases
Boston Medical Center
Boston, Massachusetts

Mary M. Sweeney, MS, PhD
Instructor
Behavioral Pharmacology Research Unit, Department of Psychiatry and Behavioral Sciences
Johns Hopkins University School of Medicine
Baltimore, Maryland

Javier Ponce Terashima, MD
Adult Psychiatry Resident
University Hospitals Cleveland Medical Center–Case Western Reserve University
Cleveland, Ohio

Jeanette M. Tetrault, MD, FACP, FASAM
Associate Professor of Medicine
Yale School of Medicine
Program Director
Addiction Medicine Fellowship
Yale Hospital
New Haven, Connecticut

Anil Abraham Thomas, MD
Assistant Professor
Psychiatry
Icahn School of Medicine at Mount Sinai
Director, Addiction Psychiatry Fellowship Program
Mount Sinai St. Luke's and West
Psychiatry
Mount Sinai St. Luke's and West
New York, New York

Chris Tremonti, BMBS
Addiction Trainee
Drug Health Services
Royal Prince Alfred Hospital
Sydney, Australia

Federico E. Vaca, MD, MPH
Professor and Vice Chair
Emergency Medicine
Yale School of Medicine
New Haven, Connecticut

Leila M. Vaezazizi, MD
Clinical and Research Fellow
Department of Psychiatry Division on Substance Use Disorders
Columbia University
New York State Psychiatric Institute
New York, New York

Nora D. Volkow, MD
Director
National Institute on Drug Abuse
National Institutes of Health
Rockville, Maryland

Trang M. Vu, MD
Assistant Professor
Department of Medicine
Icahn School of Medicine at Mount Sinai
New York, New York

Jonathan M. Wai, MD
Addiction Psychiatry Fellow
Department of Psychiatry
Columbia University
Addiction Psychiatry Research Fellow
Division on Substance Use Disorders
New York State Psychiatric Institute
New York, New York

R. Corey Waller, MD, MS, FACEP, DFASAM
Michigan State University College of Human Medicine
Spectrum Health Hospital Systems
Grand Rapids, Michigan

Alexander Y. Walley, MD, MSc
Associate Professor of Medicine
Department of Medicine
Boston University School of Medicine
Director, Addiction Medicine Fellowship
Clinical Addiction Research and Education Unit
Boston Medical Center
Boston, Massachusetts

Linda Wang, MD
Clinical Instructor
Division of General Internal Medicine
Icahn School of Medicine at Mount Sinai
Attending Physician
Department of Medicine
Mount Sinai Hospital
New York, New York

Eric M. Wargo, PhD
Health Science Policy Analyst
Science Policy Branch, Office of Science Policy and Communications
National Institute on Drug Abuse
Bethesda, Maryland

Alan A. Wartenberg, MD, FACP, DFASAM
Affiliated Faculty Member
Brown Center for Alcohol & Addiction Studies
Brown University
Providence, Rhode Island

Michael F. Weaver, MD, DFASAM
Professor
Psychiatry and Behavioral Sciences
McGovern Medical School
Medical Director
Center for Neurobehavioral Research on Addiction
University of Texas Health Science Center at Houston
Houston, Texas

Julia Megan Webb
Pain Medicine Fellowship Graduate
Department of Anesthesiology and Pain Medicine
University of California Davis
Sacramento, California

Arthur F. Weissman, MD
Clinical Assistant Professor
Family Medicine
Jacobs School of Medicine and Biomedical Sciences
Staff Physician
DART
Community Action Organization of Western New York
Buffalo, New York

Sandra P. Welch, PhD
Professor
Pharmacology and Toxicology
Virginia Commonwealth University
Richmond, Virginia

Joseph Westermeyer, MD, MPH, PhD
Professor of Psychiatry, Adjunct Professor of Anthropology
University of Minnesota
Staff Psychiatrist
Addiction Recovery Service
Minneapolis, Minnesota

William L. White, MA
Emeritus Senior Research Consultant
Lighthouse Institute
Chestnut Health Systems
Bloomington, Illinois

Ursula Whiteside, PhD
Clinical Faculty
Psychiatry and Behavioral Sciences
University of Washington
Locum Tenens
Behavioral Health Services
Kaiser Permanente Washington
Seattle, Washington

Bonnie B. Wilford, MS
Executive Vice President
Coalition on Physician Education in Substance Use Disorders (COPE)
Easton, Maryland

Jeffery N. Wilkins, MD, DFAPA, DFASAM
Lincy-Heyward/Moynihan Endowed Chair in Addiction Medicine
Department of Psychiatry and Behavioral Neurosciences
Cedars-Sinai Medical Center
Los Angeles, California

Mark Willenbring, MD
Adjunct Full Professor
Psychiatry
University of Minnesota
Minneapolis, Minnesota

Emily C. Williams, PhD, MPH
Associate Professor
Department of Health Services
University of Washington School of Public Health
Core Investigator
Health Services Research & Development
Veterans Affairs Puget Sound Health Care System
Seattle, Washington

Ken C. Winters, PhD
Senior Scientist
Oregon Research Institute
Eugene, Oregon

John J. Woodward, PhD
Professor
Neuroscience
Medical University of South Carolina
Charleston, South Carolina

Tara M. Wright, MD
Assistant Professor
Department of Psychiatry
Medical University of South Carolina
Assistant Chief
Mental Health Service Line
Ralph H. Johnson VA Medical Center
Charleston, South Carolina

Martha J. Wunsch, MD
Chief
Addiction Medicine Consultation and Liaison Service
Kaiser Permanente Hospital
San Leandro, California

Stephen A. Wyatt, DO
Adjunct Faculty
Psychiatry
University of North Carolina
Chapel Hill, North Carolina
Medical Director, Addiction Medicine
Behavioral Health
Atrium Health
Charlotte, North Carolina

Yvonne H.C. Yau, MSc
PhD Candidate
Neurology and Neurosurgery
McGill University
Montreal, Canada

Sarah W. Yip, PhD, MSc
Assistant Professor
Department of Psychiatry
Yale School of Medicine
New Haven, Connecticut

Christine Yuodelis-Flores, MD, FAPA, FASAM
Associate Professor
Department of Psychiatry and
  Behavioral Sciences
University of Washington
Harborview Medical Center
Seattle, Washington

Anne Zajicek, MD, PharmD
Deputy Director
Office of Clinical Research, Office
  of the Director
National Institutes of Health
Assistant Professor
Department of Pediatrics
Walter Reed National Military
  Medical Center
Bethesda, Maryland

Douglas Ziedonis, MD, MPH
Associate Vice Chancellor—Health
  Sciences
Department of Psychiatry
University of California, San Diego
La Jolla, California

Joan E. Zweben, PhD
Clinical Professor
Psychiatry
University of California, San
  Francisco
Staff Psychologist
Substance Abuse
Veterans Affairs Medical Center
San Francisco, California

Preface

Welcome to the third edition of *The ASAM Essentials of Addiction Medicine*. This book is a companion guide to *The ASAM Principles of Addiction Medicine*, a comprehensive reference text that reflects the state-of-the-art science and practice of addiction medicine. It was created with the goal of providing a more concise source of up-to-date and clinically relevant information.

The text is organized to allow the reader to easily switch back and forth between the companion guide and the comprehensive text, with each chapter in *Essentials* providing a distilled summary of the corresponding chapter in *Principles*. As such, each chapter lists the summary author as well as the authors of the original chapters. We are delighted that many of the original authors also contributed the summaries for this book. At the end of each chapter, three new sections have been added. Key Points highlight the most relevant information from each chapter; Review Questions allow the reader to test his or her knowledge; and Suggested Readings point toward more in-depth information about the topic.

When summarizing such a large and comprehensive textbook, information from the original text must be omitted in order to provide only succinct, relevant information to the reader. In that vein, we have not included the full list of references, a decision carried forward from the first edition of *Essentials* and made out of necessity in order to keep the book as concise as possible.

Acknowledgments

Thank you to the American Society of Addiction Medicine for the opportunity to work on this text. We are grateful to the editors and contributors of *The ASAM Principles of Addiction Medicine* for their work, which provided the foundation for this text, as well as to Christopher Cavacuiti, editor of the first edition of *Essentials*. Finally, we thank each of the authors who lent their time and talent to make *The ASAM Essentials of Addiction Medicine* possible.

Contents

Editors of *The ASAM Principles of Addiction Medicine, Sixth Edition*   v

Contributors to *The ASAM Essentials of Addiction Medicine, Third Edition*   ix

Preface   xxiii

Acknowledgments   xxv

Introduction: A Public Health Approach to Prevention: The Health Professional's Role   xxxvii
Linda Richter, Kevin Kunz, and Susan E. Foster

SECTION 1   Basic Science and Core Concepts

1   Drug Addiction: The Neurobiology of Motivation Gone Awry   2
Nora D. Volkow and George F. Koob

2   Recommended Use of Terminology in Addiction Medicine   7
Richard Saitz

3   The Epidemiology of Substance Use Disorders   11
Faye Chao

4   The Anatomy of Addiction   16
Thomas J.R. Beveridge

5   From Neurobiology to Treatment: Progress Against Addiction   22
Drew D. Kiraly and Eric J. Nestler

6   Clinical Trials in Substance-Using Populations   28
Yonina C. Mar

7   The Addiction Medicine Physician as a Change Agent for Prevention and Public Health   33
Kevin Kunz

SECTION 2   Pharmacology

8   Pharmacokinetic, Pharmacodynamic, and Pharmacogenomic Principles   40
Anne Zajicek and Lori D. Karan

9   The Pharmacology of Alcohol   44
John J. Woodward

10   The Pharmacology of Nonalcohol Sedative Hypnotics   50
Carolina L. Haass-Koffler and Elinore F. McCance-Katz

11   The Pharmacology of Opioids   55
Kimberly D.L. Parks, Coreen Domingo, and Thomas R. Kosten

12   The Pharmacology of Stimulants   60
David A. Gorelick and Michael H. Baumann

13   The Pharmacology of Caffeine   66
Mary M. Sweeney, Laura M. Juliano, Sergi Ferré, and Roland R. Griffiths

14   The Pharmacology of Nicotine and Tobacco   72
John A. Dani

15   The Pharmacology of Cannabinoids   78
Sandra P. Welch, Tricia H. Smith, Robert Malcolm, and Aron H. Lichtman

16   The Pharmacology of Hallucinogens   84
Manassa Hany

17   The Pharmacology of Dissociatives   91
Edward F. Domino and Shannon C. Miller

18   The Pharmacology of Inhalants   97
Robert L. Balster

19   The Pharmacology of Anabolic–Androgenic Steroids   102
David Lehman

20   Electronic Cigarettes   108
Thomas W. McCarry

21   Novel Psychoactive Substances: Their Recognition, Pharmacology, and Treatment   113
Kathryn Hawk, Barbara M. Kirrane, and Gail D'Onofrio

SECTION 3   Diagnosis, Assessment, and Early Intervention

22   Screening and Brief Intervention   119
Benjamin M. Clemens

Sidebar: Screening and Brief Intervention for Pregnant Women   123
Nicolas Bertholet

Sidebar: Trauma Centers, Hospitals, and Emergency Departments   125
Arthur F. Weissman

Sidebar: Implementation of Screening and Brief Intervention (SBI) in Clinical Settings Using Quality Improvement Principles   126
Emily C. Williams and Katharine A. Bradley

Sidebar: Screening for Unhealthy Alcohol Use in the Elderly   128
James W. Campbell

23   Laboratory Assessment   130
Trang M. Vu and Linda Wang

24 Assessment 136
Launette Marie Rieb

25 Environmental Approaches to Prevention: Communities and Contexts 141
Paul J. Gruenewald, Joel W. Grube, Robert F. Saltz, and Mallie J. Paschall

SECTION 4 Overview of Addiction Treatment

26 Addiction Medicine in America: Its Birth, Early History, and
Current Status (1750-2018) 147
Kevin Kunz and William L. White

27 Treatment of Unhealthy Alcohol Use: An Overview 154
Mark Willenbring and Brian Grahan

28 The Treatment of Addiction: An Overview 161
Andrea G. Barthwell, Jeffrey Allgaier, and Lawrence S. Brown Jr.

29 Integrated Care for Substance Use Disorder 166
Keith Humphreys, Mark McGovern, and A. Thomas McLellan

30 The ASAM Criteria and Matching Patients to Treatment 172
David Mee-Lee and Gerald D. Shulman

31 Linking Addiction Treatment With Other Medical and Psychiatric Treatment Systems 179
Karran A. Phillips, Peter D. Friedmann, Richard Saitz, and Jeffrey H. Samet

32 Alternative Therapies for Substance Use Disorders 186
David Y.W. Lee

33 Harm Reduction, Overdose Prevention, and Addiction Medicine 189
India Perez-Urbano, Sharon Stancliff, and Alexander Y. Walley

34 Quality Improvement for Addiction Treatment 196
James H. Ford II, Kim A. Hoffman, Kimberly Johnson, and Javier Ponce Terashima

35 Nursing Roles in Addressing Addiction 202
Deborah S. Finnell, Marianne T. Marcus, and Christine L. Savage

36 International Perspectives on Addiction Management 206
Annie Levesque

SECTION 5 Special Issues in Addiction

37 Prescription Medications: Nonmedical Use, Use Disorders, and Public Health
Consequences 211
Jack B. Stein, Wilson M. Compton, Eric M. Wargo, and Christopher M. Jones

38 Special Issues in Treatment: Women 219
Joan E. Zweben

39   Traumatic Brain Injury and Substance Use Disorders   224
David L. Pennington and Jennifer Bielenberg

40   Military Sexual Trauma   229
Joan E. Zweben

41   Alcohol, Prescription, and Other Drug Problems in Older Adults   233
Frederic C. Blow, Kristen L. Barry, and Angela M. Galka

42   Cultural Issues in Addiction Medicine   240
Joseph Westermeyer and Patricia Jean Dickmann

43   College Student Drinking   245
Frank J. Schwebel, Ursula Whiteside, Joyce N. Bittinger, Jason R. Kilmer, Ty W. Lostutter, and Mary E. Larimer

44   Understanding "Behavioral Addiction"   250
Yvonne H.C. Yau, Sarah W. Yip, and Marc N. Potenza

45   Gambling Disorder: Clinical Characteristics and Treatment   255
Jon E. Grant

46   Problematic Sexual Behaviors and "Sexual Addiction"   260
Timothy M. Hall, Simone H. Schriger, and Steven Shoptaw

47   Microprocessor-Based Disorders   267
Richard N. Rosenthal

48   Behavioral Syndromes to Consider as Forms of "Addiction"   272
Abigail J. Herron

49   Physician Health Programs and Addiction Among Physicians   278
Andrea Cole

     Sidebar: The California Diversion Program: A Cautionary Tale   283
     Abigail J. Herron

SECTION 6   Management of Intoxication and Withdrawal

50   Management of Intoxication and Withdrawal: General Principles   285
Tara M. Wright, Jeffrey S. Cluver, and Hugh Myrick

51   Management of Alcohol Intoxication and Withdrawal   290
Radha Sadacharan and Alan A. Wartenberg

52   Management of Sedative–Hypnotic Intoxication and Withdrawal   298
Jonathan M. Wai

53   Management of Opioid Intoxication and Withdrawal   304
Kenneth L. Morford and Jeanette M. Tetrault

54   Management of Stimulant, Hallucinogen, Marijuana, Phencyclidine, and Club Drug
Intoxication and Withdrawal   309
Jeffery N. Wilkins, Itai Danovitch, and David A. Gorelick

SECTION 7 Pharmacological Interventions and Other Somatic Therapies

55 Pharmacological Interventions for Alcohol Use Disorder 316
James Besante

56 Pharmacological Interventions for Sedative–Hypnotic Use Disorder 321
Prameet Singh

57 Pharmacological and Psychosocial Treatment for Opioid Use Disorder 326
David Kan

58 Special Issues in Office-Based Opioid Treatment 332
Andrew J. Saxon

Sidebar: Concerning Veterans and Office-Based Treatment of Opioid Use Disorder 336
Tim K. Brennan

59 Pharmacological Treatment of Stimulant Use Disorders 337
David A. Gorelick

60 Pharmacological Interventions for Tobacco Use Disorder 342
Jon O. Ebbert, J. Taylor Hays, David D. McFadden, Ryan T. Hurt, and Richard D. Hurt

61 Pharmacological Interventions for Other Drugs and Multiple Drug Use Disorders 347
Jeffery N. Wilkins, Mark Hrymoc, and David A. Gorelick

62 Neuromodulation for Addiction-Related Disorders 351
David A. Gorelick

SECTION 8 Psychologically Based Interventions

63 Enhancing Motivation to Change 354
James O. Prochaska and Janice M. Prochaska

64 Group Therapies 360
Dennis C. Daley and Antoine Douaihy

65 Individual Treatment 364
Harshit Sharma

66 Contingency Management and the Community Reinforcement Approach 369
Sarah H. Heil, Christopher A. Arger, Danielle R. Davis, and Stephen T. Higgins

67 Behavioral Interventions for Nicotine/Tobacco Use Disorder 374
Erika Litvin Bloom, Christopher W. Kahler, Adam M. Leventhal, and Richard A. Brown

68 Network Therapy 379
Dmitry Ostrovsky

69 Therapeutic Communities and Modified Therapeutic Communities for Co-Occurring Mental and Substance Use Disorders 384
George De Leon and Stanley Sacks

70 Aversion Therapies 389
P. Joseph Frawley

71 Family Involvement in Addiction, Treatment, and Recovery 395
Kathleen A. Gross and Maritza E. Lagos

72 Twelve-Step Facilitation Approaches 399
Tim K. Brennan

73 Relapse Prevention: Clinical Models and Intervention Strategies 402
Antoine Douaihy, Dennis C. Daley, G. Alan Marlatt, and Dennis M. Donovan

74 Digital Health Interventions for Substance Use Disorders: The State of the Science 408
Lisa A. Marsch and Jacob T. Borodovsky

75 Medical Management Techniques and Collaborative Care: Integrating Behavioral with
Pharmacological Interventions in Addiction Treatment 412
Richard N. Rosenthal

SECTION 9 Mutual Help, Twelve-Step, and Other Recovery Programs

76 Twelve-Step Programs in Addiction Recovery 419
Edgar P. Nace

77 Recent Research into Twelve-Step Programs 424
Barbara S. McCrady

78 Spirituality in the Recovery Process 429
Sonya Lazarevic

SECTION 10 Medical Disorders and Complications of Addiction

79 Medical and Surgical Complications of Addiction 433
Karsten Lunze

80 Cardiovascular Consequences of Alcohol and Other Drug Use 442
Steven Pfau and Samit Shah

81 Liver Disorders Related to Alcohol and Other Drug Use 448
Paul S. Haber and Chris Tremonti

82 Renal and Metabolic Disorders Related to Alcohol and Other Drug Use 454
Catreena Al Marj and Laith Al-Rabadi

83 Gastrointestinal Disorders Related to Alcohol and Other Drug Use 460
Paul S. Haber and Chris Tremonti

84 Respiratory Tract Disorders and Selected Critical Care Considerations Related to Alcohol
and Other Drug Use 465
Joseph Lurio

85 Neurological Disorders Related to Alcohol and Other Drug Use   470
Emmanuelle A.D. Schindler and Jason J. Sico

86 Human Immunodeficiency Virus, Tuberculosis, and Other Infectious Diseases Related to Alcohol and Other Drug Use   475
Carol A. Sulis and Simeon D. Kimmel

87 Sleep Disorders Related to Alcohol and Other Drug Use   479
Sanford Auerbach and Yelena Gorfinkel Pyatkevich

88 Traumatic Injuries Related to Alcohol and Other Drug Use: Epidemiology, Screening, and Prevention   486
Walter Green, Deepa Camenga, Gail D'Onofrio, and Federico E. Vaca

89 Endocrine and Reproductive Disorders Related to Alcohol and Other Drug Use   490
Felipe Bolivar Rincon

90 Alcohol and Other Drug Use during Pregnancy: Management of the Mother and Child   494
Michael F. Weaver, Hendrée E. Jones, and Martha J. Wunsch

91 Perioperative Management of Patients with Alcohol- or Other Drug Use   500
Daniel P. Alford

SECTION 11   Co-Occurring Addiction and Psychiatric Disorders

92 Substance-Induced Mental Disorders   507
Christine Yuodelis-Flores, R. Jeffrey Goldsmith, and Richard K. Ries

93 Co-occurring Mood and Substance Use Disorders   513
Laura Diamond

94 Co-Occurring Substance Use and Anxiety Disorders   517
Andrea L. Maxwell, Alyssa M. Braxton, and Karen J. Hartwell

95 Co-Occurring Addiction and Psychotic Disorders   522
Douglas Ziedonis, Celine Larkin, Xiaoduo Fan, Stephen A. Wyatt, and David Smelson

96 Co-occurring Substance Use Disorder and Attention Deficit Hyperactivity Disorder   525
Leila M. Vaezazizi and Frances R. Levin

97 Co-occurring Personality Disorders and Addiction   532
Adam R. Demner and Stephen Ross

98 Posttraumatic Stress Disorder and Substance Use Disorder Comorbidity   537
Colette L. Haward

99 Co-occurring Substance Use Disorders and Eating Disorders   541
Lisa J. Merlo, William M. Greene, and Mark S. Gold

SECTION 12 Pain and Addiction

100 The Pathophysiology of Chronic Pain and Clinical Interfaces With Substance
Use Disorder 548
David Son

101 Psychological Issues in the Management of Pain 553
Martin D. Cheatle

102 Rehabilitation Approaches to Pain Management 558
Abigail J. Herron

103 Nonopioid Pharmacotherapy of Pain 562
Simy K. Parikh, Michael Perloff, and James A.D. Otis

104 Opioid Therapy of Pain 566
Tim K. Brennan

105 Co-Occurring Pain and Addiction 573
Anil Abraham Thomas

106 Legal and Regulatory Considerations in Opioid Prescribing 578
Julia Megan Webb, David J. Copenhaver, and Scott M. Fishman

SECTION 13 Children and Adolescents

107 Preventing Substance Use Among Children and Adolescents 582
Kenneth W. Griffin and Gilbert J. Botvin

Sidebar: Governmental Policy on Cannabis Legalization and Cannabis as Medicine:
Impact on Youth 587
Sion Kim Harris, Julie K. Johnson, and John R. Knight Jr.

108 Translational Neurobiology of Addiction from a Developmental Perspective 591
Deborah R. Simkin and Ammar El Sara

109 Screening and Brief Intervention for Adolescents 596
Traci L. Brooks, John R. Knight Jr., and Sion Kim Harris

110 Assessing Adolescent Substance Use 602
Ken C. Winters, Andria M. Botzet, and Randy Stinchfield

111 Placement Criteria and Strategies for Adolescent Treatment Matching 607
Marc Fishman

Sidebar: Confidentiality in Dealing with Adolescents 612
Margaret R. Moon

Sidebar: Drug Testing Adolescents in School 613
J. Wesley Boyd

112 Adolescent Treatment and Relapse Prevention 615
Steven L. Jaffe and Ashraf Attalla

113 Pharmacotherapies for Adolescents with Substance Use Disorders 620
Ashwin Jacob Mathai and Samar Ali Mirzaei

114 Co-occurring Psychiatric Disorders in Adolescents 625
Kelly S. Mulé

SECTION 14 Ethical, Legal, and Liability Issues in Addiction Practice

115 Ethical Issues in Addiction Practice 630
Tim K. Brennan

116 Consent and Confidentiality Issues in Addiction Practice 636
R. Corey Waller

117 Clinical, Ethical, and Legal Considerations in Prescribing Drugs With Potential for Nonmedical Use and Addiction 642
Theodore V. Parran Jr., James W. Finch, and Bonnie B. Wilford

Sidebar: Drug Control Policy: History and Future Directions 650
John J. Coleman and Robert L. DuPont

Sidebar: Guidance on the Use of Opioids to Treat Chronic Pain 651
James W. Finch and Bonnie B. Wilford

118 Medicinal Uses of Cannabis and Cannabinoids 655
Jag H. Khalsa

119 Practical Considerations in Drug Testing 659
Gary M. Reisfield, Roger L. Bertholf, Bruce A. Goldberger, and Robert L. DuPont

Sidebar: Workplace Drug Testing and the Role of the Medical Review Officer 664
James L. Ferguson and Robert L. DuPont

120 Reducing Substance Use in Criminal Justice Populations 667
Peggy Fulton Hora

Sidebar: Treatment of Substance Use Disorders During Incarceration 671
Lori D. Karan

121 Preventing and Treating Substance Use Disorders in Military Personnel 675
Kenneth Hoffman, Robert M. Bray, and Janet H. Lenard

Sidebar: Risk Factors for Military Families 681
Joan E. Zweben and Susan A. Storti

Index 683

Introduction: A Public Health Approach to Prevention: The Health Professional's Role

Linda Richter, Kevin Kunz, and Susan E. Foster

The risky use of substances and addiction are the largest and most costly preventable cause of health problems in the United States, yet they are not adequately addressed in healthcare practice. These conditions cause and contribute to innumerable conditions requiring medical care, including cancer, respiratory disease, cardiovascular disease, HIV/AIDS, trauma, and mental illness and account for nearly one third of all hospital inpatient costs and nearly a quarter of deaths in the United States. They can exacerbate existing health conditions and complicate their treatment. Despite the indisputable link between addiction and medicine, historically, physicians' primary role in addressing it has been on the back end, once it has wreaked havoc on a patient's health and well-being, rather than on the front end when it and its many adverse and costly health and social consequences could have been averted.

There are many reasons for this state of affairs, but primary among them is that, for years, risky substance use and addiction have been mainly perceived by both the public and health professionals as moral or social problems rather than as preventable and treatable health conditions. At worst, this perspective has driven these conditions underground, clouded in a shroud of shame and stigma, whereas at best, it has driven them into the hands of law enforcement officials and a broad range of treatment providers; the majority of whom are not equipped with the knowledge, skills, or credentials necessary to provide the full range of evidence-informed prevention and treatment services for a health condition.

Physicians, even in the most technically clinical specialties, have recognized the importance of macrolevel public health and prevention efforts as they relate to other health conditions that, historically, have been considered purely treatment issues. For example, neurosurgeons are on the forefront of efforts to educate the public and transform public policy with regard to helmet wearing among bikers and among child and adult athletes who participate in contact sports. The same is true in the case of the involvement of health professionals in public education and other public health initiatives to help prevent and reduce obesity; the realization that these conditions cause and contribute to countless preventable medical conditions has spurred this commitment to primary prevention.

Although the principal responsibility of health professionals with regard to preventing risky substance use and addiction will play out within the confines of individual clinical practices via patient education, screening, early intervention services, and referrals to treatment when necessary, it is imperative for the medical profession to transcend the clinical walls and become involved in broader public health initiatives that can have a significant impact on forestalling and mitigating the damage of these devastating health conditions. This process has begun with the recognition by the American Board of Medical Specialties of addiction medicine as a multispecialty subspecialty and the newly available accreditation of addiction medicine fellowship training programs by the Accreditation Council of Graduate Medical Education (ACGME). ACGME accreditation requires training in prevention competencies as well as treatment and disease management. Addiction medicine specialists are trained to provide expert clinical care to patients and consultation services to other health professionals. They also are trained to serve as faculty to move the science and evidence-informed practice across healthcare broadly and as change agents in communities, health systems, and government.

Nearly one third of the US population, although not addicted, engages in the use of addictive substances in ways that threaten health and safety. Another 16% meet the diagnostic criteria for addiction, more than the share of the population with heart disease, diabetes, or cancer. In 2017, 72,000 people died from a drug overdose; the ongoing opioid epidemic is responsible for taking more than two thirds (49,000) of those lives. Drug overdose is now the leading cause of death among Americans under the age of 50 years. Even when it doesn't take lives, addiction can destroy them. Yet addiction remains the only disease for which available and effective preventive interventions are not routinely provided within the healthcare system. This can and must change.

RISKY SUBSTANCE USE VERSUS ADDICTION

Although both addiction and the risky use of addictive substances cause and contribute to numerous health problems, they are very different conditions and require different approaches if they are to be effectively addressed.

Addiction is a disease and, like other diseases, it can and should be diagnosed and treated in the context of the medical system in which an interdisciplinary team of physicians, nurses, and behavioral health professionals work collaboratively with auxiliary and support personnel, using available evidence-informed therapies and disease management protocols. In contrast, the risky use of addictive substances is primarily a public health problem, and tools to address it are available for use by trained healthcare professionals in a wide range of health, social services, education, criminal justice, and other sectors. These public health approaches to addressing the risky use of addictive substances strive to educate the public about it, screen for it, and intervene early to reduce it and its consequences, including the potential for it to progress to addiction.

The tendency to frame the risky use of addictive substances and addiction as the same issue varying only in intensity does not reflect the evidence. Most people who use addictive substances will not go on to develop addiction, yet the risky use of tobacco/nicotine, alcohol, and other drugs still represents a significant threat to the public's health and safety. Conflating them has hampered efforts to prevent these conditions and to offer appropriate and effective interventions that match those offered for other health conditions. It also has led health professionals who feel ill equipped to treat the disease of addiction to throw up their hands in the face of exhortations to implement public health measures to help prevent and reduce the risky use of addictive substances.

A SPECIAL FOCUS ON YOUTH

Addiction is a disease that typically originates with substance use in adolescence. Nine out of 10 people with an addiction started smoking, drinking, or using other drugs before the age of 18 years. A substantial body of evidence demonstrates that the earlier substance use begins, the greater the likelihood of developing addiction, yet the average age that high school students report starting to use an addictive substance is between 12 and 13 years of age.

Both physiologically and socially, adolescence is the critical period of vulnerability for engaging in substance use and for triggering the onset of addiction. Nevertheless, 7 in 10 high school students have used one or more addictive substances, 4 in 10 are current users, and 1 in 7 meet the diagnostic criteria for addiction.

Adolescents are more vulnerable than adults to the addictive effects of nicotine, alcohol, and other drugs. Adolescent substance use is also directly linked to the three leading causes of death in that age group—accidents, homicides, and suicides—and it is implicated in numerous other negative health and social consequences. To address it, the public, policymakers, and especially health professionals must recognize youth substance use as a health threat rather than a normal rite of passage; help young people delay all forms of substance use for as long as possible; be vigilant for signs of risk; and intervene appropriately as they do for other health conditions. In order to make any meaningful headway in reducing the prevalence of risky substance use and addiction and their consequences, preventive efforts cannot wait until a patient shows up in a doctor's office with signs and symptoms of the disease. Prevention efforts must begin early and must comprehensively address the complex interplay of biological, personal, social, and environmental risk factors.

THE ROLE OF HEALTH PROFESSIONALS IN A COMPREHENSIVE PUBLIC HEALTH APPROACH TO RISKY SUBSTANCE USE AND ADDICTION

In part because substance use has typically been seen as a cultural or social issue, rather than a health issue, and due to the newness of the addiction medicine subspecialty, the public is only now beginning to look to physicians and other healthcare professionals for information or help in preventing risky use and addiction in young people. The onus of protecting youth from addiction still falls largely on parents who are encouraged to monitor their children, communicate openly with them, and set clear and consistent rules, and on educators who are given prevention curricula to implement in schools and policies to enact to discourage students from using. However, as we learn more about the effects of addictive substances on the brain and body, we know that, despite the considerable social ramifications of substance use and addiction, these are primarily health issues which should, therefore, fall squarely under the purview of the medical profession. Health professionals can perform several functions to help prevent use from starting and from escalating or progressing to addiction if it has already begun.

Most physicians and other clinicians do not routinely educate their patients about the health risks of substance use; screen for, identify, or address risky substance use in their practices; or know what to do with patients who present with identifiable and treatable symptoms of addiction. This is in spite of the facts that 85% of adults and 93% of children in the United States have contact with a healthcare professional at least annually, that screening and early intervention strategies are increasingly being covered by insurance, and that government organizations, health associations, and medical societies have endorsed these practices.

Prevention and early intervention, including SBIRT (screening, brief intervention, and referral to treatment), involve a set of promising and increasingly well-established practices that can be performed by physicians and other qualified health professionals to address risky substance use and addiction within mainstream medical care. Although the term "screening" might connote invasive drug testing to some patients, it generally means having a confidential and authentic conversation with patients about their use of addictive substances, their motivations for use, and their awareness of the health effects of such use. Education of this nature should be offered on a routine basis and in a manner that is tailored to the age, gender, and other personal characteristics of the patient and should be coupled, when indicated, with intervention services.

Addiction medicine physicians are trained in prevention and early intervention and, as specialists, help broadly drive science-informed practice across medicine and healthcare. They can also drive public education and enhance the traditional role of families, schools, communities, religious institutions, and social service agencies in performing this role. The evidence base with regard to what works in prevention is too often confined to the academic and clinical scientific literature and is not routinely translated into practical and comprehensible terms for those

on the front lines of prevention. Health professionals can work with educators, community organizations, social service agencies, and policymakers to help ensure that prevention messaging is based on the evidence. They also can become more involved in the education, training, and support of those working in nonmedical settings to identify and appropriately manage substance-related problems in the populations they serve.

There are several accepted models for preventing unhealthy or unsafe behaviors on a public health level and intervening when early signs of those behaviors are detected. For example, the *ecological* model of prevention examines the domains of influence on an individual's behavior—including on the individual (eg, personality characteristics, personal experiences), family, peer, community, and larger societal levels—and seeks to target prevention efforts at the risk factors within each of these domains. The *spectrum of prevention* model is more procedural in that it examines specific public health approaches for preventing health risk behaviors, such as educating individuals, families, and communities; establishing coalitions and relationships among key players; modifying organizational practices; and influencing regulations and policies, all with an aim toward health promotion and disease prevention. A third model that integrates both the domains of influence and the specific actions needed to effect change is often referred to as the *public health* model of prevention. Although this latter model is framed around the population groups being targeted, it represents a comprehensive approach to preventing and reducing risky substance use and addiction. Among other things, it calls for the involvement of physicians and other health professionals in health promotion generally and specifically in intervening with populations at different levels of risk, on the primary (universal), secondary (selected), and tertiary (indicated) levels of prevention.

Health Promotion

Preventing risky substance use and addiction are critical for promoting public health. Aside from the more direct prevention measures that are to be described in the following, action on the policy level is required to truly make a dent in the pervasiveness of risky substance use and addiction in this country.

Public awareness that risky substance use and addiction are primarily health problems rather than social or moral issues is essential for transforming how these conditions are perceived and managed. Healthcare providers who, aside from families, are most often the firsthand witnesses to the damage incurred by substance use are a trusted source for the public in conveying this message and fostering a well-informed populace. As such, they should partner with health educators and public and private organizations to develop and implement awareness campaigns that translate scientific information about the nature and effects of substance use and addiction into common language while educating the public about the availability of effective interventions for those struggling with these problems.

Physicians and other health professionals also should be involved in promoting and advocating for legislative and regulatory measures that control the availability and accessibility of addictive substances, especially to youth. The effects of the easy accessibility of nicotine, alcohol, and other drugs on reducing perceptions of their harm and on their use are well documented. The involvement of health professionals in this regard is especially critical at this time when the nation seems to be moving directly down an ill-conceived path toward increasing rather than decreasing the availability of addictive substances.

With what seems like unstoppable momentum, we appear to be opening ourselves up to a largely unregulated flooding of the addictive substances market with marijuana of largely unknown potency, vaping devices that deliver nicotine as well as other drugs at dangerously high and addictive doses, and prescriptions for addictive psychoactive medications for children and adults often written for off-label use and not adequately vetted for long-term safety. Too often, physicians have played an unfortunate role in the widespread availability of these addictive substances. In the case of electronic cigarettes, mixed messages were offered for years by the medical profession with regard to their potential benefits, despite the fact that vaping devices were not subject to the testing and review process that the US Food and Drug Administration requires for smoking cessation aids and other medications. Today, we find ourselves in a situation where the commissioner of the Food and Drug Administration has declared vaping an epidemic among youth. Likewise, the relentless expansion of marijuana legalization across the country has bypassed the normal procedures for bringing a medical product to market and has been bolstered by claims of its medical benefits that far exceed the research evidence. As a result, marijuana potency, rates of marijuana use and addiction, and unintentional childhood exposures have all increased, especially in states where it has been legalized for medical use. Finally, the opioid epidemic, which began with the excessive prescribing of addictive opioid medications

to treat all types and intensities of pain, is another clear example of the significant role health professionals can play both in preventing or, unfortunately, fostering addiction.

To stem this tide and help enact a rational and evidence-informed set of policies related to these issues, physicians and other healthcare professionals should advocate for laws and regulations to:

- increase taxes on tobacco and nicotine products and alcohol, and raise the purchase age to 21 years;
- have the FDA more tightly regulate the production, advertising, and marketing of electronic cigarettes/vaping devices and other noncigarette tobacco/nicotine products, including enacting a complete ban on flavors in these products;
- further restrict the advertising and marketing of alcohol, especially to youth;
- manage the production, distribution, and marketing of marijuana in those states where it is legal, restricting sale to and possession by people under the age of 21 years, prohibiting advertising and marketing to them, and banning marijuana edibles and flavors that appeal to children;
- enact a national prescription drug monitoring program to ensure effective monitoring across state lines;
- increase the use of non–opioid-based treatment options for patients with pain, especially youth;
- implement more prescription drug take-back programs and require patient education around prescription drug misuse and proper storage and disposal of unused medication;
- ensure comprehensive insurance coverage for addiction prevention and treatment and adequate reimbursement for providers; and
- increase funding for methodologically sound research on prevention and treatment.

Healthcare professionals also should work to expand treatment capacity in the medical system and press government and private healthcare insurers to reimburse for the full range of services aimed at preventing risky substance use and treating and managing addiction.

Primary Prevention

Primary prevention involves the implementation of broad-scale programs and services to prevent the public from engaging in unhealthy behaviors and acquiring a disease. Numerous primary prevention programs exist to keep young people from using addictive substances. Most of these are school- and community-based efforts, only some of which have a solid base of evidence to back up their efficacy in preventing young people from initiating and engaging in substance use.

Physicians and other health professionals can play a larger role in the development and implementation of quality prevention programs, and in public education efforts more broadly both in and out of their clinical practices. The following are methods to accomplish this.

- Advocate for the implementation of a nationwide public health campaign to educate the public about risky substance use and addiction. Such a campaign should help the public understand that risky substance use is a health concern and inform the public about the consequences of such use, factors that increase and reduce the risk of use, the link between early use and addiction, and how best to respond if a problem is identified.
- Incorporate education, screening, and early intervention into routine healthcare practice and mandating their inclusion in health services offered through schools, social service programs, and justice systems. Screening should occur on a routine basis and be designed to identify all types of risky substance use, including tobacco/nicotine, alcohol, illicit drugs, and controlled prescription drugs, in all healthcare settings.
- Promote physician education and training in the origins of risky substance use and addiction; prevention, intervention, treatment, and management options; co-occurring conditions; and special population and specialty care needs.
- Educate professionals in non–health-related sectors about risky substance use and addiction. Those who do not provide direct addiction-related services but who come into contact with significant numbers of individuals who engage in risky substance use or who may have addiction should have a level of knowledge about these issues and how to address them that surpasses that of the lay public. These professionals include, but are not limited to, law enforcement and other criminal justice personnel, legal staff, educators, and child welfare and other social service workers. Education, screening, and when needed, brief interventions should be provided by trained professionals in all educational, mental health, developmental disabilities, child welfare, housing, juvenile justice, and adult corrections services. Patients who screen positive for risky use or a potential diagnosis of addiction should be connected with a trained health professional for intervention,

comprehensive assessment, diagnosis, treatment, and disease management.

- Invest in and conduct research designed to improve and track progress in the prevention of risky substance use and the treatment and management of addiction.

Secondary Prevention

Secondary prevention involves the early detection of risk for a health condition in a population and the provision of early interventions targeted to those at risk in order to forestall its progression or reduce its adverse consequences. Physicians and other health professionals have critical roles to play in this regard. They should:

- provide targeted prevention services to young people and other vulnerable populations at risk for substance use and addiction due to family history, the presence of mental health or behavioral conditions, trauma, or other known risk factors.
- conduct evidence-informed interventions with those who screen positive for risk. Such interventions generally include feedback about the extent and effects of patients' substance use and recommendations for how they might change their behavior. These interventions involve motivational interviewing techniques and substance-related education, and typically are more effective when parents and/or families are involved, with the exact recommended approach differing depending on the target population.

Tertiary Prevention

Tertiary prevention involves stabilizing a disease once it is established, preventing further deterioration of health, and attempting to reverse its course and maintain a patient's rehabilitation and optimal functioning. At this level of prevention, it is the healthcare professional's responsibility to treat those who evince signs and symptoms of addiction by:

- conducting a comprehensive assessment to determine the disease stage and severity as well as the presence of co-occurring health conditions and special population needs;
- stabilizing the patient via detoxification and/or medication, when necessary, as a precursor to treatment;
- consulting with addiction medicine specialists as needed, developing a tailored treatment plan that includes acute treatment via evidence-informed psychosocial and/or pharmaceutical interventions, chronic disease management as needed,

and connection to support and auxiliary services, including legal, educational, employment, housing and family supports, nutrition and exercise counseling, and mutual support programs; and

■ referring patients to addiction medicine specialists for specialty care in the case of greater disease severity or inadequate patient response to other interventions.

This level of "prevention," which essentially involves the treatment and management of disease, is what physicians and other health professionals traditionally consider to be within their realm of professional practice. Yet, although it is critical, it is rarely provided for those with addiction and, even when provided, only touches a small proportion of the population that is otherwise adversely affected by risky substance use and addiction. Failing to provide care for addiction or limiting medical knowledge and expertise to this level of care no longer suffices if we are to make significant strides in reducing the significant health problems of risky substance use and addiction.

Physicians and other health professionals should do all they can to help make prevention, brief intervention, and the treatment and management of risky substance use and addiction and their health consequences available and accessible at all points of contact with the healthcare system, including at physicians' offices, community clinics, school and college health centers, emergency rooms, trauma centers, hospitals, and other healthcare facilities.

THE NEED FOR AN EXPANDED WORKFORCE TO REFORM ADDICTION CARE

Significant barriers stand in the way of making this critical shift in the current approach to addiction care, including a profound disconnect between medical practice and the current approach to addiction treatment as well as funding limitations to expand the addiction medicine workforce. The predominant workforce that currently provides services to those with addiction operates largely outside the medical profession and lacks a capacity to provide the full range of evidence-informed practices, including necessary medical care. The need for an expanded workforce to implement what we know about addiction care can be accomplished in several ways.

Ensure That All Physicians, Regardless of Specialty, Are Trained in the Basics of Addiction Care

All medical schools and residency training programs should educate and train physicians to address risky substance use and addiction. Specifically, all physicians should be educated and trained in the risk factors for and nature of risky substance use and addiction; evidence-informed approaches for prevention, intervention, treatment, and management; co-occurring conditions; and the needs of special populations. Basic addiction medicine core competencies should become required components of all medical school curricula, medical residency training programs, medical licensing exams, board certification exams, and continuing medical education requirements, including maintenance of certification programs. As with other medical competencies for diagnosing and treating diabetes or high blood pressure, for example, these core competencies can be adapted from those developed for addiction medicine fellowship training and required by ACGME.

Ensure That Nonphysician Health Professionals Are Educated and Trained to Identify and Address Risky Substance Use and Addiction

Nonphysician health professionals, including physician assistants, nurses and nurse practitioners, dentists, pharmacists, and graduate-level clinical mental health professionals (eg, psychologists, social workers, counselors) should be trained in the core competencies (adapted from the ACGME addiction medicine core competencies) for addressing risky use and preventing and treating addiction. To ensure a well-informed healthcare workforce:

■ These core clinical competencies and specialized training should be required components of all professional healthcare program curricula, graduate fellowship training programs, professional licensing exams, and continuing education requirements.

■ All nonphysician health professionals who provide psychosocial addiction treatment services should be required to have graduate-level clinical training.

■ All pharmaceutical treatments for addiction should be provided by a physician or in accordance with a treatment plan managed by a physician.

Expand the Addiction Medicine Specialist Workforce

To promote addiction care reform, it is necessary to ensure that addiction medicine training programs are available to physicians, that training opportunities in addiction psychiatry are expanded, and that the specialty of addiction medicine is formally available in every healthcare system nationally. Across the field of medicine, it is the specialty training programs that drive evidence-informed change across healthcare, public policy, and public information. To help accomplish these goals, the following steps should be taken:

- Accelerate the work begun by the American College of Academic Addiction Medicine[1] to develop one-year full-time fellowship training programs in addiction medicine and to secure accreditation of these from ACGME. As of December 2018, there were a total of 62 fellowships, of which 33 were ACGME accredited.
- Implement a fellowship or an addiction medicine program affiliated with each of the nation's 183 medical schools and additional programs in teaching hospitals not affiliated with a medical school.
- Support the efforts of ACGME-accredited addiction psychiatry fellowships to increase the number of enrolled fellows.

Addiction medicine specialists can play three critical roles in ensuring effective care for those with at-risk use and those with an addiction: (1) provide specialty care and consultation to other medical providers; (2) train other healthcare providers in how to address these issues within the context of their practices; and (3) serve as change agents for public education and public policy reform. To that end, addiction medicine specialists must engage in outreach and collaboration efforts, partnering with established and influential organizations in the field of substance use and addiction research, prevention, and treatment, such as the Substance Abuse and Mental Health Services Administration and its subdivisions, the Center for Substance Abuse Treatment and the Center for Substance Abuse Prevention; the National Institutes of Health, including the National Institute on Drug Abuse and the National Institute on Alcohol Abuse and Alcoholism, the Office of Disease Prevention, and the National Cancer Institute; the Centers for Disease Control and Prevention; the White House Office of National Drug Control Policy; the US Department of Defense; the US Department of Veterans Affairs; as well as non-government organizations and entities devoted to these critical issues.

Certainly, no one individual, group, or service sector alone can realize the changes required in healthcare practice, policy, insurance coverage, and public understanding to bring addiction prevention and treatment and reductions in risky substance use in line with the standard of care for other public health and medical conditions. Resolute action is required by physicians and other medical and health professionals, policymakers, insurers, and the general public. It is long overdue for healthcare practice to catch up with the science about what works in the prevention and treatment of risky substance use and addiction, which constitute one of the most prevalent and costly, yet preventable, health conditions that this nation faces.

SUGGESTED READINGS

Accreditation Council for Graduate Medical Education. ACGME program requirements for graduate medical education in addiction medicine. https://www.acgme.org/Portals/0/PFAssets/ProgramRequirements/404Addiction Medicine1YR2018.pdf?ver=2018-03-30-090748-000. Accessed February 5, 2018.

Addiction Medicine: Closing the Gap Between Science and Practice. New York: The National Center on Addiction and Substance Abuse (CASA) at Columbia University, 2012.

Adolescent Substance Use: America's #1 Public Health Problem. New York: The National Center on Addiction and Substance Abuse (CASA) at Columbia University, June 2011.

Hawks D, Scott K, McBride N. *Prevention of Psychoactive Substance Use: A Selected Review of What Works in the Area of Prevention*. Geneva, Switzerland: World Health Organization, 2002.

Meyers K, Cacciola J, Ward S, Kaynak O, Woodworth A. *Paving the Way to Change: Advancing Quality Interventions for Adolescents Who Use, Abuse or Are Dependent Upon Alcohol and Other Drugs*. Philadelphia: Treatment Research Institute, 2014.

Tulchinsky TH, Varavikova EA. What is the "New Public Health"? *Public Health Rev*. 2010;32(1):25-53.

Volmert A, Sweetland J, Kendall-Taylor N. *Turning Down the Heat on Adolescent Substance Use: Findings From Reframing Research*. Washington, DC: FrameWorks Institute, 2018.

---

[1]Formerly, The Addiction Medicine Foundation.

Basic Science and Core Concepts

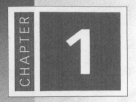

Drug Addiction: The Neurobiology of Motivation Gone Awry

Summary by Nora D. Volkow and George F. Koob

Based on THE ASAM PRINCIPLES OF ADDICTION MEDICINE, 6th edition chapter by Nora D. Volkow and George F. Koob

Drug addiction manifests as a chronic relapsing disorder characterized by a compulsive drive to take a drug despite serious adverse consequences, loss of control over intake, and the emergence of a negative emotional state during abstinence. Converging evidence shows that frequent drug misuse changes the brain in ways that can lead to the profound behavioral disruptions that are seen in addicted individuals. This is because drugs of abuse impact many neuronal circuits, including those that are involved in processing responses to rewarding stimuli, negative emotions, interoception, decision making, and cognitive control, turning drug use into a compulsive behavior. The fact that these changes are progressive, but, once developed, are long-lasting and persist even after years of drug use discontinuation is what makes addiction a chronic and relapsing disease.

Drug addiction has been conceptualized as a cycle of three stages, each representing basic neurocircuitry that is involved in motivation and each predominantly linked to a functional domain and associated brain functional networks but with the recognition that brain networks interact with one another (Fig. 1-1). The *binge/intoxication* stage via the neurocircuitry of the basal ganglia reflects the rewarding effects of drugs and how drugs impart motivational significance to cues and contexts in the environment, termed incentive salience, which is experienced as "well-being," "high," "euphoria," or "relief," depending on the degree of tolerance to the rewarding effects of the drug. The *withdrawal/negative affect* stage via the extended amygdala and habenula reflects the enhanced sensitivity and recruitment of brain stress systems and the loss of reward and motivation, termed a negative emotional state, which is experienced as dysphoria, anhedonia, and irritability. The *preoccupation/anticipation* ("craving") stage via neurocircuitry of the prefrontal cortex reflects the impulsivity and loss of control over drug taking, termed loss of executive control, and the input from the default mode network that reflects the enhanced interoceptive awareness of the desire for the drug, which is experienced as drug craving.

Drug addiction develops as a progressive process that involves complex interactions between biological and environmental factors. Important discoveries have provided a means of explaining this environmental/biological interaction via our increased knowledge of the ways in which drugs affect the epigenome, the expression patterns of specific genes, their protein products, neuronal communication and plasticity, and neural circuitry and the ways in which these biological factors might conflate to effect compulsive human drug-seeking behavior.

ADDICTION: A DEVELOPMENTAL DISORDER

Drug use and misuse often start in adolescence, as does the process of addiction, and it is well documented that the frontal lobes and connections of the frontal lobes do not fully develop until the age of 25 years. Preclinical studies with animal models and human imaging studies have begun to show that drug exposure during adolescence might result in neuroadaptations that are different from those that occur during adulthood and may explain the greater vulnerability to alcohol or other substance use disorders (eg, nicotine, cannabis) among individuals who start using alcohol or other drugs early in life.

NEUROBIOLOGY OF ADDICTIVE DRUGS: BINGE/INTOXICATION STAGE

During the *binge/intoxication* stage, large surges of dopamine and the release of opioid peptides have been consistently associated with the reinforcing

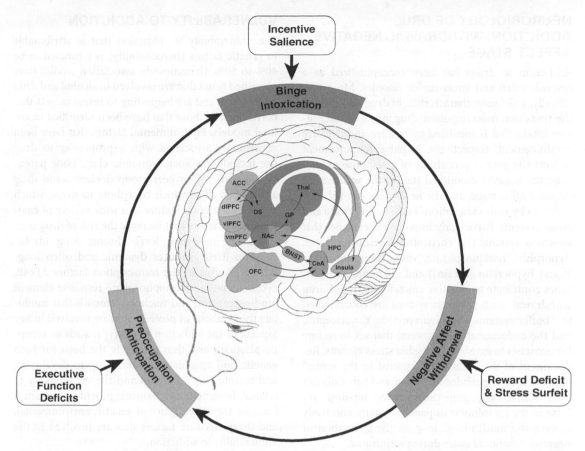

Figure 1-1. The conceptual framework for the neurobiology of addiction. The three stages of the addiction cycle are linked to three domains of neurocircuitry that mediate three domains of dysfunction: *binge/intoxication* (basal ganglia: incentive salience), *withdrawal/negative affect* (extended amygdala: negative emotional states), and *preoccupation/anticipation* (prefrontal cortex: executive dysfunction). In parallel, disruption of the default mode network that is necessary for interoceptive awareness makes it harder to ignore drug cravings and the negative emotional states that are associated with the *withdrawal/negative affect* and *preoccupation/anticipation* stages. ACC, anterior cingulate cortex; BNST, bed nucleus of the stria terminalis; CeA, central nucleus of the amygdala; dlPFC, dorsolateral prefrontal cortex; DS, dorsal striatum; GP, globus pallidus; HPC, hippocampus; NAc, nucleus accumbens; OFC, orbitofrontal cortex; Thal, thalamus; vlPFC, ventrolateral prefrontal cortex. (Modified with permission from George O, Koob GF. Control of craving by the prefrontal cortex. *Proc Natl Acad Sci U S A.* 2013;110[11]:4165-4166.)

effects of most addictive drugs. Other drugs, such as nicotine, alcohol, opioids, and marijuana, work directly or indirectly to modulate dopamine cell firing through their effects on nicotinic, γ-aminobutyric acid, opioid, and cannabinoid (predominantly CB_1) receptors, respectively, and cortical brain structures that convey different messages about stimulus response, approach behavior, learning, and decision making. This dopamine response initiates a cascade of neurochemical neurocircuitry changes. Imaging studies with individuals who are diagnosed with cocaine addiction have shown the expected, drug-induced fast dopamine increases in the striatum (including the nucleus accumbens) associated with the drug's rewarding effects and that such increases are markedly blunted compared to controls. These same subjects with drug addiction, however, show significant dopamine increases in the striatum in response to drug-conditioned cues that are associated with self-reports of drug craving and appear to have a greater magnitude than the dopamine responses to the drug. We postulate that the discrepancy between the expectation for the drug effects (conditioned responses) and the blunted pharmacological effects maintains drug taking in an attempt to obtain the expected reward, leading to the negative reinforcement of the *withdrawal/negative affect* stage.

NEUROBIOLOGY OF DRUG ADDICTION: WITHDRAWAL/NEGATIVE AFFECT STAGE

Addiction to drugs has been conceptualized as a reward-deficit and stress-surfeit disorder. More specifically, a defining characteristic of drug addiction is the transition from impulsive drug intake to compulsive intake that is mediated by positive and negative reinforcement, respectively. Negative reinforcement reflects the greater probability of a response to alleviate the negative emotional state of the *withdrawal/negative affect* stage, and the negative emotional state is driven by neuroadaptations in the brain reward and stress systems. Particularly important is evidence that prostress systems (eg, corticotropin-releasing factor, dynorphin, norepinephrine, vasopressin, substance P, and hypocretin [orexin]) and inflammatory cytokines contribute to negative emotional states of drug withdrawal. Such prostress systems are counteracted by "buffer systems" (eg, neuropeptide Y, nociceptin, and the endocannabinoid system) that act to restore homeostasis to extended amygdala stress circuits. Recruitment of the brain stress systems in the ventral tegmental area, extended amygdala, and habenula can in turn inhibit dopamine cell firing and dopamine release in the mesolimbic dopamine system, effectively closing the motivational loop on the generation of negative emotional states during withdrawal.

NEUROBIOLOGY OF DRUG ADDICTION: PREOCCUPATION/ANTICIPATION ("CRAVING") STAGE

A hallmark of addiction involves poor inhibitory control and poor executive function, which are mediated by prefrontal cortical regions. For example, for both alcohol and cocaine, regions of the prefrontal cortex are selectively damaged by chronic intermittent use and result in poor decision making that can perpetuate the addiction cycle. Impairments in prefrontal cortex areas result in the perturbed regulation of reward and stress regions and disruptions of higher order executive function (eg, self-control, salience attribution, and awareness). Indeed, gray matter volume deficits in specific medial frontal and posterior parietal–occipital brain regions are predictive of relapse risk, suggesting a significant role for gray matter atrophy in poor clinical outcomes in addiction. Preclinical studies have shown that drug-related adaptations in these prefrontal cortex regions result in perturbations of glutamatergic pathways that regulate subcortical reward and stress systems.

VULNERABILITY TO ADDICTION

The vulnerability to addiction that is attributable to genetic factors (hereditability) is estimated to be 40% to 60%. Genomewide association studies have identified genes that are involved in alcohol and drug metabolism and are beginning to reveal targets that correspond to those that have been identified in animal models. Environmental factors that have been consistently associated with a propensity to drug use include low socioeconomic class, poor parental support, within-peer-group deviancy, and drug availability, all of which contribute to stress, which may be a common feature in a wide variety of environmental factors that increase the risk of drug use.

At the molecular level, chronic drug administration itself produces dynamic and often long-lasting changes in the transcription factors ΔFosB, cyclic adenosine monophosphate response element binding protein, and nuclear factor κB that modulate the synthesis of proteins that are involved in key aspects of the addiction phenotype, such as synaptic plasticity, and thus are likely the basis for both genetic and epigenetic vulnerability to developing and maintaining addiction and the vulnerability to relapse. Epigenetic mechanisms provide a biological basis for the convergence of genetic, environmental, and drug exposure factors that are involved in the vulnerability to addiction.

COMORBIDITY WITH MENTAL ILLNESS

Different neurobiological factors are likely involved in comorbidity, depending on the temporal course of its development (ie, mental illness followed by drug use or vice versa). In some instances, mental illness and addiction appear to co-occur independently; in others, however, there might be a sequential dependency. It has been proposed that comorbidity might be attributable to the use of drugs to self-medicate the mental illness in cases in which the onset of mental illness is followed by the use of some types of drugs. When drug use is followed by mental illness, chronic and excessive drug exposure could lead to neurobiological changes, which might explain the greater risk of mental illness.

PREVENTING ADDICTION

A neurobiological basis for the greater vulnerability of adolescents to experimentation with addictive drugs, incomplete development of top-down control, and subsequent vulnerability to addiction underscores why the prevention of early exposure is such an important strategy to combat drug addiction.

Current prevention strategies include educational interventions that are based on comprehensive school-based programs and effective media campaigns and strategies that decrease access to drugs and alcohol. Such strategies also provide supportive community activities that engage adolescents in productive and creative ways. Particularly promising are the recent results of a major longitudinal study that showed a dramatic positive influence of childhood self-control on a wide range of life outcomes, including substance use risk, overall health, and financial status. Tailored interventions that take into account socioeconomic, cultural, age, and gender characteristics of children and adolescents are more likely to improve the effectiveness of the interventions.

TREATING ADDICTION

Long-term treatment will be required for most persons with addiction, just as for other chronic diseases, like hypertension, diabetes, and asthma, because the neuroadaptations in the brain that result from chronic drug exposure are long lasting. The involvement of multiple brain circuits (reward, motivation, memory, learning, stress, emotion, interoception, inhibitory control, and executive function) and the associated behavioral disruptions point to the need for a multimodal approach to the treatment of individuals with addiction and may require a combination of pharmacological and behavioral interventions. Both pharmacological and behavioral interventions can be classified according to their intended remedial function, such as to strengthen inhibitory control circuits, provide alternative reinforcers, reduce stress, improve mood, and strengthen executive function, but pharmacological interventions can also directly block the positive reinforcing effects of drugs. Dual approaches that pair cognitive–behavioral strategies with medications to compensate for or counteract the neurobiological changes that are induced by chronic drug exposure are a promising area of translational research that might, in the near future, provide more robust and longer lasting treatments for addiction than either treatment provided in isolation. Similarly, advances in brain stimulation strategies, such as transcranial magnetic stimulation and transcranial direct current stimulation, might offer alternatives in the future to rebalance the function of neurocircuits that are affected by addiction.

TREATING COMORBIDITIES

The proper management of individuals with addiction should include considerations of comorbidities of other drug misuse and/or other medical and mental illnesses because addictive drugs adversely affect virtually all organs in the body. A particularly relevant example is human immunodeficiency virus (HIV) and acquired immune deficiency syndrome, with the promising approach of the Seek, Test, Treat, and Retain paradigm. Here, one seeks out hard-to-reach/high-risk populations, including substance users and those in the criminal justice system; tests them for HIV; links those who test positive to HIV treatment and other services; and provides the necessary support to ensure these individuals remain in the care system. Similarly, the treatment of pain in patients with a substance use disorder is particularly relevant for individuals with an opioid use disorder in whom pain is more prevalent and may drive relapse if not properly controlled.

CHALLENGES FOR SOCIETY

An important challenge for society is to reduce the stigma of addiction that interferes with intervention and proper recovery and rehabilitation. Such elements as the treatment of persons with addiction in the criminal justice system, the role of unemployment in vulnerability to the use of drugs, and family dysfunctions that contribute to stress are key and might impede the efficacy of otherwise effective interventions. The recognition of addiction as a chronic disease that affects the brain is also essential for large-scale prevention and treatment programs that require participation of the medical community and thus training of the medical community, including doctors, physician assistants, dentists, nurses, and pharmacists. Other challenges include collaborations with federal agencies to facilitate translation to the public of effective screening, prevention, and treatment interventions; with the private sector for insurance reimbursement; and with the pharmaceutical industry for the development of new medications to treat addiction. The rich growing knowledge of the neurobiology of addiction provides exciting opportunities for the diagnosis, prevention, and treatment of addiction in all of these domains.

KEY POINTS

1. Drug addiction manifests as a chronic relapsing brain disorder, characterized by a compulsive drive to take a drug despite serious adverse consequences, the loss of control over intake, and the emergence of a negative emotional state during abstinence.
2. A heuristic neurobiological framework of the stages of the addiction cycle that guide the diagnosis, prevention, and treatment of substance use

disorders includes binge/intoxication, withdrawal/negative affect, and preoccupation/anticipation.

3. The three domains of dysfunction associated with the three stages of the addiction cycle are binge/intoxication (incentive salience), withdrawal/negative affect (negative emotional states), and preoccupation/anticipation (executive function).

4. Dysfunction in the corresponding neural circuits account for the pathology of addiction: binge/intoxication (basal ganglia), withdrawal/negative affect (extended amygdala), and preoccupation/anticipation (frontal cortex).

REVIEW QUESTIONS

1. Which of the following key brain structures mediates negative emotional states that are associated with abstinence from excessive drug use?
   A. Extended amygdala
   B. Hypothalamus
   C. Frontal cortex
   D. Hippocampus

2. Which of the following key brain structures mediates the reward, incentive salience, and habit components of the binge/intoxication stage of the addiction cycle?
   A. Basal ganglia
   B. Hypothalamus
   C. Frontal cortex
   D. Hippocampus

3. The dysfunction of which area of the brain is associated with impulsive and compulsive drug use?
   A. Cerebellum
   B. Hypothalamus
   C. Frontal cortex
   D. Hippocampus

4. Which of the following neurotransmitter systems mediates hormonal, sympathetic, and behavioral responses to stressors?
   A. Endorphin
   B. Corticotropin-releasing factor
   C. Dopamine
   D. Serotonin

5. Which of the following accurately describes a heuristic neurobiological framework of the stages of the addiction cycle that guides the diagnosis, prevention, and treatment of substance use disorders?
   A. Binge/intoxication, withdrawal/negative affect, preoccupation/anticipation
   B. Binge/intoxication, withdrawal/negative affect, wanting/liking sensitization
   C. Sensitization/incentive salience, withdrawal/negative affect, preoccupation/anticipation
   D. Impulsive, compulsive, craving

6. Which of the following accurately describes a key essence of addiction?
   A. Addiction is a moral failure.
   B. Addiction is a developmental disorder.
   C. Addiction is untreatable and can only be managed.
   D. All of the above.

ANSWERS

1. **A**
2. **A**
3. **C**
4. **B**
5. **A**
6. **B**

SUGGESTED READINGS

Koob GF, Le Moal M. Review. Neurobiological mechanisms for opponent motivational processes in addiction. *Philos Trans R Soc Lond B Biol Sci*. 2008;363:3113-3123.

Koob GF, Volkow ND. Neurobiology of addiction: a neurocircuitry analysis. *Lancet Psychiatry*. 2016;3:760-773.

Morgenstern J, Naqvi NH, Debellis R, Breiter HC. The contributions of cognitive neuroscience and neuroimaging to understanding mechanisms of behavior change in addiction. *Psychol Addict Behav*. 2013;27:336-350.

Volkow ND, Koob GF, McLellan AT. Neurobiologic advances from the brain disease model of addiction. *N Engl J Med*. 2016;374(4):363-371.

Volkow ND, Wang GJ, Fowler JS, Tomasi D, Telang F. Addiction: beyond dopamine reward circuitry. *Proc Natl Acad Sci U S A*. 2011;108(37):15037-15042.

Recommended Use of Terminology in Addiction Medicine

Summary by Richard Saitz

Based on THE ASAM PRINCIPLES OF ADDICTION MEDICINE, 6th edition chapter by Richard Saitz, Shannon C. Miller, David A. Fiellin, and Richard N. Rosenthal

RECOMMENDED CONCEPTS AND TERMINOLOGY BY CONSTRUCT

Avoiding Stigmatizing the Patient

Stigmatizing terms can negatively impact a patient's quality of care. For example, research demonstrates that when patients are described as having "substance abuse" instead of a "substance use disorder," clinicians are more likely to recommend punitive approaches. Although there may not be consensus on exactly which terms in and of themselves are stigmatizing versus which are not, clearly using terminology in a way that ignores the many human aspects of the patients beyond their substance use and defines them by their behavior or condition is potentially stigmatizing. Examples include use of the terms "alcoholic," "abuser," "drunk," "user," "addict," or "junkie." Although some may view the use of age-old terms such as "alcoholic" and "addict" as acceptable in addiction recovery programs or other nonmedical settings, these terms could easily be replaced with more medically defined and less stigmatizing terms that incorporate person-first language (eg, "patient with alcohol use disorder," and not "alcoholic"). Our patients are people first, who secondarily have a disease or disorder; using proper terminology can remind clinicians, families, and patients of that fact.

The Spectrum of Use

Several terms are preferred when discussing the spectrum of unhealthy alcohol and other drug use. They include low or lower risk use (and nonuse) and unhealthy use (as in drinking and drug use), which includes hazardous use or at-risk use, harmful use, and addiction and substance use disorder.

Low risk use (or lower risk) or no use refers to the consumption of alcohol or other drugs below the amount identified as physically hazardous, and use in circumstances not defined as psychosocially hazardous.

Unhealthy use covers the entire spectrum including all use that results in negative consequences to one's health, including addiction. Unhealthy alcohol and other drug (substance) use is any use that increases the risk or likelihood for negative health consequences (hazardous use), or has already led to negative health consequences (harmful use). Unhealthy use is an umbrella term that encompasses all levels of use relevant to health, from at-risk use through addiction.

The exact threshold for unhealthy use is a clinical and/or public health decision based on epidemiologic evidence for measurably increased risks for the occurrence of use-related injury, illness, or other negative health consequences. The term "unhealthy," just as with the descriptors "unsafe," "hazardous," "harmful," or "misuse," does not imply there exists an alternatively healthy, safe, nonhazardous, or harmless use, or that there is a way to use such substances properly (ie, without addiction risk).

Hazardous or at-risk use is use that increases the risk for negative health consequences. It does not include use that has already led to negative health consequences. Thresholds are defined by amount, frequency, and/or circumstances of use. The exact definitions may change with evolving epidemiologic evidence and can also vary by preferences of those making clinical or public health decisions regarding thresholds.

Harmful substance use is use that has resulted in negative health consequences. The *International Statistical Classification of Diseases and Related Health Problems*, 10th revision (*ICD-10*) definition of harmful use can be summarized as repeated use that has caused physical or mental damage. Hazardous and harmful are mutually exclusive of each other. The terms could also apply to potentially addictive behaviors.

The US Department of Veterans Affairs describes misuse as the target of alcohol screening and intervention, including disorder and addiction (which is labeled as severe misuse), and misuse is often used to describe taking nonaddictive medications incorrectly. However, the term "misuse" is not an appropriate descriptor for substance dependence, addiction, or substance use disorder because it minimizes the seriousness of the disorder. In addition, a value judgment is at least potentially implied, as if it were an accident, mistake, or even purposeful (a choice), none of which would be appropriate for describing the varied states of harmful use. As such, the term "misuse" can be seen as pejorative and stigmatizing.

"Problem use" is also not preferred because it is not well defined, is used to occasionally refer to harmful use but other times to encompass the spectrum, and can lead to a stigmatizing discussion with the patient being blamed (eg, "you have a problem," "you are a problem"). "Inappropriate use" is not well defined and also carries a pejorative nuance. The terms "binging" or "binge drinking" can be useful for public health messaging but needs to be clearly defined as it is sometimes used to mean a one-time heavy drinking episode but also can be used to mean a more lengthy episode of heavy drinking or other substance use, such as cocaine. "Moderate" drinking or use is not preferred as a term because it implies safety, restraint, avoidance of excess, and even health. Because alcohol is a carcinogen and cancer risk appears at amounts lower than those generally defined as hazardous and, for women who are pregnant, lower limit amounts harmful to the fetus are not well defined, better terms for amounts lower than the amounts defined as risky or hazardous include "lower risk" or "low risk" amounts or simply the term "alcohol use."

The Disorder

When referring to substance use disorders, terms that have been defined and agreed upon should be used. This specificity is essential for clinicians to accurately communicate with each other and for researchers and policy makers to accurately compare populations. Examples of terms that typically indicate a medical disorder and that are roughly synonymous include "person with addiction," "substance use (or gambling) disorder," and "substance dependence."

"Addiction" is a term long used by laypeople, patients, and healthcare providers to indicate a condition that is "characterized by an inability to consistently abstain," that includes "impairment in behavioral control, craving, diminished recognition of significant problems with one's behaviors and interpersonal relationships, and a dysfunctional emotional response." However, the term "addicted" can be problematic because it often incorrectly conflates addiction and physical dependence.

The American Psychological Association's (APA) *Diagnostic and Statistical Manual of Mental Disorders* (*DSM*) Committee on Substance-Related Disorders had "good agreement among committee members as to the definition of the medical condition known as addiction, but there was disagreement as to the label that should be used." "Addiction" was a consideration; however, there was concern that labeling it as such could be pejorative and invite stigma. Although there was agreement that the term "addiction" would "convey the appropriate meaning of the compulsive drug-taking condition and would distinguish it well from 'physical' dependence," the concern for stigma resulted in changing the term from "addiction" to substance "dependence." Thus "addiction" and "substance dependence" were considered as synonymous in describing the same clinical disorder. With the publication of *DSM-5* in 2013, the previous *DSM* terms "substance abuse" and "substance dependence" were made obsolete. This was after consistent findings from studies of over 200,000 study participants revealing that these two terms—"abuse" and "dependence"—were clinically and statistically recognized as representing a single disorder with varying degrees of severity, renamed in *DSM-5* as "substance use disorder" with mild, moderate, or severe severity ratings. Criteria for the disorder no longer included legal problems but did now include craving. In addition, rather than have the threshold as one or more criteria (as in "substance abuse") or three or more criteria (as in "substance dependence"), the threshold was set at two or more criteria for "substance use disorder."

Substance use disorder is well defined, and the features of addiction are carefully described. The *DSM-5* does not define addiction, nor does it exclude addiction as present in a moderate or mild substance use disorder. In addition, a diagnosis of addiction does not require that six (or more) criteria of a substance use disorder be present.

Finally, with respect to the term "dependence," if this term is used it should be clearly defined as the *ICD-10* disorder, the *DSM-IV* disorder, or as physical dependence, which does not necessarily indicate any disorder or addiction and may simply reflect a pharmacologic effect.

Treatment

Medication, including opioid agonist, treatment of addiction has previously been mislabeled "drug," "medication-assisted," "substitution," or "replacement" treatment. These terms are inaccurate; their

pejorative nature and their implicit communication that pharmacotherapy is in some way inferior to psychosocial or mutual help pathways to remission of substance use disorders may be partly responsible for the slow uptake in practice of these efficacious treatments. Such treatments do not substitute for, reproduce the effects of, or replace illicit drugs. And medications do not "assist" treatment; they are

TABLE 2-1	Recommendations for Nonstigmatizing, More Clinically Accurate Language
Avoid	**Prefer**
Abuse	Use (or specify low risk or unhealthy use; the latter includes at-risk/hazardous use, harmful use, substance use disorder, and addiction)
Addict, user, abuser, alcoholic, crackhead, pothead, dope fiend, junkie	Person with addiction, person with a substance use disorder
Addicted baby	Baby experiencing substance withdrawal
Binge[a]	Heavy drinking episode
Dirty vs. clean (drug test)	Positive or negative, detected or not detected
Drunk, smashed, bombed, messed up, strung out	Intoxicated
Fix	Dose, use
Inappropriate use	Harmful use or more accurate terms to specify what is meant
Medical marijuana	Cannabis as medicine[b]
Meth	Methamphetamine, methadone, methylphenidate
Misuse, problem[c]	At-risk or risky use, hazardous use, unhealthy use (to describe the spectrum from risky to at-risk to hazardous use)
Moderate drinking (or drug use)	Low or lower risk use
Relapse[d]	Use, return to use, or disorder vs. remission specifiers (early or sustained) as defined by *DSM-5*
Smoking cessation[e]	Tobacco use disorder treatment, reduction or cessation of tobacco use
Substitution, replacement, medication-assisted treatment	Opioid agonist treatment, medication treatment, psychosocially assisted pharmacological treatment, treatment

DSM-5, *Diagnostic and Statistical Manual of Mental Disorders*, fifth edition.
[a]Can be useful for public health messaging but needs to be clearly defined as it is sometimes not only used to mean a heavy drinking episode but also used to mean a more lengthy episode of heavy drinking or other substance use, such as cocaine.
[b]Currently, marijuana (the plant leaf, stems, and seeds) is not typically sold as medicinal grade or conclusively researched as having more benefits than risks, nor is it Food and Drug Administration (FDA) approved. Moreover, "cannabis" is the term more internationally used and is more descriptive, relating to compounds being researched to explore medical value, such as cannabidiol.
[c]Could be used if clearly defined, and most useful for prescription drug (misuse) when the nature or severity of the condition is unknown. Avoid calling the person or their use a problem.
[d]This term will likely continue to be used, but it should not imply a binary process (abstinent vs. relapse) that does not reflect a typical clinical course that can include lapses or in-between states.
[e]A similar term is not typically used for other drugs with addiction liability. This term seems to place tobacco in a category different than other drugs, which may not be helpful considering its high addiction risk and high morbidity and mortality. More favored terms for smoking include "tobacco use" or "nicotine use." Further, "cessation" or "abstinence," although highly desired, should not be the only goal. Reducing smoking, as opposed to complete cessation, may have limited health benefits but may reduce relapse rates with other substances used by the patient. However, the evidence for smoking reduction having health benefits related to smoking is low, and these results are small compared to complete abstinence.

treatments shown to be efficacious on their own, and studies often fail to show additional benefits of added psychosocial therapies. More accurate alternative terms would be "medication treatment," "treatment," "opioid agonist treatment," or even "psychosocially assisted pharmacotherapy."

During treatment, testing is often performed for addictive substances. In these cases, results should be presented like other medical tests. Results should be identified as "positive" or "negative," "detected" or "not detected" and not "dirty" or "clean," terms which are then often used to describe people in a highly stigmatizing way (eg, "I'm clean," "your urine was dirty," "I tested you today and you were dirty").

SUMMARY

This chapter does not make recommendations regarding what terms people with disorders should use. Some patients (eg, those succeeding in part with participation in social networks such as Alcoholics Anonymous) clearly find benefit in calling themselves an alcoholic or an addict even if it might reflect an internalized stigma. Other patients have strong negative associations to being labeled a drug addict or alcoholic that do not aid in their treatment engagement. Furthermore, patient acceptance of such labels has not been shown to be necessary to achieve good clinical outcomes.

In general, stigmatizing terms should be avoided in the medical profession, as should disorder-first constructions. Terms to be avoided by clinicians and scientists because they may be potentially stigmatizing or clinically unclear are outlined in Table 2-1; however, this table is not exhaustive. In general, scientific and medical terms that are clearly defined and nonstigmatizing are preferred over vague and inaccurate terms, terms that are difficult to define, and terms that have multiple meanings. Better use of terminology can improve communications in addiction science and healthcare and can improve quality of care for patients.

KEY POINTS

1. Avoid stigmatizing and ill-defined terms such as "abuse."
2. Avoid disorder-first terms, such as "addict."
3. Use "substance use disorder" or "addiction" to refer to the disorder and "at-risk" or "hazardous" to refer to use that has a risk of negative consequences.

REVIEW QUESTIONS

1. Which of the following is the most accurate and least stigmatizing term to refer to illicit drugs found in a urine test of a person with addiction?
   A. Dirty
   B. Not clean
   C. Detected, positive
   D. Altered

2. Which term is the most accurate and least stigmatizing to refer to people who use substances, have a loss of control over use, and have tolerance and withdrawal symptoms?
   A. Substance abuser
   B. Problem substance user
   C. Addict
   D. Person with a substance use disorder

3. A patient imbibes six alcoholic drinks on an occasion twice a week. She has no health conditions related to drinking; no loss of control; is not spending a great deal of time procuring, using, or recovering from the effects of drinking; has no withdrawal; and has no other criteria of a disorder except tolerance. The most accurate term to refer to this condition is:
   A. hazardous use.
   B. problem use.
   C. addiction.
   D. substance use disorder.

ANSWERS

1. **C**
2. **D**
3. **A**

SUGGESTED READINGS

Broyles LM, Binswanger IA, Jenkins JA, et al. Confronting inadvertent stigma and pejorative language in addiction scholarship: a recognition and response. *Subst Abus.* 2014; 35(3):217-221.

Kelly JF, Westerhoff CM. Does it matter how we refer to individuals with substance-related problems? A randomized study with two commonly used terms. *Int J Drug Policy.* 2010;21(3):202-207.

O'Brien CP. Addiction and dependence in DSM-V. *Addiction.* 2011;106(5):1-3.

Saitz R. Things that work, things that don't work, and things that matter: including words. *J Addict Med.* 2015;9:429-430.

Saitz R. Unhealthy alcohol use. *N Engl J Med.* 2005;352(6): 596-607.

Wakeman SE. Medications for addiction treatment: changing language to improve care. *J Addict Med.* 2017;11(1):1-2.

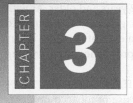

3

The Epidemiology of Substance Use Disorders

Summary by Faye Chao

▌ Based on THE ASAM PRINCIPLES OF ADDICTION MEDICINE,
6th edition chapter by Rosa M. Crum

SOME EPIDEMIOLOGIC PRINCIPLES

Epidemiology is the study of how diseases are distributed in populations as well as the study of the determinants of disease and health. *Prevalence* is the ratio of the total number of cases of a particular disease divided by the total number of individuals in a particular population at a specific time. *Incidence* refers to the occurrence of new cases of a disease divided by the total number at risk for the disorder during a specified period. Incidence is generally taken to represent the risk of disease, whereas prevalence is an indicator of the public health burden that the disease imposes.

Relative risk measures the incidence of the disease among those with a particular characteristic divided by the incidence of the disease among those without exposure to that characteristic. *Odds ratio* is also a measure of the strength of association, such as between a characteristic and disease. A relative risk or odds ratio greater than one indicates a positive association of disease with a given characteristic, whereas a ratio less than one indicates a negative association. If there is no difference in the incidence among those with and without the characteristic, the ratio is one.

Epidemiologic studies can be divided into two types: observational or experimental. In observational studies (eg, cross-sectional, case–control, cohort), the investigator observes the study participants and gathers information for analysis. Analytic studies, such as case–control or cohort studies, generally test a hypothesis of a suspected association between a particular exposure (risk factor) and a disease or other outcome. In experimental studies (eg, randomized clinical trials), study groups are selected, and often an intervention is given to one group. The study participants are followed, and the outcomes of each group are measured and compared.

Many major surveys in the United States and other countries have assessed the prevalence of addiction. Comparison of these studies sometimes is difficult because different measures and definitions of addiction are employed. Some surveys have used structured interviews according to criteria that have become universally recognized, such as the *Diagnostic and Statistical Manual of Mental Disorders*, now in its fifth edition (*DSM-5*), and the *International Classification of Diseases and Related Health Problems*, now in its 10th revision (*ICD-10*). Throughout the text, when we use the term *substance use disorder*, we are referring to substance abuse and/or dependence (diagnoses prior to *DSM-5*).

The National Epidemiologic Survey on Alcohol and Related Conditions (NESARC) was first conducted from 2001 to 2002, with a prospective follow-up between 2004 and 2005. This provided lifetime and 12-month estimates of substance use disorders based on *DSM-IV* criteria using the Alcohol Use Disorder and Associated Disabilities Interview Schedule. The NESARC-III, completed during 2012 to 2013, was an independent cross-sectional sampling of the US population based on *DSM-5* criteria. To date, it is likely the largest nationally representative survey in the United States that evaluates the prevalence of substance use disorders based on *DSM-5* criteria.

ALCOHOL USE DISORDERS

Prevalence

The overall 12-month prevalence of *DSM-5*–defined alcohol use disorder in the United States is 13.9%, with 7.3% having mild, 3.2% having moderate, and 3.4% having severe alcohol use disorder. Overall lifetime prevalence is 29.1%, with 8.6% having mild, 6.6% having moderate, and 13.9% having severe lifetime alcohol use disorder. Consistent with earlier findings and other surveys, data from the NESARC-III show that alcohol use disorder is found to be higher among males (17.6% 12-month and 36.0% lifetime prevalence) than among females (10.4% 12-month and 22.7% lifetime prevalence). Most studies have found that the prevalence of alcohol use disorder is highest among young adults and decreases among older age groups.

The most recent prior-year estimates of alcohol use disorders in the United States come from the annual National Survey on Drug Use and Health (NSDUH). Since 2000, the NSDUH has gathered information of prior-year prevalence of substance use disorders based on *DSM-IV* criteria. Data from the 2016 NSDUH indicate that 5.6% of survey participants met the criteria for *DSM-IV* alcohol use disorder (abuse or dependence) in the prior year. The highest prevalence for past year *DSM-IV* alcohol use disorder was found for young adults aged 18 to 25 years (10.7%).

Differences in estimates across surveys may be due to variations in the diagnostic instrumentation, the version of the *DSM* used, the size of the survey sample, specific methods used during data gathering, and the locale of the survey participants as well as specific characteristics of the populations surveyed.

Incidence

Prospective data gathered over time are less available; consequently, there is less information on incidence rates for substance use disorders in the general population. Generally, studies have found that the incidence of drinking problems is lower for women than for men and that the incidence for both men and women declines with age. One study found that women tended to develop problems associated with drinking later in life than did men, and women were found to have higher rates of remission across all age groups than did men. Both the Epidemiologic Catchment Area (ECA) study and the NESARC indicate that the greatest risk for alcohol use disorders occurs during young adulthood (late teens to twenties).

DRUG USE DISORDERS
Prevalence

In the NESARC-III, use of the following substances was included in drug use disorder assessments: sedatives (tranquilizers), cannabis, amphetamines, cocaine, opioids, hallucinogens, "club drugs" (eg, ketamine, ecstasy), and inhalants. Overall 12-month prevalence of *DSM-5* drug use disorders in the NESARC-III survey is 3.9%, with 1.9% being mild and 2.0% being moderate to severe. Lifetime prevalence of *DSM-5* drug use disorder is 9.9%, with 3.4% being mild and 6.6% being moderate to severe. The 2016 NSDUH found that the past-year prevalence of drug use disorders based on *DSM-IV* criteria was

2.7% among participants 12 years and older. As with alcohol use disorder, men generally are found to have a higher lifetime prevalence of drug use disorders overall, with a higher prevalence among young adults.

From the 2016 NSDUH, we know that 28.5% of the population reported use of tobacco products within the prior year. Data from the NESARC-III indicate that 20.0% of the population met the *DSM-5* criteria for nicotine use disorder in the prior year, and 27.9% had a history of nicotine use disorder during their lifetime.

Incidence

There is a relative paucity of information regarding the incidence of drug use disorders as a group, with less information available for specific drugs. Early findings from the 1-year prospective ECA data showed that the incidence of illicit drug use disorders as a group was 1.09 per 100 person-years. More recent analyses of the 3-year prospective NESARC data showed the annual incidence of drug use disorder was 0.31 per 100 person-years. In both studies, men developed drug use disorder at a higher rate than women, and the highest incidence for both was found in the 18- to 29-year-old age group. Annual incidence dropped sharply after young adulthood, and the incidence of drug use disorders among those 65 years of age and older was extremely low or zero.

Recent Trends of Alcohol, Tobacco, and Illicit Drug Use

Comparing data from the 2001-2002 and the 2012-2013 NESARC surveys, 12-month alcohol use and alcohol use disorder increased over time. Alcohol use rose from 65.4% to 72.7% and alcohol use disorder increased from 8.5% to 12.7%. The largest increases were found for women, older adults, individuals in lower socioeconomic groups, and racial minorities. These findings differ from the most recent 2016 NSDUH data, which indicate that over the past one and a half decades, the proportion of current drinkers (ie, having at least one drink in the past month) has remained essentially unchanged (51.8% in 2002 vs. 50.7% in 2016). Similarly, the rates of binge drinking and heavy drinking have not changed significantly from the 2002 to 2016 NSDUH (about 23% to 24% for binge drinking and 6% to 7% for heavy drinking).

Use of tobacco products has declined over the prior one and a half decades based on NSDUH data, from a high of 30.4% prevalence in 2002 to the current prevalence of 23.5%. However, these estimates vary by age group, gender, and race/ethnicity. Use of tobacco cigarettes has also been shown to decline by the Monitoring the Future (MTF) surveys, which annually completes a school-based sample of 8th, 9th, and 12th graders in the United States. These declines have leveled off in recent years, and new trends have emerged. For example, electronic cigarette (e-cigarette) use is more common among US youth than is traditional cigarette use.

Past-month illicit drug use has risen slightly over the past one and a half decades according to NSDUH data: 8.3% in 2002 versus 10.6% in 2016. The most commonly used illicit substance is marijuana. Synthetic marijuana has been tracked by the MTF since 2011 and prior-year prevalence among 12th graders peaked in 2011 at 11.4% then declined markedly to 3.5% in 2016.

Over the past two decades, there has been a massive increase in the use, both medical and non-medical, of opioids and in deaths related to their use. Many individuals who use heroin report earlier non-medical use of prescription opioids. Relatively large increases in heroin use and opioid use disorder have been reported among white young adults and among those with prior nonmedical use of prescription opioids. Lifetime prevalence of heroin use increased from 0.33% in the 2001-2002 NESARC to 1.6% in the 2012-2013 NESARC-III. A large proportion of recent opioid deaths has been attributed to overdose due to synthetic opioids, particularly fentanyl. A recent assessment of overdose deaths in ten US states between July and December 2016 indicated that 56.3% of the states' reported opioid overdose deaths involved fentanyl, and fentanyl was the stated cause of death in 97.1% of the medical examiners' reports.

REMISSION FROM SUBSTANCE USE DISORDERS

Remission varies by individual characteristics and subtype of disorder, and maintaining remission is dependent on consumption patterns while in remission. Using data from the NESARC, one group found that at 3-year follow-up, maintenance of successful recovery from alcohol dependence was greatest for abstainers. Only a minority of individuals with substance abuse or dependence reported using treatment services.

CORRELATES AND SUSPECTED RISK FACTORS

Gender

Alcohol use disorders are more common among men than among women, although survey data in the United States over the past 20 years provide evidence that the gender gap is narrowing. Men also have a higher prevalence and incidence of drug use disorders than do women, although gender differences vary by the specific substance and the age of use. For example, in the 2016 MTF, annual prevalence of any illicit drug use as well as for particular substances including inhalants, tranquilizers, and amphetamines was slightly higher for eighth-grade girls than for boys.

Age

The prevalence of alcohol and drug use disorders is generally lower among older adults, possibly because the incidence decreases over the life span, the duration of the disorder is reduced, or some combination of the two factors. It is also possible that the means by which a substance use disorder is identified in young adults may not be relevant to the elderly, leading to underrecognition. Prevalence and incidence rates for alcohol and drug use disorders are highest among individuals in late adolescence and young adulthood. In general, the earlier the age of first use of alcohol or illicit drugs, the greater the estimated risk associated with the subsequent development of a substance use disorder. More recent birth cohorts have been more likely to initiate drug use in childhood and early adolescence, particularly for cannabis, cocaine, and nonmedical use of drugs.

Race and Ethnicity

Evaluating the effect of race and ethnic background on addiction is complex and sometimes conflicting. African American youth begin drinking at older ages and are less likely to develop alcohol use disorder relative to whites. However, African Americans tend to suffer more medical and social consequences from drinking. The prevalence of alcohol use disorder is also lower for Hispanics relative to whites, but alcohol-related mortality is higher for Hispanic men relative to non-Hispanic white men. Asian Americans generally have the lowest prevalence of alcohol use disorders in the United States, and American Indians historically have had the highest. Less information is available for drug use disorders. Reports using data from the 2016 NSDUH indicate that the occurrence of past-year illicit drug use disorders was highest among Native Americans and lowest among Asian Americans. Similar relationships were documented in analyses of 12-month prevalence using the NESARC-III. Black, Asian, and

Hispanic subgroups were less likely than whites to report specific nonmedical prescription drug use and disorders, whereas American Indians were more likely to report this.

Family History

Alcohol use disorder clusters in families, and a family history of pre–*DSM-5* alcohol dependence may predict the severity of the disorder in probands. Although studies have indicated a possible genetic relationship for alcohol dependence, the association is complex. Evidence indicates that approximately half of the risk may be attributed to genetic influences, and environmental influences have a major role. Analyses have also indicated associations of genetic liability to drug use disorders.

Employment Status and Occupation

In the 2016 NSDUH findings, alcohol use disorder in the prior year was slightly higher among the unemployed than in full-time employed individuals (8.8% vs. 7.0%). Other associations are less clear; some studies find that labor jobs are more often associated with alcohol use disorder, whereas others find associations with employment in high occupational strata. Stressful working conditions can be associated with drinking levels, and employment status may also influence recovery. The 2016 NSDUH showed a higher proportion of illicit drug use disorders among the unemployed (8.0%) as compared with those employed full or part time (2.4% and 3.7%, respectively). Associations with employment status may differ by specific substance type. Findings from the National Comorbidity Study (NCS) indicate that high occupational strata are associated with drug use disorders.

Marital Status

Marital status has been found to be related to the occurrence of alcohol disorders and drinking behavior, but understanding the temporal relationships may be difficult. Analyses of NESARC data showed that persons in stable marriages or who cohabit had the lowest 12-month prevalence of alcohol use disorder (10.4%) as opposed to adults who had never married (25.0%) or who were widowed, divorced, or separated (11.4%). Marriage has been shown to relate to decreases in subsequent risk for alcohol use disorder, and this potentially protective association was found to be strongest for those with a positive family history of alcohol use disorder.

Individuals who had never married also had the highest prevalence of drug use disorders. Lack of marital stability and the periods of transition to and from marriage or divorce appear to influence substance use, treatment outcomes, and drug-related mortality.

Educational Level

Studies of the relationship between educational level and drinking patterns as well as the development of alcohol use disorders have yielded conflicting results. Analyses of the 2016 NSDUH data show that the proportion of those who reported drinking in the prior year increased with higher levels of education. However, individuals without a college degree have higher risks for alcohol use disorder relative to those with a college degree or more. Moreover, dropping out of high school or leaving college early is associated with an increased risk of alcohol use disorder. These associations are bidirectional, and genetic factors may be associated with both. Lifetime prevalence of drug use disorders also varies by educational level. The proportion of those with prior-year illicit drug use disorders is lowest for college graduates. One study found that high-risk youth had greater access to drugs as well as greater adverse consequences from drug use relative to students considered low risk.

COMORBIDITY OF ALCOHOL AND DRUG USE DISORDERS

Alcohol use disorders are also frequently comorbid with other drug use disorders. Analyses of the NESARC data found positive associations for mood, anxiety, and personality disorders occurring with most substances use disorders. Outcomes tend to be worse for individuals with co-occurring psychiatric and substance use disorders.

KEY POINTS

1. Numerous major surveys in the United States have assessed the prevalence of addiction. These include the Epidemiologic Catchment Area (ECA) study, the National Comorbidity Study (NCS), the National Epidemiologic Survey on Alcohol and Related Conditions (NESARC), the Monitoring the Future (MTF) study, and the annual National Survey on Drug Use and Health (NSDUH).
2. Use of tobacco products in general has shown some declines over the past one and a half

decades, although use of electronic cigarettes has risen.

3. There has been a massive increase over the past two decades in the use and misuse of opioids as well as in the rate and occurrence of deaths related to their use.

4. There are many correlates and suspected risk factors for alcohol and drug use disorders.

   a. Alcohol and illicit drug use disorders are more common in males than in females.

   b. Rates of both decrease with age.

   c. African Americans and Hispanics have a lower prevalence of alcohol and drug use disorders than whites, but when disorders do develop in these minority populations, the disorders may be more persistent and lead to more medical and social consequences. Asian Americans have the lowest prevalence of alcohol and drug use disorders, and American Indians have the highest prevalence of both.

   d. Genetics play a significant role in the development of alcohol and drug use disorders.

   e. Persons in stable marriages have a lower prevalence of alcohol and drug use disorders than do those who have never married, but stressful marriages or transitions may increase substance use.

REVIEW QUESTIONS

1. Prevalence is:
   A. The ratio of the total number of cases of a particular disease divided by the total number of individuals in a particular population at a specific time
   B. The occurrence of new cases of a disease divided by the total number at risk for the disorder during a specified period
   C. The incidence of the disease among those with a particular characteristic divided by the incidence of the disease among those without exposure to that particular characteristic
   D. A measure of the strength of association such as between a characteristic and disease

2. Which study is updated annually to assess prior-year prevalence of substance use disorders?
   A. The Epidemiologic Catchment Area (ECA) study
   B. The National Comorbidity Survey (NCS)
   C. The National Survey on Drug Use and Health (NSDUH)
   D. The National Epidemiologic Survey on Alcohol and Related Conditions (NESARC)

3. What is the association of age and gender with prevalence of alcohol and drug use disorders?
   A. Alcohol and drug use disorders are more prevalent in males than females, and prevalence increases with age.
   B. Alcohol and drug use disorders are more prevalent in females than males, and prevalence increases with age.
   C. Alcohol and drug use disorders are more prevalent in males than females, and prevalence decreases with age.
   D. Alcohol and drug use disorders are more prevalent in females than males, and prevalence decreases with age.

ANSWERS

1. **A**
2. **C**
3. **C**

SUGGESTED READINGS

Ahrnsbrak R, Bose J, Hedden SL, Lipari RN, Park-Lee E. *Key Substance Use and Mental Health Indicators in the United States: Results from the 2016 National Survey on Drug Use and Health*. Rockville, MD: Center for Behavioral Health Statistics and Quality, Substance Abuse and Mental Health Services Administration; 2017. HHS Publication No. SMA 7-5044, NSDUH Series H-52.

Grant BF, Goldstein RB, Saha TD, et al. Epidemiology of DSM-5 alcohol use disorder: results from the National Epidemiologic Survey on Alcohol and Related Conditions III. *JAMA Psychiatry*. 2015;72(8):757-766.

Grant BF, Saha TD, Ruan WJ, et al. Epidemiology of DSM-5 drug use disorder: results from the National Epidemiologic Survey on Alcohol and Related Conditions-III. *JAMA Psychiatry*. 2016;73(1):39-47.

CHAPTER 4

The Anatomy of Addiction

Summary by Thomas J.R. Beveridge

Based on THE ASAM PRINCIPLES OF ADDICTION MEDICINE, 6th edition chapter by Thomas J.R. Beveridge, Colleen A. Hanlon, and David C.S. Roberts

PRIMER ON NEUROANATOMY

The structures most often mentioned in the context of drug abuse are closely associated with the limbic system, lateral hypothalamus, basal ganglia, and frontal cortical regions.

The limbic system has been characterized as highly interconnected, phylogenetically older regions of the forebrain that appear to form the only major route for information transfer between the neocortex and the hypothalamus. The main structures denoted by the limbic system are the limbic lobe (subcallosal area, cingulate, and parahippocampal gyri), amygdala, hippocampus, parts of the basal ganglia, anterior thalamic nucleus, parts of the hypothalamus, the habenula, and the olfactory cortex (Fig. 4-1). The structures associated with the limbic system (such as the hypothalamus, hippocampus, and amygdala) are essential not only for learning and memory but also for the emotional context and the affective response to learned associations.

Many drugs of hazardous use have their sites of action within the limbic system, and the neurochemistry within these structures is altered during the addiction process. This may help explain why decisions surrounding drug seeking and drug taking seem to be driven more by emotion and instinct rather than by logic.

The basal ganglia are traditionally thought of as a motor system; however, the idea that this system deals only with motor function while the limbic system deals with reinforcement and emotion is oversimplified. As more is learned about how the basal ganglia and limbic system communicate, it is becoming increasingly clear that the two systems are jointly involved in coordinating motivated behavior. The largest mass associated with the basal ganglia is the striatum (caudate–putamen). The dorsal portion has long been considered part of the basal ganglia, whereas the ventral striatum (also called the accumbens) is considered to be part of the limbic system. Mogenson famously described the accumbens as "the place where motivation is translated into action."

The prefrontal cortex (PFC) is thought to be the "hub" of executive function in the brain. The PFC in humans is subdivided into three main regions: (1) the orbitofrontal cortex and the ventromedial areas (vm-PFC), which are thought to be involved in processing reward; (2) the dorsolateral prefrontal cortex (dl-PFC), more broadly involved in decision making; and (3) the anterior and ventral cingulate cortex, which helps to control whether a particular behavior will be performed and to what intensity.

NEUROANATOMY OF DRUG REINFORCEMENT

The "site of action" is a pharmacologic concept that defines the access point for a drug to produce a specific response. If that response is defined behaviorally (eg, anorexic effect, convulsant effect, antidepressant effect), then the site of action identifies the receptors and brain regions responsible for that particular behavioral response. In vitro experiments have shown that many drugs of hazardous use, particularly psychostimulants, interact with dopamine (DA), noradrenaline (NA), and serotonin (5-hydroxytryptamine [5-HT]) transporters. Therefore, psychostimulant drugs act as indirect agonists everywhere these transmitters are found. The projections from DA, NA, and 5-HT cell bodies are extensive; indeed, there is hardly a brain region that is not innervated by at least two of the monoamines. Given that psychostimulants have an effect at the terminal regions of each of these systems, every area of the brain would be expected to be affected to some extent by an injection of cocaine or amphetamine. It has been a considerable challenge, therefore, sorting out what transmitter in which particular area produces toxic effects and adverse reactions on the one hand and pleasurable or positive reinforcing effects on the other. Much of these data has been gleaned from preclinical studies of drug reinforcement.

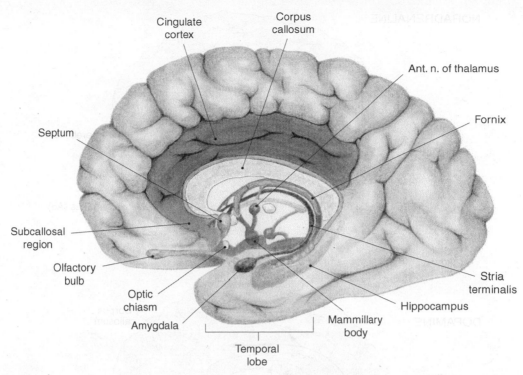

Figure 4-1. Regions of the human brain associated with the limbic system, which include a loop of cortex extending from the subcallosal region through the cingulate cortex to the parahippocampal gyrus. Also shown are the hippocampal formation, septum, amygdala, and mammillary bodies. (Reprinted with permission from Miller SC, Fiellin DA, Saitz R, Rosenthal RN. *The ASAM Principles of Addiction Medicine*. 6th ed. Philadelphia: ASAM, 2019.)

Psychostimulants

Cocaine binds to DA, NA, and 5-HT transporters and blocks the reuptake of these neurotransmitters. Amphetamine acts additionally as a releasing agent. Both of these actions result in an increased concentration of monoamine neurotransmitters in the synapse.

Figure 4-2 demonstrates how the origins and projections of the main neuronal mass are associated with NA, 5-HT, and DA. All start in the brainstem and project upward. The catecholaminergic NA fibers start in the locus coeruleus and spread diffusely. The DA system is more contained, originating in the ventral tegmental area (VTA) and the substantia nigra.

The extensive reach and overlap of the DA, NA, and 5-HT systems throughout the brain make research complex. For many years, it was thought that drug use and addiction were confined to humans and thus was attributed to the neocortex; however, subsequent research on animals demonstrated that self-administration of drugs will occur in other mammalian species such as rats, dogs, cats, rabbits, and nonhuman primates. This supports neuroanatomical findings that addiction arises in subcortical, evolutionary residual regions of the brain—that is, limbic and brainstem areas.

This anatomical understanding may help us to understand the complex nature of reinforcement. Although patients may describe the alterations in consciousness associated with a specific substance as the "reason" for ongoing use, the mechanics behind use and addiction are more complex and involve subcortical, unconscious factors.

Dopamine plays a central role in reward and drug addiction. Studies by Roy Wise demonstrated that treatment with DA antagonists produced an increase in cocaine or amphetamine intake in animals previously trained to self-administer these drugs. The use of the dopaminergic neurotoxin 6-OH-DA has been a useful tool in highlighting the role of DA. Removing the DA input to the ventral striatum (previously called nucleus accumbens, or NAcc) or destroying the DA cell bodies in the VTA resulted in diminution or abolition of cocaine self-administration in animals. Denervation of NA systems to the entire forebrain had no effect. The data demonstrate that the DA projects from the

NORADRENALINE

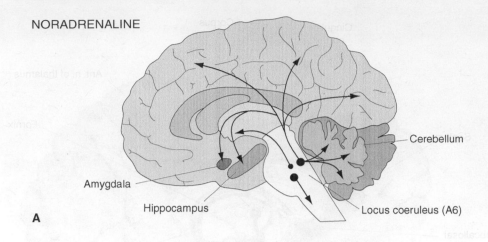

Cerebellum

Amygdala

Hippocampus

Locus coeruleus (A6)

A

DOPAMINE

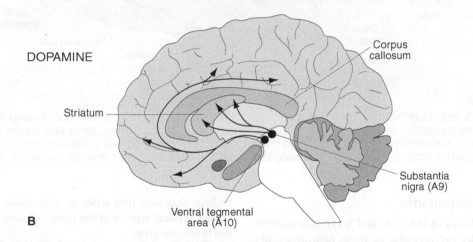

Corpus
callosum

Striatum

Substantia
nigra (A9)

Ventral tegmental
area (A10)

B

SEROTONIN

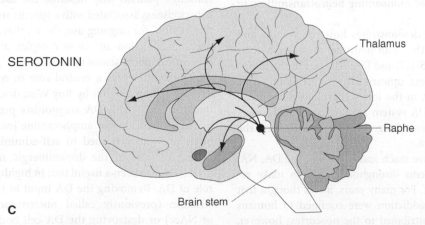

Thalamus

Raphe

Brain stem

C

Figure 4-2. Schematic diagram illustrating the distribution of the main central neuronal pathways containing noradrenaline (**A**), dopamine (**B**), and serotonin (**C**). The location of cell bodies of origin is indicated by *circles* with the projections indicated by *arrows*. (Reprinted with permission from Miller SC, Fiellin DA, Saitz R, Rosenthal RN. *The ASAM Principles of Addiction Medicine*. 6th ed. Philadelphia: ASAM, 2019.)

VTA to limbic areas are critical for the reinforcing effects of cocaine and amphetamines.

Both ablation and stimulation studies confirm that the striatum is responsible for motor behavior: the ventral area for locomotion and the dorsal for stereotypy. The appearance of parkinsonian side effects of neuroleptics confirms the involvement of DA in motor pathways involved in stereotypic repetitive motor behaviors. Any behavior can become reinforced, and the more frequently an action occurs in the setting of drug use, the more likely it will become stereotyped. As such behaviors increase, others are excluded—thus limiting the behavioral range of the animal. In the case of a person with addiction, the frequent behaviors associated with drug seeking and drug taking become repetitive and ritualistic.

The great body of research showing VTA-DA neurons' role in drug use and with primary reinforcing stimuli such as food, drinking, and sex has led to the term "mesolimbic reward pathway." Interestingly, there is no direct connection between this region and visual, auditory, or somatosensory systems. It appears instead that the VTA is a part of, and receives inputs from, a widespread collection of neurons that belong to the isodendritic core. This system is a network of neurons stretching from the brainstem to telencephalon. It would appear that this network serves an integrative function and responses to changes in the environment that are biologically significant. At present, it remains unclear whether the VTA-DA neurons respond differentially than others in the network and whether they are specifically activated by reward or more generally by any other important stimulus.

Opioids

Opioid receptors are expressed throughout the brain, especially in limbic and limbic-related structures. There are three different types of G protein–coupled opioid receptors: μ, κ, and δ, which are acted on by both endogenous and exogenously applied opioids. Selective μ agonist drugs, such as morphine, heroin, and most clinically used opioid analgesics, produce analgesia, euphoria, respiratory depression, emesis, and antidiuretic effects. Selective κ agonist drugs, such as the experimental compounds ethylketazocine and bremazocine, produce analgesia, dysphoria, and diuretic effects but no respiratory depression. There is less known about the direct role of δ receptors. Agonists at the μ receptor are more likely to have abuse liability than κ agonists.

Almost all that is known about the neurobiology of opioid reinforcement is derived from animal models. Three approaches have been used to investigate the involvement of various brain regions in opioid reward: (1) intracerebral self-administration of opioid agonists, (2) blockade of intravenous (IV) heroin self-administration by intracerebral injections of opioid antagonists, and (3) disruption of IV heroin self-administration by lesions. Generally, the focus has been on areas associated with the mesolimbic DA system (ventral striatum and VTA). Self-administration of drugs directly into various brain regions would seem to be the most straightforward test of their involvement in reinforcement processes; however, the procedures have a number of technical problems that limit their appeal. The main areas supporting opioid self-administration are the ventral striatum, NAcc, and VTA, with the latter being the most responsive. Interestingly, whereas injection of μ- and δ-opioid agonists into the VTA is strongly reinforcing, injection of antagonist into the VTA has little effect. This is especially surprising given that intracranial injections of antagonists into other areas of the brain can produce strong and predictable reactions.

When systemic naloxone is given, a compensatory increase in opioid self-administration is noticed. Similarly, increase in IV heroin self-administration is noticed when low-dose opioid antagonists are injected into the NAcc, periaqueductal gray, stria terminalis, and lateral hypothalamus but not the PFC.

Lesion studies offer further support of the key role played by the NAcc in opioid reinforcement—kainic acid injected into the NAcc correlated with impaired heroin self-administration and yet did not have this effect when injected into other areas. Further studies suggest that the NAcc core is far more responsive than the shell—namely, opioid self-administration. Similar site-specific effects have been found when β-funaltrexamine (an irreversible opioid antagonist) is injected into the caudal but not rostral NAcc.

The role of the mesolimbic DA system in opioid reinforcement is unclear. DA antagonists reduced self-administration of cocaine but not of heroin, and opioid antagonists reduce heroin but not cocaine use. However, it has been shown that opioids indirectly affect DA cell firing through inhibition of γ-aminobutyric acid interneurons in the VTA. This disinhibition can result in enhanced DA release in the NAcc. Heroin self-administration increases DA in the accumbens, and this has been argued to be the mechanisms of action for heroin reinforcement. It appears that DA innervation to the VTA is very important to opioid reinforcement, whereas altering such innervation to the NAcc has little effect. In contrast, reducing DA innervation to the NAcc results in a dramatic reduction in cocaine reinforcement.

Cannabinoids

Two cannabinoid receptors (CB1 and CB2) have been identified. Both are G protein–coupled receptors and function to inhibit adenylate cyclase. They are acted on by endogenous cannabinoids and exogenous activators such as marijuana. There remains limited understanding about the reinforcing neuroanatomy of cannabinoids—this being due to difficulties in study designs with inhaled marijuana. The use of IV Δ9-tetrahydrocannabinol for self-administration studies on animals and the use of synthetic cannabinoid agonists have shown some reinforcing effects. It appears that both opioid and DA mechanisms may interact with cannabinoid reinforcement.

NEUROANATOMY OF DRUG ADDICTION

The research questions that can be addressed by using animal models are necessarily different than those that can be asked with human subjects. The former allow for invasive interventions (ie, surgical manipulations not possible with humans), whereas the latter provide insight into the uniquely human aspects of addiction. Addiction is a disease that lives in the real world and thus encompasses many different facets, such as polydrug use, comorbidity with other disorders, predisposition, drug use history, and environmental context. Thus, the literature on human drug abuse offers quite different insights.

The neuroanatomy of addiction in human subjects has been studied using positron emission tomography (PET) and functional magnetic resonance imaging (fMRI). PET uses a radioisotope that is introduced into the body and binds to specific receptors, transporters, and enzymes. Specific ligands can be visualized, thereby offering insights into drug distribution and changes in receptor mechanism in vivo. fMRI offers much greater temporal resolution. Changes in the fMRI signal can be assessed on the order of seconds rather than minutes, making it possible to detect metabolic changes associated with transient cognitive demands or craving states.

Volkow et al. used PET to demonstrate decreased relative cerebral blood flow in the PFC of chronic cocaine users and metabolic changes varying with time from last use (increased in the first week of withdrawal). PET has also been used to show high cocaine binding in the corpus striatum in non–drug-using human subjects and to show that striatal dopamine D2 receptor binding is reduced in cocaine, heroin, and methamphetamine abusers and also in alcohol dependence. This area of work is in good concordance with nonhuman primate PET studies showing decreased D2 receptor availability in animals that are more susceptible to the reinforcing aspects of cocaine.

fMRI studies have demonstrated increased activity in the NAcc and decreased activity in the amygdala in cocaine users during cravings. Studies also showed an increase in activity in the VTA and substantia nigra, pons, basal forebrain, caudate, and cingulate that correlated with self-reported feelings of "rush" following cocaine use. Drug users also show increases in brain activity in limbic areas and the PFC following the presentation of drug-associated cues (such as pictures of drugs and drug paraphernalia) when compared with nondrug users and decreased responsiveness when presented with nondrug reinforcers (eg, sexually evocative cues).

One brain area, the insula, has been recently recognized as having an essential role in the detection of interoceptive cues. These cues can also provoke powerful cravings for drugs and are a key component in the addiction process. A recent study by Bechara et al. discovered that nicotine-dependent patients with lesions to their insula reported a disruption in smoking regularity at a far greater frequency than did patients with lesions to other brain areas. Furthermore, smokers who acquired insula damage were more likely to quit smoking easily and immediately and to remain abstinent. Remarkably, drug-associated cues can produce limbic activation in cocaine users even when these stimuli are not consciously perceived. Childress et al. presented stimuli for only 33 milliseconds. Although this short presentation was too brief for the image to be correctly identified, the drug-related stimuli nonetheless produced a strong increase in activity in the ventral pallidum and amygdala. The intensity of this response strongly predicted the magnitude of the subject's affective response when later shown visible versions of the same cues. These data suggest that drug cues can stimulate drug craving even before there is conscious awareness. Childress et al. speculate that "by the time the motivational state is experienced and labeled as conscious desire, the ancient limbic reward circuitry already has a running start." Medical imaging technology has thus provided concrete evidence of limbic involvement in drug craving that fits well with the wealth of evidence for animal studies.

KEY POINTS

1. To understand the neuroanatomy and psycho-pharmacology of addiction, we must understand the normal processes and structures involved in motivation, reward, decision making, and impulse control.
2. From here, we can examine the compulsivity, excessive consumption, and the resultant harm, which are central to addiction.

REVIEW QUESTIONS

1. Which part of the brain is most associated with the affective response to learned associations?
   A. Limbic system
   B. Lateral hypothalamus
   C. Basal ganglia
   D. Frontal cortical regions

2. What part of the brain could be described as the "hub" of executive function in the brain?
   A. Hippocampus
   B. Prefrontal cortex
   C. Nucleus accumbens
   D. Lateral hypothalamus

3. True or False: Drug reinforcement is restricted to humans because it requires alterations in conscious awareness.

4. Destroying the cell bodies associated with which transmitter system results in a diminished reinforcing effect of cocaine and amphetamine?
   A. Noradrenaline
   B. Dopamine
   C. Serotonin
   D. Endorphins

5. fMRI studies show that when drug users are shown pictures of drugs and drug paraphernalia, their brain activity is:
   A. increased in the ventral pallidum and amygdala.
   B. increased in the prefrontal cortex.
   C. decreased in the ventral striatum.
   D. Both A and B

ANSWERS

1. **A**
2. **B**
3. **False**
4. **B**
5. **D**

SUGGESTED READINGS

Breiter HC, Gollub RL, Weisskoff RM, et al. Acute effects of cocaine on human brain activity and emotion. *Neuron.* 1997;19(3):591-611.

Kalivas PW, Volkow ND. The neural basis of addiction: a pathology of motivation and choice. *Am J Psychiatry.* 2005; 162(8):1403-1413.

Phillips AG, Ahn S, Howland JG. Amygdalar control of the mesocorticolimbic dopamine system: parallel pathways to motivated behavior. *Neurosci Biobehav Rev.* 2003;27(6): 543-554.

Roberts DC, Koob GF, Klonoff P, Fibiger HC. Extinction and recovery of cocaine self-administration following 6-hydroxydopamine lesions of the nucleus accumbens. *Pharmacol Biochem Behav.* 1980;12(5):781-787.

Wise RA. Brain reward circuitry: insights from unsensed incentives. *Neuron.* 2002;36(2):229-240.

From Neurobiology to Treatment: Progress Against Addiction

Summary by Drew D. Kiraly and Eric J. Nestler

Based on THE ASAM PRINCIPLES OF ADDICTION MEDICINE, 6th edition chapter by Drew D. Kiraly and Eric J. Nestler

Drug addiction is a public health crisis that takes a tremendous toll on the health and well-being of millions of patients. Addiction is generally defined as increased or out of control drug use leading to negative social and medical consequences in the patient's life. Although there are existent medications to treat multiple types of addiction, there are no medications approved for all forms of addiction and the treatments are generally only somewhat effective for most individuals. Diverse types of chemicals (ie, drugs) cause addiction. Interestingly, the protein targets for most addictive drugs are well characterized (Table 5-1), and despite the fact that there are distinct mechanisms of action, they still create very similar behavioral syndromes. An extensive amount of research has been done to understand the brain circuits that are changed to mediate the behavioral phenotype of addiction. The most heavily implicated brain region in addiction is the nucleus accumbens, a part of the ventral striatum that receives extensive dopaminergic inputs from the ventral tegmental area as well as glutamatergic inputs from the prefrontal cortex. Other brain regions also interact with this circuit, including the hippocampus, amygdala, and locus coeruleus. Taken together, these structures represent the reward circuits of the brain and are important for how people process important natural rewards such as food, sex, and socialization. In addiction, drugs activate these regions in a supraphysiologic manner that leads to a drive and persistence to seek out drugs that is not seen in other circumstances. Indeed, prolonged exposure to drugs seems to cause these circuits to become rewired, and the rewarding effect of natural rewards can become significantly diminished. Patients who have recently become abstinent will frequently experience low mood, low energy, and a lack of interest in previously pleasurable activities. Unfortunately, many patients with substance use disorders come to feel that using their drug of choice is the only way to return to feeling normal, thus initiating a vicious cycle of use and relapse. Unfortunately, the changes caused to these reward systems are very long lasting, and patients who have had months or even years of abstinence remain vulnerable to intense periods of craving in response to stress, drugs, or even cues in the environment related to the drugs.

When conceptualizing addiction, it is important to note that addiction is distinct from a physiologic dependence in which individuals fall ill when drug intake is stopped. This dependence is neither necessary nor sufficient for the development of addiction. Some addictive drugs do not create physical dependence, and many medications that are not addictive do lead to physical dependence (eg, β-adrenergic antagonists such as propranolol). Importantly, the symptoms of physical withdrawal from a drug or medication are mediated through different brain circuits than addiction.

Although we now have very good treatments for physical dependence and withdrawal symptoms associated with several drugs of abuse (eg, opiates, alcohol), finding treatments for the core symptoms of addiction has been a much more difficult task. The broadly pursued approaches to finding medications to reduce drug cravings and relapse generally fall into three major categories: blockade of drug targets, mimicry of drug action, and blockade of the addiction process.

BLOCKADE OF DRUG TARGETS

The most conceptually simple method of reducing pathologic drug use behaviors is to find a treatment that can block the known initial target of the drug (see Table 5-1). If a medication is able to stop a drug of abuse from reaching its target, while also

TABLE 5-1	Acute Actions of Some Drugs of Abuse	
Drug	**Action**	**Receptor Signaling Mechanism**
Opioids	Agonist at μ, δ, and κ opioid receptors[a]	Gi
Cocaine	Indirect agonist at dopamine receptors by inhibiting dopamine transporters[b]	Gi and Gs[c]
Amphetamine	Indirect agonist at dopamine receptors by stimulating dopamine release[b]	Gi and Gs[c]
Ethanol	Facilitates $GABA_A$ receptor function and inhibits NMDA glutamate receptor function[d]	Ligand-gated channels
Nicotine	Agonist at nicotinic acetylcholine receptors	Ligand-gated channels
Cannabinoids	Agonist at CB_1 and CB_2 cannabinoid receptors[e] .	Gi
Phencyclidine (PCP)	Antagonist at NMDA glutamate receptor channels	Ligand-gated channels
Hallucinogens	Partial agonist at $5\text{-}HT_{2A}$ serotonin receptors	Gq
Inhalants	Unknown	

$GABA_A$, γ-aminobutyric acid A; NMDA, N-methyl-D-aspartate; $5\text{-}HT_{2A}$, serotonin 2A.

[a]Activity at μ (and possibly) δ receptors mediates the reinforcing actions of opioids; κ receptors mediate aversive actions.

[b]Cocaine and amphetamines exert analogous actions on serotonergic and noradrenergic systems, which may also contribute to the reinforcing effects of these drugs.

[c]Gi couples D_2-like dopamine receptors, and Gs couples D_1-like dopamine receptors, both of which are important for dopamine's reinforcing effects.

[d]Ethanol affects several other ligand-gated channels and, at higher concentrations, voltage-gated channels as well. In addition, ethanol is reported to influence many other neurotransmitter systems, including serotonergic, opioidergic, and dopaminergic systems. It is not known whether these effects are direct or achieved indirectly via actions on various ligand-gated channels.

[e]Activity at CB_1 receptors mediates the reinforcing actions of cannabinoids; CB_2 receptors are expressed predominantly in the periphery but may also be involved in central actions. Endogenous ligands for the CB_1 receptor include the arachidonic acid metabolites, anandamide, and 2-arachidonylglycerol.

Data from Nestler EJ. Molecular basis of long-term plasticity underlying addiction. *Nat Rev Neurosci*. 2001;2(2):119-128.

not causing any effect at this target, it might serve as a potent means to stop drug intake. The most widely used example of this approach is naltrexone. In theory, naltrexone is inactive in the absence of an opioid, but blocks opioids from binding to their receptors, and thus reduces any rewarding effects of the drug. Unfortunately, although naltrexone is effective at stopping the rewarding effects of drugs, it also blocks endogenous opiates in the body (enkephalin and endorphin), which are important for processing naturally rewarding stimuli. This effect can result in patients developing depressed mood or anhedonia, which can reduce patient compliance. Based on animal studies showing that alcohol's and nicotine's addicting actions are mediated in part via activation of endogenous opioidergic neurons (Fig. 5-1), naltrexone has been used to treat addiction to these drugs as well. Some efficacy is observed clinically, but the effects of naltrexone are relatively small in magnitude and are effective for only a subset of patients.

Unfortunately, the strategy of blocking the drug from reaching its target has not yet been effective for stimulant drugs (eg, cocaine, amphetamine). Although there have been extensive efforts to find a molecule that would prevent these drugs from binding to the dopamine transporter, they have not yet been successful. Interestingly, a similar but alternative approach has been in development in recent years. Work in laboratory animals suggested that immunization with a metabolite of cocaine coupled to another carrier molecule resulted in an immune response to cocaine in which the drug was then cleared more rapidly and was less behaviorally rewarding. Initial studies in human subjects treated with a cocaine vaccine showed a marked reduction in cocaine use, but a subsequent larger trial did not show any positive effect on reduced cocaine intake or craving. Further research is currently ongoing to continue to refine these treatments to see if a cocaine vaccine may one day be a useful strategy in reducing cocaine use in human patients.

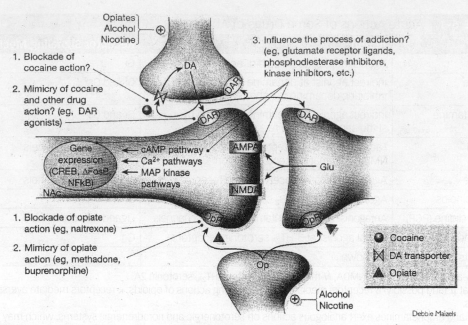

Figure 5-1. General strategies used to treat drug addiction or associated physical withdrawal syndromes. A dendritic spine of a nucleus accumbens (NAc) neuron and its innervation by terminals of glutamatergic (Glu), dopaminergic (DA), and opioidergic (Op) neurons are shown. 1: One approach is to block the ability of a drug to reach its initial protein target, for example, naltrexone's antagonism of opioid receptors (OR) or a hypothetical drug that interferes with cocaine's actions on the dopamine transporter. Not depicted is the use of immunologic methods (such as a cocaine or nicotine vaccine) to prevent a drug from entering the brain. 2: A second approach is to mimic drug action, for example, sustained activation of OR by methadone, or activation of DA receptors (DAR) by various agonists or partial agonists. 3: A third approach is to influence the process of addiction, for example, via perturbation of Glu receptors (AMPA, NMDA, metabotropic receptors) or a host of post–receptor signaling proteins (such as those involved in the cyclic adenosine monophosphate (cAMP), calcium, and mitogen-activated protein (MAP) kinase pathways and in the regulation of gene expression—ΔFosB, cAMP response element binding protein [CREB], or nuclear factor κ B [NF-κB]) that have been implicated in addiction. (From Nestler EJ. Molecular basis of long-term plasticity underlying addiction. *Nat Rev Neurosci.* 2001;2[2]:119-128; Hyman SE, Malenka RC, Nestler EJ. Neural mechanisms of addiction: the role of reward-related learning and memory. *Annu Rev Neurosci.* 2006;29:565-598; Robison AJ, Nestler EJ. Transcriptional and epigenetic mechanisms of addiction. *Nature Rev Neurosci.* 2011;12[11]:623-637.)

Cannabinoids, the active ingredients in marijuana, act through the stimulation of the cannabinoid type 1 (CB₁) receptors. Moreover, there is evidence that other drugs of abuse (eg, opioids, alcohol) may produce part of their addicting effects via the activation of endogenous cannabinoids in the brain (see Table 5-1). This has led to the speculation that CB₁ antagonists may be of use in treating various addictions. Rimonabant is a CB₁ inverse agonist. It functions as an antagonist and was previously approved in Europe for the treatment of obesity. Its potential efficacy in treating addiction remains unknown. An important cautionary note is that use of rimonabant is associated with the onset of depressive symptomatology in some patients, including the incidence of suicide, which led to withdrawal of its approval in Europe and severely limited further exploration of this pharmacologic approach.

MIMICRY OF DRUG ACTION

Although some success has been had in utilizing agents that block the effects of drugs, there has been considerable interest and progress in treating addiction by mimicking drug action. This strategy is predicated on the idea that the altered brain circuitry of a patient with an addiction will continue to lead to intense cravings in the absence of a drug. Blocking the site of action of the drug reduces the rewarding effect of the drug but may not reduce craving as dramatically. By providing a medication that mimics the effect of a drug, the brain can be allowed to slowly recover to its healthy state and for cravings to abate. Utilization of this strategy needs to be undertaken with great care because the treating provider does not want to provide another highly addictive substance that could lead to an exacerbation of the patient's symptoms. Successful medications used for this strategy need to be slowly absorbed, with longer half-lives, thus preventing the continuing cycle of highs and lows seen with many addictive drugs.

The best-established example of this approach is methadone, a particularly long-acting opioid receptor agonist. Because methadone has a much longer half-life than abused opioids, it provides for sustained, moderate activation of the opiate receptors without the daily extremes that are seen with other drugs. Ideally, this allows patients to continue with their daily activities of work and life while keeping cravings at bay. This strategy has been used successfully for many years, but it is not effective for all patients. Another variation in this theme that has become more widely used in recent years is buprenorphine. Buprenorphine is a high-affinity partial agonist that binds to opioid receptors and produces a mild agonist effect. Higher doses of the drug do not produce stronger effects because the ability of buprenorphine to activate the receptor is intrinsically low. However, buprenorphine—bound to the receptor at high affinity—can block the effects of opioid drugs, which limits the ability of a person with an addiction to obtain a drug "high" during treatment. Despite the clear utility of this general approach, and considerable success in many patients, there remains significant concern toward methadone, buprenorphine, and related treatments because the addicted person is still being exposed to opioids and may be vulnerable to certain deleterious effects of these medications.

Another example of the mimicry approach is the use of nicotine replacement strategies to treat tobacco addiction. The resulting sustained release of low levels of nicotine from patches or gum reduces craving for cigarettes and can help prolong abstinence. Despite sound theoretical footing, these approaches have limited success for most smokers. More recently, a partial agonist of nicotinic receptors, varenicline, has been developed and marketed for smoking cessation. Similar to buprenorphine, this partial agonist binds the receptor and partially activates it, while reducing the ability of cigarettes to produce rewarding effects. There is now a considerable body of evidence that this treatment can be efficacious for a significant subset of patients with tobacco use disorder.

A final example of mimicry is the use of a stimulant to treat stimulant addiction. For example, amphetamine or related drugs show some promise in treating cocaine addiction, although this clinical approach remains controversial. A related notion is the utilization of dopamine receptor agonists or antagonists to treat stimulant or other addictions. Briefly mentioned earlier is the important role of dopamine in drug addiction. Stimulation of dopaminergic transmission in the nucleus accumbens and elsewhere seems to be the most important mechanism of stimulant action and contributes to the actions of all other drugs of abuse as well (see Fig. 5-1). Despite considerable interest in modulating these circuits, efforts to date have not produced viable treatment strategies.

BLOCKADE OF THE ADDICTION PROCESS

A great deal has been learned over the past decade about the changes that drugs cause in the brain's reward pathways to produce addiction. Extensive research has been performed to see if these changes that lead to addiction can be blocked or prevented, but efforts to this point have not progressed beyond the laboratory, and the possible clinical implications should be viewed with some skepticism. An area of considerable interest is in the examination of glutamatergic signaling in the brain. Glutamate is the main excitatory neurotransmitter in the mammalian central nervous system and is important for the expression of synaptic plasticity throughout the brain. The nucleus accumbens and ventral tegmental area receive extensive glutamatergic inputs from many regions (eg, prefrontal cortex, amygdala, hippocampus), and drugs of abuse alter this glutamatergic signaling. Given the prominent role of glutamatergic mechanisms in learning and memory and increasing evidence that important aspects of addiction can be viewed as a form of memory, it is possible that glutamatergic agents, given in conjunction with behavioral therapies, might be efficacious at fundamentally altering addictive behavior. For example, we now know that extinction of a memory is not the passive process of undoing that memory but rather the formation of an active new memory that supersedes the old one. Hence, a drug that enhances glutamatergic transmission and, therefore, new memory formation, given in concert with behavioral extinction trials, might be a novel approach to treating addiction-related memories that are thought to underlie aspects of craving and relapse.

In a similar way, numerous other neurotransmitter, neuropeptide, and neurotrophic factor systems are altered by drugs and, in turn, modulate drug effects in laboratory animals, including γ-aminobutyric acid, neuropeptide Y, corticotropin-releasing factor, serotonin, norepinephrine, melanocortins, and brain-derived neurotrophic factor, to name just a few. For example, several drugs aimed at components of γ-aminobutyric acid–ergic synapses are under evaluation for the treatment of addiction. As these effects are better defined in animal models and putative treatment agents suitable for human investigation are developed, these mechanisms can be tested more definitively in clinical populations.

Drug addiction also involves adaptations at post-receptor, intracellular signaling cascades, including alterations in gene expression. Moreover, modification of particular signaling proteins can have dramatic effects on animals' responses to drugs. Examples include several proteins that regulate the function of G protein–coupled receptors: G proteins, G protein–receptor kinases, arrestins, and regulators of G protein–signaling proteins. Because the acute targets of many drugs of abuse are G protein–coupled receptors, it is possible that agents affecting these modulatory proteins could exert interesting functional effects on the receptor systems so as to treat aspects of addiction. Similarly, given the evidence for an important role of the cyclic adenosine monophosphate pathway in addiction and of the transcription factor ΔFosB, it is conceivable that novel agents directed against protein components of these pathways (such as phosphodiesterase inhibitors, which would enhance cyclic adenosine monophosphate function) might warrant investigation as clinical treatments. Still another example is inhibitors of histone deacetylases, enzymes that regulate gene expression by acetylating nearby histones. Recent evidence demonstrates that manipulation of specific histone deacetylases, or of several other chromatin-modifying enzymes, in the brain exerts a dramatic effect on drug-elicited behaviors. Drug discovery efforts should, of course, focus on subtypes of these intracellular signaling proteins that are highly enriched in the brain's reward pathways and, therefore, would represent potentially viable medication targets.

One of the central problems in approaching addiction is that truly effective treatments are not yet available. Thus, it is impossible to know what types of treatments are theoretically possible. For example, before the advent of antidepressant medications, there was considerable debate about the nature and magnitude of improvement that were possible with chemical treatments. By analogy, the addiction field now aims to identify medications that dampen drug craving or reward without interfering with motivation for natural rewards. Only as putative treatment agents are developed and tested in animals and humans will insight into the feasibility of this aim become available.

ACKNOWLEDGMENTS

Preparation of this review was supported by grants from the National Institute on Drug Abuse. Earlier versions of this chapter were adapted with permission of the publisher from Nestler EJ. From neurobiology to treatment: progress against addiction. *Nat Neurosci.* 2002;5(Suppl):1076-1079. © 2002, Nature Neuroscience, New York, NY.

KEY POINTS

1. Drugs of abuse act on the brain's reward circuitry to produce their acute rewarding effects as well as their longer lasting changes that underlie addiction.
2. Prominent brain regions that comprise this reward circuitry are the ventral tegmental area, the site of dopamine-containing neurons, and the targets of these neurons in the limbic forebrain—in particular, the nucleus accumbens.
3. All currently used medication treatments for addiction syndromes either block the acute actions of a drug of abuse or mimic those actions. An example of the former is the opioid receptor antagonist naltrexone. Examples of the latter include methadone and buprenorphine for opiates and varenicline or nicotine patches or chewing gum for smoking cessation.
4. Current research is focused on understanding the molecular changes that drugs of abuse induce in brain reward regions and on developing novel means of reversing those abnormalities.

REVIEW QUESTIONS

1. Which of the following brain regions is the site of dopamine neurons in the brain that are important contributors to the rewarding effects of drugs?
   A. Substantia nigra
   B. Locus coeruleus
   C. Ventral tegmental area
   D. Dorsal raphe
   E. Nucleus accumbens

2. Which of the following is a known direct target of drugs of abuse?
   A. Opioid receptor
   B. Dopamine transporter

C. *N*-Methyl-D-aspartate glutamate receptor
D. Nicotinic cholinergic receptor
E. All of the above.

3. Which of the following statements about drugs of abuse is *not* true?
   A. All drugs of abuse converge by producing some similar functional effects on the brain's reward pathways.
   B. Only drugs of abuse produce tolerance and dependence.
   C. Virtually all acute targets for drugs of abuse are proteins located at the synapse.
   D. Examples of putative medications that block the actions of a drug of abuse are naltrexone and rimonabant.
   E. Examples of medications that at least partially mimic the actions of a drug of abuse are varenicline and methadone.

ANSWERS

1. **C**
2. **E**
3. **B**

SUGGESTED READINGS

Bierut LJ. Genetic vulnerability and susceptibility to substance dependence. *Neuron*. 2011;69(4):618-627.

George O, Le Moal M, Koob GF. Allostasis and addiction: role of the dopamine and corticotropin-releasing factor systems. *Physiol Behav*. 2012;106(1):58-64.

Kalivas PW, Volkow ND. New medications for drug addiction hiding in glutamatergic neuroplasticity. *Mol Psychiatry*. 2011;16(10):974-986.

Kendler KS, Myers J, Prescott CA. Specificity of genetic and environmental risk factors for symptoms of cannabis, cocaine, alcohol, caffeine, and nicotine dependence. *Arch Gen Psychiatry*. 2007;64(11):1313-1320.

Robison AJ, Nestler EJ. Transcriptional and epigenetic mechanisms of addiction. *Nat Rev Neurosci*. 2011;12(11):623-637.

Clinical Trials in Substance-Using Populations

Summary by Yonina C. Mar

Based on THE ASAM PRINCIPLES OF ADDICTION MEDICINE, 6th edition chapter by Frank Vocci

Clinical trials can play an important role in the evaluation of interventions designed to prevent, assess, treat, and educate in the field of addiction medicine. The National Institutes of Health (NIH) defines a clinical trial as "a research study in which one or more human subjects are prospectively assigned to one or more interventions (which may or may not include placebo or other control) to evaluate the effects of those interventions on health-related biomedical or behavioral outcomes." Typically, study subjects are randomly allocated to one of the interventions undergoing evaluation.

ELEMENTS OF A CLINICAL TRIAL

Randomized clinical trials can provide the strongest level of evidence that an intervention has the hypothesized effect. Ideally, one hopes that results of a trial will influence clinical practice, such as showing that a new drug improves upon the previous standard of care or, conversely, that a treatment that has been used for many years does not work and is in fact harmful. For example, in a multicenter, randomized clinical trial, Ling et al. showed that buprenorphine at a dose of 8 mg/day compared to 1 mg/day resulted in better treatment retention, less evidence of illicit opioid drug use based on urine tests, less craving, and better scores on a global rating scale, thus demonstrating evidence of efficacy and safety. These results were important for the approval of buprenorphine as a pharmacotherapy for opioid use disorder.

The starting point of any clinical trial is the primary question, which should be relevant and clearly defined ahead of time. The identification of the question is fundamental because it drives the design of the trial, including all of its important components. All of the components are described in the study protocol, which is a document that justifies the study question and spells out the steps—the "how to" in addressing this question. It must be developed before the enrollment of participants. A protocol addressing a therapy involving populations with substance use disorders will typically contain the background of the study, objectives (primary and secondary questions and their corresponding outcome measures), details of the study population (both inclusion and exclusion criteria), details of the allocation process (eg, stratification, randomization method) and the interventions (dosage form, administration schedule, duration of pharmacotherapy or behavioral intervention, measures of compliance, participant discontinuation criteria, and follow-up schedule), outcome measures (assessments of both benefit and harm), proposed analyses, and sample size determination. In addition, a study protocol usually contains sections that can be considered administrative that provide information on the trial organization (eg, structure and role of study committees such as the data and safety monitoring board [DSMB]), collection and reporting of adverse events, and ethical issues. Informed consent is an essential component of a clinical trial and a proposed clinical trial, must be reviewed and approved by an institutional review board (IRB), whose role is to protect the rights and welfare of human subjects. Study subjects must provide written consent to participate in the trial prior to being assigned to an intervention.

TYPES OF CLINICAL TRIALS
Phases

There are various ways of classifying clinical trials; one common way is by phase. This has been typically used in drug development and for approval of a drug by a regulatory agency. The results from each phase of a clinical trial are used to help design the subsequent phase. However, there is not always progression sequentially through all phases for a specific agent. In a phase I trial, the toxicity of a new agent is documented and the maximally tolerated dose is determined. A phase II trial evaluates whether the drug has an effect and may estimate the rate of adverse events. It is larger than a phase I trial and is usually a single-arm trial. Occasionally, however, phase II trials can be randomized. The phase III trial compares new treatments with the best currently available treatment (the standard treatment). The hallmark of a phase III trial is that it involves the randomization of subjects. These trials are usually larger than phase II trials and expensive to carry out. Phase IV trials, sometimes referred to as postmarketing or surveillance studies, assess how the intervention works after it has been adopted into clinical practice. Often, they are used to continue to monitor the safety of a new intervention. Phase IV trials are typically conducted in the general target population, thus in a heterogeneous population that often has multiple comorbidities. There is no comparison group.

Efficacy Versus Effectiveness

Another way to consider a clinical trial is whether it is an efficacy or an effectiveness trial. Efficacy refers to what the intervention accomplishes in an ideal setting, whereas effectiveness refers to what the intervention accomplishes in actual practice under real-world conditions. Efficacy trials use carefully selected, homogeneous populations with strict inclusion and exclusion criteria. The intervention is strictly enforced and standardized, and typically, there are no concurrent interventions. Conversely, effectiveness trials use heterogeneous populations with few to no exclusion criteria. The intervention is applied with flexibility, and concurrent interventions and crossovers are permitted. It is more difficult to demonstrate the effect of the intervention in an effectiveness trial due to statistical noise (unexplained variability within a data sample), and thus, a larger sample size is required to detect an effect. Thus, efficacy trials are the most controlled and have less generalizability, and effectiveness trials are often less controlled with high generalizability to the real-world setting. In the last decade, public policy makers in the United States were concerned about the costs of healthcare. Accordingly, the concept of comparative effectiveness research (CER) was put forward. Comparative effectiveness trials directly compare interventions to each other to determine which pose the greatest benefits and harms. The core question of CER is which treatment works best, for whom, and under what circumstances.

FEATURES OF CLINICAL TRIALS

There are several key features of a clinical trial that warrant further discussion to help understand the fundamentals of a clinical trial.

Randomization

Randomization is the hallmark of the randomized controlled trial (RCT), which is considered the gold standard trial design in the assessment of efficacy. There are several advantages of the randomized design. Specifically, the randomized allocation of subjects to interventions minimizes the potential for bias in the comparison of experimental and control groups as it tends to ensure that the groups are balanced for baseline prognostic variables. Stratification is often used in randomization in order to help achieve balance for prognostic factors between treatment groups. It does this by performing allocation within each stratum.

Blinding

Blinding refers to the process of concealment of the assignment to treatment groups. Its purpose, similar to randomization, is to minimize bias. The common double-blind design masks treatment assignment from both the investigator and the study participant. This means that both the investigator and subject are not aware of treatment interventions. It is done by employing a placebo. A single-blind design, conversely, conceals the treatment assignment from the participant but not the investigator. In many RCTs, it is not possible to blind the investigator and study subject to treatment allocation.

Sample Size, Power, Effect Size, and Feasibility

Determining how many subjects to recruit is an important aspect of a clinical trial because a sufficient sample size to detect treatment differences is necessary. The sample size is calculated by considering three elements: effect size, significance level, and power. Effect size is a way of quantifying the magnitude of difference in end points between groups and needs to be estimated and specified prior to calculating the sample size. Depending on the outcome measure, the effect size may be represented as a ratio, eg, relative risk, risk ratio, hazard ratio, or the difference, eg, absolute difference in rates. The expected effect size may be based on previous knowledge from other trials. The smaller the estimated effect size, the larger the sample size required and vice versa. The significance level, referred to as α, is often set at

5% (0.05) and is the chance of finding an effect when one does not actually exist (false-positive rate or type I error). Power is the ability to detect an effect if, in fact, an effect actually exists. Power is represented as $1 - \beta$, where β is the chance of concluding that there is no difference between groups when one exists (false-negative rate or type II error). Most clinical trials use a power of 80% or 90% so that the false-negative rate is 20% or less. Formulas exist where effect size, significance level, and power are inserted to calculate sample size. Trials in populations with substance use disorders may have a higher dropout rate than trials in other disciplines. For example, in a 24-week clinical trial examining treatment retention in subjects who use opioids, the dropout rates were 26% for patients receiving methadone and 54% for those receiving buprenorphine. Trials with high dropout rates have missing data issues that can compromise the integrity of the findings and result in finding no difference between groups, when one might actually exist, ie, false negative. One way to reduce this possibility would be to increase sample sizes to compensate for the high dropout rates.

A common issue related to sample size determination faced by researchers is feasibility; ie, can sufficient numbers of patients be recruited in a reasonable time frame to meet the specified target? Often, investigators overestimate the number of patients who will fit the eligibility criteria of an RCT and the number of patients who agree to be randomized, thus resulting in an insufficient sample size.

Design

When assessing the potential efficacy of an intervention, it is necessary to postulate whether it is likely to have an improved effect or similar effect when compared to the comparison group. This concept can influence the study design. In the former case, the design specifies a superiority trial, whereas in the latter, the design specifies a non-inferiority trial or equivalence trial. There are various other designs that are used in clinical trials that are beyond the scope of this chapter. A superiority trial examines whether a new intervention is different from (ie, better or worse than) the control, whereas a non-inferiority trial examines whether a new intervention is no worse than the control, where the control group is on a standard treatment, previously shown to be effective. In a non-inferiority trial, a margin of difference (noninferiority margin or equivalence margin, δ) needs to be specified in order to establish non-inferiority. Superiority trials in the field of addiction may seek to determine whether a difference exists between a

medication and a placebo (eg, buprenorphine compared to placebo), between a medication and a standard treatment or active control (eg, buprenorphine compared to methadone), or between different doses (eg, ascending doses of buprenorphine, magnitude of monetary reinforcement in contingency management trials, frequency of counseling in medication treatment). Non-inferiority trials in the field of addiction, conversely, may seek to determine whether one type of opioid agonist treatment is noninferior to another type of opioid agonist treatment (eg, buprenorphine versus methadone) or whether a type or mode of behavioral intervention is noninferior to another type or mode. Equivalence trials, although often equated to non-inferiority trials, are in fact not the same. They assess whether the intervention is more or less equal to the control and require a larger sample size than a non-inferiority trial.

Outcomes

Clinical trials should have clearly defined outcome measures. Trials involving populations with substance use disorders have a unique set of outcomes. Abstinence and/or reduction of drug or alcohol use are often primary outcome measures of efficacy in clinical trials involving such populations. Abstinence and reduction of drug or alcohol use are examples of dichotomous variables or outcomes, which lend themselves well to comparison of rates. For example, a randomized clinical trial using abstinence as a primary outcome would compare the proportion of subjects who were abstinent versus those who were not.

For analysis, a chi-square test may be used to test for statistical significance. The measurement of drug or alcohol use can be by biological assay, self-report, or a combination of the two measures. Urine is the most common biological fluid used to test for the presence of drugs, likely due in part to the noninvasive nature of collecting urine. Alcohol and most drugs, with the exception of cannabis and phencyclidine, have detection times in urine of 2 to 4 days. Relating the measurement of drugs or alcohol in urine to use presents challenges because use may be missed if testing is too infrequent, and conversely, use may be overestimated due to carryover if testing is too frequent.

Management of withdrawal syndromes is a common secondary outcome measure in clinical trials. Craving is another commonly measured secondary outcome variable that often serves a role in the convergent validity of behavioral findings; for example, reduced craving is associated with reduced use or abstinence. Craving can be measured in real time using ecological momentary assessment techniques on mobile devices where study participants are queried on craving and its relationship to drug intake or abstinence.

Various scales are commonly utilized in clinical trials involving populations with substance use disorders and commonly include psychiatric scales such as the Structured Clinical Interview for *DSM-5* for evaluating psychiatric diagnoses, the Beck Depression Inventory, the Hamilton Depression Rating Scale, and the Hamilton Anxiety Rating Scale for assessing mood and anxiety disorders. Addiction-focused scales and reduction of HIV risk scales are also utilized. Scores on these scales are not only used as outcome measures but are also used as stratification criteria in randomization and in screening procedures for inclusion and exclusion criteria. When used as outcome measures, scale scores are examples of continuous variables or outcomes because such a variable can take on any value between its minimum value and its maximum value. A continuous outcome may be analyzed with a *t* test or an analysis of variance to test for statistical significance.

Other outcome measures that are used in the addiction literature include quality of life measures, pharmacokinetic measures (eg, plasma pharmacokinetics to determine appropriate dosing intervals), healthcare service utilization measures, cost-analysis–related measures (eg, do the benefits associated with an intervention exceed its cost), and treatment adherence measures, which can be measured in such ways as by self-report, direct measurement of medication in urine, and via a medication event monitoring system.

MONITORING AND QUALITY CONTROL

Monitoring and quality control are important in clinical trials to ensure high-quality data is collected in a safe manner that protects the rights and well-being of subjects. Quality assurance or quality control in clinical trials pertains to methods or procedures that aim to maintain or enhance the reliability and/or validity of data. Preventing problems with carrying out interventions or collecting outcomes, detecting problems, and taking appropriate and effective action to correct problems are goals of quality assurance. For example, in a trial examining behavioral interventions in populations with substance use disorders, ensuring that there is accuracy and consistency between those delivering the behavioral intervention is fundamental to maintaining quality assurance. Monitoring involves

efforts to ensure that standardized operation procedures are being followed, records are being accurately kept, and adverse events are being reported appropriately. The investigators, the IRB, DSMBs, the US Food and Drug Administration, the pharmaceutical industry (if industry sponsored), and the NIH (if the study is NIH funded) all play a role in the monitoring of clinical trials.

KEY POINTS

1. The randomized clinical trial, considered the highest quality trial design in the assessment of efficacy, examines whether an intervention has the hypothesized effect compared to a control.
2. The protocol justifies the study question and outlines the background, objectives, study population, sample size estimate, allocation process, interventions, outcome measures, proposed analyses, and trial organization.
3. Efficacy trials assess an intervention in an ideal setting, are more controlled, and have less generalizability. In contrast, effectiveness trials assess an intervention under real-world conditions, are less controlled, and have more generalizability.
4. Outcome measures should be clearly defined in a clinical trial. Abstinence and/or a reduction of drug or alcohol use are often primary outcome measures in clinical trials involving populations with substance use disorders.

ACKNOWLEDGMENTS

The author would like to acknowledge Dr. Mark Levine, Professor of Oncology, McMaster University, for his contribution to this chapter.

REVIEW QUESTIONS

A multicenter, randomized, placebo-controlled trial examining the safety and efficacy of a sublingual-tablet formulation of buprenorphine-naloxone, a buprenorphine tablet, and placebo in an office-based setting found that the proportion of urine samples that were negative for opioids was greater in both the buprenorphine-naloxone combination group and buprenorphine alone group compared to the placebo group.

1. In this example, buprenorphine in combination with naloxone is a(n):
   A. standard treatment.
   B. intervention.
   C. control.
   D. outcome.

2. This trial, as described, is an example of a(n):
   A. superiority trial.
   B. efficacy trial.
   C. phase III trial.
   D. All of the above

3. In this trial, opioid-negative urine samples are a:
   A. continuous outcome.
   B. secondary outcome.
   C. dichotomous outcome.
   D. positive outcome.

ANSWERS

1. **B**
2. **D**
3. **C**

SUGGESTED READINGS

Consolidated Standards of Reporting Trials. Welcome to the CONSORT website. http://www.consort-statement.org. Accessed February 20, 2018.

Friedman LM, Furberg CD, DeMets DL, Reboussin DM, Granger CB. *Fundamentals of Clinical Trials.* 5th ed. New York: Springer, 2015.

Guyatt G, Rennie D, Meade MO, Cook DJ, eds. *Users' Guides to the Medical Literature: A Manual for Evidence-Based Clinical Practice.* 3rd ed. New York: McGraw-Hill Education, 2015.

Hackshaw A. *A Concise Guide to Clinical Trials.* Chichester, UK: BMJ Books, 2009.

Ling W, Charuvastra C, Collins JF, et al. Buprenorphine maintenance treatment of opiate dependence: a multicenter, randomized clinical trial. *Addiction.* 1998;93(4):475-486.

PARINT. Publishing addiction research internationally. http://www.parint.org. Updated January 8, 2018. Accessed February 20, 2018.

7 The Addiction Medicine Physician as a Change Agent for Prevention and Public Health

Summary by Kevin Kunz

Based on THE ASAM PRINCIPLES OF ADDICTION MEDICINE, 6th edition chapter by Kevin Kunz

WE ARE RESPONSIBLE

There is an urgent need to translate addiction science into everyday clinical practice, while also translating it into institutional and public policies that constructively impact health. This text presents a vast array of effective evidence-based interventions, which can be applied in clinical and community settings. However, these lifesaving and life-enhancing practices are neither fully appreciated nor adequately applied. Unhealthy substance use is one of the world's largest and most costly health issues. Unhealthy substance use is prevalent on every continent and in virtually every culture, accounting for the top causes of preventable death and disability on a global scale. In the United States, unhealthy substance use and addiction cause 23% of all deaths. And the unrelenting opioid use crisis of the last two decades has brought a sharper focus on all unhealthy substance use.

Despite the availability of a large and growing body of science to guide effective care, American medicine is primarily focused on treating the complications of substance use rather than on the prevention and treatment of substance use disorders (SUDs).

It is the ethical responsibility of every physician to provide competent medical care and to incorporate current scientific knowledge into his or her medical practice. Yet SUDs have historically been the unattended orphan of the medical profession. A growing workforce of addiction medicine physicians is now positioned to join those of addiction psychiatry to drive system-level changes to improve the quality of patient care and advance population health. They can do this by serving as expert clinicians, teachers and faculty, and community- or governmental-level change agents. Addiction medicine

itself has entered a new era. The recent recognition of the subspecialty of addiction medicine by the American Board of Medical Specialties (ABMS) and the Accreditation Council for Graduate Medical Education (ACGME) has brought SUD into mainstream American medicine and has increased the opportunity for all physicians to more effectively address these disorders. There are also ongoing expansions of governmental and health system initiatives to create and fund SUD prevention, treatment, and recovery programs. Thus, medicine and healthcare at large are entering the preparation and action phases for addressing this long neglected malady. The chapter offers an introduction to the role of addiction medicine physicians in integrating science and evidence-informed practice into systems of care and public health initiatives.

PROTECTING AND PROMOTING THE PUBLIC HEALTH

American medicine and healthcare may reasonably take pride in the technical application of science and discovery, yet we rank near the bottom on a global rating of health—36th of 37 among developed nations. This is nowhere more obvious than in disease and social dysfunction caused or exacerbated by unhealthy substance use. Unhealthy substance use and addiction is America's number one health problem. Although death is a crude measure of health, it is informative that nearly a quarter of annual deaths in the United States are attributable to harmful substance use and addiction. These deaths are almost always preceded by medical, social, public health, and economic sequelae of substance use. The good news is that SUDs are not only treatable conditions but they are also responsive to well-coordinated prevention and public health initiatives, which can be informed by leaders in our field.

The current US epidemic of opioid use disorders, in which physicians and medicine are complicit, has propelled attention to the role of individual physicians, as well as medicine and healthcare systems generally, in the field of addiction medicine. All stakeholders have been sensitized by the opioid crisis rocking our national health and our collective consciousness. Calls to action to combat the opioid crisis stand in stark contrast to the relative passivity of decades of nicotine and alcohol addiction and unhealthy use of other substances.

Missing from the current approach of medicine today is what is at the front end in the continuum of healthcare practice: attention to issues of public health and illness prevention. In this space, every addiction medicine physician can incorporate new competencies into their professional practice. Prevention is a woefully neglected aspect of routine medical care for SUDs: Unhealthy substance use is a preventable condition and addiction is a preventable disease, which when unaddressed, can become chronic and more difficult and costly to treat.

Progress in prevention generally and for substance use specifically has been restricted in part by our national healthcare systems, which developed from and are sustained by an acute care disease model. There is sparse implementation of available evidence-informed prevention and treatment strategies, while there are easily accessible advanced and costly treatment options for late-stage complications of addiction, eg, trauma, organ damage, cancer, metabolic disorders, psychiatric complications. As well, late-stage "interventions" for social sequelae of substance use, such as incarceration, disability, and unemployment assistance, are more readily available than less costly and more effective prevention and public health initiatives. This situation is "upside down."

The acute care focus of American medicine has historically rewarded short-term care of back-end medical complications of substance use, while providing minimal reward for front-end and cost-effective prevention. There are many other reasons why prevention lacks broad institutional support: Success is invisible, lack of drama makes prevention less interesting, statistical lives have little emotional effect, there is usually a long delay before rewards appear, benefits often do not accrue to the payer for prevention, persistent behavioral change may be required, bias against errors of commission may deter action, avoidable harm is accepted as normal, there is a double financial standard in the evaluation of

prevention as compared to treatment, commercial interests may conflict with disease prevention, advice is inconsistent or changes, and advice may conflict with personal or religious or cultural beliefs.

In a physician's interaction with a patient, he or she is expected to engage and apply specific core competencies learned in medical school, residency, and community practice. As physicians, this is what we do. It is our passion. Yet for all the years and money spent on medical education and training, and spent annually in medical practices and healthcare systems, the profession of medicine in America has not adopted or implemented adequate competencies and strategies to systematically improve the population health of our nation's citizens.

All physicians can endeavor to weave into their practice a "red thread" of public health, disease prevention, and policy advocacy, striving to prevent illnesses from occurring or recurring through educating patients and the public, providing effective prevention and early intervention services, and when possible, recommending effective policies and conducting research. Public health services also include efforts to limit health disparities and promote healthcare equity, quality, and accessibility. A public health approach with a particular focus on prevention is essential to effectively address the health issue of unhealthy substance use as well as to prevent its costly medical and social consequences.

To address these and other concerns, the landscape of healthcare in this country needs our help to change. This will require addressing the full continuum of care from prevention and early intervention to chronic disease management, breaking down the silos of health professional education and practice, and ensuring competency rather than curricular completion.

THE ROLE OF THE ADDICTION MEDICINE PHYSICIAN

The newly recognized field of addiction medicine is embracing these needed changes in medicine as it prepares a physician workforce to ensure that all patients receive prevention and early intervention services and effective treatment and disease management for addiction and its co-occurring disorders. Addiction medicine physicians play four essential roles in this process: providing clinical expertise in direct patient care and in consultation with other providers in multispecialty and interdisciplinary settings, serving as faculty and teachers to educate and train others, performing clinical and health policy research, and functioning as change agents to secure needed reforms.

Within addiction medicine and focusing on the role of physicians as change agents, the ABMS and ACGME competencies of systems-based practice and professionalism are especially salient. Systems-based practice is the physician's ability to "demonstrate awareness of and responsibility to the larger context and systems of health care" and to "be able to call on system resources to provide optimal care." Because unhealthy substance use and addiction are influenced by societal and public policy forces, and impact most other areas and disciplines within medicine, a systems-based approach is necessary.

The core competency of professionalism includes accountability to society. Addiction medicine physicians can effectively employ this competency by bringing attention and quality care to SUDs at a level consistent with the attention medicine gives to other medical conditions. Physicians dedicated to the health of individual patients and families are also ethically obligated stakeholders in health promotion for communities and larger populations.

Some physicians eschew these aspects of physician competencies as "politics," believing that they do not apply to their own practice of medicine. However, as Virchow wisely stated, "Medicine is a social science, and politics is nothing more than medicine on a larger scale." The field of social medicine, not to be confused with socialized medicine, posits that social and economic conditions profoundly impact health, disease, and the practice of medicine; that the health of the population is a matter of social concern; and that society should promote health through both individual and social means. Conversely, a disease state such as addiction also profoundly and adversely impacts society.

One aim of social medicine is physician promotion of "social justice" through the reduction of health disparities or inequities deriving from social determinants of health—the social, environmental, cultural, and physical factors that different populations are born into and that impact childhood development and adult maturation. These factors are determinants in the use of addictive substances, the medical and social consequences of their use, and in opportunities for medical and social interventions for prevention, treatment, and recovery.

TRANSFORMATIONAL CHANGE

The old adage that a "Band-Aid approach won't fix this problem" clearly applies to the unsuccessful efforts of medicine and healthcare to attenuate the morbidity and mortality associated with unhealthy substance use and addiction. Medicine, healthcare systems, and key stakeholders are now being challenged to produce a thorough and dramatic change in the form, character, and appearance of the antiquated interventions, or complete lack thereof, necessary to address unhealthy substance use and addiction.

Transformational change derives from a radical divergence from the underlying consciousness, strategy, and processes that an organization or system has been using. It can be identified by a shift in the culture of an organization, field, or population that results in new expectations and new practices. Examples include the near-total restriction of tobacco smoking in public places, the removal of all tobacco products from major drug store chains, and the acceptance of routine vaccinations. The United States is now witnessing the emergence of another transformative shift of consciousness—that addiction is a disease and not a character, moral, or criminal problem. Addiction medicine physicians are challenged to lead, contribute to, and actualize strategies and processes driving system changes to reflect this new public and medical reality. Physicians are the ultimate purveyors of messaging and action in this arena because SUDs are medical disorders modulated by genetics and environment, and these same medical disorders significantly impact human environment and society. If not us, who?

America's current acute care health system resulted from transformative change triggered by the Flexner report a century ago. This report was the basis for a sweeping reform and renewal of medical education and practice. Physician training was increased to a minimum of 6 to 8 years of postsecondary education, medical research adhered to the scientific method, physician training itself was restructured in a scientific manner, half of all medical schools were closed, and the state regulation of physician practice was instituted. These changes, substantial and seismic at the time, are now fundamental and are today accepted as unalterable.

The need for a new shift from the acute care model to one that attends to the full continuum of care from prevention and early intervention to chronic disease management now demands a transformation of similar magnitude to that initiated by Flexner. Nowhere is this more obvious than with the prevention and treatment of SUDs described throughout this text.

Transformational change involves breakthroughs and challenges. In the last 20 years, the science of addiction and the evidence base for prevention and treatment have increased significantly. Both the need and the challenges for disseminating and implementing the science and evidence base are starkly apparent to health professionals and others. Physicians must take a lead in the campaign for modernization of care for these disorders.

A key prerequisite for transformational change is its dependence on leadership that integrates and models the change being sought. If physicians were still using tobacco in large numbers, how would that have impacted the public health campaign for reducing the prevalence of tobacco use and related disease? If physicians seek to work across traditional boundaries with other stakeholders and by working collaboratively, they can both model a winning strategy and improve the health of patients and our nation. In this, they can lead. The skills that physicians use so well in the clinical care of patients to positively accentuate and promote the benefits of personal change are needed now to advance cooperation and structural change between interdependent elements of healthcare systems.

Importantly, transformational change engages the heart. Science, economics, and critical thinking are necessary yet insufficient to produce lasting changes in the collective consciousness and behavior of society. Systems are driven by individuals who interact, cooperate, and collaborate with one another. We are not computers or robots. We are driven by our aspirations and by issues affecting people we care deeply about. This is what gives meaning to our lives.

To actualize system change, addiction medicine physicians armed with the science of addiction and knowledge of best practices for reform have much to offer. The Institute for Healthcare Improvement has promoted and validated the straightforward and effective Plan-Do-Study-Act cycle. An overview is outlined here.

A PROVEN APPROACH TO EFFECTING CHANGE IN HEALTH CARE
1. Take a Systems Approach.

A system is a set of interdependent elements interacting to achieve a common goal. Physicians know or can learn the elements and processes in the systems in which they are matriculating and can engage in interactions for improvement. Cooperation (systems interaction) across traditional boundaries is not as daunting a barrier as often perceived for physicians seeking system change. Medical specialties, other health professions, and system managers often operate in "silos of excellence." Administrators, financial stakeholders, policy makers, the public, and other interest groups also have their own "world views," goals, and preferred practices. Although a physician

entering this larger system may initially feel intimidation or hesitation, most newcomers will find this a welcoming environment. In this milieu, physicians have a unique capacity to be accepted as participants and critical leaders in improving healthcare systems and advancing the quality of care for their own patients and many others. Physician leaders holding the precept "do what is best for the patient" can bring quality of care into discussions where other outcomes may dominate. Physicians, and particularly addiction medicine physicians, have been absent or scarce in deliberations at nearly every system level due to a limited workforce, overwhelming patient care considerations, or the assumption that "someone else is working on this." Key decisions on the care of patients thus have often excluded effective input from addiction medicine physicians and defaulted to stakeholders with more parochial interests.

An effective physician leader first examines the existing situation, then imagines possibilities and seeks a process and a plan for improvement. He or she can participate in changing system shortcomings and in creating a new system. Physician leaders recognize several realities early: leadership is an action, not a position; leadership is not victimhood—you cannot be a leader and a victim simultaneously; leaders define reality with data; leaders develop and test changes; leaders take risk and have courage because complacent or threatened persons and organizations may react loudly and negatively to proposed change; leaders cross boundaries, stepping outside and letting go of defending their silo; and physician leaders seek interactions with a wide diversity of stakeholders.

2. Put Together a Diverse, Multispecialty Interdisciplinary Team.

Transformational change needs a broad set of participating stakeholders, from both the internal and external organizational environments who can collaborate with each other. It requires inclusion and collaboration by diverse and multiple stakeholders: from medicine and all disciplines, including nursing and other health disciplines; from financial, governmental, and policy players; and from patients and the public. Healthcare affects all Americans. It is central to the success of American society and culture. We all own it, and we must all participate in improving it. Every addiction medicine physician has a contribution he or she can make.

Multispecialty physicians and interdisciplinary teams provide for a group of healthcare professionals from diverse and complementary fields who work together toward a common goal: ideally, accelerating a cooperative environment. Physicians can assume the role of champion, but they do not always have to be the team leader; they can assume a mentoring role by modeling listening skills, openness to change, willingness to make suggestions, and continued participation on the team. Physicians should expect and encourage a diversity of styles—most healthcare professions have their own cultures and values, and the reality is physicians do not own the single standard. Stakeholders who are involved in the process of change are more likely to be cooperative if they sense openness instead of resistance when offering a diverse view that resets the traditionally authoritarian stance of having physicians provide the ultimate answer. When meeting with nonphysicians, the pool for ideas and suggestions can be expanded when the physician or group leader asks each person for his or her concerns and opinions. Inclusion of freely expressed and diverse ideas from a group of interdisciplinary stakeholders accelerates a cooperative environment.

3. Develop a Shared Purpose and Plan of Action.

Human systems derive their identity from a shared, common purpose. The dialogue of change thus begins with the question, "What are we trying to accomplish?" And follows this question with the equally important query, "Why is this important to you?"

It is crucial to develop and gain consensus on the purpose and aim of the desired improvement, enlisting and aligning as many stakeholders as necessary or possible to consider alternatives to the status quo. State clearly the testable objective of the plan. The "aim" of the desired improvement should be time-specific; measurable; and defines the patients, populations, and system(s) to be involved. The Institute of Medicine lists six broad categories for most desired improvements: safety, effectiveness, patient-centeredness, timeliness, efficiency, and equity.

Detail the components of the plan and remember it is prudent to start small. Develop quantitative measures as these will be used to monitor progress and will be necessary to determine whether the plan resulted in an improvement. As a physician leader, your own commitment and endurance are essential. Physicians who desire and work for change become knowledgeable and gain experience in making small improvements and in always cooperating with others. Defined rules and expectations are an attribute of cooperative environments. For those not wishing to cooperate, stay on the high road. Silent stakeholders at the beginning may influence success in the end.

This is always a group process. Persons both within and outside of the departments or organization have varying experience with the system elements involved and can suggest change concepts from which a proposed change is chosen. No change effort will succeed without cooperation. Cooperative interactions may be ethical and altruistic, yet they are a prerequisite and pragmatic strategy for engineering change in interdependent systems.

Effective leaders learn, model, and teach expertise in basic dialogue and group communication. Basic negotiation attitudes and skills are a requisite for success and can be acquired from reading or courses. Success is more likely when the decision process focuses on issues and not on individuals and empowers ownership in the change process and results. The frequently expressed complaint that nothing will change until "that person moves on" is counterproductive. There are always issues that can be win–win for all parties. Change is dependent on new solutions, not lamenting past disappointments or current shortcomings.

4. Act.

With a detailed plan in place and the assurance that the people, procedures, and processes needed to execute it are in order, and after all stakeholders—including patients if they are involved—are onboard, set a start date.

5. Set Up a Strategy for Evaluation and Improvement.

Monitor key aspects and measures of the plan, document problems and unexpected observations, and begin preliminary analysis of the data. Recall the saying "what gets measured gets done," and remember that there is no innovation without data. Take time and engage the people and system elements that the cycle will impact.

At appropriate and strategic intervals, analyze the emerging data. Compare this with your predictions and review with the team, reflecting on what was learned. Determine what modifications should be made and prepare a plan for next steps.

SUMMARY

Unhealthy substance use impacts people we work with, live with, those with whom we share a community, as well as persons we care about, and those we love. On some level, it is personal for all of us. Foremost, healthcare is much more than a calculated business venture; it is compassion and caring for all with whom we are connected. Every addiction medicine physician is needed to bring prevention, high-quality treatment, and systems improvement into reality. Addiction medicine can lead and contribute to the well-being of communities and nations as well as to our patients and their families. Whether physician contributions are made in assessing, planning, and acting on improvements in a small clinic, a large healthcare system, or at the level of governmental policy impacting public health, this is all within the mission and character of the field of addiction medicine. Addiction medicine physicians are clinical experts, faculty and teachers, researchers, and change agents. This is our work, and we can succeed.

KEY POINTS

1. As physicians, we are responsible for the systems within which we care for patients.
2. The role of the addiction medicine physician includes protecting and promoting public health.
3. Addiction medicine physicians are vital players in the transformational change needed in medicine and healthcare.

REVIEW QUESTIONS

1. When physicians engage in activities to improve the environment and processes in and through which patients receive care, they are primarily demonstrating the core competencies of which of the following?
   A. Interpersonal and communications skills
   B. Practice-based learning
   C. Systems-based practice and professionalism
   D. Administrative engagement

2. Transformative change is identifiable by:
   A. the commitment of financial and political resources.
   B. a divergence from the underlying consciousness, strategy, and processes that a system has been using.
   C. a competent and charismatic leader.
   D. a merger or buy-out by a new corporate or legal entity.

3. Which of the following is a proven method for effecting positive change within an organization?
   A. A Plan-Do-Study-Act cycle
   B. Retraining all staff in updated policies and procedures
   C. Increasing employee benefit and salary packages
   D. Recruiting younger medical and nursing staff

ANSWERS

1. **C.** The ABMS and ACGME core competencies are Practice-Based Learning and Improvement, Patient Care and Procedural Skills, Medical Knowledge, Interpersonal and Communication Skills, Systems-Based Practice, and Professionalism. All are necessary for individual patient care. The last two are essential for advancing care for populations of patients.
2. **B.** Transformative change is both deeper and more universally generated and shared than that achievable by standard business transactions.
3. **A.** A Plan-Do-Study-Act cycle is used across systems with well-documented effectiveness.

SUGGESTED READINGS

Center on Addiction. *Addiction Medicine: Closing the Gap between Science and Practice.* https://www.centeronaddiction.org/addiction-research/reports/addiction-medicine-closing-gap-between-science-and-practice. Published June 2012. Accessed August 24, 2018.

Gass R. What is transformational change? http://transform.transformativechange.org/2010/06/robertgass. Accessed October 3, 2018.

Institute for Healthcare Improvement. Plan-Do-Study-Act. http://www.ihi.org/resources/Pages/Tools/PlanDoStudyActWorksheet.aspx. Accessed October 3, 2018.

Robert Wood Johnson Foundation. Substance abuse: the nation's number one health problem. https://files.eric.ed.gov/fulltext/ED476048.pdf. Accessed October 3, 2018.

US Department of Health and Human Services, Office of the Surgeon General. *Facing Addiction in America: The Surgeon General's Report on Alcohol, Drugs and Health.* https://www.duq.edu/assets/Documents/social-justice/_pdf/_addiction/surgeon-generals-report-alcohol-drugs-health.pdf. Published November 2016. Accessed October 3, 2018.

Pharmacology

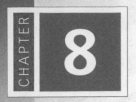
Pharmacokinetic, Pharmacodynamic, and Pharmacogenomic Principles

Summary by Anne Zajicek and Lori D. Karan

Based on THE ASAM PRINCIPLES OF ADDICTION MEDICINE, 6th edition chapter by Anne Zajicek and Lori D. Karan

Addiction medicine requires an understanding of the application of pharmacologic principles to drugs of abuse and the medications used to treat substance use disorders. Drugs of abuse produce mood alterations, which require drug penetration into the brain.

PHARMACOKINETICS

Pharmacokinetics describes the time course of drug concentrations in blood and tissues (eg, brain). Drug concentrations in blood and other sites are determined by absorption, distribution, metabolism, and elimination. The magnitude of a drug's pharmacologic effect depends upon the free (unbound) drug concentration at its site of action.

Absorption

Absorption is the process of drug movement from the site of drug delivery to the site of action. The more rapidly a psychoactive drug is delivered to its site of action in the central nervous system, the greater is its mood-altering and reinforcing effects. The more rapidly achieved and higher peak concentrations from intravenous and pulmonary (smoking) routes illustrate this point.

Bioavailability is defined as the fraction of unchanged drug that reaches the systemic circulation after administration by any route. *First-pass metabolism* is the metabolism that occurs before a drug reaches the systemic circulation and occurs most extensively for lipid-soluble drugs such as morphine, methylphenidate, and desipramine, and can significantly reduce bioavailability. Morphine, for example, requires nearly twice the dose when administered orally as compared to intravenously.

Upon absorption, when drug concentrations are graphed against time, a peak drug concentration (C_{max}) is reached at time of maximum concentration (T_{max}). The trough concentration is C_{min}.

Distribution

Once absorbed, a drug is distributed to the various organs and tissues of the body.

Most psychoactive drugs enter the brain because they are highly lipid soluble. The blood–brain barrier hinders the ability of non–lipid-soluble drugs to reach the brain tissue by diffusion. For some compounds, specific active transport systems exist. These active transport systems enable glucose, amino acids, amines, purines, nucleosides, and organic acids to gain access to the brain.

Clearance

Elimination refers to the disappearance of the parent and/or active molecule from the bloodstream or body, which can occur by metabolism and/or excretion. *Excretion* is the process of removing a compound from the body without chemically changing that compound. Metabolic capacity determines drug clearance in most cases.

Most drugs display *first-order elimination* kinetics: The *fraction* or *percentage* of the total amount of drug present in the body removed at any one time is constant and *independent* of dose. Following administration of a drug with first-order kinetics, concentrations show an exponential decline of drug concentrations. The *half-life* ($t_{1/2}$) of a drug is the amount of time it takes for a drug concentration to decrease by half or conversely achieve half of steady-state concentrations. One half-life represents a 50% change, and two, three, four, and five half-lives represent 75%, 87.5%, 93.7%, and 96.8% changes, respectively.

In contrast, for drugs with *zero-order elimination* kinetics, the *amount* of drug removed (rather than the fraction of drug removed) at any one time is constant and *dependent* on dose. The maximal rate of metabolism and/or elimination is generally due to saturation of a key enzyme. Drug dosing becomes difficult in these cases: A small increase in dose can cause a large increase in concentration, in contrast to drugs with first-order clearance where there is proportionality between dose and concentration. Aspirin, phenytoin, and ethanol are examples of drugs with zero-order elimination. Because the fraction of drug removed varies, $t_{1/2}$ is not a useful parameter for drugs with zero-order kinetics.

Drug metabolism is the process of chemical modification of drugs and other chemicals by the body, generally into less active and more hydrophilic compounds. These chemical modifications/reactions are generally performed by enzymatic systems, such as the cytochrome P450 enzyme system.

Phase I reactions are nonsynthetic reactions in which the drug is chemically altered and oxidized. Phase II reactions are synthetic reactions in which the drug is conjugated with another moiety, such as glucuronide or sulfate.

Not all metabolites are inactive or nontoxic, and active metabolites need to be considered when assessing a drug's total activity.

PHARMACOGENOMICS

Pharmacogenomics is the study of the relationship between genetic variations and drug disposition and response.

Genetic variability in drug-metabolizing enzymes can affect drug bioavailability and clearance. Single nucleotide polymorphisms may alter CYP activity. CYP 2D6, for example, which metabolizes codeine to morphine, is the best studied of the drug-metabolizing enzymes. Individuals can be genotyped for 2D6 enzyme function (with classification as poor (PM), intermediate (IM), extensive (EM), and ultrarapid metabolizers (UM). Those with poor metabolizer genotypes generally do not receive adequate analgesia due to the inability to metabolize codeine to the active morphine. Ultrarapid metabolizers, on the other hand, metabolize codeine significantly more rapidly and extensively than others, producing rare but life-threatening morphine intoxication. Breast-feeding infants of mothers who are ultrarapid metabolizers have received morphine overdoses from their mothers who are prescribed codeine for postpartum pain relief.

Drug interactions at the level of the cytochromes and other metabolizing systems are often clinically significant as well. Methadone is metabolized primarily by CYP 3A4. Inhibitors of CYP 3A4, including erythromycin, diltiazem, ketoconazole, and saquinavir, slow the metabolism of methadone and increase methadone levels. Inducers of CYP 3A4, such as carbamazepine, phenobarbital, efavirenz, and St. John's wort, speed the metabolism of methadone and decrease methadone levels. Awareness of potential interactions, clinical observation, and tailoring medication regimens and dosages are needed to optimize therapy and minimize potential toxicities.

Genetically defined differences in drug metabolism may influence the risk of addiction, with relative protection from drug use disorders for persons who experience adverse drug reactions at lower drug doses.

PHARMACODYNAMICS

Pharmacodynamics is the study of the dose–response phenomena, which are the biochemical and physiologic effects of drugs on the body, and the body's homeostatic response. Most drugs act on specific endogenous targets, or receptors, to modulate the rate and extent of the body's endogenous functions.

Potency, Efficacy, and Dose Response

When drug dose and response are plotted on a logarithmic scale, a sigmoidal curve often results. The *maximal efficacy* of a drug occurs at E_{max}, and the concentration of the drug needed to produce 50% of the maximal effect occurs at EC_{50}. *Potency* denotes the amount of drug needed to produce a given effect; the more potent the drug, the smaller the dose required to achieve maximal effect. Potency is primarily determined by the affinity of the receptor for the drug.

Antagonists have no effect upon response when used alone. Antagonists bind with equal affinity to the active and inactive conformations and prevent an agonist from inducing a response. Competitive antagonists may be reversed by adding excess agonist, but noncompetitive antagonists cannot be counteracted in this manner.

Buprenorphine is an example of a highly potent μ-opioid receptor partial agonist. The drug has a high affinity for μ receptors and displaces morphine, methadone, and other full opioid agonists from these receptors. In contrast to the full agonists, however, increases in buprenorphine dose may result in a longer duration of action but do not result in increased pharmacologic effects. Higher doses of buprenorphine can be given without respiratory depression. Buprenorphine's high receptor affinity may precipitate withdrawal in individuals who have significant physical dependence on opioids.

Some drugs, such as nalbuphine and butorphenol, act as mixed agonists and antagonists at various opioid receptor subtypes. Mixed opioid agonist–antagonists were developed in an attempt to produce analgesic drugs with less addictive potential, but this was not borne out in clinical practice.

Receptors

Receptors contain at least two functional domains: a ligand-binding site and an effector or message propagation (ie, signaling) area. Receptors can be grouped according to four common types. These are (1) ligand-gated ion channels, (2) G protein–coupled receptor signaling, (3) receptors with intrinsic enzymatic activity, and (4) receptors regulating nuclear transcription. The relatively small number of mechanisms for cell signaling is fundamental to how target cells integrate signals from multiple receptors to produce sequential, additive, synergistic, or inhibitory responses. Nicotine, benzodiazepines, phencyclidine, and ketamine work through ionotropic receptors. The opioids, cannabinoids, γ-hydroxybutyric acid, and the hallucinogens all exert their action through G_{io}. Cocaine, amphetamine, methamphetamine, and NMDA bind to transporters of biogenic amines.

Tolerance, Sensitization, and Physical Dependence

Tolerance and sensitization reflect changes in the way the body responds to a drug *when it is used repeatedly*. Tolerance is the reduction in response to a drug after its repeated administration. Sensitization indicates an increase in drug response after its repeated administration.

There are several mechanisms by which tolerance can occur. *Pharmacokinetic tolerance* most often occurs as a consequence of increased metabolism of a drug after its repeated administration, resulting in less drug being available at the receptor for drug activity. *Pharmacodynamic tolerance* refers to the adaptive changes in receptor density, efficiency of receptor coupling, and/or signal transduction pathways that occur after repeated drug exposure. *Learned tolerance* refers to a reduction in the effects of a drug because of compensatory mechanisms that are learned. *Conditioned tolerance*, which is a subset of learned tolerance, occurs when specific environmental cues such as sights, smells, or circumstances are paired with drug administration so that when the drug is taken in the presence of the specific environmental cue, a state of expectation occurs.

Cross-tolerance occurs when tolerance to the repeated use of a specific drug in a given category is generalized to other drugs in that same structural and mechanistic category. The cross-tolerance that occurs between alcohol, barbiturates, and benzodiazepines can be used to facilitate the smooth weaning of a patient from their drug of choice during detoxification.

Physical dependence is a state that develops as a result of the adaptation produced by resetting homeostatic mechanisms after repeated drug use. Withdrawal signs and symptoms can occur in a physically dependent person when drug administration suddenly ceases. Withdrawal symptoms may reflect the interactions of numerous neurocircuits and organ systems.

The conclusions in this paper represent the views of the authors and do not necessarily represent the views of the National Institutes of Health.

KEY POINTS

1. Pharmacokinetics describes the time course of drug concentrations in the blood and tissues. Drug concentrations are determined by absorption, distribution, metabolism, and elimination.
2. Drugs with high abuse liability are psychoactive and have rapid distribution into the central nervous system.
3. Pharmacodynamics is the study of dose–response phenomena, including both the activity of the drug and adaptive changes within the body. The pharmacodynamics of drugs of abuse are complex and determined by receptor interactions, tolerance, sensitization, and withdrawal.
4. Pharmacogenomics is the study of the relationship between genetic variations and drug disposition and response, including both pharmacokinetics and pharmacodynamics.

REVIEW QUESTIONS

1. Using diazepam to wean a patient from alcohol is an example of the principle of:
   A. physical dependence.
   B. cross-tolerance.
   C. learned tolerance.
   D. conditioned tolerance.
   E. sensitization.

2. Drugs with first-order elimination kinetics show an exponential decline of drug concentrations. The time to reach a steady state of drugs with first-order elimination kinetics is dependent upon:
   A. dose.
   B. frequency of drug administration.
   C. half-life.
   D. first-pass metabolism.
   E. enzyme saturation.

3. Bioavailability is the fraction of unchanged drug that reaches the systemic circulation after administration by any route. The bioavailability of drugs administered intravenously is:

A. 50%.

B. 70%.

C. 80%.

D. 90%.

E. 100%.

ANSWERS

1. **B**
2. **C**
3. **E**

SUGGESTED READINGS

Brunton L, Hilal-Dandan R, Knollmann BC. *Goodman and Gilman's The Pharmacological Basis of Therapeutics*. 13th ed. New York: McGraw-Hill, 2017.

Kelly LE, Madadi P. Is there a role for therapeutic drug monitoring with codeine? *Ther Drug Monit*. 2012;34(3):249-256.

Madadi P, Avard D, Koren G. Pharmacogenetics of opioids for the treatment of acute maternal pain during pregnancy and lactation. *Curr Drug Metab*. 2012;13(6):721-727.

Meyer MR, Maurer HH. Absorption, distribution, metabolism and excretion pharmacogenomics of drugs of abuse. *Pharmacogenomics*. 2011;12(2):215-233.

Ravindranath V, Strobel HW. Cytochrome P450-mediated metabolism in brain: functional roles and their implications. *Expert Opin Drug Metab Toxicol*. 2013;9(5):551-558.

Trevor AJ, Katzung BG, Kniudering-Hall M. *Katzung & Trevor's Pharmacology Examination and Board Review*. 11th ed. New York: Lange Medical Books/McGraw-Hill, 2015.

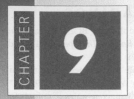

The Pharmacology of Alcohol

Summary by John J. Woodward

Based on THE ASAM PRINCIPLES OF ADDICTION MEDICINE, 6th edition chapter by John J. Woodward

DEFINITION

Alcohols are a group of related chemical compounds that contain a hydroxyl group (–OH) bound to a carbon atom. The form of alcohol most often consumed by humans is ethyl alcohol or ethanol and consists of two carbons and a single hydroxyl group (written as C_2H_5OH or C_2H_6O). Unless otherwise noted, the term *alcohol* will be used throughout this chapter to mean ethanol.

SUBSTANCES INCLUDED IN THIS CLASS

All commercially available alcoholic beverages contain ethyl alcohol with concentrations depending upon the type of beverage. Beverages made by fermentation of sugar-containing fruits and grains include beer (3% to 8% ethanol by volume) and wines (11% to 13% ethanol by volume). Spirits are produced after distillation and generally contain at least 30% ethanol. Ethanol can be concentrated by simple distillation up to approximately 95%, whereas pure ethanol requires the addition of benzene or related substances or desiccation using glycerol. Denatured alcohol contains additives or toxins to prevent human consumption. Rubbing alcohol is prepared from denatured alcohol or isopropyl alcohol and is used for topical purposes.

FORMULATIONS AND METHODS OF USE

In the United States, a standard alcoholic drink is defined as one that contains 0.6 fl oz of alcohol, the amount of alcohol typically contained in 12 oz of beer, 5 oz of wine, or 1.5 oz of distilled spirits (40% ethanol by volume). Although most alcohol is consumed orally, there are isolated cases of individuals injecting ethanol intravenously. Ethanol can also be inhaled using a vaporizer or nebulizer, and several forms of powdered alcohol have been developed (eg, Palcohol) that involve microencapsulation with a water-soluble carrier such as maltodextrin.

CLINICAL USES

In addition to its use as a topical antiseptic, alcohol has several clinical indications including treatment of accidental or voluntary ingestion of methanol or ethylene glycol. Ethanol has a higher affinity for alcohol dehydrogenase than methanol and thus reduces the formation of methanol metabolites formaldehyde and formic acid. For both indications, hemodialysis is the recommended first line of treatment.

BRIEF HISTORICAL FEATURES

Alcohol is one of the oldest used psychoactive substances. Consumption of alcohol-containing beverages predate recorded human history and written records of its use are found in Chinese and Middle Eastern texts as far back as 9000 years ago. In modern times, alcohol is second only to caffeine in incidence of use, and its manufacture, distribution, and sale are of major economic importance across the world.

EPIDEMIOLOGY

The lifetime exposure to alcohol is high, with nearly 88% of the US population reporting using alcohol at least once in their lifetime. In 2013, current alcohol use (defined as use in the past 30 days) of Americans ranged from 2.1% among 12- to 13-year-olds to nearly 70% of among 21- to 25-year-olds. Prevalence decreased among older groups, although it was nearly 54% among 60- to 64-year-olds. Rates of binge drinking (five or more drinks within a few hours) for persons aged 12 years and older approached 23% in 2013, whereas heavy drinking (five or more drinks on each of 5 or more days in the past 30) was reported by 6.3% of the US population. The latest estimate of annual alcohol-related costs (2010) in terms of lost productivity and health care was $249 billion.

Results from clinical studies of alcohol abuse and alcoholism suggest that there are several types of alcohol use disorders, based on the appearance and severity of certain alcohol-related problems. Two particularly well-known classification schemes are the type I and II forms and the type A and B forms. The type I and type A forms share several of the following similarities:

■ later onset of alcohol-related problems (>25 years old),
■ fewer childhood behavior problems,
■ relatively mild alcohol-related issues with fewer hospitalizations,
■ lower degree of novelty seeking coupled with a preference toward harm avoidance, and
■ less tendency to run in families.

PHARMACOKINETICS

Alcohol is a small, water-soluble molecule that is rapidly and efficiently absorbed into the bloodstream from the stomach, small intestine, and colon. The rate of absorption depends on the gastric emptying time and can be delayed by the presence of food in the small intestine. Alcohol is rapidly distributed throughout the body and gains access to all tissues, including the fetus in pregnant women. Because women show less gastric metabolism of alcohol than men, when body weights are equivalent, women show a 20% to 25% higher blood alcohol level than men following ingestion of the same amount of alcohol.

In the liver, alcohol is broken down by alcohol dehydrogenase (ADH) and mixed function oxidases such as P450IIE1 (CYP2E1). Levels of CYP2E1 may be increased in chronic drinkers. ADH converts alcohol to acetaldehyde, which subsequently can be converted to acetate by the actions of acetaldehyde dehydrogenase. The rate of alcohol metabolism by ADH is relatively constant because the enzyme is saturated at low blood alcohol levels and thus exhibits zero order kinetics (constant amount oxidized per unit of time). Alcohol metabolism is proportional to body weight (and probably liver weight) and averages approximately 1 oz of pure alcohol per 3 hours in adults. Clinical trials have shown that metadoxine (pyridoxal 1-2-pyrrolidone-5-carboxylate) appears to enhance the metabolic clearance of alcohol and speed the recovery of intoxicated individuals.

PHARMACODYNAMICS
Central Nervous System

Acutely, alcohol acts as a central nervous system (CNS) depressant. During the initial phase, when blood alcohol levels are rising, a period of disinhibition often occurs and signs of behavioral arousal are common. At higher blood levels, alcohol acts as a sedative and hypnotic, although the quality of sleep often is reduced after alcohol intake.

Other Organ Systems

Acute alcohol ingestion produces a feeling of warmth as cutaneous blood flow is increased, and this is accompanied by a reduction in core body temperature. Gastric secretions are usually increased, although the concentration of alcohol ingested affects this response, with high concentrations (>20%) inhibiting secretions. Long-term ingestion of high concentrations of alcohol produces deleterious effects on the gastrointestinal (GI) tract including esophageal varices and bleeding, erosive gastritis, and diarrhea and malabsorption of nutrients and vitamins. Heavy alcohol consumption increases the risk of developing tumors in the GI system as well as in other tissues including the lung and breast. Acute and chronic ingestion of alcohol generally decreases sexual performance in both men and women. Alcohol causes changes in contractility and function of the cardiovascular system, and chronic alcohol consumption increases fat accumulation in the liver that can progress to severe liver damage and cirrhosis. Low-to-moderate alcohol use is associated with a reduced risk of coronary disease.

DRUG–DRUG INTERACTIONS

Alcohol depressant actions on the CNS are additive with those produced by barbiturates, benzodiazepines, general anesthetics, volatile organic solvents, and anticonvulsants. Alcohol enhances the sedative effects of antihistamines that are commonly used in the treatment of nasal congestion. Combining these medications with alcohol can result in significant CNS depression and reduced ability to safely carry out normal functions such as automobile driving. Alcohol enhances the hepatotoxic effects of acetaminophen (Tylenol) and the gastric irritating effects of nonsteroidal anti-inflammatory drugs and increases the risk of gastritis and upper GI bleeding.

NEUROBIOLOGY (MECHANISMS OF ADDICTION)

All drugs of harmful use, including alcohol, produce reward by enhancing the release of dopamine (DA) within limbic and cortical circuits that regulate motivated behavior. The DA neurons that provide these projections are located in the midbrain ventral tegmental area, and their rate of firing is enhanced by alcohol. Chronic intake of alcohol leads to alterations in the excitability of these neurons that can persist for significant periods of time. Genetic differences in the responsiveness of these neurons and their connections may contribute to the motivational factors that drive greater alcohol-seeking behavior in certain individuals.

Molecular Sites of Alcohol Action

Psychostimulants such as cocaine and amphetamine or opiates like heroin and morphine produce their effect by binding to specific protein receptors expressed on brain neurons. In contrast, alcohol interacts with a wide variety of targets including both lipids and proteins. Although initial observations suggested that alcohol's acute actions arose from its effects on membrane lipids, the current consensus is that alcohol's behavioral actions result from interactions with a diverse set of ligand-gated and voltage-gated ion channels that regulate neuronal excitability.

GABA$_A$ and Glycine Receptors

Distinct families of subunits make up GABA$_A$ and glycine receptors, and different combinations of these give rise to ion channels with variable sensitivity to pharmacologic agents, including alcohol. In general, alcohol enhances GABA$_A$ and glycine receptor function, although in some cases, these effects may occur via increased release of GABA rather than direct effects of the ion channel itself. Stress may alter the ability of GABA receptors to control DA neurons, and this may contribute to escalations in drinking in stressed individuals.

Glutamate-Activated Ion Channels

Glutamate is the major excitatory neurotransmitter in the brain and activates three major subtypes of ion channels called α-amino-3-hydroxy-5-methyl-4-isoxazolepropionic acid (AMPA), kainate, and *N*-methyl-D-aspartate (NMDA) receptors. These channels cause depolarization of the neuronal membrane and are implicated in processes that underlie cognition, learning, and memory. NMDA receptors are readily antagonized by alcohol at concentrations associated with intoxication and sedation, whereas most non-NMDA receptors are unaffected by ethanol. Alcohol blockade of excitatory NMDA signaling may underlie its rewarding effects because more selective NMDA antagonists also increase levels of DA in reward areas of the brain. Chronic exposure to alcohol increases the density and clustering of NMDA

receptors leading to increased neuronal excitability and enhanced susceptibility to seizures that can develop during withdrawal from alcohol.

Other Ion Channel Subtypes

5-Hydroxytryptamine Type 3 Receptors

5-Hydroxytryptamine type 3 (5-HT$_3$) receptors are ligand-gated ion channels activated by serotonin. Alcohol potentiates currents carried by the 5-HT$_3$ receptor, and 5-HT$_3$ receptor antagonists block the discriminative stimulus properties of ethanol in animals. Human studies with the 5-HT$_3$ antagonist ondansetron (Zofran) report that the drug reduces drinking in certain individuals.

Acetylcholine Nicotinic Receptors

Alcohol has been shown to potentiate or inhibit acetylcholine receptors, and this seems to be related to which subtypes of nicotinic receptors are expressed. It is not clear how these effects on the nicotinic receptor are manifested at the behavioral level. However, the α4β2 nicotinic receptor partial agonist varenicline (Chantix), used in smoking cessation, reduces alcohol seeking and consumption in animal models.

Adenosine Triphosphate–Gated Ion Channels

Adenosine triphosphate (ATP) activates a variety of ion channels, some of which are sensitive to ethanol. Like nicotinic receptors, the behavioral implication of these effects are not yet fully known, but positive modulators (ivermectin) of some ATP-gated channels reduce drinking in rodent models.

Potassium- and Calcium-Selective Ion Channels

Potassium channels that are regulated by calcium (SK and BK channels) and those gated by G-proteins (GirK) channels serve as a brake on excitatory glutamatergic transmission by hyperpolarizing the membrane. The activity of some of these channels is enhanced by ethanol, and this may contribute to the inhibition of vasopressin release from neurohypophysial terminals and the resulting diuresis that accompanies alcohol ingestion. Decreased expression or changes in the location of certain potassium channels following chronic alcohol exposure may contribute to the hyperexcitability often observed during ethanol withdrawal. Enhancing SK activity with an allosteric modulator (chlorzoxazone; [Parafon Forte]) was shown to reduce alcohol consumption in rats. Alcohol inhibits certain subtypes of voltage-gated calcium channels, and this may contribute to disruptions in sleep that are commonly observed in individuals with alcohol dependence.

Pharmacologic Studies Implicating Other Neurotransmitter Systems

In addition to its effects on ion channels (discussed previously), alcohol also has important actions on various neurotransmitters. A brief review of that literature is presented as follows.

Adenosine

Adenosine is present in high concentrations in the brain and may serve as an endogenous antiepileptic because of its ability to inhibit neuronal function. Alcohol increases extracellular adenosine levels by inhibiting a nucleoside transporter.

Dopamine

Alcohol increases the firing of ventral tegmental area DA neurons leading to enhanced DA release in the nucleus accumbens, prefrontal cortex, and other areas although the mechanism underlying this effect is not precisely known.

Opioids and Other Neuropeptides

Alcohol increases the release of opioid peptides, and mice genetically modified to lack the μ-opiate receptor do not voluntarily drink alcohol and do not respond to the rewarding effects of opiates, nicotine, or cannabinoids. Naloxone and naltrexone, two opioid receptor antagonists, reduce alcohol intake in both animals and humans, and various formulations of naltrexone (ReVia), including sustained-release and depot forms (Vivitrol, Naltrel, Depotrex), are now approved for treating excessive drinking. Antagonists of κ-opioid receptors reduce alcohol self-administration in rodents, including that induced or augmented by stress. Other neuropeptides such as NPY, CRF, and orexin regulate alcohol consumption in rodents although two different corticotropin-releasing factor 1 (CRF1) antagonists (pexacerfont and verucerfont) failed to reduce cue-induced craving for alcohol in human clinical trials.

Serotonin

5-HT and 5-HT–metabolite levels are reduced in the cerebrospinal fluid of many alcohol abusers, suggesting that reduced 5-HT levels or a reduction in 5-HT–mediated neurotransmission may predispose certain people to uncontrollable drinking behavior. However, agents that enhance levels of serotonin (such as fluoxetine [Prozac] and sertraline [Zoloft]) appear to have limited efficacy in the treatment of alcohol use disorders.

Endocannabinoids

The endogenous cannabinoid system has been shown to be an important mediator of ethanol drinking. CB1 antagonists reduce ethanol preference in wild-type mice, and animals genetically lacking CB1 receptors show reduced alcohol preference.

Neuroimmune Modulators

Mediators of immune function such as the family of Toll-like receptors (TLR) and the receptor for advanced glycation end products may also influence brain systems that regulate ethanol intake. Ethanol also induces TLR4 signaling in the gut with subsequent leakage of bacterial products that are powerful stimulators of the innate immune system. Changes in gut permeability require relatively high concentrations of ethanol that are associated with binge drinking of alcoholic beverages with high alcohol content.

ADDICTION LIABILITY

Lifetime prevalence of alcohol dependence is approximately 13%, and the risk of developing alcohol dependence shows a strong inverse correlation with the age at which heavy drinking begins. Chronic use of alcohol produces several neuroadaptive changes that may be important in the development of alcohol addiction.

Sensitization

Sensitization is the increase in the pharmacologic and physiologic response to a drug after repeated exposures. Another form of sensitization is characterized by an increase in the severity and intensity of withdrawal signs after multiple episodes of alcohol intoxication and withdrawal. This form of sensitization is similar to the kindling phenomena observed after repeated brain seizures and may involve some of the same mechanisms.

Tolerance and Dependence

Tolerance is manifested as a reduced sensitivity to alcohol. In persons with an alcohol use disorder, tolerance to the sedative and even lethal effects of alcohol can be profound. For example, although the lethal dose 50% (LD50) in nontolerant humans is approximately 400 to 500 mg%, blood levels far exceeding those values are often reported in individuals arrested for drunk driving. Dependence is defined by the occurrence of symptoms that appear during withdrawal from alcohol. These symptoms include both physical (eg, tremors, convulsions) and psychological (eg, negative emotions, craving) components. Although reward mechanisms are undoubtedly important in the initiation of heavy alcohol use, processes and brain areas involved in dependence may be critical for maintaining continued drinking through negative reinforcement (eg, anxiety, stress) generated during withdrawal. Changes in these systems may also underlie the phenomena of craving that can persist long after the symptoms of alcohol withdrawal have long subsided.

Toxicity States

Alcohol is metabolized under zero order kinetics (constant amount oxidized per unit time), and blood alcohol levels fall at a rate of about 20 mg/dL/h. Alcohol produces a well-studied progression of behavioral symptoms that are highly correlated with blood alcohol levels. In nontolerant individuals,

- Low levels (10 to 50 mg%)—decreased anxiety, feelings of well-being, increased sociability
- Moderate levels (80 to 100 mg%)—impaired judgment and motor function
- Higher levels (150 to 200 mg%)—marked ataxia, reduced reaction time, blackout
- Anesthetic levels (300 to 400 mg%)—severe motor impairment, vomiting, loss of consciousness
- Lethal level (400 to 500 mg% and above)—as mentioned previously, lethal doses of alcohol in nontolerant individuals are on the order of 400 to 500 mg%, although this can vary widely.

Medical Complications

Alcohol affects nearly all tissue and organ systems studied, and heavy drinkers show skeletal fragility and damage to tissues such as the brain, liver, and heart as well as increased susceptibility to some cancers. Heavy drinkers have increases in cortical cerebrospinal fluid in both gray and white matter and diminished volume of frontal lobes and cerebellar gray matter, anterior hippocampus, and a reduced area of the corpus callosum. Individuals with alcohol use disorder often show reduced brain glucose metabolism as compared with control subjects, and brief episodes of heavy drinking, or binges, cause neuron loss in animal models of alcoholism. Despite these negative effects, light-to-moderate levels of drinking (one drink per day for women, two drinks per day for men) are associated with a reduced risk of cardiovascular disease.

ACKNOWLEDGMENTS

Development of this chapter was supported by grant R37AA009986 and P50AA010761 from the National Institute on Alcohol Abuse and Alcoholism.

KEY POINTS

1. Alcohol is among the most widely used substances in the world, and its manufacturing, distribution, and sales are of significant economic importance.
2. Nearly 90% of the US population report some use of alcohol over their lifetime, and annual costs associated with alcohol-related injury, healthcare, and lost productivity exceed $249 billion.
3. Alcohol has actions on all organ systems, and excessive consumption is associated with enhanced risk of GI pathologies, cardiovascular incidents, certain cancers, and liver and brain dysfunction.
4. Ethanol targets a variety of excitatory and inhibitory ion channels that regulate neuronal excitability, and perturbation of these channels underlies many of the behavioral effects of alcohol.
5. Acutely, alcohol engages brain reward systems and enhances the activity of midbrain DA neurons. Chronic use of alcohol induces changes in reward and stress circuits, and continued drinking may result from an attempt to minimize the negative aspects associated with withdrawal from alcohol.

REVIEW QUESTIONS

1. Which of the following statements regarding ethanol metabolism is correct?
   A. The rate of ethanol metabolism increases as more drinks are consumed.
   B. The majority of ethanol metabolism takes place in the stomach.
   C. On average, 1 oz of pure ethanol is metabolized in 3 hours in adults.

2. Alcohol is classified as a sedative–hypnotics and produces effects similar to all of the following except:
   A. benzodiazepines (eg, diazepam [Valium]).
   B. cocaine.
   C. barbiturates (eg, pentobarbital).
   D. anticonvulsants.

3. Which of the following ion channels are affected by ethanol?
   A. The NMDA receptor
   B. The GABA$_A$ receptor
   C. The 5-HT3 receptor
   D. All of the above

ANSWERS

1. **C**
2. **B**
3. **D**

SUGGESTED READINGS

Howard RJ, Trudell JR, Harris RA. Seeking structural specificity: direct modulation of pentameric ligand-gated ion channels by alcohols and general anesthetics. *Pharmacol Rev.* 2014;66(2):396-412.

Mason BJ. Emerging pharmacotherapies for alcohol use disorder. *Neuropharmacology.* 2017;122:244-253.

National Institute on Alcohol Abuse and Alcoholism. Alcohol facts and statistics. https://pubs.niaaa.nih.gov/publications /AlcoholFacts&Stats/AlcoholFacts&Stats.htm. Updated August 2018. Accessed September 25, 2018.

Pascual M, Montesinos J, Guerri C. Role of the innate immune system in the neuropathological consequences induced by adolescent binge drinking. *J Neurosci Res.* 2018;96(5):765-780.

Reilly MT, Noronha A, Goldman D, Koob GF. Genetic studies of alcohol dependence in the context of the addiction cycle. *Neuropharmacology.* 2017;122:3-21.

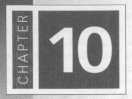

10 The Pharmacology of Nonalcohol Sedative Hypnotics

Summary by Carolina L. Haass-Koffler and
Elinore F. McCance-Katz

Based on THE ASAM PRINCIPLES OF ADDICTION MEDICINE,
6th edition chapter by Carolina L. Haass-Koffler and
Elinore F. McCance-Katz

Sedative–hypnotic drugs represent a diverse group of chemical agents that depress the function of the central nervous system (CNS). They are used in medicine as anxiolytics, sleep inducers, hypnotics, anticonvulsants, muscle relaxants, and anesthesia induction agents. Their calming (sedative) effects are dose dependent and on *a continuum* with sleep-inducing (hypnotic) effects, unconsciousness, and for some agents, coma and death. Agents discussed in this chapter include benzodiazepines, nonbenzodiazepine hypnotics, and miscellaneous related compounds.

The name *benzodiazepine* is derived from the chemical structure comprised by a benzene ring fused to a seven-membered diazepine ring. The more recent sedative–hypnotic agents include the nonbenzodiazepines (zopiclone, eszopiclone, zaleplon, and zolpidem). The chemical structure of these compounds is not similar to the benzodiazepines, their therapeutic effect is via benzodiazepine binding site at the γ-aminobutyric acid (GABA$_A$) receptor; their actions are not identical to classic benzodiazepines.

In the 1950s, the synthesis of chlordiazepoxide with hypnotic, sedative, and muscle-relaxant effects began the era of benzodiazepines. In 1960, chlordiazepoxide was marketed as Librium, a safe and effective anxiolytic agent, and in 1963, the popular drug Valium was developed. In the 1970s, benzodiazepines were found to account for 10% of all prescriptions written in the United States. Benzodiazepines have replaced barbiturates, which are less toxic in overdose, have less capacity to produce fatal CNS effects, and are associated with fewer drug interactions. At the present time, benzodiazepines are widely utilized in the management of many medical and psychiatric conditions and are often

used for long periods of time—for many patients, once started on these medications, they may be maintained on them for years. Conditions for which benzodiazepines are frequently used include acute relief of anxiety and insomnia, which may extend to long-term, chronic use. Benzodiazepines are often administered as adjuncts to anesthesia prior to surgery and as muscle relaxants in pain management (eg, the treatment of lower back pain). Further, the US Food and Drug Administration has approved the use of benzodiazepine medications for the treatment of panic disorder and generalized anxiety disorder. Benzodiazepines also remain a frequently utilized approach to the management of acute agitation in psychiatric syndromes, often in combination with antipsychotic medications.

Benzodiazepines and nonbenzodiazepines exert their clinical effects through allosteric modulation of the GABA$_A$ receptor. Because GABA is the major inhibitory neurotransmitter system in the brain, positive modulation of the receptor by benzodiazepines is responsible for sedative, anticonvulsant, hypnotic, and amnestic effects of the drug. In the human brain, the most common structure of the GABA$_A$ receptor consists of two αs, two βs, and one γ subunit. Benzodiazepines bind at the interface of the γ_2 and α subunits. GABA$_A$ receptors containing $\alpha_{1-3,5}$ subunits mediate the effects of benzodiazepines. Binding at the α_1 subunit mediates sedative and amnestic effects, whereas binding at the α_2 and possibly the α_3 subunit modulates anxiolytic and muscle relaxant effects.

Current Food and Drug Administration–approved nonbenzodiazepines are zolpidem, zaleplon, and eszopiclone (*S*-enantiomer of zopiclone, not available in the United States). Nonbenzodiazepines share many pharmacologic actions with benzodiazepines, including sedative–hypnotic, anxiolytic, myorelaxant, and anticonvulsant effects, although their selectivity for these actions differ. Benzodiazepines and nonbenzodiazepines may act through overlapping binding sites between α and β subunits of the $GABA_A$ receptor. Zolpidem, however, binds to additional sites on these subunits that are not crucial for benzodiazepine activity.

Many benzodiazepines undergo hepatic metabolism involving oxidative reactions mediated by the cytochrome P450 (CYP450) enzymes. Oxidative metabolism reactions include *N*-dealkylation or aliphatic hydroxylation. The CYP3A4 enzyme mediates the oxidative metabolism of many of the benzodiazepines and also plays a role in the biotransformation of the nonbenzodiazepine sedative–hypnotic agents. Several of the benzodiazepines are converted into active metabolites such as desmethyldiazepam, which are very slowly cleared from the body. The final phase of metabolism for most benzodiazepines consists of conjugation of either the parent drug or their metabolites with glucuronide. Zolpidem is extensively metabolized by CYP3A4, CYP2C9, and CYP2C19 to inactive hydroxylated metabolites. Also, aldehyde dehydrogenase may play a major role in the metabolism of zaleplon.

The relationship between the pharmacokinetic profile of benzodiazepines and abuse liability is complex. It is generally believed that the rapid onset of action is associated with euphoria. Lower abuse potential is more consistently predicted with prodrugs that require hepatic metabolism to form the active moiety, such as the formation of desmethyldiazepam from halazepam, which appears to have lower abuse liability than diazepam.

Pharmacogenomic investigation of benzodiazepines have focused on metabolizing enzymes; however, the impact of polymorphisms in *CYP3A4* and *CYP3A5* on benzodiazepine metabolism has produced mixed results.

The most serious drug–drug interactions occur when sedative–hypnotics are combined with drugs that depress CNS activity (ie, alcohol, opioids, muscle relaxants), potentially resulting in overdose and death. Benzodiazepines do not induce their own metabolism; however, those that are metabolized through CYP3A4 (eg, ketoconazole, itraconazole, erythromycin) are subject to altered plasma levels by agents that inhibit this metabolic pathway. Drugs that induce or inhibit CYP2C19 (eg, oral contraceptives) may influence the metabolism of some benzodiazepines. Inducers of CYP450 enzymes (eg, rifampin, carbamazepine, and phenytoin) may significantly reduce

plasma concentrations of zaleplon, zolpidem, and zopiclone or other benzodiazepines that are CYP3A4 substrates. Administration of the CYP3A4 enzyme inhibitors (eg, erythromycin or ketoconazole) can decrease the clearance of zolpidem. Compounds that inhibit CYP3A and CYP2C19 (eg, cimetidine, ketoconazole, fluvoxamine, fluoxetine, omeprazole) may lead to increased and prolonged sedation with diazepam administration.

As the unhealthy use of prescription opioids has increased, the interaction between opioids and sedative–hypnotics has become an increasing concern. There is extensive evidence implicating benzodiazepines in both fatal and nonfatal cases of opioid overdose. Pharmacodynamic interactions between benzodiazepines and opioids may lead to oversedation and impaired motor performance. High-dose diazepam also enhanced psychomotor impairment and sedation when given concurrently with either buprenorphine or methadone. Benzodiazepines have been increasingly linked to adverse events and deaths when taken with opioids. Benzodiazepines were the most frequent medication class associated with opioid overdose deaths. Although there is evidence of substantial nonmedical use of benzodiazepines, it is also the case that benzodiazepines are frequently prescribed for the treatment of pain and so may be coprescribed with opioid analgesics. However, the limited studies that have been conducted have shown little to no benefit of benzodiazepines in the management of pain. Benzodiazepine use was associated with a number of adverse effects, including reports of greater pain severity, pain interference in life, and lower feelings of self-efficacy regarding pain. Those receiving benzodiazepines in the context of pain management were more likely to be prescribed higher risk opioid doses (>200 mg morphine equivalents per day) and to be using antidepressant or antipsychotic medications. These patients were also more likely to have an alcohol use disorder, to use illicit substances, and had greater mental health comorbidity. Further, those taking opioids concomitantly with benzodiazepines had greater past month use of emergency healthcare and were more likely to experience an overdose event. As with the increasing understanding of the lack of evidence for the use of opioid therapies for chronic pain and guidance to avoid opioids as a first-line therapy, the same should apply to benzodiazepine use in pain management.

The pharmacodynamic mechanisms underlying the development of tolerance and withdrawal to sedative–hypnotics have been associated with decreased responsiveness of $GABA_A$ receptors to benzodiazepines. Another possible mechanism of tolerance may involve benzodiazepine-induced internalization of surface $GABA_A$ receptors into intraneuronal sequestration sites. The glutamatergic system may play a major role in benzodiazepine withdrawal syndrome.

Benzodiazepines occupy an intermediate position of addiction liability (Schedules 4 and 5) and nonbenzodiazepines have lower potential for addiction, although both classes of medications are controlled substances (Schedule 5). Those with the lowest positive reinforcing effects in humans are clonazepam, chlordiazepoxide, halazepam, prazepam, quazepam, and oxazepam. However, individuals at risk for sedative–hypnotic addiction (eg, those with an alcohol use disorder) may misuse any of the benzodiazepines, even those with relatively low potential for addiction. Benzodiazepines with the highest addiction potential are those that produce a rapid onset of pleasant mood, well-being, relief of dysphoria, and anxiety. Although the nonbenzodiazepines were initially thought to have little addiction liability, human laboratory studies have shown that zolpidem administration increases subjective responses such as "drug liking" and "good effects" in both those who use drugs and in healthy volunteers, indicating addiction potential.

There are certain groups of high-risk patients where long-term use and addiction are greater than in patients with anxiety disorders. Several groups reported positive mood enhancement from acute benzodiazepine doses, including moderate and heavy drinkers, abstinent alcoholics, and individuals who have strong family histories of alcoholism. Another group of individuals in which unhealthy benzodiazepine use is particularly high in both the United States and Europe are those with a history of opioid use. The most common reason such individuals use benzodiazepines is to manage anxiety and opioid withdrawal. Benzodiazepine use has also been reported to enhance euphoria or "high" when ingested concomitantly with opioids, thereby increasing the risk of coadministration. In opioid treatment programs (methadone or buprenorphine maintenance programs), urine toxicology tests positive for benzodiazepines are common. Rates of concurrent benzodiazepine use are also high for individuals receiving buprenorphine plus naloxone treatment for an opioid use disorder.

Acute doses of benzodiazepines can be associated with adverse effects that include anterograde amnesia, difficulty acquiring new learning, and sedation that may affect attention and concentration. Studies and clinical experience suggest that not all benzodiazepines produce the same type or severity of cognitive impairment. Greater impairment is seen in chronic users who are men, in the elderly, and for those taking the highest doses.

Benzodiazepines are widely prescribed in the elderly, despite the known risks in older people (eg, impaired cognition and mobility, increased risk of falls and associated injuries, increased risk of Alzheimer disease). Zolpidem also produces anterograde amnesia and has been associated with somnambulism and complex nocturnal behaviors, such as eating, shopping, and driving. Similar problems may be seen with zaleplon, especially at high doses. Several surveys in different countries have found a higher incidence of motor vehicle accidents associated with benzodiazepines. The risks of benzodiazepines during pregnancy and lactation have been the subject of controversy. Most recent studies have not found an association of in utero benzodiazepine exposure alone with major congenital anomalies. There are two other clinically important problems that may be encountered during pregnancy. Newborns who have been exposed to benzodiazepines in utero during the third trimester or during delivery may present with floppy baby syndrome and neonatal withdrawal syndromes. In nursing mothers, benzodiazepines enter the breast milk but appear in such low concentrations that they do not usually cause adverse effects in infants. There are two important exceptions to this general rule: The risk to the infant is higher if: (1) the benzodiazepine is given in high doses antepartum and continued postpartum and (2) infants have impaired hepatic function, as evidenced by hyperbilirubinemia.

The principal medical complications with benzodiazepines are related to overdose and withdrawal syndromes. When high doses of benzodiazepines are ingested, either as a therapeutic intervention or in an overdose, initial signs of toxicity are ataxia and impaired gag reflex as well as CNS depression. Respiratory depression may also occur in overdoses, and the medical approach to overdose treatment is supportive care. When administered for short periods, and at therapeutic doses, the withdrawal syndrome is usually mild, consisting of anxiety, headache, insomnia, dysphoria, tremor, and muscle twitching. After long-term treatment with therapeutic doses, the syndrome increases in severity and may include autonomic dysfunction, nausea, vomiting, depersonalization, derealization, delirium, hallucinations, illusions, agitation, and grand mal seizures. The time course of the abstinence syndrome is related to the half-life of the agent, with patients taking short half-life agents (eg, lorazepam, alprazolam, temazepam) developing symptoms within 24 hours of discontinuation, the severity of which peaks at 48 hours. With longer half-life agents such as diazepam, symptoms may develop a week after drug discontinuation and last for several weeks. In general, longer treatment periods, higher doses, sudden drug discontinuation, and psychopathology increase the severity of the withdrawal syndrome. Clinical experience has shown that there is great variability in the sensitivity of patients when discontinuing benzodiazepines. All patients who have been taking a benzodiazepine for several weeks or longer should have the medication tapered to avoid withdrawal and safely discontinue use.

CONCLUSIONS

Benzodiazepines are the most widely used and misused drugs of the sedative–hypnotic class. In patients with anxiety disorders, unhealthy use is not common; however, certain subgroups of patients, such as individuals with alcohol use disorder and those receiving opioid therapies for opioid use disorder are at a higher risk to misuse these agents. Compared to the general population, higher rates of benzodiazepine use are found in the elderly and in patients with chronic pain, with significant risks for adverse events and overdose deaths, particularly when taken in combination with opioid medications. The newer nonbenzodiazepine hypnotics may have a lower potential for tolerance or even the development of a substance use disorder, although they are not devoid of such risk. The identification of $GABA_A$ receptor subtypes and clarification of their function provide hope that drug development will lead to $GABA_A$ agonists and modulators that have fewer adverse effects, lower risks for addiction, and greater specificity of action.

KEY POINTS

1. Acute or short-term administration of benzodiazepines and nonbenzodiazepines can be useful. Chronic use should generally be discouraged as a primary means of avoiding toxicities.
2. Benzodiazepines occupy an intermediate position of addiction liability (Schedules 4 and 5), and nonbenzodiazepines (Schedule 5) have a lower potential for addiction, although both classes of medications are controlled substances.
3. Benzodiazepines with the highest addiction potential are those that produce a rapid onset of pleasant mood, well-being, relief of dysphoria, and anxiety.
4. Evidence for the benefit of benzodiazepines in acute pain management is small, and there is no evidence for the benefit of benzodiazepines in pain management when used chronically.
5. The principal medical complications with benzodiazepines are related to overdose and withdrawal syndromes.

REVIEW QUESTIONS

1. Are benzodiazepines the first-line treatment for anxiety?
   A. Yes, but always with regard to the patient's comorbid conditions.
   B. Yes; however, in patients with significant depression, tricyclic antidepressants are more likely to succeed than a benzodiazepine.
   C. Psychotherapy is preferred.
   D. The ideal treatment should be tailored to the individual and may involve a combination of both psychotherapy and pharmacotherapy.

2. Why should benzodiazepine and nonbenzodiazepine medications used for sleep be administered short term (eg, 2 to 4 weeks) versus long term?
   A. Benzodiazepines are administered for short term; nonbenzodiazepine are safer and can be administered long term without adverse events.
   B. They have the potential to become addictive or at least to induce dependence.
   C. Long-term administration can induce cardiomyopathy.
   D. Short-term benzodiazepine administration is indicated only for pediatric patients.

3. Which of the following best describes the effect of benzodiazepines in the context of pain management?
   A. There is no evidence for the benefit of benzodiazepines in pain management when used chronically.
   B. Benzodiazepines can be used with opioid therapy for pain management. There are no adverse events reported because they do no share microsomal pathways (metabolism).
   C. Evidence for the benefit of benzodiazepines in acute pain management is well-documented.
   D. People concurrently using both drugs are at a lower risk of visiting the emergency department or being admitted to a hospital for a drug-related emergencies.

ANSWERS

1. **D**
2. **B**
3. **A**

SUGGESTED READINGS

Cunningham JL, Craner JR, Evans MM, Hooten WM. Benzodiazepine use in patients with chronic pain in an interdisciplinary pain rehabilitation program. *J Pain Res.* 2017;10:311-317.

Hata T, Kanazawa T, Hamada T, et al. What can predict and prevent the long-term use of benzodiazepines? *J Psychiatr Res.* 2018;97:94-100.

Lyons PG, Snyder A, Sokol S, et al. Association between opioid and benzodiazepine use and clinical deterioration in ward patients. *J Hosp Med.* 2017;12(6):428-434.

Maldonado JR. Novel algorithms for the prophylaxis and management of alcohol withdrawal syndromes-beyond benzodiazepines. *Crit Care Clin.* 2017;33(3):559-599.

McClure FL, Niles JK, Kaufman HW, Gudin J. Concurrent use of opioids and benzodiazepines: evaluation of prescription drug monitoring by a United States laboratory. *J Addict Med.* 2017;11(6):420-426.

11

The Pharmacology of Opioids

Summary by Kimberly D.L. Parks, Coreen Domingo, and Thomas R. Kosten

Based on THE ASAM PRINCIPLES OF ADDICTION MEDICINE, 6th edition chapter by Daryl Shorter and Thomas R. Kosten

DEFINITION OF DRUGS IN THE CLASS

Three distinct G protein–coupled, opioid receptor types in the brain are the μ (MOPr), κ (KOPr), and δ (DOPr) receptors. The endogenous opioid agonists are endorphins, enkephalins, dynorphins, and endomorphins with β-endorphin, endomorphin-1, and endomorphin-2 stimulating MOPr and providing endogenous analgesic and rewarding effects.

Opium is derived from the opium poppy (*Papaver somniferum*) and stimulates the MOPr through morphine, codeine, and thebaine. Codeine is an analgesic and antitussive, and thebaine is used for producing semisynthetic MOPr ligands. Other exogenous opioids are heroin, oxycodone, meperidine, pentazocine, hydromorphone, hydrocodone, and buprenorphine as well as the synthetics methadone and levo-alpha-acetylmethadol (LAAM).

SUBSTANCES INCLUDED IN THE CLASS

Morphine

Morphine was first isolated from the poppy plant in 1817 and has been used orally, intravenously, intramuscularly, or intrathecally to treat moderate-to-severe pain. Its pharmacokinetics vary by route of administration with a favorable safety profile. Oral bioavailability is 35% to 75%, with a plasma half-life of 2 to 3.5 hours, and an analgesic effect for 4 to 6 hours. Morphine is biotransformed largely by glucuronidation to morphine-3-glucuronide and morphine-6-glucuronide (M6G), with the latter being biologically active. In liver disease, lower doses should be used, and with renal disease, accumulation of metabolites occurs as 90% are renally excreted.

Codeine

Codeine is methylmorphine. It crosses the blood–brain barrier faster and has less first-pass metabolism in the liver, giving greater oral bioavailability than morphine. It is metabolized to morphine via cytochrome 2D6 and to hydrocodone by an unknown mechanism. It is broken down into 10% morphine by demethylation, 80% codeine-6-glucuronide, and other metabolites. Most of the analgesia is thought to come from morphine with some from codeine-6-glucuronide.

Thebaine and Synthetic Compounds

Thebaine is not used clinically or recreationally because it is a potent convulsant. Modifications of thebaine result in hydrocodone (Vicodin), oxycodone (OxyContin), hydromorphone (Dilaudid), and heroin. Synthetic modifications also include antagonists such as naloxone (Narcan), naltrexone (Trexan, ReVia, or Vivitrol), and nalmefene (Revex) as well as partial agonists such as buprenorphine (Subutex).

Heroin

Heroin is derived from morphine, and its rapid onset of action and short half-life make it preferred as a drug of abuse. Heroin is a Schedule I drug, although a few countries use it for the treatment of intravenous heroin use disorder. A water-soluble prodrug that is not itself active, heroin is rapidly deacetylated to 6-monoacetylmorphine (6-MAM) and then to morphine; both are active at MOPr. It is most effective intravenously, but increasingly is used intranasally and, sometimes, smoked. Its plasma half-life is 3 minutes when given intravenously and 30 minutes for 6-MAM. Intranasal use has half the potency of parenteral routes, but intramuscular (IM), IV, and intranasal routes all have heroin and 6-MAM peaks within 5 minutes.

Oxycodone

Although oxycodone is structurally similar to codeine, it is pharmacodynamically comparable to morphine with a 1:2 equivalence. By the mid-2000s, oxycodone had become one of the most widely misused and diverted opioids in the United States, particularly in the easily crushed and administered formulation of controlled release. In 2010, the medication was reformulated and released in a tamper-resistant form, which since has decreased misuse.

Meperidine

Meperidine is a phenylpiperidine with limited potency and a short duration of action. Clinically, meperidine is used primarily for the management of acute, postoperative pain in the central nervous system (CNS) and the gastrointestinal and genitourinary systems. Meperidine is no longer used for the treatment of chronic pain owing largely to toxicity of its major metabolite, normeperidine, which can produce seizures and CNS excitation. Meperidine should not be used for greater than 48 hours or at doses greater than 600 mg/d. Its serotonergic activity can produce a serotonin syndrome when combined with monoamine oxidase inhibitors. Orally, meperidine gives analgesia within 15 minutes with both plasma and analgesic peaks at 1 to 2 hours with 50% not affected by first-pass metabolism. Total duration of analgesia lasts 1.5 to 3 hours. IM administration gives a plasma peak at 45 minutes and a range of plasma concentrations. It is metabolized by the liver with a 3-hour half-life and is 60% protein bound.

Pentazocine

Pentazocine is a weak antagonist or partial agonist at MOPr and KOPr, with some activity at the δ- and σ-opioid receptors. Pentazocine has two enantiomers with different pharmacologic profiles, but the racemic mixture provides pain reduction and is rewarding. In 1983, as an abuse deterrent, pentazocine was manufactured in combination with naloxone (Talwin Nx). Because of its psychomimetic effects due to KOPr agonism, it is not used much for chronic pain. Its half-life is 3 to 6 hours with peaks of effect at 0.5 to 1 hour for IM route and 1 to 2 hours for oral route. Pentazocine is metabolized by the liver through oxidation and glucuronidation with significant first-pass metabolism. Sixty percent is protein bound. Oral bioavailability is 10%. Small amounts are unchanged in urine.

Hydromorphone

First synthesized in the 1920s, hydromorphone is a more potent opioid analgesic than morphine. It is excreted, along with its metabolites, by the kidney. It can be given by IV, by infusion, orally, and per rectum. It is 5 times more potent than morphine when given orally and 8.5 times more potent when given by IV. Hydromorphone is morphine derived, and oral bioavailability is 30% to 40%. Analgesia effects

start at 10 to 20 minutes, peaks at 30 to 60 minutes, and lasts 3 to 5 hours.

Hydrocodone

Hydrocodone is for minor pain, such as oral/dental or osteoarthritis, and is typically combined with acetaminophen, which can produce hepatotoxicity when large doses are misused. There has been a substantial increase in the consumption of hydrocodone from 1990 (4 tons) to 2009 (39 tons). As a result, in October 2014, the Drug Enforcement Administration rescheduled hydrocodone from Schedule III to Schedule II. Subsequently, in 2015, hydrocodone prescriptions decreased by 22%. Immediate release effects peak at 0.5 to 1 hour with a duration of 3 to 4 hours. Half-life of immediate release is 3 hours roughly. Hydrocodone extended release has abuse deterrent technology and has a peak plasma level at 14 hours (range of 6 to 30 hours) and analgesic effects for about 12 hours. Its extended release formulation half-life is 6 hours. Metabolism is through 2D6 into an active metabolite hydromorphone and through 3A4 into an inactive metabolite norhydrocodone.

Methadone

Methadone is a synthetic, long-acting, full μ-opioid agonist used primarily as a maintenance treatment for heroin use disorder since 1972. Methadone is also effective in the treatment of chronic pain but has risks of accumulation and respiratory depression. Methadone consists of a racemic mixture of d(S)- and l(R)-methadone with the l(R)-methadone enantiomer having 50 times more analgesia and potential respiratory depression. Both enantiomers have a modest N-methyl-D-aspartate receptor antagonism, which retards and attenuates the development of opioid tolerance.

Methadone has >90% bioavailability with oral administration and is rapidly absorbed with delayed onset of peak levels at 2 to 4 hours after administration and sustained levels over a 24-hour dosing period. With chronic administration, methadone is stored and accumulated in the liver, and this contributes to relatively constant plasma levels due to slow release of unmetabolized methadone into the blood, where it is >90% bound to plasma proteins. Methadone is hepatically metabolized by CYP3A4, CYP2B6, CYP2D6, and CYP1A2 and equally excreted in urine and feces.

Levo-Alpha-Acetylmethadol

LAAM is a synthetic, longer acting (48-hour) congener of methadone that is also orally administered and was approved by the US Food and Drug Administration (FDA) in 1993. A black box warning was added due to postmarketing reports of prolonged QT_c intervals on electrocardiograms and is no longer available in the United States. It is processed by 3A4 to norLAAM and dinorLAAM. LAAM binds to proteins giving it a long steady state. Peak pharmacologic effect occurs at 8 hours and effects last 48 hours.

Fentanyl Derivatives

Fentanyl is a very short-acting and rapid-onset analgesic that has much higher potency than the morphine-related opioids and has significant abuse potential. Many chemical variations with potent opioid effects are possible from fentanyl, and these variations have a high resistance to the usual morphine-related antagonists and partial agonists. Reversal of overdoses from fentanyl can take 5 times greater naloxone doses than overdoses from morphine-related drugs. The receptor actions of fentanyl on MOPr are predominantly through the β-arrestin second messenger system rather than the cyclic adenosine monophosphate (cAMP) system that predominates for morphine. Specific pharmacokinetic details of these many fentanyl-related compounds can be found in more detailed pharmacology textbooks.

Buprenorphine

Buprenorphine alone, and in combination with the opioid antagonist naloxone, was FDA approved in 2002 as a Schedule III drug. Buprenorphine is not only a MOPr partial agonist but also a KOPr antagonist. Due to ceiling effect, dosing greater than 32 mg sublingually has no greater MOPr agonism, and 16 mg occupies all available MOPr. Its duration of action is 24 to 48 hours due to its slow dissociation from the MOPr. Buprenorphine is metabolized by P450–3A4 to norbuprenorphine. It has 50% to 60% bioavailability with sublingual administration and extensive first-pass metabolism. Sublingually, peak buprenorphine levels are after about 2 hours. When given via IV, it has an apparent beta-terminal plasma half-life of 3 to 5 hours. When given orally, it is relatively ineffective because of its first-pass metabolism and rapid biotransformation in the liver and small intestines. Oral administration of naloxone has limited bioavailability, whereas IV use may precipitate acute withdrawal.

EPIDEMIOLOGY OF OPIOID USE DISORDER

According to the 2014 National Survey on Drug Use and Health, there were an estimated 4.3 million current nonmedical users of prescription opioids and 914,000 past year users of heroin. Further, an estimated 1.9 million persons (aged 12 years or older) met the *Diagnostic and Statistical Manual of Mental Disorders*, 5th edition (*DSM-5*) criteria for the diagnosis of opioid use disorder related to prescription opioids, and approximately 586,000 met the criteria for heroin use disorder. The epidemiologic study, "Monitoring the Future," found that use of "narcotics other than heroin" in 12th graders peaked at 4.3% in 2004, and declined to 1.7% in 2016.

Family members and friends are the most common source of nonmedical opioids, and they were largely prescribed by physicians. Benzodiazepines are also commonly misused in combination with opioid pain medications and elevate the risk of respiratory depression, coma, and death. In 2011, 31% of opioid overdoses involved benzodiazepines. Counterfeit medications have flooded the illicit market and may be adulterated with agents that increase toxicity, such as the opioid fentanyl. Drug poisoning deaths involving synthetic opioids (except methadone) have consistently increased from 1999 to 2007.

According to the Substance Abuse and Mental Health Services Administration (SAMHSA) Treatment Episode Data Set (TEDS), annual admissions to substance abuse treatment for primary heroin use disorder slightly increased from 1995 to 2010, remaining steady at about 14% to 15% of all substance abuse treatment admissions. As the rates of prescription opioid use disorder has increased, so has treatment seeking. According to TEDS, the annual number of admissions for other opiates/synthetics grew from 1.6% of all admissions in 2000 to 8.6% of all admissions in 2010. Likewise, in 2005, the most frequently reported drug of choice in new treatment admissions to methadone maintenance changed from heroin to oral prescription opioids.

Neurobiology, Mechanisms of Action, and Relationship to Addiction Liability

Opioids are primarily agonists at the MOPr, which is a G protein–coupled 7-transmembrane protein coupled to G_i and G_o proteins. Thus, MOPr agonists inhibit adenylyl cyclase with a consequent reduction in the production of cAMP, the opening of potassium channels, the inhibition of calcium channels, and the activation of mitogen-activated protein kinase. Fentanyl-related opioids act through a β-arrestin second messenger system after binding to the MOPr, and this different pathway has significant implications for reversing fentanyl overdoses with naloxone and for overriding the FDA-approved treatments of methadone, buprenorphine, and naltrexone.

MOPr Signaling Properties and Addiction Liability

A major underlying concept in the addiction liability of MOPr agonists is their pharmacodynamic efficacy (ie, the ability to stimulate downstream second messenger systems). In general, compounds with greater efficacy (eg, fentanyl-like compounds) have greater analgesic effects and greater abuse potential than partial agonists. Furthermore, other downstream effects of MOPr agonists include producing tolerance and loss of analgesic efficacy and reinforcement. MOPr desensitization and internalization as mechanisms of tolerance are induced by morphine, but greater desensitization and internalization of receptors are induced by endogenous neuropeptide ligands and methadone. Thus, methadone maintenance can be used effectively for extended periods without further tolerance developing.

DRUG–DRUG INTERACTIONS

Other drugs can interact with opiates through hepatic metabolism by cytochrome P450–related enzymes. The major drugs potentially interacting with opiates include both inducers and inhibitors of CYP3A4, as well as inhibitors of CYP2D6, such as paroxetine. CYP3A4 inducers include rifampin, carbamazepine, phenytoin, and phenobarbital, and they typically have minimal clinical effects, but any of them may induce opioid metabolism and withdrawal symptoms. CYP3A4 inhibitors have few clinically significant drug interactions except for some HIV antiretroviral medications, which can have clinical manifestations with methadone. Methadone levels also are significantly increased by the regular consumption of more than four alcoholic drinks per day.

TOLERANCE DEVELOPMENT

Tolerance may be defined as a loss of any effect after repeated use, leading to the need for higher doses to get the desired equivalent effect. All opioid medications lead to tolerance and physical dependence, but rates of development vary by medication, different effects, and individuals. Methadone also has a modest N-methyl-D-aspartate antagonism that may attenuate tolerance.

TOXICITY STATES AND THEIR MEDICAL MANAGEMENT

Acute opioid overdose is characterized by the triad of altered mental status (ie, stupor, coma), respiratory depression, and "pinpoint" pupils. On physical examination, evidence of opioid use such as marks

signaling past or recent injection may be noted. Individualized dosing and regular clinical assessments are important because diminished respiration occurs until tolerance develops. When any opioid is used beyond its tolerance level, a reduced response to carbon dioxide centers in the pons and medulla lead to CO_2 retention. Initially depressed cough as well as nausea and vomiting disappear rapidly with tolerance. Constriction of the pupil is the result of parasympathetic excitation. In opioid overdose, convulsions have been reported, likely from inhibition of γ-aminobutyric acid (GABA) release in the CNS. Mydriasis or normal pupils may be observed with an overdose of meperidine, propoxyphene, dextromethorphan, and pentazocine. A full opioid overdose can be effectively treated with naloxone, but repeated naloxone administration is usually needed, otherwise the overdose may be only transiently reversed. Similarly, with fentanyl overdoses, higher naloxone doses than used for other opioids like morphine are needed to reverse the overdose.

MEDICAL COMPLICATIONS OF OPIOIDS

The two main effects of opioid overdose on the CNS are mental obtundation and respiratory depression, with respiratory depression as the most frequent cause of death. A suppressed gag reflex predisposes the patient to aspiration of gastric contents into the lungs. A few opioids may cause generalized seizures. Opioid overdose also can cause noncardiogenic pulmonary edema and bronchospasm in 48% to 80% of heroin overdoses. Overdose may also release histamine, leading to vasodilatation and orthostatic hypotension. Nausea and vomiting from opiates may stimulate vasovagal tone and cause bradycardia. Prolongation of the QT_c interval and torsades de pointes can occur. Opioid-induced spasms of the sphincter of Oddi can produce biliary colic.

IV opioid use can transmit HIV-1 infection, hepatitis B, hepatitis C, and bacteria leading to bacterial endocarditis, venous thrombosis, septic pulmonary emboli, pseudoaneurysms, mycotic aneurysms, and emboli of cornstarch and talc to the retina, lungs, kidney, and liver. Other infectious complications include osteomyelitis, septic arthritis, polymyositis, fibrous myopathy, cellulitis, skin and neck abscesses, and botulism. IV heroin, morphine, and pentazocine may cause rhabdomyolysis, nephropathy, and glomerulonephritis.

CONCLUSIONS AND FUTURE RESEARCH DIRECTIONS

The neuronal and molecular basis of opioid tolerance and dependence differs across different end points (eg, analgesia vs. respiratory depression vs. reward) and offers much for future research. Two specific areas for investigation are the genetics of MOPr function and relating stress responsivity to opiate function. Overall, the molecular mechanisms for partial opiate agonism, with low doses producing agonist and high doses producing antagonist responses, needs a comprehensive theory as well as data to support that theory as new opiates are developed. These contributions, as well as unique immunologic approaches such as vaccines against fentanyl, may also significantly improve our therapeutic options for the treatment of opioid addiction.

KEY POINTS

1. Among the three G protein–coupled, opioid receptor types in the brain, the mu (MOPr) provides endogenous analgesic and rewarding effects and has endogenous agonists of β-endorphin, endomorphin-1, and endomorphin-2.
2. Morphine, codeine, and thebaine from poppies and synthetics such as methadone stimulate the MOPr to inhibit cAMP formation, whereas fentanyl inhibits β-arrestin, leading to overdoses that resist reversal by naloxone.
3. The United States has had a significant opioid epidemic for at least the last 10 years, with prescription opioids more commonly abused and more often leading to overdoses than heroin since 2005.
4. Other medications can interact with opiates through hepatic metabolism by the cytochrome P450–related enzymes of CYP2D6 and CYP3A4.
5. Primary opioid overdose symptoms are mental obtundation and respiratory depression, but other symptoms and severe complications vary across specific opioids.

REVIEW QUESTIONS

1. Compared to morphine, the partial opiate agonist buprenorphine is most likely to have:
   A. more withdrawal symptoms after stopping.
   B. less respiratory depression as their doses are raised.
   C. more adenyl cyclase enzyme activity.
   D. weaker binding to the μ-opiate receptor.
   E. greater adrenergic neuronal activity after abruptly stopping.

2. In acute intoxication with opiates, the eyes of a patient will show:
   A. conjunctival injection.
   B. dilated pupils.
   C. pinpoint pupils.
   D. nystagmus.
   E. All of the above

3. A 46-year-old man is brought into the emergency room. He has been regularly using a substance, but he has not been able to buy it for 2 days. He reports feeling sad, experiencing body aches, diarrhea, yawning, and a runny nose. On your exam, you note that he has dilated pupils and is sweating. Which of the following substances is he most likely withdrawing from?
   A. Alcohol
   B. Cocaine
   C. Marijuana
   D. Opiates

ANSWERS

1. **B**
2. **C**
3. **D**

SUGGESTED READINGS

Chen LH. *Drug-Poisoning Deaths Involving Opioid Analgesics: United States, 1999-2011.* Hyattsville, MD: National Center for Health Statistics; 2014. NCHS Data Brief No. 166.

Martell BA, Arnsten JH, Ray B, Gourevitch MN. The impact of methadone induction on cardiac conduction in opiate users. *Ann Intern Med.* 2003;139:154-155.

Quillinan N, Lau EK, Virk M, von Zastrow M, Williams JT. Recovery from mu-opioid receptor desensitization after chronic treatment with morphine and methadone. *J Neurosci.* 2011;31:4434-4443.

Raehal KM, Bohn LM. The role of beta-arrestin2 in the severity of antinociceptive tolerance and physical dependence induced by different opioid pain therapeutics. *Neuropharmacology.* 2011;60:58-65.

Strang J, Groshkova T, Uchtenhagen A, et al. Heroin on trial: systematic review and meta-analysis of randomised trials of diamorphine-prescribing as treatment for refractory heroin addiction. *Br J Psychiatry.* 2015; 207(1):5-14.

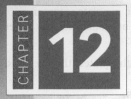

CHAPTER 12

The Pharmacology of Stimulants

Summary by David A. Gorelick and Michael H. Baumann

> Based on THE ASAM PRINCIPLES OF ADDICTION MEDICINE,
> 6th edition chapter by David A. Gorelick and Michael H. Baumann

Stimulant drugs activate central and peripheral catecholamine neuron systems, chiefly by increasing extracellular concentrations of dopamine and norepinephrine. Stimulants include both plant-derived alkaloids and synthetic compounds. All stimulants share similar psychological and physiologic effects, while differing in potency and pharmacokinetics.

FORMULATIONS AND METHODS OF USE AND ABUSE

Plant-Derived Stimulants

Cocaine

Cocaine is a tropane ester found in leaves of the coca bush, *Erythroxylon coca*, which grows in the Andean region of South America. Cocaine is available for illicit use in two forms: base and salt. The base has a low melting point (98°C) and vaporizes before pyrolytic destruction, allowing it to be smoked. In contrast, cocaine salt does not melt below 195°C, so heating destroys the drug. Cocaine salt is water soluble, making it easy to dissolve for injection. Regardless of chemical form, cocaine exerts the same actions in the brain and other target organs.

Ephedra

Ephedrine and pseudoephedrine are phenethylamines found in several *Ephedraceae* plant species. Ephedra was banned from the US market in 2006.

Khat

Khat is the common term for preparations of the *Catha edulis* plant, which is native to East Africa and the Arabian Peninsula. Fresh khat leaves contain at least two phenethylamine stimulants: cathinone and cathine (norpseudoephedrine). Synthetic analogues of cathinone are increasingly being misused in the form of "bath salts" or "research chemicals," which are marketed as innocuous "legal highs."

Synthetic Stimulants

More than a dozen synthetic stimulant medications are legally available in the United States, either by prescription or over the counter. Most represent variations on the phenethylamine structure.

Clinical Uses

Cocaine is used clinically in the United States as a local or topical anesthetic. Other prescription stimulants have various US Food and Drug Administration (FDA)-approved indications: attention deficit hyperactivity disorder (ADHD), narcolepsy and excessive daytime sleepiness, and weight loss. Prospective, longitudinal studies of children receiving stimulant treatment for ADHD found no increased risk of developing substance abuse. Over-the-counter stimulants generally are used for decongestion and bronchodilation or for weight loss. Oral stimulants are used for non–FDA-approved indications, eg, as quick-acting, short-term antidepressants.

Nonmedical Use, Abuse, and Dependence

Oral stimulants are widely used in work, school, military, and sports settings for their alerting, antifatigue, and performance-enhancing properties. These effects are well demonstrated in laboratory and field studies but are difficult to demonstrate in controlled trials. Stimulants of all types are banned by the World Anti-Doping Agency and many other sports organizations. All stimulants have a potential for misuse, abuse, and dependence. Cocaine and amphetamines have high abuse potential—one in six persons who use cocaine regularly, and one in nine who use prescription stimulants for nonmedical purposes, will become dependent. Those who use intravenous (IV) and smoked routes are more likely to become dependent.

The greater abuse liability of IV and smoked stimulants is related to faster rate of drug delivery to the brain, resulting in a faster onset of psychological effects and intense pleasurable response (the so-called "rate hypothesis" of psychoactive drug action). "Binge" stimulant use involves short periods of heavy use separated by long periods of little or no use. A small number of users may use low doses daily without dose escalation over time. Some of these users may be self-medicating an underlying neuropsychiatric disorder such as ADHD.

HISTORICAL FEATURES

Naturally occurring plant alkaloids have been used as stimulants for thousands of years. Chinese medicine has used herbal ma huang (ephedra) for at least 5,000 years. Chewing of coca leaves has been prevalent in the Andes region of South America for at least 2,000 years. Cocaine was identified as the active ingredient of the coca leaf in 1860. A nonalcoholic beverage (containing 4.5 mg of cocaine per 6 oz) was introduced in 1886 and quickly became one of the world's most popular soft drinks: Coca-Cola. In 1914, the Harrison Narcotic Act banned cocaine in the United States, except by prescription. Synthetic stimulants first appeared with the synthesis of amphetamine in 1887 and of methamphetamine in 1919. Synthetic cathinones first appeared on the US illicit drug scene in the late 2000s and were placed in Schedule I of the Controlled Substances Act starting in 2011. Nevertheless, novel synthetic cathinone analogues continue to proliferate as a means to circumvent drug control legislation.

EPIDEMIOLOGY

In 2014, there were an estimated 18.2 million cocaine users worldwide and an estimated 35.6 million nonmedical users of amphetamine-type stimulants. Cocaine is the second most widely used illegal drug in the United States, after marijuana. In 2015, an estimated 38.7 million Americans (14.5% of the US population 12 years or older) had used cocaine at some time during their lifetimes; 1.9 million (0.7%) had used in the past month. An estimated 896,000 Americans met psychiatric diagnostic criteria for cocaine use disorder, and 615,000 people received specialty addiction treatment for cocaine.

In 2015, an estimated 14.5 million Americans had used methamphetamine at some time during their lifetimes; 900,000 were past-month users. An estimated 872,000 Americans met psychiatric diagnostic criteria for methamphetamine use disorder; another 426,000 met criteria for prescription stimulant use disorder. There were 15,514 stimulant-related deaths among 15- to 64-year-olds in the United States from 1999 to 2009.

PHARMACOKINETICS
Absorption and Distribution

Smoked stimulants are rapidly absorbed by the lungs, reaching the brain in 6 to 8 seconds. The onset and peak effects occur within minutes. IV administration produces peak brain uptake in 4 to 7 minutes. A rapid decline in drug effects is experienced as a "crash" by users of smoked or IV stimulants. Intranasal and oral stimulants have a slower absorption and onset of effect (30 to 45 minutes), a longer peak effect, and a gradual decline from peak. Cocaine is well absorbed through mucus membranes but less so through skin or by passive inhalation. Stimulants distribute into most tissues, including blood, urine, hair, sweat, saliva, nails, breast milk, and across the placenta.

Metabolism

In humans, 95% of cocaine is metabolized to benzoylecgonine and ecgonine methyl ester by the action of carboxylesterases in the liver and butyrylcholinesterase in the liver, plasma, brain, lung, and other tissues. The remaining 5% is N-demethylated to norcocaine by the CYP3A4 isozyme of the liver cytochrome P450 enzyme system. Amphetamines are metabolized in the liver via three different pathways: deamination to inactive metabolites, oxidation to norephedrine and other active metabolites, and para-hydroxylation to active metabolites. Amphetamine is the N-demethylated metabolite of methamphetamine.

Elimination

Stimulants and their metabolites are largely eliminated in the urine. Benzoylecgonine is the cocaine metabolite found in highest concentration in urine for several days after cocaine use, so this substance is measured in routine urine tests for cocaine exposure. Gastrointestinal absorption and urinary elimination of amphetamines is highly pH-dependent. Because amphetamines are weak bases, acidification of the gastrointestinal tract or urine substantially decreases absorption and increases excretion.

DRUG–DRUG INTERACTIONS

The primary clinically relevant drug–drug interaction for stimulants is with other stimulants or medications that enhance catecholamine activity. A major potential for interaction is presented by monoamine oxidase inhibitors. Potent prescription stimulants should not be used within 2 weeks of monoamine oxidase inhibitor use. Stimulants should be used cautiously in conjunction with tricyclic antidepressants, which block presynaptic reuptake of catecholamines.

PHARMACODYNAMIC ACTIONS
Central Nervous System
Intoxication

All stimulants produce a similar range of effects, with intensity and duration depending on potency, dose, route of administration, and duration of use. Initial effects include increased energy, alertness, and sociability; elation or euphoria; and decreased fatigue, need for sleep, and appetite. These effects occur after 5 to 20 mg of oral amphetamines or methylphenidate, 100 to 200 mg of oral cocaine, 40 to 100 mg of intranasal cocaine, or 15 to 25 mg of IV or smoked cocaine.

With increasing potency, dose, duration of use, or more efficient route of administration, stimulant effects often progress to dysphoric effects such as anxiety, irritability, panic attacks, hypervigilance, paranoia, grandiosity, impaired judgment, and psychotic symptoms. Patients with stimulant psychosis may resemble those with acute schizophrenia. Tactile hallucinations are especially typical of stimulant psychosis. Associated behavioral effects include restlessness, agitation, tremor, dyskinesia, and repetitive behaviors such as picking at the skin or foraging for the drug. Physiologic effects include tachycardia, pupil dilation, diaphoresis, and nausea.

Chronic Effects

Chronic cocaine or amphetamine use is associated with cognitive impairment that may persist for several months of abstinence. Chronic use of amphetamines can cause a psychotic syndrome that persists for years after the last drug use, even in persons with no history of psychiatric disorders. Psychotic flashbacks have been reported up to 2 years after the last drug use.

Withdrawal

The stimulant withdrawal syndrome does not have prominent physiological features, but there can be prominent psychologic manifestations. Withdrawal symptoms generally are the opposite of those associated with stimulant intoxication, including depressed mood, anhedonia, fatigue, difficulty concentrating, increased sleep duration (with poor sleep quality), and increased appetite.

Behavioral Pharmacology

In animals, stimulants consistently produce increased motor activity, repetitive stereotyped behavior, drug discrimination, and positive reinforcement. Stimulants produce a distinctive set of subjective psychological effects in humans: euphoria, drug liking, increased energy, and increased alertness. Stimulants are readily distinguished from placebo or sedative drugs but often not from each other when given in equipotent doses.

Other Central Nervous System Effects

Stimulant use is associated with seizures, even in persons without a preexisting seizure disorder. Most cocaine-associated seizures occur within 90 minutes of drug use. Cocaine and amphetamine use are associated with cerebral vasoconstriction, cerebrovascular atherosclerosis, cerebrovascular disease, and stroke. Neurologic symptoms usually appear within 3 hours of drug use. Stimulant use is associated with certain movement disorders, including repetitive stereotyped behaviors, acute dystonic reactions, choreoathetosis, buccolingual dyskinesias, and exacerbation of Tourette syndrome and tardive dyskinesia.

Cardiovascular System

Stimulants increase heart rate, blood pressure, and systemic vascular resistance, which may lead to acute myocardial infarction. Cocaine use is a factor in about one fourth of nonfatal heart attacks in persons younger than 45 years. Frequent cocaine users are up to seven times more likely to have a nonfatal heart attack than are nonusers. Cocaine use is associated with cardiac arrhythmias and sudden death.

Other Organ Systems

Adverse effects of stimulant use on particular organ systems often depend on the route of administration. For example, smoked stimulants produce lung toxicity, injection use is associated with infectious diseases such as HIV and hepatitis C, and intranasal use is associated with damage to the nasal septum.

Pulmonary

Acute respiratory symptoms develop in up to half of cocaine users within minutes to hours after smoking. Symptoms include productive cough, shortness of breath, wheezing, chest pain, hemoptysis, and exacerbation of asthma. Standard pulmonary function tests are generally normal.

Renal

Stimulants have little direct toxic effect on the kidneys.

Gastrointestinal

Major gastrointestinal effects of cocaine include gastroduodenal ulceration and perforation, intestinal infarction and perforation, and ischemic colitis.

Concealing cocaine by swallowing large packets ("body packing") may result in severe acute toxicity if the wrapping deteriorates and allows cocaine into the gastrointestinal tract.

Liver

There is no direct evidence that cocaine is hepatotoxic in humans. Liver abnormalities reported in cocaine users can be accounted for by viral hepatitis from injection drug use, alcoholic liver disease, or other consequences of a drug-using lifestyle.

Endocrine

Acute cocaine use activates the hypothalamic–pituitary–adrenal axis, stimulating secretion of epinephrine, corticotropin-releasing hormone, adrenocorticotropic hormone, and cortisol. Acute cocaine use decreases plasma prolactin concentrations in cocaine naïve individuals, but not in experienced cocaine users. Chronic cocaine does not alter baseline levels of testosterone, cortisol, luteinizing hormone, or thyroid hormones.

Musculoskeletal

Stimulants cause rhabdomyolysis by a direct toxic effect (rare except at very high doses), indirectly by vasoconstriction resulting in ischemia, and secondary to stimulant-induced hyperthermia or seizures.

Head and Neck

Intranasal cocaine use is associated with chronic rhinitis, perforated nasal septum and nasal collapse, oropharyngeal ulcers, and osteolytic sinusitis. Cocaine or methamphetamine use by any route reduces salivary secretions and causes bruxism. Chronic use is associated with dental problems, including caries, cracked enamel, and loss of teeth.

Immune System

Cocaine use is associated with a variety of vasculitic syndromes primarily affecting skin and muscle. These may mimic rheumatologic conditions such as Henoch-Schönlein purpura, Stevens-Johnson syndrome, or Raynaud phenomenon.

Sexual Function

Stimulants are commonly thought of as aphrodisiacs, but chronic use reduces libido and impairs sexual function. Men may experience erectile dysfunction or delayed or inhibited ejaculation. Women may develop irregular menses.

Reproductive, Fetal, and Neonatal Health

Prescription stimulants are classified by the FDA in Pregnancy Category C (risk cannot be ruled out because human studies are lacking). Prenatal cocaine exposure is associated with small but statistically significant impairments in sustained attention and behavioral self-regulation among preschool- and school-aged children and in language and memory among adolescents. These impairments are modifiable by environmental factors such as prenatal care. Cocaine and amphetamines appear in breast milk and may cause irritability, sleep disturbance, and tremors in the infant.

NEUROBIOLOGY
Mechanisms of Action
Molecular Mechanisms

All stimulant drugs enhance extracellular concentrations of monoamine neurotransmitters by disrupting the function of plasma membrane transporter proteins. Stimulants can be divided into two classes based on their mechanism: transporter blockers and transporter substrates. Transporter blockers (often called *reuptake blockers*), like cocaine and methylphenidate, bind to the extracellular face of transporters and inhibit the reuptake of previously released monoamine neurotransmitters. Transporter substrates (often called *releasers*), like amphetamine and phentermine, bind to transporters, are transported into the neuronal cytoplasm, and trigger the release of intracellular monoamines by reversing the normal direction of transporter flux. Once inside the neuronal cytoplasm, transporter substrates interact with vesicular monoamine transporters to disrupt monoamine storage, thereby greatly increasing cytoplasmic concentrations of amines available for release.

Potent stimulants like cocaine and amphetamine are active at dopamine and norepinephrine transporters, whereas weaker stimulants like (-)-ephedrine preferentially target norepinephrine transporters. Many stimulant drugs have nontransporter sites of action that contribute to their pharmacologic effects. For example, cocaine blocks sodium channels and amphetamines inhibit monoamine oxidase. Ephedrine, pseudoephedrine, phenylephrine, and phenylpropanolamine are weak agonists at α-adrenergic receptors, which mediate vasoconstriction (hence their use as decongestants and antihypotensive agents). Ephedrine also acts at β-adrenergic receptors, which mediate bronchodilation.

Neural Circuits and Systems

Rewarding effects of stimulants are mediated by activation of the mesocorticolimbic dopamine system, which consists of cell bodies in the ventral tegmental area that send axonal projections to the prefrontal cortex, nucleus accumbens, and amygdala. Mesocorticolimbic dopamine neurons are part of a complex cortical–striatal–pallidal circuitry that is involved with the selection of adaptive behavioral responses. The nucleus accumbens is a critical node in the circuitry, receiving stimulatory glutamate afferents from the hippocampus, amygdala, and cortex. The primary cell type in the nucleus accumbens is the γ-aminobutyric acid-containing medium spiny neuron, which receives direct synaptic contacts from both dopamine and glutamate inputs. Natural rewards induce transient, localized changes in extracellular dopamine in nucleus accumbens that enhance stimulatory drive in spiny neurons. By contrast, stimulant drugs induce sustained supraphysiologic elevations in extracellular dopamine that cause widespread excitation of spiny neurons, and repeated drug exposure changes circuit function.

Dopamine

The cocaine-binding site on the dopamine transporter overlaps with the binding sites for dopamine and amphetamine. Acute administration of cocaine or amphetamine transiently increases brain extracellular dopamine concentrations in animals and humans. Several lines of evidence from animal studies show that increased synaptic dopamine activity in the mesocorticolimbic reward circuit mediates the behavioral effects of stimulants.

Evidence from human brain imaging studies using positron emission tomography or single-photon emission computerized tomography is largely consistent with an important role for dopamine in the acute psychological effects of stimulants. The acute euphoria or "high" response to cocaine or methylphenidate correlates in time course and intensity with drug concentration in the brain, with dopamine transporter occupancy, and with extracellular concentrations of dopamine in the striatum. Exposure to cocaine-associated cues is associated with enhanced dopamine release in the striatum.

Norepinephrine

Cocaine, amphetamines, methylphenidate, phentermine, and ephedrine enhance norepinephrine neurotransmission by acting at norepinephrine transporters. IV cocaine use increases plasma norepinephrine and epinephrine concentrations within minutes of injection. There is a significant positive correlation between potency of norepinephrine release and the oral stimulant dose that produces stimulant-like subjective effects in humans. Chronic cocaine exposure increases norepinephrine transporter function in the brain of monkeys and humans.

Serotonin

Knockout mice lacking the serotonin transporter still find cocaine rewarding, whereas double knockout mice lacking both the dopamine and serotonin transporters do not. Knockout mice lacking both the norepinephrine and serotonin transporters show increased sensitivity to cocaine reward. These findings suggest a permissive, but not obligatory, role for the serotonin transporter in cocaine reward.

Endogenous Opiates

Stimulants do not act directly on opiate receptors but do influence endogenous opiate systems in the brain. In rats, single doses of cocaine or amphetamine increase extracellular endorphin levels in the nucleus accumbens, and enkephalin and dynorphin mRNA levels in striatum. Repeated cocaine administration increases brain μ and κ opiate receptor binding in rodents. Human cocaine users show increased μ opiate receptor binding in some brain regions with positron emission tomography scanning, and this increased binding correlates with self-reported cocaine craving.

Glutamate

The acute administration of cocaine or amphetamine increases glutamate release in the ventral tegmental area, nucleus accumbens, dorsal striatum, ventral pallidum, septum, and cerebellum. Low doses of cocaine enhance glutamate-evoked neuronal firing. Chronic cocaine treatment produces persisting changes in nucleus accumbens glutamate transmission and a marked decrease in nonsynaptic extracellular glutamate levels.

Other Actions

Amphetamines and phentermine inhibit monoamine oxidase, but this action probably is not significant at the drug concentrations achieved clinically. Cocaine is unique in also blocking voltage-gated membrane sodium ion channels. This action accounts for its effect as a local anesthetic and may contribute to cardiac arrhythmias.

Neuroadaptation

Repeated exposure to stimulants results in two distinct neuroadaptations: sensitization (increased drug response) and tolerance (decreased drug response). Behavioral sensitization to stimulants has been suggested as a mechanism for drug craving and relapse and for stimulant-induced psychosis, but neither has been directly demonstrated in humans. Attempts to demonstrate sensitization prospectively in humans have yielded inconsistent results. There is significant cross-tolerance among various stimulants but not between stimulants and other drug groups, such as opiates.

Stimulant tolerance is pharmacodynamic rather than pharmacokinetic; chronic stimulant exposure does not cause substantial changes in stimulant pharmacokinetics. In clinical use, patients typically become tolerant to the appetite-suppressing effects of stimulants within several weeks of daily use, whereas the beneficial effects in narcolepsy or ADHD remain over months of treatment. In human laboratory studies, tolerance to psychological, cardiovascular, and neuroendocrine effects of cocaine and amphetamines may develop after several doses.

Neurotoxicity

In animal studies, transporter blockers like cocaine and methylphenidate do not produce neurotoxicity in dopamine or serotonin neurons. In contrast, high doses of transporter substrates like amphetamine or methamphetamine produce substantial dopamine and serotonin neurotoxicity, probably because these drugs enter nerve terminals, interact with intracellular proteins, and increase production of reactive oxygen species. Such neurotoxicity in human users has not been conclusively demonstrated.

FUTURE RESEARCH DIRECTIONS

Future research at both preclinical and clinical levels is needed to increase understanding of the mechanisms of stimulant addiction and to develop more effective prevention and treatment approaches. Productive areas for preclinical research include the neurochemical mechanisms that underlie stimulant sensitization and tolerance, the role of nondopamine neurotransmitter systems (eg, glutamate, neuropeptides) in modulating the reward circuit, the intracellular signaling cascades triggered by stimulant binding to transporter sites, and the role of various genes and transcription factors in stimulant action.

KEY POINTS

1. All stimulants have a potential for misuse, abuse, and dependence.
2. Naturally occurring plant alkaloids have been used as stimulants for thousands of years.
3. Smoked stimulants are rapidly absorbed by the lungs, reaching the brain in 6 to 8 seconds. The onset and peak effects occur within minutes. Intravenous administration produces peak brain uptake in 4 to 7 minutes. A rapid decline in

drug effects is experienced as a "crash" by users of smoked or intravenous stimulants. Intranasal and oral stimulants have a slower absorption and onset of effect (30 to 45 minutes), a longer peak effect, and a gradual decline from peak.

ACKNOWLEDGMENTS

Dr. Baumann is supported by the Intramural Research Program, National Institute on Drug Abuse, National Institutes of Health.

REVIEW QUESTIONS

1. The primary enzyme that metabolizes cocaine in humans is a(n):
    A. esterase.
    B. cytochrome P450.
    C. superoxide dismutase.
    D. glucuronidase.

2. Cocaine and amphetamines share which of the following neuropharmacologic mechanisms?
    A. Monoamine oxidase inhibition
    B. Sodium channel blockade
    C. Disruption of function of neuronal membrane transporters
    D. Blockade of dopamine receptors

3. Which of the following stimulants is not legally available in the United States?
    A. Cocaine
    B. Methamphetamine
    C. Phentermine
    D. Ephedra
    E. Methylphenidate

ANSWERS

1. **A**
2. **C**
3. **D**

SUGGESTED READINGS

Cone EJ. Pharmacokinetics and pharmacodynamics of cocaine. *J Anal Toxicol.* 1995;19(6):459-478.

Docherty JR. Pharmacology of stimulants prohibited by the World Anti-Doping Agency (WADA). *Br J Pharmacol.* 2008;154(3):606-622.

Hatsukami DK, Fischman MW. Crack cocaine and cocaine hydrochloride: are the differences myth or reality? *JAMA.* 1996;276(19):1580-1588.

Karch SB. *A Brief History of Cocaine.* 2nd ed. Boca Raton, FL: CRC Press, 2006.

Nichols T, Khondkar P, Gibbons S. The psychostimulant drug khat (*Catha edulis*): a mini-review. *Phytochem Lett.* 2015;13: 127-133.

The Pharmacology of Caffeine

Summary by Mary M. Sweeney, Laura M. Juliano, Sergi Ferré, and Roland R. Griffiths

Based on THE ASAM PRINCIPLES OF ADDICTION MEDICINE, 6th edition chapter by Mary M. Sweeney, Laura M. Juliano, Sergi Ferré, and Roland R. Griffiths

Caffeine is the most widely used mood altering drug in the world. Caffeine is a nonselective A_1 and A_{2A} adenosine receptor antagonist and mild central nervous system (CNS) stimulant at usual dietary doses. Moderate caffeine consumption is not generally associated with negative health effects, and caffeine may offer protective effects from some diseases. However, caffeine has the potential to produce clinically significant negative physiologic and psychological effects, tolerance and withdrawal, and psychiatric disorders. Furthermore, caffeine can interact with recreational and psychotherapeutic drugs and may cause increased behavioral toxicity when combined with alcohol.

DRUGS IN THE CLASS

Caffeine is the common name for 1,3,7-trimethylxanthine. More than 60 types of plants contain caffeine, including coffee, tea, cola, guarana, cacao, and yerba maté. Caffeine is a member of the methylxanthine class of alkaloids, which includes the structurally related dimethylxanthines, theophylline, theobromine, and paraxanthine. Pharmaceutical preparations of caffeine include caffeine anhydrous, caffeine sodium benzoate, and caffeine citrate.

HISTORY

The chemical structure of caffeine was identified in 1875. The use of caffeine-containing plants such as tea, coffee beans, and cacao for psychoactive effects may predate recorded history. The development of worldwide trade in the 17th and 18th centuries propagated global use of caffeinated foods and beverages. Presently, coffee, cocoa, and tea products represent major imports of the United States. Caffeinated soft drinks (eg, Coca-Cola), introduced at the end of the 19th century, and caffeinated energy drinks (eg, Red Bull), introduced at the end of the 20th century, now represent multibillion-dollar markets with hundreds of different brands available to consumers worldwide.

EPIDEMIOLOGY

Approximately 85% of the United States population age 2 years and older consumes at least one caffeinated beverage per day. Daily caffeine exposure rates are estimated to be 43% to 63% among 2- to 5-year-olds, 75% among older children and adolescents, 86% to 90% among teenagers and young adults, with rates progressively increasing with age up to 99% of those 65 years and older. More than 95% of all caffeine ingestion comes from beverages. Among adults, the primary sources of caffeine are coffee and tea, followed by soft drinks. US daily caffeine consumption is estimated to be 165 mg for all ages combined, with the greatest mean intake among consumers age 35 years and older (ie, ~200 to 225 mg caffeine/d). In general, coffee drinkers consume 3.3 eight-ounce cups per day on average and are exposed to the greatest amounts of caffeine.

SOURCES OF CAFFEINE

Sources of caffeine include beverages, foods, dietary supplements, and over-the-counter and prescription medications. Estimating caffeine exposure is challenging because of the wide variety of products that contain caffeine, large differences in serving sizes, variability in caffeine content across products of the same type, and undisclosed caffeine amounts in some products. A 12-oz cup of coffee may contain 107 to 420 mg of caffeine. Energy drinks can vary more than tenfold in caffeine content across brands. Presently, there is widespread marketing of highly caffeinated dietary supplements and energy "shots," and caffeine is added to a variety of food products (eg, potato chips, jelly beans).

THERAPEUTIC USES

Caffeine is widely used to aid energy and alertness and to prevent sleepiness. Caffeine is often added to over-the-counter and prescription analgesics because of its analgesic-enhancing effects. Caffeine administration can prevent or treat caffeine withdrawal and postoperative headache. As a respiratory stimulant, caffeine is used to treat apnea in neonates. Because of its lipolytic and thermogenic effects, caffeine is commonly added to weight loss and nutritional supplements. Caffeine and other xanthines have been used to treat postprandial hypotension.

NEUROBIOLOGY

Caffeine is a mild psychomotor stimulant drug that produces psychomotor activation as well as reinforcing and arousing effects through action at adenosine receptors and indirect effects on dopaminergic neurotransmission. Adenosine is an endogenous purine nucleoside found throughout the brain, where two of its main functions are exerting a tonic inhibitory role on central dopaminergic transmission and acting as a main mediator of homeostatic sleep. Thus, accumulation of adenosine in the extracellular space of the basal forebrain, cortex, and hypothalamus is a main mediator of sleepiness following prolonged wakefulness. Caffeine is a nonselective adenosine receptor antagonist with similar in vitro affinity for A_1, A_{2A}, and A_{2B} receptors and with lower affinity for A_3 receptors. A_1 receptors are widely expressed in the CNS, including the spinal cord, whereas A_{2A} receptors are particularly concentrated in the striatum, the main projecting area of the ascending dopamine system. Striatal adenosine receptors have been associated with the psychomotor and reinforcing effects of caffeine. On the other hand, A_1 receptors localized in the brainstem, basal forebrain, and hypothalamus (the loci of origin of ascending arousal systems) have been suggested to be involved in caffeine-induced hyperarousal. Generally, it can be concluded that striatal A_{2A} and extrastriatal A_1 receptors are preferentially involved in the psychomotor-reinforcing effects and hyperarousal induced by caffeine, respectively. Chronic caffeine consumption leads to upregulation of A_1 receptors, which seems to play an important role in the sleepiness, marked fatigue, and drowsiness of caffeine withdrawal.

Although caffeine does not directly target dopaminergic neurotransmission, experimental evidence indicates that the A_{2A}-dopamine D_2 receptor heteromer, localized in the striatopallidal neuron, is a main target for the psychomotor activating and also reinforcing effects of caffeine. Caffeine also increases dopamine neurotransmission via blockade of striatal presynaptic A_1 receptors that modulate dopamine release and postsynaptic A_1 receptors that form heteromers with dopamine D_1 receptors in the striatonigral neuron. In addition, recent evidence indicates that A_1-D_1 receptor interactions drive the effect of caffeine at the spinal level, where caffeine potentiates a spinal-generated locomotor activation.

PHARMACOKINETICS

Caffeine is rapidly and completely absorbed after oral administration, with peak levels reached in 30 to 45 minutes. It is readily distributed throughout the body, with concentrations in blood correlating with those in saliva, breast milk, amniotic fluid, fetal tissue, semen, and the brain. Caffeine is metabolized by the cytochrome P450 liver enzyme system and has several biologically active dimethylxanthine metabolites including paraxanthine, theobromine, and theophylline. On average, caffeine half-life is 4 to 6 hours, but there are wide individual differences due in large part to CPY1A2 genetic variation. Caffeine metabolism may be significantly altered by drugs or conditions that affect the cytochrome P450 liver enzyme system. Caffeine half-life is significantly decreased by cigarette smoking and significantly increased in individuals with liver disease, infants, women taking oral contraceptives, and pregnant women.

PHYSIOLOGIC EFFECTS

At moderate dietary dose levels, caffeine increases systolic and diastolic blood pressure, constricts blood vessels in the head and neck, increases urine volume, stimulates gastric acid secretions, and is a colonic stimulant. As a diuretic, caffeine also increases detrusor pressure on the bladder of patients with complaints of urinary urgency and confirmed detrusor instability. Caffeine is a respiratory stimulant and a bronchodilator at high doses. Caffeine increases plasma epinephrine, norepinephrine, renin, and free fatty acids, particularly in nontolerant individuals. It also increases adrenocorticotropic hormone and cortisol. Caffeine increases insulin levels in healthy subjects and increases postprandial glucose and insulin responses among patients with type 2 diabetes who are habitual coffee drinkers.

SUBJECTIVE EFFECTS

A single low-to-moderate dose of caffeine typically produces a profile of positive subjective effects, including increased well-being, happiness, energy, arousal, alertness, and sociability, with greater positive mood effects of caffeine for physically dependent individuals. Negative subjective effects of caffeine are more likely to be observed after acute doses of caffeine >200 mg and include anxiety, jitteriness, negative mood, upset stomach, and sleeplessness. Individual differences in use, sensitivity, and tolerance seem to play a role in the likelihood and severity of negative subjective effects. Individuals with anxiety disorders may be more sensitive to the anxiogenic effects of caffeine, and higher acute doses of caffeine can elicit panic attacks. The *Diagnostic and Statistical Manual of Mental Disorders,* 5th edition (*DSM-5*) recognizes Caffeine-Induced Anxiety Disorder, which is defined as anxiety symptoms or an anxiety disorder (eg, Generalized Anxiety Disorder) caused by caffeine use.

PERFORMANCE EFFECTS

Moderate acute doses of caffeine, usually up to 300 mg, tend to increase human performance on cognitive tasks assessing reaction time, vigilance, as well as simple and complex attention, with greater effects of caffeine for fatigued individuals. The effects of caffeine on various memory tasks, higher order executive functioning, and decision making have also been investigated, but results are mixed. Caffeine is reliably ergogenic across a variety of exercise situations, and in particular during prolonged exercise, with activity potentially mediated via multiple mechanisms, including effects on muscle contractility, reduced perception of effort, and lowered sensations of pain. A problem in interpreting the effects of caffeine on performance is that in studies that require caffeine abstinence, improved performance may simply reflect a reversal of withdrawal effects or restoration to baseline performance. However, preclinical research and some studies showing caffeine-related performance enhancements among nonwithdrawn caffeine consumers provide evidence that caffeine enhances human performance beyond reversal of withdrawal on some types of tasks (eg, vigilance), especially among nontolerant individuals. Among high-dose habitual caffeine consumers, performance enhancements above and beyond withdrawal reversal effects are perhaps modest at best.

REINFORCING EFFECTS

Circumstantial evidence for caffeine functioning as a reinforcer is compelling, given that caffeine is the most widely self-administered mood-altering drug in the world. Further, carefully controlled research studies using a variety of methodological approaches (eg, choice procedures, ad libitum self-administration) across different caffeine vehicles (eg, coffee, soft drinks, capsules) have provided unequivocal evidence for the reinforcing effects of caffeine. Doses as low as 25 mg per cup of coffee and 33 mg per serving of soft drink function as reinforcers. There is good evidence to suggest avoidance of caffeine withdrawal symptoms increases the reinforcing effects of caffeine among regular caffeine consumers.

CAFFEINE TOLERANCE

The degree of tolerance development to caffeine depends on the caffeine dose, frequency, and individual elimination rate. Complete tolerance does not occur at low daily dietary doses. Very high doses of caffeine (750 to 1,200 mg/d spread throughout the day) administered daily, produce "complete" tolerance (ie, caffeine effects are no longer different from baseline or placebo) to some but not all effects. Tolerance develops to the effects of caffeine on subjective drug effect ratings, sleep disruption, diuresis, parotid gland salivation, increased metabolic rate (oxygen consumption), increased plasma norepinephrine and epinephrine, and increased plasma renin activity. Tolerance to caffeine-produced increases in blood pressure occurs but is incomplete.

CAFFEINE INTOXICATION

Caffeine intoxication is a diagnosis in both the *DSM-5* and *International Statistical Classification of Diseases and Related Health Problems,* 10th edition (*ICD-10*). Caffeine intoxication is defined by the *DSM-5* as the presence of five or more of the following symptoms after excess ingestion of caffeine: restlessness, nervousness, excitement, insomnia, flushed face, diuresis, gastrointestinal disturbance, muscle twitching, rambling flow of thought and speech, tachycardia or cardiac arrhythmia, inexhaustibility, and psychomotor agitation. Among adults, such adverse effects are not usually observed at doses less than 250 mg, and caffeine intoxication is typically associated with higher acute doses (eg, >500 mg). Individual differences in sensitivity (eg, metabolic differences) and tolerance likely influence dose effects. Caffeine intoxication typically resolves within a day (consistent with caffeine's half-life of 4 to 6 hours) with no long-lasting consequences, but medical treatment and monitoring is necessary when significant caffeine overdose occurs. Caffeine can be lethal after ingestion of very high doses (ie, about 5 to 10 g).

CAFFEINE WITHDRAWAL

Caffeine withdrawal is characterized by symptoms conceptually grouped into five categories: (1) headache; (2) fatigue or drowsiness; (3) dysphoric mood, depressed mood, or irritability; (4) difficulty concentrating; and (5) flu-like somatic symptoms such as nausea, vomiting, and muscle pain/stiffness. The caffeine withdrawal syndrome is defined by the *DSM-5* as the presence of at least three of these five symptoms within 24 hours of abrupt caffeine reduction or cessation. Symptoms must cause clinically significant distress or impairment (eg, unable to care for children, unable to work). Headache, which is a hallmark feature of caffeine withdrawal, is likely due to rebound cerebral vasodilatation and increased cerebral blood flow during caffeine abstinence. The incidence and severity of caffeine withdrawal appears to be positively correlated with daily caffeine dose. However, caffeine withdrawal has been observed after repeated dosing as low as 100 mg/d. Withdrawal usually begins 12 to 24 hours after terminating daily caffeine intake, although onset as early as 6 hours and as late as 43 hours has been documented. Peak withdrawal intensity generally occurs 20 to 51 hours after abstinence. The duration of withdrawal ranges from 2 to 9 days, with headache possibly persisting for up to 3 weeks. Caffeine withdrawal symptoms can sometimes be misattributed to other ailments among those who are not aware of their physical dependence on caffeine.

CAFFEINE USE DISORDER

The *ICD-10* includes a diagnosis of substance dependence due to caffeine, and caffeine use disorder is now recognized by the *DSM-5* as a condition for further study. In order to fulfill the *DSM-5* research criteria for Caffeine Use Disorder, an individual must show a problematic pattern of caffeine use leading to clinically significant impairment or distress, as manifested by *all* three of the following criteria occurring within a 12-month period: (1) a persistent desire or unsuccessful efforts to cut down or control caffeine use; (2) continued caffeine use despite knowledge of having a persistent or recurrent physical or psychological problem that is likely to have been caused or exacerbated by caffeine; and (3) withdrawal, as manifested by either of the following: (a) the characteristic withdrawal syndrome for caffeine or (b) caffeine (or a closely related substance) is taken to relieve or avoid withdrawal symptoms. Other symptoms that define a substance use disorder by the *DSM-5* (such as tolerance, using more than intended) are also potential features of problematic caffeine use. However, a more restrictive set of criteria was chosen to prevent overdiagnosis. Although few studies have examined treatment for Caffeine Use Disorder, randomized controlled trials suggest a manualized

treatment that provides instructions for progressively decreased caffeine consumption over a period of weeks can help individuals with problematic caffeine use significantly reduce caffeine consumption and maintain lower consumption over long-term follow-up (eg, 1 year).

GENETICS

Relative to dizygotic twins, monozygotic twins have higher concordance rates for total caffeine consumption, heavy caffeine consumption, coffee and tea intake, caffeine intoxication, caffeine withdrawal, caffeine tolerance, and caffeine-related sleep disturbances with heritability ranging between 30% and 77%. There is evidence that a common genetic factor underlies the use of caffeine, cigarette, and alcohol use, with 28% to 41% of the heritable effects of caffeine use (or heavy use) shared with alcohol and smoking.

EFFECTS ON PHYSICAL HEALTH

Although caffeine is not associated with any life-threatening illnesses, there are some medical conditions that may be adversely affected by caffeine or coffee consumption. Epidemiologic research has also provided evidence that caffeine or coffee consumption may have some protective effects against specific diseases.

Dietary Guidelines

The dietary guidelines of the US Department of Agriculture suggest that up to 400 mg/d of caffeine from coffee is not associated with negative health effects. These guidelines do not provide recommendations for caffeine from sources other than coffee and do not encourage individuals who do not consume caffeine to start doing so. Similarly, scholarly review of the effects of caffeine on health have suggested limits of 300 mg/d for reproductive aged women, 400 mg/d for healthy adults, and 2.5 mg/d for children. For pregnant women, the American College of Obstetricians and Gynecologists concluded that consuming less than 200 mg/d of caffeine does not appear to cause miscarriage or preterm birth.

Adverse Health Effects

Caffeine can increase blood pressure, influence heart rate variability, and increase arterial stiffness, but whether such effects represent clinically significant cardiovascular risk factors is debated. Both caffeinated and decaffeinated coffees contain lipids that raise total and low-density lipoprotein cholesterol with higher levels obtained from unfiltered brewing methods (eg, French press, boiled). Coffee may exacerbate gastroesophageal reflux, but this could be due to caffeine or other coffee constituents. Caffeine is a general risk factor for urinary incontinence in women and men, and reducing caffeine intake has been shown to decrease urinary incontinence. Caffeine consumption increases urinary calcium excretion and has been linked to bone loss and fractures, but it has been suggested that the effects of caffeine on calcium loss may be offset by a relatively small intake of milk. Caffeine consumption prepregnancy and during pregnancy dose-dependently increases the rate of spontaneous abortion (miscarriage), stillbirth, low birth weight, and infants that are small for gestational age. Caffeine can also have negative effects on sleep, even when consumed early in the day. Caffeine delays sleep onset, reduces total sleep time, alters the normal stages of sleep, and decreases the reported quality of sleep. Caffeine-Induced Sleep Disorder is a diagnosis recognized by *DSM*-5, characterized by a prominent sleep disturbance etiologically related to caffeine use.

Health Protective Effects

There is an inverse association between coffee, tea, and caffeine consumption and the risk of Parkinson disease, and caffeine-derived compounds have been suggested as potential therapeutic agents for the treatment of Parkinson disease. There is some evidence suggesting protective effects of caffeine consumption against some forms of dementia and depression, but the data are more ambiguous. Increased coffee drinking is associated with reduced progression to cirrhosis for individuals with chronic liver disease, decreased mortality in individuals with cirrhosis, decreased rate of liver cancer, improved response to antiviral treatment in individuals with hepatitis C, and decreased steatohepatitis in individuals with nonalcoholic fatty liver disease. Preclinical research and systematic review provide evidence that antioxidant coffee constituents improve glucose metabolism and insulin sensitivity and consequently offer a protective effect of coffee drinking against type 2 diabetes mellitus, with similar effects for caffeinated and decaffeinated coffee.

DRUG–DRUG INTERACTIONS
Nicotine and Cigarette Smoking

Cigarette smokers consume more caffeine than nonsmokers. Caffeine can increase the reinforcing and stimulant subjective effects of nicotine, but caffeine administration has not been shown to reliably increase cigarette or nicotine self-administration. Cigarette smoking abstinence produces substantial increases in caffeine blood levels among heavy caffeine consumers, presumably because of the reversal of smoking-induced caffeine metabolism, but the clinical significance during smoking cessation has not been shown.

Alcohol

Heavy alcohol use and *DSM*-defined alcohol use disorders are associated with heavy use and clinical dependence on caffeine. One study reported substantial increases in caffeine consumption after alcohol detoxification in patients with alcoholism. A study of individuals fulfilling *DSM-IV* diagnostic criteria for substance dependence as applied to caffeine found that almost 60% had a past diagnosis of *DSM*-defined alcohol abuse or dependence.

Alcohol and Energy Drinks

Despite warnings issued by the US Food and Drug Administration, many young adults mix caffeinated energy drinks with alcohol. There is growing evidence to suggest that the coingestion of caffeinated energy drinks and alcohol may be associated with greater harms than those from alcohol consumption alone. A substantial number of studies indicate consumption of alcohol mixed with energy drinks is associated with a range of problematic behaviors such as increased alcohol consumption and alcohol-related harms, illicit drug use, sexual risk behavior, and increased drinking and driving.

Other Drug Interactions

Animal and human studies show that caffeine may potentiate the discriminative stimulus effects of cocaine. Caffeine and ephedrine have been shown to potentiate each other's discriminative stimulus effects. There is preclinical evidence to suggest that caffeine may increase the toxic effects of other stimulant drugs such as D-amphetamine, cocaine, and 3,4-methylenedioxymethamphetamine (MDMA). Animal and human studies suggest a mutually antagonistic relationship between caffeine and benzodiazepines. There is some evidence that caffeine inhibits the metabolism of the antipsychotic clozapine to an extent that might be clinically significant. Because caffeine and theophylline inhibit each other's metabolism, caffeine consumption during theophylline therapy should be monitored. Lithium toxicity may occur after caffeine withdrawal because of decreased renal clearance of lithium.

ACKNOWLEDGMENTS

Preparation of this review was supported, in part, by US Public Health Service Grant R01 DA03890 from the National Institute on Drug Abuse and by intramural funds of the National Institute on Drug Abuse.

KEY POINTS

1. Caffeine may have some health-protective effects, but caffeine also has the potential to produce clinically significant negative physiological and psychological effects, tolerance, withdrawal symptoms, and psychiatric disorders.
2. At usual dietary doses, caffeine is a mild psychomotor stimulant drug that produces psychomotor activation as well as reinforcing and arousing effects through antagonism effects at adenosine receptors and indirect effects on dopaminergic neurotransmission.
3. Caffeine metabolism is affected by a range of genetic and environmental factors, including increased metabolism in cigarette smokers and slowed metabolism in individuals with liver disease, infants, women taking oral contraceptives, and pregnant women.
4. Caffeine withdrawal symptoms (eg, headache, fatigue) can occur at daily caffeine doses as low as 100 mg/d, usually occur 12 to 24 hours after caffeine cessation, may last for 2 to 9 days, and in some instances may be severe enough to cause functional impairment.
5. Acute caffeine consumption (usually in excess of 250 to 500 mg) can cause caffeine intoxication symptoms such as nervousness (anxiety), insomnia, diuresis, gastrointestinal disturbance, psychomotor agitation, tachycardia, or cardiac arrhythmia.

REVIEW QUESTIONS

1. Which of the following symptoms is not a frequently observed caffeine withdrawal symptom?
   A. Anxiety
   B. Headache
   C. Fatigue
   D. Difficulty concentrating
   E. Depressed mood

2. The primary brain mechanism of action of caffeine is:
   A. increase in serotonin.
   B. antagonism of acetylcholine.
   C. agonism of dopamine.
   D. antagonism of adenosine.
   E. decrease in serotonin.

3. How does pregnancy affect the metabolism of caffeine?
   A. Pregnancy increases caffeine metabolism but only in the first trimester.
   B. Pregnancy speeds up caffeine metabolism.
   C. Pregnancy does not influence caffeine metabolism.
   D. Pregnancy slows down caffeine metabolism but only in the first trimester.
   E. Pregnancy slows down caffeine metabolism throughout pregnancy.

ANSWERS

1. **A**
2. **D**
3. **E**

SUGGESTED READINGS

Ferré S. Mechanisms of the psychostimulant effects of caffeine: implications for substance use disorders. *Psychopharmacology (Berl)*. 2016;233(10):1963-1979.

Juliano LM, Griffiths RR. A critical review of caffeine withdrawal: empirical validation of symptoms and signs, incidence, severity, and associated features. *Psychopharmacology (Berl)*. 2004;176(1):1-29.

McLellan TM, Caldwell JA, Lieberman HR. A review of caffeine's effects on cognitive, physical and occupational performance. *Neurosci Biobehav Rev*. 2016;71:294-312.

Meredith SE, Juliano LM, Hughes JR, Griffiths RR. Caffeine use disorder: a comprehensive review and research agenda. *J Caffeine Res*. 2013;3:114-130.

Nawrot P, Jordan S, Eastwood J, et al. Effects of caffeine on human health. *Food Addit Contam*. 2003;20(1):1-30.

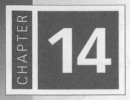

CHAPTER 14

The Pharmacology of Nicotine and Tobacco

Summary by John A. Dani

Based on THE ASAM PRINCIPLES OF ADDICTION MEDICINE, 6th edition chapter by John A. Dani, Thomas R. Kosten, and Neal L. Benowitz

Nicotine is a psychostimulant and mood modulator. It may temporarily improve alertness and relieve withdrawal as well as promote arousal, relaxation, and relief from stress and hunger. Thus, nicotine becomes a mood leveler, causing arousal during fatigue and relaxation during anxiety.

METHODS OF USE

Nicotine and tobacco come in the form of cigarettes, bidis, cigars, pipes, snuff, and chewing tobacco. Recently, electronic cigarettes (e-cigarettes or electronic nicotine delivery systems) have become widely available. Although such devices may reduce toxic compounds, they may also introduce other new toxicants while still maintaining exposure to inhaled nicotine, which may have its own long-term harmful effects. Substituting tobacco cigarettes with electronic nicotine delivery systems may substantially reduce exposure to selected tobacco-specific toxicants, but the overall safety of electronic nicotine delivery systems is still controversial.

PHARMACOKINETICS

The relatively rapid delivery of nicotine to the brain when smoking allows precise dose titration by altering puff volume, the number of puffs taken, and the depth inhaled. After nicotine is absorbed into the bloodstream, it has a volume of distribution of about 180 L, with <5% binding to plasma proteins. Based on a 2-hour half-life, nicotine accumulates during a day of regular smoking and persists for 6 to 8 hours after smoking ceases. Steady-state plasma nicotine levels in the early afternoon typically range between 10 and 50 ng/mL. Nicotine is extensively metabolized to cotinine in the liver, lung, and brain by cytochrome P450 2A6 (CYP2A6). Women metabolize nicotine faster than men. African Americans obtain, on average, 30% more nicotine per cigarette, and they clear nicotine and cotinine more slowly than do Caucasians. Chinese Americans have both a lower nicotine intake per cigarette and smoke fewer cigarettes per day than do Caucasians due to slower metabolism CYP2A6 alleles.

Nicotine obtained from tobacco reaches high initial concentrations in the arterial blood and lungs. It then distributes into the brain, storage adipose, and muscle tissue. Nicotine crosses the placenta freely and has been found in the amniotic fluid and in the umbilical cord blood of neonates. Nicotine also is found in breast milk at concentrations approximately twice those found in the blood.

Nicotine is extensively metabolized primarily in the liver and, to a lesser extent, in the lung and the brain. On average, 80% of nicotine is metabolized to cotinine, which is further metabolized to trans-3'-hydroxycotinine, the major nicotine metabolite found in the urine as well as other metabolites. About 17% of cotinine is excreted unchanged in the urine. CYP2A6 is primarily responsible both for the C-oxidation of nicotine to cotinine and for the oxidation of cotinine to trans-3'-hydroxycotinine. The ratio of trans-3'-hydroxycotinine to cotinine, which can be measured in the blood, saliva, or urine of tobacco users, is a relatively stable biomarker of CYP2A6 activity and the rate of metabolism of nicotine. The rate of metabolism can be measured as a determinant of the level of nicotine addiction and response to nicotine/tobacco use disorder treatments.

BIOCHEMICAL ASSESSMENT OF EXPOSURE TO NICOTINE AND TOBACCO

The 16-hour half-life of cotinine makes it useful as a plasma and salivary marker of nicotine intake. Salivary cotinine concentrations correlate well with blood cotinine concentrations ($r = 0.82$–0.90). The cotinine level produced by a single cigarette is 8 to 10 ng/mL. It takes several hours for the cotinine to peak after a cigarette is smoked. A cotinine value greater than 14 ng/mL typically indicates smoking. Cotinine blood levels average about 250 to 300 ng/mL in regular smokers and may persist for up to 7 days after cessation. Breath measurements of expired air that contain more than 10 ppm of carbon monoxide (CO) usually indicate tobacco smoking within the past 8 to 12 hours. Elevated CO levels in the absence of smoking may be the result of exposure to environmental pollutants, such as faulty gas boilers, car exhausts, and smog. Assays of thiocyanate are insensitive to low amounts of smoking, and thiocyanate levels can remain elevated for weeks after smoking has ceased. CO and cotinine levels generally are preferred to thiocyanate levels in the assessment of smoking.

DRUG INTERACTIONS WITH TOBACCO AND NICOTINE

Smoking accelerates the metabolism of many drugs, particularly those metabolized by CYP1A2. Cigarette smoking induces the metabolism of theophylline, propranolol, flecainide, tacrine, caffeine, olanzapine, clozapine, imipramine, haloperidol, pentazocine, estradiol, and other drugs. When people who smoke stop smoking, as often occurs during hospitalization for an acute illness, the doses of these medications may need to be lowered to avoid toxicity. Thus, stopping smoking affords patients an added benefit of potentially needing lower doses of therapeutic medications and having fewer medication-related side effects.

Several pharmacodynamic interactions arise between cigarette smoking and other drugs. Cigarette smoking and oral contraceptives interact synergistically to increase the risk of stroke and premature myocardial infarction in women. Cigarettes appear to enhance the procoagulant effect of estrogens. For this reason, oral contraceptives are relatively contraindicated in women who smoke cigarettes. Nicotine inhibits reductions in blood pressure and heart rate from β-adrenergic blockers, resulting in less sedation from benzodiazepines and less analgesia from some opioids.

PHARMACOLOGIC ACTIONS

Nicotine has a complex dose–response relationship. At low doses (such as those achieved by smoking a cigarette), nicotine acts on the sympathetic nervous system to acutely increase blood pressure, heart rate, and cardiac output and to cause cutaneous vasoconstriction. At higher doses, nicotine produces ganglionic stimulation and the release of adrenal catecholamines. At extremely high doses, nicotine

causes hypotension and slowing of the heart rate. Importantly, nicotinic acetylcholine receptors (nAChRs) are centrally involved in learning and memory functions within the human brain. Secondhand smoke exposure to the developing brain has been associated with attention deficit hyperactivity disorder.

The primary central nervous system effects of nicotine in those who smoke are arousal, relaxation (particularly in stressful situations), and enhancement of mood, attention, and reaction time. Thus, people who smoke may need regular doses of nicotine to feel normal rather than to enhance their capabilities.

The psychoactive effects of nicotine and tobacco are determined not only by the route and speed of drug administration and the pharmacokinetic parameters that determine the concentration at receptor sites over time but also by a variety of host and environmental factors.

In those who regularly smoke, nicotine's ability to cause stimulation when smoked at a low level of arousal (such as fatigue) and to affect relaxation when smoked at a high level of arousal (such as anxiety) underlies its reinforcing effects under a range of conditions. People who smoke increase their smoking under both low- and high-arousal conditions. Gender differences appear to affect nicotine responsiveness. Women have less sensitivity to changes in nicotine dose during nicotine discrimination experiments, and they may not benefit as much as men from nicotine replacement therapy during smoking cessation.

Genetics mediate differences in the development of nicotine dependence. Family linkage studies and candidate gene association studies suggest a number of loci or particular genes that are associated with smoking behavior, but the smoking phenotypes vary considerably from study to study. Candidate genes include the nicotinic acetylcholine receptor α_5 subunit, α_3 subunit, β_4 subunit, and β_3 subunit (*CHRNA5–CHRNA3–CHRNB4–CHRNB3*): the nAChR gene cluster.

The other gene that clearly affects smoking behavior and cancer risk is the *CYP2A6* gene, which codes for the primary enzyme responsible for the oxidation of nicotine and cotinine. *CYP2A6* affects cigarette smoking behavior and cancer risk. This gene is polymorphic, and reduced function variants of the gene are associated with smoking fewer cigarettes per day and a lower risk of lung cancer.

Tobacco use is most highly prevalent and more intense among psychiatric patients and among those who use other drugs. Individuals with schizophrenia, depression, and attention deficit hyperactivity disorder have a higher prevalence of cigarette smoking than the population as a whole. These groups of patients have more difficulty in quitting compared with smokers without mental illness, often experiencing greater depression after smoking cessation.

Addiction

The average age of first smoking is 15 years old. Nicotine obtained through chewing tobacco and cigarettes often precedes the use of other drugs. The earlier the age at which use begins, the more difficult it is for the user to quit. The regular use of tobacco commonly leads to its compulsive use. There have been attempts to correlate the severity of nicotine addiction with factors such as the duration of smoking, potency of cigarettes, puff frequency, puff duration, and inhalation volume. However, these variables only weakly correlate with biochemical measures, and they do not predict the intensity and extent of withdrawal symptoms. The Fagerström Test for Nicotine Dependence is one of the most widely accepted measures of the severity of nicotine physical dependence. Many studies show a relationship between the Fagerström Test for Nicotine Dependence and the ability to achieve tobacco cessation. The two items in the test that convey most predictive information are number of cigarettes smoked per day and time from waking to first cigarette of the day.

There is a high rate of relapse among individuals who try to quit smoking. Population surveys consistently find that up to 75% of adults who smoke want to stop. About one third actually try to stop each year, but less than 3% succeed unaided.

Withdrawal

Tobacco use is sustained, in part, by the need to prevent the symptoms of nicotine withdrawal, which include craving for nicotine, irritability and frustration or anger, anxiety, depression, difficulty concentrating, restlessness, and increased appetite. Performance measures such as reaction time and attention are impaired during withdrawal. Most acute withdrawal symptoms reach maximum intensity 24 to 48 hours after cessation and then gradually diminish over a few weeks. Some symptoms—including dysphoria, mild depression, and anhedonia—may persist for months.

NEUROBIOLOGICAL MECHANISMS OF ACTION

nAChRs are ligand-gated ion channels are closed at rest, are opened by nicotine, and then become desensitized for several seconds. nAChRs consist of five polypeptide subunits assembled like staves of a barrel around a central water-filled core. The intensity of the membrane depolarization, the kinetics of gating activation, the rates of desensitization and recovery from desensitization, the size of the ionic signal, the pharmacology, and the regulatory controls of the ACh response all depend on the subunit composition of the nAChRs. Genetic and neurophysiologic studies in mice indicate the alpha-4 beta-2 nicotinic receptor ($\alpha 4\beta 2^*$) nAChRs, often in combination with the α_6 subunit, are primarily responsible for the initiation of nicotine addiction. Cholinergic neurons provide diffuse and sparse innervation to practically the entire brain, including the dopamine reinforcement pathways where nicotine enhances the firing of dopamine neurons directly and through glutamatergic afferents. The withdrawal syndrome is substantially mediated by the α_5-containing nAChRs in the habenula to produce nicotine's aversive effects and the somatic symptoms of withdrawal.

Cigarette smoking is associated with reduced activity of the enzymes monoamine oxidase A and B, which might contribute to the perceived benefit of smoking by some depressed patients.

SYSTEMIC TOXICITY

Those who smoke are exposed to more than 7000 different chemicals, including at least 50 known carcinogens. The increased risk of cardiovascular disease is due to CO reductions in oxygen delivery to the heart, and oxidant chemicals are primarily responsible for endothelial dysfunction, platelet activation, thrombosis, and coronary vasoconstriction. Cigarette smoking causes an imbalance between proteolytic and antiproteolytic forces in the lung and heightens airway responsiveness and chronic obstructive lung diseases.

The agents contributing most significantly to lung cancer are thought to be the carcinogenic polynuclear aromatic hydrocarbons and the tobacco-specific N-nitrosamines, followed by polonium-210 and volatile aldehydes. As with other tobacco-related diseases, the risk of cancer of the mouth, larynx, esophagus, lung, stomach, pancreas, kidney, urinary bladder, and uterine cervix as well as leukemia is directly related to the intensity and duration of exposure to cigarette smoke and to nicotine, which is itself a tumor promoter.

Cigarette smoking is associated with skin changes, including yellow staining of fingers; vasospasm and obliteration of small skin vessels; precancerous and squamous cell carcinomas on the lips and oral mucosa; and enhanced facial skin wrinkling.

Those who currently smoke 20 or more cigarettes per day have statistically significant increases in nuclear sclerosis and posterior subcapsular cataracts compared with individuals who never smoked. Those who currently smoke more than 20 cigarettes per day also have an increased risk of age-related macular degeneration.

Cigarette smoking in women is associated with lower levels of estrogen, earlier menopause, and increased risk of osteoporosis. In men, smoking may impair penile erection, primarily in people with underlying vascular disease, through the impairment of endothelium-dependent smooth muscle relaxation. Smoking doubles the likelihood of moderate or complete erectile dysfunction associated with other risk factors, such as coronary artery disease and hypertension. Because the prevalence of erectile dysfunction in those who formerly smoked is no different from that in individuals who never smoked, erectile dysfunction is believed to improve with stopping smoking.

Nicotine both suppresses the appetite and increases metabolic rate. Patients who smoke weigh, on average, 2.7 to 4.5 kg (6 to 10 lb) less than those who do not smoke. Individuals who stop smoking typically gain weight to approximately the levels of those who have never smoked in the 6 to 12 months after smoking cessation.

Cigarette smoking is associated with the occurrence and delayed healing of peptic ulcers. Mechanisms include decreases in the mucous bicarbonate barrier in the stomach, reduction in the production of endogenous prostaglandins in the gastric mucosa, and increased proliferation of *Helicobacter pylori*.

TOBACCO AND PREGNANCY

Smoking during pregnancy and lactation has been associated with a variety of untoward child health outcomes, including preterm birth, fetal growth restriction, low birth weight, sudden infant death syndrome, neurodevelopmental and behavioral problems, obesity, hypertension, type 2 diabetes, impaired lung function, asthma, and wheezing. Nicotine itself has been implicated as at least partially causative for a number of these adverse outcomes from maternally derived exposures to smoking. Smoking during pregnancy nearly doubles the relative risk of having a low–birth-weight infant; the relative risks of spontaneous abortion and perinatal and neonatal mortality are increased by about one third. The components of tobacco smoke responsible for obstetric and fetal problems have not been definitively identified. CO clearly is detrimental because it markedly reduces the oxygen-carrying capacity of fetal hemoglobin.

The effect of smoking on lowering birth weight interacts with the metabolic genes *CYP1A1* and *GSTT1*. Infants born to mothers who smoked who had genetic variants associated with reduced *CYP1A1* activity—Aa and aa (heterozygous and homozygous variant types)—and reduced or absent *GSTT1* activity had greater reductions in birth weight than did infants born to mothers who smoked who had the normal metabolic activity genes *CYP1A1 AA* (homozygous wild-type) or *GSTT1* genotype. The CYP1A1 and GSTT1 enzymes have roles metabolizing and excreting some toxic chemicals in cigarette smoke.

In the developing fetus, nicotine can arrest neuronal replication and differentiation and can contribute to sudden infant death syndrome. Nicotine activates nicotinic cholinergic receptors in the fetal brain, resulting in abnormalities of cell proliferation and differentiation that lead to shortfalls in cell numbers and, eventually, to altered synaptic activity. Comparable alterations occur in peripheral autonomic pathways and are hypothesized to lead to increased susceptibility to hypoxia-induced brain damage, perinatal mortality, and sudden infant death.

SECONDHAND SMOKE

Secondhand smoke (SHS) is the complex mixture formed by the escaping smoke of a burning tobacco product as well as smoke that is exhaled by a smoker. Sidestream smoke contains higher concentrations of some toxins than does mainstream smoke. SHS characteristics change as it combines with other constituents in the ambient air and ages. Exposure to SHS is causally associated with acute and chronic coronary heart disease, lung cancer, nasal sinus cancer, and eye and nasal irritation in adults and with asthma, chronic respiratory symptoms, and acute lower respiratory tract infections such as bronchitis and pneumonia in children and potentially in those with certain psychiatric disorders. SHS also is causally associated with low birth weight and sudden infant death syndrome in infants. Young children's exposure to tobacco smoke comes mainly from those who smoke in the home, especially parents. Maternal smoking has the greatest effect on children's measured cotinine levels. Additional contributors include paternal smoking, smoking by other household members, and smoking by childcare personnel.

An average salivary cotinine level of 0.4 ng/mL corresponds to an increased lifetime mortality risk of 1/1000 for lung cancer and 1/100 for heart disease. Assuming a prevalence of 28% for unrestricted smoking in the workplace, passive smoking would yield 4000 heart disease deaths and 400 lung cancer deaths annually in the United States. More than 95% of SHS-exposed office workers exceeded the significant risk level for heart disease mortality and more than 60% exceeded the significant risk level for lung cancer mortality established by the Occupational Safety and Health Administration.

MORBIDITY AND MORTALITY

Each pack of cigarettes sold in the United States costs the nation an estimated $7.18 in medical care expenditures and lost productivity. Tobacco use is a leading cause of death in the United States, causing more than 480,000 deaths per year, which is about one in every five deaths. This includes ~150,000 deaths from cardiovascular causes, ~150,000 deaths from cancer, and ~100,000 deaths from nonmalignant pulmonary disease. Cigarette smoking also increases the risk of developing and the severity of respiratory tract infections, including influenza, pneumococcal pneumonia, and tuberculosis. On average, adult men and women who smoked lost 13.2 and 14.5 years of life, respectively, due to smoking. In contrast, the annual mortality attributable to passive smoking between 1995 and 1999 was estimated at nearly 40,000 deaths, including 35,000 from cardiovascular diseases, 3000 from lung cancer, and 1000 from perinatal conditions.

NICOTINE AND OTHER ADDICTIONS

There is a strong association between smoking and alcohol use disorder. People who are more severely addicted to alcohol smoke more and are less likely to quit. Tobacco also synergizes with alcohol in causing a number of medical complications. In combination, smoking and heavy drinking are associated with substantially increased rates of oral and esophageal cancers. Because lit cigarettes smolder when they fall onto upholstered furniture, alcohol use combined with smoking causes household fires that claim more than 1000 lives per year among children and adults. Persons recovering from other substance use disorders often die from tobacco-related illnesses. In a landmark population-based retrospective cohort study, death certificates were examined for 214 of 854 persons who were admitted between 1972 and 1983 to an inpatient program for the treatment of alcoholism and other non-nicotine drugs of dependence. Of the deaths reported, 50.9% were caused by tobacco use, whereas 34.1% were attributable to alcohol use. The cumulative 20-year mortality was 48.1% versus an expected 18.5% for a demographically matched control population ($p < 0.001$).

BENEFITS OF CESSATION

Most smokers (>70%) want to quit, and approximately 40% attempt to quit each year. However, without assistance, only about 2% to 5% of the attempts are successful. The good news is that stopping smoking has benefits for those who smoke at any age. The immediately decreased risk of cardiovascular death in those who stop smoking may reflect a decrease in blood coagulability, improved tissue oxygenation, and reduced predisposition to cardiac arrhythmias. Among former smokers, the reduced risk of death compared with those who continued smoking begins shortly after quitting and continues for at least 10 to 15 years. After 10 to 15 years' abstinence, the risk of all-cause mortality returns nearly to that of persons who never smoked.

KEY POINTS

1. Nicotine causes arousal during fatigue and relaxation during anxiety.
2. Blood, salivary, and plasma cotinine as well as expired breath carbon monoxide concentrations, blood carboxyhemoglobin concentrations, and plasma or salivary thiocyanate concentrations are biochemical markers of nicotine intake.
3. Tobacco withdrawal includes craving for nicotine, irritability and frustration or anger, anxiety, depression, difficulty concentrating, restlessness, and increased appetite. Symptoms reach maximum intensity 24 to 48 hours after cessation.
4. People who smoke are exposed to at least 50 known carcinogens and have an increased risk of cardiovascular disease, leading to adult men and women smokers losing 13.2 and 14.5 years of life, respectively.
5. Among those who formerly smoked, the reduced risk of death compared with those who continued smoking begins shortly after quitting and continues for at least 10 to 15 years, when the risk of all-cause mortality returns nearly to that of persons who never smoked.

REVIEW QUESTIONS

1. In most people who smoke, which of the following ranges of steady state plasma levels of nicotine are found during the afternoon?
   A. 1 to 10 ng/mL
   B. 10 to 50 ng/mL
   C. 1 to 10 mg/mL
   D. 50 to 200 ng/mL
   E. 50 to 200 mg/mL

2. The main metabolite of nicotine is:
   A. nor-nicotine.
   B. carboxy-nicotine.
   C. cotinine.
   D. nicotine glucuronide.
   E. nicotine hydroxide.

3. Daily smoking of less than five cigarettes per day would be indicated by afternoon levels of plasma cotinine above _____ and breath carbon monoxide above _____.
   A. 100 ng/mL; 10 ppm
   B. 14 ng/mL; 10 ppm
   C. 900 ng/mL; 10 ppm
   D. 50 ng/mL; 10 ppt
   E. 100 ng/mL; 10 ppt

4. Tobacco withdrawal includes all the following symptoms *except*:
   A. irritability.
   B. anger.
   C. decreased appetite.
   D. difficulty concentrating.
   E. restlessness.

5. Smoking during pregnancy increases the relative risk of having a low–birth-weight infant by:
   A. fourfold.
   B. twofold.
   C. threefold.
   D. half.
   E. one third.

ANSWERS
1. **B**
2. **C**
3. **B**
4. **C**
5. **B**

SUGGESTED READINGS

Benowitz NL. Clinical pharmacology of nicotine: implications for understanding, preventing, and treating tobacco addiction. *Clin Pharmacol Ther.* 2008;83(4):531-541.

Dani JA, Harris RA. Nicotine addiction and comorbidity with alcohol abuse and mental illness. *Nat Neurosci.* 2005;8(11):1465-1470.

15

The Pharmacology of Cannabinoids

Summary by Sandra P. Welch, Tricia H. Smith, Robert Malcolm, and Aron H. Lichtman

Based on THE ASAM PRINCIPLES OF ADDICTION MEDICINE, 6th edition chapter by Sandra P. Welch, Tricia H. Smith, Robert Malcolm, and Aron H. Lichtman

Cannabis sativa is one of the oldest and most widely used plants in the world as a source of various products including the drug Δ9-tetrahydrocannabinol (THC). More than 565 chemicals are synthesized by the cannabis sativa plant, approximately 120 of which are termed *cannabinoids*. Cannabinoids are similar in structure to THC and include several nonpsychoactive products such as cannabinol and cannabidiol. Endogenous ligands known as endocannabinoids that bind to cannabinoid receptors include *N*-arachidonoylethanolamide (anandamide [AEA]) and 2-arachidonoylglycerol (2-AG), among others. There are two known cannabinoid receptor subtypes, CB_1 and CB_2. Numerous synthetic receptor agonists and antagonists exist, including the CB_1 cannabinoid antagonist/inverse agonist, SR141716A (rimonabant), and the CB_2 receptor antagonist, SR144528. A 1:1 mixture of THC and cannabidiol has been approved by Health Canada, the United Kingdom, and other countries around the world to treat spasticity from multiple sclerosis. A mixed ratio of THC and cannabidiol in capsular formulation and a synthetic cannabinoid are also available in select countries. Numerous synthetic cannabinoids of diverse structures continue to be available for preclinical research purposes only, although the recreational use of such substances by humans has become widespread and is illegal in all 50 states in the United States.

FORMULATIONS
Natural, Plant-Derived Cannabinoids

The concentration of THC varies among three common preparations from the cannabis plant: marijuana, hashish, and hash oil. THC concentrations in marijuana containing mostly leaves and stems range from 0.5% to 5%. Sinsemilla, the flowering tops from unfertilized female plants, may have THC concentrations of 7% to 14%. Hashish, dried cannabis resin, and compressed flowers has 2% to 8% THC content. Hash oil obtained by extracting THC from hashish (or marijuana) with an organic solvent is a highly potent substance, with a THC concentration between 15% and 50%. In addition, the extraction of THC with butane produces a product called butane hash oil ("dabs"), which can contain up to 90% THC. The fibrous "hemp" form of cannabis has low THC content (typically <0.4%).

Synthetic Cannabinoids

In general, synthetic cannabinoids have a higher affinity for cannabinoid receptors than THC, have active metabolites that prolong their durations of action and increase accumulations in the body, and have increased potential for toxicity. They are sold under street names such as "Spice" and "K2," among many other rapidly changing names. A number of these compounds have not been characterized or scheduled as controlled substances by the Drug Enforcement Administration. They are not detected in standard urine drug screens, and distribution methods occur outside of traditional illicit drug sales networks. These factors have made the understanding of the epidemiology and clinical consequences of synthetic cannabinoid consumption difficult.

HISTORICAL FEATURES

The use of cannabis dates back over 12,000 years and was cultivated in early American history for its fiber. References to its medicinal uses date back to 2700 BCE. In 1842, William O'Shaughnessy, a British army physician in India, published a review on the use of cannabis in the treatment of various medical conditions; medical research on several of these conditions continues today. Cannabis was placed into Schedule I of the Controlled Substances Act in 1970.

CANNABINOID RECEPTOR NEUROBIOLOGY

Cannabinoid Receptors

Cannabinoid receptors exist in two recognized isoforms: cannabinoid receptor 1 (CB_1), highly expressed in certain brain regions, and cannabinoid receptor 2 (CB_2), associated with immune cells. Both subtypes are present in a variety of tissues.

Mechanism of Action

In 2016, x-ray crystallography revealed that the CB_1 receptor is a G protein–coupled receptor, which activates G proteins, mainly G_i/G_o. G_i/G_o protein activation inhibits adenylate cyclase; inhibition of adenylyl cyclase decreases cyclic adenosine monophosphate accumulation. CB_1-activated G proteins can couple to phospholipase C and ion channels, inhibiting voltage-dependent N- and P/Q-type Ca^{+2} channels and activating inward-rectifying K^+ channels. Collectively, the effects on ion channels serve to decrease neuronal excitability. Cannabinoid receptors are constitutively active, which means they tonically activate G proteins in the absence of an agonist. Therefore, CB_1 receptors have an intrinsic physiologic tone or rate of activation, which may be thrown out of balance when exogenous cannabinoids are used. THC is a weak agonist; maximally effective doses of THC can only activate the receptor to ~20% of its full capacity. However, many synthetic cannabinoids can fully activate the receptor (approximately 100%). Thus, synthetic cannabinoids activate significantly more G proteins than THC, which may lead to the enhanced toxicity seen during the use of these compounds.

The Endocannabinoid System

Endocannabinoids are naturally produced by the human body and bind to cannabinoid receptors. They include AEA and 2-AG. Their effects are comparable to those of other psychoactive cannabinoids. 2-AG has higher selectivity and efficacy for CB_1 and CB_2 receptors than AEA. Endocannabinoids are not stored in the body but rather are synthesized "on demand" from membrane lipids by a specific phospholipase D that hydrolyzes *N*-acyl phosphatidylethanolamine to AEA.

Endocannabinoid Signaling

The endocannabinoids bind both CB receptors. The endocannabinoids are "retrograde messengers," and they travel backward compared to classical neurotransmitters and regulate the release of neurotransmitters from the presynaptic neuron. This process begins when an action potential traveling down the presynaptic neuron causes the release of a classical neurotransmitter. After this transmitter crosses the synaptic cleft and binds to a postsynaptic receptor, postsynaptic neuronal activation causes the "on demand" synthesis and release of the endocannabinoids, AEA and 2-AG. These endocannabinoids travel back to the presynaptic neuron and bind to CB_1 receptors, resulting in a retrograde signal that attenuates presynaptic neuronal excitability. Cannabinoids reduce both excitatory and inhibitory neurotransmitter release. The net effect of the endocannabinoid system (ECS) is to function as a regulator or "rheostatic" mechanism on neuronal excitability.

CANNABINOID PHARMACOKINETICS

Marijuana inhalation (ie, smoke, vapor, or aerosol) produces the most rapid onset and intense "high." Marijuana and hashish may also be taken orally via food products. Oral absorption leads to a slower onset of the psychoactive effects and the "high" is of lesser intensity. Most synthetic cannabinoids are of high potency and short duration of action, with metabolites that are more toxic than the parent compound, making their identification via urinalysis very difficult.

CANNABINOID PHARMACODYNAMICS

Tolerance

Preclinical Studies

Tolerance develops to many pharmacologic effects of cannabinoids. Proposed mechanisms include receptor inactivation, desensitization, or decreased receptor number (downregulation).

Human Studies

Studies in humans indicate the development of tolerance to both cognitive and psychomotor effects following heavy use of cannabis. Human studies indicate that tolerance does not develop to psychomotor impairment following moderate chronic cannabis use. However, positron emission tomography scans indicate that those who chronically smoke cannabis had regional decreases in brain CB_1 receptors of approximately 12% from controls.

Cannabis Withdrawal: Human Studies

A cannabis withdrawal or abstinence syndrome is observed in human experimental studies and includes effects that are typically the opposite of those produced by the drug. Positron emission tomography studies indicate that decreases in CB_1-receptor density due to tolerance in those who chronically use are rapidly reversed upon cessation of cannabis smoking (abstinence) and associated with signs of cannabis withdrawal.

Synthetic Cannabinoids: Preclinical Studies

Synthetic cannabinoids produce profound analgesia and are associated with the development of tolerance and physical dependence, and the effects can be "reinstated" or observed again following a period of abstinence.

TOXICITY AND ADVERSE EFFECTS OF PLANT-DERIVED CANNABINOIDS AND ENDOCANNABINOIDS

Cannabinoids and the endocannabinoids have both beneficial and adverse effects on virtually every organ. Thus, the use of cannabinoids as therapeutic agents must be assessed based on the benefit-to-risk ratio for each system. Those with preexisting diseases of the cardiovascular system, liver, pancreas, and lung are particularly susceptible to the adverse effects of cannabis smoking and the less well-known effects of the numerous synthetic cannabinoids.

Psychomotor Effects

Cannabis dose-dependently impairs a variety of psychomotor functions in humans, including object distance and shape discrimination, reaction time, information processing, perceptual motor coordination, motor performance, signal detection, tracking behavior, and slowed time perception.

Behavioral Effects

Although cannabis use has been suggested to cause an "amotivational syndrome" in humans, there is little rigorous scientific evidence to support its existence. There are marked patterns of individual variability in behavioral effects due to duration, frequency, dosage, and type of cannabinoid used.

Cognitive Effects

Recent evidence in animals indicates that the ECS is a selective and rapid modulator of hippocampal synaptic function via effects on neurotransmitter release. The changes in the plasticity of the hippocampal system may explain the memory deficits observed in those who use THC.

Psychopathology

Numerous large, longitudinal studies suggest that use of cannabis increases the risk for schizophrenia,

worsens symptoms, and is associated with a poorer prognosis. Rimonabant, the CB_1 receptor antagonist/inverse agonist used in clinical trials for obesity, but which was never approved in the United States, caused a greater than twofold increase in depression, anxiety, and perceived suicidal risks. As a result, there has been increased interest in the role of the cannabinoid receptor and the use of cannabis in mental illness.

EFFECTS ON MAJOR ORGAN SYSTEMS

Respiratory

The major adverse health effect associated with cannabis smoking is damage to the respiratory system. Many of the same mutagens and carcinogens in nicotine cigarettes are found in cannabis smoke. However, clinical and epidemiologic evidence linking cannabis smoking to chronic obstructive pulmonary disease or respiratory cancer has not been shown.

Immunologic

The CB_2 receptor is expressed on cells of the immune system, bone, and in the central nervous system, leading to the hypothesis that the cannabinoid system plays a significant role in immune modulation. In preclinical tests, the effects of CB_2 receptor activation extend to include effects on most modulatory systems involved in neuropathic pain and autoimmune disorders. The role of both agonists and antagonists of the CB_2 receptor is likely to become one of the major new therapeutic fronts for drug development, especially because CB_2 agonists do not have the psychoactive effects associated with CB_1 receptor agonists such as THC.

Cardiovascular

In humans, cannabis increases the heart rate and produces orthostatic hypotension, making the drug risky in cardiac patients. Synthetic cannabinoid use has been linked to cardiovascular damage and myocardial infarction in previously healthy young people.

Liver

Cannabinoid receptors affect the pathogenesis of various liver diseases in humans. Daily cannabis use is a predictor of fibrosis progression via a steatogenic effect. The predominant liver effects of cannabis (THC, cannabidiol) in healthy human users of cannabis are inhibition of liver microsomes, thus altering the metabolism of endogenous and exogenous compounds.

Kidneys

Renal complications are rare following cannabis use. Synthetic cannabinoid use has been linked to acute kidney failure due to acute tubular necrosis, which may present as psychiatric symptoms secondary to the electrolyte changes produced.

Endocrine

Virtually no hormonal system remains unaffected by the activation of cannabinoid receptors. Clinical evidence suggests that the cannabinoids and ECS are contributors to the multifactorial effects underlying the development of diabetes, including insulin release, and the severe cardiovascular and neuropathic etiologies that accompany the disease.

Reproduction and Pregnancy

Human fertility is partially regulated by the ECS. Both male and female cannabis users show decreased fertility. Females show reduced pregnancy success and males have reduced sperm motility and counts. Cannabis use reduces the success of in vitro fertilization for both males and females. In animal models, maternal cannabinoid consumption alters the neurologic development of neurotransmission systems and can cause lifelong changes in behavior. In 2015, greater than 10% of pregnant women reported using marijuana in the past year, and about 5% of pregnant woman reported use within the past month. The lipid solubility of THC allows for its rapid transfer to the fetus through the placenta as well as rapid transfer into breast milk.

INTOXICATION AND OVERDOSE

Overdose from ingested cannabis preparations is on the rise due to an increase in availability. The major effects observed are sedation, confusion, tachycardia, chest pain, and hypotension, with the potential for severe respiratory depression. A recent large retrospective analysis of cardiovascular risk following the use of cannabis and cannabinoids found that cannabis/cannabinoid use poses a "significant cardiovascular impact," especially when used in large doses and in overdose situations. The greatest impact was on cerebral blood flow and the development of ischemic strokes.

SYNTHETIC CANNABINOIDS
Adverse Effects and Toxicity

With the regulation of synthetic cannabinoids as Schedule I drugs, numerous nonscheduled analogues have been developed. Effects include the potential for

psychotic/manic episodes and cardiovascular effects leading to cardiac arrest, stroke, and seizure induction. In addition, frequent synthetic cannabinoid use can lead to withdrawal signs upon cessation. A more ominous adverse effect of synthetic marijuana use recently reported by the Centers for Disease Control and Prevention is acute renal damage. The risk for overdose and toxicity with synthetic cannabinoids is 30-fold higher than that for cannabis alone.

Clinical Uses

Any therapeutic potential for cannabinoids is currently under investigation, including nonpsychoactive cannabinoids such as cannabidiol and numerous endocannabinoids and the modulators of their synthesis and degradation.

Antiemetic Effect

Two oral formulations described previously are approved by the US Food and Drug Administration to treat emesis refractory to conventional antiemetics as well as related cachexia.

Glaucoma

The synthetic cannabinoid nabilone is marketed in Europe for the treatment of glaucoma, but evidence is lacking that it is more effective than other agents in patients.

Ongoing Preclinical Studies
Appetite Stimulation and Control

Endocannabinoids regulate energy balance and food intake by acting at both central and peripheral sites via the limbic system (ie, the site of the desire or "craving" for food) as well as the hypothalamus and hindbrain. The ECS interacts with a number of other molecules involved in appetite and weight regulation, including leptin, ghrelin, and the melanocortins.

Anticonvulsant Effects

The therapeutic potential of cannabis as an anticonvulsant was shown in the 1940s when children, who were poorly controlled on conventional anticonvulsant medication, improved after the use of cannabis. Current clinical trials with a 99% pure cannabidiol drug show a significant reduction in seizures.

Neurologic and Movement Disorders

Several clinical trials indicate that cannabinoids ameliorate spasticity and pain and improve quality of sleep in patients with multiple sclerosis. Over 90% of patients with multiple sclerosis report improvements after taking cannabis.

Analgesia

CB_1 agonists produce analgesia by acting at several sites along pathways for pain transmission peripherally, spinally, and supraspinally. The modulators of the synthesis, transport, and degradation of the endocannabinoids have become increasingly important therapeutic targets. There is increasing evidence that the CB_2 receptor has multiple effects on inflammation, autoimmune responses, and bone density, which are all potential players in the etiology of inflammatory pain.

DRUG–DRUG INTERACTIONS

There is no rigorous scientific evidence or known neurobiologic basis for a "gateway" effect of cannabis smoking. Such an effect may be due to the increased opportunity of people who use cannabis to associate with those who use of other types of drugs or group peer pressure to use other drugs. Human studies of potential pharmacokinetic interactions of tobacco smoking, tobacco-related products, or tobacco cessation in combination with cannabinoid use reveal that cannabis smoking upregulates the liver metabolic enzymes that are also upregulated by tobacco.

CONCLUSIONS AND FUTURE RESEARCH

As described in ancient sources, cannabinoids appear to have a variety of potentially useful therapeutic effects. The major goal of cannabis researchers is to develop a cannabinoid or endocannabinoid modulator devoid of any undesirable side effects.

KEY POINTS

1. Cannabinoids have historically been shown to have therapeutic uses. The discovery of cannabinoid receptors and the endocannabinoid system has led to novel therapeutic targets.
2. Cannabinoid receptors exist in two recognized isoforms coupled to G proteins: cannabinoid receptor 1 (CB_1), which is highly expressed in certain brain regions, and cannabinoid receptor 2 (CB_2), which is associated with immune cells. Both subtypes are present in a variety of tissues.
3. Endocannabinoids are synthesized "on demand" from membrane lipids and function via "retrograde signaling" to decrease presynaptic neurotransmitter release.
4. The 2016 United Nations World Drug Report concluded that cannabis is the most widely consumed drug worldwide. In addition, increased synthesis and illicit use of novel synthetic

cannabinoids such as "Spice" leads to increased toxicity of the cannabinoids.
5. Human studies indicate that cannabis use produces tolerance, leading to cannabis use disorder, but evidence for a "gateway" to use of other drugs of abuse is lacking.

REVIEW QUESTIONS

1. THC and endocannabinoids decrease neuronal excitability in the brain by which of the following mechanisms?
   A. They bind to presynaptic CB_1 receptors, increasing the release of inhibitory neurotransmitters.
   B. They bind to membrane lipids, increasing the generation of action potentials.
   C. They bind to presynaptic CB_1 receptors, decreasing the release of endocannabinoids.
   D. They bind to presynaptic CB_1 receptors and inhibit presynaptic neurotransmitter release.
   E. They bind to presynaptic CB_1 receptors, activate ion channels, and increase action potentials.

2. CB_1 receptors are found in high densities in certain areas of the brain. How does this correlate with the effects of marijuana?
   A. THC releases endocannabinoids, leading to neuronal death and is thus a very toxic drug.
   B. THC binds to CB_1 receptors, producing alterations in the activity of these areas of the brain and causing many of the effects seen when cannabis is consumed.
   C. THC is an inhibitory neurotransmitter that induces the release of other inhibitory neurotransmitters, leading to reduced neural activity and the perception of being "high."
   D. THC opens ion channels, leading to increased action potentials in certain areas of the brain, leading to the perception of being "high."
   E. THC binds to CB_2 receptors, mobilizing the immune system to attack certain areas of the brain, leading to forgetfulness and decreased movements.

3. Marijuana use is reported in greater than 10% of pregnancies. Marijuana users who are pregnant or planning to become pregnant should be cautioned against marijuana use for all of the reasons *except*:
   A. THC easily passes into breast milk.
   B. THC easily crosses membranes and is transferred to the developing fetus.

C. only marijuana use in females is shown to impact pregnancy success.

D. human studies on the effect of prenatal THC exposure on the developing brain are preliminary but correlate with studies carried out in animals.

E. animal studies show that prenatal marijuana use impacts brain development.

ANSWERS

1. **D**
2. **B**
3. **C**

SUGGESTED READINGS

Castaneto MS, Gorelick DA, Desrosiers NA, et al. Synthetic cannabinoids: epidemiology, pharmacodynamics, and clinical implications. *Drug Alcohol Depend*. 2014;144:12-41.

Deshpande A, Mailis-Gagnon A, Zoheiry N, Lakha SF. Efficacy and adverse effects of medical marijuana for chronic non-cancer pain: systematic review of randomized controlled trials. *Can Fam Physician*. 2015;61(8):e372-e381.

National Academies of Sciences, Engineering, and Medicine. *The Health Effects of Cannabis and Cannabinoids: The Current State of Evidence and Recommendations for Research*. Washington, DC: National Academies Press, 2017.

National Institute on Drug Abuse. Monitoring the Future. https://www.drugabuse.gov/related-topics/trends-statistics/monitoring-future. Revised November 17, 2018. Released December 17, 2018.

Pertwee RG. Endocannabinoids and their pharmacological actions. *Handb Exp Pharmacol*. 2015;231:1-37.

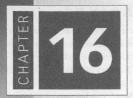

The Pharmacology of Hallucinogens

Summary by Manassa Hany

Based on THE ASAM PRINCIPLES OF ADDICTION MEDICINE, 6th edition chapter by Michael P. Bogenschutz and David E. Nichols

Hallucinogens are chemically divergent substances primarily used for their potential to alter the processing of cognitive, perceptual, and emotional understanding of self and reality. Although most hallucinogens produce alterations of perceived objects and pseudohallucinations, the term *hallucinogen* is considered not ideal because it overemphasizes perceptual changes at the expense of the often more significant changes in thought, cognition, and affectivity.

HALLUCINOGENIC SUBSTANCES

Classical hallucinogens include mescaline, psilocybin, lysergic acid diethylamide (LSD), and dimethyltryptamine (DMT). Entactogenic phenylalkylamines include methylenedioxyamphetamine, 3,4-methylenedioxymethamphetamine (MDMA), and methylenedioxyethylamphetamine. Anticholinergic dissociatives include atropine, hyoscyamine, and scopolamine. Dissociative anesthetics and miscellaneous hallucinogens include phencyclidine, ketamine, and salvinorin A.

NEUROBIOLOGY

The classical hallucinogens have high affinity for 5-hydroxytryptamine (5-HT) receptors. Phenylalkylamine hallucinogens are highly selective for 5-HT_{2A}, 5-HT_{2B}, and 5-HT_{2C} receptors, and their effects are likely exclusively 5-HT_2 mediated. Indolealkylamine hallucinogens are relatively nonselective for 5-HT receptors. The 5-HT_{2A} receptor appears to be the primary site of action. Genetic or pharmacologic inactivation of 5-HT_{2A} receptors blocks behavioral effects in preclinical models as well as subjective effects in humans. Hallucinogens enhance glutamatergic transmission in the cortex. Activation of 5-HT_{2A} leads to increased cortical glutamate levels probably mediated by thalamic afferents, which may alter corticocortical and corticosubcortical transmission. There is growing consensus that the glutamatergic

and serotonergic systems interact in complex ways and regulate each other. Most hallucinogens are partial agonists at the 5-HT_{2C} receptor. Activity at the 5-HT_{2C} receptor serves to attenuate many behavioral effects of hallucinogens. Some hallucinogens also interact with dopamine receptors and directly or indirectly activate dopamine pathways. Few studies have evaluated the dopaminergic effects of hallucinogens. There is evidence that LSD interacts with central dopamine D1 and D2 receptors. However, most hallucinogens do not significantly interact with the dopamine system. 5-HT_{2A} receptor activation in the reticular thalamic nucleus as induced by hallucinogens might increase the level of inhibitory input to relay cells, which leads to a loss of sensory-specific inhibition of thalamic nuclei. This results in relay cells recruited into thalamocortical circuits without receiving adequate sensory input and the formation of coherent assemblies of thalamocortical oscillations that would be independent of afferent sensory inputs—that is, hallucinogenic activity.

METHODS OF USE

Hallucinogenic substances influence information flow throughout the brain, thereby inducing an altered state of mind that affects conceptual cognition, affectivity, and sensory processing. Some of these actions might induce a specific matrix of brain alterations that could be beneficial for neuropsychiatric disorders. The notion that some of these substances have potential as medical and psychological treatments has emerged over the last decade. Their specific value may lie in the short-term rearrangement of brain activity, rather than in tonic long-term action as from antidepressants, psychostimulants, and neuroleptics.

Clinical Uses

More than 10,000 subjects received LSD (and other hallucinogens) from 1950 to the mid-1960s in controlled research settings, which was applied to educate psychiatric staff through the temporary self-experience of quasipsychotic states. Another important application was psychoanalytic therapy. These therapeutic approaches were later abandoned not for reasons of safety or lack of efficacy but because of criminalization of the substances.

Nonmedical Use

With the social turmoil of the 1960s student movement, use of these compounds, typically in less structured/"permissive" settings, often resulted in careless experimentation. Because of user inexperience with these drugs, a mass wave of complications resulted, which then established their new image as dangerous drugs. These complications resulted not rarely in indirect medical (eg, physical accidents) and/or psychological emergencies (eg, brief psychotic reactions, suicidality), causing emergency department visit. Hallucinogen use disorder as listed in the *Diagnostic and Statistical Manual of Mental Disorders*, 5th edition (*DSM-5*) and the *International Statistical Classification of Diseases and Related Health Problems*, 10th edition (*ICD-10*) is characterized (mild, moderate, or severe) by patterns of compulsive and repeated drug use despite the knowledge of significant harm caused by the activity. Hallucinogen use very rarely leads to the development of typical psychological (but not physical) dependence syndromes, such as seen with opiates or alcohol. As a class, the hallucinogens lack a significant direct effect on the dopamine-mediated reward system; animals cannot be trained to self-administer these compounds. In contrast to users of other substances of abuse, hallucinogen users do not experience withdrawal symptoms, and therefore, this trait is not a criterion for diagnosing hallucinogen dependence. In general, tolerance increases when hallucinogens are used with frequency, exponentially so with daily use.

EPIDEMIOLOGY

The 2010 National Survey on Drug Use and Health estimated that almost 37.5 million Americans (14.8%) over age 12 years ingested a hallucinogen at least once in their lifetime. Excluding data on the dissociative "hallucinogen" phencyclidine, less than 1% of hallucinogen users had an emergency department visit related to their hallucinogen use in 2009 (compared with 5.5% of methamphetamine users, 8.8% of cocaine users, and 35.2% of heroin users).

LSD is still the most widely used hallucinogenic drug; 23.3 million Americans used LSD at least once in their lifetime. Since the 1970s, there has been no decline in its use.

Psilocybe mushrooms appear to be the most common hallucinogen consumed in the previous year among new hallucinogen users.

Mescaline has never been synthesized and distributed for illicit purposes in the United States on a significant scale, and it is not mentioned in any drug abuse survey. The mescaline-containing peyote cactus plant is protected by the American Indian Religious Freedom Act of 1994 and is almost solely consumed in religious prayer services of the Native American Church.

DMT was never a significant drug of abuse. Since the 1960s, it was used only in tiny circles, and no significant abuse has been reported up to today.

Salvia divinorum is still legal in much of the United States. Today, an estimated 1.8 million people in the United States has tried this plant. The 2011 Monitoring the Future Survey reported an increasing trend with an annual prevalence of S. *divinorum* use in young adults of 2.5%.

Some 15.9 million Americans have tried *MDMA* at least once in their life, with 2.6 million trying it for the first time in 2010. Its use is concentrated among young adults in the age range of 15 to 25 years. In general, hallucinogens show a constant pattern of use and abuse, with MDMA showing a peak in the 1990s and a stable level since 2000.

PHARMACOKINETICS AND PHARMACODYNAMICS

Lysergic Acid Diethylamide

LSD is a semisynthetic substance derived from lysergic acid as found in the parasitic rye fungus *Claviceps purpurea*. LSD was synthesized in 1938, and its effects were discovered in 1943.

Pharmacokinetics

LSD is completely absorbed in the digestive tract; psychological and sympathomimetic effects reach their peak after 1.5 to 2.5 hours. Over the next 8 hours, plasma levels gradually fall until only a small amount of LSD is present. The half-life of LSD in humans is 175 minutes. The presence of considerable amounts in the brain and cerebrospinal fluid of rats and cats indicates that LSD may easily cross the blood–brain barrier.

Pharmacodynamics

LSD-induced sympathetic stimulation is evidenced by pupillary dilation and slight increases in heart rate (+ 5 to 15 beats per minute) and blood pressure

(10 to 15 mm Hg systolic); other more inconsistent signs are slight blood sugar elevation and, rarely, a minimal increase in body temperature. Bradycardia, hypotension, and slightly increased perspiration may occur. Respiration remains unchanged. Initial nausea, decreased appetite, temporary mild headache, dizziness, and inner trembling may occur. The most consistent neurologic effect is an exaggeration of the patellar (and other deep tendon) reflexes. No changes occur in liver and renal functions, blood cells, or electrolytes. LSD increases serum growth hormone but does not alter serum prolactin levels.

Tolerance to autonomic and psychological effects of LSD occurs after a few moderate daily doses. There have been no documented human deaths from an LSD overdose due to toxicity. The lethal dose of LSD in humans is estimated to be 1,400 mg.

Subjective Effects

A moderate oral dose (75 to 150 µg) of LSD will significantly alter the state of consciousness, including stimulation of affect, enhanced capacity for introspection, and altered psychological functioning in the direction of hypnagogia and dreams. Typical perceptual changes include illusions, pseudohallucinations, and synesthesia as well as alterations of thinking and time experience. Thinking processes can be affected at higher doses (>100 µg) of LSD. Time intervals are regularly overestimated. There is no evidence for long-lasting impairments in performance after LSD intake. The acute psychological effects of LSD last between 6 and 10 hours, depending on the dose. Traumatic experiences (called "bad trips") can have long-lasting effects, including mood swings and, more rarely, flashback phenomena. Conversely, it has been shown that under controlled and supportive conditions, the hallucinogen experience may have lasting positive effects on attitudes and personality in healthy humans.

Psilocybin

The total content of psilocybin varies with mushroom type, subspecies type, and preparation, but the most commonly used, *Psilocybe cubensis*, contains 5 to 11 mg of psilocybin per gram of dried mushroom.

Pharmacokinetics

Psilocybin and its active metabolite psilocin are substituted hallucinogenic indolealkylamines. It is readily absorbed following oral administration and is widely distributed throughout the body.

Psilocybin and psilocin are detectable in the plasma within 20 to 40 minutes following ingestion.

The full effects occur within 70 to 90 minutes following oral doses of 8 to 25 mg. The half-life of psilocybin is 163.3 ± 63.5 minutes. The mean elimination half-life of psilocin is 50 minutes. The maximum plasma concentration occurs at approximately 80 minutes, which can vary. Elimination occurs through the kidneys. Peak intoxication occurs approximately within the first 2 hours, diminishing over the subsequent 3 to 4 hours. Even though significant tolerance is known to occur with repeated daily use of psilocybin, neither physical dependence nor a withdrawal syndrome develops. There are no direct deaths from psilocybin reported in the scientific literature. Complications arising from use of psilocybin (eg, severe panic reactions, "bad trips") resulting in emergency department visits occur with less frequency than with most other hallucinogens, possibly due to its short duration of action.

Pharmacodynamics

Neurovegetative effects within the usual dose range (10 to 25 mg orally) include mydriasis, slight acceleration in heart and breathing rate, and discrete hyperglycemic and hypertonic effects. Nausea and sleepiness can occur in the initial phase of intoxication. Ingestion of *Psilocybe* mushrooms can cause nausea and vomiting, but serious toxicity has not been reported in humans. The predicted human lethal dose of psilocybin is 14,000 mg, which is equivalent to 4 kg of dried mushrooms, an amount unlikely to be consumed.

Subjective Effects

The psychopathologic phenomena induced by psilocybin are virtually identical to those of LSD. At a moderate dose (12 to 20 mg orally), psilocybin produced an altered state of consciousness marked by a stimulation of affect, enhanced ability for introspection, and altering of psychological functioning. Especially noteworthy are perceptual changes such as illusions; synesthesia; affective activation; and alterations of thought, time sense, and body experience. Most psilocybin users display an erratic pattern of use. The intense consciousness-altering/consciousness-expanding (ie, psychologically irritating) effects of psilocybin appear to limit frequency of its use. Daily consumption of psilocybin results in acute tolerance, and such users are virtually unknown in the scientific literature.

Dimethyltryptamine

DMT is derived from various plant sources and animal venoms. DMT is also produced endogenously in humans in miniscule amounts. Its physiologic functions are still unknown, although it was recently found to be an endogenous σ_1 receptor agonist.

Pharmacokinetics

DMT is quickly absorbed and distributed throughout the body and the brain. Maximal plasma levels are reached 2 minutes after intravenous administration and 107.5 minutes after oral intake of ayahuasca. DMT and its metabolites are eliminated after 30 to 70 minutes. No unchanged DMT is excreted in human urine, but 90% of its metabolites are excreted.

In contrast to other classical hallucinogens, DMT does not induce tolerance in humans.

Pharmacodynamics

After smoking or via the intravenous route, initial effects occur in 30 to 60 seconds, peaking within 2 to 3 minutes; and then clearing over the next 15 to 20 minutes. When ingested orally as the ayahuasca brew, effects commence after 30 to 60 minutes, peak within the first hour, and last for 3 to 4 hours. Ayahuasca is typically associated with a considerable amount of nausea and vomiting, which may alter its absorption. High doses may lead to seizure. Vegetative symptoms are predominant at intravenous doses of 0.05 to 0.1 mg/kg, whereas hallucinatory effects predominate at doses of 0.2 to 0.4 mg/kg. DMT significantly increases blood pressure (+ 15 to 30 mm Hg) and heart rate (+ 10 beats per minute), often combined with an oppressed feeling in the chest and a sympathomimetic excitation syndrome with mydriasis, hallucinations, and overarousal. These effects are significantly less (blood pressure: + 8 to 15 mm Hg, no change of heart rate) when DMT is ingested as ayahuasca. Respiration rates increase only slightly with oral intake. Some subjects develop slight involuntary extrapyramidal movements. There are no lethal intoxications documented in the literature.

Subjective Effects

Dysphoria or euphoria, subjective impression of breathing difficulties, and sensory disturbances resulting in impaired performance occur in multiple domains. The psychological effects can be very frightening and may lead to severe unintended injuries because of disorientation, motor incoordination, and unrealistic thoughts and behaviors. Complications are very rare, especially by the oral route, and may not appear in clinical settings because of its very short duration of action. The psychological effects of DMT are milder with orally ingested ayahuasca (than with the pure drug) and are very similar to those of LSD and psilocybin.

Mescaline

The principal hallucinogenic compound of the peyote cactus is mescaline, although over 60 other alkaloids are also found in peyote. Although mescaline is regularly mentioned as a "classical hallucinogen" in the scientific literature, its use as a recreational drug is rather limited. There have been virtually no seizures of significant amounts of synthetic mescaline in the United States, and it is almost never mentioned in statistics of emergency department visits. There are no serious physical complications or dependency syndromes from peyote or mescaline documented in the scientific literature.

Pharmacokinetics

Peyote contains, at most, 1.5% of mescaline sulfate. The cactus has a bitter, acrid taste, often inducing nausea and vomiting. The usual human dosage is 200 to 400 mg of mescaline sulfate or 175 to 350 mg of mescaline hydrochloride. The average 76-mm (3.0-in) button contains about 25 mg of mescaline. Mescaline taken orally is absorbed rapidly and completely in the gastrointestinal tract. The onset of effects is typically 30 to 45 minutes. A maximum concentration in the brain builds up in 30 to 120 minutes. Peak intoxication occurs within 2 to 4 hours, wearing off over the subsequent 4 to 6 hours. The plasma level correlates with an intensity of psychological effects. Mescaline easily crosses the blood–brain barrier. Complete tolerance develops gradually within a few days and builds with repeated usage, lasting for a few days. The lethal dose is estimated to be 6000 mg.

Pharmacodynamics

Somatic effects from mescaline intoxication include mydriasis, dizziness, diarrhea, nausea and vomiting, headache, dilated pupils, abdominal cramps, sweating, warm and cold sensations, and tremors and feelings of weakness. Somatic effects are strongest in the first 1 to 2 hours, then subside, and replaced by a dreamlike hallucinogenic state that lasts 5 to 12 hours, depending on the dose. No serious somatic side effects or lethality has been reported from mescaline. There is no evidence of lasting cognitive or psychophysical effects with mescaline.

Subjective Effects

The typical mescaline intoxication is characterized by a dreamlike state with enhanced alertness and affectivity; euphoric or dysphoric mood states; sensory–perceptual distortion; alterations of space and time sense; altered perception of color, sound, and shapes; complex hallucinations; synesthesia;

deconstructed perception; depersonalization; and ecstatic or mystical states of mind. Prominence of color is distinctive, appearing brilliant and intense. Recurring visual patterns observed during the mescaline experience include stripes, checkerboards, angular spikes, multicolored dots, and very simple fractals, which turn very complex.

Salvia Divinorum and Salvinorin A

Salvinorin A is structurally unrelated to any other hallucinogen and is found in the mint plant S. *divinorum.*

Pharmacokinetics

Most commonly inhaled by smoking, S. *divinorum* could be inhaled via volatilization or buccal absorption of tinctures. If taken orally, it has a mild effect, often compared to cannabis. Salvinorin A is only minimally absorbed through the mouth; most is degraded in the gastrointestinal tract.

Pharmacodynamics

Salvinorin A works as a κ-opioid receptor agonist, with no evidence that it works on other receptor systems, but the endocannabinoid system may play a role in its effects. More potent effects occur when smoked than when orally ingested. The psychological effects consist of mood changes and strange hallucinations that appear within seconds and may last from 30 minutes to more than 2 hours, depending on the dose. When smoked in higher concentrations, salvinorin A produces a rapid and intense hallucinogenic effect that typically lasts between 10 and 15 minutes and includes a "highly modified perception of external reality." Users become less aware of their surroundings as the dose increases, which may generate disorientation, incoordination, and potentially unrealistic self-destructive behavior. Loss of consciousness is common with higher doses. Unpleasant aftereffects include tiredness, heaviness of head, dizziness, and "mental cloudiness" lasting 24 hours or more after use. There are no reported cases of severe toxicity or deaths from overdose, and little evidence of psychiatric dysfunction lasting beyond acute effects. There are no reports of a withdrawal syndrome and no evidence that it leads to addictive behaviors.

Subjective Effects

The most commonly reported desirable psychological effects include laughter, happiness, separation from body, relaxation, and perceptual changes. There is a mild hallucinogenic effect, comparable to cannabis, from lower doses of salvinorin A and a more dissociative pattern of effects from higher doses, with serious hallucinatory effects and loosening contact with reality. There is no significant euphoria, whereas dysphoria often occurs, which may partially explain its typical erratic use pattern. Larger doses are typically aversive, and few people want to repeat the experience. The strange perceptual altering effects and lack of euphoria may also explain its pattern of intermittent use.

MDMA ("Ecstasy")

MDMA belongs to the entactogens and produces only minimal sensory effects (eg, pseudohallucinations) but consistently increases feelings of elation. It has some amphetaminelike stimulant effects mediated through the release or reuptake inhibition of dopamine and noradrenaline.

Pharmacokinetics

Maximum plasma levels after a typical oral dose of MDMA (1.6 mg/kg) are reached 1.5 to 2.5 hours after ingestion. Plasma levels decrease slowly over the following 10 hours. Excretion is more than 95% completed after 24 hours. Complex, nonlinear pharmacokinetics result from inhibition of CYP2D6 and CYP2D8 by MDMA and, in turn, results in higher-than-expected concentrations if the person takes consecutive doses. MDMA and its metabolites are excreted as conjugated glucuronides and sulfates through the kidneys, but more than 50% of MDMA is excreted unchanged in urine.

Pharmacodynamics

The first effects of MDMA are usually experienced within 30 minutes after an oral dose of 85 to 150 mg. Most individuals claim peak effects between 30 minutes to 1 hour after intake. Gender-specific sensitivity to the effects of MDMA has been reported, with stronger effects in females. Stimulant effects occur soon after ingestion, including increased energy and elevated mood. Additional side effects include nausea, jaw clenching, muscle tension, and blurred vision.

Somatic effects of MDMA (100 to 125 mg orally) include loss of appetite, diaphoresis, and bruxism. Dose-dependent increased blood pressure from MDMA is between 20 to 35 mm Hg systolic and 10 to 20 mm Hg diastolic. MDMA increases the heart rate around 10 to 20 beats per minute and body temperature by 0.3°C to 0.4°C. MDMA has significant dose-dependent effects on the endocrine system, with increases in cortisol, prolactin, vasopressin, and growth hormone. Stimulant effects, as noted previously, occur soon after ingestion, including increased energy and elevated mood. Additional side effects include nausea, jaw clenching, muscle tension, and blurred vision. A "hangover" for some hours or more can occur, with symptoms of insomnia, fatigue, sore muscles, headache, and decreased mood. Intense pleasure and increased physical stamina are sought by dance party ("rave") consumers of MDMA. Use of methamphetamine and cocaine in combination with MDMA increases the risk of serotonin syndrome.

Subjective Effects

Typical psychological reactions to MDMA in healthy, MDMA-naïve adult research volunteers include improved disposition, increased physical well-being associated with vague symptoms of derealization and depersonalization, impaired thinking, and occasional feelings of anxiety with no increase in psychomotor drive. The affective changes were, overall, positively received. Subjects described a greater attention to feelings, more openness, and an increased sense of closeness to others. MDMA ingested recreationally, however, may pose special risks to users. MDMA use may induce paranoid psychotic states, anxiety, and/or depression. In some affected individuals, symptoms may persist for days or weeks.

RELATIVE ADDICTION LIABILITY

Use of hallucinogens very rarely meets the *ICD-10* or *DSM-5* criteria for a substance use disorder. The classical hallucinogens do not induce physical dependence or a withdrawal syndrome. There are no reports of a withdrawal syndrome from salvinorin A. Additionally, all classical hallucinogens induce tolerance relatively immediately—that is, after a few days. Therefore, more frequent (eg, daily) use will lead to little or no acute intoxication after a very short period of use (days), possibly discouraging extended periods of frequent use. This is different with the entactogens like MDMA. Entactogens lead to a massive depletion of intracellular serotonin, and therefore, the serotonin storage is emptied, and no entactogenic effects will occur after a very few daily ingestions. Meanwhile, the more amphetaminelike effects from entactogens still occur: psychophysical excitation, anorexia, overarousal, restlessness, and sleeplessness. Addiction resulting from the frequent use of entactogens is consistently reported, but psychological features play a more pronounced role than physical ones. Studies suggest that addiction to entactogens may have another structure than those related to alcohol, stimulants, or opiates. The classical hallucinogens, as well as salvinorin A, have negative reinforcing properties in animal studies. Virtually all the hallucinogenic drugs do not directly affect dopamine neurotransmission. MDMA shares some pharmacologic properties with the amphetamines and, therefore, has some reinforcing efficacy but significantly less than methamphetamine and cocaine. There is behavioral evidence that the endocannabinoid system is a modulator of the rewarding/reinforcing properties of MDMA.

CONCLUSIONS AND FUTURE RESEARCH

The hallucinogens represent a heterogeneous class of substances with individually different effects as well as diverse mechanisms of action. These substances are physiologically well tolerated in medium-range doses. Their main complications result from unsupervised use and may lead to serious psychological problems. Their dependence liability is not as high as with most other psychoactive drugs. If MDMA and phencyclidine, as well as deliriants like atropine and nitrous oxide, are included in the category of hallucinogens, the spectrum of side effects and dependence potential is broader. Hallucinogenic substances stimulate neuroreceptors in a diverse and often quite nonselective fashion. Therefore, they were sometimes called "dirty ligands," that is, acting as agonists, partial agonists, or even antagonists on a vast range of receptors. Their "diffuse" mode of action may be due to their multiple receptor interactions. These multiple actions may imply a more "holistic" action, which leads to psychophysically useful and, in some cases, consciousness-expanding, enjoyable, and insightful states that may be useful in a therapeutic context. Because research with these agents was interrupted in the mid-1960s, their potential was not thoroughly evaluated. Renewed research may open new avenues for psychiatric and other therapies. Recently published studies used psilocybin and LSD or bromo-LSD for cluster headaches, MDMA in the psychotherapy of posttraumatic stress disorder, psilocybin in end-of-life anxiety, and ketamine in depression. Hallucinogens may also be used for research into experimentally induced psychotic states.

KEY POINTS

1. Hallucinogens are a heterogeneous class of substances with individually different effects as well as diverse mechanisms of action that are not fully understood.
2. Their dependence liability is not as high as with most other psychoactive drugs.
3. Because research with these agents was interrupted in the mid-1960s, their potential was not thoroughly evaluated.
4. Renewed research may open new avenues to utilize them for psychiatric and other therapies.

REVIEW QUESTIONS

1. Which of the following is true about the effects of MDMA that are usually experienced within 30 minutes after an oral dose of 85 to 150 mg?
   A. Effects are stronger in males.
   B. Effects include increased energy and elevated mood.
   C. A "hangover" occurs for hours or more, whereas symptoms of insomnia never occur.
   D. Systolic blood pressure is decreased by 10 to 20 mm Hg.

2. The 2010 National Survey on Drug Use and Health estimated that almost 37.5 million Americans (14.8%) over age 12 years ingested a hallucinogen at least once in their lifetime. Which of the following statements is true?
   A. Mescaline is the most common hallucinogen in the previous year among new users.
   B. *Psilocybe* mushrooms are still the most widely used hallucinogenic drug.
   C. There has been no decline in LSD use.
   D. DMT has been a significant drug of abuse.

3. Which of the following is true concerning the mint plant *Salvia divinorum*, which is structurally unrelated to any other hallucinogen?
   A. It is illegal in much of the United States.
   B. It works as a μ-opioid receptor agonist.
   C. It has more potent effects when orally ingested than smoked.
   D. There are no reports of withdrawal syndromes and no evidence that it leads to addictive behavior.

ANSWERS

1. **B.** Its effects include increased energy and elevated mood, which explains using MDMA at "raves." Its effects are stronger in females, it can have a "hangover" effect, and it can lead to an increase in blood pressure.

2. **C.** According to the 2010 National Survey on Drug Use and Health, there has not been a decline in LSD use. LSD still is the most widely used hallucinogenic drug. *Psilocybe* mushrooms are the most common hallucinogen consumed in the previous year among new hallucinogen users. DMT has never been a significant drug of abuse.

3. **D.** *S. divinorum* is still legal in much of the United States. It works as a κ-opioid receptor agonist, and it has more potent effects when smoked rather than ingested orally.

SUGGESTED READINGS

Grinspoon L, Bakalar JB. *Psychedelic Drugs Reconsidered*. New York: Basic Books, 1979.

Hoffer A, Osmond H. *The Hallucinogens*. New York: Academic Press, 1967.

Passie T. *Healing with Entactogens: Therapist and Patient Perspectives on MDMA-Assisted Group Psychotherapy*. Santa Cruz, CA: MAPS, 2012.

Sessa B. *The Psychedelic Renaissance: Reassessing the Role of Psychedelic Drugs in 21st Century Psychiatry and Society*. London: Muswell Hill Press, 2012.

CHAPTER 17

The Pharmacology of Dissociatives

Summary by Edward F. Domino and Shannon C. Miller

Based on THE ASAM PRINCIPLES OF ADDICTION MEDICINE,
6th edition chapter by Edward F. Domino and Shannon C. Miller

DEFINITION (DRUGS IN THIS CLASS)

A simplified view suggests that dissociatives and hallucinogens share common features. However, dissociatives are distinguished pharmacologically and clinically from hallucinogens. Hallucinogens affect primarily 5-HT$_{2A}$ receptors, and dissociatives affect glutamic acid N-methyl-D-aspartate (NMDA) receptors. Hallucinogens are associated with a different 5-HT$_{2A}$–associated clinical syndrome of intoxication (whereby dissociation or impaired reality testing is less typically involved and visual hallucinations are more commonly involved). Dissociatives include various arylcyclohexylamines (of which phencyclidine [PCP] and ketamine are best known), dizocilpine (MK-801), dextromethorphan (DXM), and the gaseous anesthetic, nitrous oxide. Nitrous oxide or "laughing gas" is not typically classified as a dissociative (more commonly considered an inhalant); however, given its NMDA antagonist and dissociative-like clinical effect, it merits inclusion in this chapter. Dissociatives share the clinical effect of causing a dissociative state of intoxication, which is desired by the user.

SUBSTANCES INCLUDED IN THIS CLASS

PCP and ketamine are the principal illicit drugs. DXM is the principal over-the-counter drug. Ketamine is a racemic mixture of D- and L-isomers. The (S)-isomer is more potent and is claimed to have less dysphoric effects. Other members of this class that are less commonly used include cyclohexamine (N-ethyl-1-phenylcyclohexylamine, CI 400), 1-(1-(2-thienyl)cyclohexyl)piperidine, 1-(1-phenylcyclohexyl)pyrrolidine, and 4-methyl pip PCP (1-(phenylcyclohexyl)-4-methylpiperidine). DXM (DM, D-3-methoxy-N-methylmorphinan) is the D-isomer of a codeine analogue, methorphan. In contrast to the L-isomer, which is an opioid analgesic, DXM is not. The PCP-derived designer drug N-(1-phenylcyclohexyl)-3-methoxypropanamine and the ketamine analogue methoxetamine should also be included in this class.

US FOOD AND DRUG ADMINISTRATION–APPROVED FORMULATIONS

Ketamine (Ketalar) is available as a sterile solution for use in general anesthesia in both animals and humans. It has also been used for prehospital analgesia, anesthesia, and conscious sedation and is currently being researched as a rapid-acting agent to reduce suicidal ideation (non-FDA approved).

PCP is no longer available as a medical commercial preparation approved by the FDA. It is available in many illicit preparations and has many of the pharmacologic effects of ketamine but is more potent, longer acting, and more likely to produce seizures. Doses of only 120 mg of PCP may cause death.

When taken as directed, DXM has a low toxicity and high therapeutic index. Capsules, tablets, lozenges, or solutions of DXM are available alone or in combination with many other substances as cough, cold, and flu relief preparations. Larger doses of DXM are used in unhealthy ways to achieve dissociation and may result in addiction. The additional ingredients in over-the-counter preparations make for additional hazards: decongestant/pseudoephedrine (cardiac toxicity), antihistamine/chlorpheniramine (antihistamine toxicity), pain/acetaminophen (liver toxicity), and bromides (bromide toxicity).

HISTORICAL FEATURES

PCP was developed as an intravenous anesthetic. The unique anesthesia it produced was complicated by a prolonged emergence delirium, which led to its demise as a clinically useful agent. PCP is associated with symptoms that model both the positive (delusions, hallucinations) and negative (blunted affect, autistic-like effects) symptoms of schizophrenia.

Years later, PCP was rediscovered by the recreational drug use community and has also been known as "angel dust," "hog," and "crystal."

The desirable anesthetic properties of PCP were retained in the short-acting arylcyclohexylamine derivative ketamine, which produced a more brief emergence delirium. The term *dissociative anesthetic* was coined to emphasize that the anesthetized patient was psychologically "disconnected" from his or her environment. Ketamine subsequently was discovered by the recreational drug use community, where it is known as "K," "super K," "special K," and "cat Valium," among others. Ketamine has the reputation among users as being medically safe to use because it is made by pharmaceutical companies, most often for veterinary use.

Because the drugs are easy to synthesize, they are relatively inexpensive substitutes for many street drugs. The user may not realize that he or she has used an arylcyclohexylamine because the drugs frequently are misrepresented as LSD-25, amphetamine, or synthetic marijuana. Moreover, they may be added to marijuana by the user to enhance marijuana's desired effects.

The history of DXM begins with the synthesis of racemethorphan (deoxydihydrothebaiodine) or methorphan (Dromoran). After the D- and L-isomers were isolated, it was discovered that the D-isomer was antitussive and had less analgesic- and narcotic-like properties. DXM is nearly equal to codeine as an antitussive. However, unlike codeine, DXM is fairly devoid of other opioid effects such as analgesia, central nervous system depression, and respiratory suppression. DXM is metabolized to dextrorphan (DXO), an NMDA receptor antagonist, which is the more psychoactive form. DXO binding sites in the brain include more than the NMDA receptor. DXM's mechanism in low doses as an antitussive is unknown. In doses of 300 to 1,800 mg (20 to 120 times the recommended dose), DXM produces PCP-like mental effects. Recreational DXM use has been a concern since at least the 1960s. Although recreational use of DXM began originally with liquid cough syrup (known to hamper the use of large doses of DXM because of the distasteful nature of cough syrup), more convenient consumer products have since been developed, including both high-dose (30 mg) tablets as well as high-dose gel capsules, which are preferred by those who use DXM recreationally. Acid–base extraction techniques have been developed by users to "free base" the DXM alone.

Nitrous oxide has been known for more than 225 years. It is widely used today in anesthesia. In addition, its recreational use as "laughing gas" has been well described since it was first discovered. Ketamine and nitrous oxide still are medically used in humans as anesthetic agents. Ketamine is used in circumstances in which other anesthetic agents are relatively contraindicated. In contrast, nitrous oxide is widely used today as part of the mixture of anesthetics used to achieve "balanced anesthesia."

EPIDEMIOLOGY

Unhealthy or recreational PCP use is more of a problem in larger cities. Ketamine is often used with other drugs; however, sole use of ketamine has been reported and is increasing in areas such as Asia. Although ketamine has often been self-administered by insufflation, there is an emerging problem in youth of injecting ketamine. Such youth are more likely to engage in multiple injections, shared bottles of ketamine, and use of syringes obtained from secondary sources—practices that increase risk for hepatitis C, HIV, and other infectious diseases.

DXM is considered one of the most commonly abused over-the-counter medications in the United States. American Association of Poison Control Centers data support increasing DXM recreational use, particularly among adolescents.

PHARMACOKINETICS

The pharmacokinetics of PCP in humans have never been well studied with psychoactive doses using modern methods. Blood PCP concentrations from 7 to 240 ng/mL (mean, 75 ng/mL) were found in arrested persons intoxicated in public or driving under its influence. The blood/plasma concentration ratio is 1. The plasma half-life ($t_{1/2}$) of PCP has been reported to vary from 7 to 46 hours, suggesting the influence of dose and/or multiphase elimination processes. PCP is biotransformed in the liver to several metabolites and excreted in the urine as both free and glucuronide conjugates. Acidification of the urine increases its renal clearance because PCP is a base. However, this maneuver is no longer recommended clinically because of the risk of increasing urinary myoglobin precipitation.

Ketamine's greater lipophilicity than PCP accounts for its rapid onset, short anesthetic duration of action, and shorter period of emergence delirium. Plasma concentrations of ketamine vary widely depending on the dose, route, and time elapsed since administration. Anesthetic doses produce plasma or serum concentrations of 1.0 to 6.3 μg/mL, and nonanesthetic psychoactive blood concentrations of ketamine are in the low nanogram per milliliter range (100 to 400 ng/mL). Ketamine follows a three-phase plasma pharmacokinetic model when given intravenously. There is a brief initial (alpha) phase with $t_{1/2}$ of about 7 minutes because of rapid redistribution, followed by a longer elimination (beta) phase with $t_{1/2}$ of 3 to 4 hours. As used in general anesthesia, an intravenous dose of 2.0 mg/kg produces rapid induction. This dose produces an onset in 30 seconds, with the coma lasting for 8 to 10 minutes. The intramuscular injection of ketamine has a latency of 3 to 5 minutes and a duration of 10 to 20 minutes or more, depending on the dose administered.

DXM is readily absorbed from the gut. Peak serum levels are reached at 2 to 3 hours for immediate release and 6 hours for sustained release preparations. DXO levels peak at 1.6 to 7 hours. Humans have a genetic polymorphism for the biotransformation of DXM. Rapid metabolizers have a plasma elimination $t_{1/2}$ of about 3.4 hours, and slow metabolizers may have $t_{1/2}$'s exceeding 24 hours. Slow metabolizers of DXM represent about 10% to 15% of the population. Phenotypic "slow" metabolizers of DXM report fewer intoxication effects than normal subjects. Thus, clinically slow metabolizers might be at higher risk for developing DXM use disorder/addiction.

PHARMACODYNAMICS

Depending on the dose and specific arylcyclohexylamine ingested, patients who have taken PCP or ketamine present with varying neurologic and psychiatric signs and symptoms. These signs and symptoms can be generally subdivided into three major clinical pictures: (1) confusion, delirium, and psychosis; (2) semicoma and coma; and (3) coma with seizures. Patients may become progressively more obtunded and eventually comatose, or the reverse, with the patient emerging from coma and showing emergence delirium. Most PCP users do not grossly overdose themselves to the point of semicoma and coma. Hence, most patients intoxicated with PCP show a clinical picture of confusion, delirium, and psychosis. Tolerance occurs with PCP and to a greater degree with continuous dosing. Human evidence remains limited regarding dissociative withdrawal.

The clinical effects of ketamine are akin to PCP and include analgesia, dissociation, hallucinations, and anesthesia. Agitation and cardiovascular and respiratory stimulation tend to be less than with PCP. Violence and unintended trauma may also result. Long-term chronic effects include dysphoria, impaired memory and cognition, apathy, and irritability as well as distortion in the subjective experience

of time. Chronic ketamine use has been associated with increased serum levels of brain-derived neurotrophic factor. Some anecdotal evidence supports the potential for tolerance and physical dependence with ketamine, but this needs further study.

DXM has significant serotonergic properties, including increasing the synthesis and release of serotonin, as well as inhibiting the reuptake of serotonin from the synaptic cleft. DXM in clinical therapeutic doses produces relatively few side effects. These include body rash, itching, nausea, and vomiting and are most likely when DXM is combined with the other ingredients in cough preparations. Depending on the dose, the drug can cause drowsiness, dizziness, altered vision, and cardiovascular and significant central nervous system effects that may resemble PCP intoxication. Euphoria and hallucinosis can occur within 15 to 30 minutes of ingestion of intoxicating doses, with peak effects experienced after roughly 2.5 hours. An intoxication state can persist in varying degrees for about 3 to 6 hours (called a "plateau"). DXO is a stronger NMDA receptor antagonist than DXM. DXO is relatively inactive at μ-, κ-, and δ-opioid receptor sites; thus, it is essentially devoid of the more conventional opioid properties, although respiratory depression has been reported with massive ingestion.

DRUG–DRUG INTERACTIONS

Many centrally acting drugs can produce an additive pharmacodynamic interaction with all of the agents described herein. Therapeutic combinations of ketamine with benzodiazepines reduce its emergence delirium, depending on the pharmacokinetics of the drug involved. Clonidine and related α-adrenergic agonists such as dexmedetomidine have been given clinically with ketamine to reduce its dissociative effects.

DXM can induce a serotonin syndrome when taken with monoamine oxide inhibitors, selective serotonin reuptake inhibitors, or other serotonergically active substances. Genetic polymorphism in the biotransformation of DXM via CYP2D6 may enhance the toxicity of the former by inhibitors of the latter.

NEUROBIOLOGY

Recent imaging data show that ketamine-induced antagonism of the NMDA receptor is directly correlated with negative symptoms of schizophrenia, suggesting that dissociatives may induce negative symptoms via NMDA antagonism. It has also been hypothesized that dissociatives induce positive symptoms via enhancing glutamate release. NMDA antagonists block excitation of γ-aminobutyric acid (GABA) interneurons, resulting in removal of GAB-Aergic inhibition of cholinergic, serotonergic, and glutamatergic afferents to the posterior retrosplenial cingulate cortex. This suggests a mechanism for triple excitotoxicity and the subsequent posterior cingulate pyramidal cell neurodegeneration. Subsequent studies using in vivo microdialysis confirmed that the administration of NMDA antagonists increased glutamate release in the frontal cortex.

Ketamine administration induces a rapid, focal decrease in ventromedial frontal cortex regional blood oxygenation level–dependent (BOLD) functional magnetic resonance imaging signals that strongly correlates with its dissociative effects. This results in significantly increased BOLD activity in the midposterior cingulate, thalamus, and temporal cortical regions—increases correlated with Brief Psychiatric Rating Scale psychosis scores. Pretreatment with lamotrigine (a sodium channel blocker that decreases glutamate release) prevented many of the BOLD changes and increases in Brief Psychiatric Rating Scale psychosis scores. Thus, dissociatives may induce positive symptoms via enhancing glutamate release. There may be other mechanisms at play that relate to the association of positive and negative symptomatology with dissociative exposure. Although ketamine and dissociatives remain a promising area of research for depression, limitations remain (very few randomized controlled trials exist, an active placebo is typically lacking, long-term data are scant, and risks remain uncertain), and this approach remains experimental. Proposed mechanisms for the rapid antidepressant action of ketamine include ketamine-mediated blockade of NMDA receptors at rest, resulting in the release of brain-derived neurotrophic factor via desuppression of its translation. Previous studies suggest increased brain-derived neurotrophic factor function as one possible mechanism of action for traditional antidepressants.

The action of nitrous oxide as an NMDA antagonist is another major advance in our knowledge. Nitrous oxide is thought to stimulate the neuronal release of an endogenous opioid peptide or dynorphins; the molecular aspects of this process are as yet unknown. Nitrous oxide may have an excitatory action on neurons via $GABA_A$ receptor–mediated disinhibition.

Addiction Liability

Why these substances are reinforcing is difficult to understand, except in the context of individuals who wish to experience the feelings of dissociation and sensory isolation that dissociatives provide. Dissociatives are self-administered by animals. Rhesus monkeys self-administer PCP, and social stimulation among monkeys in adjoining cages enhances the reinforcing strength of PCP. Changes in dopaminergic or cyclic adenosine monophosphate signal cascades induced by single or repeated PCP doses in mice likely play a role in the development of PCP-induced rewarding effects. Rodent and primate animal studies of DXM support reinforcement by DXO, akin to PCP. DXM is also strongly self-administered. Very little work has been done to develop medications to treat dissociative addiction. An anti-PCP monoclonal antibody for PCP addiction is under development.

Toxicity/Adverse Effects

NMDA antagonists have remarkable effects on brain neurons, including toxicity, which can be reduced or prevented. Not all species of animals evidence these changes. The relationship of such neurotoxicity to humans who recreationally use NMDA antagonists remains unclear. Such neurotoxic changes are reduced by pretreatment with benzodiazepines, further supporting the mechanism of NMDA antagonists blocking GABA interneuron activity, resulting in disinhibition of cholinergic, serotonergic, and glutamatergic afferents, resulting in excitotoxicity. Repeated high-dose administration of DXM during adolescence in rats may induce permanent deficits in cognitive function; increased expression of NMDA receptor AR 1 subunits in the prefrontal cortex and hippocampus may play a role in these DXM-induced memory deficits. This has troublesome implications in the setting of the increasing prevalence of recreational DXM use in adolescents coincident with a remarkable period of brain growth during this age period. Human studies show impairments in working and episodic memory, among other cognitive problems, correlating with ketamine exposure levels. Human chronic ketamine users, compared to controls, show less bilateral dorsal prefrontal grey matter, with duration of use negatively correlating with grey matter volume, and estimated total lifetime consumption of ketamine negatively correlating with grey matter volume in the left superior frontal gyrus. White matter abnormalities in bilateral frontal and left temporoparietal cortices have been found with anisotropy values negatively correlating with the total lifetime ketamine consumption (indicating pathology of white matter/axons in these brain regions). Studies using dissociative drug intoxication as a model of cognitive dysfunction in schizophrenia to develop new pharmacotherapies may also reveal solutions for the cognitive consequences of chronic dissociative use.

Intoxication and Overdose

Although a preliminary diagnosis of arylcyclohexylamine intoxication can be made on the basis of history, clinical signs, and symptoms, only a drug-positive blood or urine specimen will unequivocally establish it. Most clinically used drug screening panels include PCP, but not the other agents discussed herein; thus, a request may be required for specialized testing.

Psychotic manifestations of arylcyclohexylamine poisoning can be confused with catatonic schizophrenia, an acute toxic psychosis induced by other hallucinogens, and various acute organic brain syndromes. Arylcyclohexylamine intoxication can induce an organic brain syndrome, as well as cardiovascular and renal complications that are seldom, if ever, seen with other psychiatric syndromes. Lower urinary tract symptoms are common. Body image loss, especially numbness of the entire body; feelings of being in outer space; and less commonly, visual hallucinations suggest arylcyclohexylamine exposure, as opposed to classic hallucinogens such as LSD-25 or related agents. DXM is associated with psychosis at doses >300 to 600 mg or in fast metabolizers of DXO. Psychosis may occur at lower doses when DXM is combined with other drugs such as alcohol. Folate deficiency may also be associated with recreational DXM use. DXM use may result in brain damage, seizures, loss of consciousness, irregular heartbeat, and death. Respiratory depression from DXM may be reversed with naloxone.

CONCLUSIONS AND FUTURE RESEARCH

Dissociatives include an array of compounds sharing antagonist activity at the NMDA receptor (among other actions on the human brain) and resulting in a clinical syndrome involving dissociation or disconnection of the brain from its external and internal environments. Such a disconnection is described by users as the desired end state when abusing these compounds; however, it is not uncommon for users to exceed the dosing required for these effects, resulting in untoward psychiatric and medical effects. It is often only then that such patients present for medical assistance. Antidotes or other effective treatments do not yet exist for these compounds, making supportive care the basic treatment modality. The addiction liability of these drugs requires further exploration, particularly in light of current

off-label use as an antidepressant in psychiatrically compromised patients.

The evaluation of this drug class for its neuroprotective qualities may prove increasingly fruitful as the world population increases in average life span, and the need for such agents increases as well. The possible rapid antidepressant qualities of ketamine infusion are a recent discovery resulting in increased research, with interest in extending this research to DXM. A possible future expanded clinical use of ketamine as an antidepressant raises the concern for future ketamine/dissociative unhealthy use from a not-so-novel group of people already at risk for substance use disorders—depressed individuals.

Finally, the increasing prevalence and significance of recreational/unhealthy DXM use is alarming, particularly for the concentrated involvement of young people who appear unaware of its potential toxicities. Preliminary data suggest neuronal toxicity, and resultant neuropsychological impairment may result from DXM exposure, particularly in the developing adolescent brain. Public policy may be increasingly directed toward controlled access to DXM versus its current over-the-counter or behind-the-counter availability.

KEY POINTS

1. Dissociatives are a unique pharmacologic class of substances, with NMDA antagonism as their shared pharmacodynamic effect.
2. PCP, ketamine, and DXM are the drugs most commonly recreationally used in this class; however, nitrous oxide also shares similar pharmacodynamics.
3. Only DXM is available over-the-counter and typically must be used at doses well outside those directed to achieve a dissociative state.
4. All dissociative drugs discussed herein have a significant potential for medical and psychiatric complications.
5. Currently, there are no FDA-approved pharmacotherapies or psychotherapies to treat substance use disorders relating to these drugs.

REVIEW QUESTIONS

1. Choose all that apply. The active isomer of ketamine now being proposed for the treatment of depression is:
   A. more effective.
   B. less addicting.
   C. less dissociative.
   D. rapid acting.

2. Choose all that apply. Nitrous oxide is an anesthetic agent that should also be described as dissociative because:

A. in low anesthetic concentrations, it produces dissociative effects.

B. it produces Olney retrosplenial cortex lesions.

C. the Drug Enforcement Administration schedules it the same as ketamine.

D. it is easily injectable.

3. Choose all that apply. Dextromethorphan:

A. acts via μ-opioid receptors.

B. is an NMDA antagonist.

C. is the D-isomer of morphine.

D. is antitussive.

ANSWERS

1. **A and D**
2. **A and B**
3. **B and D**

SUGGESTED READINGS

Bobo WV, Miller SC, Martin BD. The abuse liability of dextromethorphan among adolescents: a review. *J Child Adolesc Subst Abuse*. 2005;14(4):55-75.

Domino EF, Miller SC. Dissociatives. In: Miller SC, Fiellin DA, Saitz R, Rosenthal R, eds. *The ASAM Principles of Addiction Medicine*. 6th ed. Philadelphia: Wolters Kluwer, 2018: 252-262.

Sibley DR, Hanin I, Kuhar M, Skolnick P, eds. *Handbook of Contemporary Neuropharmacology*. Hoboken, NJ: Wiley, 2007.

The Pharmacology of Inhalants

18

Summary by Robert L. Balster

Based on THE ASAM PRINCIPLES OF ADDICTION MEDICINE,
6th edition chapter by Robert L. Balster

DEFINITION

Abused inhalants are breathable chemicals that can be self-administered as gases or vapors. Drugs such as crack cocaine, which is aerosolized, and cannabis, which is smoked, are consumed by inhalation but are not generally, or usefully, classified as inhalants. Also not included in this class is inhaled nicotine from e-cigarettes.

SUBSTANCES INCLUDED IN THIS CLASS

Three subdivisions of inhalants are useful, as shown in Table 18-1. This subclassification is based on common pharmacologic effects.

Volatile Alkyl Nitrites

The prototypic alkyl nitrite is amyl nitrite, used medically as a vasodilator for the treatment of angina. Amyl nitrite is available in ampules that are broken open and the vapor inhaled. At one time, the ampules were available over the counter, and abusers would "pop" them open, hence the street name "poppers." Other alkyl nitrites produce similar effects and are typically sold as "odorizers." It seems likely that they are used because of their ability to produce syncope secondary to venous pooling in the periphery and because of their effects on tumescence and smooth muscles, making them popular as aids to sexual activity.

Nitrous Oxide

It is popular to divert anesthetic nitrous oxide for illegitimate use. Tanks can be used to fill balloons for ready sale at concerts or parties. With balloons, users typically breathe almost 100% nitrous oxide. Nitrous oxide can also be used as an aerosol propellant and is available in some food products. It can produce euphoria and feelings of intoxication, thus the common name "laughing gas." Use of nitrous oxide can

lead to anoxia, which contributes to the intoxicating effects that come on very rapidly but also dissipate rapidly.

Volatile Solvents, Fuels, and Anesthetics

This category includes a large collection of chemicals that further research may reveal to have different profiles of acute effects as well, but the state of the science is insufficient at this point to propose a further subclassification. Among the prototypic chemicals for this class are toluene and other alkyl benzenes; butane and other alkanes; R134a (1,1,1,2-tetrafluoroethane), R152a (1,1-difluoroethane), and other haloalkanes; and various ketones, alcohols, and ethers. It has been hypothesized that many of these commercial chemicals share profiles of acute effects with subanesthetic concentrations of volatile anesthetics such as sevoflurane and isoflurane and can produce a rapid-onset, short-lived alcohol-like intoxication. The abuse of these solvents, fuels, and anesthetics could be viewed clinically as special instances of unhealthy use of depressant drugs by an inhalation route.

HISTORICAL FEATURES

The unhealthy use of inhalants has a long history. Perhaps the best known instances are the use of anesthetics for purposes of intoxication that began with their discovery over 200 years ago. The euphoric-like effects of nitrous oxide were noted by Sir Humphry Davy, who synthesized the substance in 1799 and began calling it "laughing gas." Some inhalants, such as nitrous oxide and amyl nitrite, are under control of the US Food and Drug Administration as prescription medications, although forms of nitrous oxide are available commercially. Commercial sales of volatile alkyl nitrites are regulated in

TABLE 18-1	Pharmacologic Classification of Inhalants	
Class	Examples	Sources
Volatile alkyl nitrites	Amyl nitrite	Antianginal medication ampules
	Cyclohexyl nitrite	Room odorizers, video head cleaners
Nitrous oxide		Whipped cream chargers, cylinders for anesthesia
Solvents, fuels, and anesthetics	Toluene	Adhesives, paint removers and thinners (toluol), inks, nail polish and remover, industrial solvents and degreasers
	Xylene	Adhesives and printing inks, paints and varnishes, pesticides
	Difluoroethane (R152), tetrafluoroethane (R134a), dichlorodifluoromethane	Compressed air dusters for computers, refrigerants, and other uses
	Trichloroethane	This compound has almost entirely been removed from commercial use and not available for un-healthy use, but much of the research in this class has used it as a prototype.
	Chloroethane (ethyl chloride)	Topical anesthetic/freezing spray, also sold on the Internet as "popper-like" products
	Methylene chloride	A solvent in water repellants, automotive cleaners, primers and paints, adhesives and silicone lubri-cants, correction fluids, spray paints and paint removers, rust and spot removers, and other cleaning products
	Tetrachloroethylene	A solvent in water repellants, brake and carburetor cleaners, paints, adhesives and silicone lubricants, correction fluids, paint removers
	Butane, isopropane	Cigarette lighter fuel, aerosol propellant, bottled gas
	Ether, isoflurane	Anesthetics
	Ketones (methyl butyl ketone [MBK], methyl ethyl ketone [MEK])	Solvents, adhesives

the United States by the Consumer Product Safety Commission, a step that has greatly reduced the availability and abuse of most of these substances. However, nitrites are still advertised for sale on Internet sites. Many other types of inhalants used in unhealthy ways can be found in homes or workplaces or are readily purchased at retail establishments. Gasoline, a very complex mixture of volatile compounds, is available everywhere, and butane lighter fluid is easy to obtain. Although inhalants are not regulated under the Controlled Substances Act or by international treaty, several states have enacted restrictions on the sale and distribution to minors of certain products that are commonly used as inhalants. Some states have introduced fines, incarceration, or mandatory substance use treatment for the sale, distribution, use, and/or possession of inhalant chemicals. There have been discussions of strategies to prevent access to inhalants, to change their labeling, or to reformulate products to limit their potential for unhealthy use.

EPIDEMIOLOGY

More than 22 million Americans aged 12 years or older have used inhalants, and every year, about 750,000 use them for the first time. Results of national surveys suggest that the prevalence of inhalant use is greatest among 12- to 17-year-olds compared to other age groups. The use of inhalants by this age group is exceeded only by alcohol, tobacco, and cannabis. About 1 in 20 youths used inhalants sometime in their life, and 2.1% used them in the past year. Among older youth and adults, the prevalence of inhalant use falls considerably below that of marijuana, cocaine, and heroin, but current users remain a significant minority of substance abusers.

It is particularly prevalent among juvenile justice–involved youth. Although many inhalant users quit as they reach young adulthood, it is incorrect to characterize this problem as a passing fad in youth. For about half of current users, duration of use exceeds 1 to 2 years, with about 10% using inhalants for 6 years or more.

PHARMACOKINETICS

Inhalants include compounds that are self-administered as gases, vapors, and aerosols. These three forms of inhalants have somewhat different absorption characteristics and require different methods of use (eg, balloons for gases and bags or rags for volatile liquids). In the case of aerosol products such as spray paint, the likely "active ingredient" for abuse is the propellant.

Gases and vapors rapidly penetrate deep into the lung and, because of their high lipophilicity, are rapidly absorbed and distributed into arterial blood. Inhalants easily cross the placenta in pregnant women and expose the fetus as well.

Elimination of inhalants is very rapid once the source is removed from the inhaled air. For most of these chemicals, expired air is the major route of elimination. Most inhalants are metabolized to some extent, but this metabolism probably plays a greater role in determining their hepatic toxicity than their central nervous system effects.

Intoxication with inhalants is often of much shorter duration than with other drugs of abuse, with the result that many healthcare providers, as well as friends and family of users, rarely see an inhalant abuser who is grossly intoxicated.

PHARMACODYNAMICS

The neuropharmacologic mechanisms by which inhalant intoxication occurs are poorly understood. Although it is presumed that the inhalants disrupt normal neural function, it is not clear which systems are most affected and the mechanism by which such disruption occurs. Even the question of whether specific receptors are affected by these agents remains unresolved. The best current evidence is that acute solvent intoxication is probably associated with enhancement of $GABA_A$ and antagonism at the N-methyl-D-aspartate (NMDA) receptors.

ADDICTION LIABILITY

All of the vapors that have been tested produce clear, reversible, drug-like behavioral effects in animal studies. In addition, self-administration studies in

rodents, primates, and humans have shown several inhalants to have reinforcing properties.

Little is known about the development of tolerance and physical dependence with inhalants, but, in general, they do not appear to be prominent features. In animal studies, abused inhalants do not readily produce a significant degree of tolerance to their behavioral effects; however, a mild withdrawal syndrome can be observed with some. Ethanol and barbiturates can suppress these withdrawal signs, suggesting a cross-dependence within this depressant class. Unhealthy inhalant use typically is episodic in nature and thus generally would not occur with sufficient frequency and intensity to maintain a constant exposure throughout a day, much less the weeks or months it might take for physical dependence to develop. Thus, it is not surprising that significant physical dependence on inhalants is not seen in clinical settings.

Although few, if any, clinical facilities will routinely conduct tests for the presence of inhalants, such tests can be ordered through special services provided by commercial laboratories. Typically, these tests are performed on blood or urine and appear to be available mainly for solvents such as toluene, benzene, and methyl ethyl ketone. Because inhalants are eliminated so rapidly after acute exposure, such tests would be expected to have a high probability of producing false negatives.

TOXICITY/ADVERSE EFFECTS

Inhalants represent a wide and varied class of drugs, and their toxicity differs depending on which of the broad array of chemicals and chemical mixtures is being abused. It is difficult for toxicologists to ascertain the specific etiology of any adverse health effects seen in inhalant users because

1. Few chronic users confine themselves to a single inhalant.
2. Many abused inhalant products are complex mixtures.
3. Some adverse effects may be secondary to the lifestyles seen in inhalant abusers, not the chemicals themselves.

Deaths related to the acute effects of inhalants are well documented. There are two primary sources: behavioral toxicity and overdose. Overdose occurs when users lose consciousness while being continually exposed, allowing lethal concentrations to accumulate in the brain resulting in respiratory depression. At least some of the inhalants appear capable of producing acute cardiotoxicity, even in otherwise healthy young users.

Components of some abused inhalant products are well-characterized neurotoxicants. Among these are hexane and methyl-n-butyl ketone, which produce axonopathies. Most of the information on neurotoxicity of inhalants comes from case reports or small series of patients. It is not known what percentage of users have detectable brain damage nor whether the inhalants alone were responsible for the observed effects. Brain scanning, neurologic and neuropsychological assessments, or autopsy reports of inhalant users show many types of neuropathologies, including loss of white matter, brain atrophy, and damage to specific neural pathways. Of particular concern are the effects of inhalants on the developing nervous system—animal studies have revealed evidence for developmental delays and reversible changes in white matter maturation, suggesting that the prenatal period through adolescence may be particularly vulnerable periods for inhalant exposures.

There is a high rate of psychiatric disorders among inhalant abusers. For example, 70% of inhalant users in a recent study met criteria for at least one lifetime mood, anxiety, or personality disorder, and 38% experienced a mood or anxiety disorder in the past year. Conduct disorder, mood disorders, and suicidality are common among adolescent inhalant users.

Many chronic inhalant users develop irritation of the eyes, nose, and mouth and exhibit rhinitis, epistaxis, conjunctivitis, and a localized dermatitis. Inflammation of the lungs can result in coughing and may compromise respiration.

Hepatotoxicity is a concern for many inhalants, especially those that undergo hepatic metabolism. Of particular concern are some of the halogenated hydrocarbons. Renal damage also has been reported, in the form of glomerulonephritis, nephrolithiasis, and renal tubular acidosis. Some abused inhalants are known carcinogens.

It has been estimated that as many as 12,000 women use inhalants while pregnant in the United States alone. The research on inhalant use and pregnancy suggests that decreased fertility and spontaneous abortions in some women may be related to inhalant use. Clinical reports of adverse effects in the offspring of inhalant users include low birth weight, facial and other physical abnormalities, microcephaly, and delayed neurologic and physical maturation. Because certain features seen in these children resemble fetal alcohol syndrome, a "fetal solvent syndrome" has been proposed.

KEY POINTS

1. Inhalant abuse is most common among young teens.
2. There is a diverse array of chemicals that can be abused by inhalation, with volatile nitrites producing much different effects than solvents such as toluene.
3. Most inhalants produce very rapid-onset, short-acting, alcohol-like intoxication, and regular use is often associated with damage to the brain and other organs.
4. Prenatal exposure to inhalants probably can produce a "fetal solvent syndrome."

REVIEW QUESTIONS

1. Many abused inhalants produce an intoxication that most closely resembles that produced by which of the following?
   A. Alcohol
   B. Cocaine
   C. Cannabis
   D. LSD
   E. Heroin

2. What is most likely the basis for the intoxication resulting from the inhalation of alkyl nitrites?
   A. Effects on adenosine receptors regulating adenylate cyclase
   B. Sympathomimetic activation producing pressor effects and increases in heart rate
   C. Vasodilatation resulting in brain anoxia
   D. Effects of nitrites on serotonin receptors
   E. Enhancement of the actions of caffeine commonly used in the dance scene

3. Which of the following abused inhalants is most commonly available as a gas?
   A. Toluene
   B. Amyl nitrite
   C. Methylene chloride
   D. Nitrous oxide
   E. Ether

ANSWERS

1. **A**
2. **C**
3. **D**

SUGGESTED READINGS

Balster RL, Cruz SL, Howard MO, Dell CA, Cottler LB. Classification of abused inhalants. *Addiction.* 2009;104(6):878-882.

Bowen SE. Two serious and challenging medical complications associated with volatile substance misuse: sudden sniffing death and fetal solvent syndrome. *Subst Use Misuse.* 2011;46(suppl 1):68-72.

Bowen SE, Batis JC, Paez-Martinez N, Cruz SL. The last decade of solvent research in animal models of abuse: mechanistic and behavioral studies. *Neurotoxicol Teratol.* 2006;28(6): 636-647.

Dell CA, Gust SW, MacLean S. Global issues in volatile substance misuse. *Subst Use Misuse.* 2011;46(suppl 1):1-7. (Note: the entire issue of this journal is devoted to international inhalant abuse research.)

Garland EL, Howard MO. Volatile substance misuse: clinical considerations, neuropsychopharmacology and potential role of pharmacotherapy in management. *CNS Drugs.* 2012;26(11):927-935.

Howard MO, Bowen SE, Garland EL, Perron BE, Vaughn MG. Inhalant use and inhalant use disorders in the United States. *Addict Sci Clin Pract.* 2011;6(1):18-31.

Ridenour TA, Halliburton AE, Bray BC. Does DSM-5 nomenclature for inhalant use disorder improve upon DSM-IV? *Psychol Addict Behav.* 2015;29(1):211-217.

19 The Pharmacology of Anabolic–Androgenic Steroids

Summary by David Lehman

Based on THE ASAM PRINCIPLES OF ADDICTION MEDICINE, 6th edition chapter by Scott E. Lukas

Anabolic–androgenic steroids (AASs) are the most commonly used performance-enhancing and skeletal muscle-building drugs. The prototype is testosterone, from which there are greater than 100 synthetic derivatives. The federal Anabolic Steroid Control Act of 2004 classifies testosterone and its many analogues as Drug Enforcement Administration Schedule III. Individual states may attach additional restrictions on federally scheduled drugs and enact limitations on newer unregulated compounds.

DRUGS IN THE CLASS

AASs were introduced in the United States after revelation of their successful use by Russian contenders in the 1954 World Wrestling Championships. Testosterone was the drug of choice in the 1950s until synthetics were developed to augment the anabolic component of these synthetics while minimizing their masculinizing effects. However, the anabolic and androgenic component effects have never been completely separated. Testosterone can be modified to create oral and parenteral compounds. The parenteral drugs are formulated in oil and therefore can only be given intramuscularly. Testosterone gel and patches for topical administration are available, although not commonly used by strength athletes. Testosterone also comes in buccal mucoadhesive tablets and implantable pellets. There are no intravenous formulations or smokable products.

NEW-GENERATION "PERFORMANCE ENHANCERS" AND ANCILLARY DRUGS

Recombinant human growth hormone or somatotropin is a subcutaneously administered endogenous peptide used to increase performance, sprint capacity, and posttraumatic healing of bone, collagen, and soft tissue injuries. It may enlarge muscle mass by increasing protein synthesis, reduce fat by increasing lipolysis, as well as improve cardiac function. AAS users may also include low-dose recombinant

human growth hormone in cycles to prevent testicular atrophy.

Dehydroepiandrosterone is a endogenous precursor of testosterone, estrogen, and progesterone that is made in the adrenal cortex. Many athletes use it for its androgenic and anticatabolic effects. Androstenedione is another endogenous androgen precursor that was formerly available as a legal dietary supplement. Androstenedione was reclassified in 2005 as a Schedule III controlled substance.

Exogenous AASs decrease the body's own testosterone production by negative feedback of the hypothalamic–pituitary–gonadal axis. Human chorionic gonadotropin (hCG), by mimicking luteinizing hormone (LH) and helping to restore testosterone production, is used to mitigate testicular atrophy caused by AAS-induced negative feedback. Clomiphene (Clomid) and tamoxifen are oral selective estrogen receptor modulators. Clomiphene negatively inhibits hypothalamic estrogen receptors resulting in increased pituitary release of LH, which increases testosterone production, and follicle stimulating hormone, which increases sperm production. Tamoxifen mitigates undesired AAS-induced gynecomastia by blocking effects at estrogen receptors in the breast.

Erythropoiesis-stimulating agents such as recombinant erythropoietin (Procrit, Epogen), darbepoetin (Aranesp), and the longer acting continuous erythropoietin receptor activators increase the body's own production of red blood cells, which deliver more oxygen to muscles and thus improve endurance.

Opioid analgesics are frequently used to mitigate the pain of excessive training and injuries. In addition to the more readily available oxycodone and hydrocodone, use of butorphanol (Stadol), a κ partial agonist/μ antagonist, and nalbuphine (Nubain), a κ agonist/μ antagonist, has been seen. Chronic opioid use causes decreased testosterone levels.

The veterinary β_2 agonist, clenbuterol, which is banned from food-producing animals, has been used as a weight loss and performance-enhancing drug.

It also has been identified as an adulterant in numerous atypical heroin overdoses presenting with mydriasis, agitation, tremors, tachycardia, and chest pain.

Thyroid hormone (thyroxine) has been used to enhance recovery and ameliorate fatigue. Diuretics have been used as masking agents to pass urine drug testing and for rapid weight loss before competitions. Their use may predispose one to dehydration and hypokalemia. Vaptan drugs, vasopressin V2 receptor antagonists, were added to the diuretic class of prohibited drugs in 2014.

Patient requests to treat moderate-to-severe acne, especially in 18- to 26-year-old males, should trigger the clinical consideration of underlying AAS usage because the incidence of acne is about 50% in AAS users. Adolescents and young adults also use prescription stimulants such as Adderall (amphetamine aspartate, amphetamine sulfate, dextroamphetamine saccharate, dextroamphetamine sulfate) not only for academics but also as athletic performance enhancers.

Approximately one fourth of users obtain phosphodiesterase type 5 inhibitors such as sildenafil to treat erectile dysfunction associated with AAS. Finasteride and dutasteride, 5-alpha-reductase inhibitors, can be obtained to self-medicate male pattern alopecia caused or aggravated by AAS use. Their use should be discouraged because they may worsen AAS hypogonadic side effects.

AT-RISK POPULATIONS

1. *Athletes* use AASs to improve their performance. They believe that AAS-assisted training allows the user to increase both frequency and intensity of workouts, which augment the direct actions of the drugs. These combined effects increase muscle capacity, reduce body fat, increase strength and endurance, and hasten recovery from injury.
2. *Aesthetes.* Another group of users is composed of adult nonathletes, young boys, and girls who use these drugs primarily to increase their weight or to improve their physical appearance. This group might be the most common but is extremely underreported.
3. *Fighting elite.* Competitive fighters, bouncers at bars, security personnel, military, and law enforcement officers have been reported to take these drugs to increase their strength and enhance aggressiveness in order to elevate job performance.

It is difficult to estimate the true prevalence of steroid abuse in the United States, which varies with age, gender, and athletic environment. Rates of use in gym subcultures are much higher than in the general population. Anabolic steroid abuse among athletes may range from 1% to over 20% among individuals engaged in power sports and/or weight lifting. One analysis of multiple surveys revealed that AAS use begins later than most other drugs, with only 22% of users starting before the age of 20 years. They estimated that among Americans currently age 13 to 50 years, between 2.9 and 4 million Americans have used AAS, and roughly 1 million may have experienced AAS dependence. Steroid use appears to decline with advancing age, but we may begin to see long-term consequences in the large number of older men that harmfully used AASs in the 1970s and 1980s.

The National Institute on Drug Abuse's Monitoring the Future 2017 survey of drug use among adolescents in middle and high schools across the United States reported annual prevalence rates were 0.6%, 0.8%, and 1.4% for boys in grades 8, 10, and 12, respectively, compared with 0.6%, 0.5%, and 0.5% for girls. Use is now down about two thirds among 8th and 10th graders, and three fifths among 12th graders from recent peak levels; however, perceived risk from using hit a record low of 49% of 12th graders in 2017.

THERAPEUTIC USE AND MISUSE
Therapeutic Use

The main indications for AAS include the following:

- Primary male hypogonadism caused by genetic conditions, undescended testes, mumps orchitis, trauma, and cancer treatment
- Hereditary angioedema prophylaxis
- Acquired aplastic anemia and myelofibrosis treatment
- Muscle wasting secondary to starvation, weight loss following extensive surgery, chronic infections (AIDS-associated wasting), or severe trauma
- Secondary treatment of bone metastases from breast cancer in postmenopausal women
- Menopause with methyltestosterone combined with estrogen to alleviate symptoms
- Patients on dialysis to increase lean body mass
- Female-to-male gender change

Misuse

1. *Stacking* is the use of combinations of multiple drugs at the same time.
2. *Cycling* is the use of steroid combinations for weeks to months with abstinent rest periods before resumption of different steroid or combinations in order "to avoid tolerance."

3. *Pyramiding* involves starting with a low dose and gradually increasing the dose until peak levels are achieved a number of weeks before a competition and then tapering so the individual will be drug free when tested.

Testosterone replacement is usually satisfied by 75 to 100 mg/wk intramuscularly, but weight lifters and bodybuilders may use doses equivalent to 1000 to 2000 mg/wk.

ADVERSE EFFECTS

Only a small percentage of users experience very serious and deadly outcomes. For others, the side effects are largely reversible, whereas the physical benefits are ongoing. Because persons who hazardously use AAS rarely seek treatment for their "abuse" of these drugs, they tend to present with the side effects.

Most persons who use AASs experience at least one side effect. The approximate frequencies of some of these adverse effects are acne (50%), testicular atrophy (45%), gynecomastia (50%), polycythemia (40%), cutaneous striae (35%), injection-site pain (35%), and sexual dysfunction (25%). Side effects are usually dose related and may vary with age and gender.

In males, AAS use causes feminization from aromatase conversion of testosterone to estradiol. Early on, gynecomastia may be reversible, but if it persists for more than a year, it is unlikely to respond to nonsurgical medical treatment. Men may get erectile dysfunction, impaired spermatogenesis, and testicular atrophy. Benign prostatic hyperplasia can cause difficulty urinating. There is always the risk for progression of an occult prostate cancer. Baldness, cutaneous striae, and acne are significant concerns for those taking AAS to improve their physical appearance. In females, there is virilization with facial hair growth (hirsutism), male pattern baldness, voice deepening, and breast atrophy (smaller breasts). They may also get menstrual disturbances and clitoromegaly. Adverse effects common to both males and females are acne, hair loss, cutaneous striae, libido changes, subfertility, hand/feet swelling, and rapid weight gain.

Different steroids have varied effects on lipid dynamics, but most are generally considered to be unhealthy due to increasing the risk of coronary artery disease. AASs cause an increase in low-density lipoprotein (LDL) cholesterol and apolipoprotein B (apoB). AASs diminish the antiatherogenic high-density lipoprotein cholesterol and apoA1. Total cholesterol may remain unchanged because the increased low-density lipoprotein is offset by a decreased high-density lipoprotein.

Myocardial infarctions secondary to endothelial dysfunction, vasospasm, or thrombosis can result in sudden cardiac death. Structural variations in the conduction pathways and genetic abnormalities, illicit drug use, and strenuous exercise may also contribute to arrhythmias and death in users without coronary artery disease. Arterial hypertension may occur acutely with AAS abuse.

Persons who hazardously use AASs may present with manifestations of thromboembolic disease such as deep venous thrombosis and pulmonary embolism, stroke, limb arterial thrombosis, branch retinal vein occlusion, and superior sagittal sinus thrombosis. The effects on the clotting cascade are complex with procoagulant (eg, increased thrombin) and fibrinolytic (eg, increased plasmin) pathway activation. The net effect is increased platelet aggregation and elevated hematocrit, favoring thrombotic events. Concurrent use of epoetin and its analogues exacerbates the risk.

Hepatic complications occur much more commonly with oral administration (eg, 17-alkylated androgens) than from intramuscular injections. Intrahepatic cholestasis allows accumulated bile to spill over, such that bodybuilders may titrate to just having jaundice. Toxic hepatitis induced by AASs with predominantly hepatocellular necrosis is rare. Peliosis is a potentially reversible condition with multiple blood-filled cavities ranging from a few millimeters to 3 cm. Peliosis hepatis occurs more frequently than pulmonary and splenic peliosis. Although pathologically benign when these blood-filled spaces are at the surface of an organ, there is risk of life-threatening hemorrhage. Hepatocellular adenomas, which may be single or multiple, likely have a risk of development similar to oral contraceptives, which is related to dose and length of use. They also create a risk of serious hemorrhage. Hepatic adenomas may not only regress after stopping AASs but may also have a risk of malignant transformation to hepatocellular carcinoma. Monitoring with α-fetoprotein and sonography every 6 to 12 months is prudent. Much rarer are occurrences of hepatic angiosarcoma and cholangiocarcinoma.

AAS use is a risk factor for tendon rupture. The clinician should strongly suspect AAS use in a muscular man presenting with a ruptured upper body tendon. There is also a case report of bilateral quadriceps tendon rupture resulting from training beyond one's limits.

Adverse effects in adolescents may be more severe and enduring than adults, which is contrary to what a significant number of adolescents believe. Epiphyseal growth plates can close prematurely and actually stunt growth, resulting in short stature. Precocious puberty may be caused in younger adolescents. Young users also may be particularly sensitive to the increased sexual and aggressive behavior resulting from AAS use.

Psychiatric side effects from AAS dose combinations have been reported to correlate with the severity of abuse. Persons dependent on AASs appear to have a higher incidence of psychiatric illness, the majority of which being anxiety and major depression disorders. Unfortunately, there is a lack of well-controlled prospective studies connecting AAS use and psychiatric disorders. Ethical constraints preclude conducting double-blind assessments with supraphysiologic doses of these drugs. Psychiatric side effects generally resolve in 1 to 2 weeks in psychiatrically healthy individuals.

Body image disorders may have some influence on an individual's decision to use AASs. Although a significant number of bodybuilders have anorexia nervosa, others may have "reverse anorexia," where they view themselves as being too small and weak when they are actually large and strong.

"Roid rage" is the controversial extreme AAS-induced psychiatric effect that may occur during a cycle of high-dose AASs. More frequently, the constellation of symptoms appears to resemble those of hypomania or mania. At the far end of the spectrum, mania may lead to delusions and even hallucinations. Individuals with body dysmorphic disorder may present with delusions as well. The energized person who uses AASs talks faster, has more energy, sleeps less, and is more impulsive. Persons who use AASs may become paranoid and hostile, with verbal aggression and physical assault. Interestingly, animal models have confirmed that AAS administration increases aggressive behavior.

ADDICTION LIABILITY

Because the anabolic effects of AASs can be profound but slow to develop, it has been difficult to separate these "desired" muscle-building effects from direct reinforcement. Humans cannot tell whether they have been given an active AAS or placebo. No controlled studies have demonstrated immediate reinforcing positive mood effects or euphoria. Any possible direct reward is small compared to other substances, such as cocaine, heroin, alcohol, or nicotine, allowing noncompulsive AAS use patterns (eg, once per week).

AASs are not one of the ten separate classes of drugs for which there are specific *Diagnostic and Statistical Manual of Mental* Disorders, 5th edition (*DSM-5*) criteria. AAS use disorder is coded as "other substance use disorder," with the specific substance indicated (eg, 305.90 [F19.10] mild anabolic steroid use disorder). Patients meet criteria for *DSM-5* use disorder by displaying a maladaptive pattern of consumption despite medical, psychological, and social consequences. Developing actual physical dependence is more insidious than with other drugs and typically requires prolonged use of extremely high doses.

The evidence supporting tolerance development is not strong, although there is a belief among users that cycling is a necessary practice to avoid its development. Doses are increased slowly to minimize the side effects or to allow time to acclimate to them, a behavior some users are likely to confuse with tolerance. The constellation of withdrawal symptoms includes craving more steroids, fatigue, depression, restlessness, anorexia, insomnia, decreased libido, and headaches. Some of these symptoms may be related to anabolic steroid–induced hypogonadism (ASIH). Fear of withdrawal with anticipation of ensuing muscle loss and hypogonadism is the major driving force for continuing illicit AAS use. There have been no reported withdrawal effects in female athletes or among patients who have been prescribed high doses for legitimate medical purposes.

TREATMENT CONSIDERATIONS

Treatment should be nonjudgmental and provided with a multidisciplinary team approach. Medical workup includes a history and physical, and blood work (eg, free testosterone, sex hormone-binding globulin, estradiol, LH, follicle-stimulating hormone, prolactin level, prostate-specific antigen, lipids, comprehensive metabolic panel, and complete blood count). The initial recommendation is discontinuation of AASs, ancillary medications, and supplements. Psychosocial treatments, possibly with psychopharmaceuticals, should address anhedonia, depression, body image issues, craving management, and relapse prevention. Patients with symptomatic ASIH may benefit from a month-long testosterone taper with simultaneous selective estrogen receptor modulator administration. ASIH may be lifelong, requiring long-term testosterone replacement therapy.

ABSORPTION AND METABOLISM

Testosterone has low oral bioavailability, with only about half of an oral dose available after hepatic first-pass metabolism. Some analogues of testosterone (eg, methyltestosterone, oxandrolone, stanozolol) resist such metabolism, so they can be orally given in smaller doses. Oral AAS preparations have the highest incidence of liver complications because of prolonged hepatocellular and cholangiocellular exposure from first-pass liver metabolism.

Testosterone is both an active hormone and a prohormone, about 95% of which is synthesized in the interstitial cells of Leydig. The remaining 5% comes from the adrenal cortex, which by itself is insufficient to sustain male sexuality. Women secrete small amounts of testosterone from their ovaries and adrenal glands.

Testosterone is metabolized by the rate-limiting $5\alpha/\beta$-reductase to the more active 5α-dihydrotestosterone, which binds the androgen receptor two to three times more powerfully than testosterone. Testosterone may also be metabolized by an aromatase enzyme to estradiol. Males who use high doses of AAS can have circulating estrogen levels of normally cycling women. Compounds that resist aromatization (eg, mesterolone, stanozolol) may not result in the feminizing effects.

FUTURE VISTAS

The World Anti-Doping Agency (WADA) is a private law foundation based in Canada that produces independent antidoping policies under the auspices of the United Nations Educational, Scientific and Cultural Organization. It is a unique partnership between governments and organizations in all sports, even setting the standards for the International Olympic Committee. WADA annually updates a list of prohibited substances and methods as new doping threats emerge. WADA has been developing the Athlete Biological Passport for monitoring each athlete's own individualized long-term profile of numerous hematologic and urinary steroid parameters. A panel of experts interprets the data and profiles, similar to a medical record, validating that the results are consistent with "doping" and not a medical condition.

Gene doping or performance-enhancing genetics has been defined by WADA as "the nontherapeutic use of genes, genetic elements and/or cells that have the capacity to enhance athletic performance." Performance-enhancing drugs may alter the expression of specific genes by epigenetic mechanisms, such as DNA methylation and histone modifications. Current targets of gene doping involve transferring genes encoding for erythropoietin production, growth hormone, and growth factors (eg, insulin-like growth factor 1), or for silencing the expression of the myostatin gene, the product of which inhibits muscle growth. Areas of future study include genomics, transcriptomics, proteomics, and metabolomics.

KEY POINTS

1. AASs, the most commonly used performance-enhancing and skeletal muscle–building drugs, include a diverse group of synthetic and testosterone-derived agents. The anabolic and androgenic component effects have never been completely separated.
2. AAS misuse with supraphysiologic doses may result in masculinization, hepatotoxicity, and neuropsychiatric changes.
3. Unlike other drugs of abuse, AASs do not produce a significant immediate direct reward allowing for noncompulsive use, with reinforcement developing over a longer period of time.

REVIEW QUESTIONS

1. Which of the following is *not* a side effect of anabolic–androgenic steroid use in men?
   A. Impaired spermatogenesis
   B. Benign prostatic hyperplasia with difficulty urinating
   C. Male pattern baldness
   D. Decrease in low-density lipoprotein and apolipoprotein B
   E. Decrease in high-density lipoprotein and apolipoprotein A1

2. Which of the following is *not* a side effect of anabolic–androgenic steroid use in women?
   A. Facial hair growth and male pattern baldness
   B. Voice deepening
   C. Breast atrophy (smaller breasts)
   D. Subfertility, menstrual disturbances, and clitoromegaly
   E. Weight loss

3. True or False. Anabolic–androgenic steroids cause anemia.

4. Which of the following is a potential hepatic side effect of anabolic–androgenic steroids?
   A. Intrahepatic cholestasis with jaundice
   B. Hepatocellular necrosis
   C. Peliosis hepatis
   D. Hepatocellular adenomas
   E. Hepatic cholangiocarcinoma
   F. All of the above

ANSWERS

1. **D.** There is an increase in LDL and apolipoprotein B, which may help in building muscle. The increased cardiac risks from higher LDL might be mitigated by those users who also exercise and maintain low body fat.
2. **E.** Weight gain occurs with AAS use, especially during the first weeks. Stimulation of mineralocorticoid receptors results in sodium and water retention. There may be swelling of the ankles, feet, or body. Anabolic–androgenic steroids are Pregnancy Category X.
3. **False.** AASs stimulate erythropoietin synthesis and red cell production. AASs may be used to treat acquired aplastic anemia, myelofibrosis, and bone marrow failure in Fanconi anemia. Severe polycythemia may require phlebotomy.
4. **F**

SUGGESTED READINGS

Barceloux DG, Palmer RB. Anabolic-androgenic steroids. *Dis Mon.* 2013;59(6):226-248.

Duntas LH, Popovic V. Hormones as doping in sports. *Endocrine.* 2013;43(2):303-313.

Momaya A, Fawal M, Estes R. Performance-enhancing substances in sports: a review of the literature. *Sports Med.* 2015;45(4):517-531.

Pope HG Jr, Kanayama G, Athey A, et al. The lifetime prevalence of anabolic-androgenic steroid use and dependence in Americans: current best estimates. *Am J Addict.* 2014;23(4):371-377.

Rahnema CD, Lipshultz LI, Crosnoe LE, Kovac JR, Kim ED. Anabolic steroid-induced hypogonadism: diagnosis and treatment. *Fertil Steril.* 2014;101(5):1271-1279.

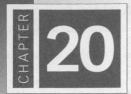

Electronic Cigarettes

Summary by Thomas W. McCarry

Based on THE ASAM PRINCIPLES OF ADDICTION MEDICINE,
6th edition chapter by Gideon St. Helen and Neal L. Benowitz

E-CIGARETTE, THE PRODUCT

Electronic cigarettes (e-cigarettes) are devices used to deliver a nicotine-containing aerosol, known as vaping, to users. E-cigarettes contain a battery, a heating element called an atomizer, and a solution of vegetable glycerin (VG) and/or propylene glycol (PG) containing nicotine and/or flavorants. The atomizer is a coil made of metal alloys around which a wick is wound. The invention of the e-cigarette is attributed to a Chinese pharmacist, Hon Lik, in the early 2000s.

Current e-cigarettes can be grouped into three main types: *first generation*, cig-a-likes; *second generation*, pen-style tank e-cigarettes; and *third generation,* advanced personal vaporizers (APVs) (Fig. 20-1). Cig-a-likes are the approximate size and shape of a cigarette, can be disposable or rechargeable, contain a low-capacity battery, and are puff activated. Pen-style tank e-cigarettes are larger than a conventional cigarette, contain a prefilled cartridge or refillable tank with a higher capacity battery, and most are activated by a switch. AVPs come in multiple shapes with high-capacity batteries. Regulated mods are an advanced subset of AVPs that can control voltage and/or power output. More recent APVs include automatic temperature-control devices that some classify as fourth-generation e-cigarettes.

CONSTITUENTS OF E-CIGARETTES AND THEIR AEROSOLS

Propylene Glycol and Vegetable Glycerin

The liquid solution used in e-cigarettes, referred to as e-liquid or e-juice, contains PG and/or VG, nicotine, flavorants, and contaminants. PG is an odorless, colorless, and tasteless synthetic liquid that produces the "smoke" and the sensory response of the aerosol produced. VG is an odorless, colorless, and sweet-tasting viscous liquid. Although both PG and VG are generally recognized as safe for use in food and oral consumption by the US Food and Drug Administration (FDA), there is no such safety assessment or rating when aerosolized and inhaled directly into the respiratory system. Additionally, heating PG and VG at high temperatures can produce toxic byproducts such as acrolein, formaldehyde, and benzene.

Nicotine

Nicotine levels in e-liquids range from low to high, with some e-liquids marketed as zero nicotine. However, studies have shown poor concordance of labeled and actual nicotine content. The amount of nicotine delivered per puff is highly dependent on the power applied to the atomizer, resulting coil temperature, and the consumer's use of the device.

Flavorants (Flavorings)

Over 7700 different e-liquid flavors have been identified in the US marketplace. Several flavorants used in e-cigarettes are known to cause bronchiolitis obliterans (referred to as popcorn lung) in humans exposed in occupational settings in addition to various toxic effects to cells in in vitro studies. Other known flavorants thermally decompose to carcinogenic aldehydes.

Contaminants

Contaminants in e-liquids and e-cigarette aerosols include known human carcinogens such as tobacco-specific nitrosamines, polycyclic aromatic hydrocarbons (PAHs), heavy metals, and minor tobacco alkaloids. Although contaminants in e-cigarette aerosols are found to be present at much lower levels compared to conventional cigarette smoke, implications of lower contaminant levels for respiratory and cardiovascular disease risks are still uncertain.

Volatile Organic Compounds

Volatile organic compounds (VOCs) are a class of compounds produced from the incomplete combustion of organic materials. Because of their abundance in cigarette smoke and their known carcinogenicity, risk assessment models indicate that VOCs account for the majority of cancer, cardiovascular, and

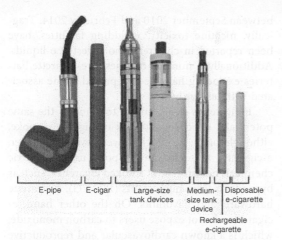

Figure 20-1. Types of e-cigarettes: E-cigarette products. From right to left, disposable and rechargeable e-cigarettes are also known as cig-a-likes or 1st-generation e-cigarettes; medium-size tank devices are also referred to as pen-style or 2nd-generation e-cigarettes; and large-size tank devices, e-cigar, and e-pipe are also referred to as advanced personal vaporizers. Source: 2016 Surgeon General's Report on E-cigarette use among youth and young adults.

respiratory risks from tobacco smoke. Adding concern, studies found that under certain conditions, VOCs are emitted in e-cigarette aerosol within the range of that achieved from smoking conventional cigarettes.

Particles

Epidemiologic studies have long associated exposure to particles—particularly, fine particles and ultrafine particles—in ambient air to an increased risk of various cancers and cardiovascular and respiratory diseases. Studies have found that the aerosol produced by e-cigarettes has a similar particle size as conventional cigarette smoke while also containing lower concentrations of ultrafine nanoparticles. Exposure to e-cigarette aerosol nanoparticles is of particular concern because they can penetrate more deeply into the lungs where particle clearance is slower.

NICOTINE DELIVERY AND ADDICTION POTENTIAL

Based on the type of e-cigarette and vaping behavior of the user, maximum blood nicotine levels can be comparable to that from conventional cigarettes. The basic shape of the e-cigarette plasma nicotine concentration-time curve after single administration is also comparable to conventional cigarettes

(rapid increase in blood nicotine levels followed by quick decline). This indicates that e-cigarette use has the potential to initiate and sustain nicotine addiction. Data from the Population Assessment of Tobacco and Health study collected in 2013 and 2014 found that 77% of adults who exclusively used e-cigarettes perceived themselves to be addicted versus 94% of those who exclusively smoked conventional cigarettes.

Nicotine intake and vaping behavior should be considered when assessing the addictiveness of e-cigarettes. For instance, a common practice among e-cigarette users is to modify the device in a way that permits dripping e-liquid directly onto the atomizer coil, thus increasing the concentration of nicotine consumed. One quarter of adolescent e-cigarette users reported "dripping" in a recent survey, and manufacturers have begun to make coils more accessible to enable this practice.

SECONDHAND AND THIRDHAND EXPOSURE

Unlike conventional cigarettes, e-cigarettes do not generate sidestream emissions, but bystanders can be exposed to constituents in the aerosol exhaled by the user. A study examining secondhand smoke found that air nicotine concentration in homes where e-cigarettes were used were lower than in homes where tobacco cigarettes were used but were higher than smoke-free homes.

Thirdhand tobacco smoke refers to the creation of secondary pollutants in indoor and outdoor environments over time caused by the presence of nicotine. Despite a lack of human health studies on the health effects of thirdhand smoke exposure, animal and in vitro studies show that it has toxic effects on organs and is genotoxic.

PREVALENCE OF E-CIGARETTE USE

The latest US national data on e-cigarette use among adults are derived from the Population Assessment of Tobacco and Health study collected in 2013 and 2014. Overall, 6.7% of adults had used e-cigarettes at least once in the previous 30 days compared to 22.5% who had smoked cigarettes. Current regular use of e-cigarettes was 5.5% in comparison to current use of cigarettes (18.1%), cigars (7.8%), or hookahs (4.2%). Among tobacco users, 62.2% used one product, 22.5% used two products, and 15.3% used three or more tobacco products. Among multiple-product users, the most common combination was conventional cigarettes plus e-cigarettes (23%).

Additional national data on e-cigarette use among adults were obtained from the 2014 National Health Interview Survey, which found that men were more likely to have tried e-cigarettes than women. The prevalence of ever using e-cigarettes among adults aged 18 to 24 years was 20%, and prevalence decreased with age. Current use was not different by sex and was higher among American Indian or Alaska natives (10.7%) and White adults (4.6%) than among Hispanic (2.1%), Black (1.8%), and Asian (1.5%) adults.

The 2015 National Youth Tobacco Survey found that 27.1% of US youth reported using e-cigarettes at least one time, which included 13.5% of middle school and 37.7% of high school students. Among middle school and high school students, ever using e-cigarettes was not different by sex. The prevalence of current (past 30-day) use among middle and high school students was 5.3% and 15.5%, respectively—an increase from 3.9% and 13.4% in 2014.

E-CIGARETTES AS A POSSIBLE GATEWAY TO COMBUSTIBLE CIGARETTES

There is concern among researchers and policy makers that nonsmokers, particularly youth, who use e-cigarettes might become users of combustible tobacco products. Use of e-cigarettes among youth is strongly associated with use of other tobacco products. For example, the 2015 National Youth Tobacco Survey found that 58.8% of high school cigarette smokers and smokers of other combustible tobacco products also used e-cigarettes in the past 30 days. Conversely, current cigarette use among US high school students dropped from 22.6% to 13.6% in 2007 when e-cigarettes entered the US market and continued declining to 7.0% in 2015. It is reassuring that while e-cigarette use in the United States has increased markedly in recent years, the prevalence of cigarette smoking has steadily declined, arguing against any large gateway effect.

HEALTH EFFECTS OF E-CIGARETTES

Few studies are available on the effects of e-cigarette use on the incidence of disease in people. Such studies are difficult to conduct because most e-cigarette users are current or former smokers and most e-cigarette-only users have not vaped for very long. The most common acute side effects of e-cigarettes are throat irritation and cough.

E-cigarettes are associated with unintentional injuries; the US Poison Control Centers reported 2405 calls concerning possible e-liquid toxicity

between September 2010 and February 2014. Tragically, nicotine toxicity, including fatalities, have been reported in children who ingested e-liquids. Additionally, a number of cases of e-cigarette batteries exploding have been reported, some associated with serious burns.

E-cigarettes expose users to some of the same potentially toxic constituents of cigarette smoke, although often in much lower levels. However, e-cigarette aerosols may expose users to toxic chemicals not present in smoked cigarettes, such as byproducts from humectants (PG, VG), e-cigarette hardware, and flavorants. On the other hand, e-cigarettes do not expose users to carbon monoxide, which is a known cardiovascular and reproductive toxin. Interestingly, studies of smokers with hypertension showed a reduction in blood pressure when they switched to e-cigarettes compared to baseline. Additional studies are needed to better understand the carcinogenic potential of e-cigarettes, as well as the association between e-cigarette use and cancer risk, and the effect of e-cigarette nicotine exposure during fetal development.

E-CIGARETTE USE AND SMOKING CESSATION
Use of E-Cigarettes as a Clinical Tool

Smokers report that they use e-cigarettes for several reasons, including curiosity, a perception of less harm, to vape in places where smoking is forbidden, and to help quit or reduce smoking. Using e-cigarettes to aid in stopping smoking has been studied in a few clinical trials and in population studies where e-cigarettes were purchased by consumers for self-managed cessation. Three randomized clinical trials have been published. However, due to the small number of subjects and low quit rates, these trials have been assessed in a Cochrane Review to be of low quality.

E-Cigarette Use and Smoking Cessation at the Population Level

There is evidence that use of e-cigarettes is associated with increased smoking cessation at the population level. An analysis of repeated cross-sectional data from five waves of a large, nationally representative survey in the United States found that e-cigarette users were more likely than nonusers to attempt to quit (65.1% vs. 40.1%) and were more likely to succeed in quitting (8.2% vs. 4.8%). The available evidence regarding e-cigarette use to aid in tobacco treatment is promising but requires more studies to establish the optimal role and methods of use in tobacco treatment.

WHAT TO TELL PATIENTS

The most important action a cigarette smoker can take to improve health is to stop smoking, and the proven pharmacologic aids for tobacco treatment are nicotine replacement therapy products, varenicline, and bupropion. The following recommendations are supported by the American Heart Association: If a smoker has failed initial treatment, has been intolerant of or refuses to use approved medications and psychotherapies, and wishes to use e-cigarettes to aid in quitting, that attempt should be supported. Smokers should be informed that although e-cigarettes are likely to be less harmful than cigarette smoking, their long-term health effects are unknown. Furthermore, the benefit of e-cigarettes for quitting smoking has not been proven by controlled clinical trials, the standard used for regulatory approval. Smokers who use e-cigarettes to quit should be encouraged to quit smoking completely and urged to set a quit date for the e-cigarette.

OTHER ELECTRONIC NICOTINE DELIVERY SYSTEMS

The tobacco industry is developing and marketing newer electronic nicotine delivery systems, such as heat-not-burn (HNB) devices that heat a modified tobacco cigarette without combustion. An example of an HNB product is the IQOS (I-Quit-Ordinary-Smoking) made by Philip Morris S.A. IQOS is sold in about 20 markets worldwide, and in January 2017, IQOS accounted for 7.6% of Japan's cigarette market. The first independent study of HNB aerosols found the presence of 8 VOCs and 13 PAHs. Although almost all VOCs and PAHs were found at vastly lower amounts in the HNB aerosol, a PAH called acenaphthene was found a levels far exceeding combusted cigarette smoke. Carbon monoxide and nicotine was also found in HNB aerosols but at lower levels than combusted cigarettes. Additional research is needed to assess health risk implications for users of HNB products.

OTHER SUBSTANCE USE WITH E-CIGARETTES

Vaporizers that heat cannabis without combustion have been marketed even before the popularization of nicotine e-cigarettes. Although e-cigarette design is not optimized for delivery of drugs such as cannabis, reports confirm that they are being used for this reason. A popular method of vaping an illicit drug is "dabbing" wax infused with tetrahydrocannabinol directly onto the heating coils. E-cigarettes are also used to deliver γ-butyrolactone known as "gleeb" and a synthetic amphetamine-like cathinone designer drug referred to as "flakka."

A survey of high school students in Connecticut revealed that 26.5% of dual e-cigarette/cannabis users had used e-cigarettes to vaporize cannabis. Studies also suggest that adult e-cigarette users are using e-cigarettes to vape cannabis. No studies have characterized tetrahydrocannabinol intake, pharmacokinetics, and effects from vaping cannabis and other illicit drugs with e-cigarettes.

REGULATION OF E-CIGARETTES

In May 2016, the FDA Deeming Rule extended its authority to e-cigarettes and e-cigarettes became subject to FDA regulation. The rule required that manufacturers of all products covered by the new regulations apply for marketing authorization. Since then, the FDA announced a delay in premarket tobacco product application submission deadline from 2018 to 2022, thus allowing products that were on the market as of August 8, 2016, to remain without FDA marketing authorization.

Given the potential health risks associated with e-cigarettes, including uptake by youth, we recommend the following policy approach to e-cigarettes:

- Include e-cigarettes in smoke-free air laws, prohibiting the use of e-cigarettes in the same locations as conventional cigarettes.
- Prohibit the sale of e-cigarettes to minors or anyone who cannot legally purchase cigarettes.
- Prohibit cobranding e-cigarettes with conventional cigarettes in ways that promote dual use.
- Subject e-cigarettes to the same level of marketing restrictions as cigarettes.
- Prohibit marketing claims that e-cigarettes are effective smoking cessation aids.
- Regulate product ingredients, components, and functioning for safety concerns.

KEY POINTS

1. Because nicotine levels and the basic shape of the plasma nicotine concentration-time curve can be comparable to that from conventional cigarettes, e-cigarette use has the potential to initiate and sustain nicotine addiction.
2. E-cigarettes expose users to some of the same potentially toxic constituents of cigarette smoke, although often in much lower levels than those found in cigarette smoke.
3. The available evidence regarding e-cigarette use to aid in tobacco treatment is promising but requires more study.

4. Additional studies are needed to better understand the carcinogenic potential and the health risks associated with the use of e-cigarettes, newer electronic nicotine delivery systems such as HNB products, as well as the use of e-cigarettes to vape cannabis and other illicit substances.

REVIEW QUESTIONS

1. The e-liquids used in e-cigarettes typically contain which of the following? (Select all that apply.)
   A. Vegetable glycerin
   B. Propylene glycol
   C. Nicotine
   D. Contaminants

2. True or False: The use of e-cigarettes should never be supported as a method for tobacco cessation.

3. What associations have been demonstrated among youth since the introduction of e-cigarettes? (Select all that apply.)
   A. Use of conventional cigarettes has increased.
   B. Use of e-cigarette products has increased.
   C. There is a strong correlation between the use of e-cigarettes and conventional cigarettes.
   D. E-cigarettes are being used to vape cannabis.

ANSWERS

1. **A, B, C,** and **D**
2. **False.** Use of e-cigarettes as a tobacco cessation aid should be supported in treatment under certain circumstances.
3. **B, C,** and **D.** Use of conventional cigarettes among high school students has decreased substantially.

SUGGESTED READINGS

Know the Risks, E-cigarettes & Young People. The facts on e-cigarette use among youth and young adults. https:// e-cigarettes.surgeongeneral.gov. Accessed July 16, 2018.

McNeill A, Brose LS, Calder R, Bauld L, Robson D. *Evidence Review of E-cigarettes and Heated Tobacco Products 2018. A Report Commissioned by Public Health England.* London, United Kingdom: Public Health England, 2018.

US Department of Health and Human Services. *E-cigarette Use Among Youth and Young Adults. A Report of the Surgeon General.* Atlanta: US Department of Health and Human Services, Centers for Disease Control and Prevention, National Center for Chronic Disease Prevention and Health Promotion, Office on Smoking and Health, 2016.

US Food and Drug Administration. Tobacco products. https:// www.fda.gov/TobaccoProducts. Accessed July 13, 2018.

Zernike K. 'I can't stop': schools struggle with vaping explosion. *New York Times.* April 2, 2018. https://www.nytimes .com/2018/04/02/health/vaping-ecigarettes-addiction-teen .html. Accessed July 16, 2018.

21

Novel Psychoactive Substances: Their Recognition, Pharmacology, and Treatment

Summary by Kathryn Hawk, Barbara M. Kirrane, and Gail D'Onofrio

Based on THE ASAM PRINCIPLES OF ADDICTION MEDICINE, 6th edition chapter by Kathryn Hawk, Barbara M. Kirrane, and Gail D'Onofrio

Although classic illicit substances such as cocaine and heroin were traditionally agents of concern and regulation, novel psychoactive substances (NPS) or designer drugs have been developed in clandestine laboratories at an alarming rate over the past several decades. Typically, these drugs are designed to mimic already existing substances such as cannabis, amphetamines, or opioids and are manufactured specifically to circumvent laws related to the sale and trafficking of controlled substances. The designation of NPS includes synthetic cannabimimetics, synthetic cathinones, phenylethylamines, piperazines, ketamine- and phencyclidine-type substances, tryptamines, benzofuranes, and synthetic opioids. Two of the better understood novel drug categories include synthetic cathinones or "bath salts," which are derivatives of cathinone, a naturally occurring amphetamine analogue found in the leaves of the *Catha edulis* plant, and synthetic cannabinoids, marketed as Spice and K2, that bind to cannabinoid receptors. Another category of NPS includes nonpharmaceutical synthetic opioids, such as acetyl fentanyl, acrylfentanyl, 3-methyl fentanyl ("China White"), butyrfentanyl, U-47700, and carfentanil, that bind μ receptors and have been reported to be between 15 and 10,000 times more potent than morphine. Little is known about the mechanisms of action, pharmacologic effects, and toxicologic profile for many other NPS, although specific details for kratom, krokodil, and salvia are explored later in this chapter, and resources with information on NPS are constantly being updated.

Some types of NPS are frequently promoted as "legal highs" and are easily accessible in gas stations, convenience stores, "head shops," and on the Internet. These substances are a particular concern for teenagers and young adults because they are easily available and affordable, often packaged in colorful wrappers that do not appear dangerous, and are typically given fun, catchy names to draw attention. They are sold as "legal highs," "herbal highs," "bath salts," "plant food," "insect repellent," "research chemicals," and "air fresheners," with disclaimers that they are "not for human consumption" or "for research purposes only" to circumvent regulation and controlled substances legislation. NPS are largely undetectable using traditional methods for drug screening, which may be a perceived benefit for individuals who anticipate monitoring for illicit substance use. Importantly, NPS use is not always intentional; there have been a number of reports of designer drugs, including high potency fentanyl and analogues or other novel synthetic opioids such as U-47700 ("Pink"), detected in counterfeit black market prescription opioids and other traditional illicitly used drugs such as heroin and cocaine.

Designer drugs are typically created when clandestine chemists modify the structure of an existing drug, for example, adding a methyl group to the compound, thereby creating an analogue drug with similar properties but not necessarily subject to regulation. Legislative attempts both within and outside of the United States, including the federal Synthetic Drug Abuse Prevention Act of 2012, have been passed in an attempt to regulate the sale and use of specific substances, with limited impact given the targeted development of novel compounds specifically developed to skirt controlled substance regulations. The European Monitoring Centre for Drugs and Drug Addiction has been following the development of hundreds of new compounds since 2010, with more than 50% of the 560 substances categorized as NPS having been identified since 2013.

TREATMENT

Different chemical structures ultimately mean different physiologic effects, and with no oversight or regulation in the production of these substances, the resulting clinical picture can show wide variation across doses and individuals even when individuals use the same amount of substance with the same label. Acute intoxication with synthetic cathinones and synthetic cannabinoids predominantly presents clinically with a sympathomimetic toxidrome that often includes tachycardia, hypertension, tachypnea, hyperthermia, agitation, tremors, and/or seizures, although somnolence and hypotension have also been reported. Synthetic cannabinoids have been associated with nephrotoxicity, rhabdomyolysis, acute psychosis, and cardiac arrest, and synthetic cathinones have been associated with acute psychosis, hallucinations, paranoia, suicidality, and respiratory depression. Daily use of synthetic cannabinoids has been associated with the development of a profound withdrawal syndrome, which can include seizures, tachycardia, chest pain, palpitations, anxiety, insomnia, diaphoresis, and anorexia, and is managed by the administration of benzodiazepines and second-generation antipsychotics.

Acute clinical care for patients with toxicity related to NPS ingestion can be challenging as a wide variety of toxicologic effects have been reported, and batch-to-batch variability in potency, chemical composition, and adulterants may limit the utility of patient-reported substance use history. Toxicologists and emergency medicine physicians have traditionally focused on treating the poisoned or intoxicated patient based on the clinical presentation and characteristics, rather than based on the specific poison or drug. Based on the clinical presentation, including toxidrome and the best available history, emergency care frequently includes supportive care, including intravenous fluids; electrolyte repletion; evaluation for end-organ damage to the kidneys, lungs, heart, and brain; treatment with benzodiazepines and antipsychotics as needed; and observation. Naloxone administration should be considered for patients presenting with the opioid toxidrome of miosis, respiratory depression, and depressed mental status, even if a clear history of opioid use is not obtained, and high-dose naloxone should be considered if clinically indicated or if there is a suspicion for fentanyl or high-potency fentanyl analogues. In the United States, Poison Control Centers provide 24 hours per day, 7 days per week access to trained toxicologists who are available to answer questions and provide consultations for clinical management, and can be reached by calling (800) 222-1222.

SPECIFIC EXAMPLES OF NOVEL PSYCHOACTIVE SUBSTANCES

See Chapters 11, 12, and 15 for more information about opioids, cathinones, and synthetic cannabinoids, respectively.

Nonpharmaceutical Fentanyl Analogues

Fentanyl is a short-action opioid with 50 to 100 times the potency of morphine, initially synthesized in 1960 by Janssen Pharmaceutica. The synthesis of multiple analogues for pharmaceutical use, including sufentanil and alfentanil, soon followed. Although nonmedical use of pharmaceutical fentanyl and fentanyl analogues (fentanyls) has been reported, surveillance data suggest that increases in fentanyl-involved fatalities are related to illicitly manufactured fentanyls produced by clandestine laboratories primarily outside of the United States. A Centers for Disease Control and Prevention analysis of 27 states with consistent death certificate reporting of substances involved in opioid overdoses found a high degree of correlation (r = 0.95) between synthetic opioid-related deaths and increased fentanyl seizures reported to the National Forensic Laboratory Information System (NFLIS). Notably, no changes in fentanyl prescribing rates were observed. Between 2013 and 2014, the Drug Enforcement Administration (DEA) reported a 354% increase in fentanyl-related submissions to the NFLIS and identified at least 15 unique fentanyl-related compounds in seized samples. Fentanyls associated with numerous regional outbreaks of fatal overdose include α-methyl fentanyl, 3-methyl fentanyl, acetyl fentanyl, carfentanil, butyrylfentanyl, ocfentanil, and furanylfentanyl. Previously, regional outbreaks of exposure to fentanyls were largely thought to be related to contamination of the heroin supply, although recent reports highlight the existence of a specific market for fentanyls with increasing reports of intentional use, sometimes purchased over the Internet or dark Web.

Fentanyl is a synthetic μ-opioid receptor agonist, with a potency 50 to 100 times greater than morphine and 30 to 50 times greater than heroin. Fentanyl analogues range in potency from acetyl fentanyl (15 times more potent than morphine) to carfentanil (10,000 times more potent than morphine). Fentanyl is well absorbed transmucosally, accounting for the lozenge and lollipop routes of administration for pharmaceutical fentanyl, and is available in a transdermal delivery system (Duragesic). In 2015, the DEA issued warnings to law enforcement and first responders about the possibility of fentanyl being absorbed through the skin and accidental inhalation of airborne powder. The American College of Medical Toxicology and American Academy of Clinical Toxicology acknowledged in 2017 the possibility of weaponized aerosolized fentanyl toxicity but concluded that incidental dermal absorption or inhalation is unlikely to cause opioid toxicity to first responders and law enforcement officers exposed during routine civic service.

Clinically, fentanyl is used in general and regional anesthesia and in the management of chronic and postoperative pain. Recreationally, fentanyls are used for their euphoric effects. Fentanyls cause a typical opioid toxidrome with respiratory depression, miosis (constricted pupils), drowsiness, and euphoria, and at high doses, respiratory arrest and pulmonary edema. The most common side effects include nausea, dizziness, vomiting, fatigue, headache, and constipation; repeated use leads to the development of tolerance and dependence. Opioid overdose, the combination of decreased respiratory rate, decreased mental status, and miosis, can be reversed with the μ-opioid receptor antagonist naloxone, which can be administered via intranasal, intramuscular, or intravenous routes. Fentanyl is not included in many hospital urine toxicology screens, so exposure is often undetected. Like many exposures, source identification may be delayed or never occur; therefore, presentation and patient toxidrome should guide acute management.

Kratom

Kratom is a plant product derived from *Mitragyna speciosa* Korth, a leafy tree that is a member of the coffee family and native to Southeast Asia, although it is now cultivated elsewhere. Kratom was used in Thailand and Malaysia as early as the 1800s by manual laborers for euphoria, stimulation, and analgesia and to prevent withdrawal from opium. Traditionally, the kratom leaves are chewed or brewed into a tea; they are rarely smoked. Kratom has become increasing popular in the United States over the past several years given its wide availability in stores and on the Internet, along with its current legal status as an unscheduled substance. Kratom is commonly used today to self-treat chronic pain, prevent opioid withdrawal, and for its hallucinogenic effects, although other reported beneficial effects include antipyretic, antihypertensive, antidiarrheal, anti-inflammatory, and for prolonging sexual intercourse.

The primary alkaloid in Kratom, mitragynine, is an agonist of multiple receptors, including the opioid μ and δ receptors, as well as postsynaptic α-adrenergic, dopamine, and serotonin receptors. Mitragynine is reported to have a μ-opioid receptor potency approximately 10 times that of morphine, a key reason why kratom is used to prevent opioid withdrawal. Kratom has dual properties that result in both stimulation and analgesia, depending on the exposure dose. At low doses, kratom acts primarily as a stimulant, producing a sympathomimetic toxidrome; at higher doses, effects are predominantly consistent with an opioid toxidrome. Effects begin between 5 and 10 minutes after exposure and typically last for 1 hour. Symptoms of acute intoxication reported to poison centers include tachycardia, agitation, drowsiness, nausea, and hypertension. Published case reports have associated kratom exposure with psychosis, seizures, coma, and death. A withdrawal syndrome has been reported in regular users and include symptoms such as nausea, vomiting, diarrhea, insomnia, hot flashes, and abdominal pain. There is no antidote for kratom, and the treatment is primarily supportive.

Krokodil

"Krokodil" is a common name for desomorphine, an injectable opioid derivative created as a less expensive alternative to heroin. Its name is derived from the word "crocodile" (*krokodil* in Russian) and refers to the scaly, green-black ulcerated skin discoloration frequently seen in users. Desomorphine, the intended ingredient in krokodil production, is a μ-opioid receptor agonist with a potency approximately 10 times that of morphine. Krokodil is easily synthesized in homes and clandestine labs from codeine, which is available over the counter in Russia, and combined with other easily available, low-cost chemicals such as hydrochloric acid, red phosphorous, iodine, gasoline, or paint thinners. Due to its crude production and lack of a purification process, the final product is typically contaminated with high concentrations of corrosive chemical byproducts, and extensive skin necrosis has been reported after its injection.

Clinical symptomatology resembles that of the opioid toxidrome. However, additional significant damage occurs to the area of injection, which starts with swelling and pain and progresses to green-black discolored scaling and large-scale necrotic ulceration. This ulceration can progress to involve the muscle and tissue to decay and expose the underlying bone. Furthermore, complications such as meningitis, speech and motor impairments, multi-organ injury, thrombophlebitis, venous ulcers, and skin eschar have been reported. Like other opioids, withdrawal syndromes are possible with cessation of use. Treatment includes opioid antagonism for acute intoxication and supportive care for skin and systemic sequela.

Salvia Divinorum

Salvia divinorum is a member of the mint family and endemic to a limited area of the highlands of the Mexican Oaxaca state. Other names for *Salvia divinorum* include "Diviner's Sage," "Mystic Sage," "Magic Mint," "Maria Pastora," and "Sally D." Long recognized for its hallucinogenic properties, the indigenous Mazatec people of Mexico ingest fresh leaves or leaf preparations to promote visions and experiences for divinatory rituals, healing ceremonies, and medicinal purposes. Of the known salvia species, only *S. divinorum* is known to contain salvinorin A, the component responsible for its hallucinogenic properties. Since the late 1990s, salvia has had a surge in popularity due to its reputation as a "legal high," its wide availability on the Internet and in head shops, its lack of detection on drug screens, as well as its perceived safety. In the United States, it is most commonly used in young adults aged 18 to 25 years.

Salvinorin A is a highly selective agonist of the κ-opioid receptor, but unlike other hallucinogens, it does not demonstrate binding affinity for the serotonin 5-HT 2A receptor. Typically, stimulation of the κ-opioid receptor results in hallucinations, diuresis, and spinal analgesia, but does not result in respiratory depression. Classically, the plant is smoked or chewed. Effects are seen rapidly, often between 30 seconds and 10 minutes depending on the route of administration. Hallucinations are intense and many users report visual distortions of body images; out-of-body, dream-like experiences; and synesthesia, although dysphoria and frightening hallucinations have also been reported. Hallucinations are brief and typically dissipate within 30 minutes. Other symptoms include confusion, dizziness, flushed sensation, and tachycardia. Treatment for salvia toxicity is primarily supportive.

IDENTIFYING AND ACCESSING INFORMATION ON NEWLY EMERGING AND NOVEL PSYCHOACTIVE SUBSTANCES

A variety of organizations conduct surveillance and collate information to inform the public and clinicians and for the development of public health and

TABLE 21-1	Online Resources for Information on Emerging, Novel Psychoactive Substances
National Institute on Drug Abuse	www.drugabuse.gov
Drug Enforcement Administration	www.dea.gov
Monitoring the Future (University of Michigan)	www.monitoringthefuture.org
American Association of Poison Control Centers	www.aapcc.org
European Monitoring Centre for Drugs and Drug Addiction	www.emcdda.europa.eu
Substance Abuse and Mental Health Services Administration	www.samhsa.gov/data/

law enforcement policy (see Table 21-1). In the United States, poison control centers collect national surveillance data on drug exposures and provide toxicology support 24 hours per day, 7 days per week for lay people and clinicians. The DEA enforces the controlled substance laws and regulations of the United States, collaborates with local law enforcement and health professionals regarding seizures and poisonings, and maintains the NFLIS to collect, analyze, and disseminate drug intelligence information. The European Monitoring Centre for Drugs and Drug Addiction conducts similar data collection, registration, and analyses of both licit and illicit substances, including wastewater and seized material chemical analyses, and analyses of global market and trade patterns for the European Union. The Substance Abuse and Mental Health Services Administration and the National Institutes of Health fund periodic large-scale, population-based epidemiologic studies that collect self-reported data on substance use that are available to the public.

KEY POINTS

1. Novel psychoactive substances are clandestinely manufactured substances that often mimic traditional drugs of abuse that often circumvent federal laws on the sale and trafficking of controlled substances.
2. NPS includes a broad array of substances including more commonly known synthetic

cannabimimetics ("Spice" and "K2"); synthetic cathinones ("Bath Salts"); synthetic nonfentanyl opioids (U-4770 or "Pink") and fentanyls (acetyl fentanyl and carfentanil); as well as kratom, krokodil, salvia, phenylethylamines, piperazines, tryptamines, benzofuranes, and ketamine- and phencyclidine-type substances.

3. Emergency medical care should be directed by the patient's clinical presentation and toxidrome with evaluation for end-organ damage and intravenous fluids, electrolyte repletion, benzodiazepines, and antipsychotics given as needed, with a low threshold for naloxone administration because a detailed accurate exposure history is often unavailable or unknown.

REVIEW QUESTIONS

1. A 32-year-old male presenting to your office with a scaly, necrotic skin ulceration near an injection site on his left arm has most likely been using:
   A. salvia.
   B. acrylfentanyl.
   C. kratom.
   D. krokodil.

2. A police officer presents to your emergency department feeling lightheaded and concerned that he may be having a reaction to fentanyl after accidentally touching a white powder suspected to be fentanyl on a scene. His vital signs and clinical exam are unremarkable. What would your course of action be?
   A. Reassure him that fentanyl is not absorbed through the skin and that his symptoms are unlikely to be due to a fentanyl exposure.
   B. Administer naloxone (Narcan).
   C. Admit to the hospital for monitoring.

3. A Centers for Disease Control and Prevention analysis of overdose fatalities in 27 states, drug seizures reported to a national database, and prescribing practices concluded that the fentanyl involved with US overdose fatalities is most likely:
   A. manufactured by pharmaceutical companies in the United States.

   B. manufactured by pharmaceutical companies outside of the United States.
   C. illicitly manufactured.

ANSWERS

1. **D.** Chemical by-products associated with the crude production process of krokodil can lead to black-green skin discoloration with extensive damage, including skin ulceration and muscle damage.

2. **A.** The American College of Medical Toxicology and American Academy of Clinical Toxicology released a statement in 2017 that incidental dermal absorption or inhalation is unlikely to cause opioid toxicity to first responders and law enforcement officers exposed during routine civic service.

3. **C.** A Centers for Disease Control and Prevention analysis of overdose fatalities in 27 states, drug seizures reported to a national database, and prescribing practices found that changes in synthetic opioid-involved overdose deaths were highly correlated with fentanyl seizures but not correlated with fentanyl prescribing, supporting the argument that illicitly manufactured fentanyl is driving increases in fentanyl deaths.

SUGGESTED READINGS

American College of Medical Toxicology. *ACMT and AACT Position Statement: Preventing Occupational Fentanyl and Fentanyl Analog Exposure to Emergency Responders*. Phoenix: Author; 2017. https://www.acmt.net/cgi/page.cgi/_zine.html/The_ACMT_Connection/ACMT_Statement_on_Fentanyl_Exposure. Accessed July 22, 2017.

Banks ML, Worst TJ, Rusyniak DE, Sprague JE. Synthetic cathinones ("bath salts"). *J Emerg Med*. 2014;46(5):632-642.

Baumann MH, Solis E Jr, Watterson LR, et al. Baths salts, spice, and related designer drugs: the science behind the headlines. *J Neurosci*. 2014;34(46):15150-15158.

European Monitoring Centre for Drugs and Drug Addiction. *New Psychoactive Substances in Europe. An Update from the EU Early Warning System (March 2015)*. Luxembourg City, Luxembourg: Publications Office of the European Union, 2015.

Gladden RM, Martinez P, Seth P. Fentanyl law enforcement submissions and increases in synthetic opioid-involved overdose deaths—27 states, 2013-2014. *MMWR Morb Mortal Wkly Rep*. 2016;65(33):837-843.

Diagnosis, Assessment, and Early Intervention

Screening and Brief Intervention

Summary by Benjamin M. Clemens

Based on THE ASAM PRINCIPLES OF ADDICTION MEDICINE,
6th edition chapter by Suena H. Massey, Nicole A. Hayes,
Michael F. Fleming, and Aleksandra E. Zgierska

A large proportion of patients seen in hospital or primary care settings have or have had problems with alcohol and other drugs. Rates are higher among those presenting in emergency settings or with mental health problems. Physicians provide medical care to patients with unhealthy alcohol or drug use and related medical symptoms or conditions, including liver failure, hypertension, obesity, glucose intolerance, memory loss, and a variety of mental health conditions directly related to unhealthy alcohol use.

Screening and brief intervention (SBI) is a tool that is well suited for use in primary care; evidence suggests that patients prefer to address alcohol use with their own physicians over self-help groups or specialty addiction treatment centers. It was designed to be used in primary care settings and has been shown to reduce excessive alcohol use in those without alcohol use disorder via a harm reduction model that seeks to reduce the negative consequence as opposed to seeking abstinence. Adoption has not been widespread, leading to research on delivering SBI via smartphone or online.

NATIONAL RECOMMENDATIONS ON THE IMPLEMENTATION OF UNHEALTHY SUBSTANCE USE SCREENING AND TREATMENT IN MEDICAL CARE SETTINGS

Studies over almost five decades have demonstrated the potential benefits of SBI for tobacco and unhealthy alcohol use in a variety of settings, and as a result, structured efforts have been made to encourage implementation in clinical practice.

The US Preventive Services Task Force (USPSTF) recommends routine SBI for alcohol use for all adults and strongly recommends that clinicians screen all adults for tobacco use and provide tobacco cessation interventions. The USPSTF concludes that the evidence is insufficient to recommend for or against

routine SBI to prevent or reduce alcohol misuse or tobacco use among children and adolescents and has found insufficient evidence to recommend universal SBI for illicit drug use.

Numerous professional medical organizations have adopted policies calling on their members to be knowledgeable, trained, and involved in all phases of prevention and SBI for tobacco and unhealthy alcohol use. Organizations recommend screening for alcohol and tobacco use in adults and adolescents. The National Quality Forum recommends alcohol and tobacco SBI services for patients 10 years and older and the National Institute on Alcohol Abuse and Alcoholism recommends alcohol screening starting at age 9 years. Recommendations for screening for marijuana reflects the evolving view of marijuana, which varies by state.

Implementation of these recommendations has been modest; however, adoption of billing codes by the American Medical Association and adoption of tobacco as well as alcohol/other drug use–structured SBI services by the Centers for Medicare & Medicaid Services represents a step toward this goal.

SCREENING AND BRIEF INTERVENTIONS: CLINICAL GUIDELINES

Clinical Approaches to Screening and Brief Intervention Services in Primary Care Settings

A commonly recommended framework for the delivery of SBIs, particularly for tobacco use, is the five A's:

- *Ask*: Screen and assess the level of the risk. Intervention is provided on the basis of the level of risk identified.
- *Advise*: Provide direct personal advice about substance use. Patients should hear clearly that a

change in their behavior is recommended that is based on a review of results with the patient and to learn about their personal substance use and its effects on health. Facts should be presented in an objective way, using strong and personalized language.

- *Assess*: Evaluate the severity of the patient's problem and the patient's readiness to change. Clinicians should restate the substance use–related health concerns if the patient is not ready to change and reiterate a willingness to help when the patient is ready, as well as developing the discrepancy of the benefits of continued use versus reducing use.
- *Assist*: Develop a treatment plan that incorporates the patient's goals. Behavior change techniques like motivational interviewing should be used to assist the patient in pursuing the patient's goals. The treatment plan is most useful when it is actionable and measurable by the patient and follows progressive steps that build on each other toward the patient's ultimate goal. Considerations should be made for medical addition treatment like detoxification or medication, assessment and treatment for comorbid physical or mental health problems, safe sex counseling, as well as testing for human immunodeficiency virus and sexually transmitted diseases for sexually active patients, and human immunodeficiency virus and hepatitis testing for patients who inject drugs.
- *Arrange*: Make follow-up appointments and consider specialty referrals for those who screened positive. Follow-up appointments should be arranged for all patients who screened positive to provide ongoing assistance and adjust the treatment plan as needed. Patients should also be encouraged to see an addiction specialist and participate in self-help groups.

Approaches to Screening and Brief Interventions for Unhealthy Substance Use (Alcohol, Drugs, Tobacco)

Unhealthy Substance Use Screening

There are a variety of screening and intervention options to screen for unhealthy substance use. The National Institute on Drug Abuse's (NIDA) recommendation is a progressive screening process that starts with one question about substance use in the last year. An affirmative answer on this question would lead to a more questions to assess substance use to help determine the risk level and to determine if a brief intervention is appropriate. A negative response would end the screening process.

Drug Screening and Brief Interventions

Assessment of Severity: At-Risk Use or Disorder

Those with a positive screen for drugs (ie, yes to any use) should have an assessment for severity via a tool like the NIDA-Modified ASSIST (NM-ASSIST). When using the NM-ASSIST, a score is generated to determine the level of risk for drug use. In cases where more than one substance is being used, the questions are repeated to determine a risk level for each.

Clinical judgment should be used to decide if or when to intervene on drug use. When more than one substance has been identified, a decision should be made about which is focused on. Criteria of either highest risk or greatest motivation for change can be considered, and addressing all substances may be appropriate as well.

Alcohol Screening and Brief Intervention for Adults

Adult Alcohol Screening

Screening for heavy drinking can be accomplished via a single question, like the one recommended by the NIDA, or via a short questionnaire like the AUDIT-C (Alcohol Use Disorders Identification Test—Concise). Positive screens should lead to a further assessment to determine severity.

Assessment of Severity in Adults: At-Risk Drinking and Alcohol Use Disorder

Patients who exceed recommended drinking limits or cutoffs based on assessment scores but who do not meet the *Diagnostic and Statistical Manual of Mental Disorders,* 5th edition (*DSM-5*) criteria for an alcohol use disorder are considered to be "at risk." Those identified as such are most likely to benefit from a brief intervention, whereas those who meet the criteria for an alcohol use disorder should receive more intensive intervention.

Brief Interventions for Alcohol Use in Adults

Brief interventions for unhealthy drinking should provide an objective assessment of drinking and its consequences. Personalized advice on behavior changes should be provided in a clear and specific way. Abstinence is recommended for those with alcohol use disorder or specific comorbid medical or psychiatric disorders. For those not willing to abstain, a reduction in drinking can decrease the health risks associated with drinking.

Screening and Brief Interventions for Youth

Substance Use in Youth: General Considerations

Research shows that one in three children has had an alcoholic beverage by the end of 8th grade, with half becoming intoxicated. Drinking is also, at times, a factor in the leading causes of death in adolescents: unintentional injury, homicide, and suicide.

Although USPSTF guidelines state insufficient evidence to recommend routine screening, many professional organizations do recommend SBIs. The National Institute on Alcohol Abuse and Alcoholism recommends screening for all children ages 9 to 18 years and particularly for those who present with other risk factors, like commonly co-occurring mental health disorders (eg, depression, anxiety, attention deficit hyperactivity disorder, schizophrenia), or health conditions that might be alcohol related (eg, sleep, gastrointestinal or eating problems, sexually transmitted infections, unintended pregnancies).

Confidentiality and Parental Involvement

Confidentiality may help strengthen trust between the clinician and minor. Communication with the minor patient on the boundaries of confidentiality and when it might be broken is best delivered prior to screening. When substance use is identified, information about parental awareness should be gathered, and the clinician should encourage the minor patient to disclose the substance use to parents or guardians, particularly if consent has not been granted for direct communication with them. Clinicians should consider breaking confidentially to ensure safety, like in the presence of acute risk factors, a need for a treatment referral, or negative health consequences. Clinicians should utilize their medical judgment in their decision to break confidentiality as well as consult with organization guidelines and state laws.

Alcohol Screening in Youth

Establishing time alone with an adolescent during a visit and explaining confidentiality are central to building a good rapport with them. Explaining the purpose of asking about substance use is key to encourage honest answers. The NIDA recommends two age-appropriate questions that vary with age that assess the patient's and their friends' alcohol use.

Assessment of Severity in Youth: At-Risk Drinking and Alcohol Use Disorder

All youth who endorse drinking should be further assessed for severity. Those who do not drink should have that behavior reinforced via praise and should be counseled on plans to maintain their nondrinking status. Those who do drink should be evaluated for an alcohol use disorder via additional questions.

Substance Use Assessment Questionnaires for Youth

Several questionnaires can be used to clarify risk in an adolescent's substance use. The AUDIT may be used, but the threshold should be lowered to identify unhealthy alcohol use in adolescents. The NIDA and American Academy of Pediatrics recommend the CRAFFT (Car, Relax, Alone, Forget, Friends, Trouble), which evaluates drug and alcohol use in different contexts. The results of these assessments help the consideration of whether there is a substance or alcohol use disorder. Care should be taken to clarify the definition of a "single" drink, and additional risk factors should be considered, including family history and other environmental factors.

Alcohol Brief Intervention in Youth

All youth using alcohol should receive brief interventions, with those with low and moderate risk without the presence of an alcohol use disorder being advised to stop drinking, or at minimum to reduce their use. Those with an alcohol use disorder or who are at higher risk should be referred for addiction treatment. Follow-up appointments are more likely to be kept when other problems are also being addressed at that appointment.

CURRENT EVIDENCE ON SCREENING AND BRIEF INTERVENTIONS: A BRIEF SUMMARY

Screening and Brief Interventions for Unhealthy Alcohol Use

A meta-analysis of screening and brief interventions estimated a 10% risk reduction in risky drinking, a health impact that has been compared to other preventative interventions like screening for colorectal cancer or hypertension, and immunization for influenza. Notably, SBIs are delivered at much lower rates. Evidence for use in emergency department settings is mixed, but there is some evidence that it can reduce morbidity and mortality, and electronic SBIs have shown some promising results in different contexts.

Screening and Brief Interventions for Unhealthy Drug Use

The USPSTF has indicated that there is currently insufficient evidence to weigh the costs and benefits of SBIs. Despite a number of randomized trials, there is not evidential support for widespread implementation of SBIs for unhealthy drug use.

Screening and Brief Interventions for Prescription Opioid Misuse

Prescription and illicitly manufactured opioid use are on the rise, and deaths related to use are increasing. Tools for SBIs for opiate use are currently being studied and thus far have focused on drug-seeking behavior and toxicology results. Although there is no tool that has been validated for universal screening in primary care settings, the NIDA recommends the NM-ASSIST and the Substance Abuse and Mental Health Services Administration has noted the use of the CAGE questionnaire for these purposes.

Technology-Based Interventions for Unhealthy Drug Use

There is substantial evidence supporting the use of computer-, Internet-, text message-, or phone-based interventions for alcohol and tobacco use, but there is not strong evidence around drug use.

SYSTEMATIC REVIEWS AND META-ANALYSES OF SCREENING AND BRIEF INTERVENTIONS FOR UNHEALTHY ALCOHOL USE

Literature in the form of systematic reviews and meta-analyses indicate evidence in support of SBIs for alcohol. It is shown to be effective in primary care and emergency department settings, that multiple contact brief interventions provide the most benefit for both adults and adolescents, and that it can reduce binge drinking as well as the amount of alcohol consumed. Systematic reviews have also served, at times, to highlight the need for additional research.

INDIVIDUAL STUDIES OF SCREENING AND BRIEF INTERVENTIONS FOR UNHEALTHY ALCOHOL USE

Primary Care Settings

SBIs have been shown to be effective in primary care settings for unhealthy alcohol use that does not yet meet the criteria for an alcohol use disorder. Delivered in this setting, it allows for an integrated care for substance use, which can benefit related medical problems and can be cost-effective compared to "treatment as usual." Studies have shown that follow-up appointments are a critical component of SBIs and that when multiple sessions of brief interventions are provided, it can have an impact on drinking for years. The delivery of SBIs in dental clinics has also shown promising initial results in one study.

Adolescents and Young Adults

Research for SBIs for adolescent alcohol use is limited but encouraging. Studies focusing on screening in adolescents detected alcohol misuse more often than routine care and found that intervention with motivational interviewing can be effective for change around alcohol use. Motivational interviewing interventions have also been found to impact substance use behavior across a variety of substances. For adolescents, a decrease in risky alcohol or substance use can have a downstream positive impact in the form of fewer emergency department visits, motor vehicle accidents, and arrests.

Older Adults

A trial in older adults indicated decreased alcohol use 2 years after SBIs in a primary care setting.

College Students

Strong evidence exists for counselor- or psychologist-delivered SBIs, and interventions by primary care physicians in college health centers have shown moderate reductions in alcohol use.

INDIVIDUAL STUDIES OF SCREENING AND BRIEF INTERVENTIONS FOR UNHEALTHY DRUG USE

The evidence for SBIs for illicit drug use is limited, although some research has shown that computerized interventions for some substances and in some populations has also been effective.

Studies Suggesting a Benefit of Brief Interventions for Drug Use

Peer educators have been successfully utilized to reduce cocaine and heroin use in one study, but other research looking at both self-reports and biological outcomes demonstrated decreasing self-report scores and unchanging biological outcomes, indicating a component of social desirability impacting the results.

Studies Suggesting No Benefit of Brief Interventions for Unhealthy Drug Use Versus Treatment as Usual

A multinational study showed small substance changes for the sample overall, but when broken out by country, no change was observed for patients in the United States for those who received brief interventions versus those who received treatment as usual.

Other research with both single intervention and multiple intervention designs has found no efficacy for drug SBIs.

SUMMARY

SBIs in primary care settings have been shown to reduce self-reported alcohol use. In addition, SBIs are perceived as low cost and having little risk for harm, which is also why multiple professional organizations have recommended the use of SBIs. Good evidence exists for the effectiveness of SBIs in adolescents for both alcohol and tobacco use. Although implementation of SBIs can be challenging, it has become a high priority for federal funding initiatives.

KEY POINTS

1. Screening and brief intervention is an evidence-based intervention for alcohol use in general clinical settings.
2. Screening and brief intervention has shown efficacy for tobacco use but has inconsistent results for drug use interventions.
3. Motivational interviewing is an effective brief intervention that is best delivered over multiple visits.

REVIEW QUESTIONS

1. Brief intervention has been shown to be most effective when delivered in:
   A. writing.
   B. an hour-long session.
   C. multiple sessions.
   D. one session.

2. What should always be factored into planning next steps when reviewing screening tool scores?
   A. Toxicology results
   B. Clinical judgment
   C. Blood pressure
   D. Comorbid medical problems

3. Screening and brief intervention is supported by strong evidence for decreasing:
   A. drug use.
   B. tobacco use.
   C. alcohol use.
   D. both B and C.

ANSWERS

1. **C.** Brief interventions, like motivational interviewing, have been shown to work best and impact substance use behavior the most when delivered in multiple sessions.
2. **B.** Clinical judgment is always part of determining a plan for addressing substance use with a patient.
3. **D.** Strong evidence does not support SBIs for decreasing drug use.

SUGGESTED READINGS

Babor T, Higgins-Biddle JC. *Brief Intervention for Hazardous and Harmful Drinking: A Manual for Use in Primary Care*. Geneva: World Health Organization, 2001.

National Institute on Alcohol Abuse and Alcoholism. *Alcohol Screening and Brief Intervention for Youth: A Practitioner's Guide*. Rockville, MD: National Institute on Alcohol Abuse and Alcoholism, 2015. https://www.niaaa.nih.gov/publications/clinical-guides-and-manuals/alcohol-screening-and-brief-intervention-youth. Revised October 2015. Accessed July 5, 2018.

National Institute on Alcohol Abuse and Alcoholism. *Helping Patients Who Drink Too Much: A Clinician's Guide*. Rockville, MD: National Institute on Alcohol Abuse and Alcoholism, 2005. https://pubs.niaaa.nih.gov/publications/Practitioner/CliniciansGuide2005/clinicians_guide.htm. Updated 2007. Accessed July 5, 2018.

National Institute on Drug Abuse. Resource guide: Screening for drug use in general medical settings. https://www.drugabuse.gov/publications/resource-guide-screening-drug-use-in-general-medical-settings/introduction. Updated March 2012. Accessed July 5, 2018.

Substance Abuse and Mental Health Services. Screening, Brief Intervention, and Referral to Treatment. https://www.samhsa.gov/sbirt. Updated September 15, 2017. Accessed July 5, 2018.

Screening and Brief Intervention for Pregnant Women

Summary by Nicolas Bertholet

Based on THE ASAM PRINCIPLES OF ADDICTION MEDICINE, 6th edition sidebar by Nicolas Bertholet and Richard Saitz

ALCOHOL

Alcohol has harmful effects on the fetus that are completely preventable (by not drinking) and can be responsible for lifelong consequences such as fetal alcohol syndrome. Alcohol is teratogenic, and because of the absence of a developed blood filtration system, the fetus is unprotected from alcohol. Research suggests a linear association between prenatal alcohol exposure and birth defects and growth deficiencies, without evidence of a threshold. The current recommendation for pregnant women and women who might be pregnant is

Continued

to abstain from alcohol. Physicians should inform patients of this recommendation.

Women of childbearing age, including pregnant women, should be screened using validated tools (eg, T-ACE, TWEAK). Screening instruments developed for general populations may not perform as well in women and in women of childbearing age, which is why instruments have been developed specifically for this population. The T-ACE questionnaire, based on the CAGE questionnaire, is a four-question instrument involving the following:

- T (Tolerance): How many drinks does it take to make you feel high?
- A (Annoyed): Have people annoyed you by criticizing your drinking?
- C (Cut down): Have you ever felt you ought to cut down on your drinking?
- E (Eye opener): Have you ever had a drink first thing in the morning to steady your nerves or get rid of a hangover?

Affirmative answers to questions A, C, or E are 1 point each. Reporting tolerance to more than two drinks (T question) is scored 2 points. A score of 2 or more is considered positive.

The TWEAK questionnaire, also derived from the CAGE, is a five-question instrument and asks about the following points:

- T (Tolerance): How many drinks can you hold? (positive if ≥ six drinks), or How many drinks does it take before you begin to feel the first effects of alcohol? (positive if ≥ three drinks)
- W (Worry): Have close friends or relatives worried or complained about your drinking in the past year?
- E (Eye opener): Do you sometimes take a drink in the morning when you first get up?
- A (Amnesia): Has a friend or a family member ever told you about things you said or did while you were drinking that you could not remember?
- K ("Kut down"): Do you sometimes feel the need to cut down on your drinking?

Affirmative answers to question E, A, and K are 1 point each. Affirmative answers to questions W and T are 2 points each. The cutoff score is 2. Women positive by screening should then receive a brief intervention.

Although not specifically developed to screen pregnant women, the three-question AUDIT-C (Alcohol Use Disorders Identification Test—Concise), could also be used:

1. How often do you have a drink containing alcohol? Response options: *Never (0 points), monthly or less (1 point), two to four times a month (2 points), two to three times a week (3 points), four or more times a week (4 points)*
2. How many drinks containing alcohol do you have on a typical day when you are drinking? Response options: *One or two (0 points), three or four (1 point), five or six (2 points), seven to nine (3 points), ten or more (4 points)*
3. How often do you have six or more drinks on one occasion? Response options: *Never (0 points), less than monthly (1 point), monthly (2 points), weekly (3 points), daily or almost daily (4 points)*

Scoring is obtained by adding points of the three questions, with possible scores from 0 to 12 points. The cutoff score is ≥3 to screen for at-risk drinking (sensitivity: 95%; specificity: 85%) and alcohol use disorders (sensitivity: 96%; specificity: 71%).

Early intervention strategies are especially recommended. Unhealthy alcohol use should be identified before pregnancy to allow for behavior change. Pregnancy itself, or an assessment of alcohol use, may lead women to decrease or stop drinking. In addition to that effect, brief interventions can decrease risky use in young women (pregnant or not). Although not extensively confirmed in the literature to date, brief interventions can also decrease drinking during pregnancy and the risk of alcohol-exposed pregnancy, may increase abstinence, and may improve fetal outcomes. Even if brief interventions are effective predominantly in those in the highest risk category among those who drink, screening, advice to abstain from alcohol during pregnancy and before a planned pregnancy, and feedback on consequences of alcohol use on the fetus as well as medical complications related to alcohol use during pregnancy should be included in routine practice, because preventing alcohol use is the only way to prevent fetal alcohol syndrome and other alcohol-related effects on infants. Depending on resources available, the intervention can be repeated over a few sessions and/or include the partner because partner involvement may have beneficial effects.

OTHER DRUGS

Use of illicit drugs during pregnancy has a negative impact on the course of pregnancy and on the fetus. There is currently insufficient evidence to determine the benefits and harms of screening for illicit drug use among pregnant women. Nevertheless, given its potential preventive benefits, it seems reasonable, if not ethically required, for physicians to at least give feedback on consequences of use as well as advice to abstain. The Committee on Ethics of the American

College of Obstetricians and Gynecologists recommends universal screening and brief interventions for alcohol and illicit drug use based on an ethical rationale. This should be done with protection of confidentiality.

CONCLUSION AND RECOMMENDATIONS

Even in the absence of scientific data on screening and brief intervention efficacy among pregnant women, one should ask about medications, illicit drug use, and alcohol and tobacco use as part of a prenatal exam. If a substance use disorder is suspected, women should be referred for a comprehensive assessment in order to address substance use severity and associated psychosocial issues. As for alcohol, information on consequences of illicit drug and tobacco use on the fetus should also be provided to women of childbearing age. It should be noted that the specific context of pregnancy and the potential legal consequences will impact the accuracy of the screening and necessary ingredients of brief intervention, and clinicians will face the ethical challenges of having to balance principles of beneficence and respect for autonomy as they apply to both women and their children.

Trauma Centers, Hospitals, and Emergency Departments

Summary by Arthur F. Weissman

Based on THE ASAM PRINCIPLES OF ADDICTION MEDICINE, 6th edition sidebar by Arthur F. Weissman and Richard D. Blondell

Patients with substance use disorders are overrepresented in trauma, acute medical, and emergency settings. Untreated comorbid substance use problems generate worse clinical outcomes and increased costs, suggesting an important target for screening.

CASE FINDING AND SCREENING

Validated screening instruments for unhealthy ethanol use include single questions ("how many times in the past year have you had X or more drinks in a day," where X is four for women, and five for men), and the three-item AUDIT-C (Alcohol Use Disorders Identification Test—Concise). Modified versions are available for illicit drug use. A state prescription monitoring program report can suggest a substance use disorder. Routine toxicology testing is useful in trauma patients due to the high rate of alcohol and illicit drug use in this population. Clinicians should be aware of confidentiality and insurance issues regarding toxicology. In some states, insurers can deny payment for trauma costs if there has been a positive alcohol or drug test.

CLINICAL ASSESSMENT FOR RISK OF WITHDRAWAL

Withdrawal syndromes may be life threatening, particularly with alcohol or sedative–hypnotic medications. Regular heavy drinking or sedative use should prompt monitoring for withdrawal. The best predictor of severe alcohol withdrawal syndrome (AWS) is a prior history of complicated alcohol withdrawal, including delirium tremens or alcohol withdrawal seizures.

INITIAL MANAGEMENT OF WITHDRAWAL SYNDROMES

Parenteral thiamine should be administered to patients with an alcohol use disorder or a history of heavy drinking before glucose-containing intravenous fluids are given to prevent Wernicke encephalopathy. Long-acting benzodiazepines are the medications of choice to prevent and treat AWS. Dexmedetomidine and propofol have been used to control refractory alcohol withdrawal symptoms; both should be used with intensive care unit monitoring. Evidence is insufficient to support the routine use of anticonvulsants for the treatment of AWS. Phenobarbital has no proven advantages over long-acting benzodiazepines for treatment of AWS and has a less favorable safety profile. Opioid withdrawal, which can be life threatening, should be treated, for example, with long-acting opioids such as methadone or buprenorphine.

Continued

NEW CHALLENGES

Patients misusing new synthetic cannabinoids, "bath salts," and synthetic hallucinogens may present with tachycardia, anxiety, agitation, and psychosis. Potent synthetic opioids such as U-47700 ("Pink") and carfentanil may cause profound respiratory depression, noncardiogenic pulmonary edema, and hemoptysis. Commercially available toxicology screens are usually unable to detect these drugs. Physicians should continue to screen patients, and especially young patients, for cannabis use due to significant health risks (including cannabis use disorder, impaired driving, and associations with poor educational and occupational performance), notwithstanding the enthusiasm for legalization of cannabis in the United States.

EFFICACY OF BRIEF INTERVENTIONS

Brief interventions for unhealthy alcohol use are associated with modest reductions, at best, in alcohol consumption and health consequences. Research showing any benefit of brief interventions for illicit drug use has been elusive. A large, multisite, randomized controlled trial of screening and brief intervention for adult illicit drug use in the emergency department showed no evidence of efficacy.

THE PHYSICIAN'S ROLE

In these high prevalence settings, patients should be screened for unhealthy substance use, for example, with brief validated tools, prescription monitoring reports, and toxicology, and should be counseled to cut down or quit in the context of a teachable moment. The absence of a proven benefit for screening and brief intervention for illicit drug use does not mean that identifying unhealthy substance use is not important. Brief interventions may have an improved effect when repeated over time, and treatment should be offered if the patient is ready. Physicians can demonstrate an important leadership role by screening their patients for unhealthy substance use behaviors.

SUGGESTED READINGS

Choo E, Ranney M, Wetle T, et al. Attitudes toward computer interventions for partner abuse and drug use among women in the emergency department. *Addict Disord Their Treat*. 2015;14(2):95-104.

Gurmankin AD, Baron J, Hershey JC, Ubel PA. The role of physicians' recommendations in medical treatment decisions. *Med Decis Making*. 2002;22(3):262-271.

Haskins BL, Davis-Martin R, Abar B, et al. Health evaluation and referral assistant: a randomized controlled trial of a Web-based screening, brief intervention, and referral to treatment system to reduce risky alcohol use among emergency department patients. *J Med Internet Res*. 2017;19(5):e119.

Mello MJ, Bromberg J, Baird J, et al. Translation of alcohol screening and brief intervention guidelines to pediatric trauma centers. *J Trauma Acute Care Surg*. 2013;75(4 suppl 3): S301-S307.

Seale JP, Shellenberger S, Clark DC. Providing competency-based family medicine residency training in substance abuse in the new millennium: a model curriculum. *BMC Med Educ*. 2010;10:33.

Implementation of Screening and Brief Intervention (SBI) in Clinical Settings Using Quality Improvement Principles

Summary by Emily C. Williams and Katharine A. Bradley

Based on THE ASAM PRINCIPLES OF ADDICTION MEDICINE, 6th edition sidebar by Emily C. Williams and Katharine A. Bradley

Despite evidence-based recommendations that alcohol screening and brief intervention (SBI) be routinely implemented in primary care settings, efforts to implement SBI have been disappointing. However, some integrated healthcare systems are making progress toward implementation. One example is the Veterans Administration (VA). We provide a retrospective analysis of VA's implementation based on a comprehensive conceptual model of dissemination of innovations in healthcare settings (Fig. 22-1).

Greenhalgh and colleagues' model outlines the importance of the nature of an *Innovation* as well as the characteristics of both the *User System* and *Innovators* and the *Linkage* between the two. *Innovations* are more likely to be successfully implemented if they are simple, relevant to the user, and easily transferable. The setting in which

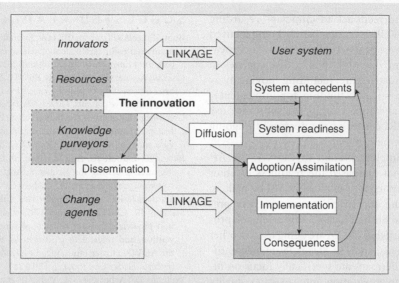

Figure 22-1. Factors that influence the success of implementing innovations. (Adapted from Greenhalgh T, Robert G, Macfarlane F, Bate P, Kyriakidou O. Diffusion of innovations in service organizations: systematic review and recommendations. *Milbank Q* 2004; 82[4]:581-629.)

implementation occurs—the *User System*—is also central to the success of innovations. Important components of *User Systems* that help determine the success of innovations include system antecedents (eg, quality improvement resources), system readiness (eg, institutional pressures for change), characteristics of adopters (eg, motivation, values, understanding of the innovation), the implementation process (eg, support from leadership), and evaluation and feedback that allows the system to address consequences of implementation. *Innovators* typically consist of formal or informal "teams" of experts ("knowledge purveyors") and leaders able to actualize change ("change agents") with access to resources required to implement an innovation. Efforts to implement innovations are also most successful when there is strong *Linkage* between the innovators and the user system, both during the development of an innovation and throughout the implementation process.

The VA healthcare system had undergone a number of quality improvement initiatives, which served as system antecedents that provided an essential foundation for SBI implementation. These include a nationwide electronic medical record (EMR) with embedded clinical reminders, a system of nationwide performance measures that incentivize recommended care and are linked to financial incentives for network directors, and data systems (medical record reviews and patient satisfaction surveys) to monitor performance. The VA

also had condition-specific Quality Enhancement Research Initiative centers, including one focused on substance use disorders (SUD QUERI). These centers developed research programs to identify important gaps in the quality of VA care, evaluate interventions to address identified gaps, and develop and evaluate strategies for implementation. Findings from the VA's Large Health Study of Veterans suggesting an unmet need among patients with unhealthy alcohol use created pressure from the US Congress for VA leadership to do more to recognize and treat unhealthy alcohol use and served as the impetus for *linkage* between VA quality managers and SUD QUERI researchers. Via this linkage, the VA built upon its existing quality improvement structures to implement national performance measures and electronic clinical reminders to prompt and document both screening and brief intervention. The QUERI infrastructure provided ongoing core funding for implementation research after initial funding of innovations by research (ie, development and pilot testing of EMR clinical reminders). However, clinician education regarding SBI was delegated to local quality and clinical leaders with variable expertise and interest. Initially, the QUERI infrastructure—with a rapid grant-funding mechanism coupled with core funding—enabled formative evaluations that identified gaps in SBI quality. Formative evaluations also highlighted the importance of ongoing attention to the educational needs of clinicians

Continued

("adopters") and feedback to clinicians regarding performance. While attention is now being focused on identifying best practices and performance measures that incentivize high-quality SBI, changes in the QUERI infrastructure, including moving away from condition-specific funding for implementation research (and thus closing the substance use disorders QUERI center), have decreased ongoing quality improvement research.

Since SBI implementation in the VA, the Affordable Care Act increased the readiness of other US healthcare systems to implement SBI by making alcohol screening and brief intervention core preventive benefits. Similar quality improvement processes to those used in the VA are being used in other healthcare systems, such as Kaiser Permanente. Efforts in Kaiser Permanente specifically focus on incorporating implementation into existing quality improvement structures, such as performance monitoring and "Plan Do Study Act" or "PDSA" cycles that are currently used by local clinics to optimize care quality. Cross-system implementation research could enable identification of key determinants of implementation success, as measured by delivery and quality of care provided.

SUGGESTED READINGS

Bobb JF, Lee AK, Lapham GT, et al. Evaluation of a pilot implementation to integrate alcohol-related care within primary care. *Int J Environ Res Public Health*. 2017;14(9):E1030.

Chi FW, Weisner CM, Mertens JR, Ross TB, Sterling SA. Alcohol brief intervention in primary care: blood pressure outcomes in hypertensive patients. *J Subst Abuse Treat*. 2017;77:45-51.

Greenhalgh T, Robert G, Macfarlane F, Bate P, Kyriakidou O. Diffusion of innovations in service organizations: systematic review and recommendations. *Milbank Q*. 2004;82(4):581-629.

Jonas DE, Garbutt JC, Amick HR, et al. Behavioral counseling after screening for alcohol misuse in primary care: a systematic review and meta-analysis for the U.S. Preventive Services Task Force. *Ann Intern Med*. 2012;157(9):645-654.

Mertens JR, Chi FW, Weisner CM, et al. Physician versus non-physician delivery of alcohol screening, brief intervention, and referral to treatment in adult primary care: the ADVISe cluster randomized controlled implementation trial. *Addict Sci Clin Pract*. 2015;10:26.

Williams EC, Achtmeyer CE, Young JP, et al. Local implementation of alcohol screening and brief intervention at five Veterans Health Administration primary care clinics: perspectives of clinical and administrative staff. *J Subst Abuse Treat*. 2016;60:27-35.

Williams EC, Johnson ML, Lapham GT, et al. Strategies to implement alcohol screening and brief intervention in primary care settings: a structured literature review. *Psychol Addict Behav*. 2011;25(2):206-214.

Screening for Unhealthy Alcohol Use in the Elderly

Summary by James W. Campbell

Based on THE ASAM PRINCIPLES OF ADDICTION MEDICINE, 6th edition sidebar by James W. Campbell

EPIDEMIOLOGY

The 2010 census projects nearly 50 million Americans older than 65 years by 2020. Current projections are that by 2050, 83 million Americans will be elderly. Alcoholism is present in 6% to 11% of older persons admitted to hospitals. Alcoholism is estimated to be the third most common psychiatric disorder among elderly persons.

Definitions are confounded in this population, and screening tools have to be appropriate for the biopsychosocial reality of elderly persons. The older cohort is especially adverse to the label of person with an alcohol use disorder and is more amenable to accepting that their alcohol intake is negatively impacting their health. Screening for unhealthy alcohol use is a more appropriate goal for primary care. Elders are more likely to be widowed, retired, and socially isolated, all contributing to poor alcohol use detection rates. The presence of alcohol use disorder is significantly impacted by pharmacokinetic changes with aging, which cause more consequences at lower quantities and frequency of alcohol intake.

Older individuals are less likely to be screened and are more likely to have their symptoms attributed to aging or to diseases common in elders rather than suspected as an alcohol problem. In addition, alcohol's impact on etiology or exacerbation of common diseases is likely to be overlooked in older persons. Many older people with alcohol use disorders present as a new medical diagnosis or an exacerbation of a chronic medical condition.

TABLE 22-1   Test Sensitivity and Specificity for Alcohol Use Disorder when Used in Older Individuals

Tool	Sensitivity	Specificity
MAST	1.0	0.83
AUDIT[a,b]	0.83	0.91
GMAST short version	0.94	0.78
CAGE (1 of 4 considered positive screen)	0.91	0.48
Alcohol-related problems survey (short version)	0.92	0.51

[a]AUDIT-C had similar psychometric properties to AUDIT.
[b]Hager-Johnson G, Sabia S, Brunner EJ, et al. Combined impact of smoking and heavy alcohol use on cognitive decline in early old age: Whitehall II prospective cohort study. *Br J Psychiatry*. 2013;203(2):120-125.
Data from Buchsbaum DG, Buchanan BA, Welsh MA, et al. Screening for drinking in the elderly using the CAGE questionnaire. *J Am Geriatr Soc*. 1992;40:662; and Widlitz M, Marin DB. Substance abuse in older adults: an overview. *Geriatrics*. 2002;57:29.

Screening is improved by the use of geriatric-specific screening instruments or standard tools that are age adjusted for a number of responses that indicate a positive screen. Table 22-1 summarizes a few of the more common tools. The Alcohol Use Disorders Identification Test—Concise is helpful for primary care screening where time is limited. A brief screen facilitates primary care intervention.

Impact of Alcohol Use Disorder on Health

In elders, the negative consequences of alcohol use disorder are even more severe than in younger populations. The neurocognitive impairment that is already common in this population is worsened by an alcohol use disorder. It is estimated that as many as 10% of patients with diagnosed Alzheimer disease may have an alcoholic dementia or a dementia presentation worsened by an alcohol use disorder. Many health and sensory realities of aging also make manifestations of alcohol use disorder more severe. A classic example, hip fracture, is associated with alcohol use disorder through not only an increase in falls but also a direct effect by exacerbating osteoporosis.

INTERVENTION

Mechanisms to guide a patient into treatment are similar to other age groups, and brief office or urgent care/emergency department intervention can be effective, at least for those without a moderate-to-severe disorder. The value of an elderly-specific treatment milieu or group is debated. Although logical, no evidence exists to support the differential benefit of an elderly-specific treatment environment or group.

SUMMARY

In summary, the age wave is upon us, and rates of alcohol use and other drug abuse—especially prescription drug abuse—in elders approach the rates in younger populations. The diagnosis is often missed as a result of poor screening techniques, cohort underreporting, age bias, and misattribution of alcohol-related health issues to either aging or diseases common in elders. Appropriate screening tools do exist and are useful, although markedly underused. In addition, brief intervention and standard treatment strategies, including Alcoholics Anonymous, are effective. The health yield of sobriety is tremendous because alcohol use disorder is even more dangerous when it occurs in older persons. Finally, alcohol recovery rates are at least as favorable in elders as in younger populations.

Laboratory Assessment

Summary by Trang M. Vu and Linda Wang

Based on THE ASAM PRINCIPLES OF ADDICTION MEDICINE,
6th edition chapter by Jessica S. Merlin, Elizabeth A. Warner, and
Joanna L. Starrels

Laboratory testing can help identify substance use, assist in the diagnosis and management of substance use disorders, and monitor for safety and pattern of use in patients prescribed controlled substances.

APPROACH TO TESTING

Clinicians should learn how to effectively interpret results within the clinical context while recognizing the limitations of testing, such as false-positive and false-negative results.

Commonly used testing sources include urine and blood, with urine being the most common. Urine specimens can be easily adulterated or substituted, but valid specimens typically are between 90° and 100°F within 4 minutes of collection, have a specific gravity over 1.003, and creatinine concentrations greater than 5 ng/mL. Blood specimens are less likely to be altered, can be more accurate than urine in assessing recent substance use, and are useful when patients cannot easily produce urine (ie, dialysis). However, alcohol and other substances are usually present in urine longer than in blood.

Oral fluids can also be used as a testing source; substance concentrations mirror that in blood. However, contamination of oral fluids from recent smoking, gum, citric acid candy, or mouthwash can affect results. Oral fluid collection is noninvasive and can be done in the presence of an examiner, thereby reducing the risk of adulteration. Similar to blood, substances may not be present in oral fluids as long as in urine.

Proper specimen collection and processing are critical for accurate results. Clinicians should note the timing of the collection and when the last dose of the substance was taken in order to interpret results in the appropriate context. Chain-of-custody regulations in forensic or workplace testing are used to prevent misidentification but are not routinely done in clinical practice.

The initial ordered test is usually a screening urine immunoassay. It is inexpensive, yields rapid results, and often tests for multiple commonly used substances. Immunoassays utilize antibodies to detect a target, which might be a specific substance class, parent substance, or a metabolite. They are limited, however, by antibody cross-reactivity with other substances that can yield a false-positive result (Table 23-1). Another limitation is immunoassays have variable sensitivities for detecting different substances within the same class. Confirmatory testing by gas or liquid chromatography followed by mass spectroscopy can specifically identify and quantify the concentration of substances or metabolites but is often expensive and not widely available. In clinical practice, confirmatory testing is necessary to specifically identify substances when there is an unexpected immunoassay result.

A cutoff or threshold is a defined concentration of an analyte in a specimen at or above which the test result in an immunoassay is reported as positive. If a substance is detected in concentrations lower than the set cutoff, the test result is reported as negative. If this occurs with a screening immunoassay, additional confirmatory testing can be helpful. Lower cutoff levels are associated with high sensitivity and longer detection times but cause more false-positive results. Table 23-2 lists approximate duration of detection time from the time of last use.

Point-of-care (POC) or on-site testing refers to tests performed outside of a central laboratory and include rapid immunoassay kits that test urine or oral fluid for commonly used substances. Although studies show that POC test results are comparable to those of immunoassays, their interpretation can be subjective and operator dependent. Moreover, cutoffs are not standardized, subjecting these tests to false-positive and false-negative results. As such, they remain screening tests, and unexpected results should be verified with confirmatory testing.

Federal guidelines govern the drug testing of federal and Department of Transportation (DOT)

TABLE 23-1 Substances Reported to Cause False-Positive Results in Urine Immunoassays Due to Cross-reactivity

Amphetamines/ Methamphetamines	Barbiturates	Marijuana	Oxycodone
• Benzphetamine (Didrex)	• Phenytoin	• Dronabinol	• Naloxone
• Bupropion	**Benzodiazepines**	• Sativex	**Phencyclidine**
• Chloroquine	• Oxaprozin	• Efavirenz	• Dextromethorphan
• Chlorpromazine	• Sertraline	• Pantoprazole	• Diphenhydramine
• Ephedrine	• Lysergic acid	• Quinacrine	• Thioridazine
• Fenfluramine	diethylamide (LSD)		• Venlafaxine
• Labetalol	• Amitriptyline	**Methadone**	
• Mexiletine	• Chlorpromazine	• Quetiapine	**Propoxyphenes**
• N-Acetylprocainamide	• Doxepin		• Cyclobenzaprine
• Phentermine	• Fluoxetine	**Opiates**	• Diphenhydramine
• Phenylephrine	• Haloperidol	• Ciprofloxacin	• Doxylamine
• Phenylpropanolamine	• Metoclopramide	• Gatifloxacin	• Imipramine
• Propranolol	• Risperidone	• Levofloxacin	• Methadone
• Pseudoephedrine	• Sertraline	• Lomefloxacin	
• Quinacrine	• Thioridazine	• Moxifloxacin	
• Ranitidine	• Verapamil	• Norfloxacin	
• Selegiline		• Ofloxacin	
• Trazodone		• Papaverine	
• Tyramine		• Pefloxacin	
• Vicks inhaler		• Rifampicin	
		• Poppy seeds	

TABLE 23-2 Approximate Detection Time Using Screening Urine Immunoassays (with Commonly Used Cutoffs)

Drug	Duration of Detection[a] (Approximate)
Amphetamine	1–3 d
Methamphetamine	3 d
Barbiturate	
Short acting	1–4 d
Long acting	Several weeks
Cocaine	3 d
Marijuana	
Single joint (using 50 ng/mL cutoff)	2 d
Heavy use (using 20 ng/mL cutoff)	Up to 27 d
Opioids	
Heroin, codeine, morphine	1–2 d
Methadone (using a specific assay for methadone)	2–3 d
PCP	7 d

[a]The duration of detection is variable and depends on dose, route of administration, pattern of use, laboratory cutoff, and individual metabolism.

workers, which must be done in nationally certified laboratories. Workplace urine drug testing includes marijuana metabolites (tetrahydrocannabinol [THC]), cocaine metabolites, opiate metabolites, phencyclidine (PCP), and amphetamines. Clinical laboratories perform substance testing for diagnostic purposes and can select which substances to include in their immunoassay screens. Specimens obtained for clinical use are not subject to the same collection and testing requirements used in the federal workplace. Consulting with the laboratory's clinical toxicologist can be helpful for interpretation.

SUBSTANCE-SPECIFIC TESTS
Alcohol

Recent alcohol intake can be assessed using blood and breath tests, but these measurements cannot determine impairment because some individuals develop tolerance to the effects of alcohol. Blood alcohol concentration (BAC) reflects alcohol ingestion in the preceding few hours. Gas chromatography is considered the gold standard for measuring ethanol in forensic labs, but many clinical laboratories use enzymatic methods. The enzymatic analysis measures the amount of nicotinamide adenine dinucleotide formed during oxidation of ethanol. The presence of isopropanol, such as when acetone produced in diabetic ketoacidosis or starvation states is metabolized into isopropanol, can falsely elevate readings.

Although clinical laboratories measure ethanol in serum or plasma, most states define intoxication based on whole-blood alcohol levels of either 80 or 100 mg/dL. The water content of serum is higher than that of whole blood; therefore, serum samples will have a higher ethanol level than whole blood samples. An estimated ratio of serum to whole blood is 1.14/1.00; serum or plasma specimens for alcohol must be corrected appropriately.

Breath alcohol testing, usually done in traffic law enforcement and Department of Transportation testing, analyzes the alveolar concentration of ethanol in the last third of a deep breath. Failure to obtain a deep breath can lead to an underestimation of BAC. The ratio of blood-to-breath concentration of alcohol is approximately 2,100:1. In the United States, breath alcohol concentration is reported in grams per 210 L, so a breath level of 0.1 g/210 L is equivalent to a whole-blood level of 100 mg/dL.

POC oral fluid tests that approximate serum ethanol levels are available, but salivary alcohol levels do not correlate as well with breath tests in measuring BAC. Urine testing for alcohol offers a qualitative marker of recent alcohol ingestion in the preceding 8 hours but is difficult to interpret given variable urine concentrations that are affected by length of time urine has been in the bladder. Ethyl glucuronide and ethyl sulfate are metabolites of ethanol that can be detected in urine from 24 hours up to 5 days later depending on the amount of alcohol ingested but have high false-positive rates.

Certain biomarkers in the blood can be used to predict alcohol-related health problems, including γ-glutamyltransferase (GGT), erythrocyte mean cell volume (MCV), and serum aminotransferases. GGT is the most sensitive marker for detecting alcohol use disorder (AUD), its levels being elevated in approximately 75% of persons with diagnosed AUD, in approximately 50% of patients hospitalized for alcohol-related problems, and in approximately 30% of people who drink heavy amounts and have alcohol-related problems. However, GGT is not specific for AUD and can be elevated in patients with fatty liver or obstructive liver disease and in those using anticonvulsant medications. It can be used to monitor abstinence—levels can return to normal over 2 to 4 weeks after abstinence. MCV, a measurement of red blood cell (RBC) size, increases with chronic heavy drinking but is not specific for detecting alcohol-related conditions because RBC size can be increased in chronic liver

disease, hypothyroidism, folate deficiency, and megaloblastic disorders. MCV can decline with abstinence but can take at least 3 months to see an improvement due to the life span of an RBC. Serum aminotransferases such as aspartate amino transferase (AST) and alanine aminotransferase (ALT) may be elevated in patients with AUD, with AST is typically more elevated than ALT in the setting of alcohol use. Although elevations in AST and ALT can suggest alcohol-related liver disease, they are not sensitive markers for AUD or intoxication.

Phosphatidylethanol, a phospholipid in cellular membranes that is produced in the presence of alcohol, is a newer alcohol biomarker. When tested in blood, a level ≥8 ng/mL can be used to identify heavy alcohol use in the preceding 2 to 3 weeks; however, it has limited accuracy, and further study is warranted before it can be widely implemented.

Despite the availability of these tests, it is important to remember that patients with a low pretest probability of AUD are likely to have false-positive results, and none of the biomarkers are sensitive or specific enough to be used in screening for unhealthy alcohol use or AUD.

Amphetamines

Amphetamines include stimulants such as amphetamine, methamphetamine, 3,4-methylenedioxymethamphetamine (MDMA), 3,4-methylenedioxyamphetamine (MDA), and 3,4-methylenedioxy-N-ethylamphetamine (MDEA). Screening tests for amphetamines usually target methamphetamine and have variable cross-reactivity with MDMA, MDEA, and MDA. Amphetamine is a metabolite of methamphetamine and can be differentiated using confirmatory testing. Compared with other commonly tested substances, amphetamines have the most false-positive test results as many sympathomimetic amines are structurally similar and cross-react with the immunoassays. Selegiline and benzphetamine are metabolized to either amphetamine or methamphetamine, and medications for attention deficit hyperactivity disorder, including Adderall (mixture of L-amphetamine and D-amphetamine), will give a positive amphetamine test. Methylphenidate is not metabolized to amphetamine or methamphetamine and is not detected on confirmatory testing for either.

Amphetamines can be detected in a urine immunoassay between 1 and 3 days after last use; however, daily use of methamphetamines can prolong the detection period to 3 days in urine and 1 day in oral fluids. Urine pH can influence the excretion of amphetamines; ingestion of large quantities of bicarbonate can reduce the amount of amphetamines excreted.

Barbiturates

Barbiturates are central nervous system depressants that vary in duration of action. Most urine immunoassays detect the parent substance secobarbital using a cutoff of either 200 or 300 ng/mL, and with the exception of phenobarbital, only small amounts of the parent substance are detectable in urine. The duration of detection in urine is variable and depends on the dose; short-acting barbiturates are detected from 1 to 4 days after use and long-acting barbiturates can be detected for several weeks after use.

Benzodiazepines

Benzodiazepines comprise multiple substances with diverse potencies and metabolites, making urine, immunoassay interpretation complicated. The parent substance is seldom present in the urine, and many benzodiazepines cross-react poorly with common immunoassays, leading to false-negative results. Clorazepate, chlordiazepoxide, and diazepam are metabolized to nordiazepam and oxazepam. Clonazepam is metabolized to 7-aminoclonazepam. Alprazolam, lorazepam, and triazolam are excreted as glucuronide conjugates. Many benzodiazepine immunoassays are designed to detect nordiazepam or oxazepam and are less likely to detect clonazepam, lorazepam, or triazolam unless present in high doses. The cutoff for these immunoassays is typically 200 or 300 ng/mL, which may not detect therapeutic doses.

Cocaine

Cocaine is available as either cocaine hydrochloride, a powdered, water-soluble form that can be snorted or injected, or as "crack," an alkaloid, non–water-soluble form that can be smoked. Urine immunoassays specifically detect benzoylecgonine, the major urinary cocaine metabolite, using a cutoff of 300 ng/mL. Detection is variable based on the amount ingested, and the usual detection time after use is 2 to 3 days, but some reports suggest positive immunoassays up to 22 days after periods of prolonged and heavy use. Ingestion of coca tea can result in positive immunoassays.

Lysergic Acid Diethylamide

The hallucinogen lysergic acid diethylamide (LSD) metabolizes to *nor*-LSD (*N*-desmethyl-LSD), and less than 1% of the parent LSD is present in urine. Most immunoassay panels do not include LSD,

which can be detected for 2 to 5 days after use at a cutoff of 0.5 ng/mL. False-positive results can occur with amitriptyline, chlorpromazine, doxepin, fluoxetine, haloperidol, metoclopramide, risperidone, sertraline, and verapamil.

Marijuana

Marijuana's psychoactive component, THC, is quickly absorbed into circulation and stored in fat tissues. Its inactive metabolite, 11-nor-9-carboxy-Δ9-tetrahydrocannabinol (THC-COOH or THCA), is what most laboratories measure in urine immunoassays at cutoffs of 20, 50, or 100 ng/mL. The federally mandated cutoff is 50 ng/mL. Detection time varies based on assay sensitivity, amount ingested, and whether an individual uses marijuana intermittently (detectable up to 2 to 4 days later) or chronically (detectable up to 27 days later). Hemp seed oil and dronabinol (Marinol), a synthetic THC, can result in positive urine test results for marijuana. Cannabis products that include cannabidiol (CBD) or other cannabinoids do not contain THC and are not likely to test positive. Passive exposure to marijuana smoke is unlikely to result in positive screening tests.

Opiates and Opioids

Opiates, which include morphine, codeine, and heroin, are derived from seeds of the opium poppy. The term *opioid* encompasses these natural opiates as well as all agonists and antagonists with morphine-like activity, such as semisynthetic opioids (eg, hydrocodone, hydromorphone, oxycodone, oxymorphone) and synthetic opioids (eg, methadone, buprenorphine, meperidine, fentanyl).

Opiate screening immunoassays detect opiates using morphine for the target and have little to no cross-reactivity with synthetic opioids and variable cross-reactivity with semisynthetic opioids. A patient taking oxycodone is likely to have a negative urine opiate screen, whereas someone taking morphine or codeine is likely to have a positive urine opiate screen. Ingestion of poppy seeds, which contain morphine and codeine, can result in a positive urine opiate screen. As a result, in 1997, the federal government raised the screening cutoff for opiate testing in workplace programs from 300 to 2,000 ng/mL to reduce the number of false-positive results, although many clinical laboratories still use a cutoff value of 300 ng/mL. Immunoassays specific for semisynthetic and synthetic opioids are available, including for oxycodone, methadone, fentanyl, carfentanil, and buprenorphine. Some screening panels may assess for these substances.

TABLE 23-3 Monitoring Opioid Therapy: Expected Results on Urine Opiate Screening and Confirmatory Testing

Prescribed Opioid	Opiate Immunoassay	GC/MS or LC/MS-MS
Morphine	Positive	Morphine
		Codeine
Codeine	Positive	Codeine
		Morphine
		Hydrocodone (minor metabolite)
Hydrocodone	Positive	Hydrocodone
		Hydromorphone (minor metabolite)
Hydromorphone	Positive	Hydromorphone
Oxycodone	Positive/negative[a]	Oxycodone
		Oxymorphone (minor metabolite)
Oxymorphone	Negative	Oxymorphone
Methadone	Negative	Methadone
Fentanyl	Negative	Fentanyl

GC/MS, gas chromatography/mass spectrometry; LC/MS-MS, liquid chromatography with tandem mass spectrometry.
[a]Depends on the cross-reactivity of the opiate assay with the prescribed drug; varies among assays.

If they are not included, skip directly to confirmatory testing.

Knowing opioid metabolic pathways is crucial to being able to accurately interpret opioid screening and confirmatory testing (Table 23-3). Heroin is metabolized to a short-acting metabolite, 6-monoacetylmorphine, which is rapidly hydrolyzed to morphine and further to hydromorphone. 6-Monoacetylmorphine is a specific byproduct of heroin metabolism, but is not routinely tested for. Codeine metabolizes to morphine and subsequently to hydromorphone or hydrocodone, which further breaks down to hydromorphone. Oxycodone metabolizes exclusively to oxymorphone.

Methadone

Methadone is not detected in opiate immunoassays and requires a separate immunoassay that has little cross-reactivity with other opioids and can detect methadone at a cutoff of 300 ng/mL about 2 to 3 days after use.

Phencyclidine

PCP can be snorted or smoked in powdered form ("angel dust") or ingested in tablet form. The federal government requires PCP testing for all federal employees. Urine immunoassay results can detect PCP at a cutoff of 25 ng/dL approximately 7 days after a single dose and up to 21 days after chronic use.

Lab Testing for Newer Substances

Newer substances, which include synthetic cannabinoids and "bath salts," ketamine, γ-hydroxybutyic acid (GHB), salvia, and flunitrazepam (Rohypnol), are used recreationally and not routinely tested for in clinical settings.

Synthetic cannabinoids refer to a growing group of substances found in herbal products such as "Spice" or "K2" that are structurally related to that of THC and are agonists at cannabinoid receptors. Despite being structurally similar, these compounds are not detected by routine THC screening, but specific immunoassays and confirmatory tests are being developed and increasingly available. "Bath salts" are synthetic stimulants derived from the khat plant. Ketamine, an N-methyl-D-aspartate receptor antagonist, is being explored as a rapid antidepressant but is also increasingly used recreationally. Ketamine is metabolized to norketamine, which is not detected on standard urine toxicology screens. Commercially available immunoassays can detect ketamine for approximately 3 days after use; more sensitive gas chromatography/mass spectrometry testing can detect ketamine for a week or more, depending on the amount used.

GHB is an agonist at GHB and γ-aminobutyric acid (GABA$_B$) receptors and cause central nervous system depression. GHB can be detected on gas chromatography/mass spectrometry testing but has a window of detection of less than 12 hours in urine after a single episode of use and even shorter detection time in plasma. Flunitrazepam (Rohypnol) is a powerful benzodiazepine also used recreationally and in sexual assault. It can be detected in most urine immunoassays for benzodiazepines for up to 12 days.

Ethical Considerations

Drug testing to aid in the diagnosis or treatment of substance use disorder is recommended and associated with improved outcomes. Routine laboratory screening is not currently a standard of care. There are limits and implications to drug testing. Care must be taken when interpreting test results to not draw premature or incorrect conclusions about substance use. Clinicians should adhere to regulations about obtaining consent, disclosure of medical records, and federal substance use disorder confidentiality.

KEY POINTS

1. Laboratory testing in clinical settings can identify substance use, support the diagnosis and treatment of substance use disorders, and monitor for safety and adherence in patients prescribed controlled substances.
2. Urine opiate screening immunoassays test for morphine and codeine and do not reliably detect semisynthetic and synthetic opioids such as oxycodone, fentanyl, or methadone.
3. Urine benzodiazepine immunoassays do not reliably detect clonazepam unless present in high doses.
4. Marijuana detection in the urine depends on whether the person is an occasional versus a chronic user.
5. Many newer substances, including synthetic marijuana, are not detected in routine urine screening.

REVIEW QUESTIONS

1. Which of the following is not detected on urine opiate drug immunoassays?
   A. Codeine
   B. Morphine
   C. Fentanyl
   D. Heroin
   E. Hydrocodone

2. What is the most appropriate initial screening test for drug use?
   A. Urine gas chromatography with mass spectroscopy
   B. Blood levels for specific drugs
   C. Saliva test for specific drugs
   D. Urine immunoassay that may include a panel of drugs

3. Which of the following is not routinely detected in standard urine drug immunoassays?
   A. Cocaine
   B. Amphetamines
   C. Opiates
   D. Benzodiazepines
   E. Synthetic marijuana

ANSWERS

1. **C.** Most urine opiate drug immunoassays detect natural opiates (morphine, codeine, heroin), have little to no cross-reactivity with synthetic opioids (fentanyl), and have variable cross-reactivity with semisynthetic opioids (oxycodone).
2. **D.** The initial ordered test is usually a screening urine immunoassay. It is inexpensive, yields rapid results, and often tests for multiple commonly used substances.
3. **E.** Newer substances, which include synthetic cannabinoids and "bath salts," ketamine, GHB, salvia, and flunitrazepam (Rohypnol), are used recreationally and are not routinely tested for in screening immunoassays.

SUGGESTED READINGS

Dolan K, Rouen D, Kimber J. An overview of the use of urine, hair, sweat and saliva to detect drug use. *Drug Alcohol Rev.* 2004;23(2):213-217.

Jaffee WB, Trucco E, Levy S, Weiss RD. Is this urine really negative? A systematic review of tampering methods in urine drug screening and testing. *J Subst Abuse Treat.* 2007;33:33-42.

Meyer MR, Peters FT. Analytical toxicology of emerging drugs of abuse—an update. *Ther Drug Monit.* 2012;34(6):615-621.

Smith HS. Opioid metabolism. *Mayo Clin Proc.* 2009;84(7): 613-624.

Starrels JL, Becker WC, Alford DP, et al. Systematic review: treatment agreements and urine drug testing to reduce opioid misuse in patients with chronic pain. *Ann Intern Med.* 2010;152(11):712-720.

Swotinsky RB, Smith DR, eds. Alcohol and specific drugs. In: *The Medical Review Officer's Manual: MROCC's Guide to Drug Testing.* 4th ed. Beverly Farms, MA: OEM Press, 2010:217-267.

Assessment

Summary by Launette Marie Rieb

Based on THE ASAM PRINCIPLES OF ADDICTION MEDICINE,
6th edition chapter by Theodore V. Parran Jr., Mark Bondeson,
Richard A. McCormick, and Christina M. Delos Reyes

ASSESSMENT OF PATIENTS WITH SUBSTANCE USE

Addiction affects the behavioral control areas in the brain, impacting the intrapersonal sense of self and relationships, avocations and hobbies, financial status, legal standing, and employment or school performance and can progress to physical or end-organ damage. The assessment process is a critical aspect of the approach to the disease of addiction and ensures the accuracy of diagnosis, helps with patient safety, and identifies the most effective and efficient care.

Primary Care Assessment Needs and Tools

The primary care provider (PCP) should perform a brief patient assessment in one or more office visits to quickly verify the diagnosis, gauge the severity of the disease from the perspective of psychosocial morbidity, end-organ damage, and physical dependence; gauge the patient's readiness for behavior change; and screen for immediately important medical or psychiatric comorbidities, including level of suicide risk. This needs to be done through patient interview, physical examination, use of one or more validated tools, laboratory testing including toxicology, query of the Prescription Drug Monitoring Program (PDMP) database, and, if possible, corroboration from collateral sources after informed consent and release of information requests are signed.

Validated *screening tools* can provide assessment information and positive answers can be used for follow-up questions to elicit information about patterns of use, past attempts at controlling use, adverse consequences of use, possible physiologic dependence, and quantity/frequency data. Screening tools can also be utilized with a lower cutoff score to screen for unhealthy use in the absence of addiction.

The PCP should inquire about prior success or failure with abstinence, attempts at controlled use,

harm reduction concepts, prior treatment experience, and affiliation with the 12-step or mutual/self-help community. Brief depression and anxiety screening are important, as are a medical history review and review of systems to identify illnesses and symptoms that may be related to substance use. Brief tools to assess readiness to change can be used.

Any primary care assessment should include a physical examination, laboratory evaluations including toxicology, complete blood count, and liver profile, along with HIV, hepatitis C, and pregnancy testing when appropriate. Review of the PDMP database is key.

Standardized assessment tools can be self-administered on a variety of platforms including websites, apps for smart phones, computer tablets provided in waiting rooms, or the patient's home. These applications can be linked to the electronic health records, making the results of the evaluation immediately available to the provider and permitting the trending of scores over time. Emerging research indicates that Web- or app-based interventions are well accepted and often an effective option for some patients, particularly those at the hazardous stage of use. Assessments should be repeated over time to identify treatment response and needs for changes in strategy.

Addiction Specialist Assessment Needs and Tools

The addiction medicine or psychiatry specialist will do a more in-depth diagnostic interview than the PCP and will utilize tools for *staging* the disease and *quantifying* the severity, evaluating medical detoxification needs, and reviewing all prior assessments. In addition, formal depression and anxiety screening with tools, such as the Beck Depression Inventory (BDI) or the Hamilton Anxiety Scale, are often utilized along with assessing for a new emergence of or change in symptoms of other psychiatric disorders. A thorough review of prior treatments, length and characteristics of remissions, patterns and triggers for relapse, and current supports and resources available for treatment is essential. Assessing the readiness for behavior change, level of commitment to a recovery program, and possibilities for pharmacotherapy are necessary as is a careful evaluation for withdrawal issues. Interviewing significant others about the patient in order to corroborate the history is even more essential. The assessment should include a physical examination for the stigmata of substance use and the signs of related disease, along with further laboratory investigations and toxicology screenings as indicated.

Substance Use Disorder Treatment Provider Needs and Tools

Assessment within the treatment program setting is designed to individualize treatment approaches and must use formalized processes for quality control and accreditation reasons. A full medical history and physical exam are mandatory for focusing on the aforementioned areas, but a structured interview such as the Addiction Severity Index (ASI) or even the Substance-Related and Addictive Disorders module of the Structured Clinical Interview for *DSM-5* (SCID-5), the Mini International Neuropsychiatric Interview (MINI), or the Composite International Diagnostic Interview Substance Abuse Module (CIDI-SAM) should also be used. Both the SCID and the MINI have been updated to *DSM-5*. Assessing treatment readiness and treatment resistance as well as relapse patterns and coping skills is typically a part of this assessment process.

Substance Use Disorder Researcher Needs

The substance use disorder or evaluation researcher typically focuses on elucidation of accumulated morbidities in the patient's life, treatment-matching efforts, predictors of response to treatment, and subtypes of addiction disorders. Well-validated diagnostic tools and measures of change over time, administered in ways that minimize errors, are key.

TASKS OF THE ASSESSMENT PROCESS

Tools used in an assessment may change depending upon the clinical situation, the competency of and resources available to the clinician, and the specific characteristics of patient presentation, but the basic areas to be assessed remain fairly constant and are indicated in Table 24-1.

TABLE 24-1	Major Areas for Addiction Assessment
1. Diagnostic criteria
2. Presence and level of intoxication
3. Suicidal or homicidal ideation
4. Physiologic dependence and withdrawal potential
5. Level of addiction-associated morbidity by domain: self-image, close significant others, social, financial, legal, work or school, physical
6. Co-occurring medical diagnoses
7. Co-occurring psychiatric diagnoses
8. Readiness for behavior change
9. Prior treatment successes and relapse patterns

Assessment of a substance use disorder is generally utilized for one or more of the following tasks: diagnostic verification, assessing for physiologic dependence, staging disease severity, identifying the domains of life affected by the disease, evaluating for additional medical or psychiatric diagnoses, quantifying the disease-associated morbidity, identifying characteristics of the disease that are important from a prognostic or possibly from a treatment-matching perspective, quantifying the impact of treatment on disease-associated morbidity, or attempting to determine subtypes of addiction.

Pretreatment assessments focus on identifying the treatment needs of the patient, identifying positive and negative predictive factors for treatment retention, quantifying the pretreatment level of morbidity and impairment of functioning, and screening for urgent co-occurring medical, psychiatric, and psychosocial issues. *Intratreatment* assessment updates should be performed at periodic intervals during the formal treatment and aftercare phase in such a way as to inform the ongoing treatment planning and patient diagnostic process. A *posttreatment* assessment is performed at the end of formal addiction treatment to summarize the treatment experience; inform aftercare and follow-up monitoring; focus on relapse prevention; reorder the problem list; and focus attention on additional, new, or previously deferred problems.

SOURCES OF ASSESSMENT INFORMATION

Sources that commonly are utilized in assessing addictive disease include patient history (eg, licit and illicit drug use history, legal history, educational and occupational history), physical exam, laboratory results, toxicology testing, family interview, PDMP data, and readiness for behavior change evaluation. Due to the stigmatization of substance use disorders in our society, it is important to interview patients in ways that avoids shaming and minimizes defensiveness about the behaviors resulting from their addictive disease. Patient self-report reliability can be improved by using questions that progress from general and open-ended to specific information sought in a more closed-ended question form and by utilizing family or significant other interviews whenever possible. Owing to high rates of psychiatric symptomatology, a specific screening for suicidal and homicidal ideation is required. Rates of interpersonal violence are quite high in patients with chemical dependence, so assessing for physical, emotional, and sexual abuse history is necessary. Cultural background, spiritual inclination, and belief systems that the patient holds regarding substance use disorders are also essential areas of assessment.

ASSESSMENT TOOLS

The natural history of addiction involves progressive dysfunction and disability in the major life domains in a cascade pattern, often starting with the intrapersonal, advancing to the interpersonal, and eventually progressing to the physical in the later stages. This is why assessment strategies must be sensitive to the natural history of the disease of addiction. The instruments highlighted previously and in the following paragraphs have been shown to be reliable and valid for the purposes suggested.

Screening Tool Results Can Provide Assessment Information

Screening tool results can be used as a bridge to the assessment process. Positive answers on validated *screening tools* like the single screening questions, Alcohol Use Disorders Identification Test (AUDIT), AUDIT—Consumption Items (AUDIT-C), and Drug Abuse Screening Test (DAST) can be further elaborated on to gain more detailed information. Longer questionnaires like the Alcohol Smoking and Substance Involvement Screening Test (ASSIST) and other tests no longer recommended for screening (eg, CAGE/CAGE-AID, family-CAGE [F-CAGE]) can be used instead as brief assessment tools for psychosocial morbidity, risk of withdrawal, need for detoxification, and indication for specialized treatment.

A second way to use screening is to use the screening test "score" to begin a rough estimate of the severity of the disease. For example, the AUDIT-C can

indicate low-risk use, risky use, or *DSM-5*–defined substance dependence depending on the score. Some formerly used tools for screening are probably better suited for disease staging or the assessment process. Realize that although screening tools may be adapted for use as an aid in assessing and diagnosis, they are not endorsed by the *DSM-5* as a substitute for the gold standard, which is a diagnostic interview and examination performed by a clinician trained in addiction-related disorders.

Diagnostic Assessment Tools

Semistructured clinical interviews designed for administration by trained evaluators are considered the "gold standard" for establishing reliable diagnoses of substance use disorders. The Substance-Related and Addictive Disorders module of the *SCID-5* utilizes questions that parallel *DSM-5* diagnostic criteria and establishes lifetime and current disorder diagnoses for alcohol and each psychoactive substance included in the *DSM-5*. Age of onset and an estimate of current severity are also obtained. The CIDI-SAM, a detailed interview designed to ascertain specific diagnoses of *DSM-IV* substance abuse and dependence, is also frequently utilized; updates to *DSM-5* are anticipated. Alternatively, the diagnostic portion of the Substance Abuse Outcomes Module has been shown to correlate well with the CIDI-SAM, has the advantage of being considerably shorter to administer, and can be self-administered and implemented in routine clinical practice. Alternatively, the MINI can be used. It has been validated in both the United States and Europe as a shorter alternative to the SCID and the CIDI.

Intoxication and Withdrawal Assessment

Intoxication

Both the patient history and the results of toxicology testing are essential in the assessment of intoxication and withdrawal. Toxicology testing can be used to verify recent use, involvement of more than one substance, and current levels of intoxication. High levels found on toxicology testing, with a relative absence of obvious physical impairment, are a strong indicator of high levels of tolerance and of physical dependence.

Often, the first step in conducting an addiction assessment is to establish the degree of risk associated with withdrawal. The Revised Clinical Institute Withdrawal Assessment for Alcohol Scale (CIWA-Ar) is a brief 10-item scale that can be administered in less than 3 minutes. It quantifies the severity of the alcohol withdrawal syndrome by rating 10 common alcohol withdrawal symptoms and can be clinically useful in monitoring progress over time. The Clinical Institute Narcotic Assessment (CINA) scale and the Clinical Opiate Withdrawal Scale (COWS) have been developed to quantify opioid withdrawal symptoms.

Assessment Tools for Comorbid Conditions and Functioning

Patients with substance use disorders often present with co-occurring psychiatric disorders that require concomitant or sequential treatment. The full SCID has modules for each of the other major syndrome groups, anxiety disorders, affective disorders, and psychotic disorders as well as other comorbidities that are common in people with substance use disorders—most notably the other disorders of impulse control, such as eating disorders and pathologic gambling, and the personality disorders. Each module may stand alone for the assessment of a particular diagnostic syndrome. Administration of the full SCID can take 2 or more hours. The CIDI or the MINI can be shorter alternatives.

Short self-report instruments are available to measure some of the most common comorbidities. The 18-item Brief Symptom Index (BSI) assesses psychological distress severity and includes scales for somatization, depression, and anxiety. It has been shown to be a powerful predictor of poor treatment outcomes among people with substance use disorders.

The Patient Health Questionnaire 9 (PHQ-9) assesses symptoms of depression and is highly correlated with more comprehensive assessments of current major depressive disorder. It includes one question assessing *suicidal ideation*. The BDI and the Beck Anxiety Inventory (BAI) are both relatively short (21-item) instruments that take about 10 minutes to administer and can be readministered over time to monitor progress. Special versions for children (ages 7 to 14 years) are also available. Gambling disorder can be effectively screened for and assessed using the South Oaks Gambling Screen (SOGS).

The ASI provides a reliable measure of lifetime use and use within the past 30 days for a full range of commonly used substances. It also assesses additional key dimensions of functioning: medical status; vocational; legal; family, including family history and social issues; and psychiatric status. For each dimension, the ASI yields both composite scores, which are mathematically calculated based on selected quantifiable items and a rater-generated severity score. The scores are based on structured interviews that take approximately 1 hour to administer. The ASI sections can be readministered to assess progress over time.

The Drinker Inventory of Consequences (DrInc) measures the adverse consequences of alcohol use in five domains: physical, social, impulsive, interpersonal, and intrapersonal. The 50-item self-administered test takes only about 10 minutes, yielding lifetime and last 3-month scores for each domain, and an overall score. A companion instrument, the Inventory of Drug Use Consequences (InDUC), provides similar information for a broader population of patients using drugs or drugs and alcohol. Finally, the SIP-AD (Short Inventory of Problems—Alcohol and Drugs) is a brief 15-item self-report test that measures physical, social, intrapersonal, impulsive, and interpersonal consequences of alcohol and drug consumption. Versions of the SIP also exist for alcohol only or drug only.

It is important to assess the *motivational level* of the patient for engaging in treatment. Self-report instruments are available, including the Stages of Change Readiness and Treatment Eagerness Scale (SOCRATES). The 19-item short form of the self-report instrument assesses motivation to change drinking behavior. A drug use version is also available. Based on the transtheoretical model of change, it assesses the patient's level of recognition of a problem, ambivalence or uncertainty about changing, and whether the patient is taking steps to change. It has been employed to monitor motivational levels and to predict compliance with and outcomes of treatment. A similar instrument, the University of Rhode Island Change Assessment (URICA), is slightly longer (32 items) and can readily be modified to assess motivation for change across a range of behaviors, including alcohol, other drugs, or concomitant unhealthy behaviors.

When a more comprehensive assessment of *resistance to treatment* is needed, the Recovery Attitude and Treatment Evaluator (RAATE) provides both a 35-item semistructured clinical interview option (RAATE-CE) and a 94-item self-report version (RAATE-QI). They both measure five constructs: resistance to initial treatment, resistance to continuing care, severity of biomedical problems, severity of psychiatric/psychological problems, and social/environmental support for recovery. Both take approximately 30 minutes to complete.

Assessment instruments can be valuable aids in constructing a *relapse prevention* plan. The Inventory of Drinking Situations is a 100-item self-report instrument that allows a patient to assess his or her tendency to drink in a variety of situations.

A number of instruments are available to assess coping repertoire. The Coping Response Inventory (CRI) is a relatively short (48-item) self-report instrument that assesses four types of avoidant coping and four types of approach coping methods. A youth version is also available. Self-efficacy for alcohol-related situations can be measured using the Situational Confidence Questionnaire (SCQ), a 39-item self-report instrument, or the abridged 8-item version. A companion instrument, the Drug Taking Confidence Questionnaire, assesses self-efficacy for drug-related situations.

As with many of the domains of assessments highlighted, comorbidities can first be screened for with relatively brief self-report instruments, and then those who screen positive can be further assessed with more comprehensive instruments. The ASAM Patient Placement Criteria provide further guidance on how to match assessment results to the appropriate level of care. Ironically, many individuals cannot access all levels of care, and many communities lack the resources to fund and sustain all levels of care. This is the "art" of creating a workable treatment plan and also an ongoing call to action to advocate for adequate funding of treatment, including treatment on demand.

KEY POINTS

1. A quality assessment permits the development of a comprehensive problem list and a thorough treatment plan.
2. Screening instruments can be expanded on by the clinician after an initial assessment of quantity, frequency, and impact of substance use.
3. In addition to the history, physical, and toxicology screenings, reliable and validated assessment tools exist for self-administration or administration by a health professional to confirm a diagnosis and to assess for risk of withdrawal, physical and mental comorbidities, social factors influencing use, motivation, triggers, and resistance to match for treatment placement and to monitor follow-up.
4. Repeating the assessments over time can track patient progress and assist with further treatment planning.

REVIEW QUESTIONS

1. Which of the following is an example of a screening tool that can be expanded on for assessment of an alcohol use disorder?
   A. SCID
   B. ASI
   C. AUDIT
   D. CIDI

2. Which instrument is *not* used in withdrawal management?
   A. SOGS
   B. CIWA
   C. CINA
   D. COWS

3. All of the following items may be helpful in assessing recent ingestion of a substance, except:
   A. urine toxicology.
   B. state or provincial Prescription Drug Monitoring Program records.
   C. a physical examination.
   D. RAATE.
   E. a patient history.

ANSWERS

1. **C.** The others are all "gold standard" assessment tools, not screening tools.
2. **A.** SOGS is used for pathologic gambling. The others are used for either alcohol or opioid withdrawal.
3. **D.** RAATE assesses resistance to treatment.

SUGGESTED READINGS

Allen JP, Wilson VB, eds. *Assessing Alcohol Problems: A Guide for Clinicians and Researchers*. 2nd ed. Bethesda, MD: National Institute on Alcohol Abuse and Alcoholism, 2003. NIH publication No. 03-3745, revised 2003.

McLellan AT, Kushner H, Metzger D, et al. The fifth edition of the Addiction Severity Index. *J Subst Abuse Treat*. 1992; 9(3):199-213.

Miller WR, Tonigan JS. Assessing drinker's motivations for change: the Stages of Change Readiness and Treatment Eagerness Scale (SOCRATES). *Psychol Addict Behav*. 1996; 10(2):81-89.

Opiate.com. Using the clinical opiate withdrawal scale to assess opiate withdrawal. http://www.opiate.com/withdrawal /using-the-clinical-opiate-withdrawal-scale-to-assess-opiate-withdrawals/. Accessed February 2, 2018.

Sullivan JT, Sykora K, Schneiderman J, Naranjo CA, Sellers EM. Assessment of alcohol withdrawal: the Revised Clinical Institute Withdrawal Assessment for Alcohol Scale (CIWA-Ar). *Br J Addict*. 1989;84(11):1353-1357.

25 Environmental Approaches to Prevention: Communities and Contexts

Summary by Paul J. Gruenewald, Joel W. Grube, Robert F. Saltz, and Mallie J. Paschall

Based on THE ASAM PRINCIPLES OF ADDICTION MEDICINE, 6th edition chapter by Paul J. Gruenewald, Joel W. Grube, Robert F. Saltz, and Mallie J. Paschall

At the end of prohibition in 1933, the Twenty-first Amendment to the US Constitution delegated control over the production and sales of alcoholic beverages to the states, territories, and possessions. States were given powers to license or monopolize alcohol production, wholesale distribution, and retail sales; restrict use to certain social contexts and groups; limit production; prohibit sales; preclude sales on specific days or times; and restrict sales to certain retail outlets. States began regulating alcohol sales and use and now largely determine the social, economic, physical, and legal environments in which alcohol can be used. Over subsequent years, the grand experiment of prohibition was followed by another less grand but more important experiment: a progressive deregulation of alcohol sales that allowed use in more contexts, at reduced costs, with greater retail availability, and with the exception of the minimum legal drinking age, fewer restrictions on use. As a consequence, illegal production has been almost eliminated, whereas many health problems related to use have increased. Deregulation continues to be actively pursued as a goal by alcohol beverage and social hosting industries.

Although state laws and regulations determine the environments where alcohol can be sold and used, the impacts of deregulation are felt at local community and neighborhood levels. For example, a state regulation that allows special use permits for summer wine festivals enables festivals to operate in communities across the state. State restrictions on the number of outlets may generally limit numbers but allow for overconcentration in some neighborhoods. State alcohol taxes may raise average retail prices but leave unaffected the costs of alcohol at neighborhood stores. In response, many communities want to

push back against deregulation and use community resources to decrease neighborhood alcohol problems. Physicians and other health professionals can act at the community level to reduce health impacts associated with expanding community environments for alcohol use (and, of course, other addictive substances such as tobacco and marijuana). By focusing on the very local impacts of secondhand smoke on nonsmokers, young adults, and infants, important gains have been made to restrict environments in which tobacco can be used. Similar gains can be made with respect to alcohol and other drugs. Communities can take control of drug use environments, and community-based environmental prevention programs can effectively reduce problems related to use and use disorders.

In this chapter, we outline some effective environmental approaches to reduce alcohol problems in community settings that complement those used to reduce problems related to tobacco and other substance use. We state the scope of the problem, distinguish environmental from other approaches to prevention, review the scientific bases for these efforts, and summarize current knowledge and best practices for community prevention efforts.

SCOPE OF THE PROBLEM

Alcohol use and abuse is a serious public health issue. Nearly 88,000 people die in the United States from alcohol-related causes each year, making alcohol use the third leading preventable cause of death. This corresponds to 2.5 million years of potential life lost at an estimated cost of $249 billion each year. Excessive underage drinking is responsible for more than 4300 deaths at an estimated cost of $24 billion each year. Overall social and health costs attributable to alcohol far exceed those of all other illicit drugs, with large disparities across communities.

Alcohol-related motor vehicle crashes account for many fatalities related to alcohol use. It is estimated that more than 29% of traffic crashes involve some degree of alcohol impairment; 10,265 people died in 2015 due to alcohol-involved traffic crashes at an estimated cost of $44 billion. Of US drivers aged 16 years and older, 11% reported driving while under the influence (DUI) of alcohol at least once each year, which is 28.7 million people. Because alcohol use alters motor skills, reaction time, and judgment, it also increases risks of injury to the drinker and others and is involved in a substantial percentage of drownings, burns, and falls. Thus, it has been concluded that "no safe level of consumption appears to exist in relation to injury risk."

Finally, alcohol use is also related to violence and crime. Alcohol is estimated to be involved in 28% to 43% of violent injuries and 47% of homicides, with much of this violence taking place among youth between the ages of 15 and 29 years, including both interpersonal violence and suicide. Alcohol intoxication, with blood alcohol levels (BAC) in excess of 0.08%, is involved in 24% of suicides, and alcohol use is involved in about 27% of hospital discharges recording the survival of a suicide attempt. Crimes attributable to alcohol are estimated to cost $84 billion a year—more than twice the $38 billion attributable to illegal drugs.

ENVIRONMENTAL VERSUS INDIVIDUAL APPROACHES TO PREVENTION

Although essential to ameliorating alcohol-related problems, treatment alone cannot stem the flow of new problem drinkers. Alcohol markets help ensure that susceptible at-risk drinkers continue to drink, drink despite problems, and sometimes progress to alcohol dependence and addiction. These populations remain stable because despite treatment, relapse rates are high. Treatment would have to be nearly universal to reduce alcohol use disorders in drinking populations. Of greater concern than problems related to heavy and dependent drinking, however, is the observation that most alcohol problems and healthcare costs arise among moderate drinkers with no alcohol use disorder. Treatment is not indicated for these drinkers and prevention efforts are essential to reduce risks in this population.

Many prevention programs have been implemented over the past decades to educate people about the effects of alcohol and consequences of use, to encourage individuals to abstain from use, or to promote the development of social norms that discourage risky use. Largely due to their narrow focus to the exclusion of other prevention alternatives, educational programs that inform about risks and consequences, or that encourage the development of refusal skills, have had limited success. Recent interventions that have focused on correcting misperceptions about alcohol use norms have shown some success at reducing use among young people, but critical reviews continue to conclude that there is little evidence that individual prevention programs alone lead to long-term reductions in alcohol problems. Perhaps it is unreasonable to expect individual approaches alone to be effective when drinkers are immersed in an environment in which alcohol is readily available and heavily marketed.

Environmental approaches acknowledge that alcohol problems result from interactions among individuals in community environments and note that some features of these environments can be changed to the benefit of the community. Designed to complement individual approaches, environmental interventions can be implemented without directly intervening with the individual. These programs share a common heritage with policy, regulatory, and enforcement interventions that reduce problems by changing the economic, physical, or social environments in which alcohol or drugs are obtained and used. The focus on neighborhoods and communities recognizes that interventions at this level are most effective. It is at the levels of neighborhoods and cities that modifiable components of community systems bear on alcohol use and consequences, including families, schools, neighborhoods, alcohol and drug markets, enforcement agents, and treatment systems.

Environmental approaches contrast with individual approaches in five key respects. First, they change components of community systems that make substance use problems more likely (eg, reducing hours and days of alcohol sales, enforcing social host laws prohibiting provision of alcohol to underage youth). Second, media efforts are not intended to inform individuals but rather to motivate gatekeepers to pursue prevention goals that extend routine activities (eg, enforcement of social host laws) and motivate support for prevention efforts (eg, underage sales compliance checks). Third, environmental approaches target broader environments and affect whole populations, including people who use and do not use alcohol or other drugs. Thus, a workplace intervention may alter workplace policies toward alcohol to reduce use in the workplace and thus provide greater safety for all employees. Fourth, unlike efforts of educational programs to reduce individual demand for drugs, environmental approaches focus on the supply-side of substance use. These approaches can include increasing the social costs for obtaining alcohol among youth, reductions in availability through interdiction efforts, limiting the provision of legal drugs in retail environments (eg, responsible beverage service [RBS] programs), harm reduction efforts (eg, needle exchange programs), and efforts to change drug distribution to ameliorate problem hot spots. Fifth, environmental approaches often focus on problems related to use rather than to use itself. Thus, an RBS program may reduce sales to intoxicated patrons in bars and subsequently reduce driving while intoxicated but need not have an overall effect on drinking.

EFFICACY TRIALS

Over the past three decades, community-based environmental prevention research has moved from establishing that these approaches can work to reduce problems to asking questions about what works, for whom, and why. Using quasi-experimental case-comparison research methods, the early phases of this research demonstrated the following:

1. Community action encouraged by media, education, and enforcement campaigns can reduce drinking and DUI.
2. Community monitoring of alcohol sales to youth, compliance checks to detect sales at alcohol outlets, keg registration, shortened hours of alcohol sales, RBS training, and educational programs to mobilize youth and adults can reduce alcohol sales to and purchases by underage youth, drinking, and DUIs.
3. Media mobilization, RBS programs, compliance checks to reduce retail sales to underage youth, greater enforcement of DUI laws, and reduced access to alcohol can lead to reductions in alcohol-involved motor vehicle crashes, injuries due to assaults, heavy drinking, and DUIs.

Because communities have different structures, needs, problems, and concerns, each requires adaptation of environmental approaches to its own circumstances. The application of these adaptive processes is illustrated by the following recent studies.

A DUI enforcement program was begun at the United States/Mexico border to reduce the number of young people crossing the border to drink in the city of Tijuana (across the border from San Diego). The program included increased enforcement of drinking and driving laws through sobriety checkpoints, border

checkpoints to prevent minors from entering Mexico without parents or other adult guardians, and publicity demonstrating the extent of the problem to gain public support. These interventions led to a 32% reduction in the number of late-night border crossings back into the United States, a 29% decrease in the proportion of pedestrians with BACs $\geq$.08%, and a 45% decrease in the number of 16- to 20-year-old drivers involved in alcohol-related motor vehicle crashes.

A program in a major American city implemented neighborhood-specific environmental interventions to reduce youth and young adult access to alcohol, risky drinking, and related consequences in two low-income ethnically diverse neighborhoods. Focusing on youth and young adults between the ages of 15 and 29 years, the interventions included (1) community mobilization to make neighborhood residents aware of intervention efforts and goals, (2) an RBS component to reduce sales to minors, and (3) a law enforcement component to prevent sales to minors and service to intoxicated patrons. The interventions led to a 3.9% reduction in police calls related to assaults and a 33.4% reduction in emergency medical system responses related to motor vehicle crashes in the first intervention site, followed by corresponding 36.5% and 37.4% reductions in these outcomes in the second intervention site.

A program in a city in Europe focused on preventing risky alcohol use in restaurants, bars, and night clubs by implementing community mobilization, RBS training and practices to prevent overserving alcohol, and enforcement activities to reinforce these efforts. The program increased rates of service refusal to apparently intoxicated patrons from 5% prior to the program to 70% 5 years later, demonstrated a 29% decrease in violent crimes reported to the police, and significantly increased the likelihood that doormen would refuse entrance to apparently impaired patrons. Taking implementation costs into account, the program was estimated to save the city €31 million over 10 years through reductions in judicial, healthcare, and other costs.

A college-based program targeted college students living in off-campus settings to reduce the incidence of student intoxication on college campuses. Using a randomized case-comparison design, the project implemented five intervention activities across seven experimental sites: (1) nuisance party enforcement to reduce problems related to off-campus parties, (2) compliance checks at on- and off-premise outlets to reduce underage sales and sales to intoxicated patrons, (3) roadside sobriety checkpoints, (4) implementation of local ordinances to discourage nuisance parties and the provision of alcohol to minors in social gatherings, and (5) campus and local media to increase the visibility of these environmental strategies. Significant reductions were observed in the incidence of intoxication at off-campus parties and bars/restaurants. Importantly, stronger intervention effects were observed at campuses with the highest intensity of implementation.

Each of these studies targeted different populations in different sites, relied on different community development and implementation models for environmental prevention, and used different evaluation tools. Each also involved the careful collection of baseline data, targeted well-defined problems, involved long-term implementation and monitoring, and documented success at reducing problems. They collectively demonstrate, across a variety of research and community settings, that interventions targeting physical, economic, social, and legal aspects of the alcohol environment can reduce problems related to drinking. In short, environmental approaches to prevention work. What works best and why, however, remain important questions.

THE EMERGENCE OF ECOLOGIC RESEARCH

The search for ways to develop effective and efficient environmental prevention interventions has recently led prevention scientists down two independent paths. One path explores local ecologic interactions that reinforce problem drinking and may serve as critical intervention points in community settings. The other develops logic models of intervention structure, action, and goals to focus community resources on those critical points.

It has long been known that the availability of alcohol in the home, among peers, and through alcohol outlets is correlated with youth access to and use of alcohol. But locations where alcohol may be obtained and used vary a great deal by environmental circumstance and age. Some use contexts (eg, drinking in others' homes) are associated with much greater risks than others (eg, with family at home), and different forms of social or parental control are needed to moderate unhealthy alcohol use in these contexts.

ENVIRONMENTAL PREVENTION AND THE ROLE OF THE MEDICAL PROFESSIONALS

Although environmental prevention is often contrasted with medical treatment, its relevance to medical practice can be substantial, ranging from impacts on patient treatment in clinical settings to advocacy and advancement of broader community health policy initiatives. Perhaps the most obvious and recent concern is the gatekeeper role served by medical practitioners with respect to prescription opioid abuse. Here, medical practitioners are not only responsible for prescriber practices but also advocate for the regulation of prescribed access through the development of effective prescription drug monitoring programs. As part of their social function, medical practitioners can advise their patients on harms related to the use of many different drugs, especially alcohol because this drug affects so many in the United States, but also other newly legal drugs like cannabis, and the many illegal drugs that lead to overdose, accidents, injuries, and death. Well-informed medical professionals can advocate for effective local policy practices and community-based preventive interventions to reduce alcohol and drug use problems.

KEY POINTS

1. Following the end of prohibition in 1933, the Twenty-first Amendment delegated control over production and sales of alcoholic beverages to the states, territories, and possessions of the United States. Since that time, all US states have deregulated many aspects of their alcohol control systems, enabling greater access to all forms of alcoholic beverages at much lower prices.

2. Today, alcohol use is the third leading cause of preventable death in the United States, with most problems attributed to moderate drinking; no safe level of consumption appears to exist in relation to injury risk.

3. US communities and public health researchers in the Unites States have responded to deregulation by developing individual and environmental prevention programs to reduce alcohol-related problems.

4. Although individual-oriented preventive interventions have demonstrated limited success, environmental interventions have a track record of proven success and have been successfully tailored to special populations and neighborhoods most at risk.

5. In order to enhance the effectiveness of environmental prevention programs, recent community-based research has begun to focus on the ecologic contexts in which drinkers are most at risk for problems.

ACKNOWLEDGMENTS

Preparation of this chapter was supported by grant number P60-AA06282 (Environmental Approaches to Prevention) from the National Institute on Alcohol Abuse and Alcoholism of the National Institutes of Health. The content is solely the responsibility of the authors and does not necessarily represent the official views of the National Institute on Alcohol Abuse and Alcoholism or the National Institutes of Health.

REVIEW QUESTIONS

1. Which of the following is an example of an environmental intervention?
   A. Prescribing disulfiram to a patient in a substance use disorder clinic.
   B. Dispensing a clean syringe to a patient in a substance use disorder clinic.
   C. Dispensing rescue naloxone to the family member of a patient with an opioid use disorder.
   D. Decreasing the alcohol sales hours from 24/7 to 12 pm to 10 pm at stores that sell alcohol.

2. Which of the following is *true* regarding alcohol?
   A. It is the leading cause of death in the United States.
   B. It is the third leading cause of death in the United States.
   C. It is the fifth leading cause of death in the United States.
   D. It is the eighth leading cause of death in the United States.

3. Which of the following is *incorrect* regarding environmental preventive interventions?
   A. Environmental preventive interventions are designed to complement individual prevention programs.
   B. Environmental preventive interventions are targeted to both people who do and do not drink.
   C. Environmental preventive interventions are tailored to inform drinkers about ways they can help reduce their own drinking.
   D. Environmental preventive interventions are directed at components of community systems.

ANSWERS

1. **D**
2. **B**
3. **C**

SUGGESTED READINGS

Babor T, Caetano R, Casswell S, et al. *Alcohol No Ordinary Commodity: Research and Public Policy*. 2nd ed. Oxford: Oxford University Press, 2010.

Cook PJ. *Paying the Tab: The Costs and Benefits of Alcohol Control*. Princeton: Princeton University Press, 2008.

Gruenewald PJ. Regulating availability: how access to alcohol affects drinking and problems in youth and adults. *Alcohol Res Health*. 2011;34(2):248-256.

Saltz RF, Paschall MJ, McGaffigan RM, Nygaard PM. Alcohol risk management in college settings: the Safer California Universities Randomized Trial. *Am J Prev Med*. 2010;39:491-499.

Wallin E, Gripenberg J, Andréasson S. Overserving at licensed premises in Stockholm: effects of a community action program. *J Stud Alcohol*. 2005;66(6):806-814.

Overview of Addiction Treatment

Addiction Medicine in America: Its Birth, Early History, and Current Status (1750-2018)

Summary by Kevin Kunz and William L. White

Based on THE ASAM PRINCIPLES OF ADDICTION MEDICINE, 6th edition chapter by Kevin Kunz and William L. White

The recent recognition of the subspecialty of addiction medicine by the American Board of Medical Specialties and the Accreditation Council of Graduate Medical Education presents a timely backdrop to this condensed history of American physicians' involvement in the prevention and treatment of alcohol and other drug-related problems. Shakespeare's quote, "What is past is prologue," has prescient value in medicine and public health: This chapter represents a still evolving history, one in which the reader is a participant. The modern field of addiction medicine can trace its lineage from the scholars of ancient civilizations, through Drs. Benjamin Rush, Ruth Fox, and Robert Smith, and the American surgeons general, to include today some 5000 practicing addiction physician specialists and thousands more health professionals across disciplines who have brought the field to its new standing in mainstream medicine and healthcare.

THE BIRTH OF ADDICTION MEDICINE

Although this chapter focuses on addiction medicine in America, it should be noted that the roots of addiction medicine can be traced as far back as the ancient world. Special methods to care for persons addicted to alcohol were developed in ancient Egypt, and references to chronic intoxication as a sickness date to Herodotus (fifth century BC). In North America, the earliest medical responses to alcoholism emerged from the systems of medicine practiced by American Indian tribes, which included both individual and public health approaches. American Indians used botanical agents to suppress cravings for alcohol, to induce an aversion to alcohol, and to facilitate personal transformation within

sobriety-based cultural mores and revitalization activities. In the 18th and 19th centuries, however, alcohol-related problems rose dramatically among native populations all over the globe as alcohol became increasingly used as a tool of economic, political, and sexual exploitation. For instance, it was common for alcohol to be used to purchase enslaved Africans to work the fields of America's thriving new export—tobacco.

Annual per capita alcohol consumption nearly tripled in the colonies between 1780 and 1830, along with a shift in preference from fermented to more potent forms of distilled alcohol. It was in this changing context that several prominent Americans "discovered" the phenomenon of addiction. In 1774, the philanthropist and social reformer Anthony Benezet observed that intoxication had a tendency to self-accelerate: "Drops beget drams, and drams beget more drams, till they become to be without weight or measure." Benezet's warning was followed by Dr. Benjamin Rush's 1784 pamphlet, *Inquiry Into the Effects of Ardent Spirits on the Human Mind and Body*. This first American treatise on alcoholism almost single-handedly launched the American temperance movement. Rush claimed that many persons with alcohol addiction could be restored to full health through proper medical treatment and care in "sober houses."

By the late 1820s, the concepts of inability to abstain, loss of control, craving ("an insatiable desire for drink"), and a "morbid alteration" in nearly all the major structures and functions of the human body were outlined. Dr. William Sweetser viewed this syndrome as the product of a devastating paradox: "The poison (alcohol) was itself its only antidote." Soon, the collective observations of physicians, clergy, and social activists led to the view that chronic intoxication was a problem with biologic roots and consequences and thus was the province of the physician. The major elements of an addiction disease concept were in place: biologic predisposition, drug toxicity, pharmacologic tolerance, disease progression, morbid appetite (craving), loss of volitional control, chronicity, and the pathophysiologic consequences of sustained alcohol and opiate ingestion. Recovery, however, was viewed as a climactic decision.

Addiction medicine then expanded to include treating the addiction itself and acknowledging that substances in addition to alcohol, notably opioids, also had addictive potential. Three events between the early and mid-19th century profoundly altered the future of narcotic addiction in America: the isolation of morphine from opium, the introduction of the hypodermic syringe, and the emergence of a patent drug industry. Drugs of greater potency were produced, with a more efficient and euphorigenic method of ingestion accompanied by increased drug availability and promotion.

EARLY PROFESSIONALIZATION AND MEDICAL ADVANCEMENTS (1830 TO 1900)

Physician-directed asylums for persons with severe alcohol addiction began proliferating in the mid-19th century. Also at this time, Dr. Samuel Woodward at the Hospital for the Insane in Massachusetts broke with Rush, who advised that abstinence from only distilled alcohol was sufficient, declaring that "the grand secret of the cure for intemperance is total abstinence from alcohol in all its forms." A series of clinical contributions to the understanding of chronic intoxication followed that exerted considerable influence on the emerging field of addiction medicine. The science of addiction had begun.

Magnus Huss's 1849 text, *Chronic Alcoholism,* presented an extensive review of the chronic effects of intoxication. Huss declared, "These symptoms are formed in such a particular way that they form a disease group in themselves and thus merit being designated and described as a definite disease . . . ," and he coined the clinical term "alcoholism" that became and remains popular in medical and public use.

A multibranch treatment field emerged in the mid-19th century, with homes and cure institutions for persons who are chronically inebriated arising from public and for-profit private entities. The later institutions generated considerable controversy over

their claim to have a cure for addiction. Simultaneously, bottled and patented "medicinal" addiction cures (most containing alcohol, opium, morphine, or cocaine) were promulgated by some physicians and many entrepreneurs.

The central organizing concept of 19th century addiction medicine specialists was that of inebriety. Inebriety was viewed as a disease that manifested itself in many ways, all of which were meticulously detailed by clinical subpopulation and drug choice. Addiction medicine texts were often organized under such headings as "alcoholic inebriety," "opium inebriety," "cocaine inebriety," and "ether inebriety." By the 1880s, the problem of posttreatment relapse for all substances was also recognized.

Understanding the potential physiologic foundations and consequences of addiction increased during the last two decades of the 19th century. For instance, Carl Wernicke's 1881 discovery of a psychosis with polyneuritis and Sergei Korsakoff's 1887 description of an alcoholism-induced psychosis underscored the organic basis of behavior in persons with chronic alcoholism. And there was considerable discussion about the potential hereditary transmission of inebriety.

The field of addiction medicine experienced professionalization and specialization between 1830 and 1900. The practice of addiction medicine shifted from the private physician's practice to the institutional setting. Within this institutional practice, there began a growing understanding of the physiologic consequences of chronic alcoholism and an extension of the concept of inebriety to embrace dependence on opium, morphine, cocaine, chloral hydrate, chloroform, and ether. There was now a well-articulated addiction disease concept with elaborate protocols for detoxification and rehabilitation.

The field of addiction medicine was infused with optimism by the century's end. The disease was defined by the concept of inebriety and two addiction-related medical organizations were established that embraced science and treatment—the American Association for the Cure of Inebriety, founded in 1870, and the American Medical Temperance Association, founded at the American Medical Association (AMA) in 1891. But forces outside the medical profession that were stirring would drive a wedge between physicians and patients with addiction.

DEMEDICALIZATION AND THE COLLAPSE OF ADDICTION TREATMENT (1900 TO 1935)

The proliferation of science-based addiction literature and practice could not withstand America's shifting response to addiction. By the early 1900s, a new national policy on alcohol and drug control, rising pessimism in therapy, and economic austerity triggered by unexpected depressions shifted and then reversed the gains of the previous century. In the eyes of the nation, prohibition became the solution to addiction and drug use.

In 1919, the year prohibition laws began to go into effect, treatment programs closed in tandem with the spread of local and state prohibition laws, and persons with alcoholism were relegated to the "foul wards" of large city hospitals and aging local and state psychiatric asylums, all of which did everything possible to discourage the admission of persons with addiction. Public hospitals stepped up where they could. Wealthy persons sought discrete detoxification in a new genre of private establishments. For all but the most affluent, the management of alcoholism shifted from a strategy of treatment to a strategy of control and punishment via inebriate penal colonies. The shift from viewing those with substance use disorders as persons with a disease in need of help to persons of weak and questionable moral character was reflected in the medical literature of the early 20th century. Kurtz and Kraepelin coined the term "alcohol addiction" to depict those whose will was "not strong enough to abandon the use of alcohol even if drinking causes them serious economic, social and somatic changes." After passage of the National Prohibition Act, also known as the Volstead Act, which promulgated prohibition in keeping with the 18th Amendment, there was a subsequent sharp decline in demand for treatment. Alcohol-related problems decreased dramatically in the early 1920s but rose to pre-Prohibition levels by the decade's end. Cultural ownership of alcohol and drug problems transferred from physicians to law enforcement authorities.

A premonition of today's opioid crisis can be seen in Dr. Foster Kennedy's 1914 declaration that narcotic addiction was "a disease, in the majority of cases, initiated, sustained and left uncured by members of the medical profession." With the passage of the Harrison Anti-Narcotic Act of 1914, treatment of persons with addiction was dramatically altered by the designation of physicians and pharmacists as the gatekeepers for the distribution of opioids and cocaine. The 1919 Supreme Court case *Webb v. United States* declared that prescriptions of narcotics for maintenance treatment was not within the discretion of physicians, not privileged under the Harrison Narcotics Act, not "good faith" medical practice, and thus was an indictable offense for which loss of license and incarceration could result.

Despite this intrusion of government into medical practice, between 1919 and 1924, physicians in 44 communities operated morphine maintenance clinics, some of which were sponsored by local health departments and even local police departments. All eventually closed under federal threat. The Harrison Act effectively transferred responsibility for the care of persons with addiction from physicians to criminal syndicates and the criminal justice system. Rapid detoxification of persons with addiction became the rule. Physician culpability in the problem of addiction to opioids made it difficult for the AMA to oppose this restriction of medical practice, and the AMA passed a resolution opposing ambulatory treatment, in effect opposing medication management as treatment. Having or treating addiction became illegal.

The influence of psychiatry on the characterization and treatment of addiction increased in tandem with the decline of a specialized field of addiction medicine. Karl Abraham's 1908 essay, "The Psychological Relations Between Sexuality and Alcoholism," marked the shift from seeing alcoholism as a primary medical disorder to seeing the condition as a symptom of underlying psychiatric disturbances. In the mid-1920s, Public Health Service psychiatrist, Dr. Lawrence Kolb, published a series of articles challenging earlier physiologic explanations of narcotic addiction and portraying addiction as a product of defects in personality—persons with addiction were characterized as psychopathic and constitutionally inferior. The first *American Standard Classified Nomenclature of Disease* (1933) classified "alcohol addiction" and "drug addiction" as personality disorders.

Few institutional resources existed for the treatment of alcoholism and narcotic addiction during the 1920s and 1930s, but the growing visibility of these problems began to generate new proposals for their management. The opening of the California Narcotics Hospital at Spadra in 1928 marked the beginning of state support for addiction treatment. Physicians working within the federal prison system also wrote about the problems posed by a growing population of incarcerated persons with addiction and advocated more specialized treatment of these individuals.

Medical treatments for addiction to narcotics in the first three decades of the 20th century focused on managing narcotic withdrawal. Heroin was briefly used for detoxification from morphine, and its subsequent emergence as the drug of preference among persons addicted to opioids was instructive. The fear of exposing patients to other addicting agents led to experimentation with a wide variety of nonnarcotic withdrawal procedures. These procedures included various belladonna treatments (scopolamine and hyoscine); peptization treatments (sodium thiocyanate) that could induce long-lasting psychosis; sleep treatments (sodium bromide) that had a 20% mortality rate; and insulin treatments that had no effect on the withdrawal process. The first decades of the 20th century were marked by a profound therapeutic pessimism regarding treatment of alcoholism and narcotic addiction. Biologic views of addiction fell out of favor and were replaced by psychiatric, characterological, moral, and criminal models that argued for control and sequestration of this group of citizens.

THE REBIRTH OF ADDICTION TREATMENT (1935 TO 1970)

After the early 20th century collapse of systems of care for those addicted to alcohol and other drugs, addiction medicine was revived within the larger context of two movements. One was an emerging new scientific approach to alcohol problems in post–Repeal America led by the Research Council on Problems of Alcohol, the Yale Center of Alcohol Studies, and by a national recovery advocacy effort led by the National Committee for Education on Alcoholism in 1944. Goals of these movements were to encourage local hospitals to detoxify patients dependent on alcohol and to encourage local communities to establish posthospitalization alcoholism rehabilitation centers. The modern alcoholism movement was ignited by the founding of Alcoholics Anonymous in 1935. The establishment of this successful, community-based, and noninstitutional mutual support organization for alcohol use disorders was cofounded by Dr. Robert Smith, a physician in recovery from severe alcohol dependence. This "12-step" prototype and burgeoning movement of broader institutional and community attention to alcoholism spawned new resources for treatment from the mid-1940s through the 1960s. These included "AA wards" in local hospitals, model outpatient clinics for alcoholism, and model community-based residential programs pioneered in Minnesota at Hazelden (1949) and other locales. The Minnesota Model was adapted for community hospitals and replicated by innumerable hospital-based programs.

The spread of these models nationally was aided by efforts to legitimize the work of physicians in the treatment of alcoholism. Early milestones included resolutions on alcoholism passed by the AMA (1952-1967) and the American Hospital Association (1944-1957) that paved the way for hospital-based treatment. Midcentury alcoholism treatments included nutritional therapies; brief experiments with chemical and electroconvulsive therapies; psychosurgery; and new drug therapies, including the use of disulfiram, stimulants, sedatives, tranquilizers, and lysergic acid diethylamide.

A mid-20th century reform movement advocating medical rather than penal treatment of people with opioid dependence also helped spawn the rebirth of addiction medicine. This began with the founding of state-sponsored addiction treatment hospitals and led to the creation of two US Public Health Hospitals within the Bureau of Prisons—one in Lexington, Kentucky, and the other in Fort Worth, Texas. The documentation of relapse rates after community reentry from Lexington and Fort Worth confirmed the need for community-based treatment. Three replicable models of treatment emerged: therapeutic communities directed by persons in sustained recovery, methadone maintenance pioneered by Drs. Marie Nyswander and Vincent Dole, and outpatient drug-free counseling.

State and federal funding for alcoholism and addiction treatment increased in the 1940s through the 1960s and was followed by landmark legislation that created the National Institute on Alcohol Abuse and Alcoholism (NIAAA) and the National Institute on Drug Abuse (NIDA)—the beginning of the federal, state, and local community partnership that has since been the foundation of modern addiction research and treatment. The expansion of insurance coverage for alcoholism and other drug dependencies in the 1960s and 1970s and the establishment of accreditation standards for addiction treatment programs by the Joint Commission on Accreditation of Hospitals set the stage for the dramatic growth of hospital-based and private freestanding addiction treatment programs in the 1980s. NIAAA and NIDA also made heavy investments in research that led to dramatic breakthroughs in understanding the neurobiology of addiction that encouraged more medicalized approaches to severe alcohol and other drug problems. The growing sophistication of addiction science was aided by other key organizations, including the College on Problems of Drug Dependence and the Research Society on Alcoholism, both of which hold an annual conferences and publish scientific journals.

ADDICTION MEDICINE COMES OF AGE (1970 TO 2018)

Insights from basic, clinical, and epidemiologic science and the availability of evidence-based prevention and treatment interventions provided new understanding and tools and led to the modernization of organized addiction medicine practice. Pioneering brain imaging studies demonstrated even to the casual observer that addiction was more than a moral failing or a behavioral or criminal problem. An emerging consensus arose that substance use disorder is a unified etiologic and diagnostic disease state and that subclassifications based on the particular substances used, although useful, are insufficient. The unified view of substance use disorders is exemplified in the 2016 *Surgeon General's Report on Alcohol, Drugs and Health: Facing Addiction in America*. Previous US Surgeon General reports had focused only on tobacco/nicotine and most reports from the National Institutes of Health were also substance specific.

Whereas physician culpability in the previous opioid epidemic made it difficult for organized medicine to oppose a criminal justice solution in the early 1900s, in 2016 to 2017, organized medicine responded to addressing the complicity of physicians in the modern opioid epidemic by advancing physician credentialing and training in addiction medicine. Thus, the current response of medicine has brought physicians into the solution, rather than defaulting to a historically ineffective and flawed criminal justice approach. Thus, addiction medicine has gained renewed relevance in medicine and public health.

ORGANIZED ADDICTION MEDICINE TODAY

Addiction medicine as an organized clinical subspecialty of medical practice has been significantly advanced by six entities. The American Academy of Addiction Psychiatry (AAAP) was established in 1985 with the goal of elevating the quality of clinical practice in addiction psychiatry. AAAP successfully advocated for the American Board of Psychiatry and Neurology (ABPN) to recognize addiction psychiatry as a subspecialty in 1991. Between 2006 and 2016, there were 1189 ABPN diplomates holding active subspecialty certification in addiction psychiatry. It is the pioneering and enduring work of ASAM and AAAP that set the stage for all physicians to meet medicine's responsibility in the prevention and treatment of substance use disorders.

The ASAM, founded by Dr. Ruth Fox in 1954, is a membership organization that advocates for advancing physician education, patient care, and treatment access. ASAM's organizational priority has been the acceptance of addiction medicine within the "house of medicine" for nearly three decades. The ASAM leadership understood that if patients were to have access to qualified addiction medicine physicians and that if health systems and insurers were to offer and compensate addiction medicine services, then training and credentialing standards would need to be established as they are for other medical fields. Addiction medicine would thus have to become part of the American Board of Medical Specialties (ABMS), and fellowship training would have to eventually become accredited by the Accreditation Council for Graduate Medical Education (ACGME). In 2006, the ASAM directors unanimously voted to "encourage and assist" in the establishment of a new independent entity to bring addiction medicine into formal recognition by ABMS.

Thus, in 2007, the American Board of Addiction Medicine (ABAM)—a freestanding, independent organization—was incorporated. ASAM transferred the addiction medicine certification examination to ABAM, which added clinical relevance testing and a full multispecialty content. ABAM certified just over 4000 physicians between 2009 and 2016. A watershed moment for addiction medicine occurred in 2015 to 2016, when the board of directors of ABMS officially recognized addiction medicine as a subspecialty. The American Board of Preventive Medicine (ABPM), an ABMS member board, became the sponsoring board and home to the new addiction medicine subspecialty. With the formal ABMS recognition of addiction medicine, ABAM discontinued its certification exam, and (as in the case of all medical specialties) the exam passed to the sponsoring ABMS board. The first annual ABMS level certification exam was given in late 2017 by ABPM, and the first cohort of 1230 subspecialists in addiction medicine was announced in February 2018. In March of 2018, ACGME gave final approval for the program requirements and accreditation application for addiction medicine fellowships. It is anticipated that several dozen current and emerging programs will receive accreditation in 2018 and more in 2019.

Another certifying entity is the American Osteopathic Association (AOA). In 2017, the AOA began granting addiction medicine (ADM) status to active AOA certificants who held active ABAM diplomate status. As of the date of this publication, approximately 100 physicians hold AOA ADM certification.

Equally important to physician certification was the creation of formal physician education in addiction medicine. One doesn't simply decide that one is a cardiologist, and likewise, addiction medicine needed to create a formal pathway for fellowship education. The Addiction Medicine Foundation (formerly the ABAM Foundation) was incorporated in 2007 as a nonprofit entity to support the advance of addiction medicine. The Addiction Medicine Foundation (TAMF) guided the acceptance of the field by the AMA and has fostered the development of the nation's first addiction medicine fellowship programs. Currently, there are 52 US fellowships and 3 Canadian fellowships of 12-month or longer duration that have been accredited by TAMF. Most graduated fellows are family medicine physicians and internists and yet also include pediatricians, obstetrician/gynecologists, preventive medicine physicians, anesthesiologists, and other specialists. TAMF has estimated that 125 ADM fellowships will be needed to train an adequate workforce of addiction medicine subspecialists. TAMF has received major funding from numerous philanthropies such as the Conrad N. Hilton Foundation, without which the acceptance and advance of the field in organized medicine and healthcare would likely not have occurred.

The Addiction Medicine Fellowship Directors Association (AMFDA) was incorporated as an independent nonprofit organization in 2016. Its mission is "to promote excellence in the education and training of current and future generations of physicians in evidence-based practices in the prevention and treatment of substance related-complications including addiction."

Finally, several other historical initiatives should be mentioned that have advanced addiction-related medical education. The NIAAA and NIDA created the Career Teacher Program (1971 to 1981) that developed addiction-related curricula for the training of medical students. In 1976, Career Teachers and others involved in addiction-related medical education and research established the interdisciplinary Association for Medical Education and Research in Substance Abuse (AMERSA). AMERSA draws its members primarily from American health professional school faculty, hosts an annual meeting, and publishes the journal *Substance Abuse*.

As this history has reviewed, addiction medicine has been around for millennia and was first practiced in North America by American Indians, rose to prominence in the United States in the mid-19th century, collapsed in the opening decades of the 20th century, yet reemerged and became increasingly professionalized in the late 20th century. Now, at the opening of the 21st century, addiction medicine has been formally recognized and accepted within the "house of medicine." The field is now positioned to nationally integrate the prevention and treatment of unhealthy substance use and addiction into healthcare and public health systems. Patients, families, and our nation will all be the beneficiaries.

KEY POINTS

1. Addiction medicine was first practiced in North America by American Indians.
2. Addiction medicine has gone through several iterations in the United States.
3. Addiction medicine is now a recognized medical specialty by the ABMS, and the sponsoring board is the ABPM.

REVIEW QUESTIONS

1. Benjamin Rush first identified alcoholism as a disease and:
   A. advocated the use of American Indian remedies such as hop tea and the root of the trumpet vine.
   B. believed that fermented spirits were not causative and that only distilled spirits were.
   C. considered alcoholism as both moral and biologic in etiology.
   D. is known as the father of addiction medicine.
   E. was an atheist.

2. Which of the following shifted the focus of addiction from a disease to a legal issue?
   A. The 18th Amendment
   B. The Volstead Act
   C. The Harrison Anti-Narcotic Act
   D. The Supreme Court case *Webb v. United States*
   E. All of the above

3. Addiction medicine is:
   A. a primary specialty of both the American Board of Medical Specialties and the American Osteopathic Association.
   B. available only to physicians certified in a primary care specialty (eg, internal medicine, pediatrics, emergency medicine).
   C. a multispecialty subspecialty of the American Board of Medical Specialties, sponsored by the American Board of Preventive Medicine.
   D. a field with eligibility limited to those who complete a 12-month addiction medicine fellowship.
   E. focused primarily on the pharmacologic treatment of addiction and substance use disorders.

ANSWERS

1. **B**
2. **E**
3. **C**

SUGGESTED READINGS

American Board of Preventive Medicine. Web site. www.the abpm.org. Musto D. *The American Disease: Origins of Narcotic Controls*. New Haven, CT: Yale University Press, 1973.

O'Connor PG, Sokol RJ, D'Onofrio G. Addiction medicine: the birth of a new discipline. *JAMA Intern Med*. 2014; 174(11):1717-1718.

Rush B. *An Inquiry Into the Effect of Ardent Spirits Upon the Human Body and Mind, With an Account of the Means of Preventing and of the Remedies for Curing Them*. 8th rev ed. Brookfield, MA: E. Merriam & Co, 1814.

US Department of Health and Human Services, Office of the Surgeon General. *Facing Addiction in America: The Surgeon General's Report on Alcohol, Drugs and Health*. Washington, DC: US Department of Health and Human Services, 2016.

Volkow ND, Koob GF, McLellan AT. Neurobiologic advances from the brain disease model of addiction. *N Engl J Med*. 2016;374(4):363-371.

White WL. *Slaying the Dragon: The History of Addiction Treatment and Recovery in America*. Bloomington, IL: Chestnut Health Systems, 1998.

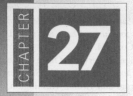

27

Treatment of Unhealthy Alcohol Use: An Overview

Summary by Mark Willenbring and Brian Grahan

Based on THE ASAM PRINCIPLES OF ADDICTION MEDICINE, 6th edition chapter by Mark Willenbring and Brian Grahan

For millennia, alcohol has been one of the most popular and dangerous substances ingested by humans. Inevitably, some individuals drink too much, causing themselves and society harm. However, other than purely custodial care, professional treatment only began in the middle of the 20th century. Since then, knowledge of the nature, course, and treatment of unhealthy alcohol use rapidly evolved. Consequently, the evidence base upon which alcohol treatment rests is considerable and broad, as good as or better than that for many other common complex disorders.

Unfortunately, there is scant evidence that any of this evidence base has made it into practice. Most programs offer little more than low-level counseling and Alcoholics Anonymous for a short period of time. Programs offer nothing different for repeat offenders, leading to a cycle of repeat admissions and failure. Efforts to integrate treatment for alcohol use disorders (AUDs) into mainstream medical care have failed almost completely. There is a pressing need for new treatment models.

THE SPECTRUM OF SEVERITY IN UNHEALTHY ALCOHOL USE

Recent research has provided a new and more complete view of the range of drinking, AUDs, and alcohol-related harms in the community. In the United States, a standard drink is defined as the amount of ethanol in 1.5 oz (45 mL) of 80-proof spirits, 12 oz of beer, or 5 oz of table wine, each containing about 14.5 g of absolute ethanol.

The National Institute on Alcohol Abuse and Alcoholism recommends that men drink no more than 4 drinks per day and 14 drinks per week and that women (and those 65 years and older) drink no more than 3 drinks per day and 7 drinks per week. Drinking within these limits is considered lower-risk drinking. Lower limits or abstinence may be indicated in the presence of coexisting medical or psychiatric disorders, in older people, or when medication

interactions are a concern. Women who are pregnant or at risk of becoming pregnant are advised to abstain. A day on which the limit is exceeded is considered a "heavy drinking day," and heavy drinking is defined as drinking more than the maximum limits on a regular basis, such as exceeding the daily limits weekly or more often. Drinking more than advised itself is not considered a disorder. Instead, to make a diagnosis, the *Diagnostic and Statistical Manual of Mental Disorders*, 5th edition (*DSM-5*) requires that drinking causes "clinically significant impairment or distress" and that an individual endorses at least 2 out of 11 diagnostic criteria for an AUD. Drinking more than the recommended limits in the absence of a disorder is considered at-risk drinking.

MODERN APPROACHES TO TREATMENT

Professional treatment for AUD that is supported by a base of basic and clinical research is a relatively new field compared to other areas of medicine. The 12 steps of Alcoholics Anonymous, counseling, and education were combined to create the Minnesota Model of treatment. The Minnesota Model has been adopted internationally, and it is the most prevalent form of treatment available in the United States. For most US residents, programs based on the Minnesota Model are the only available approach to treatment. This is true despite decades of research that provide little support for it.

The fields of psychology and psychiatry have undergone substantial development and expansion as well. Specific therapies for AUD based on these earlier psychological theories include therapeutic communities, aversion therapy, cognitive–behavioral therapy, skills training, community reinforcement, and contingency management. More recently, William Miller and colleagues developed motivational enhancement therapy based on stages of change and encouraging a motivation to change. Manualization and monitoring of the application of behavioral techniques have allowed true comparisons of efficacy with a high degree of confidence in the validity of the trials. The main conclusion from this work is that a variety of validated therapy approaches and techniques all produce similar outcomes. Thus, the best therapy approach is to use the most relevant aspects of all available therapies, rather than focusing on one type over others.

Pharmacotherapy for AUDs has experienced halting advancement. Although initial open-label studies for many older medications reported efficacy, subsequent research for all except disulfiram failed to substantiate those early claims. Disulfiram was approved for use in the United States in 1949. It took until 1995 for naltrexone to be approved for treatment of AUDs. Since then, acamprosate and an injectable depot formulation of naltrexone have been approved by the US Food and Drug Administration, and other agents, including topiramate, varenicline, baclofen, and gabapentin, have demonstrated variable degrees of efficacy in randomized controlled trials. Available antirelapse medications have a degree of efficacy in reducing the risk of recurrences like antidepressants for major depression, statins for prevention of coronary events, and nonsteroidal anti-inflammatory drugs for arthritis pain. Potentially novel targets, such as the central brain stress response system, endocannabinoid receptors, modulators of α-amino-3-hydroxy-5-methyl-4-isoxazolepropionic acid (AMPA) receptors, and the immune system, have been identified. It is likely that we will continue to see new medications and treatment modalities brought to market in the next decade.

Research on the nature, causes, consequences, and course of AUDs has also grown. Major advances have been made in identifying genetic, developmental, and environmental risk factors for AUDs, describing its natural history and treatment response as well as biopsychosocial consequences of heavy drinking and AUDs. Excellent animal models continue to underpin research on the biological mechanisms underlying behavior. The clinical criteria defining an AUD and its relationship to the timing, frequency, and quantity of heavy drinking have evolved. However, it has become apparent that we understand little about the underlying processes of behavior change in drinking or other behaviors.

DEFINING THE PROBLEM: WHAT ARE TREATMENT OUTCOMES?

The primary goal of treatment for AUDs is a reduction of alcohol use. Commonly considered outcomes are drinking behavior, the number of positive diagnostic criteria of an AUD, functional consequences of drinking, and "recovery" versus abstinence or remission. Controlled drinking may be a reasonable treatment outcome for people with a milder AUD. Nonabstinent recovery is characterized by drinking within the lower risk limits and endorsing no criteria for an AUD. As the heterogeneity and trajectories of drinking behaviors among people with a lifetime diagnosis of AUD have been better defined, it has become clear that nonabstinent recovery is a common outcome, especially among people who do not seek treatment. The likelihood of achieving nonabstinent recovery is inversely related to the severity of AUD. That is, people who endorse 6 or more of the 11 criteria for an AUD seldom achieve stable, low-risk drinking.

The impact of alcohol use on all-cause mortality seems closely tied to the frequency and quantity consumed. A recent study on the global burden of disease found that alcohol was the sixth leading cause of disability globally, including a 41% increase in attributable mortality and a 31% increase in disability-adjusted life-years since 1990. More premature deaths are due to acute events related to alcohol intoxication (56%), with the remainder due to sequelae of chronic heavy alcohol use. Even among people with moderate-to-severe AUD, all-cause mortality is reduced with decreases in alcohol consumption. These studies do not support a dualistic view of outcomes. They suggest that working with patients to achieve any reduction in drinking is better than doing nothing.

Compared to measures of consumption, the presence or absence of *DSM-5* diagnostic criteria for AUD are less frequently discussed as a measure of treatment success. Indeed, nonabstinent remission turns out to be the most common outcome 20 years after the onset of *DSM-IV*–diagnosed alcohol dependence, followed by abstinence, regardless of treatment status.

MEASURING DRINKING OUTCOMES

Methods for measuring drinking behavior has advanced significantly, with structured retrospective self-reporting being the most common tool. This approach is used in most treatment trials, and research supports its validity and reliability. Paradoxically, reporting drinking behaviors daily may independently lead to reductions in use.

Some laboratory tests are promising. Serum or exhaled alcohol concentrations continue to be useful markers of alcohol consumption in the hours before the test is performed. The refinement of biosensors that transcutaneously measure blood alcohol concentrations may improve accuracy in the assessment of drinking behavior but may also cause decreases in drinking. Other traditional lab tests such as γ-glutamyltransferase, mean corpuscular volume, and the ratio of aspartate aminotransferase to alanine aminotransferase all have poor test characteristics and may be elevated or altered by other common liver conditions. They should not be relied upon in clinical practice to detect or monitor unhealthy alcohol use. More promising clinical measures include ethyl glucuronide, ethyl succinate, percent carbohydrate deficient transferrin, and phosphatidylethanol. However, caution must be observed in using any of these tests, particularly ethyl glucuronide/ethyl succinate and phosphatidylethanol. High-quality studies of sensitivity and specificity by multiple investigators at different sites are badly needed.

In early treatment studies of AUD, drinking behavior was grouped into dichotomous categories of abstinence or drinking. Over time, these simple categories were supplanted by more complex variable-based approaches, where average values of a continuous drinking variable were compared among groups using increasingly sophisticated statistical techniques. "Percent days abstinent" and "percent days heavy drinking" are common examples.

Trajectory analyses have the capacity to characterize groups who have a differential response to treatment. One such analysis examined three different trajectories through the follow-up period: stable remission, stable nonremission, and unstable, and another considered both the duration of abstinence and the rate of risky drinking after a relapse. Comparing the likelihood of being in various trajectories for different treatments is easier for most people to grasp, compared to a change in a continuous variable such as "mean percent days abstinent." Moreover, trajectory analyses allow for consumption measures to be linked to more abstract concepts such as quality-of-life metrics.

TAILORING TREATMENT TO THE CONTINUUM OF SEVERITY

Multiple treatment modalities have been shown to be effective in the treatment of AUDs. However, the best way to match the type and intensity of treatment to the individual needs of a patient with AUD remains unclear. For example, no systematic outcome advantage has been demonstrated for residential or intensive day program treatment compared to once or twice weekly outpatient treatment. No behavioral treatment has been shown to be better than others

that are conceptually distinct and use different behavioral techniques. Several medications are efficacious in reducing relapse or heavy drinking during early recovery, but none are clearly better than others, and there is not yet a way to predict how likely a patient is to respond to one rather than another. Finally, approximately 10% of people with AUDs have a severe chronic form of the disorder, yet most treatment programs offer a few weeks or months of treatment, and information on the management of AUD as a chronic illness is limited with mixed results. In summary, current recommendations and practice regarding the selection and sequencing of treatments are based on clinical experience and expert consensus and not randomized controlled trials. In practical terms, the addiction treatment offered depends on patient preference, availability, access, coercion, urgent needs such as imminent withdrawal or suicide risk, and clinician orientation rather than on scientific evidence. One of the key research challenges ahead is to develop methods to compare the effectiveness of different stepwise or adaptive strategies for deploying treatment modalities with demonstrated efficacy.

People Who Abstain, People Who Drink at Lower-Risk Levels, and People With At-Risk Use

Those who abstain and those at lower risk require health promotion, such as education about the recommended maximum limits adjusted for that person's individual situation. The goal for those who are at risk with their drinking is to reduce consumption, preferably below recommended maximum limits to reduce the risk of future harm. Those at risk respond fairly well to facilitated self-change and brief counseling by physicians in primary care, with about a 25% overall reduction in drinking 1 year later, and a greater decrease in heavy drinking. However, implementation has proved to be difficult, if not impossible.

People With Alcohol Use Disorder

Treatment of mild AUD as defined by the *DSM-5* is not well studied. Most studies on the treatment of *DSM-IV*–defined alcohol dependence have been done on middle-aged, treatment-seeking adults, especially white males and veterans, who have severe AUDs. Thus, findings from most treatment studies cannot be generalized to most adults with an AUD. There is a pressing need is to develop and test treatment approaches for people with mild-to-moderate AUD and relatively few comorbidities. In one study, treatment with oral naltrexone plus brief behavioral support by healthcare clinicians is at least as effective as state-of-the-art outpatient addiction therapy.

These findings suggest that pharmacotherapy with medical management may be an effective approach for patients with similar characteristics. If so, making this treatment available in primary care and general psychiatry settings would substantially increase access to effective care.

About two thirds of individuals who develop *DSM-IV*–defined alcohol dependence do so in adolescence or young adulthood. However, only about half of them go on to a chronic course. Those who do are more likely to have a family history of alcohol dependence and antisocial personality traits and to have started drinking in early adolescence. About 40% of people with dependency have a midlife onset of mild-to-moderate AUD, and those who do are more likely to have coexisting psychopathology and/or a family history of AUDs. This suggests that primary care and general psychiatry may be ideal settings in which to evaluate strategies to identify and treat this group.

For those who do not respond to self-change efforts and nonintensive or brief treatment, the appropriate next steps are unclear. Because 12-step rehabilitation is the only available treatment option in most places, clinical practice is to refer to one. The American Society of Addiction Medicine Criteria describe how patients can be triaged to various intensities of rehabilitation programs and medical care. Although this has helped rehabilitation programs and payers to agree on placement, the criteria merely reflect current practice and have no scientific basis. For example, we have known since 1977 that intensive outpatient and/ or residential treatment offers no outcome advantage for patients with an AUD over nonintensive outpatient care. In general, the length of engagement in treatment is a better predictor of outcome than intensity.

At the most severe end of the spectrum are those unfortunate individuals with severe recurrent AUD. In this group, coexisting substance use, mental and physical disorders, and social disabilities are common, including antisocial personality, as is a family history of AUDs and very early onset. Not surprisingly, they are the most likely to seek and receive treatment, often due to overt coercion. Even though most of this group has a chronic or recurrent course, addiction treatment programs typically offer treatment for only a few weeks or months. Furthermore, few programs are staffed to address the serious comorbidities present, and they are often ignored or dealt with through referral. The effectiveness of treatment programs for this group is difficult to evaluate because there are many factors present that may be driving change. For example, serious physical illness, legal mandates, homelessness, unemployment, poverty, and family

pressure frequently cause or contribute to a decision to seek treatment. Many of these factors are quite powerful and could account for much of whatever change occurs. More research is needed on the mechanisms of behavior change among those who drink heavily across the spectrum of AUD severity.

Research on long-term care management strategies, like those used for other chronic disorders, is promising, especially for people with severe AUDs and serious mental or physical disorders. These studies suggest that for those with a harmful drinking habit with serious medical or psychiatric illnesses, addressing drinking directly in the context of medical or psychiatric treatment is preferable to referral to standard addiction treatment programs, which are not staffed to be able to address serious medical or psychiatric illnesses. There are no treatment approaches shown to be effective with severe and persistent AUDs in the absence of comorbidities that cause serious dysfunction. Because this group with severe AUDs are frequently heavy consumers of healthcare, social, and criminal justice services, the development of more effective treatments is a priority. It may be that external motivating factors, such as skillful application of legal coercion or contingency management may be effective with this group, especially when combined with "wraparound" services that integrate addiction, psychiatric, and medical care as well as social services and sober housing. What is clear is that treatment for these individuals needs to be structured with the goal of providing services intermittently or continuously for years to decades rather than weeks or months.

To summarize, recent research has shown that drinking and associated symptoms and problems occur along a continuum ranging from none to mild, moderate, and severe. A majority of US adults abstains or drinks at lower risk levels. Many of those with at-risk drinking behaviors are without current symptoms or problems but are at an increased risk for physical, mental, and substance use disorders developing over time. In contrast to popular belief, most people who meet AUD criteria do not have a chronic course and most recover without professional treatment or even attendance at mutual help groups. It appears that most people, upon recognizing a problem, attempt to change alone or with informal help, and the majority are eventually successful, albeit after several years of active disorder. Seeking help from mutual help groups or nonaddiction professionals (about 25%) and/or professional treatment programs (10%) occurs when informal attempts to change fail or an external contingency is applied, such as a legal charge for driving while intoxicated or family demands. A significant proportion of those who seek treatment respond with improvement or remission, although this often takes years, with multiple quit attempts and recurrences prior to achieving stable remission. There is a small but important group with severe and persistent AUDs. This continuum of drinking and associated symptoms and problems suggests a corresponding continuum of care.

TREATMENT AND BEHAVIOR CHANGE

The outcome of treatment varies based on the diagnostic severity or stage of illness. In a typical treatment study, about one third of subjects will be in full abstinent or nonabstinent remission for the following year, 30% to 40% will show substantial improvement but will have at least some episodes of heavy drinking, and 20% to 30% will not show an effect. However, over the course of the ensuing 5 to 10 years, most will suffer at least some recurrences. No one technique has proven to be overall more effective than others, thus raising the question of what the mechanisms of change really are. In fact, many people start reducing their drinking prior to treatment entry, and both study protocols and treatment programs require that someone be abstinent at treatment entry. One study qualitatively examined the process leading to seeking help in study subjects. They identified a "catalyst system" consisting of increasing problems and distress related to drinking, pressure from others, and a trigger event, which in turn led to the realization, "I can't do this on my own." Factors outside the treatment context continued to be important throughout the recovery process, especially after the discontinuation of treatment services. These findings suggest that the process of deciding to seek help is itself part of the change process and is arguably the most important, although it is not well understood.

Treatment seeking is strongly associated with increased odds of achieving full remission, but those who seek help differ systematically from those who do not seek help. Those who do seek help, on average, are older and have more severe AUDs and more coexisting mental and physical disorders as well as less social support. For those who do seek help, both professional treatment and 12-step participation are associated with an increased likelihood of full remission, especially abstinent remission. For individuals older than 35 years of age, abstinence is a much more stable outcome than even light drinking without problems, whereas in younger persons, lower-risk drinking without problems (ie, nonabstinent remission) is similar to abstinence in predicting continued remission 3 years later. Thus, full remission, whether abstinent or nonabstinent, should

be the goal of treatment for dependence, tempered with the recognition that full recovery cannot always be achieved.

SYSTEMS OF CARE

An ongoing opportunity within the field of addiction medicine is how and where tailored treatments should be provided to catalyze behavior change. Historically, rehabilitation programs independent of the healthcare system have been the cornerstone of care for people with AUDs. About two thirds of these programs are publicly funded. Most care for AUDs occurs in programs where it is uncertain whether a medical professional would be involved in their care, despite legislative and reimbursement efforts promoting a medical model of care. From 2002 to 2004, only 30.7% of publicly funded programs had a physician on staff compared with 50.7% of privately funded programs, whereas a slightly higher percentage of publicly funded programs (35.4%) employed a physician on contract compared with private programs (26.1%). Average utilization of medical staff by substance use disorder treatment programs increased by 26% from 2007 to 2010, a trend encouraged by the implementation of the Affordable Care Act. However, uptake of antirelapse medication treatment remains very low. The most strongly endorsed barriers to their use were regulatory prohibitions due to the program's lack of medical staff, funding barriers to implementation, and lack of access to medical personnel with expertise in prescribing them. The lack of physicians familiar with both pharmacologic and psychotherapeutic treatment modalities for AUDs, even among those working for treatment programs, is a formidable barrier to quality care. This limitation is accentuated by the time-limited care standard of most treatment programs, whereby patients are often discharged to follow-up with providers unfamiliar with how to support recovery, if they are discharged to follow-up with healthcare providers at all.

INTEGRATING THE EVIDENCE AND PERSONALIZING PRACTICE

Given the proliferation of new research, it is a challenge to understand and incorporate new findings into practice. Unfortunately, although studies of the efficacy of various treatments may help determine how one treatment compares to another treatment or to no treatment, there are few studies that directly address questions of central importance to clinicians. For example, should one recommend a few sessions of motivational enhancement therapy or an intensive day program for the treatment of an AUD?

If a person with at-risk alcohol use does not respond to brief motivational counseling, what is the appropriate next step? Is the stepped care strategy, where the least restrictive and expensive option for a situation is offered first, the best approach? How much evidence is required before recommending a new treatment? How much evidence is required before failure to offer or recommend a treatment based on personal taste or ideology is ethically indefensible?

Although it is not possible to provide definitive answers for these questions, certain conclusions emerge from available evidence. Although there is no systematic advantage for one type of behavioral therapy over another, the quality of the behavioral treatment provided is important. Specifically, empathic and skillful therapy is more effective than confrontation and education. Furthermore, it is more important to engage someone with an AUD in treatment than which treatment is used. Therefore, it makes sense to offer a variety of treatment options because patients are likely to vary in their preferences. The same holds true for the setting of treatment. Unless someone is unable to abstain while living in the community, there is no advantage of residential versus outpatient treatment or of intensive versus less

intensive outpatient treatment. Second, antirelapse medications offer a clinically important benefit in early recovery, and therefore, patients should routinely be made aware of them and offered the opportunity to use them. Current evidence provides no guidance, however, on choosing one medication over another, or what the sequence of subsequent antirelapse medications should be. There is no evidence that combining medications is more beneficial than monotherapy. For appropriate patients (ie, moderate levels of AUD, little or no coexisting psychopathology, socially stable and motivated to change drinking patterns), medication with medical care management and encouragement to abstain, adhere to treatment, and attend mutual help groups is as effective as specialized alcohol counseling. Third, a social network supportive of abstinence is at least as important as whatever treatment occurs in determining outcomes. Except for referral to mutual help groups, this aspect of treatment tends to be neglected to the detriment of our patients. Finally, for any given diagnosis (eg, at-risk drinking versus an AUD), there is not yet a way to identify patient characteristics that reliably predict differential responses to different treatments, although research in this area is promising (Fig. 27-1).

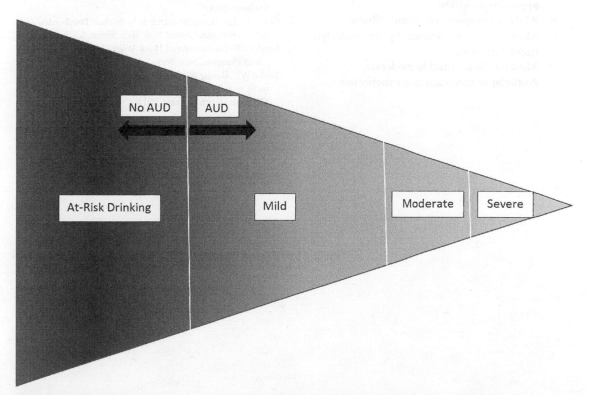

Figure 27-1. Continuum of severity of alcohol use disorder. A small minority fall into the category of severe alcohol use disorder.

KEY POINTS

1. Alcohol use disorder is common, affecting nearly 30% of the population. People who drink heavily but without dependency are also harmed by acute intoxication.

2. AUD exists on a spectrum, from mild to severe. Most people with AUD have a single episode of AUD and remain functional. Few receive treatment, but almost all recover eventually.

3. Severe, chronic AUD occurs in about 30% of people with AUDs. About half of this group will receive some treatment, or roughly one eighth of the total population with AUDs.

4. Community treatment models providing low-level counseling, lectures, and Alcoholics Anonymous groups for a brief period are most commonly available. They are likely ineffective. Treatment models do not conform to the natural history of the illness.

5. Antirelapse medications are about as effective as antidepressives or antihypertensives but are seldom prescribed.

REVIEW QUESTIONS

1. Which of the following statements is *true*?
   A. Alcoholics Anonymous is the most effective approach to AUDs.
   B. AUD is a progressive, chronic illness
   C. Most AUDs are caused by an underlying mental disorder.
   D. Most AUDs are mild to moderate.
   E. Antirelapse medications are ineffective.

2. Which of the following best describes the course of an AUD?
   A. There are multiple trajectories for AUDs.
   B. It is inexorably progressive if not treated.
   C. It waxes and wanes over decades.
   D. It is typically short lived.
   E. Most people with AUDs never recover.

3. Which of the following represents the best outcome for AUDs?
   A. Experts cannot agree on the answer.
   B. Abstinent and nonabstinent recovery
   C. Abstinent recovery is the only option.
   D. Abstinent recovery through Alcoholics Anonymous
   E. Controlled drinking is the ideal option.

ANSWERS

1. **D**
2. **A**
3. **B**

SUGGESTED READINGS

Fletcher AM. *Inside Rehab: The Surprising Truth About Addiction Treatment—And How to Get Help That Works*. New York: Penguin, 2013.

Foote J, Wilkens C, Kosanke N, Higgs S. *Beyond Addiction: How Science and Kindness Help People Change*. New York: Scribner, 2014.

Glaser G. *Her Best-Kept Secret: Why Women Drink—And How They Can Regain Control*. New York: Simon & Schuster, 2014.

Kandel ER. *The Disordered Mind: What Unusual Brains Tell Us About Ourselves*. New York: Farrar, Straus and Giroux, 2018.

White WL. *Slaying the Dragon: The History of Addiction Treatment and Recovery in America*. 2nd ed. Bloomington, ID: Chestnut Health Systems, 2014.

28 The Treatment of Addiction: An Overview

Summary by Andrea G. Barthwell, Jeffrey Allgaier, and Lawrence S. Brown Jr.

> Based on THE ASAM PRINCIPLES OF ADDICTION MEDICINE, 6th edition chapter by Andrea G. Barthwell, Lawrence S. Brown Jr., and Megan E. Crants

GOALS OF SUBSTANCE USE TREATMENT

In the United States, over 11,000 specialized substance use treatment facilities provide rehabilitation, counseling, behavioral therapy, medication, case management, and other types of services to persons with substance use disorders (SUDs). Care of individuals with SUDs includes assessing needs, providing treatment for intoxication and withdrawal, and developing, with appropriate support, a treatment plan that may consist of referrals to psychosocial care.

TREATMENT SETTINGS

Decisions regarding the site of care should be based on the patient's ability to cooperate with and benefit from treatment offered and to refrain from illicit use of substances as well as the need to avoid high-risk behaviors and the need for structure and support. Patients move from one level of care to another based on these factors and an assessment of their ability to benefit from a different level of care. Access to appropriate levels of care vary depending on the available resources in each community as well as state and federal laws. Although some hospitals have inpatient addiction medicine consultation services with specialty-trained clinicians, other hospitals limit their management of SUDs to basic detoxification and referral.

Although Federal Parity Legislation, the Affordable Care Act, and the Comprehensive Addiction and Recovery Act of 2016 have led to expanded access to addiction treatment, there are still impediments that prevent these permissive federal legislations from having the intended effects of increased access to addiction treatment. For example, many states have not expanded the use of Medicaid

funding to improve access to addiction treatment, and some states regulate midlevel practitioners in manners that prevent them from providing evidence-based addiction treatment that includes the use of US Food and Drug Administration–approved medications.

SPECIAL CONSIDERATIONS IN THE EMERGENCY DEPARTMENT

In recent years, more and more individuals with SUDs are entering the healthcare delivery system through emergency departments (EDs) following an overdose from unintentional overdosing. Because patients may present in the ED for the management of sequelae of use, the emergency physician should be prepared to intervene when the patient is stable regarding their use. The ED physician or health educators should be familiar with the technique of screening, brief intervention, and referral to treatment as well as pharmacotherapy for the treatment of SUDs, nearly all of which can be commenced in the ED. Buprenorphine has shown particular promise when started in the ED as far as increasing engagement in addiction treatment.

Hospital Settings

Hospitalization is appropriate for patients whose assessed need cannot be treated safely in an outpatient or ED setting due to:

- severe or medically complicated withdrawal potential,
- co-occurring medical or psychiatric conditions that complicate detoxification or impair treatment,
- failure to engage in treatment at a lower level of care,
- life- or limb-threatening medical conditions that would require hospitalization,

- psychiatric disorders that make the patient an imminent threat to self or others, or
- failure to respond to care at any level such that the patient endangers others or poses a self-threat.

Partial Hospital Programs and Intensive Outpatient Programs

Partial hospitalization is considered for patients who require intensive care but have a reasonable chance of making progress on treatment goals in the intertreatment interval, including maintenance of abstinence. It is often provided to individuals who still require frequent and concentrated contact with treatment professionals to monitor their behavior and manage their risk of continued use or relapse and who need to develop support for their recovery-focused efforts beyond the treatment system. The difference between partial hospital programs and intensive outpatient programs is seen in intensity, number of hours per day, the program setting, and the program's structure.

Outpatient Programs

Outpatient programs vary in structure and intensity. They are less expensive than residential or inpatient treatment and may be more suitable for individuals with less severe symptoms and a high degree of predicted compliance and those with a supportive structure in their home environment. High rates of attrition can be problematic, particularly in the early phase.

Outcomes are highly correlated with time in treatment, and as a result, retention should be one focus of treatment, along with self-efficacy regarding adherence to the abstinence plan. In many outpatient programs, as in much of treatment in general, group counseling is emphasized.

RESIDENTIAL PROGRAMS, INCLUDING THERAPEUTIC COMMUNITIES

Residential programs have the following characteristics:

- Provide care 24 hours a day
- Are generally conducted in nonhospital settings
- Are generally provided to patients who do not meet the clinical criteria for hospitalization
- May include short-term programs that provide intensive but relatively brief residential treatment based on 12-step facilitation
- Includes a duration of treatment determined by the clinical response to therapy
- Includes a duration of treatment that varies on the length of time necessary for the patient to meet specific criteria predictive of success

One residential treatment model is the therapeutic community (TC). TCs are residential programs with planned lengths of stay from 6 to 12 months. TCs focus on the "resocialization" of the individual and use the program's entire "community"—including other residents, staff, and the social context—as active components of treatment. Treatment is highly structured and can at times be confrontational, with activities designed to help residents examine damaging beliefs, self-concepts, and patterns of behavior and to adopt new, more harmonious, and constructive ways to interact with others. Recently, with pressure from reimbursement sources, the elements of TCs have been incorporated into shorter term residential programs and institutional criminal justice settings.

Community residential rehabilitation facilities include "halfway houses" or "sober living facilities," with the former providing more structure and supervision. Individuals referred to these settings are generally deemed to be at risk for relapse without such support. This setting is offered to the individual whose environmental risk is great or those needing several services after primary treatment to address deficits in vocation, employment, and social supports.

Case Management

Case management is a collaborative process that assesses, plans, implements, coordinates, monitors, and evaluates the options and services to meet an individual's health needs. Case management is provided to individuals whose social situation and complex needs would impair their ability to adhere to a prescribed treatment plan and follow-up care.

Aftercare Programs

Aftercare generally follows an episode of care and is focused on maintaining gains made in treatment over a prescribed period. Many professionals view the term "aftercare" as outdated in that it suggests that care has somehow ended. As such, some prefer the use of the term "outpatient addiction rehabilitation treatment" or follow-up.

Sober Coaches, Recovery Coaches, and Other Support Services

Sober coaches, recovery coaches, and other such aides provide nonprofessional supervision and guidance to individuals going through the recovery process. They are meant to encourage healthy structures and rituals and may also be able to help their clients build responsibility and develop an improved sense of judgment.

Treatment in the Physician's Office, Including Screening and Brief Interventions

The screening and brief interventions technique is one of the most popular clinical tools utilized by primary care providers who employ screening and brief intervention basics with nearly every patient to facilitate a trusting, healing relationship and change a variety of harmful behaviors including smoking, overeating, poor medication compliance, or sedentary lifestyle. It is one of the many treatment methods available to help patients with unhealthy substance use.

CRIMINAL JUSTICE SETTINGS FOR MANDATED TREATMENT, INCLUDING DRUG COURTS

As referenced elsewhere in this book, research has shown that combining criminal justice sanctions with substance use treatment can be effective at decreasing substance use and related crime. Individuals under legal coercion tend to stay in treatment for a longer period and do as well as or better than others not under legal pressure. Several treatment options exist for those who are incarcerated, including didactic drug education classes, self-help programs, and treatment based on TC or residential milieu therapy models. Research shows that relapse to substance use and recidivism to crime are significantly lower if the offender continues treatment after returning to the community. Several criminal justice alternatives to incarceration have been tried with offenders who have SUDs, including limited diversion programs, pretrial release conditional on entry into treatment, and conditional probation with sanctions. The drug court is a promising approach. Drug courts mandate and arrange for substance use treatment, actively monitor progress in treatment, and arrange other services for people involved in using substances.

TREATMENT SERVICES

Treatment services often include a combination of medical management combined with psychosocial treatments to help individuals suffering with the pathophysiologic effects and other clinical manifestations of addiction. Some of these services include clinical monitoring, managing intoxication and withdrawal, as well as a multitude of behavioral treatments.

Clinical monitoring is extremely important in achieving successful clinical outcomes. Self-reporting is a type of monitoring that is most useful in the context of a nonconfrontational, nonjudgmental, and empathetic clinical setting. However, because of the limitations of self-reporting in the initial assessment and during clinical monitoring, substance use testing represents an important tool for addiction medicine specialists.

Pharmacotherapy is the cornerstone for patients with either intoxication or withdrawal, although the effective treatment for intoxication typically requires a hospital setting, whereas withdrawal can be treated in either an inpatient or outpatient setting. Medications are available for detoxification or tapering from opioids, nicotine, benzodiazepines, alcohol, and other sedatives. Detoxification is a commonly used approach in responding to patients with clinical signs of intoxication or withdrawal.

Talk Therapy

Numerous studies have demonstrated that talk therapy or counseling can be an effective treatment for some SUDs, especially alcohol and stimulants. For opioid use disorder, medication management is the mainstay of treatment, whereas counseling may be helpful for some patients.

In general, therapies attempt to arrest compulsive substance use through modification of behaviors, feelings, social functioning, and thoughts. Because no form of psychotherapy has proven superior to another for all patients, a successful referral to services is more important than physician determination of the most appropriate approach.

Cognitive–behavioral therapy is based on the theory that learning processes play a critical role in the development of maladaptive patterns of behavior. Motivational enhancement therapy is a patient-centered counseling approach that attempts to initiate behavior change by helping patients resolve their ambivalence about engaging in treatment and stopping substance use. A community reinforcement approach is an intensive outpatient therapy employed for cocaine dependence with dual goals: to achieve cocaine abstinence long enough for patients to learn new life skills that will help sustain abstinence and to reduce alcohol consumption for patients whose drinking is associated with cocaine use. Voucher-based reinforcement therapy helps patients achieve and maintain abstinence from illicit substances by providing them with a voucher each time they provide a substance-free urine sample. Individualized counseling focuses directly on reducing or stopping the patient's illicit substance use. It also addresses related areas of impaired functioning—such as employment status, illegal activity, and family/social relations—as well as the content and structure of the patient's recovery program. Multidimensional family therapy is an outpatient, family-based substance use treatment approach for adolescents. It approaches adolescent substance use in terms of a network of influences (individual, family, peer, and community) and suggests that reducing unwanted behavior and increasing desirable behavior occur in multiple ways in different settings.

Computer-Assisted Therapy and Telemedicine

There is a growing body of literature that supports the use of technology in the treatment of addiction, using both computer-assisted therapy (CAT) and telemedicine. CAT is developing rapidly and includes online counseling, self-help resources, and text messaging. Several randomized controlled trials have been conducted in recent years examining the efficacy of CAT for addiction to a number of substances, with some of these demonstrating that this intervention approach may significantly reduce substance use behavior and biochemical measures of substance use. Formal CAT programs are usually clinician facilitated, although some are developed to be used independently by the individual. Telemedicine via real-time video conference is a promising healthcare delivery method currently utilized for a number of chronic diseases. There is increasing evidence to support this modality in addiction treatment, including for opioid agonist treatments. Most state Medicaid programs have adopted coverage of telemedicine into their policies.

Pharmacologic Therapies

Pharmacotherapies are increasingly being utilized to treat SUDs. With the exception of methadone, all US Food and Drug Administration–approved pharmacotherapies for alcohol and opioid use disorder can be prescribed from a physician's office. In the case of buprenorphine, a special "waiver" is required from the Drug Enforcement Administration. Recent federal legislation has been implemented for the purposes of expanding this waiver program.

KEY POINTS

1. Care of individuals with SUDs includes assessing needs, providing treatment, and developing an individualized treatment plan.
2. The site of care for a patient is dependent not only on a patient's ability to refrain from the use of illicit

substances but also on their needs for structure and support along with their ability to cooperate with and benefit from the treatment offered.
3. Pharmacotherapies can offer patients a similar result: a sustained, stabilized recovery from an SUD.

REVIEW QUESTIONS

1. Which of the following best represents our current understanding of patients with addictive disorders?
   A. Patients can often be cured with a short duration of treatment.
   B. Patients with addictive disorders usually differ in disease chronicity from patients with hypertension, diabetes, or asthma.
   C. Patients often require prolonged treatment for their chronic disease of addiction.
   D. Patients are usually cured by appropriate and robust detoxification.
   E. Patients are best treated with one mode of treatment to minimize confusion.

2. Clinicians treating patients for opioid use disorder using buprenorphine must understand which of the following?
   A. Buprenorphine represents trading one addiction for another.
   B. Preventing withdrawal and craving are important when determining the correct dose.
   C. Medication management alone should not be used without requiring counseling.
   D. Most patients should be tapered quickly to prevent the development of tolerance.
   E. Rapid detoxification off pure opioids using buprenorphine followed by intense nonmedication therapy represents the standard of care.

3. A relatively new evidence-based treatment for opioid withdrawal includes which of the following?
   A. Naltrexone followed by intense therapy
   B. Clonidine and ondansetron followed by prompt referral to an addiction specialist
   C. Cognitive–behavioral therapy followed by buprenorphine or methadone
   D. Starting buprenorphine immediately in the emergency department
   E. Sedation along with naloxone infusion to minimize the duration of withdrawals

ANSWERS

1. **C**
2. **B**
3. **D**

SUGGESTED READINGS

American Society of Addiction Medicine. *The ASAM National Practice Guideline for the Use of Medications in the Treatment of Addiction Involving Opioid Use.* Chevy Chase, MD: ASAM, 2015.

Center for Substance Abuse Treatment. *Medication-Assisted Treatment for Opioid Addiction in Opioid Treatment Programs.* Rockville, MD: Substance Abuse and Mental Health Services Administration, 2005. Report No. (SMA) 12-4214.

Center for Substance Abuse Treatment. *Substance Abuse Treatment for Adults in the Criminal Justice System. Treatment Improvement Protocol (TIP) Series, No. 44.* Rockville, MD: Substance Abuse and Mental Health Services Administration, 2005.

D'Onofrio G, Chawarski MC, O'Connor PG, et al. Emergency department-initiated buprenorphine for opioid dependence with continuation in primary care: outcomes during and after intervention. *J Gen Intern Med.* 2017;32(6):660-666.

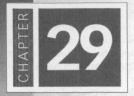

Integrated Care for Substance Use Disorder

Summary by Keith Humphreys, Mark McGovern, and A. Thomas McLellan

Based on THE ASAM PRINCIPLES OF ADDICTION MEDICINE, 6th edition chapter by Keith Humphreys, Mark McGovern, and A. Thomas McLellan

In the United States, the majority of activity and cost of healthcare delivery involves chronic, nonacute healthcare problems. These include diseases across all systems, including cardiovascular (hypertension), musculoskeletal (pain), metabolic (diabetes), and infections (hepatitis C and HIV). Alongside these problems, chronic depression, substance use, and serious mental illnesses account for significant disease burden and cost.

The general model in healthcare access involves a front-end primary care physician (PCP) who identifies a problem, treats identified cases to the scope of his or her practice, and then refers more severe cases to specialists until either the patient is stabilized—in which case the patient returns to the PCP—or if not, all care is assumed by the specialist for an extended period.

This model is standard practice, efficient, guideline and protocol driven, and widely accepted as the status quo in the medical care of chronic physical conditions. But this model has not yet been brought to scale for the care of persons with substance use disorders (SUDs).

This chapter describes an approach, as well as implementation and sustainment considerations, to deploy modern, empirically grounded techniques for integrated chronic disease management for persons with substance use concerns or SUDs.

AN UNPRECEDENTED HISTORICAL MOMENT FOR SUBSTANCE USE DISORDER TREATMENT

For decades, specialty addiction treatment has been marginalized and isolated, in part by its own design. To some extent driven by stigma, it was perceived as a rather peculiar type of nonmedical activity for people who may be more criminal than sick. In recent years through the present, we are witnessing and perhaps shaping an unprecedented opportunity to integrate SUD treatment into the rest of the healthcare delivery system. There are at least five primary drivers to the current zeitgeist:

1. Improvements in insurance benefits for SUD treatment: Medicare Improvement for Patients and Providers Act of 2008, Mental Health and Addiction Parity Act of 2008, and the Affordable Care Act of 2010;
2. The expansion of evidence-based addiction treatments, both psychosocial and pharmacologic, that are effective and feasible for routine delivery;
3. A subtle but palpable shift in societal perception from the moral and sociopathic to the health and well-being model of substance use and addiction;
4. Changes in privacy regulations and information technology, at one time designed to protect patient confidentiality and privacy, but instead limiting full participation and care coordination in the healthcare delivery system; and
5. Evolutions in the structure of healthcare organization, driven by the complexity of practice and also healthcare economics, with fewer solo practitioners, who have been replaced by patient-centered medical homes, large group practices, and financial risk–sharing healthcare systems such as accountable care organizations.

Furthermore, the recent opioid epidemic has opened up interest across general practice settings and primary care for training in integrated care for opioid use disorders with addiction medications, changes in opioid prescribing practices, and gaining competency in overdose prevention. In this new healthcare environment, these factors converge so that people with SUDs can finally interact with the healthcare system just as do people with other conditions that vary in severity and chronicity.

TOWARD INTEGRATED CARE FOR THE POPULATION OF PEOPLE WITH SUBSTANCE USE DISORDERS

As with any incurable medical condition, the chronic care management (CCM) model can conceptualize and organize an approach to service delivery for SUDs. The CCM model is a long-term, proactive strategy involving team-based care, not just a single physician. Methods include standardized protocols and metrics, measurement-based processes, patient registries to support panel and population health, and the expectation of a long-term relationship.

The goal of CCM is to engage and activate patients and their collaterals in their own care; share decision making about treatment options; and, in addition to good outcomes and quality of life, move toward increased autonomy, self-empowerment, and illness self-management. Instead of providing reactive, acute care responses, often resulting in high emergency department and hospitalization utilization, the CCM model is proactive and collaborative, and harnesses preemptive strategies that anticipate signs of prodromal or actual relapse and deterioration.

The CCM model is increasingly adopted by healthcare systems from the private (eg, Kaiser Permanente) to the public (eg, Veterans Affairs) sectors. The evidence for CCM is robust for depression and physical illnesses, preferred by patients and providers, and has favorable cost outcomes. Although more studies are underway, the existing findings for randomized controlled trials evaluating CCM for SUDs have been less than compelling (eg, AHEAD, SUMMIT). We assert that the lessons learned in the CCM approach based on this research, both in terms of clinical conceptualization and implementation/sustainment factors, will significantly enhance its scalability.

A STAGE MODEL OF CHRONIC CARE MANAGEMENT FOR SUBSTANCE USE DISORDERS

Within the CCM, we delineate four linked stages to organize a clinical model for SUDs. Each stage has a specific clinical purpose that is related to the overall goal: patient empowerment through self-management to maximize functioning and reduce relapse risk.

The stages are Early Identification/Intervention, Stabilization, Clinical Monitoring/Management, and Patient Self-Management (Table 29-1).

Five introductory points are important to consider prior to the discussion of stages of CCM for SUDs. First, PCPs will observe that the activities and goals of this stepped care model are similar to the routine management of other chronic conditions. Two, the stages are appropriate to the management of SUDs ranging in severity and complexity from no problem to a severe problem (ie, addiction). Thus, the approach is objective, individualized, and optimizes patient preference and choice. Third, because the stages are conceptually linked, many treatment practices will have a role in more than one stage (eg, naltrexone for craving reduction in the Stabilization *and* Clinical Monitoring/Management stages). Fourth, there are, as of this writing, no standardized rules to guide decisions and transitions from stage to stage. Although there are both biological (eg, urine drug screens, liver function tests) and behavioral measures (eg, motivation level, distress tolerance), these metrics still need to be systematized for care monitoring protocols. The fifth and final point is that these four stages are not isomorphic with models of traditional addiction treatment settings, ie, detoxification, rehabilitation, outpatient, peer recovery support groups, but instead are stages organized by goals and activities independent of setting and of provider type.

The Early Identification/Intervention Stage of Care

The main goal at this stage is to engage and activate the person whose substance use is affecting his or her health and well-being. Screening; patient education; observing the connection among substance use, its consequences, and goal attainment; and instituting a behavioral experiment–type monitoring plan are all components of this stage. Based on a patient's success or lack thereof at the "experiment," a more severe problem (and diagnosis) may be obvious. The goal at this stage is to develop an accurate

TABLE 29-1	Four Stages of Chronic Care Management for Substance Use Disorders	
Stage	**Goals**	**Clinical Methods**
Early Identification/ Intervention	Identify "medically harmful" substance use	Screening instruments (verbal or electronic)
	Educate and motivate the patient to reduce substance use	Brief motivational interviewing
	Engage the patient in healthy alternative behaviors and continuing self-management	Office-based and off-site (through electronic media) monitoring with consequences
Stabilization	Eliminate substance use	Medications to manage withdrawal, craving
	Safe reduction of withdrawal symptoms; improve patient health	Initiate medication maintenance if needed
	Educate/manage patient to accept problem	Brief motivational interviewing
		Individual therapy
Clinical Management/ Monitoring	Maintain reductions in use and related medical consequences	Medications—maintenance medications
	Educate the patient and family to maintain no/low-level use	Brief motivational interviewing
	Engage the patient in health behaviors and continued self-management	Family and couple therapy
		Individual therapy
		Monitoring (on-site and off-site) with consequences
Personal Management	Maintain reductions in use and related consequences	Medications—maintenance medications
	Prevent emotional or social threats that reinitiate use	Self-help groups and activities
		Individual, family, and couple therapy as needed

(and shared) appreciation of the nature and severity of the substance use issue and what may be necessary to address it. In some cases, the patient goal may be continued use without consequences, whereas the physician's goal might be total abstinence.

The clinical practices at this stage involve collaborating, or coinvestigating, alongside the patient to assess the presence, type, and potential severity of the substance use. This includes standardized screening, a review of functional domains for potential consequences, and brief motivational interventions to help the patient examine and solidify a plan for change. At this stage, it is important for the provider to empathize with the patient, including the awareness of any shame, guilt, or fear about the struggle to control his or her substance use. Stigma, discrimination, and remnants of a judgmental viewpoint that substance

use problems constitute weakness or sociopathy can be undermining attitudes festering within either patient or provider.

This stage encompasses the Screening, Brief Intervention, and Referral to Treatment (SBIRT) approach. SBIRT is a workflow that has been tested extensively in over 100 trials with individuals who are dependent on alcohol or other drugs. SBIRT and brief interventions generically have been studied in emergency and primary care settings. The findings of the effectiveness of SBIRT and brief interventions are attenuated by variation in participant motivation, substance type, SUD severity and complexity, and, of course, who delivers the intervention. When the patient fails at his or her goal, or brief interventions fail, this is suggestive of a more serious disorder.

The Stabilization Stage of Care

Alcohol and other substances with addictive potential often cause significant physical and psychological impairment, directly due to physiologic toxicity and neurobiological changes and indirectly due to sleep disturbance, poor nutrition, and general lack of personal care. The primary goal at the stage of stabilization is to keep the patient safe and comfortable through a period of withdrawal and also prepare him or her for the clinical monitoring/management stage. Stabilization alone is insufficient to produce lasting change. It is a necessary step (but not a sufficient one) toward the next stage of rehabilitation.

The major clinical components of Stabilization include medications to relieve physical and emotional distress symptoms during withdrawal and also to reduce craving. Often but not always delivered in the safety of a residential or hospital setting, psychosocial therapies to promote motivation and transition to the next stage are important. In less severe cases, stabilization may occur in less structured environments such as outpatient or office-based settings. The American Society of Addiction Medicine Patient Placement Criteria offers guidance as to the appropriate setting or level of care.

Regardless of setting, the goal is to help the patient develop the capability, probably with professional help, to manage their substance use. Patients who suffer serious withdrawal would seem less likely to achieve "control" through moderation but may still insist on this option. It is important to negotiate frankly about the realistic possibility for maintaining controlled use and to develop a close monitoring plan for the next stage. Other patients will accept the goal of abstinence and may accurately or underestimate the challenges in meeting this objective. In most all cases, patients exiting the Stabilization phase and entering (or reentering) the Clinical Monitoring/Management Stage will require a rather intensive combination of psychosocial therapies and one or more medications. Critical at this transition is the assessment of, stabilization of, and treatment planning for any comorbid physical and psychiatric conditions that could complicate and undermine even the highest quality addiction-focused therapies.

The Clinical Monitoring/Management Stage of Care

This stage may be the most variable—in time, procedure, and patient eligibility—of all the stages of care. It is appropriate for patients who are physically and emotionally stabilized and who have at least gained some capacity for distress tolerance, self-regulation, and control over cravings. Clinical goals are to maintain the reductions or eliminations of substance use; to address complicating factors in medical, social, family, and psychiatric domains; and to continue to build skills and monitor for relapse. Environmental factors, including housing, work, and relationships, may require structural attention (eg, sober living facility), intervention (marital or family therapy), or careful monitoring (examining risks and supports in social network). Maintaining motivation to make behavioral and lifestyle changes compatible with recovery is also critical. Clinical practices include the pharmacologic (eg, anticraving, maintenance or relapse prevention, US Food and Drug Administration–approved medications) and psychosocial (eg, cognitive–behavioral therapies, behavioral marital therapy, 12-step facilitation therapy, acceptance and commitment therapy, mindfulness and contingency management).

Addressing co-occurring psychiatric problems in this phase is crucial for the focused addiction therapies to work. Psychotropic medications, such as for mood, anxiety, or psychotic spectrum disorders, and evidence-based psychosocial therapies are effective options.

Team-based care provides the workforce model to deliver this assortment of therapies. Although it is possible, seldom does a single physician provide the entire range of treatment options. Thus, good coordination across the team, including communication and cohesion, is a sustainable approach to delivering the full range of pharmacologic, psychotherapy, case management, and systems-based therapies.

Although important in all earlier stages, monitoring substance use through biologic tests and patient self-report is critical. Evaluating treatment response and adjusting dose, intensity, or level of care is determined by these markers. Further, patient and provider shared decisions about transition back to Stabilization or on to the next stage of Self-Management are based on these objective data.

The Patient Self-Management Stage

This stage involves the transition from some/any form of clinically directed care and monitoring toward self-management by the patient, likely with the informed support of family, friends, and other community resources (eg, peer recovery support groups). There is substantial research support for the positive role of peer recovery support participation and favorable outcomes. In addition, simply contacting, supporting, and monitoring previously treated patients has also shown benefit. Likewise, the value of technologies for recovery self-management with or without therapist involvement has shown some promise. All of these components are, at minimum, a hedge against relapse and reutilization of expensive healthcare resources but even more so can play a transformative role in a patient's quality of life and recovery.

The goals at this stage include the maintenance of physiologic and emotional improvements made during earlier stages, developing the capacity to self-monitor relapse threats, practicing effective coping behaviors and self-care, and maintaining healthy relationships and social behaviors.

Continuing care may involve medications, less frequent group or individual check-ins, random toxicologic monitoring, and ongoing care for psychiatric and physical health comorbidities.

Conceptualizing the integrated care of SUDs within a CCM model, organized by pragmatic stages, may assist routine healthcare providers in how to structure services and may also assist researchers in how to categorize patients and interventions within and across clinical trials. The CCM model is a familiar approach to common conditions encountered in medical practice and for which there is no cure, yet for which effective evidence-based treatments are available and with clinical outcome and cost benefits. However, this is clearly more so a framework to be modified than a sacred relic.

IMPLEMENTATION AND SUSTAINABILITY

The CCM model has more recently been applied to the management of substance use and addiction in routine medical practice settings. Although it is clinically reasonable, and stands to deliver a valuable service, barriers to implementation are significant. For example, outside of special funding, efforts to implement simple practices such as SBIRT or more complex practices such as medications for opioid use disorders, have been challenging. For integrated care of SUDs to be brought to scale, implementation and sustainment issues must be at the forefront. For chronic medical conditions, the CCM model is flexible to accommodate a variety of diseases, for example hypertension and diabetes, either alone or in combination. Protocols are not additive but are braided and integrated. The CCM model for depression has been widely adopted but has also experienced a decline in effectiveness in

routine practice settings because of patient heterogeneity and complexity. For these reasons, an implementable and sustainable CCM model for SUDs must capitalize on the same workflow, workforce, and whenever possible the financing and reimbursement for other chronic disease management from diabetes to depression. This approach would account for the stages described previously and includes the same workforce and workflow, patient registries for population health management, and metrics for primary care consultation/referral/coordination with specialists. A unified CCM model that builds upon and braids the evidence-based approaches for the most commonly encountered conditions is needed to guide providers and patients across the stages outlined in this chapter. Especially if we consider general medical settings such as primary care, a unified model is both implementable and sustainable within typically existing workflows and workforces, unlike the more single disorder approaches in clinical research. Such a unified model would incorporate the evidence from specific disorder findings but more realistically address the typical patient, the typical provider, and the typical setting within which integrated healthcare is to take place.

CONCLUSION

A variety of factors—legislative, financial, a growth in effective treatments, changes in societal attitude, and a public health epidemic—have converged to create an unprecedented opportunity for the integration of addiction medicine into general primary healthcare settings. Although progress has been made, the evidence for any single model of integrated care has not yet emerged. We propose building upon the existing chronic care management model, using a stage approach to the care of substance use issues, and considering a priori factors that influence the scalability of any approach to integrated care.

ACKNOWLEDGMENTS

Development of this chapter was supported by the Veterans Affairs Health Services Research and Development Service (Humphreys) and the National Institute on Drug Abuse (McGovern).

KEY POINTS

1. There is an unprecedented opportunity to implement integrated approaches for substance use disorders in routine general primary care settings.

2. The chronic care management (CCM) model is a promising approach, particularly if organized by a clinical conceptualization of stages from Early Identification/Intervention, Stabilization, Clinical Monitoring/Management, and Patient Self-Management.

3. Because routine general primary care settings have enormous challenges implementing any new practice, regardless of effectiveness and/or benefit, the CCM model for SUDs must consider implementation and sustainment factors in the design phase.

REVIEW QUESTIONS

1. The chronic care management model involves:
   A. the physician only.
   B. a nurse and behavioral health counselor.
   C. members of a full treatment team.
   D. only a physician and a nurse.

2. At the first stage of Early Identification/Intervention, select the practice that is *least likely* to occur for a patient with no expressed concern about his alcohol use and no prior SUD treatment experience.
   A. Having the patient complete a self-assessment screening measure such as the AUDIT
   B. Reviewing the patient's liver profile and discussing the pros and cons of his level of alcohol use
   C. Signing the patient up for the relapse prevention group offered on Tuesday evenings
   D. Obtaining a urine toxicology

3. What statement is most true about the Stabilization stage?
   A. After the Stabilization stage, it is expected that patients have completed treatment for a severe SUD.
   B. The Stabilization stage involves preparing the patient for the Clinical Monitoring/Management stage.
   C. Because patients are too sick during withdrawal, no motivational or behavioral interventions should be offered.
   D. Patients in the stabilization phase still typically do not require anticraving medication.

ANSWERS

1. **C**
2. **C**
3. **B**

SUGGESTED READINGS

Korthuis PT, McCarty D, Weimer M, et al. Primary care–based models for the treatment of opioid use disorder. *Ann Intern Med.* 2017;166(4):268-278.

McGovern M, Dent K, Kessler R. A unified model of behavioral health integration in primary care. *Acad Psychiatry.* 2018;42(2):265-268.

McLellan AT, Lewis DC, O'Brien CP, Kleber HD. Drug addiction as chronic medical illness: implications for treatment, insurance and evaluation. *JAMA.* 2000;284(13):1689-1695.

Saitz R, Cheng DM, Winter M, et al. Chronic care management for dependence on alcohol and other drugs. *JAMA.* 2013;310(11):1156-1167.

Watkins KE, Ober AJ, Lamp K, et al. Collaborative care for opioid and alcohol use disorders in primary care: the SUMMIT randomized clinical trial. *JAMA Intern Med.* 2017;177(10):1480-1488.

30

The ASAM Criteria and Matching Patients to Treatment

Summary by David Mee-Lee and Gerald D. Shulman

Based on THE ASAM PRINCIPLES OF ADDICTION MEDICINE, 6th edition chapter by David Mee-Lee and Gerald D. Shulman

The ASAM Criteria: Treatment Criteria for Addictive, Substance-Related, and Co-Occurring Conditions has its roots in the mid-1980s and was designed to help clinicians, payers, and regulators use and fund levels of care in a person-centered and individualized treatment manner. To increase access to care and improve the cost-effectiveness of addiction treatment, the ASAM Criteria represents a shift from:

- One-dimensional to multidimensional assessment—from treatment based solely on diagnosis to treatment that addresses multiple needs;
- Program-driven to clinically and outcome-driven treatment—from placement in a program often with fixed lengths of stay to person-centered, recovery-oriented, individualized treatment responsive to specific needs and progress and outcomes in treatment;
- Fixed length of service to a variable length of service, based on patient needs and outcomes; and
- A limited number of discrete levels of care to a broad and flexible continuum of care in a chronic disease management system of care.

UNDERSTANDING THE ASAM CRITERIA

Four features characterize the ASAM Criteria: (1) comprehensive, individualized treatment planning; (2) ready access to services; (3) attention to multiple treatment needs; and (4) ongoing reassessment and modification of the plan.

Functionally, the criteria are used to match services, interventions, and treatment settings to each individual's particular problems and (often changing) treatment needs as well as his or her strengths, skills, and resources. By expanding the criteria to incorporate more use of outpatient care, especially for those in the early stages of readiness to change, providing five levels of withdrawal management,

and encouraging flexible lengths of stay, the ASAM Criteria is designed to assist in reducing waiting lists for residential treatment and thus improve access to care.

To be effective, treatment must address any associated medical, psychological, social, vocational, legal, and recovery environment problems. Through its six assessment dimensions, the ASAM Criteria underscore the importance of multidimensional assessment and treatment.

Principles Guiding the ASAM Criteria

Goals of Treatment

The goals of intervention and treatment determine the methods, intensity, frequency, and types of services provided. The healthcare professional's decision to prescribe a type of service, and the subsequent transfer of a patient from a level of care, is based on how that treatment and its duration will help resolve dysfunction and positively alter the prognosis for the patient's long-term outcome. Thus, in addiction treatment, services usually extend beyond simple resolution of observable signs and symptoms to the achievement of overall healthier functioning—the difference between abstinence alone and recovery.

Individualized Treatment Plan

Effective treatment is tailored to the needs of the individual and guided by an individualized treatment plan that is developed in collaboration with the patient. Such a plan is based on the patient's goals for treatment and a comprehensive biopsychosocial assessment of the patient and, when possible, a comprehensive evaluation of the family. As with other disease processes, length of service is linked directly to the patient's response to treatment rather than a predetermined time frame based on the length of the treatment program or available reimbursement.

Choice of Treatment Levels

For both clinical and financial reasons, the preferred level of care is the least intensive level that meets treatment objectives, while providing safety and security for the patient. Moreover, although the levels of care are presented as discrete levels, in reality, they represent benchmarks or points along a continuum of treatment services that could be used in a variety of ways, depending on a patient's needs and response. A patient could begin at a level of care and move to a more or less intensive level, depending on his or her individual needs and progress in treatment. For patients who have been previously treated and have relapsed, the choice of level of care should be based on an assessment of the patient's history and current functioning, not automatic placement in a more intensive level of care.

Continuum of Care

In order to provide the most clinically appropriate and cost-effective treatment system, a continuum of care must be available. Such a continuum may be offered by a single provider or multiple providers. For the continuum to work most effectively, it is best distinguished by three characteristics: (1) seamless transfers between levels of care, (2) philosophical congruence among the various providers of care, and (3) timely arrival of the patient's clinical record at the next provider. It is most helpful if providers envision admitting the patient into the continuum *through* their program rather than admitting the patient *to* their program.

Progress Through the Levels of Care

As a patient moves through treatment in any level of care, his or her progress in all six dimensions should be continually assessed. Certain problems and priorities are identified as justifying admission to a particular level of care. The resolution of those problems and priorities determines when a patient can be transferred to a different level of care or discharged from treatment. The appearance of new problems may require services that can be effectively provided at the same level of care or that require a more or less intensive level of care.

Length of Stay

The length of stay (LOS) or service is determined by the patient's progress toward achieving his or her treatment plan goals and objectives. Fixed LOS or program-driven treatment is not individualized and does not respond to the particular problems of a given patient.

Clinical Versus Reimbursement Considerations

The ASAM Criteria describes a wide range of levels and types of care that may not be available in all locations, nor do all payers cover them. Clinicians should make placement decisions using their own clinical judgment and their knowledge of the patient and the available resources. The ASAM Criteria are not intended as a reimbursement guideline but rather as a clinical guideline for making the most appropriate placement recommendation for an individual patient with a specific set of symptoms and behaviors.

"Treatment Failure"

Two incorrect assumptions are associated with the concept of "treatment failure." The first is that addiction is acute rather than chronic, leading to the idea that the only criterion for success is total and complete cure and elimination of the problem. Such expectations are inappropriate in the treatment of other chronic disorders, such as diabetes, asthma, or hypertension. The second assumption is that responsibility for treatment "failure" always rests with the patient (eg, "the patient was not ready"). However, poor treatment outcomes may also be related to a provider's failure to provide evidence-based services tailored to the patient's needs.

Finally, there is a concern that some managed care guidelines require that a patient "fail" at one level of care—for instance, outpatient treatment as a prerequisite for approving admission to a more intensive level of care like residential treatment. Such a strategy potentially puts the patient at risk because it delays care at a more appropriate level of treatment and potentially increases healthcare costs if restricting the appropriate level of treatment allows the addiction disorder to progress.

ASSESSMENT DIMENSIONS

The ASAM Criteria describes six assessment areas or dimensions that are used to identify patient needs and inform placement decisions across levels of care. Table 30-1 outlines the six dimensions and the assessment and treatment planning focus of each one.

LEVELS OF CARE

The ASAM Criteria contains descriptions of treatment programs at each level of care, including the setting, staffing, support systems, therapies, assessments, documentation, and treatment plan reviews typically found at that level. It conceptualizes treatment as a chronic disease management continuum

TABLE 30-1	ASAM Criteria Assessment Dimensions
Assessment Dimensions	**Assessment and Treatment Planning Focus**
1. Acute intoxication and/or withdrawal potential	Assess for intoxication or withdrawal management. Manage withdrawal in a variety of levels of care and preparation for continued addiction services.
2. Biomedical conditions and complications	Assess and treat co-occurring physical health conditions or complications. Treatment is provided within the level of care or through coordination of physical health services.
3. Emotional, behavioral, or cognitive conditions and complications	Assess and treat co-occurring diagnostic or subdiagnostic mental health conditions or complications. Treatment is provided within the level of care or through coordination of mental health services.
4. Readiness to change	Assess the stage of readiness to change. If not ready to commit to full recovery, engage into treatment using motivational enhancement strategies. If ready for recovery, consolidate and expand action for change.
5. Relapse, continued use, or continued problem potential	Assess readiness for relapse prevention services and teach where appropriate. Identify previous periods of sobriety or wellness and what worked to achieve this. If still at early stages of change, focus on raising consciousness of consequences of continued use or continued problems as part of motivational enhancement strategies.
6. Recovery environment	Assess the need for specific individualized family or significant other, housing, financial, vocational, educational, legal, transportation, and childcare services. Identify any supports and assets in any or all of the areas.

marked by five basic levels of care, which are numbered from Level 0.5 through Level 4 as follows:

Level 0.5: Early intervention
Level 1: Outpatient services
Level 2: Intensive outpatient/partial hospitalization services
Level 3: Residential/inpatient services
Level 4: Medically managed intensive inpatient services

Within each level, a decimal number (ranging from 0.1 to 0.9) expresses gradations of intensity within that level of care. For more detail on each of the gradation levels of care, see Table 30-2.

SELECTING APPROPRIATE SERVICES

In individualized, assessment-driven treatment, service priorities are identified in the context of the patient's severity of illness and level of function (Fig. 30-1). Treatment services are matched to the patient's needs over a continuum of care. Ongoing progress assessments and treatment response influences further service recommendations and length of treatment.

PLACEMENT DILEMMAS
Co-Occurring Disorders

Clinical reality suggests that programs and practitioners must be able to meet the needs of people with co-occurring and complex disorders, either directly or through referral or consultation. The ASAM Criteria incorporate criteria for co-occurring capable (able to treat both unstable substance use and mental disorders), co-occurring enhanced (capable of accepting and assessing patients with co-occurring substance use and mental disorders), and complexity capable services (able to treat patients with complex physical, mental health, and addiction needs). Because co-occurring disorders are so prevalent, the ASAM Criteria encourage all programs to be at least co-occurring capable.

Assessment of Imminent Danger

Residential treatment has often been used for patients with chronic relapse problems, those with poor recovery environments, those who are homeless, and those in need of motivational strategies to "break through denial." In the ASAM Criteria, residential treatment is reserved for stabilization of those in imminent danger. Such patients need a residential program that offers clinical staff and services 24 hours a day in order to respond to the patient's issues that pose the imminent danger—that is, that there is a strong probability certain behaviors such as continued use will occur, that such behaviors will present a significant risk of adverse consequences to the individual and/or others, and that such adverse events will occur in the very near future (ie, within hours or day, not week or months).

TABLE 30-2	ASAM Criteria Levels of Care	
ASAM Criteria Level of Withdrawal Management Service for Adults[a]	**Level**	**Description**
Ambulatory withdrawal management without extended on-site monitoring	1-WM	Mild withdrawal with daily or less than daily outpatient supervision; likely to complete withdrawal management and to continue treatment or recovery
Ambulatory withdrawal management with extended on-site monitoring	2-WM	Moderate withdrawal with all-day withdrawal management support and supervision; at night, has supportive family or living situation; likely to complete withdrawal management
Clinically managed residential withdrawal management	3.2-WM	Minimal to moderate withdrawal but needs 24-h support to complete withdrawal management and to increase the likelihood of continuing treatment or recovery
Medically monitored inpatient withdrawal management	3.7-WM	Severe withdrawal and needs 24-h nursing care and physician visits as necessary; unlikely to complete withdrawal management without medical, nursing monitoring
Medically managed inpatient withdrawal management	4-WM	Severe, unstable withdrawal and needs 24-h nursing care and daily physician visits to modify the withdrawal management regimen and manage medical instability
ASAM Criteria Levels of Care[b]	**Level**	**Description**
Early intervention	0.5	Assessment and education for at-risk individuals who do not meet diagnostic criteria for substance-related disorder
Outpatient services	1	Less than 9 h of service per week (adults); <6 h/wk (adolescents) for recovery or motivational enhancement therapies/strategies
Intensive outpatient	2.1	9 h of service or more per week (adults); 6 h or more per week (adolescents) in a structured program to treat multidimensional instability
Partial hospitalization	2.5	20 h of service or more per week in a structured program for multidimensional instability not requiring 24-h care
Clinically managed low-intensity residential	3:1	24-h structure with available trained personnel with emphasis on reentry to the community; at least 5 h of clinical service per week
Clinically managed population-specific high-intensity residential	3.3	24-h care with trained counselors to stabilize multidimensional imminent danger; less intense milieu and group treatment for those with cognitive or other impairments unable to use a full active milieu or therapeutic community
Clinically managed high-intensity residential	3.5	24-h care with trained counselors to stabilize multidimensional imminent danger and prepare for outpatient treatment; able to tolerate and use a full active milieu or therapeutic community
Medically monitored intensive inpatient	3.7	24-h nursing care with physician availability for significant problems in Dimensions 1, 2, or 3; 16 h/d for counselor ability
Medically managed intensive inpatient	4	24-h nursing care and daily physician care for severe, unstable problems in Dimensions 1, 2, or 3; counseling available to engage the patient in treatment
Opioid treatment program	OTP	Daily or several times weekly opioid medication and counseling available to maintain multidimensional stability for those with opioid use disorder

ASAM, American Society of Addiction Medicine; WM, withdrawal management; OTP, opioid treatment program.
[a]There are no separate withdrawal management services for adolescents.
[b]Same levels of care for adolescents except Level 3.3.

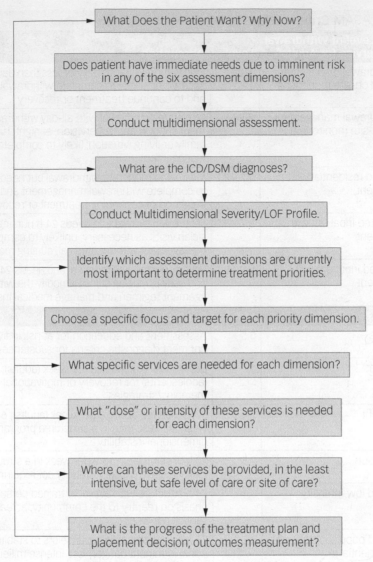

What Does the Patient Want? Why Now?

Does patient have immediate needs due to imminent risk in any of the six assessment dimensions?

Conduct multidimensional assessment.

What are the ICD/DSM diagnoses?

Conduct Multidimensional Severity/LOF Profile.

Identify which assessment dimensions are currently most important to determine treatment priorities.

Choose a specific focus and target for each priority dimension.

What specific services are needed for each dimension?

What "dose" or intensity of these services is needed for each dimension?

Where can these services be provided, in the least intensive, but safe level of care or site of care?

What is the progress of the treatment plan and placement decision; outcomes measurement?

Figure 30-1. Decision tree to match assessment and treatment/placement assignment. ICD, *International Classification of Diseases*; DSM, *Diagnostic and Statistical Manual of Mental Disorders*; LOF, level of function. (Reprinted with permission from the *American Society of Addiction Medicine Criteria* [2013, p 124].)

Mandated Level of Care or Length of Service

In some cases, an individual is referred for treatment at a specific level of care and/or for a specific length of service (eg, a person in the criminal justice system may be given a choice of a prison term or a fixed LOS in a treatment center). A mandated or court-ordered referral not based on clinical considerations may be inconsistent with a placement decision arrived at through the ASAM Criteria. In such a case, the provider should make reasonable attempts to have the order amended to mandate assessment and treatment adherence.

If the court order or other mandate cannot be amended, the individual may be continuing treatment at a level of care or for an LOS more intense than is clinically indicated. The patient's readiness for discharge or transfer and the staff's attempts to implement a clinically appropriate placement should be noted in the clinical record, and the treatment plan should be updated in a manner that provides the patient with the opportunity to continue the recovery process at the same level of care even though it could be continued at a less intensive level of care.

Logistical Impediments

Logistical problems are significant in rural and underserved inner city areas. When logistical considerations are an impediment to the indicated services (eg, lack of available transportation as a barrier to accessing an outpatient program), an outpatient service combined with unsupervised/minimally supervised housing may be an appropriate treatment intervention.

Ensuring Individualized Treatment

There are at least three efficient ways for auditors of quality to determine whether a program is providing truly individualized treatment:

1. Take ten closed clinical case records and compare the treatment plans. If the auditor cannot clearly distinguish patients by their treatment plans, the treatment is not individualized.
2. Review the progress notes and determine whether they relate back to the objectives or strategies in the treatment plan.
3. For programs that receive reimbursement from multiple payers, compare LOS by sources of payment. If the lengths of stay correspond to payer type, then the program is payment driven rather than offering individualized treatment.

THE ASAM CRITERIA SOFTWARE

A software product authorized by ASAM implements every admission decision rule of the ASAM Criteria and is designed to be user-friendly and to serve as the authorized, standard implementation named CONTINUUM.

This software presents the opportunity, for the first time, to permit both providers and payers to speak the same language and to arrive at the same level-of-care determinations. It enables payers and providers to decrease the time necessary for utilization review decisions.

KEY POINTS

1. *The ASAM Criteria: Treatment Criteria for Addictive, Substance-Related, and Co-Occurring Conditions* was designed to help clinicians, payers, and regulators use and fund levels of care in a person-centered and individualized treatment manner.
2. The ASAM Criteria describes six assessment areas or dimensions that are used to identify patient needs and to inform placement decisions across levels of care.

3. The ASAM Criteria conceptualizes treatment as a chronic disease management continuum marked by five basic levels of care: Level 0.5, Early intervention; Level 1, Outpatient services; Level 2, Intensive outpatient/partial hospitalization services; Level 3, Residential/inpatient services; and Level 4, Medically managed intensive inpatient services.

REVIEW QUESTIONS

1. The six assessment dimensions of the ASAM Criteria:
   A. help assess an individual's comprehensive needs in treatment.
   B. provide a structure for assessing severity of illness and level of function.
   C. require that there be access to medical and nursing personnel when necessary.
   D. can help focus the treatment plan on the most important priorities.
   E. All of the above

2. A multidimensional assessment in addiction treatment:
   A. should include psychosocial factors such as readiness to change.
   B. is ideal, but not necessary within a managed care environment.
   C. should include biomedical and psychiatric problems, but not motivation or relapse potential.
   D. is best done after withdrawal management is completed.
   E. should be completed by the primary therapist only.

3. The best treatment system for addiction is:
   A. a 28-day stay in inpatient rehabilitation with much education.
   B. a broad continuum of care with all levels of care separated to maintain group trust.
   C. a broad range of services designed as seamless as possible for continuity of care.
   D. short stay inpatient hospitalization for psychoeducation.

ANSWERS

1. **E.** The ASAM Criteria six assessment dimensions provide for a comprehensive, holistic multidimensional assessment that covers all life areas affected by addiction.
2. **A.** Medical necessity in managed care is often focused just on acute withdrawal and physical or mental illness severity in what is an acute care

model. But in the ASAM Criteria, all six assessment dimensions are important in an assessment.

3. **C.** Because addiction is a chronic disease for many, ongoing disease management is needed in a flexible, seamless continuum of care through which a patient moves.

SUGGESTED READINGS

Fishman MJ, Shulman GR, Mee-Lee D, et al. *The ASAM Patient Placement Criteria: Supplement on Pharmacotherapies for Alcohol Use Disorders*. Philadelphia: Lippincott Williams & Wilkins, 2010.

Gastfriend DR, ed. *Addiction Treatment Matching: Research Foundations of the American Society of Addiction Medicine (ASAM) Criteria*. Binghamton, NY: Haworth Medical Press, 2003.

Mee-Lee D, ed. *The ASAM Criteria: Treatment Criteria for Addictive, Substance-Related, and Co-Occurring Conditions*. 3rd ed. Rockville, MD: American Society of Addiction Medicine, 2013.

Mee-Lee D, Gastfriend DR. Patient placement criteria. In: Galanter M, Kleber HD, Brady KT, eds. *Textbook of Substance Abuse Treatment*. 5th ed. Washington, DC: American Psychiatric Publishing, 2015:111-128.

Mee-Lee D, McLellan AT, Miller SD. What works in substance abuse and dependence treatment. In: Duncan BL, Miller SD, Wampold BE, Hubble MA, eds. *The Heart & Soul of Change*. 2nd ed. Washington, DC: American Psychological Association, 2010:393-417.

31

Linking Addiction Treatment With Other Medical and Psychiatric Treatment Systems

Summary by Karran A. Phillips, Peter D. Friedmann, Richard Saitz, and Jeffrey H. Samet

Based on THE ASAM PRINCIPLES OF ADDICTION MEDICINE, 6th edition chapter by Karran A. Phillips, Peter D. Friedmann, Richard Saitz, and Jeffrey H. Samet

Persons with substance use disorders (SUDs) are at substantial risk for coexisting medical and mental health problems and may present to medical, mental health, and/or addiction treatment settings. In both medical and addiction treatment settings, the provision of comprehensive care for individuals with SUDs presents challenges to clinicians who traditionally have focused only on issues reflecting their own training and perspectives. For the patient, these issues are inseparable and often interrelated; yet, many clinicians operate in distinct systems of care, each with its own—often exclusive—focus. Patients with SUDs and psychiatric or medical illnesses are sometimes bounced between systems and given contradictory recommendations that can lead to continued substance use or that can be dangerous (eg, told that they must be abstinent before they can receive treatment for their psychiatric and medical problems, that they cannot receive treatment if they are taking particular medications, that they are too sick [medically or psychiatrically] to get into an addiction treatment program), resulting in a clinical "Catch-22."

The Patient Protection and Affordable Care Act includes addiction as an "essential health benefit" and increased the number of individuals with an addiction presenting to primary care and other healthcare settings. The establishment of the new subspecialty of board-certified physicians in addiction medicine joining the ranks of addiction psychiatry physicians will greatly help to close some of these treatment gaps. However, given that many systems still lack access to certified addiction physicians, further training of generalist clinicians about addiction issues and their acceptance to take on role responsibility for addiction care and linkages across the systems of medical, mental health, and addiction care will be needed to improve the quality of care delivered to patients with an addiction.

POTENTIAL BENEFITS OF LINKED SERVICES

Effective linkage may benefit individuals who use substances in the following common scenarios: when issues related to use and addiction are not addressed in primary care and mental health settings, when medical and mental health issues are not addressed in addiction treatment, and when the patient is seen in two or more of these settings but no effective communication between or within the systems occurs (Table 31-1).

BARRIERS TO OPTIMAL LINKAGE
Medical Training

Many barriers impede a better linkage of services. One well-documented problem has been the perspective of many medical practitioners that addressing alcohol and other drug use issues is not providing medical care and thus is outside his or her purview. This viewpoint is changing due to efforts by the Health Resources & Services Administration and the Center for Substance Abuse Treatment and the creation of the Coalition on Physician Education in Substance Use Disorders. Furthermore, the American Board of Medical Specialties officially recognized addiction medicine as a subspecialty in October 2015. These efforts were energized by the

TABLE 31-1 Potential Benefits of Linking Addiction Treatment With Other Medical and Psychiatric Services

From the Patient's Perspective

- Is provided in a structured format
- Improves overall quality of care
- Facilitates access to addiction treatment for patients in medical care settings
- Enhances access to primary medical care for patients receiving addiction treatment
- Improves patient well-being in terms of addiction severity and medical problems
- Provides care that may be easier to access
- Increases patients' satisfaction with their healthcare

From the Primary Care Provider's Perspective

- Promotes screening of all patients for alcohol problems
- Facilitates inclusion of alcohol and drug causes when considering a differential diagnosis
- Allows more achievable access to the addiction treatment system
- Supports the prevention of relapse to alcohol and drug use
- Encourages other mental health services for primary care patients
- Enhances adherence with appointments and medical regimens
- Provides addiction training opportunities for personnel

From the Addiction Treatment Provider's Perspective

- Improves addiction treatment outcomes
- Reduces the stigma about addiction issues among medical providers
- Provides training opportunities about addiction-related medical problems
- Promotes healthier behaviors
- Enhances medical providers' appreciation of the value of addiction treatment
- Creates support for reimbursement parity for addiction services
- Develops ongoing quality improvement efforts within addiction programs

From a Societal Perspective

- Reduces costs of healthcare, criminal activity, and loss of productivity
- Reduces duplication of services and administrative costs
- Improves health outcomes of specific populations

emergence of the American Board of Addiction Medicine and the American Board of Addiction Medicine Foundation and should continue as addiction medicine physicians work together with addiction psychiatrists to treat this population and model excellent care to medical students and residents.

In practice, medical clinicians generally report having received minimal training in SUDs, and they screen inadequately for preclinical cases. Because they neither find patients with less severe addiction nor follow up those who have had success in treatment, most physicians have experienced few successes. This latter product of poor linkages biases the spectrum of medical clinicians' clinical experience and further

discourages physician involvement. The recent highly visible opioid overdose epidemic and complex issues surrounding pain and opioid prescribing have served as opportunities to expand addiction education, including some related to prescribing that is required in some states for licensure.

Payment and Service Linkage Issues

In the past, payment for addiction treatment and mental healthcare has been limited compared to payments for other medical services. In recent years, there have been successes in the effort to achieve parity for healthcare benefits; nonetheless, parity has not yet been fully realized in practice. Many managed behavioral health plans have "carved out" addiction benefits, separating the financing of care for mental health and addiction from that for the rest of the patient's ailments. Efforts to improve parity for addiction services include the Mental Health Parity and Addiction Equity Act of 2007 (HR 1424) and the Affordable Care Act, which mandated inclusion of substance use treatment among the essential health benefits for all insured Americans.

Some current systems of payment often do not cover addiction services provided by primary care physicians; however, as payment systems evolve, this will likely change. In 2007, the White House Office of National Drug Control Policy announced new healthcare codes for substance use screening and brief intervention. The American Medical Association's Level I Current Procedural terminology codes (99408 and 99409) went into effect in 2008 and allow healthcare providers to report and be reimbursed for structured screening and brief intervention. Now that these codes exist, their success is largely dependent on their uptake and utilization by healthcare providers.

Stigma and Concerns About Confidentiality

Stigma remains a fundamental barrier in the treatment of any patient with alcohol or drug use. Stigma may prevent a person from acknowledging his or her addiction and seeking care and may also result in medical clinicians' disinclination toward spending time addressing drug and alcohol issues. Well-meaning concerns about patient confidentiality can be barriers to effectively linked medical, mental health, and addiction care. Although the protection of patient confidentiality is noble, in some cases, it can impede integrated care. Intended to protect patients with SUDs, special addiction information protection may also inadvertently reinforce a stigma against patients.

The dissemination of electronic health records has resulted in a major revolution in information sharing across systems. The incorporation of screening, brief intervention, and referral to treatment; substance use screening and assessment tools; and data into electronic health records may increase the utilization of these tools and standardize their implementation across settings and clinicians. The increase of Internet-based systems in the addiction treatment sector will need an influx of resources, as occurred in the healthcare sector (but not in the specialty addiction treatment sector) with the American Recovery and Reinvestment Act of 2009.

Further expansion of health information technology, including patient portals, brings additional opportunities to integrate patients with SUDs and psychiatric disorders into primary care. Regulators and clinicians will continue to struggle to balance protections against discrimination with the need for information sharing among healthcare providers in integrated systems of care.

MODELS OF LINKED SERVICES

Patients with alcohol and drug use consume services in "inefficient" ways (eg, emergency department presentations rather than outpatient clinic visits), and they do not receive care in the continuous, longitudinal, and comprehensive manner that is often essential for high-quality preventive care and for the management of any chronic disease. Two basic models have been proposed to bring the system of care for patients with SUDs closer to a primary care or chronic disease management (CDM) model (Table 31-2). One model uses a centralized approach in which treatment of addiction, primary medical care, and mental health services are all located at a single site. A second model uses a distributive approach to facilitate effective patient referrals to services at different sites.

Centralized Models

Centralized or on-site models bring primary care, mental health, and/or addiction services together at a single site. This fully integrated "one-stop shop" model has been best described in primary care medical clinics and in addiction treatment programs. In addition to overcoming the substantial political, bureaucratic, attitudinal, and financial barriers that separate addicted persons from needed services, centralized delivery overcomes the problems of geographic separation, patient disorganization, and poor motivation that inhibit patients with addiction from keeping outside appointments.

Recent studies have demonstrated the effectiveness of incorporating pharmacologic treatment for alcohol use and opioid use disorders in the primary care setting. Sublingual buprenorphine and a combination of buprenorphine and naloxone have been used for opioid use disorder treatment in the United States since 2003. Several studies have found that buprenorphine works as well as methadone for patients with opioid use disorders of mild-to-moderate severity. In addition to achieving positive treatment outcomes, office-based buprenorphine has been well received by patients. With the development and dissemination of new pharmacologic therapies

TABLE 31-2	Features of Centralized and Distributive Integrated Service Models
Centralized Models	
• Addiction treatment and pharmacotherapy in primary medical care and mental health services sites	
• Addiction providers located in group HMOs, private practices, or clinics	
• Behavioral medicine and primary medical provider offices colocated in shared space	
• Addiction treatment delivered at public health clinics (eg, sexually transmitted infections, HIV, or tuberculosis care)	
• Addiction treatment delivered in a general hospital with proximate medical and mental health clinics	
• Addiction treatment and primary care services colocated in a community mental health setting	
• Addiction-trained nurse practitioner or physician available in a primary care practice to prescribe and monitor naltrexone, to prescribe and monitor buprenorphine, and to initiate and manage detoxification	
• Addiction and mental health specialty teams present in medical care sites (eg, consult teams in EDs or hospitals)	
• Smoking cessation counseling and pharmacotherapy delivered as part of primary care	
• Brief interventions and advice for unhealthy substance use in doctors' offices, EDs, and hospitals	
• Primary medical care and mental health services delivered at addiction treatment sites	
• Medical and mental health providers or clinic located at a methadone treatment program	
• Collocated primary care and addiction care	
• An integrated alcohol and medical clinic	
• An addiction medicine physician with medical and psychiatric skills	
• A multiservice community agency with a central location	
Distributive Models	
• HMOs or preferred provider organizations with defined, yet decentralized, referral networks	
• Addiction triage and referral or central intake and assessment centers that perform medical and mental health assessments and referrals for multiple addiction treatment programs	
• Community-based case management	
• Evaluation at addiction treatment sites with external referral for ongoing medical and mental healthcare	
• Defined networks of providers with facilitated communication and financial/contractual links and systems	
• Informal links between clinicians or agencies facilitated by releases of information, transportation, and case management	
• A multiservice community agency with a single owner but several locations	

HMO, health maintenance organization; ED, emergency department.

for alcohol and other SUDs, the impetus for addiction services in the primary care setting will only increase. Although methadone is an effective treatment for opioid use disorder, federal law relegates its dispensing to clinics separate from the general healthcare system. There is evidence that medical methadone treatment involving stabilized methadone patients in a medical setting results in good treatment outcomes (ie, high rates of 1-year retention in treatment and abstinence) and high physician and patient satisfaction rates.

Centralizing primary medical care, SUD treatment, and psychiatric services has also proven to be an effective way to manage concomitant medical conditions such as hepatitis C, tuberculosis, and human immunodeficiency virus (HIV). Centralized models of primary medical and mental healthcare in addiction treatment settings may also improve access to these services for patients with addiction. The integration of addiction treatment and community mental health services has been shown to reduce relapse and improve social stability for patients dually diagnosed with addictions and mental illness.

The integration of buprenorphine into HIV primary care settings has been funded by the US Department of Health and Human Services. Studies have shown that individuals in an HIV clinic receiving on-site buprenorphine have increased access to opioid agonist treatment and improved addiction treatment outcomes.

In general, patients with nicotine use, at-risk drinking, and low-severity illicit drug use can be managed in primary care settings without subspecialty addiction medicine consultation. Conversely, patients with severe SUDs generally should be cared for in collaboration with addiction specialists and/or treatment counselors (whether integrated in a primary care office or located elsewhere). However, it is uncertain, except in more severe cases and in cases where treatment response is not seen, when such specialty care must be invoked. Recent advances support and encourage a major role for primary care physicians and office-based psychiatrists in the pharmacologic management of patients with opioid or alcohol use disorder while at the same time recognizing the need for substantial collaboration and coordination with addiction treatment providers in some cases.

All patients should have primary and preventive healthcare—again, where this care is delivered will depend on the system of care. An ideal centralized model of care can provide addiction, mental health, and medical care at a single site. Whether specialty addiction medicine or addiction psychiatry services are delivered at an addiction specialty treatment site or within the primary care setting, the key is that systems should be integrated to deliver the most appropriate and efficient care.

The Chronic Disease Management Model

CDM, also referred to as chronic care management, is a care delivery approach based on the chronic care model described by Wagner that links, integrates, and coordinates primary and specialty care. It is also sometimes described as a collaborative care model. The key components are an informed and motivated patient, a proactive team, and an established delivery system resulting in maximized CDM and outcomes. Such an approach has been successfully applied to many chronic diseases, but has not yet been applied to SUDs. It has been hypothesized that strong CDM linkages within and between systems of care and integrated case management will increase access to, receipt of, and retention in effective SUDs and medical treatment that in turn will improve utilization and health outcomes. It is possible that despite the logic and possible effectiveness of the approach, that CDM also requires the health system at large to improve facilitation of care for patients with complex chronic conditions.

Additional guidance may be found in implementation science, which studies the best methods to promote the systematic uptake of clinical research findings and other evidence-based practices into routine practice. Studies using implementation indices (eg, the Behavioral Health Integration in Medical Care index) to measure integration capability at baseline and follow-up may help to target technical assistance and resources. Additional studies of how to integrate substance use interventions in the medical care setting are ongoing. It has been difficult to demonstrate benefits of CDM on SUD outcomes. This difficulty suggests that attention to focused approaches based on specific diagnoses, patient needs and severity, and implementation details will be important if benefits are to be achieved.

Distributive Models

Given the lack of parity in reimbursement for the treatment of SUDs and the absence of unified budgets for medical and behavioral health services, most providers lack resources to provide comprehensive, centralized services for patients with addiction. Moreover, patients (especially those in long-term recovery) may object to long-term primary care in settings primarily identified as addiction treatment programs. Therefore, the development and dissemination of effective decentralized or distributive models is an important step toward service integration in the current healthcare environment.

Successful referral is the central task of the distributive model. Anecdotes and limited data suggest that simple referral alone cannot integrate the care of patients with addiction in primary care settings. The substantial interorganizational distance between addiction treatment programs and mainstream healthcare presents great barriers to successful referrals. Because people with SUDs can have disorganized lifestyles and poor motivation, contemporary distributive models typically use case management to facilitate referrals. Community-based case management can effectively link patients to needed services.

The hospital setting serves as another point of contact with patients where linkages can be established between traditional medical care and addiction treatment. In addition to establishing linkages between the inpatient setting and addiction treatment, there is some evidence that linkage between the emergency department and addiction treatment services may also be beneficial.

In addiction treatment programs, distributive arrangements are commonly used to link patients to medical and mental health services. Distributive arrangements range, for example, from an addiction treatment unit that contracts with a local group practice to provide physical examinations and routine medical care to its patients, to one that makes ad hoc referrals to a local community mental health center. The advantage of this model is that it makes use of existing healthcare systems, and there is evidence that case management or transportation assistance can facilitate these referrals. This model requires no rearrangement of existing healthcare delivery systems; however, it does require efforts (and therefore costs) to ensure that linkage is facilitated.

There is evidence for the efficacy of a model utilizing a combination of centralized and distributive approaches. Another model that has emerged to improve access to addiction treatment is called ECHO (Extension for Community Healthcare Outcomes) in which teams of specialists at academic centers provide clinical expertise for specific cases using videoconferencing, an approach particularly useful for rural areas.

Vulnerable Populations

Integrated models may be most germane and show the most benefit to vulnerable populations including those with HIV, those who are homeless, those who have been incarcerated, veterans and active military, and young adults. Integrated models have been found to promote delivery of HIV-related care, medication adherence, and outpatient medical services. Further research is needed to determine which of these models will be most feasible and effective and whether they can be replicated.

SUMMARY

In summary, several effective models of centralized and distributive linkage in primary care and specialty addiction treatment settings have been developed. Addiction interventions in medical settings are appropriate for a spectrum of patients: those who drink and are considered at risk and those with SUDs of mild-to-moderate severity; medically ill patients who are dependent on substances who refuse formal treatment referral; and patients with SUDs who receive rehabilitative counseling elsewhere yet would benefit from addiction-related pharmacotherapy and management of their medical problems. With adequate support, primary care physicians also can have a productive role in outpatient detoxification. Minimally motivated patients who will accept only harm-reduction interventions can benefit from management in the primary care setting as well. For patients in formal addiction treatment, linkage

to needed medical and psychological services may improve access to healthcare, improve physical and mental health, and reduce relapse.

Both centralized and distributive models show promise for integrating care across these systems. The distributive model predominates in the United States. Although it can be less effective than the centralized model in linking patients who use substances to needed services, its relatively low cost, flexibility, and adaptability (especially its integration with secondary and tertiary care services) suggest that the distributive model, with further refinements, is likely to remain the method of coordinated services in the future. Although with the advent and increasing adoption of office-based addiction treatments using pharmacotherapy, the impact of integrated systems of care within primary care will be of great interest to patients, doctors, and other providers as well as policy makers and researchers.

KEY POINTS

1. Effective linkage of addiction treatment with primary and mental healthcare may benefit individuals with substance use in the following common scenarios: when issues related to use and addiction are not addressed in primary care and mental health settings, when medical and mental health issues are not addressed in addiction treatment, and when the patient is seen in two or more of these settings but no effective communication between or within the systems occurs.

2. Barriers to an integrated system of care for patients with SUDs are manifold and include issues of professional responsibility, education among clinicians, financial disincentives, concerns about confidentiality, and stigma, among others. Although the barriers can appear to be extensive, they are not insurmountable.

3. Two basic models have been proposed to bring the system of care for patients with SUDs closer to a primary care or CDM model; one model uses a centralized approach in which treatment of addiction, primary medical care, and mental health services are colocated at a single site, and the other uses a distributive approach to facilitate effective patient referrals to services at different sites.

4. Integrated models may be most germane and show the most benefit to vulnerable populations including those with HIV, those who are homeless, those who have been incarcerated, veterans and active military, and young adults.

REVIEW QUESTIONS

1. The two models of care linkage are:
   A. the centralized approach, in which treatment of addiction, primary medical care, and mental health services are colocated at a single site, and the distributive approach, in which effective patient referrals to services at different sites is facilitated.
   B. the centralized approach, in which treatment of addiction is central and primary medical care and mental health services are off site, and the distributive approach, in which primary medical care is central and addiction and mental health services are off site.
   C. the commutative approach, where addiction, primary medical care, and mental health service coverage can be swapped, and the distributive approach, where addiction, primary care, and mental health service coverage is distributed equally throughout the community.
   D. the commutative approach, where addiction, primary medical care, and mental health service coverage can be swapped, and the associative approach, where addiction, primary care, and mental health service coverage is grouped differently in different communities.

2. True or False: Medical clinicians in practice generally report having received minimal training in substance use disorders, and they screen inadequately for preclinical cases.

3. Which model of care is the most common in the United States?
   A. Centralized
   B. Distributive
   C. Chronic disease management model or chronic care management
   D. Commutative

ANSWERS

1. **A**
2. **True**
3. **B**

SUGGESTED READINGS

Druss BG, von Esenwein SA. Improving general medical care for person with mental and addictive disorders: systematic review. *Gen Hosp Psychiatry*. 2006;28(2):145-153.

Friedmann PD, Zhang Z, Hendrickson J, Stein MD, Gerstein DR. Effect of primary medical care on addiction and medical severity in substance abuse treatment programs. *J Gen intern Med*. 2003;18(1):1-8.

Institute of Medicine. *Improving the Quality of Health Care for Mental and Substance-Use Conditions. The Quality Chasm Series*. Washington DC: National Academies Press, 2006.

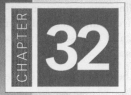

32

Alternative Therapies for Substance Use Disorders

Summary by David Y.W. Lee

> Based on THE ASAM PRINCIPLES OF ADDICTION MEDICINE,
> 6th edition chapter by David Y.W. Lee

Addiction is a complex process with physiologic, behavioral, psychological, and social components; therefore, treatment is usually multifaceted. There are two fundamental approaches: prevention of the onset of compulsive use and prevention of relapse and the craving that leads to relapse. In the past, much medical attention has been directed at the symptoms of acute abstinence (detoxification), and these symptoms can be treated with available therapies and medications. However, relapse, which may be precipitated by withdrawal and/or craving even after prolonged abstinence, poses the most serious therapeutic challenge. In view of the current opioid epidemic in the United States, the complexity of substance use disorders (SUDs), and the limited number of effective treatments, it is conceivable that certain selected alternative pharmacotherapies may have important clinical significance. This chapter reviews traditional herbal medicines and therapies for the prevention of drug and alcohol relapse.

HERBAL REMEDIES WITH ANTIADDICTIVE POTENTIAL

Herbal remedies, which usually consist of a complex mixture of herbs, have been used in China for thousands of years to treat human disease. Poppy has been known in China for 12 centuries and for its medicinal use for 9 centuries. Opiates—alkaloids derived from poppy—effectively activate the endogenous opioid system in the body. This activation produces many cardiovascular, endocrine, immune, and neuropsychological effects including euphoria, analgesia, and addiction. It has been clear that the effects of opioids are mediated through interaction with specific opioid receptors. Moreover, studies of the binding of various related opioid compounds in the brain indicate the existence of at least three opioid receptor types such as μ, κ, and δ (with multiple subtypes). Because the rewarding effects of opioids are mediated primarily through action at μ opioid receptors, interference with actions at these receptors presents a rational strategy for developing medications for the treatment of opioid use disorder. Specifically, medications that block the activation of μ opioid receptors (eg, naltrexone) might reduce drug-seeking behaviors.

The Chinese remedies developed during the Opium Wars era (mid-19th century) were combinations of more than a dozen herbs; thus, a mixture of herbs may well represent a multitargeted approach, perhaps acting on opioid receptors, that would have the benefits of improved overall efficacy with reduced toxicity. However, it is necessary to isolate and characterize the bioactive compounds as well as elucidate the mechanisms of action for the further development of safe and complementary natural medications for SUDs. Few original remedies have been investigated scientifically. YGT (NPI-025) consists of five herbs—qiang huo, gou teng, chuan xiong, fu zi, and yan hu so—and is most frequently used for SUD treatment in China. One study observed YGT effects among 300 individuals with "drug addiction" over a 10-year period and reported that NPI-025 was significantly associated with reduced withdrawal symptoms (−48%) compared to addicted individuals without treatment. Follow-up visits of many "cured" patients 1 to 3 years after treatment suggested that the use of NPI-025 may have been associated with overcoming cravings for drugs.

YGT, used clinically in Hong Kong, was subjected to bioactivity-guided fractionation and showed that the alkaloids, such as L-tetrahydropalmatine (L-THP), isolated from one of the components (yan hu so) shows potent opioid receptor–binding activities. These studies provide important evidence for further development of such natural products.

DOPAMINE RECEPTORS AND PHARMACOLOGIC ACTIONS OF L-THP

Despite extensive research for new approaches, there is currently no effective pharmacotherapy for cocaine or methamphetamine addiction. *Corydalis yanhusuo* is one of the five Chinese medicinal plants in NPI-025. Chemical fractionation resulted in the isolation and characterization of L-THP as one of the bioactive components. Some effects of L-THP on cocaine and methamphetamine self-administration have been demonstrated, suggesting potential, but not yet proven, clinical utility. Similar to LEK-8829, plant-derived L-THP has both D1 receptor agonist and D2 receptor antagonist actions. Its effects on cocaine and methamphetamine addiction are suggested.

Uncaria rhynchophylla, another component of NPI-025, is an important traditional Chinese medicine used in the treatment of pain, infantile convulsions, headaches, dizziness, hypertension, and rheumatoid arthritis.

REDUCTION OF ALCOHOL DRINKING BY THE EXTRACT OF *PUERARIA LOBATA*

Isoflavone compounds naturally occurring in the root of the kudzu plant (*Pueraria lobata*) have been used historically to treat alcohol-related problems. Early research showed that the herbal formula NPI-028, which contains *P. lobata*, reduced acute alcohol consumption in two strains of alcohol-preferring rats when administered parenterally or orally without affecting water intake. Several studies have systematically explored the ability of three major isoflavones of kudzu root—daidzin, daidzein, and puerarin—to reduce alcohol consumption in animals and humans.

TRANSCUTANEOUS ELECTRICAL ACUPUNCTURE STIMULATION

In a serendipitous observation in 1972, a physician in Hong Kong noted that electroacupuncture relieved a patient's withdrawal symptoms from opium. In a subsequent study of 40 individuals with an addiction to heroin and/or opium, acupuncture combined with electrical stimulation was effective at relieving withdrawal symptoms. This method was later adopted in many clinical settings in Western countries.

OPIOID DETOXIFICATION WITH TRANSCUTANEOUS ELECTRICAL ACUPUNCTURE

Systematic studies have revealed that the mechanism of acupuncture analgesia is attributed mainly to the increased release of endogenous opioid peptides in the central nervous system. A rational extrapolation would be that the activation of the endogenous opioid system by acupuncture should ease opioid withdrawal symptoms. Transauricular electrostimulation was reported to suppress the naloxone-induced morphine withdrawal syndrome in mice and rats. Human studies are ongoing.

PREVENTION OF CRAVING AND RELAPSE TO OPIOID USE

SUDs are a chronic and recurrent condition. A high rate of relapse after prolonged drug-free periods characterizes the behavior of experienced users of heroin and other drugs. Once addiction is established, craving can last for a long period of time. The protracted withdrawal syndrome and the craving for drugs often drive the patient to relapse. Recently, electrical acupuncture has been shown to reduce craving and postpone or prevent relapse.

ACUPUNCTURE AND UNHEALTHY ALCOHOL USE

Acupuncture was considered promising for the treatment of alcohol use disorder in the 1980s. A recent randomized placebo-controlled clinical trial of auricular acupuncture ($N = 503$) was unique in that aside from the "specific" ear acupuncture group, "nonspecific" ear acupuncture group, and conventional treatment group, there was a symptom-based acupuncture group for which the acupuncturists were not constrained to the four ear points stipulated for the other acupuncture groups, and the point prescription could be changed from day to day according to the patients' discomfort. Six treatments per week were given for as long as 3 weeks to maximize the effect. All four groups showed significant improvement, with few differences associated with treatment assignment and no treatment difference on alcohol use measures, although 49% of subjects reported that acupuncture reduced their desire for alcohol. The authors concluded that ear acupuncture did not make a significant contribution over and above that achieved by conventional treatment in the reduction of alcohol use.

CONCLUSION

Traditional Chinese medicines have been used for the treatment of human disease for more than 2000 years. It is estimated that roughly half of current pharmaceuticals originally were procured from plants. Examples include foxglove leaf (digitalis), belladonna tops (atropine), poppy herb (morphine), white willow tree bark (salicin), and cinchona bark (quinine). It is therefore reasonable that medication development for unhealthy drug and alcohol use should seek active isolates from traditional herbal remedies. Although acupuncture and related acupoint therapies are most commonly recognized for their analgesic effects, their medical applications extend beyond pain treatment and might include treatment of SUDs. Although alternative therapies may provide new treatments for existing drug treatments, rigorous studies to evaluate both the risks and the benefits of such treatments are needed. Biologic investigations that couple in vitro and in vivo pharmacologic models to characterize the mechanism of action and the possibility of synergistic effects of components are crucial to further the development of successful complementary and alternative therapies for SUDs and related conditions.

KEY POINTS

1. Traditional Chinese medicines have been used to treat human disease for more than 2000 years. It is estimated that roughly half of current pharmaceuticals originally were procured from plants.
2. Although acupuncture and related acupoint therapies are most commonly recognized for their analgesic effects, their medical applications extend beyond pain treatment.
3. None of the treatments discussed in this chapter are approved by the US Food and Drug Administration approved for any SUD.

REVIEW QUESTIONS

1. Which of the following products are approved by the US Food and Drug Administration for the treatment of opioid withdrawal?
   A. Acupuncture
   B. Ibogaine

C. LEK-8829
D. None of the above.

2. Which of the following therapies has shown promise in the treatment of alcohol use disorder?
   A. Acupuncture
   B. Equine therapy
   C. Aqua therapy
   D. Dancing therapy

3. Which of the following is the proposed mechanism for the treatment of opioid detoxification with acupuncture?
   A. Increased vagal tone
   B. Increased release of endogenous opioid peptides in the central nervous system
   C. Decreased release of norepinephrine in the central nervous system
   D. Increased release of serotonin

ANSWERS

1. **D**
2. **A**
3. **B**

SUGGESTED READINGS

Han JS, Terenius L. Neurochemical basis of acupuncture analgesia. *Annu Rev Pharmacol Toxicol*. 1982;22:193-220.

Han JS, Trachtenberg AI, Lowinson JH. Acupuncture. In: Lowinson JH, Ruiz P, Millman RB, Langrod JG, eds. *Substance Abuse: A Comprehensive Textbook*. 4th ed. Philadelphia: Lippincott Williams & Wilkins, 2004: 743-782.

Kreek MJ, LaForge KS, Butelman E. Pharmacotherapy of addictions. *Nat Rev Drug Discov*. 2002;1(9):710-726.

Yang MMP, Yeun RCF, Kwok JSL. Effect of certain Chinese herbs on drug addiction. In: Chang HM, Yeung H W-C, Tso WW. *Advances in Chinese Medicinal Materials Research*. Singapore: World Scientific Publishing, 1985: 147-158.

33 Harm Reduction, Overdose Prevention, and Addiction Medicine

Summary by India Perez-Urbano, Sharon Stancliff, and Alexander Y. Walley

Based on THE ASAM PRINCIPLES OF ADDICTION MEDICINE, 6th edition chapter by Alexander Y. Walley, Sharon Stancliff, and India Perez-Urbano

HARM REDUCTION DEFINITION AND PRINCIPLES

Harm reduction is a person-centered public health approach to reducing the harms of substance use to individuals and communities. Through practical and evidence-based interventions, harm reduction engages individuals who use substances as fully enfranchised collaborators to make their lives healthier. Fundamentally, harm reduction approaches are built for, and by, individuals who use substances, with an emphasis on their human rights and the destigmatization of people who use substances. Overall, harm reduction interventions improve the health of people who use substances by increasing engagement with, and access to, healthcare resources and substance use treatment; assisting individuals in accessing and navigating social services to ensure basic needs; and reducing the risk of life-threatening illnesses and events such as human immunodeficiency virus (HIV), hepatitis C, and fatal overdose.

Table 33-1 includes examples of tangible harm reduction strategies that are discussed throughout this chapter.

THE INTEGRATION OF HARM REDUCTION AND ADDICTION TREATMENT

The integration of harm reduction and addiction treatment offers benefits for the full continuum of people who use substances, from those who are not yet willing to reduce or stop their use as well as those who are committed to abstinence but are at risk of relapse.

High-quality, person-centered harm reduction programs share several principles with addiction treatment programs. These principles include culturally competent, nonjudgmental care that respects individual dignity, addresses the socioeconomic and physical consequences of substance use, incorporates outreach strategies to engage and motivate people who use substances, and offers specific services that reduce the harms of substance use for those who continue to use substances. Care providers should not stigmatize a person who relapses as a failure. Additionally, they should not restrict access to medical, psychiatric, or addiction treatment due to the receipt of medication treatment (eg, medical and residential addiction treatment settings should be open to people treated with opioid agonists). Finally, they should recognize that collaboration between service programs makes the continuum of care stronger.

INTERVENTIONS THAT REDUCE THE HARMS OF SUBSTANCE USE

Overdose Risk Education and Naloxone to Prevent Overdose

Naloxone is an opioid antagonist that reverses the effects of opioid overdose by displacing opioid agonists (eg, heroin, fentanyl, oxycodone) from opioid receptors. Naloxone has minimal to no adverse effects and is the standard overdose treatment used by emergency medical personnel. Prescribing or distributing naloxone alongside overdose reversal and prevention education has become integral to community harm reduction programs. Laypersons with the potential of being bystanders to an overdose are a primary target of these programs, allowing for prompt revival and increased survival rates by mitigating barriers such as a fear of calling 911 due to illegal activities, delays in arrival by first responders, and the absence of medical care. Overdose responder training often includes how to recognize signs of overdose, seek help, rescue

TABLE 33-1	Harm Reduction Strategies and Mechanisms of Reducing Harm			
	Reducing the Acute Harms of Use (eg, overdose)	Reducing the Complications of Use (eg, infection, trauma)	Reducing Harm by Reducing Use	Reducing Harm by Engaging in Care
Overdose education and take-home naloxone rescue kits	X			
Drug checking	X			
Preexposure HIV prophylaxis (PrEP)		X		
Postexposure HIV prophylaxis (PEP)		X		
Syringe needle access programs	X	X		X
Supervised drug consumption venues	X	X		X
Heroin treatment	X	X		X
Opioid agonist or antagonist medication	X	X	X	X
Alcohol medication	X	X	X	X
Designated drivers		X		
Housing first		X		X
Managed alcohol programs	X	X	X	X

breathing and/or chest compressions, administer naloxone, and stay with the person who is overdosing. Studies have found no evidence of compensatory drug use behavior among individuals who use heroin after being trained in overdose response and given a take-home naloxone rescue kit. Overdose prevention programs have been established in many venues, including syringe access programs, HIV prevention outreach programs, methadone maintenance clinics, inpatient detoxification programs, emergency department settings, and community meetings. See Table 33-2 for a list of online resources.

Studies of community and office-based naloxone initiatives have demonstrated a reduction in community-wide fatal overdose rates, a reduction in opioid-related emergency visits and cost-effectiveness, increased knowledge and skills, and a reduction in fatal overdoses after the initiation of community naloxone rescue programs.

Access to Clean Injection Equipment to Reduce Infection Risks

Syringe needle access programs (SNAPs) provide risk reduction education, resources, and tools to reduce the sharing and reuse of injection equipment among their participants. SNAPs typically complement these services with syringe disposal services, sexually transmitted infection testing, viral hepatitis and tuberculosis

TABLE 33-2	Overdose Prevention Online Resources	
Website		**Resource**
Prescribe to Prevent (https://prescribetoprevent.org)		Information on naloxone rescue kits for prescribers and pharmacists, including patient materials, continuing education courses, and research reviews
Prescription Drug Abuse Policy System (http://PDAPS.org)		Updated interactive map of state laws, including Good Samaritan laws, related to prescription drug abuse
Substance Abuse and Mental Health Services Administration (https://www.samhsa.gov/capt/tools-learning-resources/opioid-overdose-prevention-toolkit)		Opioid Overdose Prevention Toolkit for healthcare providers, first responders, treatment providers, and those recovering from opioid overdose
Harm Reduction Coalition (https://harmreduction.org/issues/overdose-prevention/)		Resources including guides to developing and managing overdose prevention programs

screening, on-site referral to substance use treatment, safe sex education, case management, and increasingly, overdose education and naloxone distribution. Studies of SNAPs have demonstrated decreases in HIV and hepatitis C virus prevalence among people who inject drugs (PWIDs). Studies show no evidence of increases in drug use frequency or initiation among individuals who participate in SNAPs. SNAPs involvement in syringe disposal and syringe pick-up efforts have been shown to decrease the prevalence of improperly disposed hypodermic needles on the street as well as reduce needlestick injuries among first responders.

Complementary initiatives, such as programs that allow pharmacies to sell syringes and needles without a prescription, have played an important role in increase syringe access, particularly in geographic areas in which SNAPs are inaccessible, limited in capacity, or nonexistent. Barriers to pharmacy-based syringe procurement include pharmacy staff attitudes and lack of training (that perpetuate the discrimination of PWID), requirements to show identification, cost and unaffordability of syringes, and the lack of engagement in risk reduction education for PWID. Table 33-3 discusses ways to educate patients who inject drugs on safer methods.

Clean injection equipment can also be distributed via public syringe dispensing machines 24 hours a day, 7 days per week, without the fixed overhead and staffing costs of SNAPs and without the requirement of walking into a pharmacy. Syringe dispensing machines have been shown to attract PWID who would otherwise not go to SNAPs or pharmacies, including younger people, people who more recently started injecting, and people with no contact with addiction service providers.

Supervised Drug Consumption Venues to Reduce Infection Risks and Overdose

Supervised injection facilities (SIFs), or drug consumption venues, are facilities where people may go to consume drugs (obtained elsewhere) under trained supervision in a hygienic environment, both with appropriate equipment and without a fear of arrest. SIFs are a harm reduction response to the public health issues that surround overdose deaths, high-risk injection practices, and public injection (eg, in parks, empty lots, public restrooms). The first SIF opened in Switzerland in 1986. Today, there are more than 100 legally sanctioned sites in at least eight countries; yet, there are none in the United States.

SIFs are strongly associated with reductions in overdose fatalities in the vicinity of the facility, with

TABLE 33-3	Discussing Safer Injection Practices With People Who Inject Drugs

Educating patients on safer injection techniques can reduce the risks of injection and improve the patient–provider relationship.

Key Techniques

Equipment

- Use a sterile needle/syringe or a new needle/syringe with each injection.
- Use your own clean cooker or spoon.
- Use sterile or clean water.
- Use a clean cotton filter. Ideally, a prepilled dental filter, rather than cotton swabs. Avoid lint or cigarette filters.
- Avoid sharing equipment.
- Keep used needles/syringes in a sturdy container until disposed of in a biohazard box.

Hygiene

- Wash your hands with soap and water.
- Use alcohol wipes to clean the injection site.
- Use clean surfaces for preparation.

Injection site

- Veins on the arms and hands are safest. Avoid injecting into the groin or neck.

A video by Canadian organization CATIE demonstrates safer injection techniques: http://www.catie.ca/en/resources/safer-injection-demo

no reported overdose deaths within the facilities. They have not been associated with increases in drug use or drug crimes but have been associated with a cessation of drug injection, increased substance use treatment uptake, and a reduced time to entry into substance use treatment. They reduce public disorder, including public injection and public syringe disposal. They have also been found to reduce risk behaviors for blood-borne infections such as reusing and sharing injection equipment, while increasing access to drug treatment and timely access to healthcare. Modeling studies have found that SIFs are likely to reduce HIV and hepatitis C infections, would be cost-effective, and potentially cost saving.

Pre– and Post–HIV Exposure Prophylaxis Medication to Reduce HIV Infection

HIV transmission risk can be reduced by taking anti-HIV medication within 24 hours before an unsafe exposure (preexposure prophylaxis [PrEP]) or within 72 hours after an unsafe exposure (postexposure prophylaxis [PEP]). People who use drugs are at risk of HIV transmission through high-risk sexual practices and the sharing of injection equipment. High-risk sexual practices include having a sexual partner who is HIV positive, having recent bacterial sexually transmitted infections, having multiple sexual partners, inconsistent or no condom use, or engaging in transactional sex work. PrEP has been shown to be efficacious in reducing the risk of HIV transmission by up to 74% and is a recommended HIV prevention tool by the Centers of Disease Control and Prevention for high-risk patients. Guidelines for PEP and PrEP are available, and there is a national hotline for immediate consultation.

Medications to Prevent Injection and Overdose Risks

Medication to treat substance use disorders can be considered a harm reduction strategy when it results in reduced complications of substance use. The best evidence for addiction medication as a harm reduction strategy exists for methadone and buprenorphine treatment for opioid use disorders. Studies have shown that opioid agonist treatment reduces injection frequency, HIV transmission, overdose, and criminal activity, even among those who continue to use and inject opioids and other substances. The American Society of Addiction Medicine's guidelines on the use of medications recommend that "the use of marijuana, stimulants, or other addictive drugs should not be a reason to suspend opioid use disorder treatment." The guidelines acknowledge that concurrent use is associated with poorer outcomes and recommend that the overall harms and benefits of continuing treatment must be weighed against concurrent use of other substances. In Europe, Canada, and Australia, slow-release morphine, diacetylmorphine (heroin), and hydromorphone have reduced illicit heroin use and the complications of injection for people who continue high-risk heroin use while taking methadone.

Alcohol: Targeted Use of Opioid Antagonists

Daily use of opioid antagonists has been shown in randomized controlled trials to reduce the number of drinks per day among people with daily alcohol consumption. Relative to daily use, targeted use has the potential to reduce episodes of alcohol intoxication and the consequences that follow while also reducing the risks of side effects of daily medication use (eg, hepatotoxicity). One study demonstrated

greater reductions in alcohol use from a targeted naltrexone strategy rather than a daily naltrexone strategy. Although the effect sizes were small, three randomized trials of nalmefene in Europe have demonstrated improvements in multiple alcohol-related outcomes over placebo. Targeted nalmefene is approved for the treatment of people with alcohol use disorders in Europe.

Managed Alcohol Programs

People with severe alcohol use disorder who are actively drinking and homeless are commonly restricted from housing due to ongoing alcohol use. Managed alcohol programs provide individuals who are unstably housed and living with an alcohol use disorder with alcohol of known quality with the goals of stabilizing alcohol use and improving the health and well-being of this target population. Longitudinal observational evaluations of managed alcohol programs have reported fewer emergency department visits, fewer police contacts, reduced alcohol consumption within the program over time, less nonbeverage alcohol use, reductions in tests of liver inflammation, an improved perception of quality of life, and housing stability. Peer-reviewed, published descriptions and evaluations of managed alcohol programs have come from only Canada at this point. Randomized controlled trials have not been conducted but are warranted because current evaluations are promising.

Consumer Drug Testing to Reduce the Risk of Contaminant Ingestion

In response to a burgeoning "rave" and "techno" culture, a number of harm reduction initiatives emerged to introduce "drug checking" services as a means to warn partygoers of harmful or unexpected substances. Programs conduct on-site chemical analyses at dance parties and raves to inform individuals of the contents of their drug supply. Some programs, such as Dance Safe in the United States, sell test kits online, allowing individuals to perform their own tests at home. Programs in the Netherlands, Austria, France, Spain, Belgium, Germany, and Switzerland have spearheaded pill-testing initiatives across the European Union, some of which are part of the national drug policy.

In the midst of the emergence of illicitly made fentanyl in North America, harm reduction programs in British Columbia checked urine samples of participants and found that 29% of samples tested positive for fentanyl; yet, the majority did not report any known fentanyl use. In the United States, syringe/needle access programs are increasingly engaging in drug checking efforts in which participants are offered fentanyl test kits to test their heroin for the presence of fentanyl.

CONCLUSION

Harm reduction, as an approach to improve the lives of people who use substances, emerged in the midst of widespread stigmatization and criminalization of substance use. Several specific harm reduction interventions that were developed by and for people who use substances have been proven effective and lie at the core of the public health strategy to address the complications from substance use. Comprehensive approaches to substance use and its complications have evolved to incorporate harm reduction, bringing harm reduction into the mainstream, and improving the reach of prevention and treatment efforts to reach many individuals who are at high risk. Effective harm reduction efforts will require ongoing innovation and adaptation in response to the evolving impact of substances and their complications on public health.

KEY POINTS

1. Harm reduction is a set of principles and strategies aimed at reducing the harms of drug use.
2. Harm reduction considers drug use risk on a spectrum, from safer use, to managed use, to abstinence. Harm reduction strategies work alongside individuals who use drugs (ie, "meeting them where they are at") to move along this continuum by taking steps to reduce harm, with the objective of improving patients' health and quality of life.
3. Providers can integrate pragmatic harm reduction strategies in their practices such as recommending and prescribing opioid agonists/antagonists (eg, methadone, buprenorphine, naltrexone, nalmefene) to treat opioid dependency, naloxone for overdose prevention, sterile hypodermic needles/syringes to reduce needle sharing and reuse, safe injection and drug use practices, PrEP or PEP for HIV prevention, and more.
4. Nonprofit organizations, healthcare and public health entities, and local governments can champion and implement harm reduction interventions in their communities via syringe/needle access programs, opioid overdose prevention program (naloxone distribution efforts), supervised injection facilities, drug testing/checking programs, housing first programs, managed alcohol programs, and more.

REVIEW QUESTIONS

1. Which of the following are tools for *preventing* fatal and nonfatal overdoses? (Select all that apply.)
   A. Preexposure prophylaxis
   B. Naloxone
   C. Fentanyl test kits
   D. Benzodiazepines
   E. Buprenorphine

2. Which of the following is the single best example of a harm reduction approach?
   A. A person who is seeking shelter attempts to stay at an emergency shelter for the night; however, she is turned away because the shelter requires that all residents demonstrate a blood alcohol content of 0.00 on a breathalyzer test and have not had an alcoholic drink in the last 3 months.
   B. A local emergency department implements a new policy that for all patients presenting with opioid overdose symptoms, the department will apply to the court to hold the patient without their consent for medically managed withdrawal treatment (detoxification).
   C. A patient discloses to his healthcare provider that he is HIV positive and injects heroin. He also shares that he does not share his syringes among his friends, but he sometimes shares with his girlfriend. His provider suggests that his girlfriend gets tested for HIV, discusses PrEP and PEP with his patient, and recommends a local syringe services program.
   D. An individual is recently hired after a few months of unemployment. Looking to decrease his heroin usage so that it does not interfere with his new job, he asks his physician about buprenorphine. He tells his physician that he still wants to be able to use heroin a few nights a week. His physician refuses to initiate the patient on buprenorphine because he requires that all of his patients practice abstinence while on long-term buprenorphine treatment.

3. Which of the following is a risk associated with drug use that can be mitigated through harm reduction interventions?
   A. Bacterial and viral infections such as HIV, hepatitis C, endocarditis, cellulitis, and abscess
   B. Overdose and overdose-related death
   C. Legal problems related to illegal drug use, drug acquisition, and/or trafficking, including driving under the influence of drugs
   D. Physical, emotional, and behavioral consequences of drug withdrawal
   E. All of the above.

4. Which of the following best describes harm reduction?

A. Harm reduction is the philosophy that criminalizing illicit drug use will decrease drug abuse and addiction prevalence overall.

B. Harm reduction is the approach of addressing harmful drug use by adopting abstinence-based models of care, in which services are conditional upon the individual abstaining from all drug use and does not accept other alternatives.

C. Harm reduction refers to the practice of taking legal action against multinational pharmaceutical companies to hold them accountable for the harm that their pharmaceutical products have instilled on the health of communities.

D. Harm reduction refers to targeted policies, programs, and practices that aim primarily to reduce the adverse health, social, and economic consequences of the use of legal and illegal drug use.

E. Harm reduction is the ideology that practitioners should cease prescribing all potentially addictive substances to patients, particularly opioid analgesics.

ANSWERS

1. **B, C, and E.** PrEP is an HIV prevention tool (ie, when people at high risk of HIV take HIV medications daily to significantly reduce their chances of getting infected). Benzodiazepines (eg, alprazolam [Xanax], diazepam [Valium]) are psychoactive drugs that are commonly used to treat anxiety and insomnia. They do not reduce the risk of overdose; in fact, if used in conjunction with opioids, alcohol, or cocaine, they can increase the chance of overdose. Naloxone is an opioid antagonist that is used to treat opioid overdose; this medication is used nationwide as an opioid antidote to revive people who overdose and reduce the risk of overdose death. Fentanyl test kits test the presence of fentanyl (a potent synthetic opioid that is highly associated with overdose death) and can be used as a preventative measure to overdose by assessing the potency or purity of one's drug supply. Buprenorphine is a partial opioid agonist that is commonly used to treat opioid dependency; studies have shown that buprenorphine is associated with a reduced overdose risk.

2. **C.** A harm reduction approach is not contingent upon abstinence, which is why A and D are incorrect. Harm reduction is a movement for social justice built on a belief in, and respect for, the rights of people who use drugs. B exemplifies a violation of these basic rights and potentially inflicts gratuitous harm on the patient, which is why this response is incorrect. C is correct because the provider is being nonjudgmental toward the patient's health behaviors and is recommending tools and strategies that can mitigate the harms of his drug use.

3. **E.** A, B, C, and D are all examples of risks associated with drug use that can be mitigated through harm reduction efforts. Syringe/needle access programs are examples of harm reduction interventions that can prevent bacterial and viral infections by reducing the need to reduce and share injection equipment (answer A). Naloxone is a harm reduction intervention proven to prevent nonfatal and fatal opioid overdose (answer B). Supervised injection facilities reduce the need to inject in public, further reducing adverse interactions with law enforcement and possible prosecution. Buprenorphine treatment has also shown to decrease rates of recidivism (answer C). Medication-assisted treatment allows individuals to reduce or stop illicit drug use while also reducing withdrawal symptoms and their harmful effects (eg, drug-seeking behaviors, criminal activity, discomfort, physical harm) (answer D).

4. **D.** D is the definition of harm reduction. A is incorrect because harm reduction calls for the destigmatization and decriminalization of substance use disorders. B is incorrect because harm reduction recognizes abstinence as one method, but not the only method, of reducing the harms of drug use. C and E are not aligned with the principles of harm reduction.

SUGGESTED READINGS

American Society of Addiction Medicine. *The ASAM National Practice Guideline for the Use of Medications in the Treatment of Addiction Involving Opioid Use.* Chevy Chase, MD: American Society of Addiction Medicine, 2015. http://www.asam.org/docs/default-source/practice-support/guidelines-and-consensus-docs/asam-national-practice-guideline-supplement.pdf. Accessed November 13, 2018.

American Society of Addiction Medicine. Terminology related to addiction, treatment, and recovery. http://www.asam.org/docs/default-source/public-policy-statements/1-terminology-atr-7-135f81099472bc604ca5b7ff000030b21a.pdf?sfvrsn=0. Published July 2013. Accessed November 13, 2018.

Amlani A, McKee G, Khamis N, et al. Why the FUSS (Fentanyl Urine Screen Study)? A cross-sectional survey to characterize an emerging threat to people who use drugs in British Columbia, Canada. *Harm Reduct J.* 2015;12:54.

Aspinall EJ, Nambiar D, Goldberg DJ, et al. Are needle and syringe programmes associated with a reduction in HIV transmission among people who inject drugs: a systematic review and meta-analysis. *Int J Epidemiol.* 2014;43(1):235-248.

Centers for Disease Control and Prevention. *Preexposure Prophylaxis for the Prevention of HIV Infection in the United States—2014: A Clinical Practice Guideline*. Atlanta: Centers for Disease Control and Prevention, 2014.

Coffin PO, Behar E, Rowe C, et al. Nonrandomized intervention study of naloxone coprescription for primary care patients receiving long-term opioid therapy for pain. *Ann Intern Med*. 2016;165(4):245-252.

Coffin PO, Sullivan SD. Cost-effectiveness of distributing naloxone to heroin users for lay overdose reversal. *Ann Intern Med*. 2013;158(1):1-9.

Crawford ND, Amesty S, Rivera AV, et al. Randomized, community-based pharmacy intervention to expand services beyond sale of sterile syringes to injection drug users in pharmacies in New York City. *Am J Public Health*. 2013;103(9):1579-1582.

DeBeck K, Kerr T, Bird L, et al. Injection drug use cessation and use of North America's first medically supervised safer injecting facility. *Drug Alcohol Depend*. 2011;113(2):172-176.

Duplessy C, Reynaud EG. Long-term survey of a syringe-dispensing machine needle exchange program: answering public concerns. *Harm Reduct J*. 2014;11:16.

Ferri M, Davoli M, Perucci CA. Heroin maintenance for chronic heroin-dependent individuals. *Cochrane Database Syst Rev*. 2011;7(12):CD003410.

Ferri M, Minozzi S, Bo A, Amato L. Slow-release oral morphine as maintenance therapy for opioid dependence. *Cochrane Database Syst Rev*. 2013;5(6):CD009879.

Freeman K, Jones CG, Weatherburn DJ, et al. The impact of the Sydney Medically Supervised Injecting Centre (MSIC) on crime. *Drug Alcohol Rev*. 2005;24(2):173-184.

Gjersing L, Bretteville-Jensen AL. Is opioid substitution treatment beneficial if injecting behaviour continues? *Drug Alcohol Depend*. 2013;133(1):121-126.

Groseclose SL, Weinstein B, Jones TS, et al. Impact of increased legal access to needles and syringes on practices of injecting-drug users and police officers—Connecticut, 1992-1993. *J Acquir Immune Defic Syndr Hum Retrovirol*. 1995;10(1):82-89.

Hagan H, McGough JP, Thiede H, et al. Reduced injection frequency and increased entry and retention in drug treatment associated with needle-exchange participation in Seattle drug injectors. *J Subst Abuse Treat*. 2000;19(3):247-252.

Havnes I, Bukten A, Gossop M, et al. Reductions in convictions for violent crime during opioid maintenance treatment: a longitudinal national cohort study. *Drug Alcohol Depend*. 2012;124(3):307-310.

Hernandez-Avila CA, Song C, Kuo L, et al. Targeted versus daily naltrexone: secondary analysis of effects on average daily drinking. *Alcohol Clin Exp Res*. 2006;30(5):860-865.

Hurley SF, Jolley DJ, Kaldor JM. Effectiveness of needle-exchange programmes for prevention of HIV infection. *The Lancet*. 1997;349(9068):1797-1800.

Jones JD, Campbell A, Metz VE, Comer SD. No evidence of compensatory drug use risk behavior among heroin users after receiving take-home naloxone. *Addict Behav*. 2017;71:104-106.

Kriener H, Billeth R, Gollner C, et al. *An Inventory of On-Site Pill-Testing Interventions in the EU*. Lisbon, Portugal: European Monitoring Centre for Drugs and Drug Addiction; 2001.

Lloyd-Smith E, Wood E, Zhang R, et al. Determinants of hospitalization for a cutaneous injection-related infection among injection drug users: a cohort study. *BMC Public Health*. 2010;10:327.

Marlatt GA, Blume AW, Parks GA. Integrating harm reduction therapy and traditional substance abuse treatment. *J Psychoactive Drugs*. 2001;33(1):13-21.

Marshall BD, Milloy MJ, Wood E, Montaner JS, Kerr T. Reduction in overdose mortality after the opening of North America's first medically supervised safer injecting facility: a retrospective population-based study. *Lancet*. 2011;377(9775):1429-1437.

Martin M, Vanichseni S, Suntharasamai P, et al. Risk behaviors and risk factors for HIV infection among participants in the Bangkok tenofovir study, an HIV pre-exposure prophylaxis trial among people who inject drugs. *PLoS One*. 2014;9(3):e92809.

Niciu MJ, Arias AJ. Targeted opioid receptor antagonists in the treatment of alcohol use disorders. *CNS Drugs*. 2013;27(10):777-787.

Oviedo-Joekes E, Guh D, Brissette S, et al. Hydromorphone compared with diacetylmorphine for long-term opioid dependence: a randomized clinical trial. *JAMA Psychiatry*. 2016;73(5):447-455.

Pauly BB, Gray E, Perkin K, et al. Finding safety: a pilot study of managed alcohol program participants' perceptions of housing and quality of life. *Harm Reduct J*. 2016;13(1):15.

Podymow T, Turnbull J, Coyle D, Yetisir E, Wells G. Shelter-based managed alcohol administration to chronically homeless people addicted to alcohol. *CMAJ*. 2006;174(1):45-49.

Potier C, Laprévote V, Dubois-Arber F, Cottencin O, Rolland B. Supervised injection services: what has been demonstrated? A systematic literature review. *Drug Alcohol Depend*. 2014; 145:48-68.

PrEP: pre-exposure prophylaxis. Clinical Consultation Center Web site. http://nccc.ucsf.edu/clinician-consultation/prep-pre-exposure-prophylaxis/.

Reich W, Compton WM, Horton JC, et al. Injection drug users report good access to pharmacy sale of syringes. *J Am Pharm Assoc (Wash)*. 2002;42(6 Suppl 2):S68-S72.

Schwartz RP, Gryczynski J, O'Grady KE, et al. Opioid agonist treatments and heroin overdose deaths in Baltimore, Maryland, 1995-2009. *Am J Public Health*. 2013;103(5):917-922.

Stancliff S, Phillips BW, Maghsoudi N, Joseph H. Harm reduction: front line public health. *J Addict Dis*. 2015;34(2-3):206-219.

Strathdee SA, Ricketts EP, Huettner S, et al. Facilitating entry into drug treatment among injection drug users referred from a needle exchange program. *Drug Alcohol Depend*. 2006;83(3):225-232.

Vallance K, Stockwell T, Pauly B, et al. Do managed alcohol programs change patterns of alcohol consumption and reduce related harm? A pilot study. *Harm Reduct J*. 2016;13(1):13.

Walley AY, Doe-Simkins M, Quinn E, et al. Opioid overdose prevention with intranasal naloxone among people who take methadone. *J Subst Abuse Treat*. 2013;44(2):241-247.

Walley AY, Xuan Z, Hackman HH, et al. Opioid overdose rates and implementation of overdose education and nasal naloxone distribution in Massachusetts: interrupted time series analysis. *BMJ*. 2013;346:f174.

Wolfson-Stofko B, Bennett AS, Elliott L, Curtis R. Drug use in business bathrooms: an exploratory study of manager encounters in New York City. *Int J Drug Policy*. 2017;39:69-77.

Wood E, Kerr T, Small W, et al. Changes in public order after the opening of a medically supervised safer injecting facility for illicit injection drug users. *CMAJ*. 2004;171(7):731-734.

34 Quality Improvement for Addiction Treatment

Summary by James H. Ford II, Kim A. Hoffman,
Kimberly Johnson, and Javier Ponce Terashima

Based on THE ASAM PRINCIPLES OF ADDICTION MEDICINE,
6th edition chapter by James H. Ford II, Kim A. Hoffman,
Kimberly Johnson, and Javier Ponce Terashima

Addiction treatment services have traditionally been provided under the auspices of an acute rather than chronic care model despite evidence that addiction behaves much like other chronic conditions such as hypertension, diabetes, and asthma. Through a series of four reports published between 2000 and 2012, the Institute of Medicine (IOM) has called for significant changes to how addiction and mental health services are provided. This chapter provides an overview of this framework for change and highlights ongoing efforts to improve the quality and effectiveness of addiction treatment services. These efforts fall into four general categories: (1) defining and measuring expected treatment outcomes, (2) accreditation of programs that deliver substance use disorder (SUD) treatment, (3) building the capacity for efficient and effective treatment delivery, and (4) integrating substance use treatment with primary care.

FRAMEWORK FOR CHANGE

A series of reports from the IOM (now the National Academy of Medicine) and the implementation of the Patient Protection and Affordable Care Act (ACA) as well as the final rules associated with the Mental Health Parity and Addiction Equity Act (MHPAEA) provide a framework for change in the field of SUD treatment. The IOM reports identified the need for better healthcare and outlined strategies to improve the quality of healthcare in the United States. One of the reports, *Improving the Quality of Health Care for Mental Health and Substance Use Conditions* (2005) recommends that alcohol, drug, and mental health treatment systems emphasize the six dimensions of quality of care first identified in the IOM 2001 report titled *Crossing the Quality Chasm: A New Health System for the 21st Century.* This 2001 IOM report indicated that care should be

safe, effective, patient centered, timely, efficient, and equitable. The 2005 IOM report also recommended that public agencies and payers promote the development of process and outcome measures that track quality of care. Another IOM report, *Substance Use Disorders in the U.S. Armed Forces* (2012) recognizes the effect of combat on veterans' substance use and strongly recommends the full implementation of the Department of Defense evidence-based guideline for treating SUDs. One common theme across the series of published IOM reports is that system design, reimbursement processes, and service delivery have more impact on treatment results (patient outcomes) than variation in individual practitioner knowledge or behavior. The most recent National Academy of Medicine report, *Psychosocial Interventions for Mental and Substance Use Disorders* (2015), places the patient at the center of a process to identify important outcomes; to utilize research methods that identify key elements of interventions and translation efforts that ensure fidelity; and to identify implementation strategies that promote the use of evidence-based psychosocial interventions.

One important common theme that carried across all five IOM/National Academy of Medicine reports on quality is that system design, reimbursement processes, and service delivery have more impact on treatment results (patient outcomes) than variation in individual practitioner knowledge or behavior. In other words, improved outcomes will come more readily from improved research and delivery systems than from additional training. Although human resource development is important, better system design trumps improvement of skills as a leverage point for improving outcomes for populations.

In November 2016, the Surgeon General released the report *Facing Addiction: The Surgeon General's*

Report on Alcohol, Drugs, and Health, presenting "a call to action to end the public health crisis of addiction." The report calls for more fully integrating SUD treatment with the healthcare delivery system to improve both access and quality. It also calls for the treatment system to increase the adoption of health information technologies including electronic health records, clinical decision support systems, and patient support mobile apps to increase data-driven decision making and improve patient and population outcomes. Other recommendations related to quality improvement include a wider use of medications to treat alcohol and opioid use disorders and greater adoption of evidence-based psychosocial interventions.

DEFINING AND MEASURING QUALITY TREATMENT AND OUTCOMES

The use of standardized quality measures has not been widely adopted in addiction treatment. In response, organizations such as the Washington Circle Group, the National Quality Forum (NQF), and the American Society of Addiction Medicine are leading efforts to develop, implement, and use standardized measures.

Washington Circle Measures

The Washington Circle Group (http://www.washingtoncircle.org) is composed of experts in SUD policy, research, and performance management who have developed and evaluated six quality measures related to SUD treatment in private and public payer systems. The measures focus on treatment identification, initiation, engagement, and continuity of care. The identification, initiation, and engagement measures are included in the Health Plan Employer Data and Information Set that health plans submit annually to the National Commission for Quality Improvement. The applicability of the measures has been assessed by more than 16 states and the US Department of Veterans Affairs. Public sector studies indicate that initiation and engagement in treatment predicts future arrests or incarcerations and treatment continuity predicts 3-month treatment recovery as measured by substance use. However, studies conducted in the Department of Veterans Affairs using the Washington Circle measures show mixed results.

National Quality Forum

The NQF is a congressionally chartered membership organization charged with using an empirically based consensus process to define and disseminate standards and measures for the healthcare system.

- Identification
  - Screening and Case Finding (2)
  - Diagnosis and Assessment (1)
- Initiation and Engagement
  - Brief Intervention (1)
  - Promoting Engagement (1)
  - Withdrawal Management (1)
- Therapeutic Interventions
  - Psychosocial (1)
  - Pharmacotherapy (3)
- Continuing Care Management (1)

Figure 34-1. National Quality Forum treatment practice domains. The numbers correspond to how many treatment practices are in each of the subdomains or domains.

The NQF report *National Voluntary Consensus Standards for the Treatment of Substance Use Conditions* identifies 11 treatment practices, organized into 4 domains and subdomains, as evidence-based treatments for alcohol, tobacco, and drug use disorders (Fig. 34-1). The numbers in Figure 34-1 correspond to the treatment practice distribution across the domains. Endorsement by NQF members of these practices is the first formal consensus on evidence-based practices for the treatment of substance use conditions. The NQF continues to define, test, and disseminate operational measures for these sanctioned practices in the field of mental health and SUD care. Eligible professionals must report on these measures in order to receive incentive payments or avoid penalties in the final rule for stage 2 criteria for meaningful use of electronic health record systems. The NQF developed measures and an associated framework intended to address the multiple chronic conditions present in many individuals seeking treatment for these conditions.

The Health Plan Employer Data and Information Set and NQF measures can be organized in a cascade of care framework where system success in identification, initiation, engagement, and continuation in treatment are steps in a treatment process that are the measures of the performance of a system of care. Current efforts to use this framework focus in identifying which data sources and measures are best able to populate a cascade of care framework for addiction.

ASAM Standards Workgroup

The American Society of Addiction Medicine has released two reports: *Standards of Care for the Addiction Specialist Physician* and *Performance Measures for the Addiction Specialist Physician.* The documents outline the standards of care and how to measure performance in meeting the standards for addiction specialists.

ACCREDITATION FOR TREATMENT PROGRAMS

Accreditation requires an organization to conduct an extensive internal analysis of its performance against standards that focus on multiple domains (eg, use of clinical interventions or governance). The standards are aimed, at minimum, to promote patient safety and, optimally, to improve patient outcomes. Three organizations—the Joint Commission, the Commission on Accreditation of Rehabilitation Facilities, and the Council on Accreditation for Children and Family Services—are the primary entities that provide peer-reviewed accreditation for alcohol and drug treatment programs. The accreditation process requires a significant investment of resources; the 2016 National Survey of Substance Abuse Treatment Services indicates that approximately 55% of all SUD treatment programs have received accreditation, and 51% of non-opioid treatment programs are accredited.

An exception to the limited accreditation of treatment programs are outpatient opioid treatment programs. Federal regulations (42 CFR Part 8) require that opioid treatment programs receive certification from a national accreditation organization (eg, Commission on Accreditation of Rehabilitation Facilities, Joint Commission, or the National Commission on Correctional Health Care) or a Substance Abuse and Mental Health Services Administration–authorized state agency. These accrediting bodies review opioid treatment programs to confirm that the services comply with federal quality standards.

EVALUATING POLICY IMPACT ON TREATMENT

In 2006, the Center for Substance Abuse Treatment (CSAT) published the results of an evaluation of the shift from an enforcement model administered by the US Food and Drug Administration to a regulatory model administered by the CSAT and carried out by approved accrediting bodies. Of the programs that responded to a survey conducted as part of the evaluation, 86% reported that accreditation improved their service quality. Survey respondents identified improved quality assurance activities as the single largest effect on the shift from enforcement to accreditation.

A 2016 task force evaluation of whether insurers were following the 2008 MHPAEA and the ACA found that the primary violations of the two laws that limit access to services and medications for SUD are what are called "nonquantitative treatment limits," such as requirements to fail in outpatient counseling before being able to obtain medication or residential treatment services, or prior authorization requirements that are different from those for other health conditions. Federal government limits, such as the institutions of mental disease, limit on the use of Medicaid to reimburse for inpatient psychiatric or SUD treatment were also raised, and, as a result, there are efforts underway to allow for waivers for reimbursement of short-term inpatient care for emergency purposes.

BUILDING SYSTEM CAPACITY TO DELIVER EFFECTIVE TREATMENTS

Since 2003, behavioral health providers as well as other community-based treatment providers have been using the NIATx process improvement model (NIATx Model) to improve treatment quality. The NIATx Model (www.niatx.net) integrates the work of quality improvement pioneers such as Edward Deming and Joseph Juran with key process-improvement principles that facilitate organizational changes. In most cases, the change should help address issues that impede the organization's achievement of its strategic plan or affect revenue and costs. Executive leadership should also take an active role in selecting a powerful change leader. This individual is an integral part of the successful change effort in the organization and must have the necessary skills, aptitude, and interest. Change leaders should have the respect of their peers and of staff and access to agency management, effective project management skills, and be comfortable with using data to guide improvement efforts.

Although change ideas may come from within an organization, the NIATx Model encourages change leaders and teams to seek ideas from other behavioral health providers or even outside the field. For example, an organization might be able to learn from the airline industry about how to sequence and hand off clients within or across organizations. Likewise, retailers may have transferrable ideas on how to manage an influx of new customers and how to avoid long queues. Leveraging ideas requires an ability to recognize that other organizations experience similar problems and adapt their solutions to the specific situation in a particular organization.

Plan–Do–Study–Act cycles are a central component of process improvement. Planning includes specifying the problem that will be fixed, collecting data to assess the extent of the problem, selecting a goal, and identifying solutions to test. Process improvement is about action. Change teams test the proposed change (Do): The test is for a limited time and a limited number of patients. A few simple but key measures are collected and analyzed (Study): Did a change occur in the frequency or extent of the problem? Were there any unintended outcomes? Based on the planning, doing, and studying, the change team decides what to do next (Act). The change can be abandoned if it does not work. It may be modified to enhance the effect. If the pilot was successful, it can be expanded to include more patients and more staff or more sites and eventually institutionalized through policy and procedure manuals. Plan–Do–Study–Act cycles are best when they are rapid. Two weeks or less is usually sufficient to learn whether a change is viable and if additional time and resources should be invested. The NIATx Model requires few resources, can be learned quickly, and can be applied to achieve any of the quality standards identified by previously mentioned standards-creating bodies.

ENSURING PRIMARY CARE PROVIDERS CAN IDENTIFY, TREAT, OR REFER AND MONITOR SUBSTANCE USE DISORDER

There is an increasing recognition that general medical practitioners should be able to screen, monitor, and provide medication for SUDs. A study found a high prevalence of harmful alcohol (30%) and drug use (5%) among patients of primary care practices. Patients with SUDs have a higher prevalence of heart, liver, and gastrointestinal disorders. The White House Office of National Drug Control Policy 2015 National Drug Control Strategy asserts that SUDs are medical conditions and that treatment should be integrated into mainstream healthcare and suggests concrete steps toward the goal of improved access to addiction treatment services, including the integration of Screening, Brief Intervention, and Referral to Treatment (SBIRT) into all healthcare settings. The Health Resources and Services Administration has taken steps to promote the use of SBIRT, such as including brief intervention codes in the Uniform Data Systems to track activity in federally qualified health centers. States are encouraged to adopt SBIRT as a reimbursable service and train more service providers in SBIRT. Lastly, the American College of Obstetrics and Gynecologists calls for screening and early intervention in women's healthcare settings including obstetrics and gynecologists offices because it has the potential to reduce the estimated 400,000

to 440,000 infants affected by prenatal alcohol or drug exposure.

With new research into how alcohol and drugs affect the body and the brain, more doctors are coming to an understanding of addiction as a medical problem and addressing it as a chronic disease. Until recently, there have been no national standards for training in addiction medicine, and medical students received little addiction training. In 2016, the American Board of Medical Specialties recognized addiction medicine as a new subspecialty under the American Board of Preventative Medicine. This has replaced the American Board of Addiction Medicine's subspecialty process that primary care providers used to become certified in addiction medicine.

One requirement of the specialty boards is that physicians implement a performance in practice project for recertification and licensing. Launched in 2006, the Improving Performance in Practice initiative uses quality improvement tools. Techniques like NIATx outlined in this chapter provide an approach that physicians could use to achieve their maintenance of certification requirements. Studies suggest that specialists such as addiction psychiatrists can leverage the maintenance of certification process to improve clinical care.

A number of tools exist for physicians to ensure quality in office-based addiction treatment. CSAT offers treatment improvement protocols (TIPs), three of which are for prescribers treating either alcohol or opioid addiction. Each of these manuals comes with a knowledge application program key that is a short version of the critical clinical information outlined in the TIP. In 2017, TIP 40 (on guidelines for prescribing buprenorphine) and TIP 43 (on medication use in opioid treatment programs) have been combined into one manual, *Medications for Opioid Use Disorder: TIP 63*, and updated to include the new formulations of medications recently made available.

Buprenorphine prescribing requires an 8-hour training for physicians and 24 hours for nurse practitioners and physician assistants and an application for a waiver from the Drug Enforcement Administration. The Provider's Clinical Support System for Medication-Assisted Treatment (PCSS-MAT) provides these prescribers with training, support, and mentoring in treating patients with opioid use disorder. The training, waiver process, and PCSS-MAT are all part of a federal effort to ensure quality in the treatment of patients with opioid use disorder. Although training is required only for those seeking to prescribe buprenorphine, all three currently available medications (methadone, buprenorphine, and naltrexone) are mandated to be included in the training so that practitioners are knowledgeable about the choices available to their patients and the rationale for prescribing one medication over another for specific patients.

INTERNATIONAL EFFORTS: THE INTERNATIONAL CENTRE FOR CREDENTIALING AND EDUCATION OF ADDICTION PROFESSIONALS

Established in February 2009, The International Centre for Credentialing and Education of Addiction Professionals (ICCE) is a global initiative funded by the Bureau of International Narcotics and Law Enforcement Affairs, within the US Department of State. ICCE's mission is to train, professionalize, and expand the drug demand reduction workforce globally. ICCE was formed in response to inadequate evidence-based programs and lack of trained addiction professionals. It is an international certified education provider of the Association of Addiction Professionals.

ICCE collaborates with international experts to develop training curricula in the areas of substance use prevention and the treatment of SUDs. The Universal Prevention Curricula and the Universal Treatment Curricula are multimodule training programs designed to equip prevention and addiction treatment professionals with knowledge, skills, and competencies to efficiently deliver drug demand reduction services. Both curricula were developed by a team of experts in the field and approved by three international organizations, namely, the United Nations Office on Drugs and Crime, the Organization of American States, and the Colombo Plan. Each curriculum is piloted, adapted, and adopted by the region or country implementing the initiative. The curriculum content of both curricula have been found to meet the national and international certification standards set by the US National Certification Commission of Addiction Professionals.

CONCLUSIONS

Quality improvement efforts are affecting the organization and delivery of treatment for SUDs. Delivery system design and quality processes have a greater effect in ensuring patient outcomes than increasing physician knowledge. Therefore, health systems that provide addiction treatment, whether integrated or a separate specialty care, need to ensure quality improvement systems are in place. Quality interventions that build on the foundation of the NIATx Model may be especially promising and have a growing body of

research that supports them. Outcome studies suggest that process changes can lead to reductions in days to admission and to improvements in retention in care, which are key indicators of positive outcome.

Continuing medical education is evolving to be more practice oriented in general, focusing less on information provision and more on supporting change in practice and in the development of skills. As physicians are asked to demonstrate their ability to institute change and ensure quality treatment, demonstration of the use of the tools of quality management, including the institutionalization of a quality improvement mechanism, becomes an essential component of a medical practice.

KEY POINTS

1. Quality is still being defined.
2. Current standards involve a cascade framework including access, engagement, and retention with evidence that increased treatment retention is related to improved outcomes. However, similar evidence for quicker access to treatment and improved outcomes is mixed.
3. Screening and early intervention has the potential to address SUDs early on and to prevent the progression of the disease.
4. The ACA and MHPAEA, as well as the availability of medications, are driving the integration of SUD treatment into primary care, which may change how quality is defined.

REVIEW QUESTIONS

1. True or False: The ASAM workgroup has identified standards for addictions specialist physicians that address their role in direct patient care and improving systems outcomes, giving priority to standards that have the highest impact on quality, are feasible, and reduce costs.

2. Which of the following is not a tool that physicians could use to ensure quality in office-based addiction treatment?
   A. SAMHSA's treatment improvement protocols
   B. Physician clinical support system
   C. Prescription drug monitoring programs
   D. Improving performance in practice

3. What are the current elements that are being measured for quality in substance use disorder care?
   A. Identification including screening, diagnosis, and assessment
   B. Initiation and engagement including measures of access, retention, and continuation in care

C. Impact of therapeutic interventions including psychosocial and pharmacotherapy

D. All of the above

ANSWERS

1. **True**
2. **D**
3. **D**

SUGGESTED READINGS

Drye EE, Altaf FK, Lipska KJ, et al. Defining multiple chronic conditions for quality measurement. *Med Care*. 2018;56(2):193-201.

England MJ, Butler AS, Gonzalez ML, eds. *Psychosocial Interventions for Mental and Substance Use Disorders: A Framework for Establishing Evidence-Based Standards*. Washington, DC: National Academies Press, 2015.

Gustafson DH, Johnson KA. *The NIATx Model (Process Improvement in Behavioral Health)*. Madison, WI: University of Wisconsin-Madison, 2012.

Pincus HA, Spaeth-Rublee B, Watkins KE. Analysis & commentary: the case for measuring quality in mental health and substance abuse care. *Health Aff (Millwood)*. 2011;30(4):730-736.

Socías ME, Volkow N, Wood E. Adopting the 'cascade of care' framework: an opportunity to close the implementation gap in addiction care? *Addiction*. 2016;111(12): 2079-2081.

Substance Abuse and Mental Health Services Administration. *Medications for Opioid Use Disorder. Treatment Improvement Protocol (TIP) Series 63*. Rockville, MD: SAMHSA; 2018. HHS Publication No. (SMA) 18-5063FULLDOC.

Williams AR, Nunes E, Olfson M. To battle the opioid overdose epidemic, deploy the 'cascade of care' model. https://www .healthaffairs.org/do/10.1377/hblog20170313.059163/full/. Published March 13, 2017. Accessed February 3, 2018.

35 Nursing Roles in Addressing Addiction

Summary by Deborah S. Finnell, Marianne T. Marcus, and
Christine L. Savage

Based on THE ASAM PRINCIPLES OF ADDICTION MEDICINE,
6th edition chapter by Deborah S. Finnell, Marianne T. Marcus, and
Christine L. Savage

HISTORY OF DEVELOPMENT OF NURSING ROLES IN ADDICTION CARE

Content on alcohol and associated health risks, and recommended nursing care of late-stage alcohol use disorder first appeared in nursing textbooks in the 1950s. Efforts to increase nursing education were stimulated by federal funding, especially from the National Institute on Alcohol Abuse and Alcoholism. A nursing text on alcoholism by Estes and Heinemann was published in 1977 and was among the first to promote education of nurses on alcohol disorders, the health and social consequences, and interventions.

Despite these national efforts, translation of content related to the prevention and treatment of substance use disorders into nursing curricula did not occur across schools of nursing and, when it did, it was included only minimally. Recent funding from federal agencies, including the Health Services Research Administration and the Substance Abuse and Mental Health Services Administration (SAMHSA) has resulted in increased substance use–related content in nursing curricula in general and the integration of evidence-based screening and brief interventions in particular. Model nursing curricula now exist on how to address the full spectrum of substance use, including prevention, detection, and treatment—a shift from the focus primarily on treatment of these as disorders. This expanded view of substance use along a continuum has required that nurses at all levels of practice broaden their skill set from treatment of substance use disorders to include screening for substance use and further assessments when that use increases the risk for adverse health outcomes.

CURRENT TRENDS IN SUBSTANCE USE

Emerging trends in at-risk substance use have serious implications for nursing practice, underlining the importance of developing a nursing workforce with the knowledge and skills to actively participate in the prevention of adverse consequences related to at-risk use as well as treatment of those with a substance use disorder. There is increased recognition of and focus on the increasing global burden of disease related to substance use with tobacco and alcohol as two of the top three causes of preventable death.

The opioid epidemic has raised alarms worldwide. Opioid overdose deaths are associated with the use of heroin and fentanyl as well as taking amounts higher than the prescribed opioid. Opioid dependence is associated with use of illicit opioids and can occur with even short-term use of prescription opioids for acute pain. Spurred by former President Obama and the Office of National Drug Control Policy, numerous professional nursing organizations pledged to be part of the solution in reversing the opioid epidemic, including such efforts as prescriber education and those directed to improving access to treatment. In 2016, a barrier to access to medication treatment for persons with an opioid disorder was removed with the enhancement of the Comprehensive Addiction and Recovery Act (P.L. 114-198). This legislation allowed nurse practitioners (NPs) (and physician assistants) to be eligible to prescribe buprenorphine, a medication that previously only qualified physicians could prescribe.

Although the future nursing workforce will be the beneficiary of curricula aimed at increasing the knowledge and skills necessary to address the burden of disease associated with substance use, efforts also need to be directed to the current nursing workforce. The number of easily accessible online educational programs has increased to ensure that the current nursing workforce has the requisite knowledge and competencies to provide evidence-based interventions across the continuum of use and the life span for all levels of practice and all practice settings.

LEVELS OF NURSING EDUCATION AND PRACTICE

Most nurses are registered nurses (RNs) who receive an associate degree from a 2-year program at a community college or a baccalaureate degree from a 4-year university. Graduates of both levels of nursing education are required to pass the same nationally standardized licensing examination. Although all RNs provide direct patient care in various healthcare settings, baccalaureate nursing education includes additional preparation in leadership, research utilization, and population health. Master's degrees in nursing prepare nurses for administration, clinical leadership, faculty positions, or advanced practice in a specialty area. Advanced practice registered nurse roles include the NP, the clinical nurse specialist, the certified nurse anesthetist, and the certified nurse-midwife.

The NP is prepared to obtain histories and conduct physicals, diagnose and treat illnesses, prescribe medications, order and interpret x-rays and other diagnostic tests, and provide patient education and counseling. The scope of practice for NPs is regulated by individual states, and there is a wide variation in limitations imposed by the states. The full practice provision allows the NP to assess, diagnose, interpret diagnostic tests, and prescribe medications independently.

The clinical nurse specialist provides advanced care in hospitals and other clinical sites, develops quality improvement programs, and serves as educator and consultant. Certified nurse anesthetists safely administer anesthesia in a variety of settings. Certified nurse midwives provide primary care to women including gynecology, family planning, prenatal care, low risk labor and delivery, and neonatal care.

Doctoral programs in nursing fall into two principal types: research focused and practice focused. Most research-focused programs grant the doctor of philosophy degree (PhD); however, a small percentage offer the doctor of nursing science degree (DNS, DSN, or DNSc). These doctorally prepared nurses develop the science, steward the profession, educate the next generation of nurses, define its uniqueness, and maintain its professional integrity. The practice-focused doctoral degree is the doctor of nursing practice (DNP), which builds upon generalist education acquired through a baccalaureate or advanced generalist master's degree in nursing. DNP graduates are prepared for advanced practice roles and leadership in clinical settings.

The 2011 Institute of Medicine report, *The Future of Nursing: Leading Change, Advancing Health*, specified four key messages relevant for nurses at all levels. (1) Nurses should practice to the full extent of their education and training. (2) Nurses should achieve higher levels of education and training through an improved education. (3) Nurses should be full partners, with physicians and other health professionals, in redesigning healthcare in the United States. (4) Effective workforce planning and policy making require a better data collection and an improved information infrastructure. This report has profoundly impacted all levels of the profession. Nurse educators seek to accommodate seamless academic progression to higher levels of education, and nursing groups advocate for a broader scope of practice regulations for NPs. The lack of sufficient education in the past and present nursing curricula means that the current and future nursing workforce is not fully equipped to address the nation's alcohol and drug crises. Nurses specializing in substance use and substance use disorders are critically needed to lead the change and advance the health of individuals, families, and populations affected by alcohol, tobacco, and other drugs as well as maladaptive behaviors that may lead to substance use disorders.

GENERALIST'S ROLES RELATED TO ADDICTIONS

Considering the pervasive nature of at-risk substance use and substance use disorders and the associated serious health consequences, it is imperative that nurses at all educational levels have basic competencies to address this phenomenon. The core nursing competencies for the generalist nurse related to substance use were last identified in 2002 as a component of discipline-specific recommendations outlined in the *Strategic Plan for Interdisciplinary Faculty Development* by the Association for Medical Education and Research in Substance Abuse. Since the development of these competencies in 2002, significant changes in the field of substance use have emerged and have impacted nursing. In addition to the emerging trends previously discussed, evidence-based treatments including pharmacotherapy are also now available. In 2017, with funding support from SAMHSA, work began to update these core nursing competencies for the generalist nurse (ie, RN) and the advanced practice nurse. The framework for these competencies is aligned with the Standards of Professional Nursing Practice and Standards of Professional Performance set forth by the American Nurses Association. The Strategic Plan was updated in 2018 to provide competencies for nurses, physicians, physician assistants, pharmacists, and social workers and is available at amersa.org. The nursing competencies can be used to inform nurse educators and nurse leaders on preparing the current and future nursing workforce to meet the challenge of substance use.

Advances in neuroscience have informed the understanding of substance use disorders and addictive disorders as brain-based disorders, shifting from a moral view to a science-based perspective. This paradigm shift can help diminish the blame and shame that is associated with addiction and hopefully remove barriers to available lifesaving treatments. With sufficient knowledge and competence, nurses can (1) identify those at risk; (2) conduct further assessment and based on the assessment; (3) provide evidence-based interventions and, if within their scope of practice, prescribe evidence-based medications to support abstinence and recovery; and (4) ensure continuing care through referral to treatment for those needing specialty treatment. Additionally, nurses across all settings and specialties can teach patients and colleagues alike about the biologic mechanisms underlying substance use and how behavioral and pharmacologic treatments promote abstinence and recovery. Finally, the shift in the global focus from treatment of substance use disorders to a focus on reducing harm related to the continuum of use changes how nursing approaches competencies and the leveling of those competencies across levels of practice.

Screening, Brief Intervention, and Referral to Treatment (SBIRT) is an example of a set of practice strategies that should be provided by all generalist nurses. Screening determines the extent of the substance use and signals the need for additional assessment and interventions as indicated. Brief intervention is a nonconfrontational, patient-centered approach to addressing unhealthy alcohol and tobacco use and other drug use. It is intended to raise awareness of the consequences related to the substance use and motivate a patient toward behavior change (ie, reduction in or cessation of use). Referral to treatment provides those patients who need more extensive substance-related treatment with referral to specialty care. SBIRT has emerged as a valuable tool as an evidence-based practice for detecting risk as well as substance use disorders and initiating appropriate clinician response. SBIRT has been shown to be effective in primary care patients with nondependent alcohol use but to have limited effectiveness for drug use. Despite a lack of conclusive evidence about the effectiveness of SBIRT in various settings, in 2012, the Joint Commission put forward four optional performance measures related to tobacco and alcohol screening for hospitalized patients. This directive underscores the need for all nurses in all settings to have the knowledge and skills to address the use of alcohol and other drugs that places a person at risk for harm to self or others.

THE ADDICTION NURSE

The *Scope and Standards of Addictions Nursing Practice* relays that the addiction nurse possesses knowledge of the fundamental biologic, behavioral, environmental, psychological, social, cultural, and spiritual aspects of human responses to the use of substances and engagement in behaviors that can lead to substance use disorders. The competencies for each standard are identified for the RN specializing in addiction and the advanced practice or graduate-level addiction nurse. The highest standards of addiction practice are reflected by the Certified Addictions Registered Nurse (CARN) and the graduate-level certification (CARN-AP).

ADDICTION NURSING WORKFORCE

The International Nurses Society on Addictions (IntNSA) is a specialty professional organization for nurses engaged in addiction nursing practice. The stated mission of the organization is "to advance excellence in nursing care for the prevention and treatment of addiction for diverse populations across all practice settings through advocacy, collaboration, education, research and policy development." The official journal of IntNSA is the *Journal of Addictions Nursing*, an international peer-reviewed quarterly publication. IntNSA also publishes the *Core Curriculum of Addiction Nursing*, a comprehensive overview of the specialty intended for clinicians, educators, and researchers, and, in conjunction with the American Nurses Association, the *Scope and Standards of Addictions Nursing Practice*.

As substance use–related knowledge and competency has been increasingly sought after by nurses, special interest groups are emerging and expanding. For example, the Addictions Council of the American Psychiatric Nurses Association advocates for comprehensive, evidence-based interventions for substance use and substance use disorders that are patient centered, population focused, and delivered in a continuum of care, from prevention to recovery. Since its inauguration in 1997, the Expert Panel on Psychiatric, Mental Health and Substance Abuse has undertaken policy-related initiatives to improve the public's mental health and the delivery of high-quality mental/behavioral healthcare, and to inform policy makers about nursing's contributions to mental/behavioral healthcare. One such policy publication relates to removing barriers to increase the use of SBIRT for reducing the risks associated with alcohol.

In conjunction with developing the knowledge and skills of all nurses across all healthcare settings and specialty areas is the need to build the nursing workforce in the specialty of addiction nursing. To meet the demands across the spectrum of care related to substance use, the need for nurses certified at the generalist or advanced practice level in addiction nursing is growing. For example, to meet the American College of Surgeons' and Joint Commission standards, hospitals need nurses with the specialty background to implement and evaluate these programs and provide the needed training. Nurses are acquiring a stronger voice in the field of addiction at the state and national levels through the leadership of addiction nursing. To strengthen this voice, developing educational programs at the advanced practice level in schools of nursing should be a priority.

KEY POINTS

1. Nursing standards of practice and associated competencies are defined for the generalist and advanced practice levels.
2. All nurses should have generalist competencies related to the continuum of substance use, from at-risk use to substance use disorder.
3. Nurses across all levels are instrumental in addressing the global burden of disease associated with alcohol and other drug use.
4. Holding the CARN or the CARN-AP certifications demonstrates a commitment to advancing one's knowledge and skills related to the continuum of substance use.

REVIEW QUESTIONS

1. Nurse educators engaged in designing, implementing, and evaluating substance use–related curricula:
   A. must have federal funding support to do so.
   B. can utilize or tailor existing curricular models.
   C. should integrate all content into the psychiatric mental health course.
   D. should focus exclusively on substance use disorders.

2. Which US legislation lifted the restriction on nurse practitioners to prescribe buprenorphine?
   A. The Harrison Narcotic Act
   B. The Substance Abuse and Mental Health Services Act
   C. The Comprehensive Addiction and Recovery Act
   D. Proposition 215

3. The set of clinical strategies, screening, brief intervention, and referral to treatment can be *only* delivered by:
   A. healthcare providers with the skills to do so.
   B. advanced practice nurses with the skills to do so.
   C. registered nurses with the skills to do so.
   D. all of the above.

ANSWERS

1. **B**
2. **C**
3. **D**

SUGGESTED READINGS

American Nurses Association. *Addictions Nursing: Scope and Standards of Practice.* Silver Spring, MD: Author, 2013.

Finnell DS, Savage CL, Hansen BR, et al. Integrating substance use content in an "overcrowded" nursing curriculum. *Nurse Educ.* 2018;43(3):128-131.

Fioravanti MA, Hagle H, Puskar K, et al. Creative learning through the use of simulation to teach nursing students screening, brief intervention, and referral to treatment for alcohol and other drug use in a culturally competent manner. *J Transcult Nurs.* 2018;29(4):387-394.

Puskar K, Kane I, Lee H, et al. Interprofessional Screening, Brief Intervention, and Referral to Treatment (SBIRT) education for registered nurses and behavioral health professionals. *Issues Ment Health Nurs.* 2016;37(9):682-687.

Savage CL, Daniels J, Johnson JA, et al. The inclusion of substance use-related content in advanced practice registered nurse curricula. *J Prof Nurs.* 2018;34(3):217-220.

36 International Perspectives on Addiction Management

Summary by Annie Levesque

Based on THE ASAM PRINCIPLES OF ADDICTION MEDICINE, 6th edition chapter by Nady el-Guebaly, Vladimir Poznyak, and Gilberto Gerra

International efforts to reduce the health and social burden attributable to psychoactive substance use are gaining momentum. In recent years, more emphasis has been placed on public health measures, including prevention and treatment of substance use disorder (SUD). This chapter focuses on different topics relevant to the field of addiction medicine internationally, including (1) global data about psychoactive substance use; (2) international policy frameworks for psychoactive substances; (3) the role of the United Nations (UN) system, including the World Health Organization (WHO) and the United Nations Office on Drugs and Crime (UNODC); and (4) the different international medical organizations addressing public health aspects of substances use.

WORLDWIDE PREVALENCE OF PSYCHOACTIVE SUBSTANCE USE AND SUBSTANCE USE DISORDERS

Alcohol is the most widely used psychoactive substance, with about 2.6 billion people using alcohol beverages worldwide. According to WHO estimates, the number of people with harmful use of alcohol or alcohol dependence as defined by the *Diagnostic and Statistical Manual of Mental Disorders* (4th edition, text revision; *DSM-IV-TR*) reached 283 million worldwide in 2010. Nicotine is the second most widely used psychoactive substance, with greater than 1 billion people using tobacco products worldwide. Based on the 2016 UNODC's World Drug Report, around 247 million people have used a psychoactive drug other than alcohol or tobacco at least once in 2014, and 29 million of them fulfilled the criteria for an SUD. Cannabis was the most widely used drug, followed by amphetamine-type stimulants, "ecstasy," opioids, and cocaine.

UNODC estimates indicate more than 200,000 drug-related deaths in 2014, at least one third of which were attributable to overdose, mostly from opioids. Other significant health consequences of substance use include HIV and hepatitis C infections that can result from sharing of contaminated injection equipment among people who inject drugs (PWID). Globally, there are approximately 13.1 million PWID, and >10% of all HIV infections result from sharing contaminated injection paraphernalia.

INTERNATIONAL POLICY FRAMEWORKS FOR PSYCHOACTIVE SUBSTANCES

All current international policy frameworks for psychoactive substances were negotiated and concluded under the auspices of the UN. The framework of the present international drug control system is based on the three landmark conventions: (1) the Single Convention on Narcotic Drugs of 1961 (as amended by the 1972 Protocol), (2) the Convention on Psychotropic Substances of 1971, and (3) the UN Convention Against Illicit Traffic in Narcotic Drugs and Psychotropic Substances of 1988. These conventions provide the international legal basis for regulating the supply and the demand for a wide range of psychoactive drugs with the objective to ensure their availability for medical and scientific purposes only.

Particularly relevant to addiction medicine, these conventions specify that signatory countries are required to do the following:

- Take all practicable measures for the prevention, identification, treatment, education, aftercare, rehabilitation, and social reintegration of people who use drugs.
- Promote the training of personnel involved in delivering these interventions and facilitate an understanding of the problems of unhealthy drug use among professionals and in the general public.

- Provide treatment, education, aftercare, rehabilitation, and social reintegration either as an alternative or as an addition to criminal conviction for drug offenses.
- Promote harm reduction measures, including measures that may decrease the sharing of needles among PWID.
- Treatment programs that include agonist medications and maintenance treatment do not breach current treaties.

The WHO Framework Convention for Tobacco Control (FCTC) entered into force in 2005 and has been ratified by 180 countries to date. WHO FCTC advocates for six effective tobacco control policies: (1) raising taxes and prices; (2) banning advertising, promotion, and sponsorship; (3) protecting people from secondhand smoke; (4) warning everyone about the dangers of tobacco; (5) offering help to people who want to quit; and (6) carefully monitoring the epidemic and prevention policies.

Alcohol is the only commonly used psychoactive substance with significant potential for unhealthy use that is not currently covered by a legally binding international treaty. As an alternative, a global strategy to reduce the harmful use of alcohol, a nonbinding global policy framework, was endorsed by the World Health Assembly in 2010. This framework promotes increased access to affordable and effective preventive and treatment services for individuals and families affected by harmful alcohol use.

Overall, the international policy frameworks for psychoactive substance use have a substantial impact on the type of addiction services delivered in different jurisdictions. In recent years, drug control treaties have shifted from measures promoting predominantly supply reduction toward measures aimed at promoting prevention, treatment, and social reintegration of people with SUDs. Health professionals, including addiction medicine specialists, have an important role to play in supporting the development and the implementation of such policies.

THE ROLE OF WHO AND THE UNODC

WHO is a directing and coordinating authority for health within the UN system, whereas the UNODC is the leading UN entity for dealing with drug problems. Prevention and management of substance use and SUDs are integral components of both organizations' activities.

The UNODC-WHO Program on Drug Dependence Treatment and Care is a collaboration between the two organizations with the overall goal of promoting and supporting worldwide strategies and interventions to reduce the health and social burden caused by substance use and SUDs. This collaboration resulted in the development and worldwide dissemination of several publications addressing key topics relevant to addiction medicine, including opioid overdose prevention, standards for the treatment of SUDs, discussions on the interaction between health and the criminal justice systems, and recommendations on how to approach substance use in the education sector.

UNODC Addiction Medicine Initiatives

The UNODC initiatives to support member states in improving their drug prevention and treatment systems include the following:

- *Family skills training*: The UNODC has published guidelines on how to implement family-based prevention of SUDs. The organization has piloted evidence-based family skills training programs in more than 20 countries, targeting the behavior of children, parents, and families to strengthen protective factors and to prevent substance use.
- *The International Standards of Drug Use Prevention* is a 2013 publication based on a systematic review of evidence on SUD prevention that was conducted in an effort to support the healthy and safe development of children and youth.
- *Treatnet* is a large UNODC program offering guidance and training to support the improvement of addiction treatment policies worldwide. Treatnet has been active in more than 40 countries and has published important resources such as the Treatnet Training Package and "From Coercion to Cohesion," a publication promoting evidence-based, ethical, and volunteer treatment of SUDs as an alternative to involuntary confinement of substance users in prisons or in treatment centers.

WHO Addiction Medicine Initiatives

One of the core functions of WHO is to monitor and assess international health situations and trends. Initiatives of WHO regarding SUDs include the following:

- *Global Burden of Disease (GBD) Study*: This WHO conducted study was implemented to quantify the burden of different diseases and health conditions. Estimates of mortality and of disease burden expressed in disability-adjusted life years lost provided a better understanding of the impact of psychoactive substance use on populations' health.

- *The Global Information System on Alcohol and Health (GISAH)* is a tool that collects, compiles, analyzes, and disseminates data regarding a wide range of alcohol-related health indicators globally.
- *The ATLAS on Substance Use (ATLAS-SU)* project was implemented to monitor available resources for the prevention and treatment of SUDs at a global level.
- *Screening and brief intervention:* WHO has been advocating for years for the implementation of screening and brief intervention procedures for hazardous and harmful use of alcohol using the Alcohol Use Disorders Identification Test (AUDIT), which was found to be effective and inexpensive. In line with the AUDIT-based screening and brief interventions for alcohol problems, WHO has developed the Alcohol, Smoking and Substance Involvement Screening Test (ASSIST), a screening instrument for hazardous and harmful use of any psychoactive substance.
- *The Mental Health Gap Action Program Intervention Guide (mhGAP)* was developed and disseminated in many countries with the objective to promote the identification and management of mental illness, neurologic problems, and SUDs in primary healthcare and other nonspecialized settings.
- *Neurobiological basis of SUD:* WHO produced the report "Neuroscience of Psychoactive Substance Use and Dependence," which provides an overview of the biological factors related to SUDs. The concept of SUD as a neurobiological disorder is also reflected in the ongoing work of WHO on a new revision of the *International Statistical Classification of Diseases and Related Health Problems.*

In addition to the aforementioned initiatives, WHO has also produced a number of guidelines on different topics related to addiction medicine, including pharmacotherapy for opioid use disorder, management of substance use in pregnancy, and management of opioid overdose.

THE EVOLVING ROLE OF INTERNATIONAL MEDICAL ASSOCIATIONS

The founding of international medical associations created opportunities for addressing issues of global concern by medical professionals. International medical associations help bolster the perception of addiction as a treatable disease by disseminating information about empirically based treatment practices. The stigma associated with addiction often influences addiction care providers. Medical associations can help battle the stigma that exists both in the general public and in the medical profession.

The World Medical Association has several position statements in relation to the use of substances, and the World Psychiatric Association currently includes sections on both addiction psychiatry and dual disorders. The International Society of Addiction Medicine (ISAM) was founded in the late 1990s. Currently, ISAM has committed itself to advancing knowledge about addiction as a treatable disease, advocating for the major role of physicians worldwide in addiction management, enhancing the credibility of their role, and developing educational activities including consensus guidelines. ISAM has a membership spanning 73 countries.

The development of a medical field with specialized expertise must be accompanied by an accreditation process. Since 2005, an International Certification in Addiction Medicine with an international editorial board has been held with applicants from 15 countries and 119 certifications so far.

Policies addressing the use of various substances including alcohol and tobacco vary between countries. The management of opioid use disorder may, arguably, arouse the most polarizing divide among national drug policies. The support or denial of the need for opioid agonist therapy varies widely from country to country and even from region to region within countries. Organizations like ISAM must strive to promote empirically based practices while at the same time accounting for local culture and economic resources. One of the goals of international collaborations and structures is to reduce the use of ineffective practices and policies as well as to promote evidence-based solutions.

CONCLUSIONS

The complementary efforts of major international institutions such as WHO and the UNODC supported by research funding organizations and by international associations of physicians such as the World Medical Association, World Psychiatric Association, and ISAM all contribute to increasing the evidence-based interventions required to counteract the global public health consequences of psychoactive substances use.

KEY POINTS

1. Alcohol followed by nicotine are the most widely used psychoactive substances worldwide.
2. International policy frameworks regarding psychoactive substances were elaborated under the auspices of the UN.
3. Within the UN system, both WHO and UNODC implemented initiatives supporting the prevention and management of SUD.
4. The World Medical Association, the World Psychiatric Association and the International Society of Addiction Medicine are medical societies addressing addiction medicine related issues on a global level.

REVIEW QUESTIONS

1. Signatory countries to the current international conventions for psychoactive substances are required to promote the following *except*:
    A. measures for the prevention, identification, treatment, and rehabilitation of drug users.
    B. measures that reduce the harm associated with drug use.
    C. programs that include agonist medications and maintenance treatment.
    D. alternatives to "needle exchange programs."

2. Which psychoactive substance is the most widely used worldwide?
    A. Tobacco
    B. Cannabis
    C. Alcohol
    D. Amphetamine-type stimulants

3. Which of the following measures is *not* one of the most effective tobacco control policies advocated by WHO?
    A. Raising taxes and prices
    B. Controlling advertisements to youth in particular
    C. Protecting people from secondhand smoke
    D. Offering help to people who want to quit

ANSWERS

1. **D.** Governments need to adopt measures to reduce the sharing of hypodermic needles to limit the spread of HIV and hepatitis C.
2. **C.** Worldwide, 2.6 billion people use alcoholic beverages, followed by 1 billion for tobacco. Additionally, 247 million people use other psychoactive substances.
3. **B.** WHO advocates for a ban on advertisements for all age groups.

SUGGESTED READINGS

Degenhardt L, Whiteford HA, Ferrari AJ, et al. Global burden of disease attributable to illicit drug use and dependence: findings from the Global Burden of Disease Study 2010. *Lancet.* 2013;382(9904):1564-1574.

United Nations Office on Drugs and Crime. *World Drug Report 2016.* Vienna, Austria: United Nations Office on Drugs and Crime, 2016.

WHO ASSIST Working Group. The Alcohol, Smoking and Substance Involvement Screening Test (ASSIST): development, reliability and feasibility. *Addiction.* 2002;97(9):1183-1194.

World Health Organization. *Global Status Report on Alcohol and Health 2014.* Geneva, Switzerland: World Health Organization, 2014.

World Health Organization. *WHO Framework Convention on Tobacco Control.* Geneva, Switzerland: World Health Organization, 2003.

Special Issues
in Addiction

37 Prescription Medications: Nonmedical Use, Use Disorders, and Public Health Consequences

Summary by Jack B. Stein, Wilson M. Compton, Eric M. Wargo, and Christopher M. Jones

Based on THE ASAM PRINCIPLES OF ADDICTION MEDICINE, 6th edition chapter by Wilson M. Compton, Christopher M. Jones, Maureen P. Boyle, and Eric M. Wargo

Use of pharmaceuticals in a manner or for a purpose not directed by a physician (ie, nonmedical use or misuse) has been a problem as long as such products have existed, and the current patterns in the United States represent the newest iteration. The primary categories of medications misused are opioids, stimulants, and sedatives–hypnotics (Fig. 37-1). Prescription opioid misuse has been implicated as a major component in the nearly fourfold increase in drug overdose deaths in the United States between 2000 and 2016. Most recent data show that in 2016, drug overdose deaths stood at a record 63,632 persons (Fig. 37-2), with 17,087 of these deaths attributed to opioid analgesics.

Nonmedical use of prescription drugs presents unusual difficulties for clinicians for two reasons. First, the medical system itself is the origin of the substances that are misused in most cases. Second, boundaries between therapeutic use, nonmedical use, and a use disorder or addiction can be quite vague. (A prescription drug use disorder is a medical illness that occurs when ongoing nonmedical use of prescription drugs leads to clinically and functionally significant impairment, such as health problems, disability, and failure to meet major responsibilities at work, school, or home; a moderate-to-severe substance use disorder is commonly called an addiction.) Overall, prescribers are in a unique situation of having to optimize medication dosage to minimize symptoms of the disease being treated while also monitoring their prescribing practices to reduce, as much as possible, the risk of nonmedical use and addiction in their patients as well as diversion to the larger community.

EPIDEMIOLOGY OF NONMEDICAL USE OF PRESCRIPTION MEDICATIONS

Approximately 6.9% or 18.7 million persons in the United States aged 12 years or older (see Fig. 37-1) reported past-year nonmedical use of prescription drugs in 2016. Analgesics were the most common class of medication used nonmedically, followed by sedatives–hypnotics and stimulants. Hydrocodone and oxycodone are the most commonly reported opioids used nonmedically, but virtually all the opioids, especially higher potency agents such as oxymorphone, hydromorphone, and fentanyl (both prescription and illicitly manufactured versions), are reported frequently by treatment-seeking populations.

Nonmedical use of prescription drugs was most prevalent in young adults (aged 18 to 25 years), followed by adolescents (aged 12 to 17 years), and adults (aged 26 years and older). Nearly 70% of high school seniors who use prescription drugs nonmedically also reported use of alcohol, marijuana, and other substances, suggesting that prescription drug misuse is a potential indicator for broader substance use problems in this population. In 2016, over 2.5 million Americans met the criteria for a prescription drug use disorder, including over 1.75 million due to opioid analgesics, 618,000 due

Conflict of Interest Disclosures: Compton reports ownership of stock in General Electric Co., 3M Co., and Pfizer Inc., unrelated to the submitted work. Other authors report no conflicts to disclose.

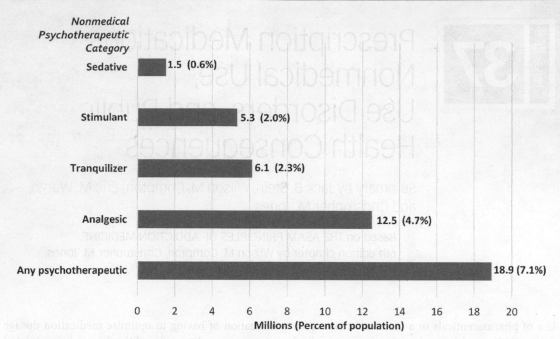

Figure 37-1. Past-year nonmedical use of prescription psychotherapeutics among US persons aged 12 years and older, 2016. (Source: https://www.samhsa.gov/data/sites/default/files/NSDUH-DetTabs-2016/NSDUH-DetTabs-2016.pdf, accessed November 5, 2018.)

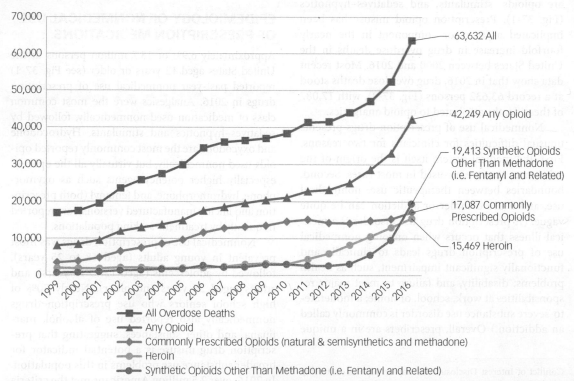

Figure 37-2. Overdose deaths in the United States, 1999 to 2016. (Source: Hedegaard H, Warner M, Miniño AM. Drug overdose deaths in the United States, 1999–2016. NCHS Data Brief, no 294. Hyattsville, MD: National Center for Health Statistics. 2017.)

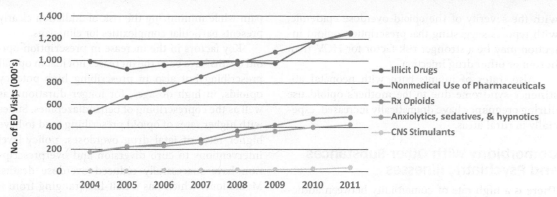

Figure 37-3. Rates of prescription drug-related emergency department visits, 2004 to 2011. (Source: Substance Abuse and Mental Health Services Administration, Drug Abuse Warning Network, 2011: National Estimates of Drug-Related Emergency Department Visits. HHS Publication No. [SMA] 13-4760, DAWN Series D-39. Rockville, MD: Substance Abuse and Mental Health Services Administration, 2013.)

to tranquilizers, 540,000 due to prescription stimulants, and 205,000 due to sedatives.

Prescription drug–related emergency department visits more than doubled between 2004 and 2011, from 535,447 to 1,244,872 (Fig. 37-3). Treatment admissions related to prescription opioids also more than doubled between 2004 and 2014. Rates of overdose mortality associated with prescription opioids (Fig. 37-4) have increased markedly throughout the United States between 1999 and 2016. The coingestion of benzodiazepines with opioids is responsible for an increasing percentage of overdose deaths. More than 53% of overdose deaths involving benzodiazepines also involved prescription opioids, and 33% of prescription opioid overdose deaths involved benzodiazepines in 2016. Interactions between opioids and some

antidepressant medications—specifically, selective serotonin reuptake inhibitors—may also increase the risk for overdose by increasing the risk for serotonin syndrome.

The sharing of needles and syringes by people who misuse prescription opioids via injection has also been associated with increased transmission of infectious diseases including hepatitis C (HCV) and human immunodeficiency virus (HIV), especially among young people in suburban and rural areas. Annual incidence of HCV infection among young people who inject drugs is between 8% and 25%. HCV is roughly ten times more infectious than HIV and lives longer outside of the body, which translates to an increased risk for infection among people who inject drugs. Regional rates of HCV are correlated

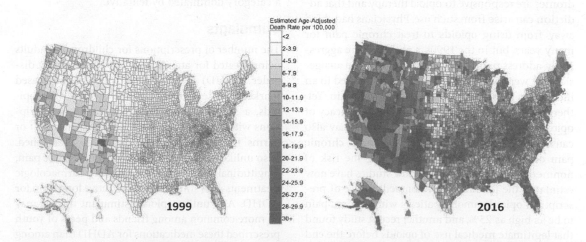

Figure 37-4. Estimated age-adjusted death rates per 100,000 for drug poisoning by county in the United States in 1999 and 2016. (Source: Rossen LM, Bastian B, Warner M, Khan D, Chong Y. Drug poisoning mortality: United States, 1999–2016. National Center for Health Statistics. 2017 [available from: https://www.cdc.gov/nchs/data-visualization /drug-poisoning-mortality/, accessed March 2, 2018].)

with the severity of the opioid overdose epidemic, with reports suggesting that prescription opioid injection may be a stronger risk factor for HCV than heroin or other drug injection.

Also, rates of infants born with neonatal abstinence syndrome due to the mother's opioid use during pregnancy have dramatically increased, especially in rural areas.

Comorbidity With Other Substances and Psychiatric Illnesses

There is a high rate of comorbidity between addictive disorders and psychiatric disorders. Abuse and/or dependence on one type of prescription drug (especially an opioid), as defined by the *Diagnostic and Statistical Manual of Mental Disorders,* 4th edition, text revision (*DSM-IV-TR*) is highly predictive of a clinically significant drug use disorder related to another prescription drug, to an illicit drug, and/or to alcohol. Common mental health disorders and unhealthy drug use are associated with nonmedical use of prescription drugs. Clinicians need to carefully assess for co-occurring mental health and substance use disorders whenever a patient is found to be misusing prescription drugs.

THE MAJOR CLASSES OF NONMEDICALLY USED PRESCRIPTION MEDICATIONS

Opioids (Analgesics)

Chronic pain is highly prevalent in the United States, and opioids are a common treatment despite long-standing recognition that not all pain syndromes are responsive to opioid therapy and that addiction can arise from such use. Physicians had shied away from using opioids to treat chronic pain for many years, but in the 1990s, a push to more aggressively address pain, coupled with new opioid analgesics that were promised to be less addictive, led to an increase in prescribing opioids for chronic pain. Yet, there remains a dearth of evidence on the efficacy of opioids for treating chronic pain; opioids may also cause hyperalgesia and exacerbate some chronic pain conditions, in addition to raising the risk of nonmedical use or addiction. Some studies have now estimated the prevalence of nonmedical use of prescription opioids among patients with chronic pain to be as high as 25%, and another recent study found that legitimate medical use of opioids before the end of high school was independently associated with future misuse of opioids. However, patients with severe debilitating pain may be undertreated due to concerns about addiction. The difficulty of treating pain while minimizing the risk of addiction clearly presents particular complexities for clinicians.

Key factors in the increase in prescription opioid deaths have been the increases not just in opioid prescribing but also in prescribing high-potency opioids, in high dosages, for longer durations, as well as the coprescribing of benzodiazepines. States with higher rates of opioid prescribing tend to have higher rates of fatal drug overdoses; policy-level interventions to curb diversion and overprescription have successfully reduced overdose deaths. Methadone, which has a half-life (ranging from 8 to 59 hours) substantially longer than the duration of its analgesic effects (4 to 8 hours), has been disproportionately involved in overdose mortalities in some states, and reductions in prescribing methadone for pain have led to decreased diversion and overdose deaths.

The availability of high-purity, low-cost heroin has driven a transition to heroin use among a subset of people who misuse prescription opioids, with a transition rate of about 1% to 3% per year. Heroin initiation is predicted by more frequent nonmedical use of prescription opioids, the presence of a prescription opioid use disorder, injecting prescription drugs, and polysubstance use.

Heightening the urgency of addressing this problem is the recent increase in the use of illicitly produced fentanyl, a synthetic opioid 50 to 100 times more potent than morphine that is commonly mixed with heroin or sold alone in powder form or as counterfeit tablets. Between 2013 and 2016, there was a 525% increase in overdose deaths involving synthetic opioids other than methadone, a category dominated by fentanyl.

Stimulants

The number of prescriptions for children and adults being treated for attention deficit hyperactivity disorder (ADHD) in the United States has increased markedly since 1990, but unlike the case with opioids, a specific association of increasing prescriptions with changes in rates of nonmedical use of or harms from stimulants has not been established. Also unlike opioids in the treatment of chronic pain, longitudinal studies have shown that pharmacologic treatments with stimulants are effective long term for ADHD. And unlike opioids, stimulant misuse may be more common among friends and peers of youth prescribed these medications for ADHD than among those with a prescription. Adolescent patients with ADHD show lower rates of stimulant misuse than their peers but still may be part of a sharing or diversion pathway for friends and classmates.

National data show that stimulants are among the only substances used more by college students than by their same-age peers who do not attend college. The reasons for using stimulant medication nonmedically in college include weight loss, improving attention, partying, reducing hyperactivity, and improving grades. Because these are prescription substances, they are perceived by students to be "safe." Further, they are falsely perceived as enhancing academic performance; the opposite is actually found when they are used nonmedically.

Sedatives–Hypnotics

Prescription sedatives–hypnotics, including older agents such as the barbiturates and chloral hydrate and the benzodiazepines available since the 1960s, pose a high risk for misuse and addiction. Some (eg, methaqualone, the short-acting barbiturates) are no longer accepted as standards of care except in limited circumstances; newer agents like zolpidem and zopiclone, although somewhat safer, have also been associated with nonmedical use. Increases in the prescribing of benzodiazepines may account for increases in the nonmedical use of these drugs.

Although benzodiazepines alone do not typically cause overdoses, they may be lethal when combined with other respiratory depressants, including alcohol or opioids. A large study of nonfatal opioid overdoses found that 56% of patients obtained a benzodiazepine prescription in the 90 days before the overdose.

Discontinuation of sedatives should be medically monitored because withdrawal from these medications can pose significant health risks, including seizures.

EVIDENCE-BASED PREVENTION AND HARM REDUCTION STRATEGIES

Prevention Programs

Broad-based prevention approaches, including universal family-based interventions such as the Strengthening Families Program: For Parents and Youth 10–14, a family-based program for younger adolescents, and PROSPER (Promoting School–Community–University Partnerships to Enhance Resilience), a system for delivering evidence-based interventions during grades 6 and 7, have been demonstrated to reduce nonmedical use of prescription drugs. These approaches target families as key agents to address a range of adolescent-onset risk behaviors. The 2016 *Surgeon General's Report on Alcohol, Drugs, and Health* highlights the need to increase the implementation of evidence-based prevention practices both in the community and throughout healthcare systems.

Prescriber Education

In March 2016, the Centers for Disease Control and Prevention released a Guideline for Prescribing Opioids for Chronic Pain (see Table 37-1 for a summary of recommendations). This guideline provides recommendations to limit short-term opioid prescriptions and summarizes recent research on the use of opioids in the treatment of chronic pain. Opioid analgesic metabolism varies markedly between individuals, however; therefore, doses should be adjusted based on individual patient response. In addition, although opioid equivalency tables enable general comparison of the potency of various opioids, there is significant interindividual variation. Therefore, prescribers should exercise caution with initial dosing when shifting from one opioid to another.

Prescription Drug Monitoring Programs

Prescription drug monitoring programs (PDMPs) have been implemented in almost every US state to identify risky prescribing patterns and to alert prescribers, pharmacists, and, in some states, law enforcement officials to potential problems with the prescribing and use of controlled substances. PDMP data can inform clinicians about other controlled substances that may have been prescribed to their patients and thereby change prescribing practices when these systems are implemented fully. States with PDMPs that monitored all drug schedules (II through IV) and update data at least weekly had lower opioid-related overdose death rates compared to other states with less robust PDMPs.

Naloxone

Naloxone can safely and quickly reverse an opioid-induced coma or respiratory depression because of its rapid action as a μ-opioid receptor antagonist. Increasing ready access to naloxone—for instance, through opioid overdose education and naloxone distribution—shows promise in reducing overdose mortality among individuals who use heroin and in communities hard hit by overdoses. Coprescribing naloxone self-injection kits or nasal spray to persons receiving high-dose opioids for chronic pain is associated with a reduced risk of emergency department treatment for opioid complications.

However, current formulations of naloxone may not be sufficient to reverse an overdose on fentanyl or other highly potent opioids; multiple doses may

TABLE 37-1	Summary of Centers for Disease Control and Prevention's Guideline for Prescribing Opioids for Chronic Pain

When Prescribing Opioid Pain Relievers for Acute Pain:

- Providers should prescribe the lowest effective dose possible.
- Providers should prescribe no greater quantity than needed for the expected duration of pain severe enough to require opioid pain relievers (3 or fewer days will usually be sufficient).

When Prescribing Opioid Pain Relievers for Chronic Pain:

- Nonopioid therapies are preferred for chronic pain.
- If opioids are prescribed, they should be used in combination with nonopioid therapy such as cognitive–behavioral therapy, exercise therapy, and/or nonopioid pharmacologic therapy such as NSAIDs and acetaminophen; avoid concurrent prescribing of other opioids and benzodiazepines if possible.
- Prior to beginning prescription opioid therapy, establish treatment goals and discuss risks and realistic benefits.
- Reassess risks and benefits throughout treatment; only continue prescription opioids if pain and functioning meaningfully improve.
- Use PDMPs to determine whether patients are using other opioids.

Prescription Opioid Selection, Dosage, and Follow-Up:

- Prescribe immediate-release opioids instead of long-acting/extended-release opioids.
- Start low and go slow: Prescribe opioids with the lowest possible effective dose; reassess individual benefits and risks when considering increasing dosage to ≥50 MME/day; avoid increasing dosage to ≥90 MME/day unless justified.
- Evaluate benefits and harms within 1 to 4 weeks of starting opioid therapy for chronic pain or after dose escalation and discuss considerations for discontinuation of opioid therapy.

Assessing Risk and Addressing Harms of Opioid Use:

- Prior to beginning opioid therapy and periodically during therapy, evaluate risk factors for opioid-related harms. Risk factors include sleep-disordered breathing, pregnancy, kidney disease, ≥65 years of age, mental health conditions, substance use disorder, or prior nonfatal overdose.
- Incorporate strategies to mitigate risk; offer naloxone when patient is at increased risk of opioid overdose.
- Ask patients about their drug and alcohol use with a validated screening tool such as the single-question screener, the Drug Abuse Screening Test (DAST), or the Alcohol Use Disorders Identification Test (AUDIT).
- Use urine drug test screening to test for concurrent illicit drug use.
- Offer evidence-based treatment for opioid use disorders.

NSAID, nonsteroidal anti-inflammatory drug; PDMP, prescription drug monitoring program; MME, morphine milligram equivalent.

Source: Dowell D, Haegerich TM, Chou R. CDC Guideline for Prescribing Opioids for Chronic Pain — United States, 2016. MMWR Recomm Rep 2016;65(No. RR-1):1–49.

be needed. Patients should be monitored for up to 12 hours after resuscitation. More research is needed to develop new naloxone formulations tailored to higher potency opioids and to find the best ways to link persons who have been resuscitated to substance use treatment.

Syringe Services Programs

One policy that has repeatedly been proven effective for reducing the spread of infectious diseases is access to sterile syringes and other injection equipment. In addition to reducing infectious disease transmission, syringe services programs also offer counseling services, HIV testing, and referral to substance use disorder treatment services as well as safe disposal of injection equipment.

HIV Prevention and Treatment

The seek, test, treat, and retain model of care, also known as the HIV care continuum, involves reaching out to high-risk, hard-to-reach populations who use substances who have not been recently tested for HIV; engaging them in HIV testing; initiating, monitoring, and maintaining combined antiretroviral therapy for those who test positive; and retaining patients in care. Implementation of the seek, test, treat, and retain model may decrease the rate of HIV transmission by more than half, both by decreasing viral load and by increasing access to medical care.

Prescription Take-Back Programs

Major sources for nonmedically used prescription opioids are family and friends who have their own prescriptions. Take-back programs show promise in removing unwanted, common nonmedically used medications from people's medicine cabinets, where they may not only remain available for nonmedical use by the intended recipient but may also be found and taken by family members and visitors. They also serve as an opportunity to amplify public messages about appropriate use, storage, and disposal of medications.

EVIDENCE-BASED TREATMENT FOR PRESCRIPTION MEDICATION USE DISORDERS

The class of medication being used (eg, opioid, stimulant, sedative–hypnotic) determines the appropriate type of care for an individual with a prescription drug use disorder. The opioid-agonist medication methadone and the opioid–partial agonist medication buprenorphine are effective for the treatment of all opioid use disorders and have been shown to decrease opioid use, opioid overdose deaths, infectious disease transmission, and justice system involvement, while increasing social functioning and retention in treatment. The extended-release version of the opioid-antagonist medication, naltrexone, which blocks opioid interaction with the μ-opioid opioid receptor but does not reduce cravings or withdrawal symptoms, also has demonstrated efficacy at reducing illicit opioid use. In recent trials, it has performed as well as buprenorphine once patients could overcome the initial "detox hurdle" necessary for induction. Methadone or buprenorphine may be used to manage opioid use during pregnancy; some research suggests buprenorphine may decrease the length of the hospital stay of infants with neonatal abstinence syndrome compared to methadone. The safety of naltrexone in pregnancy requires study. Just as for heroin use disorder, tapers and drug-free approaches for prescription opioid use disorder show a significant risk of relapse. Implementing medication-assisted opioid addiction treatment in correctional systems has been shown to dramatically reduce overdose deaths following release. Although there are no medications currently approved by the US Food and Drug Administration to treat stimulant or sedative use disorders, these can be treated with the same behavioral therapies used for other substance use disorders.

CONCLUSION

When it comes to the nonmedical use of prescription drugs, physicians find themselves on the horns of a dilemma. They are the principal "supply" of these substances, while also being the first line of defense against their diversion and nonmedical use. These complexities require the exercise of caution when prescribing in addition to compassion. Physicians need to be knowledgeable about the conditions addressed by these medications (eg, pain, anxiety, ADHD, withdrawal) as well as the potential of these medications to lead to substance use disorders both in their patients and in the wider community. This requires physicians to keep up to date with the latest prescribing guidelines and with the current and evolving body of evidence-based strategies to prevent and treat addiction.

ACKNOWLEDGMENTS

This work was jointly sponsored by the National Institute on Drug Abuse, a component of the National Institutes of Health, and the Substance Abuse and Mental Health Services Administration, US Department of Health and Human Services. The sponsors supported the authors who were responsible for preparation, review, and approval of the manuscript and the decision to submit the manuscript for publication. The sponsors had no role in the design and conduct of the study; in the collection, management, analysis, and interpretation of data; in the preparation and review of the manuscript; or in the decision to submit the manuscript for publication. The sponsors reviewed and approved the manuscript.

REVIEW QUESTIONS

1. What is the most common class of nonmedically used medications?
   A. Sedatives–hypnotics
   B. Stimulants
   C. Opioid analgesics

2. Regional rates of _____ are correlated with the severity of the opioid overdose epidemic.
   A. human immunodeficiency virus (HIV)
   B. hepatitis C virus (HCV)
   C. human papilloma virus (HPV)

3. Fentanyl is _____ times more potent than morphine.
   A. 10 to 20
   B. 25 to 50
   C. 50 to 100

4. Which of the following has been demonstrated to be useful in randomized studies for use to manage opioid use disorder during pregnancy?
   A. Methadone
   B. Buprenorphine
   C. Naltrexone
   D. A and B only.
   E. A and C only.
   F. A, B, and C.

ANSWERS

1. **C**
2. **B**
3. **C**
4. **D**

SUGGESTED READINGS

Blanco C, Compton WM, Han B, Jones CM, Johnson K. Prevalence and correlates of benzodiazepine use, misuse, and use disorders among adults in the US. *J Clin Psychiatry*. 2018;43:638.

Compton WM, Boyle M, Wargo E. Prescription opioid abuse: problems and responses. *Prev Med*. 2015;80:5-9.

Compton WM, Han B, Blanco C, Johnson K, Jones CM. Correlates of prescription stimulant use, misuse, use disorders, and motivations for misuse among adults in the U.S. *Am J Psychiatry*. 2018;175:741-755.

Han B, Compton WM, Blanco C, et al. Prescription opioid use, misuse, and use disorders in U.S. adults: 2015 National Survey on Drug Use and Health. *Ann Intern Med*. 2017;167(5):293-301.

Special Issues in Treatment: Women

CHAPTER **38**

Summary by Joan E. Zweben

Based on THE ASAM PRINCIPLES OF ADDICTION MEDICINE, 6th edition chapter by Joan E. Zweben

For more than two decades, treatment providers have worked to define and address the unique needs of women. This chapter discusses treatment issues specific to women, including the relationship of drug and alcohol use problems to psychiatric and medical conditions, and reviews new findings on gender-specific treatment.

EPIDEMIOLOGY

Gender Differences With Alcohol and Other Drug Use

Several large-scale epidemiologic studies document gender differences in the use of alcohol and almost all other drugs, with higher rates found in men. However, more recent studies are showing a smaller gender difference for all age groups except adolescents aged 12 to 17 years. With these young people, the gap virtually disappeared for alcohol, marijuana, cocaine, and cigarettes. Stimulants such as cocaine and methamphetamine have a particular appeal for women. Their use is associated with a loss of appetite and desirable weight loss, and the stimulating effects are often initially perceived as alerting and beneficial with all the work and household tasks that confront them. An increasing number of non-Hispanic white women are using opioids, possibly reflecting the changing demographics of the opioid use epidemic.

Common Psychiatric Disorders in Women With Addictive Disorders

Most adults in treatment for addictive disorders have at least one coexisting psychiatric disorder, but the pattern differs for women. Prominent studies have found that women were more likely to have an affective disorder than men (with the exception of mania, for which rates were the same). Women also had a higher lifetime and 12-month prevalence of three or more disorders.

MEDICAL CONSIDERATIONS

Alcohol

The influence of alcohol on women's health has been much more carefully studied than other substances. When women drink heavily or even moderately, they are more vulnerable to alcohol-related liver damage, cardiovascular disease, and brain damage. Negative consequences occur at lower levels of consumption and after much shorter periods of drinking. This is referred to as the "telescoped course" in women.

Researchers have explored the mechanisms by which women achieve higher blood alcohol concentrations than men after drinking equivalent amounts of alcohol, even when doses are adjusted for body weight. Women tend to have lower levels of alcohol dehydrogenase and lower volumes of distribution, leading to an increased effect of alcohol from an equivalent exposure in a man. Alcohol consumption raises breast cancer risk even after adjusting for age, family history, and other known dietary and reproductive risk factors. The increased risk appears to be modest and dose related, and the form of alcohol appears to be irrelevant.

Prenatal Alcohol Exposure

Drinking during pregnancy remains a serious concern. Fetal alcohol syndrome encompasses a set of birth defects considered the single leading nonhereditary cause of intellectual disability. Growth deficiencies and the characteristic set of facial traits tend to become less significant over time, but the alcohol-induced damage to the developing brain is enduring. These mental impairments include deficits in general intellectual functioning and specific difficulties with learning, memory, attention, and problem solving, in addition to manifestations in psychosocial arenas. The impairments are dose related and may be evident in children without the distinguishing physical features of fetal alcohol syndrome. The effects of lower levels of alcohol exposure prenatally are still unclear, and thus, the prevailing view is that there is no demonstrated safe level of alcohol consumption during pregnancy.

Drugs

The evidence of gender differences in the effects of drug use is not as extensive at this time as it is for alcohol. Several studies suggest that some women may have greater vulnerability to the effects of cocaine relative to men. Mechanisms including female steroid hormones, estrogen, menstrual cycle phase, and differences in receptor function have all been suggested. The prescription drug epidemic has fueled an upsurge in heroin use as supplies become more expensive or less available. Women constitute a significant segment of new heroin users.

Methadone is considered the gold standard maintenance treatment for pregnant women with an opioid dependence. It is important that the dose be adequate. Higher doses are not associated with increased risks of neonatal abstinence. Likewise, women who are stable on methadone should not be discouraged from breastfeeding.

Buprenorphine is now an option for pregnant women. The Maternal Opioid Treatment Human Experimental Research study demonstrated that buprenorphine is effective and can be used safely. At this time, follow-up data indicate that it does not appear to have negative consequences for the child, and may reduce neonatal hospital time. To avoid in utero exposure to naloxone, buprenorphine alone is usually chosen over the combination buprenorphine/naloxone. Buprenorphine provides the opportunity to expand treatment access in rural areas and other circumstances where methadone is unavailable or unacceptable to the pregnant patient. The overall goal is to reduce early treatment dropout in pregnant women because it is well known that participation in treatment is associated with better maternal and neonatal outcomes. Buprenorphine requires intense medical monitoring, and it is not known how many private medical practices can provide this. Large, definitive randomized controlled trials of buprenorphine in pregnant women have not been conducted.

Domestic Violence

A large number of women are treated in hospital emergency departments for violence-related injuries, usually inflicted by an intimate partner. Women who have been battered report that their general health is fair or poor and that they have needed medical care that they have not received. Chronic headaches, hearing, vision, and concentration problems can reflect neurologic damage, and a host of other stress-related symptoms can manifest. Therefore, psychosocial treatment efforts must integrate good medical care to be fully comprehensive.

Human Immunodeficiency Virus/Acquired Immune Deficiency Syndrome

Acquired immune deficiency syndrome (AIDS) cases are composed of more women than ever before. Complications from human immunodeficiency virus (HIV) infection, AIDS, is the leading cause of death for African American women aged 25 to 34 years. Latinas are also disproportionally affected. Heterosexual sex with a man with HIV is the most common mode of transmission, followed by sharing injection drug needles used by someone with HIV. Similar patterns of increase are also beginning to be apparent in the distribution of reported hepatitis C cases. Condoms remain the major method to reduce sexual transmission of HIV. Women with an addiction are at disadvantage when attempting to practice safer sex and may fear emotional or physical abuse if they insist on safe sex.

Women with an HIV infection also struggle with how to address their health issues and their possible deaths. Women who have given birth to children who are HIV positive have an added layer of anxiety and guilt. All of these women require as much support and counseling as possible.

PSYCHIATRIC DISORDERS

Women have high rates of co-occurring disorders, and it is preferable to address multiple disorders with an integrated approach. Psychotropic medications are increasingly viewed as compatible with recovery, especially when prescribed by physicians who are knowledgeable about addiction.

Anxiety Disorders

Anxiety disorders constitute the most common psychiatric disorders among women, with a total lifetime prevalence of 30.5% and a 12-month prevalence of 22.6%. Women in early recovery will experience heightened distress as they try to cope with situations that they previously relied on alcohol and other drugs to endure, and also as they more clearly see the impact of their self-destructive behaviors. However, overwhelming anxiety is debilitating, interferes with new learning, and contributes to relapse as well as premature dropout. Psychosocial strategies are beneficial for the management of anxiety regardless of whether it is normal or excessive. Fortunately, the first-line medications for anxiety and panic disorders are no longer the benzodiazepines; instead, selective serotonin reuptake inhibitors are utilized. When anxiety symptoms do not resolve with abstinence, a variety of psychosocial interventions can be used, which are selected to address the tasks specific to the woman's stage of recovery.

Benzodiazepines, commonly prescribed for anxiety disorders, can be problematic for those with a personal or family history of addiction. Nonreinforcing alternatives, such as sedating antidepressants or buspirone (BuSpar) for anxiety or trazodone (Desyrel) for insomnia, are recommended. Anticonvulsants, antihypertensives, or the newer atypical neuroleptic medications can also be used.

Posttraumatic stress disorder is the most difficult and complex anxiety disorder to manage. The relationship between female gender and post-traumatic stress disorder is robust across patient populations. Rape and sexual molestation were the most frequently reported "most upsetting event," with childhood parental neglect and childhood physical abuse reported more frequently by women. Participants in addiction treatment have much higher rates of traumatic experiences and posttraumatic stress disorder than the general population. Treatment providers must equip themselves to meet these complex needs to avoid common outcomes such as early dropout and increased difficulty in obtaining positive outcomes from treatment.

Mood Disorders

In assessing for depression, it is important to rule out the direct effects of alcohol, illicit drugs, or medications as well as general medical conditions, such as hypothyroidism, that can lower mood. This is especially true in the identification of mood disorders in pregnant women because these women tend to do worse on drug use outcomes than with other disorders.

Negative mood states that are the direct result of alcohol or illicit drugs generally clear within 2 to 3 weeks, with symptoms of longer duration suggesting an independent mood disorder. A sad or depressed mood is only one of many signs and symptoms of a clinically significant depression and may not be the most prominent feature. Other indications include disturbances in emotional, cognitive, behavioral, or somatic regulations. The mood disturbance itself can include apathy, anxiety, or irritability along with, or instead of, sadness. Not all patients who are clinically depressed feel sad, and many who feel sad are not clinically depressed. Women with mood disorders may have a markedly reduced interest in or capacity for pleasure or enjoyment, making it difficult for them to experience rewards in recovery or to invest in new social relationships with others who do not drink or use drugs.

Eating Disorders

Eating disorders are more prevalent among women with a substance use disorder than in the general population, with bulimia being more common than anorexia. Stimulants and over-the-counter diet preparations are particularly appealing to women seeking to lose or control weight.

There are many possible relationships between substance use and eating disorders. Some patients report that heroin is appealing because it facilitates vomiting. Stimulants are attractive because they make women feel capable and energetic and suppress the appetite. Alcohol can be used to suppress the panic associated with bingeing and vomiting or to quash the shame that follows an episode.

Because secrecy is a feature of both disorders, careful inquiry is important during the initial assessment, and observation by staff members is necessary throughout treatment. A thorough medical evaluation should assess possible problems and be part of a plan for nutritional stabilization, including strategies to stop aberrant eating behaviors, as well as medication planning and discharge planning that actively addresses both disorders. Both cognitive–behavioral approaches and psychotherapy are well supported by evidence to assist in the management of eating disorders.

Borderline Personality Disorder

A misdiagnosis of borderline personality disorder is quite common because of confusion of borderline characteristics with the behaviors exhibited during active alcohol and drug use and early recovery. Persistent characteristics of borderline personality disorder include unstable mood and self-image; unstable, intense interpersonal relationships; extremes of overidealization and devaluation; and marked shifts from baseline to impulsive outbursts, anxiety states, or other extreme moods. Women constitute about 75% of those with the diagnosis.

In summary, the prevalence of co-occurring disorders in women underlines the importance of offering psychiatric services. In addition to education about addiction, programs should include material on co-occurring mental health disorders and how they can influence relapse and recovery.

SPECIAL POPULATIONS

Variations in cultural groups and sexual orientation play important roles in addiction treatment. The use of alcohol and other drugs may be taboo for women; therefore, recognition of their use or seeking treatment for those who do use may be impossible. Those from patriarchal cultures can face strong taboos about disclosing family secrets, especially around interpersonal violence. Many women also fear institutions such as the police, social services, and mental health agencies.

Sexual minorities, especially lesbians, are at particular risk partly because of an extensive use of alcohol and drugs in a segment of the culture. Historically, gay bars were seen as gathering places and safe arenas for self-expression. Clearly, socializing patterns built around bars and drug sharing increase the risk of addiction. Even when problems are recognized, sexual minorities, including women, may avoid treatment if they fear discrimination.

ADDITIONAL TREATMENT ISSUES

Women tend to seek help in medical or mental health settings; thus, it is important to improve diagnosing and referrals to treatment for women with substance use disorders. At this time, it appears that gender is not a significant predictor of outcomes overall, but specific treatment elements improve outcomes for specific groups. Barriers clearly exist, including a lack of pregnancy services and childcare, fear of losing custody, and inadequate services for women with co-occurring disorders. Treatment retention has been shown to improve with the inclusion of children in residential treatment and other key factors.

Management and Retention Issues

The finding that women have high rates of three or more co-occurring disorders has consequences for treatment. It is useful to focus on the most immediate or threatening problems a woman identifies at admission. Thus, women with addictive disorders who are in domestic violence situations are relatively resistant to addressing their alcohol and drug use. They are preoccupied with achieving greater safety and see their alcohol and other drug problems as secondary. Treatment providers need to be willing to start by addressing the problem the woman is most ready to change while cultivating readiness in other areas.

It is generally agreed by providers that women-only programs or activities are an important aspect of effective treatment, particularly those associated with pregnancy and parenting. Women-only programs also were more likely to assist with housing transportation, job training, and practical skills training. These programs also were more likely to be funded through the Medicaid system instead of through fees or private insurance. It appears that gender-specific treatment is also associated with higher rates of continuing care. There is also reason to think that women-only groups tend to foster greater interaction, greater emotional and behavioral expression, and more variability in style than mixed-gender groups. Both Lisa Najavits and Shelly Greenfield have developed evidence-based treatment manuals specifically for women.

Physical and Sexual Abuse and Domestic Violence

Trauma-related difficulties can impair parenting in a variety of ways. Women with histories of childhood trauma can have attachment problems that impact their own parenting. They often lack appropriate role models, leading to reliance on physical punishment, difficulties setting appropriate boundaries, and neglect. Current alcohol and other drug use will exacerbate these vulnerabilities.

Children with battered mothers experience posttraumatic stress reactions themselves. Preschool children are more vulnerable to the effects of domestic violence than older children. The extensive variety and complexity of children's reactions to domestic violence argues for the routine assessment and case management for such families.

Treatment Culture

The male-dominated treatment culture characteristic of some programs is not conducive to meeting women's needs. Female leadership at all levels is important to provide role models.

An emphasis on harsh confrontation is particularly problematic in populations with a high frequency of traumatic experiences. Women with severe psychiatric disorders can decompensate and leave treatment if confrontation is too intense.

Both the National Institute on Drug Abuse and the Center for Substance Abuse Treatment have funded specialized research and treatment demonstration programs focused on women, and these programs have enhanced the development of provider groups committed to improving women's treatment.

Women and the Criminal Justice System

Women constitute the fastest growing segment of the national criminal justice population and yet have the fewest appropriate social services available to them. They are more likely than men to serve time in prison for drug offenses. Half of women reported committing their crimes while under the influence of drugs or alcohol, and about 40% reported using drugs daily before arrest. Women who are incarcerated were overwhelmingly confronted with obstacles such as absent parents, poor education, poverty, drug accessibility, and minimal social resources. Many were victims of childhood sexual or physical abuse and traumatic experiences as adults. They had high rates of depression and other psychiatric disorders and suffer from low self-esteem, addiction, and shame. HIV infection rates in women who are incarcerated are several times higher than those found in the community.

CONCLUSIONS

Biomedical effects of gender differences are far better understood for alcohol than for illicit drugs. Research and treatment funding incentives over the past 20 years have provided a much better understanding of women's treatment needs and preferences. Removing barriers, such as lack of transportation and childcare services, increase women's participation in treatment. Treatment for women must be comprehensive. For the children of women with substance use disorders, attention to physical, social, and emotional states is necessary to reduce the negative effects of their parent's addictive disorders. Programs need to be capable of addressing co-occurring mood and anxiety disorders, and research in the last decade continues to identify effective interventions. Women report that women-only groups and activities and women role models at all levels of decision-making are important to them.

Going forward, it is important to develop and test effective treatment for subpopulations such as those who use prescription drugs, those with eating and substance use disorders, and various ethnic groups. It is important to continue to examine the effective elements in gender-specific and mixed-gender programs, including costs. Finally, it would be useful to be able to identify the characteristics of women who can benefit from mixed- versus single-gender programs.

KEY POINTS

1. There are biomedical and psychosocial gender differences that shape women's treatment needs.
2. It is necessary to recognize epidemiologic patterns and address co-occurring mental health disorders in an integrated treatment approach.
3. It is important to continue to examine the effective elements in gender-specific and mixed-gender programs, including costs.

REVIEW QUESTIONS

1. Recent epidemiologic studies show:
   A. women are less likely to use stimulants.
   B. a smaller age difference for all age groups except adolescents.
   C. older women smoke more marijuana.
   D. younger women drink less alcohol.

2. Which of the following disorders are women more likely to have?
   A. Antisocial personality disorder
   B. Substance use disorder
   C. Affective disorder
   D. Schizophrenia

3. Women-only programs:
   A. have consistently been shown to have better outcomes for women.
   B. should avoid having male staff.
   C. do not exist in the criminal justice system.
   D. are more likely to provide transportation, child care, and job training and assistance with housing.

ANSWERS

1. **B**
2. **C**
3. **D**

SUGGESTED READINGS

Greenfield SF. *Treating Women with Substance Use Disorders: The Women's Recovery Group Manual.* New York: Guilford Press, 2016.

Najavits LM. *A Woman's Addiction Workbook: Your Guide to In-Depth Healing.* Oakland, CA: New Harbinger Publications, 2002.

Najavits LM. *Seeking Safety: A Treatment Manual for PTSD and Substance Abuse.* New York: Guilford Press, 2002.

Substance and Mental Health Services Administration. *Substance Abuse Treatment: Addressing the Specific Needs of Women. Treatment Improvement Protocol (TIP) Series, No. 51.* Rockville, MD: Substance Abuse and Mental Health Services Administration, 2009. DHHS Pub. No. (SMA) 13-4426.

39

Traumatic Brain Injury and Substance Use Disorders

Summary by David L. Pennington and Jennifer Bielenberg

Based on THE ASAM PRINCIPLES OF ADDICTION MEDICINE, 6th edition chapter by David L. Pennington, Tatjana Novakovic-Agopian, and Steven L. Batki

Traumatic brain injury (TBI) is a major cause of death and disability in the United States. The Centers for Disease Control and Prevention estimate that TBIs account for approximately 2.5 million annual hospital emergency department visits in the United States. Costs for TBI hospital care, extended care, and other medical care and services, coupled with indirect costs such as lost productivity, are estimated to exceed $75 billion annually. Those who serve in the military are at significant risk for TBI. Internationally, continuing conflicts have increased the likelihood of exposure to high energy blasts and explosions, resulting in TBIs and mental health problems. Repeated TBIs among athletes in contact sports also increase the risk for the development of chronic traumatic encephalopathy (CTE) and mental health problems.

Mental health comorbidities are common in patients with TBIs and often include substance use disorders (SUDs). There is a growing body of literature indicating that as many as 60% of persons with TBIs have significant problems with alcohol and/or other substances, and existing research suggests the relationship between TBIs and SUDs is bidirectional. Knowing about TBI and the clinical strategies required to address it appropriately is a needed skill set for addiction medicine professionals.

DEFINITION OF TRAUMATIC BRAIN INJURY

A TBI is an injury that disrupts the normal function of the brain caused by a hit, explosive blast, jolt to the head, or a penetrating injury. The US Department of Defense and the US Department of Veterans Affairs have defined TBI as any traumatically induced injury and/or physiologic disruption of brain function that involves new onset or worsening of at least one of the following clinical signs, immediately following the event:

- Any period of **loss of** or a **decreased level of consciousness**;
- Any **loss of memory** for events immediately before or after the injury;
- Any **alteration in mental state** at the time of the injury (eg, confusion, disorientation, slowed thinking);
- **Neurologic deficits** (eg, balance disturbance, change in vision, other sensory alterations, aphasia) that may or may not be transient; and/or
- **Intracranial lesion** secondary to head trauma (excluding other acquired conditions, eg, stroke, tumor).

Classification of Traumatic Brain Injury

Regardless of injury mechanism, TBI severity grade at the time of the injury (mild, moderate, or severe) is determined using four indices and may be supported with neuroimaging findings (Table 39-1).

Diagnosis of Traumatic Brain Injury

Acute-stage injury parameters of loss of consciousness (LOC), posttraumatic amnesia (PTA), and Glasgow Coma Scale (GCS) are strongly predictive of long-term recovery and form the basis for establishing a diagnosis of TBI. In cases of moderate or severe TBI, the diagnosis is readily assessed through history and examination in the emergency medical setting. TBI diagnosis may be complicated in cases of closed head injury, particularly in the case of mild TBI (mTBI). TBI symptoms may be physical (eg, fatigue, headache, vertigo, dizziness, disordered sleep), cognitive (eg, deficits in attention or memory), or emotional (eg, depression, anxiety, affective lability, apathy, other changes in personality) and are commonly referred to as postconcussional disorder or postconcussion syndrome. Behavioral, cognitive, and emotional

TABLE 39-1	Classification of Traumatic Brain Injury[a]		
Severity Index	**Mild TBI/Concussion**	**Moderate TBI**	**Severe TBI**
Neuroimaging Findings	Normal structural imaging	Normal *or* abnormal structural imaging	Normal *or* abnormal structural imaging
Initial Glasgow Coma Scale (GCS)	13-15	9-12	<9
Loss of Consciousness (LOC)	0-30 min	>30 min and <24 h	>24 h
Length of Alteration of Consciousness (AOC)	A moment up to 24 h	AOC >24 h (use other criteria)	
Length of Posttraumatic Amnesia (PTA)	0-1 d	>1 and <7 d	>7 d

[a]US Department of Defense, US Department of Veterans Affairs, and American Congress of Rehabilitation Medicine consensus-based classification of traumatic brain injury (TBI) severity.

symptoms can be nonspecific and therefore must not be used in isolation to establish a TBI diagnosis.

Military Populations

Diagnosis of mTBI in military populations is more complex due to reluctance to report brain injuries for fear of removal from duty, delays between time of TBI and discharge from military service, and because of the unique mechanisms of injury, often including repeated blast exposure. Blast-induced TBI (bTBI) is considered the "signature wound" of modern warfare. Primary blast injury is caused by exposure to a blast wave, a sudden change in atmospheric pressure. Primary blast injury is often accompanied by blunt or penetrating trauma from material propelled by the blast wave (secondary blast injury); by the body being thrown to the ground or against an object (tertiary blast injury); or from other injury mechanisms attributable to the blast such as burns, wounds, broken bones, or breathing toxic fumes (quaternary blast injury). All of these injuries may contribute to symptom development following bTBI and add to the complexity of diagnosis and treatment.

High-Impact Sports

Repeated exposure to primary mTBIs in military veterans and more commonly from repeated mTBIs in contact sport athletes have been associated with the development of a progressive, neurodegenerative disease called chronic traumatic encephalopathy (CTE). Symptoms associated with CTE include disruptions in mood, behavior, cognition, and motor function; typically take 8 to 10 years after repeated exposures to present; and can range in severity from mild to those that produce a parkinsonian-like syndrome. Currently, CTE can be diagnosed only via postmortem examination. Increased attention in the media and medical research has resulted in more studies that may soon provide a pathway for diagnosing CTE in

living patients. Ultimately, prevention may prove to be the most beneficial approach to reducing CTE.

Mild TBIs can be assessed using the Ohio State University TBI Identification Method, the Boston Assessment of Traumatic Brain Injury-Lifetime (BAT-L), the VA TBI Identification Clinical Interview, the Warrior-Administered Retrospective Casualty Assessment Tool (WARCAT), and the Structured Interview for TBI Diagnosis. The most widely researched and used tool for the assessment of concussion (mTBI) in athletes is the Sports Concussion Assessment Tool 3 (SCAT-3).

EPIDEMIOLOGY OF TRAUMATIC BRAIN INJURY

Approximately 80% of patients who sustain TBIs have a mild case. Currently, there is no standard for assessing for or reporting of substance use for patients presenting with TBIs. Thus, rates of substance use at the time of injury remain largely unknown. However, it is estimated that alcohol intoxication at the time of a TBI is common and may be as high as 50% of all cases. There is over two times greater risk of having SUD among US veterans with a positive TBI screen compared to those with a negative screen. TBIs also increase service members' risk of being diagnosed with alcohol use disorder in the 12 months following a head injury by 50%. Conversely, rates of head injury in populations with an SUD range as high as 68%.

RISK FACTORS INFLUENCING CO-OCCURRENCE OF TRAUMATIC BRAIN INJURY AND SUBSTANCE USE DISORDER

There is an increased likelihood of high-risk behavior in those with unhealthy substance use, which results in TBIs (eg, motor vehicle accidents, falls, blunt trauma from violent acts). There is also substantial literature demonstrating that substance use often declines immediately following brain injury but later increases commensurate with improvement in functional status. However, not all subpopulations of patients with TBIs and SUDs exhibit this immediate drop in substance use. For instance, TBI increases the risk of heavy drinking immediately following head injury in young men with a previous history of SUD problems and a diagnosis of depression.

Traumatic Brain Injury Increases Risk of Developing a Substance Use Disorder

TBI alone can result in an increased risk for substance-related problems postinjury. Patients with a TBI are more likely than individuals without a TBI to be treated with potentially addictive opioid medications. Risk for SUD following TBIs may be greater in those with mild-to-moderate TBIs than in those with severe TBIs. Increased rates in substance- and alcohol-related problems in those with mild-to-moderate TBIs can be partially attributed to psychiatric comorbid disorders such as depression, posttraumatic stress disorder, and physical discomfort of postinjury chronic pain. The *decreased* risk of SUD among those with a *severe* TBI is likely due to the inability to seek or access drugs and alcohol because of the debilitating nature of the head injury. There is also early evidence showing that this increased SUD risk is related to the neurobiological and related neurocognitive mechanisms underlying TBIs.

Dopaminergic Neurocircuitry in Animal Models of Traumatic Brain Injury

Many of the neurologic deficits that result from severe TBIs are a result of direct anatomic damage. However, changes in neurotransmitter systems, particularly in the long axonal projections of the dopamine pathways (easily injured by acceleration and deceleration shearing force), appear to be vulnerable to mild-to-moderate TBIs. Animal models consistently show a reduction in dopaminergic neurons postinjury associated with blood–brain barrier breakdown and microglial activation accompanying inflammatory processes. Evidence of disruption of the dopamine system in humans is limited, but imaging studies show altered dopamine transporter and D2 receptor binding varying by brain region.

Traumatic Brain Injury–Related Neurobehavioral Risks of Developing Addiction

The orbitofrontal cortex (OFC) is a component structure of the prefrontal cortex, which underlies the reflective control system implicated in addiction. The OFC is also especially vulnerable to direct blunt trauma to the head and to shearing along the sharp edges of the orbital surface of the skull that can occur following percussive shock waves to the brain. TBI structural damage to the OFC can result in organic personality changes including impaired empathy, interpersonal problems, antisocial behavior, poor distress tolerance, apathy, increased mood lability, hostility, and impulsive responding. Patients with TBI with frontal brain damage may be impaired in their ability to delay gratification and seek immediate rewards related to substance use. There may be a subset of patients with TBIs that have disrupted executive function, leaving them at risk for the development of psychological disorders including unhealthy substance use following injury. Identifying these patients and providing treatment aimed at reducing executive dysfunction may aid in decreasing the risk for development or reemergence of SUDs.

HARMS ASSOCIATED WITH CO-OCCURRENCE OF TRAUMATIC BRAIN INJURY AND SUBSTANCE USE DISORDER

Excessive alcohol use, younger age, previous histories of substance use or head injuries, and risk of suicide are elevated in patients with TBIs and comorbid SUD. Preexisting alcohol use disorder and other SUDs are also associated with lower scores on the GCS and increased brain tissue atrophy. TBIs and SUDs have both discrete and overlapping negative impacts on cognitive performance. There is an increased risk of violent behavior following a head injury in individuals with SUDs compared to those without SUDs. Comorbid TBIs and SUDs have also been associated with decreased productivity, life satisfaction, and ability to return to work postinjury compared to those without preinjury heavy alcohol or substance use.

Chronic pain is also associated with both TBIs and SUDs. Treatments focusing on patient acceptance of chronic pain can be beneficial for reducing disability and improving quality of life in patients with problematic alcohol use and mTBIs. Collaboration among specialists in pain management, SUD treatment, and neurology is recommended.

ASSESSMENT OF TRAUMATIC BRAIN INJURY AND SUBSTANCE USE DISORDER

Screening, Brief Intervention, and Referral for Treatment (SBIRT) for at-risk alcohol use as part of general medical care is highly efficacious and results in large reductions in alcohol use, increased healthcare utilization, economic savings, and fewer motor vehicle accidents. The Substance Abuse and Mental Health Services Administration recommends SBIRT for medical settings (eg, inpatient settings, emergency departments, ambulatory settings, primary and specialty healthcare settings, community health clinics), and the National Institutes of Health recommends the inclusion of SUD evaluation and treatment in rehabilitation programs for TBIs. Screening patients with TBIs acutely after injury for both the presence of preinjury substance use along with the development of new-onset substance use may promote early detection and facilitate adequate follow-up healthcare.

Few studies have examined and identified appropriate and standardized screening instruments that adequately assess for substance use in patients with TBIs despite their shared impacts on cognitive function, mood, and disinhibition. Future research will need to develop uniformity in assessments, reporting, and development of screening tools specific for populations with TBI. Until then, we recommend that clinicians use the following standard tools: Brief Michigan Alcoholism Screening Test (MAST), the Substance Abuse Subtle Screening Inventory, and Alcohol Use Disorders Identification Test (AUDIT).

TBI screening should also be considered part of a routine intake process to facilitate the early detection of head injury in SUD treatment settings. Uncovering a self-reported head injury may provide an indicator that other mental health and cognitive problems are present and that the patient may need a proper evaluation and management. Reliance on a singular self-report question (eg, LOC) to identify brain injury and failure to classify the degree and extent of injury is a common mistake. Therefore, properly trained clinicians are advised to use the standard measures of TBI screening and assessment as mentioned previously.

Early detection can identify patients with TBI treatment needs, allowing clinicians to provide education regarding symptoms of both conditions, coping strategies to minimize their impact, and reducing risky behavior. Upon identification of a TBI, SUD clinicians can offer treatment that emphasizes preventing risk-taking behaviors that may lead to reinjury, the resumption of work, social and other interpersonal obligations, and accommodation strategies for limitations related to poor cognitive function. Neurocognitive testing and/or neuroimaging may be used to establish the presence of and track changes in the associated symptoms of a TBI, and may also be used to support a TBI diagnosis to the extent that these symptoms cannot be accounted for by causes other than TBI itself. In general, routine clinical imaging is not sensitive enough to diagnose most mTBIs.

FACTORS INFLUENCING RECOVERY FROM TRAUMATIC BRAIN INJURY

Persons with higher levels of preinjury cognitive functioning often preserve more functional capacity after a TBI. Social and environmental factors, such as social support, caregiver and family functioning, and socioeconomic status, can influence the effectiveness of rehabilitation treatments. Comorbidities such as preexisting psychological adjustment and social difficulties, learning disabilities, history of previous neurologic or psychiatric disorders, and preinjury use of alcohol or drugs can complicate the assessment and treatment of TBI. Social functioning, including well-functioning caregivers and available financial and social supports, contributes to better recovery and outcomes.

SPECIAL TREATMENT APPROACHES FOR TRAUMATIC BRAIN INJURY AND SUBSTANCE USE DISORDER

Cognitive rehabilitation training can improve processes such as attention, memory, and executive functions after brain injury. Compensatory interventions, such as electronic or prosthetic memory book devices and electronic alerting systems, also help improve functional skills. Furthermore, cognitive rehabilitation therapy techniques have been successfully applied to the problems of social integration and vocational training. The most effective therapy occurs when cognitive training is conducted in real-life situations and has a high interest to the individual.

Specific techniques to directly restore neuropsychological processes are being identified, and augmentation of cognitive therapy with pharmacologic treatments is a promising option in the future. Unfortunately, no cognitive rehabilitation strategies have been tested in patient populations with dual SUD and TBI. There is little published information regarding the pharmacologic treatment of SUDs in individuals with TBIs.

KEY POINTS

1. SUDs and TBIs are highly comorbid and associated with significant functional harms and mortality rates than either diagnosis alone.
2. Providers should routinely screen for both SUDs and TBIs in order to identify individuals at risk of negative outcomes.
3. Treatment may include a reduction of risk-taking behaviors; accommodation strategies for

limitations related to poor cognitive function; and support for the resumption of work, social, and other interpersonal obligations.

REVIEW QUESTIONS

1. Which of the following is the best method for determining TBI severity?
   A. The presence of abnormal neuroimaging results
   B. LOC
   C. Length of altered consciousness, GCS, LOC, and PTA
   D. Degree of impairment from specific behavioral, cognitive, and emotional symptoms following injury

2. Which of the following medications are US Food and Drug Administration approved for the treatment of TBI?
   A. Acamprosate
   B. Disulfiram
   C. Naltrexone
   D. Baclofen
   E. None of the above

3. Which of the following statements is incorrect?
   A. Healthcare providers should screen for TBI for patients seeking SUD treatment.
   B. Asking a single question related to LOC is sufficient in TBI screening.

C. Harm reduction interventions are appropriate for patients with comorbid SUDs and TBIs.
D. Specialty consultation and modified treatment approaches should be considered to accommodate individual needs in SUD treatment.

ANSWERS

1. **C**
2. **E**
3. **B**

SUGGESTED READINGS

Corrigan JD, Bogner J, Hungerford DW, Schomer K. Screening and brief intervention for substance misuse among patients with traumatic brain injury. *J Trauma.* 2010;69(3): 722-726.

Defense Centers of Excellence for Psychological Health and Traumatic Brain Injury, Veterans Brain Injury Center. *Mild Traumatic Brain Injury Pocket Guide (CONUS).* Washington, DC: US Department of Defense, 2010.

Miller SC, Baktash SH, Webb TS, et al. Risk for addiction-related disorders following mild traumatic brain injury in a large cohort of active-duty U.S. airmen. *Am J Psychiatry.* 2013;170(4):383-390.

Weil ZM, Corrigan JD, Karelina K. Alcohol abuse after traumatic brain injury: experimental and clinical evidence. *Neurosci Biobehav Rev.* 2016;62:89-99.

West SL. Substance use among persons with traumatic brain injury: a review. *NeuroRehabilitation.* 2011;29(1):1-8.

40

Military Sexual Trauma

Summary by Joan E. Zweben

Based on THE ASAM PRINCIPLES OF ADDICTION MEDICINE,
6th edition chapter by Joan E. Zweben

Community treatment providers serving returning military veterans need to be aware of their special characteristics and needs to serve them appropriately. Although the US Veterans Affairs (VA) Medical Centers can offer excellent comprehensive care in many communities, there are those who have experienced sexual trauma in the military who may refuse to seek help there because of the complex feelings surrounding such trauma. With over 2.2 million active duty military returning to the US since the beginning of the wars in Iraq and Afghanistan, community treatment providers will inevitably need to provide some care for those seeking help for unhealthy substance use. Military sexual trauma (MST) is an important risk factor for substance use problems in these veterans. When these men and women appear in community settings or seek out private practitioners, it is essential that they are met by professionals with some understanding of not only their issues around trauma, but also the distinctive features of their military background. They also need to know what is available from the VA, as this integrated system of care provides many services that are not available in most community medical centers. The VA also offers a model of how to address MST that can be useful for programs wishing to enhance their services in community settings.

It can take a few months or years for a veteran to decide that their alcohol, nicotine, and/or other drug use is actually a problem, and they may be moved along by clinicians treating them for depression, post-traumatic stress disorder (PTSD), or other conditions causing them distress. A significantly higher percentage of women are assaulted, but men outnumber women in the military. Although the percentage of men reporting an assault are lower, the actual numbers are almost equal. Outside of the VA, males may be less likely to be screened for sexual trauma than women.

Despite the strong commitment of the US Department of Defense (DOD) to address sexual assault, both men and women continue to report devastating experiences of sexual assault and subsequent betrayal by their command when they seek accountability. Emerging data support the view that the problem is complex. These include barriers to reporting, failure to hold perpetrators accountable, and retaliation against victims. Currently, the DOD is making comprehensive prevention and intervention efforts, but the legacy will remain for some time.

According to the VA, "MST is sexual harassment and/or sexual assault experienced by a military service member regardless of the geographic location, the gender of the victim, or the relationship to the perpetrator. Both men and women can experience MST, and the perpetrator can be of the same or of the opposite gender. Perpetrators may or may not be service members themselves."

Since 2012, the DOD has devoted a great deal of attention to preventing and appropriately addressing sexual harassment and assault and have demonstrated steady improvement. The estimated number of service member victims was 26,000 in fiscal year 2012, 20,300 in 2014, and 14,900 in 2016. The DOD began implementing strategies to reduce barriers to reporting, and since 2012, there was a significant increase in victim reports of sexual assault. Service members have several pathways open to them. A restricted report allows victims to confidentially access medical care and advocacy services without triggering an investigation. An unrestricted report is provided to command and/or law enforcement for investigation. Service members may reclassify their report as unrestricted at any time and participate in the military justice process. Over time, the rate of unrestricted reports has risen, and restricted reports have converted more quickly.

According to a 2014 RAND study, there was a decline in the percentage of active duty women who experienced unwanted sexual contact from an estimated 6.1% (26,000) in 2012 to an estimated 4.3% (18,900) in 2014. Approximately 72% of those who reported their assault said they would make the same decision if they had to do it again. The DOD continues its efforts to prevent MST through systematic efforts at prevention and checks and balances once reports are made.

BARRIERS TO REPORTING SEXUAL ASSAULT

Many of the barriers to reporting are common to other victims of sexual assault; some are more characteristic of military members. Service members may minimize the seriousness of the experience or be too embarrassed to report it. They may fear not being believed, being blamed, or having their reputation suffer. In the military, they may have a well-founded fear of harm or retribution if they report it; there unfortunately are numerous examples of this often shared by military members among themselves and discussed in the media. They may fear for their career. They may also be concerned that their own behavior, such as alcohol and other drug use and fraternization offenses, may undermine their efforts to hold perpetrators accountable. For all these reasons, victims of sexual assault may seek help in community settings once they leave active duty.

MILITARY CULTURE

Clinicians are beginning to acknowledge that the military has a distinctive culture as complex as others routinely discussed under the theme of cultural competence. It is important to make an effort to learn on your own and also let your patient teach you about what was important to him or her. What branch did the patient serve in, and what are the distinctive features of that branch? Did the patient serve in peace time or war time? What was the patient's job? There are great differences between Vietnam-era US veterans and those who served in Afghanistan and Iraq. Because of the nature of the wars in Afghanistan and Iraq, it is safe to assume that all veterans who served there are combat veterans, even if that is not in their official job description.

Cultural values in the military include a strong emphasis on honor, respect, and obeying the chain of command. These can be positive forces in treatment. Community programs working with homeless veterans have noted a heartening level of follow-through once treatment plans have been agreed upon. The value placed on "leave no one behind" can be a positive factor in recognizing the value of cohesion in treatment groups and working to promote it. However, military values can also be impediments to seeking and utilizing help. The value placed on protecting yourself may add to the shame the patient feels about the sexual assault, and this may make it more difficult for them to report it. They may feel like they "should have been able to fight my perpetrator off." This is particularly true for men, who are even more likely to feel they should have been able

to overpower the assailant and prevent the assault. Respect for authority turns to a profound sense of betrayal when officers higher up actively discourage reports, avoid investigating, and fail to impose serious consequences on perpetrators.

CLINICAL ISSUES

It is important to screen for MST when patients seek care for physical or psychiatric conditions. This is now standard practice in the VA and should be in community medical care as well. This requires creating a comfortable, unhurried climate for disclosure with adequate privacy. Interruptions should be minimized as much as possible. In general, patients are willing to answer specific questions if the clinician is perceived as nonjudgmental and potentially helpful. Questions can be asked as part of the social history, explaining to the patient that these experiences are sufficiently common in the military and that the questions are routine. There are two questions that should be asked as recommended by VA protocols:

- Did you receive uninvited and unwanted sexual attention, such as touching or cornering, pressure for sexual favors, or verbal remarks?
- Did someone ever use force or the threat of force to have sexual contact with you against your will?

It is important to manage and limit the initial disclosure process, to assess current status and safety, and to be prepared to offer mental health services or make an appropriate referral. One of the most prominent issues these patients will present with is substance use and PTSD. There are high rates of childhood trauma among veterans in general, particularly those who experience MST. Multiple traumatic experiences in childhood and adulthood exacerbate PTSD and often increase the severity of substance use. In the military, as in other situations, a victim may be continually seeing and working with the perpetrator during workplace or other military settings, adding to the difficulty. Often, the risk is ongoing.

Treatment with these patients is often tempestuous. They are often highly anxious and irritable and may be prone to angry outbursts. It can be difficult to establish a therapeutic alliance, particularly if the therapist is of the same gender as the perpetrator. Working with a treatment team is helpful because multiple treatment contacts with different individuals may be necessary for engagement, and these patients may need a higher level of care than a solo practitioner in the community can provide. These patients can be highly crisis prone, and a treatment team can help sort out their many complexities and arrive at a viable plan. A treatment team can also help the clinician avoid becoming too self-critical and discouraged, while utilizing a forum for self-examination.

Given the potential for severe PTSD symptoms and the high suicide rates of military members, clinicians must address the issue of guns. It is appropriate to assume that the patient, whether male or female, has at least one weapon in the home and that this weapon is an important part of his or her identity. Ask specific questions about how he or she stores the weapon and the bullets. If lethality is an issue, attempt to negotiate storing ammunition with a friend or getting a trigger lock. All VA patients are eligible to receive gun locks at no charge, and they may be available to other veterans upon request. Weapons may be turned in to the VA police. It is advisable to put comparable arrangements in place for patients to surrender their weapon if they express willingness to do so.

Women with MST present with a variety of medical problems. They may report chronic pain, such as headaches and back or pelvic pain. They can have a variety of gynecologic problems such as sexual dysfunction, menstrual abnormalities, menopausal symptoms, or reproductive symptoms. Gastrointestinal symptoms include diarrhea, indigestion, nausea, and difficulty swallowing. Other complaints can include chronic fatigue, sudden weight changes, and heart palpitations. These may be the vehicle through which the woman asks for help because a nurse or primary care physician may be less threatening. It is important to rule out organic causes prior to ascribing the symptoms to MST.

Men who reported either sexual harassment or assault were more likely to have a history of sexual trauma and alcohol-related problems as well as poorer baseline physical and mental health. Men with MST are more likely to have sexually transmitted diseases, such as HIV/AIDS, syphilis, and herpes as well as disorders of sexual desire and arousal. They are also more likely to report symptoms of PTSD and depression. They report stronger symptoms at the beginning of treatment and perceive their general health as more damaged.

Conducting a physical examination or doing medical procedures can also present challenges. It is important to make the medical encounter as safe as possible by providing a private, calm setting and explaining what to expect. If the patient becomes upset or begins to dissociate, it is important to stop touching the patient or discontinue the procedure and then reorient and soothe the patient. A well-established pathway for mental health referrals and a "warm hand off" is part of good care because these patients may be reluctant to seek help and give up easily if the referral is not guided at each point that obstacles might occur.

GETTING HELP AT THE VETERANS ADMINISTRATION

Many women, in particular, will emphatically refuse to go to the VA; however, it is important for them to know what it has to offer, particularly if other resources in the community are scarce. A pioneer in the use of electronic records in the 1980s, the VA has used them to identify the factors involved in good outcomes and then formulate and disseminate protocols to improve care across the system. The result is that VA care produces better outcomes for chronic conditions such as diabetes and hypertension than Medicaid and the private sector. All veterans seen in VA healthcare settings are asked if they experienced MST. All treatment for physical or mental health conditions related to MST is free. Every VA health care facility has a designated MST coordinator who serves as the contact person for MST-related issues. Many veterans are confused about their eligibility for benefits and should be encouraged to get into the system (Table 40-1), in case they lose their current insurance or later need care they cannot access in the community.

CONCLUSIONS

Community treatment providers can expect to see veterans who are victims of MST in their programs and should prepare to address their complex needs. Many will have highly conflicted feelings about their military experience and may not even share they are a veteran unless specifically asked. Although the VA has worked hard to provide excellent services to these patients, many will not consider seeking help in that setting. Community providers who are knowledgeable about the culture of the military will be better able to engage them. Their traumatic experiences will influence their efforts to address their physical and emotional problems because it affects

TABLE 40-1	Resources
HOW TO APPLY FOR VETERANS AFFAIRS BENEFITS	
• Phone: (877) 222-VETS (8387) • Visit http://www.va.gov/healthbenefits/online • Apply in person at your local VA hospital	
NATIONAL CRISIS LINE FOR MENTAL HEALTH EMERGENCIES: (800) 273-8255, option #1 for veterans	

everything from their ability to tolerate a physical exam to their emotional stability and participation in a recovery process. Expertise in addressing PTSD is a must for substance use disorder treatment to be effective for this group. Their training often enhances the character assets they bring to the recovery process, and veterans can be very rewarding to work with.

ACKNOWLEDGMENTS

The author thanks John Straznickas, MD, associate clinical professor, University of California, San Francisco, and team leader, Substance Use Post-traumatic Stress Disorder Team, San Francisco Veteran's Affairs Medical Center.

KEY POINTS

1. Women veterans have a high incidence of MST and are screened and appropriately referred when they seek help at the VA.
2. Women veterans should be screened when they seek help in the community by providers who have familiarity with the culture of the military and its barriers to seeking help.
3. Medical practitioners should be familiar with ways to ease the stress of a physical examination.

REVIEW QUESTIONS

1. Military sexual trauma:
   A. is limited primarily to women.
   B. is defined as when both victim and perpetrator are military members.
   C. can be experienced by any military member.
   D. must occur in a military installation.

2. Community treatment providers:
   A. can assume the patient will bring up the MST if it is relevant.
   B. should ask all patients if they have served in the military and if they have ever been forced or threatened with force to have sexual contact against their will.
   C. can conduct a physical exam on current or former service members without any modifications.
   D. should carefully document the trauma in detail as soon as possible.

ANSWERS

1. **C**
2. **B**

SUGGESTED READINGS

Association of VA Psychologist Leaders. Fact sheet: comparison of VA to community healthcare summary of research 2000-2016. https://advocacy.avapl.org/pubs/FACT %20sheet%20literature%20review%20of%20VA%20vs%20 Community%20Heath%20Care%2003%2023-16.pdf. Published March 23, 2016. Accessed October 16, 2018.

Morral AR, Gore K, Schell TL, eds. *Sexual Assault and Sexual Harassment in the US Military. Volume 2. Estimates for Department of Defense Service Members From the 2014 RAND Military Workplace Study*. Santa Monica, CA: RAND Corporation, 2015.

O'Toole M. Military sexual assault epidemic continues to claim victims as Defense Department fails females. *Huffington Post*. https://www.huffingtonpost.com/2012/10/06/military -sexual-assault-defense-department_n_1834196.html. Published October 6, 2012. Updated December 6, 2017. Accessed October 16, 2018.

US Department of Defense. *Department of Defense Annual Report on Sexual Assault in the Military. Fiscal Year 2017*. Washington, DC: US Department of Defense, 2017.

41 Alcohol, Prescription, and Other Drug Problems in Older Adults

Summary by Frederic C. Blow, Kristen L. Barry, and Angela M. Galka

Based on THE ASAM PRINCIPLES OF ADDICTION MEDICINE, 6th edition chapter by Frederic C. Blow and Kristen L. Barry

Many of the medical and psychiatric disorders experienced in aging are greatly influenced by the unhealthy use of alcohol, prescription medications, and other drugs. Compared to earlier cohorts, the unhealthy use of substances is more common in the Baby Boomer generation (persons born between 1946 and 1964). The excessive use of alcohol and/or drugs combined with age-related comorbid diseases have resulted in a generation in need of more age-specific interventions and treatment options. Due to the physiologic changes that take place during the natural aging process, older adults are more vulnerable to the effects of alcohol and drugs, putting them at an increased risk of adverse consequences such as drug interactions, injury, depression, memory problems, liver disease, cardiovascular disease, cognitive changes, and sleep problems. Yet many of these comorbid conditions and adverse events are often not immediately recognized as being associated with substance use. Even when there is recognition, issues such as shame, stigma, and ageist beliefs prevent many older adults from experiencing lifesaving treatment.

SCOPE OF THE PROBLEM IN OLDER ADULTHOOD

Alcohol

The most common substance use problems seen in older adults are at-risk or harmful alcohol use. Although at-risk drinking increases the potential for developing health problems, many older adults have drinking issues that go undetected by their healthcare professional. Any changes in life events (eg, bereavement, serious illness, retirement, change in income, etc.) can affect alcohol use patterns.

Alcohol and Prescription Medications

Older adults who drink alcohol have an increased likelihood of being prescribed alcohol-interactive (AI) medications. Taking AI medications on a regular basis and/or taking multiple AI medications further increases the risk of adverse reactions, including falls, heart problems, and liver damage, especially among frequent drinkers. It is imperative that physicians discuss the potential risks of combining alcohol with AI prescription medications with their patients, especially if the patient has a past or current history of alcohol problems.

Nonmedical Use of Prescription Medications

Although there are older adults who use prescription drugs to get high, the vast majority become problematic users unintentionally due to medications for pain, anxiety, and sleep concerns. Other factors such as being female, social isolation, a history of substance use or mental health disorders, and medical exposure to prescription drugs with problematic potential are associated with prescription medication disorders. The medications of most concern for older adults are the ones that affect brain function, resulting in changes in perception, pain, mood, consciousness, cognition, and behavior. This includes medications for pain, such as opioids, and sedative–hypnotics for anxiety or insomnia, such as benzodiazepines. Both have a high addiction potential and interact with alcohol, increasing the risk of negative outcomes.

Illegal Drugs

Rates of illegal drug use disorders are generally very low in older adults. However, with the increased legalization and availability of marijuana (cannabis)

as medicine, as well as recreational marijuana, rates of marijuana use are on the rise and are expected to increase as the Baby Boomer generation ages. Many older adults are using marijuana to treat pain and promote relaxation. Although the extent to which marijuana interacts with specific prescription drugs is not well known, it can intensify the effects of alcohol. Studies have shown that cannabis affects both the central nervous system and peripheral processes, anxiety, depression, cognition, learning, and motor coordination. Its use is associated with increased injury and short-term memory deficits.

Nicotine

Nicotine/tobacco use disorders remain prevalent across age groups. Older adults who smoke face numerous health consequences, and recent research has suggested a relationship between smoking and decreased cognitive functioning. Persistent older adult smokers have significantly higher levels of psychological distress when compared to quitters, which should be kept in mind when implementing a smoking cessation intervention. For older adults, there remains little information specific to ideal dosing, adherence, and adverse events for nicotine replacement therapy. However, interventions aimed to reduce the prevalence of smoking among people as they age can have tremendous health benefits.

ISSUES UNIQUE TO OLDER ADULTS

Given the high utilization of general medical services by older adults, primary care physicians and other healthcare professionals are essential for identifying those with substance use problems in need of treatment, especially because few older adults seek help in specialized addiction treatment settings.

Other venues in which to detect substance-related problems in older adults include specialty care settings, home healthcare, elder housing, and senior center programs. Older individuals have unique patterns of drinking and nonmedical use of prescription medications, substance-related consequences, social issues, and treatment needs. However, the criteria for classifying older adults with an alcohol or substance use disorder remain a concern. For example, the American Psychiatric Association's *Diagnostic and Statistical Manual of Mental Disorders*, 5th edition (*DSM-5*) criteria for a substance use disorder (SUD) may not apply to older adults because, for example, they may not experience a use of substances that results in a failure to fulfill major role obligations at work, school, or at home.

Older adults have increased sensitivity to substances as they age, resulting in lowered rather than increased tolerance, particularly when combined with the use of some over-the-counter (OTC) or prescription medications. In addition, patients with co-occurring aberrant medication-taking behaviors and chronic pain often find it hard to accept that they have, or are developing an SUD. Rather than finding treatment, they seek alternative ways to obtain medication. See Table 41-1 for signs and symptoms of potential alcohol and substance use problems in older adults.

Older adults present challenges in applying strategies for reducing use. Because of stigma, older adults who drink at at-risk levels often find it particularly difficult to acknowledge their own risky use. In addition, chronic medical conditions may make it more difficult for clinicians to recognize substance misuse, in particular, and its impact on decreased functioning and quality of life. These issues present barriers for both clinicians and older adults in identifying

TABLE 41-1 Signs and Symptoms of Potential Alcohol and Substance Use Problems in Older Adults: Time to Ask Questions		
Mental/Cognitive/Relationship Changes	**Physical Health**	**Alcohol and Medication**
Anxiety	Poor hygiene	Increased alcohol tolerance
Depression	Falls, bruises	Unusual medication response
Social isolation	Poor nutrition	
Excessive mood swings	Incontinence	
Disorientation	Sleep problems	
Memory loss	Increased heart rate	
New decision-making problems	Elevated blood pressure	
Idiopathic seizures	Falls/injuries	

Adapted from Barry KL, Oslin D, Blow FC. *Alcohol Problems in Older Adults: Prevention and Management.* New York: Springer, 2001.

the need for change. When working with resistant patients who do not recognize a problematic level of alcohol or drug use, clinicians can begin by teaching about normative changes in metabolism with aging, the interactions between alcohol/drugs and specific medications (especially sedatives), the potential for falls, and the relationship between alcohol/drugs and medical problems (eg, hypertension, anxiety). The use of nonjudgmental, motivational approaches can be key to successfully engaging these patients in appropriate care.

CO-OCCURRING DISORDERS IN OLDER ADULTHOOD

Patients with co-occurring disorders can be more difficult to diagnose and treat because each illness may complicate the other. It is important to note that alcohol and other drugs can affect emotional health long before psychiatric diagnoses are made, and early interventions can be the key to maintaining mental and physical health. Illnesses, bereavement, job loss, and retirement can all worsen depressive responses and increase alcohol/drug use. Chronic pain, difficulty sleeping, and anxiety are other factors that can increase alcohol/drug use.

Sleep

Although physiologic changes in sleep–wake patterns can occur as part of normal aging, sleep problems that lead to impairments in daytime functioning, mood, and fatigue are not. Although psychological interventions such as cognitive–behavioral therapy have been shown to improve perceived sleep in older adults, sedative–hypnotic medications are the most commonly prescribed treatment approach for insomnia in this group. However, according to the 2012 American Geriatric Society Beers Criteria (see Suggested Readings), benzodiazepines should not be used to treat insomnia in older adults due to the increased risk of cognitive and psychomotor impairments, falls, fractures, and motor vehicle accidents.

Comorbid Depression and Other Psychiatric Disorders

Psychiatric comorbidities complicate interventions, treatments, and relapse prevention. Mental health issues such as depression are a major public health concern in older adults and can lead to serious consequences. Although depression is not a normal part of aging, depression and alcohol use are the most commonly cited co-occurring disorders in older adults. Co-occurring addiction and psychiatric disorders among older adults are associated with poor health outcomes, higher healthcare utilization,

increased complexity, poorer prognosis of mental illness, heightened mortality, higher rates of active suicidal ideation, and social dysfunction compared to individuals with either disorder alone. Although pharmacotherapies are common for depression in older adults with co-occurring disorders, long-term data on the effectiveness and safety of psychotropic drugs in older populations are scarce. Selective serotonin-reuptake inhibitors are considered first-line therapy, but older adults may be at an increased risk of side effects, such as falls, cognitive issues, and hospitalizations. Psychotherapy and, to some extent, lifestyle changes such as moderate-intensity exercise, improving nutrition, and engagement in pleasurable activities and social interactions are all effective psychosocial treatments for depression in older adults.

Comorbidity and Suicidality

Among all ages, the co-occurrence of diagnosed alcohol use disorders (AUDs) and mood disorders is associated with a greater suicide risk than either diagnosis alone. Research has indicated that at-risk and even drinking within National Institute on Alcohol Abuse and Alcoholism guidelines can aggravate affective disorders, such as depression, among some older adults. This all points out the importance of conducting systematic screening for alcohol issues and comorbid psychiatric conditions, especially in the context of a suicide assessment protocol.

Weighing the Positive and Negative Aspects of Alcohol Use

With the mixed opinions regarding the detrimental effects and potential benefits of alcohol use, clinicians may feel confused as to whether they should recommend no change in consumption or a reduction in consumption for older adults who do not meet the criteria for an SUD. For older adults who are more susceptible to both the physiologic and the psychosocial effects of substance use, erring on the side of caution with nonconfrontational messages about the guidelines and following up if there are concerns is generally the most practical and effective approach.

SCREENING AND DETECTION OF ALCOHOL, PRESCRIPTION AND OTHER DRUG PROBLEMS IN OLDER ADULTS

The overall model and approach to the process of screening and intervening with older adults who may have at-risk or problem use of alcohol and/or the nonmedical use of prescription medications is called SBIRT (screening, brief intervention, and referral to treatment; see Chapter 22). Clinicians should screen for alcohol use (frequency and quantity), drinking consequences, use of prescription medications, levels of use, and alcohol/medication interactions. Screening can be done as part of routine mental and physical checkups and should be updated annually, before prescribing any new medications, or in response to physical or mental health changes. The Substance Abuse and Mental Health Services Administration's and Center for Substance Abuse Treatment's TIP 26: *Substance Abuse Among Older Adults* (see Suggested Readings) recommends screening all adults aged 60 years or older on a yearly basis and when there are changes that warrant additional screening (eg, major life events, retirement, loss of partner/spouse, changes in health). Clinicians can obtain more accurate histories by asking questions about the recent past, embedding the alcohol, medication, or substance use questions in the context of other health behaviors (eg, exercise, diet, weight, smoking, alcohol use), and asking straightforward questions in a nonjudgmental manner.

Additionally, a "brown bag approach," where the clinician asks the patient to bring in all medications, OTC preparations, and herbal remedies in a bag to the next clinical visit, is one potential means of getting reliable information about all medication use. Most states allow physicians or pharmacists to query a state database of controlled substance prescriptions without a patient's consent. This can reveal multiple prescribers for controlled substances, such as opioid analgesics or benzodiazepines. It is also important to ask about any use of cannabis, including any recommendations or prescriptions for marijuana use. Used together, these strategies allow the provider to determine what the patient is taking and what, if any, interactions these medications, OTC medications, and herbal remedies may have with each other and with alcohol/drugs. OTC preparation use often remains unevaluated in clinical settings and the use of some OTC preparations (particularly anticholinergic agents) can be problematic in combinations with alcohol or prescriptions.

Screening Process

The first step in the screening process is to simply ask a few questions to rule out the majority of individuals who do not need more systematic screening and to determine the extent of the problem. Screening generally identifies at-risk and harmful substance use. More extensive assessments are used to measure the severity of the substance use symptoms and consequences associated with use, factors

that may be contributing to an SUD, and other characteristics of the problem. The screening process should help determine if a patient's substance use is appropriate for brief advice/interventions or if it warrants a more intense approach.

Screening Instruments

Screening for alcohol use is not always standardized, and not all standardized instruments show good reliability and validity with older adults. In addition to quantity/frequency questions, the Michigan Alcoholism Screening Test–Geriatric version and the Short Michigan Alcoholism Screening Test–Geriatric version (Table 41-2) were developed specifically for use with older adults. In addition, the Alcohol Use Disorders Identification Test is well validated in adults younger than 65 years in primary care settings and has had initial validation in a study of older adults.

Broad-Based Assessment

Clinicians can follow-up the brief questions about consumption and consequences such as those in the Michigan Alcoholism Screening Test–Geriatric version, the Short Michigan Alcoholism Screening Test–Geriatric version, and the Alcohol Use Disorders Identification Test, with a few more in-depth questions about consequences, health risks, and social/family issues. To assess an AUD, questions should be asked about alcohol- or drug-related problems, a history of failed attempts to stop or cut back, or withdrawal symptoms such as tremors. Clinicians should refer patients thought to meet the criteria for an AUD for a diagnostic evaluation and possible brief or formal specialized treatment. If there is evidence of a prescription drug use disorder, the patient should also be referred to a specialist to obtain a further assessment. For older adults with SUD symptoms, assessments are needed to confirm the problem, to characterize the dimensions of the problem, and to develop individualized treatment plans. For insurance reimbursement purposes, the assessment should follow the criteria in the *DSM-5* or other relevant criteria, keeping in mind that these criteria may not apply directly to planning older adults' treatment.

The use of validated SUD assessment instruments can be of great help to clinicians by providing a structured approach to the assessment process as well as a checklist of items that should be evaluated with each older adult. Despite limitations with criteria used to assess older adults, a general psychiatry structured assessment instrument that has been widely used (and updated) over many years is the

TABLE 41-2	Short Michigan Alcoholism Screening Test–Geriatric Version (SMAST-G)		
		YES (1)	NO (0)
1. When talking with others, do you ever underestimate how much you actually drink?		_____	_____
2. After a few drinks, have you sometimes not eaten or been able to skip a meal because you didn't feel hungry?		_____	_____
3. Does having a few drinks help decrease your shakiness or tremors?		_____	_____
4. Does alcohol sometimes make it hard for you to remember parts of the day or night?		_____	_____
5. Do you usually take a drink to relax or calm your nerves?		_____	_____
6. Do you drink to take your mind off your problems?		_____	_____
7. Have you ever increased your drinking after experiencing a loss in your life?		_____	_____
8. Has a doctor or nurse ever said they were worried or concerned about your drinking?		_____	_____
9. Have you ever made rules to manage your drinking?		_____	_____
10. When you feel lonely, does having a drink help?		_____	_____
TOTAL SMAST-G SCORE (0–10)		_____	

Scoring: Two or more "yes" responses are indicative of alcohol problem.
For further information, contact Frederic C. Blow, PhD, at the University of Michigan Department of Psychiatry, 4250 Plymouth Road, Ann Arbor, MI 48109; (734) 232-0270, fredblow@med.umich.edu.
© The Regents of the University of Michigan, 1991.

Structured Clinical Interview for *DSM-5* (SCID-5). It takes a trained clinician approximately 30 minutes to administer the 35 SCID questions that probe for an AUD.

Laboratory Tests

Although self-reporting is the primary tool used to assess alcohol consumption, biological markers for alcohol use may be useful for physicians. Such tests can be used to identify current alcohol consumption status, facilitate discussions with patients about adverse health outcomes associated with their alcohol intake, as well as provide prognostic information for follow-up. However, alcohol biomarkers have their pros and cons and should be interpreted with caution.

INTERVENTION STRATEGIES FOR OLDER ADULTS

Brief Alcohol Interventions

Studies have shown that older adults can be engaged in brief motivational interventions in a variety of healthcare and social settings. In general, brief interventions with older adults have seen statistically significant changes in alcohol use, but the actual

number differences are small. This could, in part, be that older adults in primary care studies are at-risk drinkers and not harmful drinkers. Those with harmful drinking patterns generally require continuity of care and support to maintain changes.

FORMAL ADDICTION TREATMENT IN OLDER ADULTHOOD

There have been few systematic studies of formal addiction treatment outcomes for older adults, mainly because residential and intensive outpatient SUD treatment programs provide services to very few older individuals. Naltrexone and acamprosate have been approved for treatment of *DSM-IV*–defined alcohol dependence and have shown to improve alcohol consumption outcomes. However, these treatments are underutilized in the treatment of older adults with AUDs.

Because traditional residential SUD treatment programs generally provide services to few older adults, there have been only limited studies with large enough populations of older adults to determine the effectiveness of residential programming in this age group. There are a few naturalistic studies that suggest older adults who do engage in treatment have better outcomes when compared with younger adults. Older adults also seem to do best in programs that offer age-appropriate care with providers who are knowledgeable about aging issues. Studies have shown that age-specific programming improved treatment completion and resulted in higher rates of attendance at group meetings compared to mixed-age treatment. In addition, older adults with SUDs were significantly more likely to complete treatment than younger patients.

LIMITATIONS OF TREATMENT OUTCOME RESEARCH

Major limitations remain in the treatment adherence literature, and studies on the effect of age of onset on treatment compliance have yielded mixed result. More carefully controlled, prospective treatment outcome studies that include sufficiently large numbers of older subjects who meet the criteria for AUDs and other SUDs are needed to address the methodologic limitations of prior work.

RELAPSE REDUCTION

Older adults have age-related risks for relapse that need to be considered. Studies show that psychosocial factors such as social isolation, loneliness, loss and grief, and depression can become antecedents to alcohol use, and older drinkers tend to report using alcohol to alleviate negative emotional states. Comorbid medical conditions, such as pain, also put older adults at higher risk for relapse (see Barrick and Connors under Suggested Readings).

CONCLUSIONS

From both a public health standpoint and from a clinical perspective, with the aging of the Baby Boomer cohort, there is a critical need to implement effective alcohol and drug screening and intervention strategies in older adults who are at risk for more serious health, social, and emotional problems. Because of the complexity of medical and psychosocial intervention and treatment issues, older adults present unique challenges to the healthcare system. Fortunately, there are a number of venues in which to detect substance-related problems in older adults as well as strategies for working with older adults. The development of short, effective techniques to address substance use issues in the growing population of older adults continues to be an important focus for the alcohol and drug field. If successfully implemented, the evidence-based screening techniques, brief interventions, and brief treatments will be key steps in the process of ensuring that current

and future generations have the opportunity for improved physical and emotional health. The challenge to the system will be moving from the development of these evidence-based programs specific to older adults to actually implementing them in the real world—the "bench to bedside" dilemma.

KEY POINTS

1. Older adults are more vulnerable to the effects of alcohol and medications, have unique patterns of drinking and nonmedical use of prescription medications, substance-related consequences, social issues, and treatment needs. They require screening and intervention procedures specific to older adults.

2. Given the high utilization of general medical services by older adults, primary care physicians and other healthcare professionals are essential for identifying those in need of treatment. However, most older adults experiencing issues related to their drinking are unidentified by healthcare personnel, and few older adults seek help on their own. Other venues in which to detect substance-related problems in older adults include specialty care settings, home healthcare, elder housing, and senior center programs.

3. Co-occurring addiction and psychiatric disorders among older adults are associated with poor health outcomes, higher healthcare utilization, increased complexity, poorer prognosis of mental illness, heightened mortality, higher rates of active suicidal ideation, and social dysfunction compared to individuals with either disorder alone. This all points out the importance of conducting systematic screening for alcohol/drug problems and comorbid psychiatric conditions.

4. The use of nonjudgmental, motivational approaches are key to successfully engaging older adults with alcohol or drug problems. In working with resistant patients who do not recognize a problematic level of alcohol or drug use, clinicians can begin by teaching about changes in metabolism with aging, the interactions between alcohol and specific medications (especially sedatives), the potential for falls, and the relationship between alcohol and some medical problems (eg, hypertension).

5. Older adults do better in treatment programs that offer age-appropriate care administered by providers who are knowledgeable about aging issues. Strategies for working with older adults who use alcohol and/or other drugs at at-risk levels include minimal advice, structured brief

intervention protocols, formalized treatment, and specialized relapse prevention programs provide useful tools to begin to address this growing issue.

REVIEW QUESTIONS

1. Your older adult patient reports that she drinks wine every night to help with her back pain and sleep issues. She also says it calms her nerves. What would be your next step?
   A. Determine what medications she's taking, assess her level of alcohol use using the Short Michigan Alcohol Screening Test–Geriatric version, and then determine your next steps.
   B. Let her know that the drinking is okay, as long as she limits it to one or two glasses a night.
   C. Obtain more detail from the patient about her back pain, sleep issues, and possible anxiety issues.
   D. Both A and C

2. The misuse of alcohol and/or drugs by older adults is associated with which of the following?
   A. Depression
   B. Bipolar disorder
   C. Medical problems
   D. All of the above

3. A new patient is seen in your office for a broken ankle. You learn that his wife recently passed away and he's in the process of grieving. How would you proceed?
   A. Find out how he's coping with the grieving process.
   B. Learn more about how he broke his ankle. Were substances involved?
   C. Give your condolences and provide a course of treatment for his ankle.
   D. All of the above

ANSWERS

1. **D**
2. **D**
3. **D**

SUGGESTED READINGS

American Geriatric Society 2012 Beers Criteria Update Expert Panel. American Geriatrics Society Updated Beers Criteria for Potentially Inappropriate Medication Use in Older Adults. *J Am Geriatr Soc.* 2012;60(4):616-631.

Barrick C, Connors GJ. Relapse prevention and maintaining abstinence in older adults with alcohol-use disorders. *Drugs Aging.* 2002;19(8):583-594.

Center for Substance Abuse Treatment. *Substance Abuse Among Older Adults: Treatment Improvement Protocol (TIP) Series, No. 26.* Rockville, MD: Substance Abuse and Mental Health Services Administration, 1998. HHS Publication No. (SMA) 12-3918.

Kuerbis A, Sacco P, Blazer DG, Moore AA. Substance abuse among older adults. *Clin Geriatr Med.* 2014;30(3):629-654.

Wu LT, Blazer DG. Illicit and nonmedical drug use among older adults: a review. *J Aging Health.* 2011;23(3):481-504.

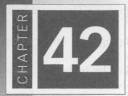
Cultural Issues in Addiction Medicine

Summary by Joseph Westermeyer and Patricia Jean Dickmann

Based on THE ASAM PRINCIPLES OF ADDICTION MEDICINE,
6th edition chapter by Joseph Westermeyer and Patricia Jean Dickmann

Cultural factors can serve as either pathogenic agents or therapeutic resources for substance use disorders (SUDs). Clinicians who can apply cultural concepts to SUD care possess "clinical cultural competence." Our clinical goal consists of enabling patients to resume their health and cultural competence.

Other people teach us about substance use and misuse via their communications, behaviors, and interactions. We learn about substances on numerous levels: information, skills, attitudes, values, experience, and personal history. Once taught, individuals can expand or reorganize what they have learned about substances in new, idiosyncratic ways. For example, a child might observe that substance-related values taught at home or school are rarely practiced. An adolescent may discover that substance use apparently eases developmental transitions. Adults can learn that substance misuse may aid in performing a dreaded task.

Subgroups within a culture can alter values, customs, and substance use over time. For example, college attendance in the United States once lowered the risk of substance use disorder, whereas today, college attendance increases SUD risk. Two thirds of college students report a high-risk drinking pattern characterized by five drinks or more for men (four drinks or more for women) in one drinking session over the last two weeks.

Cultural values can affect psychoactive substance use in populations. For example, alcohol consumption increases in cultures that value personal autonomy over collective obligation, and egalitarianism over hierarchy. Sociocultural disruption and armed conflict have led to widespread addiction in some cultures, whereas peace, stability, and progress have generally reduced SUD rates. Many national governments are devoting more attention to culture and behavioral health epidemics, including SUDs, smoking, sexually transmitted infections, violence, gambling, obesity, and physical inactivity—so-called "syndemics" due to their propensity to co-occur.

CULTURAL DEFINITIONS RELATED TO SUBSTANCE USE

Culture encompasses the sum total of shared values, attitudes, beliefs, customs, technology, environment, and lifeway that distinguishes a people with a common identity. Although subject to change over time, and largely learned, culture tends to persist across generations via language, the arts, social institutions, and informal associates. Psychoactive substances produced (or imported), distributed, and consumed comprise one element of a people's culture. Elected officials, traditional leaders, celebrities, teachers, parents, mass media, and other culture arbitrators promulgate models of use and abstinence.

Most nations encompass numerous cultures, or *ethnicities*, with varying national origins, language, dress, religious/spiritual beliefs, kinship, and ceremonies. Within a nation, *ethnic groups* can differ greatly in their use of alcohol and other psychoactive substances. These ethnicities may share a common government, healthcare system, educational systems, and mass media, while differing in norms, values, traditions, rituals, and beliefs.

Groups of people with close ties, shared beliefs, and common goals comprise *subcultures*. Examples include people with mutual occupations (eg, physicians), hobbies (eg, golf), political beliefs, or communal concerns (eg, Mothers Against Drunk Driving). Subcultures may evolve from local substance use venues, specific drugs, or the need for privacy or security (eg, neighborhood taverns, "crack" cocaine houses, "shooting galleries" for parenteral injection, college "party houses"). Although subcultures can furnish environments for spreading addiction, recovery subcultures can impart settings for escaping addiction. Affiliating with Alcoholics Anonymous, Narcotics Anonymous, Gamblers Anonymous, and SMART Recovery can reinforce healthy norms and reduce relapse risk.

Norms consist of attitudes, values, beliefs, and behaviors within a culture that possess positive or negative valance. Preferences or choices having moral overtones are especially apt to involve norms. Cultures prescribe *ideal norms* for decisions with moral import, including substance use (eg, type, dose, frequency, context, or rationale for use vs. abstinence). *Behavioral norms* consist of what people actually do within a culture, regardless of its ideals. *Norm gap*, *dissonance*, or *conflict* occurs if an ideal norm and behavioral norm diverge. Substance use disorders predictably ensue in cultures with norm conflicts regarding substance use. Although norm conflicts may exist outside of awareness, skilled ethnographers can reliably obtain data on *self-reported ideal norms* versus *observed behavioral norms*. Clinicians working across cultural boundaries in a significant way can become insightful regarding ideal versus behavioral norms.

CULTURE AND PATTERNS OF SUBSTANCE USE

When ideal and behavioral norms regarding substance use match up, SUDs rarely exists. Conversely, groups that prohibit the use of a substance in theory and yet foster its use in practice invite individuals to invent unique use patterns. Such a circumstance results in some people abstaining, others engaging in nonhazardous use, and some adopting risky use practices. Recent examples of norm conflict fostering increased SUDs in the United States include legalizing marijuana at the state level despite it remaining illegal at the federal level, widespread opioid prescribing for chronic symptoms, and college binge drinking. Parenthetically, SUD subcultures seldom manifest norm gaps within their group because ideal and behavioral norms both prescribe heavy use, thereby easing the task of recruiting novitiates. Development of norm dissonance in a person with an unhealthy substance use may signal initial interest in reduced use, abstinence, or recovery.

SUD rates can change over generations. Sociocultural changes within ethnic groups can affect the pattern of substance use and SUD over time. For example, some people join abstinence-oriented religious sects to overcome SUDs. Ethnic groups with no previous norm conflict have manifested norm conflict over time or after migration into a multiethnic culture that allows or promotes use of certain substances.

CULTURAL ASPECTS OF CLINICAL ASSESSMENT

Taking a Cultural History

The first step in conducting a cultural history consists of asking the patient about the ethnic origins of his or her parents and grandparents or their surrogates. Relevant information includes their place of birth, national origin, language learned at home, migrations, roles and affiliations in the ethnic community, and roles and affiliations in the community at large. Educational experiences and marital history may be relevant depending on the case. The next step consists of assessing the family's enculturation of the patient. Parental SUD threatens healthy identity formation, undermines cultural competence, and increases SUD risk.

Adapting to life in an unfamiliar culture can precipitate an SUD. Relocation for college, the military, or a distant job can alter previously learned substance use norms. Optimal environmental conditions in adoptive or foster home placement may not counter increased genetic risk from biologic parents.

Substance-Specific History

Cultural groups *ensocialize* youth into psychoactive substance use. Inquiry into patients' unique learning experiences can guide clinicians in understanding patients' substance use decisions. Relevant queries include the following:

- *Observations of role models*: What substances did parenting adults use? Was the use excessive or disruptive to the family?
- *Socialization into psychoactive substance use*: Who guided the patient's early substance use? Did this occur with family or peers? At what age?
- *Early substance use experience*: Did early use enhance coping or alter mood? What consequences occurred in association with substance use?
- *Association with other developmental tasks and life stressors*: Was the patient learning new anxiety-provoking academic, social, or performance skills? Did a major life stressor or loss prompt heavy or binge substance use?

ADDICTION AND PATIENTS' CULTURAL COPING

Psychoactive substance use may foster social coping, at least initially. For example, use of stimulants may enhance studying, athletics, working long hours, or functioning despite lack of sleep. Similarly, ecstasy and GHB (γ-hydroxybutyrate), sometimes referred to as club drugs, appear to foster sociability, feelings of acceptance, and transient intimacy. Once dependence ensues, drugs that previously enhanced performance undermine it. Initial doses fail to relieve anxiety as tolerance grows. Sustaining symptom relief may require higher doses over time, leading to unintended emotional, behavioral, financial, mental, or physical complications.

Achieving a certain social status followed by its loss may also herald an SUD. These crises may affect marital status, employment, housing, community participation, and/or social network. Legal or financial problems may restrict a patient's ability to address these crises.

SUD subcultures may welcome new members estranged from family and other groups. These subcultures do not impose the pressures of societal "goals" such as career advancement, achievement in sports, or devotion to family and community. Youth struggling to attain cultural competence may drift toward SUD subcultures.

CULTURE, TREATMENT, AND RECOVERY

Addiction, Recovery, and the Intimate Social Network

The normal "intimate social network" (ISN) of any one person (or "proband") consists of 20 to 30 people organized into four or five subgroups (Table 42-1). Typical subgroups include a face-to-face living group, relatives, friends, coworkers, and perhaps another group or two (eg, neighbors, association members, gymnasium, church, recreational or Internet group). If the proband and another ISN member become estranged, their subgroup fosters rapprochement, thereby enhancing maturation, intimacy, and trust over time. Healthy ISN relationships are reciprocal: The proband exchanges work, time, or resources with other ISN members. Exchanges necessarily limit ISN size to around 20 to 30 people (rarely more than 40). SUDs can diminish ISN size through inability or disinterest in reciprocity. Recovery can further

reduce ISN size as the proband avoids people who may rekindle the SUD.

Progressive dysfunctions reduce ISNs to less than 20 people with two or three groups (eg, family and relatives) plus some one-on-one relationships. The "connectedness" of the ISN falls as short-lived, one-on-one relationships replace longer lasting subgroups. The proband assumes client roles vis-à-vis other ISN members (eg, drug dealers, bartenders, clergy, social workers, health professionals). People with depleted ISNs may report deceased persons, pets, or people who were close friends years ago.

The ISN can decline down to ten or fewer people, most of whom know one another only through the proband. Their common link involves nonreciprocal relationships with the proband. For example, a parent, social worker, homeless shelter manager, and policeman may all know one another through their respective efforts to help the proband. Eventually, the alienated proband may become isolated to the point of not having anyone to call upon—a grave prognostic sign.

ISN reconstruction offers a potent means for intervening and supporting recovery. A key element involves eliminating companions who use drugs from the ISN, with retention of only those committed to the patient's ultimate recovery. Sober communities, halfway houses, and shelters employ this powerful strategy. Return to a full-sized, reciprocal ISN occurs over years.

Patients should undergo several months' sobriety and emotional recovery before initiating a process that could be stressful and result in rejections. Choosing an initial group highly likely to invite the person in (eg, a mutual-help group) provides a favorable beginning. Accreting additional subgroups should be a careful, deliberate process.

TABLE 42-1	Characteristics of the Intimate Social Network in Relation to Clinical Category				
Clinical Categories (and Clinical Locus)	**Number of People**	**Subgroups**	**Reciprocity**	**Connectedness**[a]	**Other Characteristics**
Healthy, normal	20–30	4–5	Symmetric	80%	Stable, durable
Dysfunctional and/or discomforted (clinic)	10–19	2–3	Symmetric	60%	May include pets, caregivers, deceased
Disabled (residential, day program)	1–9	1	Asymmetric	100%	Overly reliant on one group
Isolated (inpatient setting, jail, homeless, emergency room)	0	0	Absent	0%	Crisis, suicidal, high mortality

[a]Likelihood that any one person in the proband's intimate social network (ISN) knows anyone else in the ISN.

Cultural Recovery in Addictive Disorders

ISN reconstruction poses challenges because most healthy people have a full complement of people with whom they have stable relationships. Useful strategies for rebuilding one's ISN include the following:

- Joining a recovery group
- Residing in a sober-living facility
- Participating in a sports, exercise, or occupational association
- Volunteering at a clinic, hospital, nursing home, or social agency
- Returning to an ethnic association or church group
- Starting a new job

More difficult obstacles await building bridges back to relatives and family members. Previous SUD-related affronts may have alienated them. Delaying these efforts until achieving 6 to 24 months' sobriety may be wise. If the recovering person suffers slips or recurrences—common in the early months or recovery—this can reaffirm the family's worst fears. Twelve-step work covers several early steps that prepare the recovering person for making amends to estranged family and former friends.

Resuming former affiliations can give rise to emotionally warm and spiritually uplifting experiences. These journeys back can also give rise to pain, regret, shame, and guilt. Rejection can encourage affiliations with new relationships.

Internet-based social media comprises an increasingly popular means for recovering people to engage with like-minded people via messaging, posting stories, sharing photos, playing competitive games, beginning new relationships, and even attending mutual-help groups. For some, social media can serve as a valuable source of support, such as receiving "likes" and supportive comments after posting an achievement. However, overuse, risky use, or too trusting use of the Internet can precipitate relapse. A lonely person might buy into the illusion of real relationships, which turn out to be Internet fictions or scam artists. Having 400 "friends" on an online social network cannot mimic the commitment, continuity, and reciprocity existing within a flourishing face-to-face ISN.

Evolution of Sociocultural Interventions

Sociocultural therapies outside of traditional clinics and hospitals have evolved over decades and centuries, as individuals, communities, clinicians, and researchers grapple with the lengthy duration and extensive rehabilitation necessary for recovery. Some of these interventions survive and are used internationally (eg, mutual help groups, day hospitals, workplace programs).

Culture-Specific Treatment

Therapies specific to particular cultures can contribute to recovery from SUDs. Participation aids the recovering person in several ways: by providing a sober environment, engaging in meaningful work, receiving emotional support from others, and building a new identity as a recovering person. Some interventions are ceremonial in nature, symbolizing spiritual rebirth or successful healing.

CONCLUSIONS

Across history, cultural groups have fostered specific norms with regard to type, amount, frequency, location, and even demography of substance use. Cultural dissension regarding tobacco, alcohol, opioids, cannabis, and other substances aspires fundamentally at evolving a common cultural consensus—a difficult task in complex, multiethnic cultures that value individuality, autonomy, and egalitarianism.

Clinicians can increase their effectiveness by inquiring about the cultural elements that accompany patients into the consultation room. Assessing the patient's ISN can instruct us on the severity of the disorder, social resources at hand, and formulation of realistic treatment goals. Cultural factors have contributed greatly to SUD transmission, but cultural resources and traditions can also guide clinicians and patients during recovery.

REVIEW QUESTIONS

1. Which of the following is *not* an example of a norm gap?
   A. Cannabis is illegal under federal law but legal according to certain state laws.
   B. Gangs requiring cocaine use as part of new member initiation
   C. Widespread opioid prescribing for chronic pain despite limited evidence of its efficacy
   D. Binge drinking on "dry" college campuses
   E. None of the above

2. Which of the following clinical categories is characterized by an intimate social network (ISN) involving 10 to 19 people; two or three longstanding subgroups; plus more recent one-on-one relationships; 60% connectedness; reciprocity; and

possible reporting of pets, caregivers, or deceased persons?

A. Normal, healthy
B. Dysfunctional and/or discomforted
C. Disabled
D. Isolated
E. A and B

3. Eliciting a culturally competent substance use history should include inquiry regarding which of the following?

A. Socialization into psychoactive substance use disorder
B. Association of substance use with developmental tasks and life stressors
C. Observations of role models
D. Early substance use experience
E. All of the above

ANSWERS

1. **D**
2. **B**
3. **E**

SUGGESTED READING

Carstairs GM. Daru and bhang; cultural factors in the choice of intoxicant. *Q J Studies Alcohol*. 1954;15(2):220-237.

Dumont MP. Tavern culture: the sustenance of homeless men. *Am J Orthopsychiatry*. 1967;37(5):938-945.

Favazza A, Thompson JJ. Social networks of alcoholics: some early findings. *Alcohol Clin Exp Res*. 1984;8(1):9-15.

Galanter M. *Network Therapy for Alcohol and Drug Abuse*. New York: Basic Books, 1993.

Hingson RW, Zha W, Weitzman ER. *Magnitude of and trends in alcohol-related mortality and morbidity among U.S. college students ages 18-24, 1998-2005. J Stud Alcohol Drugs Suppl.* 2009;(16):12-20.

College Student Drinking

Summary by Frank J. Schwebel, Ursula Whiteside, Joyce N. Bittinger, Jason R. Kilmer, Ty W. Lostutter, and Mary E. Larimer

> Based on THE ASAM PRINCIPLES OF ADDICTION MEDICINE, 6th edition chapter by Frank J. Schwebel, Ursula Whiteside, Joyce N. Bittinger, Jason R. Kilmer, Ty W. Lostutter, and Mary E. Larimer

PREVALENCE AND CONSEQUENCES

The US Department of Health and Human Services and the Surgeon General have classified college student heavy episodic (or binge) drinking as a major public health problem. Annually, an estimated 1825 college student deaths between 1998 and 2005 involved alcohol. Despite ongoing research and administrative efforts directed toward decreasing college student binge drinking, problems and consequences such as driving under the influence, academic and relationship consequences, and student deaths due to alcohol-related injuries and suicide continue to occur at relatively high rates.

Drinking Rates and Disorders Among College Students

Approximately four of five college students (81%) have consumed alcohol, and 68% have been drunk at least once in their lives. Approximately 18% to 21% of college students meet *Diagnostic and Statistical Manual of Mental Disorders*, 4th edition (*DSM-IV*) criteria for an alcohol use disorder (with 8% to 13% classified as abuse and 7% to 13% classified as dependence). For college students, 38% reported having been drunk in the past month, 31% reported having engaged in heavy episodic drinking in the past 2 weeks (defined by the National Institute on Alcohol Abuse and Alcoholism as reaching a blood alcohol concentration of 0.08% or higher, usually by consuming five or more drinks for men or four or more for women over a 2-hour period), and 3% reported drinking daily. An estimated 43% of students diagnosed with an alcohol use disorder during early college continue to meet criteria (ie, are not in remission) after college.

Alcohol-Related Problems and Consequences

The National Institute on Alcohol Abuse and Alcoholism (NIAAA) Task Force on College Drinking categorized college student drinking consequences as damage to self, others, or the institution.

Damage to Self

The most commonly reported negative physical effects of alcohol in college populations are nausea, vomiting, and hangovers. Approximately 25% of college students report negative academic consequences due to drinking such as missing or falling behind in class, and higher levels of drinking are associated with a lower grade point average. Additionally, college students risk legal consequences by driving under the influence (29%) and/or may be involved with local or campus police due to drinking (5%).

Damage to Others

Damage to others due to heavy alcohol use include motor vehicle accidents, noise, fighting, public urination, and problematic encounters with drunken individuals. Among students living on campus, 60% experienced interrupted study or sleep due to other students' drinking, 48% took care of a drunk student, and almost 20% had a serious argument or experienced an unwanted sexual overture (for females) involving alcohol. An estimated 646,000 students experience physical assault by another drunken student and 97,000 experience alcohol-related sexual assaults. Sexual assaults tend to occur at colleges with high rates of binge drinking and approximately three out of four students who reported a sexual assault were under the influence of alcohol during the assault.

Damage to the Institution

Damage to the institution includes problems such as violence, vandalism, and property damage. Those who sporadically and frequently binge drink are 4 and 10 times more likely, respectively, to report having damaged property than those who do not binge drink, and it is estimated that 50% to 80% of the violence that occurs on campuses is alcohol related.

Risk Factors for College Student Drinking

Identified risk factors for heavy drinking among college students include demographic and environmental influences, cognitive and motivational factors, and affective factors. However, college student drinking is predominantly considered a contextually limited pattern of use characterized by high rates of alcohol use that does not typically persist past students' transition to postcollege roles.

Demographics

Sex

College men drink more often, consume greater quantities of alcohol, experience more alcohol-related problems, and are more likely to engage in heavy episodic drinking than college women. However, current measures of alcohol-related problems may be biased toward detecting consequences more common in men (eg, externalizing behavior) than women (eg, internalizing behavior).

Ethnicity

White college students are the most likely to engage in heavy episodic drinking. White, American Indian, and Alaskan native college students tend to experience more problems related to drinking. African American students are least likely to engage in heavy drinking and are less likely to experience alcohol-related problems, followed by Asian American students.

Team Athletics and Fraternity and Sorority Membership

Involvement in college athletics is associated with more frequent drinking and other risky behaviors. Students in team sports report higher drinking and binge drinking rates than individual sports.

Fraternity and sorority organizations can be environments in which heavy drinking is considered normative. Members of the Greek system consume alcohol at greater frequencies and quantities than their non–fraternity/sorority peers, and membership has consistently been shown to be a risk factor for heavy episodic drinking. However, there can be a great deal of variability in drinking rates within a fraternity or sorority, and not all Greek organization members drink heavily or at all.

VETERANS AND MILITARY SERVICE MEMBERS

Many veterans will return from deployment with physical and psychological challenges that may impede their academic success. In average, veterans have high rates of alcohol use and psychiatric disorders that can interfere with class attendance, decrease grades and tests scores, and lead to withdrawal or dropout from college.

Individual and Environmental Risk Factors

Drinking Expectancies and Motives

Alcohol outcome expectancies are the set of beliefs one carries about the positive and negative effects of alcohol consumption. Expectancies likely develop into motives—a person's stated reason for drinking or not drinking over time. The most commonly reported drinking motives are conformity (ie, drinking to avoid social costs or rejection), enhancement (ie, drinking to enhance a positive mood), social (ie, drinking to obtain positive social rewards), and coping (ie, drinking to regulate a negative affect).

Social Norms and Misperceptions

College students consistently overestimate the rates at which other college students drink, the amount they consume when drinking, and the extent to which other students support heavy drinking. The degree to which students overestimate other students' drinking predicts their own increased consumption (ie, the higher the overestimation, the higher the drinking level). Identification with a specific reference group (eg, same sex, Greek status) is a moderator of the relationship between perceived group drinking norms and own drinking levels such that the greater the group identification, the more similar the individual drinking levels.

Environmental Risk and Protective Factors

Environmental factors such as the cost and accessibility of drinking venues can influence alcohol consumption. As the cost of alcohol around a university increases, consumption decreases. When multiple drinking venues exist, short- and long-term drinking problems increase. Students in a setting where many people are intoxicated were found to be 13 times more likely to report consuming five or more drinks. Consuming alcohol prior to departing for one's intended social activity or eventual destination (eg, prepartying, pregaming) is associated with an increased blood alcohol concentration and a higher incidence of consequences, particularly for women. Drinking games are a common form of prepartying and have been identified as a risk factor for "problematic" drinking and have been associated with heavy drinking episodes. Additionally, the culture surrounding collegiate sporting events seems to be influenced by alcohol. However, some environmental variables can serve as protective factors against high-risk drinking. These include designated substance-free housing and 12-step recovery groups on campus. Research suggests that living in a designated substance-free housing environment, even for those who drink, is a protective factor for negative consequences and is associated with increased use of preventive behaviors.

PREVENTION STRATEGIES AND INTERVENTIONS
College Drinking Prevention Strategies

The NIAAA's 2002 Task Force Report on College Drinking represented the joint efforts of researchers and college presidents to address the harms of and solutions to college drinking. The task force report designated four tiers of prevention strategies:

- Tier I interventions have documented, replicated evidence of efficacy in college populations. Interventions may be delivered in an individual or group setting with a facilitator.
- Tier II interventions have documented evidence of efficacy in general populations and could be adapted for college students.
- Tier III interventions show logical and theoretical promise but need more research.
- Tier IV interventions show no evidence of effectiveness.

In 2015, the NIAAA created the College Alcohol Intervention Matrix (CollegeAIM) to help college administrators review cost and effectiveness findings of college drinking interventions.

Individually Focused Interventions

Each Tier I intervention of the NIAAA Task Force Report on College Drinking has an individually focused intervention component. Research supporting the efficacy of these approaches has typically evaluated their use with high-risk students. Studies have also examined peer versus professional delivery and the efficacy and benefits of Web-based delivery of interventions.

Multicomponent Skills-Based Interventions

Multicomponent skills-based interventions (eg, the Alcohol Skills Training Program) typically combine cognitive–behavioral skills training with norms clarification, using a motivational interviewing (MI) style to reduce resistance and promote change. The CollegeAIM matrix reported that 20 of 32 studies including a multicomponent skills intervention produced statistically significant reductions in alcohol use, harmful consequences due to drinking, or both.

Expectancy Challenge Interventions

Expectancy challenge interventions are a Tier I cognitive–behavioral intervention, typically delivered experientially or didactically, aimed at changing students' positive expectations for alcohol intoxication via the alcohol placebo effect. Experientially, students experience the alcohol placebo effect directly to demonstrate how expectations influence experiences. Didactically, students are educated about the placebo effect and alcohol expectancies. Experiential interventions are typically found to be more effective; however, there also are positive effects associated with didactic interventions.

Brief Motivational Interventions

The Brief Alcohol Screening and Intervention for College Students is listed in the task force report as a Tier I intervention. It includes a comprehensive assessment followed by a 1-hour personalized feedback interview. The interview uses an MI style (ie, a nonjudgmental, nonconfrontational approach that emphasizes meeting people where they are with regard to their readiness to change) and is structured around a review of graphic feedback generated from the assessment.

Brief MI approaches to college drinking, such as Brief Alcohol Screening and Intervention for College Students, have been found to reduce alcohol use, consequences of alcohol use, or both across follow-up periods of up to 4 years. Studies have successfully employed brief MI approaches in both group and individual formats, with men, women, mixed genders, and high-risk volunteers as well as mandated or judicially referred students. Additionally, brief MIs have been successfully implemented in a variety of settings, including campus health clinics and fraternities. Thus, this type of intervention appears to be flexible and robust, reliably producing drinking reductions in a wide segment of the campus population in efficacy studies.

Feedback-Only Interventions

Written, mailed, or Internet-based assessment and feedback interventions provide an inexpensive and less resource intensive method of delivering motivational feedback. The CollegeAIM matrix found that 26 of 31 feedback-only interventions were associated with significant reductions in alcohol use, albeit less significant than in-person brief MIs. Four of five studies investigating self-monitoring or self-assessment of alcohol use and/or consequences in the absence of other intervention strategies reported significant reductions in alcohol use and/or consequences.

Pharmacotherapy

There is a lack of research on the use of pharmacotherapy with college students for the treatment of alcohol use disorder. This may in part be caused by the lack of college students who self-refer for treatment. A large proportion of college students receiving treatment are mandated and either may not be aware of or may not be interested in pharmacotherapy or may be reluctant to use a medication that can cause them to experience unpleasant sensations (eg, nausea) while drinking. Early findings on pharmacotherapy are promising for decreasing the amount of drinking. However, the challenge remains in motivating college students to seek pharmacotherapy.

Structural Interventions

Due to the important interaction between context and drinking, the NIAAA Task Force Report and the CollegeAIM matrix outlined several environmentally focused approaches. Environmental strategies had varying amount of empirical data and were found to fall in either Tier II or III. They are recommended for use as part of an overall multicomponent strategic plan. Strategies include

- increased enforcement of minimum drinking age laws (Tier II),
- increased publicity about and enforcement of underage drinking laws on campus and eliminating "mixed messages" (Tier III),
- restrictions on alcohol retail outlet density (Tier II), and
- consistently enforcing disciplinary actions for policy violations (Tier III).

Another study identifies environmental change as one of four key areas for intervention to decrease alcohol misuse. They suggest five subcategories of strategic interventions:

1. Promoting alcohol-free options;
2. Creating an environment that supports health-promoting norms;
3. Limiting alcohol availability on and off campus;
4. Restricting alcohol promotion and marketing on and off campus; and
5. Developing and enforcing policies and laws surrounding alcohol consumption.

CONCLUSIONS AND FUTURE DIRECTIONS

Advances have been made in identifying effective strategies to reduce alcohol consumption and associated consequences. It is important to recognize that alcohol use does not occur in a vacuum, and attention should be paid to the context of college student alcohol use. In addition to reported alcohol use, 41% of college students also report use of an illicit drug in the past year, 38% of students report past-year use of marijuana, and 19% of students report past-year use of any illicit drug other than marijuana. Another trend is for individuals to combine alcohol use with over-the-counter caffeinated energy drinks.

Future research efforts will need to more consistently measure the impact on other drug use when alcohol is the focus of prevention or intervention efforts and will need to identify effective strategies for working with polysubstance-using college students. Also related to the context of student alcohol use are co-occurring mental health problems. In a national survey of counseling center directors conducted in 2014, 94% of directors felt that psychological problems were becoming more severe. Given success with brief interventions focused on depression and alcohol, future research must consider strategies to address the overlap of mental health issues and substance use.

Brief MIs utilizing assessments and individualized, in-person feedback are consistently efficacious at reducing alcohol use across a number of college student settings, and effectiveness trials on college campuses have supported these findings. In addition, cognitive–behavioral skills-based interventions have clear evidence of efficacy. Given the difficulties with engaging students in in-person interventions on college campuses, integration of these resources into existing points of contact (eg, academic courses, residence halls, Greek social organizations, student services, and campus health and mental health settings) holds promise for reaching students in need of services.

Although it may seem intuitive to screen for alcohol problems in a campus health setting, the data suggest that this is not a widespread practice. Approximately one third of health centers at 4-year colleges or universities routinely screen for alcohol problems; however, only 17% of these used standardized instruments as part of their screening. Thus, in addition to integrating services into points of contact, reliable and valid screening strategies should be used.

There is also evidence to suggest mailed and computerized feedback can be effective and feasible on college campuses. Several commercially available computerized screening and intervention products exist, and many are reviewed in the CollegeAIM matrix. Although there are documented barriers to dissemination, adoption, implementation, and maintenance of empirically tested approaches, these barriers are clearly surmountable.

College student alcohol use and consequences are not unique problems on any one campus. Rather, there are shared challenges across campuses and increasingly shared successes. As colleges move toward developing campus–community coalitions and cooperative statewide coalitions, efforts to impact student health move beyond the responsibility of the individual campus that allows for shared knowledge and resources.

ACKNOWLEDGMENTS

Portions of this chapter were written with grant support from the National Institutes of Health/National Institute on Alcohol Abuse and Alcoholism, F31 AA025531, awarded to Frank J. Schwebel, and R01 AA012547 and T32 AA07455-29, awarded to Mary E. Larimer, and from the Alcoholic Beverage Medical Research Foundation, the Foundation for Alcohol Research awarded to Ty W. Lostutter, and with fellowship support from the Group Health Foundation, awarded to Ursula Whiteside.

KEY POINTS

1. Heavy episodic drinking by college students is a major public health and safety problem impacting both the individuals that drink and the environment around them. However, college drinking is also predominantly considered a contextually limited pattern of use that does not typically persist beyond students' transition to postcollege roles.

2. Individually focused interventions, multicomponent skills-based interventions, expectancy challenge interventions, brief motivational interventions, feedback-only interventions, pharmacotherapy, and structural/environmental interventions are tools and strategies that have been developed to help address the issue of heavy episodic drinking among college students.

3. It is important to take into account changing methods of reaching young people (eg, Internet-, text message-, and app-based interventions) as well as ever-evolving demographic and structural changes.

REVIEW QUESTIONS

1. Which of the following is not a Tier I intervention?
   A. Brief motivational interventions
   B. Structural interventions
   C. Individually focused interventions
   D. Expectancy challenge interventions

2. Which of the following is not an environmental risk factor for college student drinking?
   A. Pregaming
   B. Tailgating
   C. Cost of alcohol near campus
   D. Drinking to cope

3. Which of the following pharmacotherapies is specifically designed for college-aged students?
   A. Disulfiram
   B. Extended release naltrexone
   C. Acamprosate
   D. None of the above.

ANSWERS

1. **B**
2. **D**
3. **D**

SUGGESTED READINGS

Cronce JM, Larimer ME. Brief individual-focused alcohol interventions for college students. In: White HR, Rabiner DL, eds. *College Drinking and Drug Use.* New York: Guilford Press, 2011.

Hingson RW, Zha W, Weitzman ER. Magnitude of and trends in alcohol-related mortality and morbidity among U.S. college students ages 18-24, 1998-2005. *J Stud Alcohol Drugs Suppl.* 2009;(16):12-20.

National Institute on Alcohol Abuse and Alcoholism. *Planning Alcohol Interventions Using NIAAA's College AIM Alcohol Intervention Matrix.* Rockville, MD: National Institutes of Health, 2015. NIH Publication No. 15-AA-8017.

Task Force of the National Advisory Council on Alcohol Abuse and Alcoholism. *A Call to Action: Changing the Culture of Drinking at US Colleges.* Rockville, MD: National Institutes of Health, 2002. NIH Publication No. 02-5010.

Wechsler H, Lee JE, Kuo M, et al. Trends in college binge drinking during a period of increased prevention efforts: findings from 4 Harvard School of Public Health College Alcohol Study surveys: 1993-2001. *J Am Coll Health.* 2002;50(5):203-217.

44 Understanding "Behavioral Addiction"

Summary by Yvonne H.C. Yau, Sarah W. Yip, and
Marc N. Potenza

Based on THE ASAM PRINCIPLES OF ADDICTION MEDICINE,
6th edition chapter by Yvonne H.C. Yau, Sarah W. Yip, and
Marc N. Potenza

The term *addiction* is derived from the Latin word *addicere*, meaning "bound to" or "enslaved by." Addiction is often described as having four defining components: (1) continued engagement in behavior despite adverse consequences, (2) diminished self-control over engagement in the behavior, (3) compulsive engagement in the behavior, and (4) an appetitive urge or craving state prior to engagement in the behavior. In its original formulation, the term was not linked to substance use but gradually became primarily associated with substance use behaviors. More recently, the term addiction has been increasingly applied to describe excessive engagement in nondrug behaviors, such as gambling, sex, and eating. Aided by data from neurobiological studies, this view is gaining momentum and has led to the renaming of the substance-related disorders diagnostic category to substance-related and addictive disorders in the *Diagnostic and Statistical Manual of Mental Disorders*, 5th edition (*DSM-5*). Currently, only gambling disorder (previously referred to as pathologic gambling) has been included in this category by the American Psychiatric Association, which concluded that there is presently insufficient research to warrant the consideration of other behavioral addictions in the main section.

IMPULSE CONTROL DISORDERS: BEHAVIORAL ADDICTIONS?

Several disorders that may be considered as behavioral addictions have been traditionally categorized in the *DSM* as impulse control disorders (ICDs) not elsewhere classified. Among issues being considered within research workgroups are whether ICDs might be best categorized separately, with substance use disorders (SUDs) as addictions, or with obsessive-compulsive disorders as obsessive-compulsive spectrum disorders.

GAMBLING DISORDER

Gambling disorder (GD) and SUDs share similar clinical characteristics and diagnostic criteria. Individuals with GD often experience withdrawal, craving, tolerance, and failed attempts to reduce or abate gambling behaviors, all of which are common features of SUDs. They also share phenomenological features: both often begin in adolescence and young adulthood, prevalence estimates tend to decrease across adulthood, and the phenomenon of "telescoping," whereby the time between initiation and problematic engagement in the addictive behavior is shorter in females than males, is observed in both conditions. These commonalities, in addition to high comorbidity rates for GD and SUDs, suggest common vulnerability factors for both disorders.

Neurocognitive research provides evidence for dysregulation of the ventromedial prefrontal cortex and orbitofrontal cortex in individuals with GD. Impaired performance on risk/reward decision-making tasks, and on neurocognitive tasks involving inhibition, time estimation, cognitive estimating, and planning tasks has been observed among individuals with GD and in individuals with SUDs.

Individuals with GD often make disadvantageous decisions, selecting small immediate rewards over larger delayed rewards. The rapid temporal discounting of rewards has been termed *delay discounting* because rewards are more steeply discounted as a function of delay duration. Poorer performance on delay discounting measures (ie, more rapid discounting of rewards) has been observed in multiple populations, including in those with SUDs and GD. Delay discounting involves aspects of reward evaluation, and multiple brain regions contribute to reward processing in humans. Among the most widely implicated brain regions in subjective reward valuation is the nucleus accumbens (NAc), situated in the ventral striatum, and the ventromedial prefrontal cortex, both of which are also frequently implicated in SUDs. An effective functional balance between these reciprocally connected neural regions may underlie appropriate and advantageous behavioral responses to varying reward contingencies.

Research suggests that dysregulation of the mesocorticolimbic dopamine system (often referred to as the reward pathway and frequently implicated in SUDs) may contribute to GD. In particular, corticostriatal and forebrain neuromodulatory systems are frequently implicated. In recent years, multiple studies have investigated the neurostructural correlates of psychiatric disorders using either diffusion tensor imaging or voxel-based morphometry to assess white and gray matter structures, respectively. Findings from diffusion tensor imaging studies indicate similar alterations in white matter microstructure—encompassing regions of callosal, association, and projection fiber tracts among individuals with GD and SUDs. Preliminary voxel-based morphometry data suggested no alteration in grey matter macrostructures in GD, although more recent data indicate smaller amygdalar and hippocampal volumes, as have been reported in SUDs.

A number of neurotransmitters have also been implicated in GD, with studies suggesting possible roles for serotonin (5-HT), dopamine (DA), and norepinephrine (NE). Serotonin neurons project from the raphe nucleus of the brain stem to multiple brain regions, including the hippocampus, amygdala, and prefrontal cortex. It has been hypothesized that dysregulated 5-HT functioning may underlie behavioral inhibition and impulsivity in GD. Data from studies of cerebrospinal fluid, pharmacologic challenge, and preclinical investigations together suggest a role for 5-HT in GD. Selective serotonin reuptake inhibitors (SSRIs) have been found to improve social functioning and reduce gambling behaviors and thoughts about gambling in GD, although clinical trial findings involving SSRIs have generally been mixed.

DA is involved in the encoding of rewarding and aversive stimuli and is implicated in the neurobiology of drug addiction particularly those involving stimulant use. Mixed data exist for a role for DA in GD, and clinical treatments for GD have yet to emerge based on DA, perhaps given inconsistencies in findings linking DA to aspects of GD.

Dysregulation of NE (a neurotransmitter implicated in arousal, attention, and sensation-seeking behaviors) has been reported in individuals with GD. Data suggest that there may be an elevation of NE activity (as indexed by elevated urinary concentration and cerebrospinal fluid levels of a metabolite of NE) among individuals with GD, and this elevation may be potentiated by gambling behaviors.

Pharmacologic challenge studies suggest a dysregulation of the opioid system in GD. Naltrexone and nalmefene, both opioid receptor antagonists, have been found to reduce gambling-related thoughts and behaviors in individuals with GD.

Family and twin-based studies of addiction indicate that genetic factors are important in the development of both SUDs and GD. Twin data suggest similar heritability rates to SUDs, with roughly 50% of the probability of developing GD attributable to inherited factors. Molecular genetic research has identified specific genetic alleles involved in the encoding of DA- and 5-HT–related moieties that are associated with GD, although negative results have also been observed.

BINGE EATING DISORDER

Data suggest that both substance use and eating behaviors may be modulated by the same motivational neurocircuitry, leading to the conceptualization of "foods as drugs." Binge eating disorder (BED)—distinct from bulimia nervosa because it does not include compensatory behaviors such as purging—is associated with obesity and other negative sequelae.

Previously listed as an eating disorder not otherwise specified, BED has its own diagnostic code in the *DSM-5*. The new diagnostic features are very similar to those for SUDs and ICDs: recurrent episodes, impaired control, and marked distress in relation to binge eating. There have been multiple and diverse attempts at treatment interventions, including preventive, pharmaceutical, and the more invasive surgical interventions.

Lesions in the hypothalamus, which plays an important role in the maintenance of energy homeostasis via regulatory neuropeptides such as leptin, cholecystokinin, and ghrelin, can result in hypophagia. Leptin, an adipose-derived hormone, has been implicated in other reward-seeking behaviors, including SUDs. Administration of leptin replacement treatment in individuals with leptin deficiency syndrome, a rare condition in humans, has decreased hyperphagia and reduced activation of reward centers such as the NAc during feeding conditions, suggesting that leptin may help encode palatability.

In addition to its metabolic function, leptin may help modulate mesolimbic DA reward circuits. For example, exogenous leptin administration to the ventral tegmental area results in a decrease in food consumption and reduces the firing of DA neurons.

The mesocorticolimbic reward pathways contribute importantly to eating behaviors. For example, increased activation of these brain regions have been observed subsequent to both the presentation and consumption of palatable food. Preclinical research has demonstrated that knockdown of striatal DA D2-receptors rapidly accelerates the development of addictionlike reward deficits and the onset of compulsivelike food-seeking behaviors.

Partially modulated by adipose-derived hormones such as leptin and ghrelin, orexins are important modulators for eating behavior and help to maintain energy homeostasis. Orexin administration has been demonstrated to increase feeding behaviors and reinstate substance-using behavior, whereas the opposite is observed with orexin receptor antagonists. Preclinical research suggests orexin may directly influence DA pathways, although further research investigating their relationship in clinical populations is needed.

Unlike leptin and orexin, ghrelin is orexigenic and increases food intake and body weight. Ghrelin levels appear inversely correlated with a patient's body mass index and have also been positively associated with synapse formation and DA turnover in the NAc, which in turn modulates the rewarding properties of food.

Stimulation of NAc opioid receptors enhances palatability and food intake, whereas opioid receptor antagonists extinguish previously established preferences for hyperpalatable foods. The NAc may also be important in general habit formation or basic motor control of feeding behaviors, independent of palatability. Cannabinoid receptors in the NAc have been implicated in appetitive behavior, and endogenous cannabinoids may contribute to the experience and encoding of food-associated rewards. Cannabinoid receptor antagonists have demonstrated some positive results for the treatment of BED, although they have been associated with adverse psychiatric effects.

Aside from mesolimbic areas, frontal regions also play an important role in food cravings, gluttony, and weight. Within the prefrontal cortex, the activation of dorsal regions has been associated with reductions in food craving and weight loss success, whereas activation of ventral regions, including the orbitofrontal cortex, has been negatively correlated with greater dietary restraint. Individuals with BED, anorexia nervosa, or bulimia nervosa typically perform poorer on decision-making tasks, indirectly suggesting a frontal lobe dysfunction.

Increases in both exogenous and endogenous 5-HT is associated with reductions in food intake and weight gain and increases in energy expenditure. Hypothalamic 5-HT may, in part, mediate the experience of satiety and has been implicated in the management of eating behavior, in particular with meal termination. Preclinical research suggests 5-HT may contribute to food preference and carbohydrate intake. Some research suggests that SSRIs are effective at targeting binge eating, psychiatric, and weight symptoms, although the effectiveness and duration of these medications remain under debate.

COMPULSIVE SEXUAL BEHAVIOR

Characterized by excessive engagement in normative sexual behavior, compulsive sexual behavior (CSB) or problematic sexual behavior can be divided into paraphilic (ie, disturbance in object selection) and nonparaphilic (ie, engaging in sexual behavior in an excessive, obsessive, or compulsive manner) behaviors. Although it is estimated that 5% to 6% of the US adult population match the criteria for CSB, systematic examinations are lacking and most studies predominantly investigate male clinical populations. CSB frequently co-occurs with multiple psychiatric disorders where high impulsivity is implicated (eg, SUDs, ICDs, attention deficit hyperactivity disorder), as well as with mood disorders. Nonparaphilic CSB is not specifically listed in the *DSM-5*; it can be classified as either ICD not otherwise specified or a sexual disorder not otherwise specified. Seven distinct CSB categories have been proposed, each with its own constellation of symptoms. When assessing sexual behaviors, some criteria are based on frequency of orgasms, whereas others more closely resemble the diagnostic criteria for SUDs and ICDs, including impaired control and maladaptive preoccupation with sexual behavior and/or thoughts.

Structural studies suggest bilateral temporal lobe and amygdala lesions have been associated with Klüver-Bucy syndrome, of which a symptom is hypersexuality. However, Klüver-Bucy syndrome is extremely rare in humans. There has been one small-scale diffusion tensor imaging study of white matter microstructures in CSB, suggesting higher mean diffusivity in the superior frontal region among individuals with CSB compared to healthy controls.

Open-label prescriptions of various antidepressants and antipsychotics have been used to treat CSB, but their efficacy remains to be systematically examined. These include treatments targeting serotonergic, opioid, and dopaminergic systems, which may influence sexual functioning and desire.

However, there is mixed evidence to support the efficacy of these pharmacologic interventions in treating CSB symptoms.

PROBLEMATIC INTERNET USE

Problematic Internet use (PIU) or Internet addiction is characterized by excessive or poorly controlled urges and a maladaptive obsession with the Internet. As with other ICDs, PIU involves excessive engagement in socially normative activities. Although considered for inclusion in the *DSM-5*, it was concluded there is currently insufficient evidence to warrant the addition of PIU. Definitions of PIU have therefore often been based on the *DSM-IV* criteria for GD. However, the lack of a universal assessment tool may contribute to the wide range of prevalence estimates among adolescents and adults. PIU frequently co-occurs with SUDs as well as other psychiatric conditions.

Although evidence remains scarce, emerging research suggests increased resting-state regional homogeneity in frontal areas among individuals with PIU. Other evidence suggests differences in brain function, such as in the anterior and posterior cingulate cortices, during cognitive tasks that may reflect a sensitization to reward and desensitization to loss. Structurally, decreased grey matter density in brain areas implicated in decision making and widespread impairments in white matter microstructures have been reported among individuals with PIU although further research is needed.

Currently, two small-scale ligand-based studies of dopaminergic functioning among individuals with PIU exist. Together they indicate that individuals with PIU may have reduced dopamine transporter expression and dopamine D2-receptor availability in striatal regions.

Specific genetic alleles related to encoding for 5-HT and nicotinic acetylcholine–related moieties have also been implicated in PIU. However, replication of these findings is needed. Data suggest that attention deficient hyperactivity disorder, depression, and aggression may be vulnerability factors for PIU. However, certain factors (such as aggression) were associated with increased severity in PIU but only among males. Moreover, some data suggest that men are more likely to have PIU, although this gender gap may be diminishing.

PROBLEMATIC VIDEO GAME PLAYING

Problematic video game playing (PVG) or video game addiction is both similar to and distinct from other behavioral addictions in its availability and use of visual and auditory rewards. Previous research on PVG has often included online games; thus, video game findings cannot be clearly separated from Internet findings based on existing data.

Although no *DSM*-based diagnostic criteria exist, similar to PIU, assessment tools for PVG are often based on the *DSM-IV* definitions for SUDs and GD. Prevalence estimates have ranged from 4.2% to 20.0% for adolescent populations and roughly 11.9% for adult populations. Psychiatric comorbidities remain poorly researched, although preliminary findings suggest links with attention deficit hyperactivity disorder, mood disorders, and SUDs. Criteria for Internet gaming disorder have been introduced into section III of the *DSM-5*, and this has facilitated research into this phenomenon.

Structural and functional differences in the ventral striatum are demonstrated when comparing frequent versus infrequent gamers. Other brain regions have also been implicated in other studies. In particular, the orbitofrontal cortex, striatum, and anterior cingulate—all of which are involved with subjective reward valuation—have been found to be hyperactivated among individuals with PVG.

Playing video games may increase the release of DA, particularly in the ventral striatum, at levels comparable to that induced by psychostimulant drugs. Moreover, bupropion (a drug with dopaminergic/noradrenergic reuptake blocking properties) administration decreased craving, time spent playing, and cue-induced brain activity in individuals with PVG. Polymorphisms of alleles related to encoding for DA receptors have been implicated in preliminary studies.

Although adolescent boys were more likely to endorse video gaming, no associations between video gaming and negative health measures were observed, suggesting that video gaming may be a normative behavior among boys. Research pertaining to gender-related differences in adults has yielded mixed results.

COMPULSIVE BUYING DISORDER

Although compulsive buying disorder (CBD) has long been recognized, little is known regarding its pathophysiology. Findings in an initial imaging study suggest individuals with CBD find shopping cues more rewarding (ie, increased NAc activation) and have poorer cognitive control (attenuated insula and anterior cingulate activation) while making purchasing decisions.

Results have been mixed with regard to the efficacy of pharmacologic treatment using SSRIs for CBD. Moreover, substantial placebo effects have been observed, raising questions regarding the clinical utility of SSRIs in treating CBD. There have been several case reports of successful naltrexone treatment (typically of high dosage) in patients with CBD.

CONCLUSION

Research on the neurobiology of behavioral addictions, particularly in GD, has increased in recent years. Whether we consider the neurobiological overlap between the two diagnostic criteria (eg, similarities between ICDs and SUDs as with the categorical *DSM* approach) or individual differences in different domains (eg, overlap in dimensional traits, such as impulsivity, with the research domain criteria approach), there is growing evidence suggesting multiple shared features between ICDs and SUDs. This has led to the consideration of these conditions as behavioral addictions, although alternate conceptualizations also warrant consideration. Additional research is needed to determine how specific disorders are related to one another and to specific SUDs, and how an improved understanding of the biology of these disorders may be translated into improved prevention and treatment strategies.

KEY POINTS

1. Research suggest similarities between substance addiction and excessive engagement in nondrug behaviors.
2. This has led to growing support for the conceptualization of *behavioral addictions*.
3. Disordered gambling has been recategorized under substance-related and addictive disorders in the *DSM-5*.
4. Internet gaming disorder has been introduced into section III of the *DSM-5* as an entity warranting further attention.
5. Behavioral addiction remains a debated topic and merits further research.

REVIEW QUESTIONS

1. Which of the following is categorized in the *DSM-5* as a substance-related and addictive disorder?
   A. Binge eating disorder
   B. Gambling disorder
   C. Internet gaming disorder
   D. Compulsive sexual behavior disorder

2. Which of the following statements is *false*?
   A. Dopamine has been implicated in the processing of rewards across disorders.
   B. Frontal cortical mechanisms have been implicated in gambling disorder and other behavioral addictions.
   C. Knowledge of the biological mechanisms underlying gambling disorder has been translated into effective pharmacotherapies with US Food and Drug Administration approval.
   D. One or more medications are available with US Food and Drug Administration indication for binge eating disorder.

3. Leptin has been most widely implicated in which of the following conditions?
   A. Gambling disorder
   B. Internet gaming disorder
   C. Binge eating disorder
   D. Compulsive sexual behavior disorder

ANSWERS

1. **B**
2. **C**
3. **C**

SUGGESTED READINGS

American Psychiatric Association. *Diagnostic and Statistical Manual of Mental Disorders*, 5th ed. Arlington, VA: American Psychiatric Association, 2013.

Grant JE, Potenza MN, Weinstein A, Gorelick DA. Introduction to behavioral addictions. *Am J Drug Alcohol Abuse.* 2010;36(5):233-241.

Holden C. Psychiatry. Behavioral addictions debut in proposed DSM-V. *Science.* 2010;327(5968):935.

45 Gambling Disorder: Clinical Characteristics and Treatment

Summary by Jon E. Grant

Based on THE ASAM PRINCIPLES OF ADDICTION MEDICINE,
6th edition chapter by Jon E. Grant and Brian L. Odlaug

Gambling disorder, also called pathologic gambling, is a psychiatric disorder characterized by persistent and recurrent maladaptive patterns of gambling behavior, which is associated with impaired functioning; reduced quality of life; and high rates of bankruptcy, divorce, and incarceration. Defined broadly as wagering money or something of value on an event with an uncertain outcome, gambling and excessive gambling behaviors have been reported for millennia across cultures and have been discussed in the medical literature since the early 1800s. Gambling disorder, however, was recognized by the American Psychiatric Association only in 1980 in their 3rd edition of the *Diagnostic and Statistical Manual of Mental Disorders* (*DSM-III*).

Currently classified in *DSM*, 5th edition (*DSM-5*) as a "substance-related and addictive disorder," the diagnosis of gambling disorder recommends that a person meet four of the possible nine criteria listed for the disorder. These criteria include (1) a preoccupation with gambling; (2) the need to gamble with higher amounts of money (tolerance); (3) has tried unsuccessfully to stop or reduce time spent gambling; (4) feels restless or irritable when not able to gamble; (5) gambles to escape from a mood or problems; (6) chasing losses; (7) lies to family, friends, others about amount or extent of gambling; (8) has lost or put into jeopardy a job, educational, or other opportunity due to gambling; and (9) has needed others to pay for finances due to gambling losses. Further, the gambling must not be better accounted for by a manic episode. The term *problem gambling* has been used to describe forms of disordered gambling, sometimes inclusive and at other times exclusive of gambling disorder. Problem gambling, like problem drinking, is not an officially recognized disorder by the American Psychiatric Association.

EPIDEMIOLOGY

A range of prevalence estimates have been reported for gambling disorder depending upon the time frame of the study, the instruments used to diagnose the disorder, and the population examined. In the general population of the United States, however, only four national studies and one meta-analysis of state and regional surveys have examined prevalence estimates of gambling disorder. The first national study in 1976 noted that 0.8% of 1749 adults contacted via telephone survey had a significant gambling problem. Twenty years later, the National Opinion Research Center at the University of Chicago conducted a national telephone survey (requested by the National Gambling Impact Study Commission) of 2417 adults and found a lifetime prevalence estimate of 0.8% of gambling disorder and an additional 1.3% of problem gambling. The National Epidemiologic Survey on Alcohol and Related Conditions, however, found that only 0.4% of adults in a community sample met current criteria for gambling disorder. A meta-analysis of 120 prevalence estimate surveys completed in North America from the late 1970s to the late 1990s found that the lifetime estimate of gambling disorder was 1.6% and the estimate of problem gambling was 3.9%, for a combined rate of 5.5% for some kind of disordered gambling; however, gambling exposure may influence prevalence rates of gambling disorder.

Subpopulations, including military veterans, young adults, and adolescents, have also demonstrated remarkable rates of problem gambling or gambling disorder. A recent study of 3157 US veterans noted that 2.2% met the criteria for at-risk or problem gambling. Young adult (ages 18 to 22 years) and adolescent (ages 14 to 18 years) studies have also illustrated that problem gambling is relatively common.

The incidence of gambling disorder appears higher in clinical samples. In individuals seeking treatment for substance use disorders, lifetime estimates of gambling disorder range from 5% to 33%. In studies of psychiatric inpatients, estimates of lifetime gambling disorder have ranged from 4.9% in adolescents to 6.9% in adults. There has been an accelerated proliferation of gambling venues since 2000, particularly with online gaming, American Indian casinos, and state-legalized forms of gambling such as riverboat gambling and casinos. With increased opportunity to gamble, some research suggests that we can expect greater rates of gambling disorder in the future.

Assessment

Gambling behavior and expenditures can be reliably measured with a timeline follow-back interview adapted from a method used for individuals who have problems with alcohol. A range of self-report and interview-based measures to screen for a gambling disorder have been developed.

Clinical Characteristics

Gambling disorder often begins in adolescence or early adulthood, with males tending to start at earlier ages. Although prospective studies are largely lacking, gambling disorder appears to follow a trajectory similar to that of substance use disorder, with high rates in adolescent and young adult groups, lower rates in older adults, and periods of abstinence and relapse. Gambling disorder can be a serious psychiatric disorder, but there is recent evidence that approximately one third of individuals with gambling disorder experience natural recovery (ie, without formal treatment). The research on natural recovery, however, is based on retrospective reports, and there is no data regarding whether these individuals who are symptom free for 1 year remain free of symptoms beyond that time or whether they relapse or change addictions.

Significant clinical differences have been observed in men and women with gambling disorder. Men with gambling disorder are more likely to be single and live alone as compared to women with the disorder. Males with gambling disorder are also more likely to have sought treatment for substance abuse, have higher rates of antisocial personality traits, and have marital consequences related to their gambling. Although men seem to start gambling at earlier ages and have higher rates of gambling disorder, women, who constitute approximately 32% of those with gambling disorder in the United States, seem to progress more quickly to severe consequences than do men. But women with gambling disorder are more likely to recover from and to seek treatment for their gambling problem.

The types of gambling preferred by men tend to be different from those preferred by women. Men with gambling disorders have higher rates of "strategic" forms of gambling, including sports betting, video poker, and blackjack. Women, on the other hand, have higher rates of "nonstrategic" gambling, such as slot machines or bingo. In regard to gambling triggers, though, both men and women report that advertisements trigger their urges to gamble, but men tend to report gambling for reasons unrelated to their emotional state, whereas women report gambling to escape from stress or owing to depressive states. Higher rates of sensation-seeking or action-seeking behavior in men have been suggested as a possible reason for this difference in gambling preference.

Functional Impairment, Quality of Life, and Legal Difficulties

Individuals with gambling disorder suffer significant impairment in their ability to function socially and occupationally. Many individuals report intrusive thoughts and urges related to gambling that interfere with their ability to concentrate at home and work. Work-related problems such as absenteeism, poor performance, and job loss are common. The inability to control behavior about which a person has mixed feelings may lead to feelings of shame and guilt. Gambling disorder is also frequently associated with marital problems and diminished intimacy and trust within the family. Financial difficulties often exacerbate personal and family problems; 44% of those with gambling disorder report loss of savings or retirement funds and 22% report losing homes or automobiles or pawning valuables owing to gambling.

With the functional impairment that these individuals experience, it is not surprising that they also report poor quality of life. In three studies systematically evaluating quality of life, individuals with gambling disorder reported significantly poorer life satisfaction compared to general, nonclinical adult samples. Gambling disorder is also associated with greater medical comorbidity (eg, cardiac problems, liver disease, obesity) and increased use of medical services. Possible reasons for the association of gambling disorder with health problems might be the sedentary nature of gambling, reduced leisure and exercise time, reduced sleep, increased stress, and increased nicotine and alcohol consumption.

Many individuals with gambling disorder report the need for psychiatric hospitalization owing to the depression and, at times, suicidality they feel was brought on by their gambling losses. Research on individuals in gambling treatment centers has found that 48% of individuals report having had gambling-related suicidal ideation at some time. The often overwhelming financial consequences, such as bankruptcy, associated with gambling disorder may also contribute to attempted or completed suicide. A study of Gamblers Anonymous participants (recruited through a gambling telephone hotline) found that 17% to 24% reported having attempted suicide owing to gambling.

In addition to the emotional impact of problem gambling, many individuals with gambling disorder have faced legal difficulties related to their gambling. Problem gambling or gambling disorder may lead people to engage in illegal behavior including embezzlement, stealing, and writing bad checks in order to either finance the gambling behavior or to compensate for past losses related to the excessive gambling.

Psychiatric Comorbidity

Psychiatric comorbidities are common in individuals with gambling disorder. Frequent co-occurrence has been reported between substance use disorders (including nicotine use disorder) and gambling disorder, with the highest odds ratios generally observed between gambling and alcohol use disorders.

Among clinical samples, 52% of Gamblers Anonymous participants reported either alcohol or drug use and 35% to 63% of individuals seeking treatment for gambling disorder also screened positive for a lifetime substance use disorder, rates notably higher than those found in the general population (26.6%). Similarly, a recent study of 84 treatment-seeking individuals with gambling disorder noted lifetime rates of attention deficit hyperactivity disorder in 26.3% of the sample, much higher than general population rates of 4% to 5%. Other studies clinically assessing co-occurring disorders in treatment-seeking individuals with gambling disorder have also noted high estimates of mood disorders (34% to 78%). These studies raise the question of whether co-occurring mood disorders may be secondary to gambling disorder.

High prevalence estimates of co-occurring anxiety disorders (28% to 40%) also exist in those with gambling disorder, but not all anxiety disorders are seen with equal frequency. Research suggests that estimates of co-occurring generalized anxiety disorder range as high as 40% among patients with a gambling disorder, whereas those of obsessive-compulsive disorder may be as low as 1%.

Significantly fewer data are available regarding the frequencies of personality disorders in those with pathologic gambling disorders. Borderline (3% to 70%), narcissistic (5% to 57%), avoidant (5% to 50%), and obsessive-compulsive (5% to 59%) personality disorders are most commonly reported. One of the best studied personality disorders in gambling disorder, antisocial personality disorder, has been found in 15% to 40% of gambling disorder patients; a frequency higher than the 0.6% to 3% estimate reported for the general population.

Family History

High frequencies of psychiatric disorders are seen in first-degree relatives of those with a gambling disorder. Commonly reported conditions include mood, anxiety, substance use, and antisocial personality disorders. Studies have also found that 20% of first-degree relatives of those with a pathologic gambling disorder also have a gambling disorder. Recent research examining possible familial aggregation of gambling disorder found that individuals with a parent who has a problem with gambling were at a 3.3 times higher risk of also having a gambling disorder.

TREATMENT
Psychologically Based Treatments

Although there is a great deal of literature with case reports using psychodynamic psychotherapy for gambling disorder, there are no randomized controlled trials supporting its use. Similarly, although some evidence exists that Gamblers Anonymous and self-exclusion contracts may be beneficial for those with a pathologic gambling disorder, limited and conflicting data assessing the long-term efficacy for these interventions have been published.

A variety of psychosocial treatments have been examined in controlled studies for the treatment of gambling disorders. Cognitive strategies have traditionally included cognitive restructuring, psychoeducation, and irrational cognition awareness training. Behavioral approaches focus on developing alternate activities to compete with reinforcers specific to the gambling disorder as well as the identification of gambling triggers. Although no data support its use for gambling disorders, contingency management has been used successfully in the treatment of individuals with substance use disorders who also gamble and has not worsened the gambling behavior in these individuals.

Assessment of Psychologically Based Treatments

Empirical studies of cognitive–behavioral therapy (CBT) and using various elements of CBT (ie, cognitive or behavioral therapy, motivational interviewing, and CBT workbooks) support the efficacy of using CBT for those with a gambling disorder because the majority of trials found reductions in gambling disorder symptomatology compared to the control conditions. However, these trials are insufficient to provide information about the optimal treatment duration and the level of training needed by the therapy administrator. Both brief and longer treatments have been found effective, but no study has randomized subjects into psychotherapeutic treatments of varying durations to determine the most efficacious treatment length. In addition, few studies have long-term follow-up, highlighting the need for future studies to include long-term follow-up visits to assess maintenance of therapeutic gains.

Pharmacotherapy

No medication is currently approved by the US Food and Drug Administration or indicated for the treatment of gambling disorders. However, 20 randomized, placebo-controlled trials of pharmacotherapy treatment in those with a gambling disorder have been conducted, and these studies suggest that medications may be beneficial in treating gambling disorder.

Assessment of Pharmacotherapy

Due to the promising results of the double-blind trials of naltrexone and nalmefene, opioid antagonists appear to be the most promising pharmacologic treatments for gambling disorders. Similar to the nalmefene, however, empiric trials of naltrexone should be conducted at additional research sites to examine the efficacy of naltrexone in varying patient populations. Results from trials investigating the glutamate modulator *N*-acetylcysteine and lithium suggest these medications may also be effective, but with only one trial completed for lithium and two for *N*-acetylcysteine, additional research is needed to bolster support. Antidepressants have been the most widely examined with findings providing indefinite results. Currently, no evidence supports the use of atypical antipsychotics. No randomized, placebo-controlled studies have been completed comparing pharmacotherapy treatments or comparing pharmacotherapy to psychotherapy. These trials would provide insight into which individuals may respond best to a certain class of medication or to psychotherapeutic treatment.

Treatment Recommendations

Gambling disorder is a common, disabling psychiatric disorder that is associated with high rates of co-occurring disorders, particularly substance use disorders, and high rates of illegal activities. Psychotherapy and pharmacotherapy have shown promise in the treatment of gambling disorder. In terms of psychosocial treatments, CBT appears promising. There are several manualized forms of this therapy. Although the stronger evidence suggests eight sessions of CBT should be considered, some data suggest that even fewer sessions or brief interventions may be effective. With a manualized treatment, counselors with a background in addiction counseling should be able to deliver the treatment with minimal training.

KEY POINTS

1. Gambling disorder is a common psychiatric problem with prevalence rates similar to or higher than most other mental health conditions.
2. Gambling disorder is associated with significant personal and interpersonal costs (eg, unemployment, divorce, poverty) as well as social and public health problems (eg, bankruptcy, crime).
3. There are several evidence-based approaches to gambling disorder that have demonstrated benefits, most notably cognitive–behavioral therapy.

REVIEW QUESTIONS

1. Gambling disorder has been associated with all of the following *except*:
   A. financial difficulties such as bankruptcy.
   B. work-related problems such as absenteeism.
   C. improved overall health.
   D. high rates of nicotine dependence.

2. The following psychosocial interventions have demonstrated benefit for gambling disorder in controlled studies *except*:
   A. cognitive therapy.
   B. interpersonal psychotherapy.
   C. behavioral therapy.
   D. imaginal exposure therapy.

3. Which of the following medications are FDA approved for the treatment of gambling disorder?
   A. Olanzapine
   B. Paroxetine
   C. Naltrexone
   D. Lithium
   E. None of the above

ANSWERS

1. **C.** Gambling disorder has been associated with a range of health problems such as obesity, hypertension, and liver disease.
2. **B.** There are no controlled studies assessing the benefits of interpersonal psychotherapy for gambling disorder.
3. **E.** There is no FDA-approved pharmacotherapies for gambling disorder.

SUGGESTED READINGS

Grant JE, Potenza MN, eds. *Pathological Gambling: A Clinical Guide to Treatment*. Washington, DC: American Psychiatric Publishing, 2004.

Hodgins DC, Stea JN, Grant JE. Gambling disorders. *Lancet*. 2011;378(9806):1874-1884.

National Research Council. *Pathological Gambling: A Critical Review*. Washington, DC: National Academy Press, 1999.

Petry NM. *Pathological Gambling: Etiology, Comorbidity, and Treatment*. Washington, DC: American Psychological Association, 2005.

CHAPTER 46

Problematic Sexual Behaviors and "Sexual Addiction"

Summary by Timothy M. Hall, Simone H. Schriger, and Steven Shoptaw

> Based on THE ASAM PRINCIPLES OF ADDICTION MEDICINE, 6th edition chapter by Timothy M. Hall, Simone H. Schriger, and Steven Shoptaw

HISTORICAL AND CULTURAL CONTEXT

Sexual behaviors that are perceived as compulsive and distressing to the patient, their partners, or other persons, and the patient may come to clinical attention at the initiative of the individual or their partner or through involvement in the legal system. Such distressing behaviors include concerns for excessive sexual desires and high-volume sexual behaviors (HVSBs), paraphilias and paraphilic disorders, and the combination of compulsive sexual behavior with the use of psychoactive drugs.

Proposals to interpret these phenomena as strongly analogous to substance addiction have not been well supported by research. Suggested diagnostic criteria for both sexual addiction and hypersexual disorder were rejected by the *Diagnostic and Statistical Manual of Mental Disorders,* 5th edition (*DSM-5*) for lack of empirical support. Research on these and related constructs has been limited by small sample sizes, lack of replication, disagreement over how best to operationalize and measure symptoms, and by arbitrary cutoffs for identifying excessive amounts of sexual behavior.

With patients distressed over their sexual behaviors or fantasies, clinicians should conduct a careful biopsychosocial assessment to understand the specific content of their sexual fantasies and behavior (which may suggest a more specific paraphilic disorder or specific internal conflicts), and the personal and social context in which they are occurring. Such patients tend to be quite heterogeneous. Labeling patients with sexual addiction or hypersexual disorder risks medicalizing problems in their primary relationships or exacerbating negative cultural or individual attitudes toward sexuality—negative attitudes that have been found to better predict a self-diagnosis of sexual addiction than the actual sexual behavior. Labeling may also distract from identifying and treating primary mood, personality, substance use, or obsessive-compulsive disorders presenting as concerns about sexual behaviors.

This chapter uses *problematic sexual behavior* (PSB) as a more theory-neutral term that is deliberately broad. Patients may present because of ego-dystonic distress over the content or frequency of their fantasies or behaviors, because their partner or family members are distressed by them, or because their behaviors have incurred legal or other disciplinary sanctions.

HIGH-VOLUME SEXUAL BEHAVIORS: HYPERSEXUAL DISORDER AND SEXUAL ADDICTION

Several theoretical perspectives have proposed diagnostic criteria for problematic HVSB. *Hypersexual disorder,* potentially related to impulse-control disorders, would describe recurrent, intense sexual fantasies and behaviors that cause distress, are inappropriately used to cope with stress, cannot be voluntarily curtailed, and risk or cause harm to oneself or others. At least two different criteria sets for *sexual addiction* have been proposed, modeled after substance use disorders (SUDs) and operationalizing analogues of tolerance and withdrawal.

HVSB shares some behavioral features with SUDs. Individuals with HVSB may engage in sexual behaviors that they experience as compulsive, despite knowledge of adverse medical, legal, and/or interpersonal consequences, and may neglect social and recreational activities and role responsibilities. They spend large amounts of time planning, engaging in, or recovering from the behavior. Some authors note the gradual development of a need for increased sexual activities to get the desired effects, parallel to the concept of tolerance, although this is based on case reports rather than systematic trials.

Others have noted mood changes related to sexual activity (euphoria) or sexual abstinence (depressed mood).

Negative self-evaluations are often part of the clinical picture, including feeling abnormal or sick; guilty or ashamed; and regret, depression, or emotional numbness. Indeed, an individual's negative attitudes toward sexuality predict self-identification with sexual addiction better than objective measures of sexual acts, sexual partners, or time spent thinking about sex, suggesting that preexisting conflicts about sexuality may lead a person or their partner to identify sexual behavior as problematic.

Psychometrically, studies suggest HVSB is dimensional rather than categorical, ie, there is no obvious cut point in the absence of distress, risk, or harm to distinguish HVSB from normal behavior on criteria such as frequency of orgasm or intercourse. This complicates estimating population prevalence. Some authors have proposed cut points of greater than two or three standard deviations above the median in terms of frequency of sexual behavior, although others see this as arbitrary.

Etiology of High-Volume Sexual Behavior

Our understanding of the etiology of HVSB relies heavily on theoretical models rather than empirical data. There are no systematic studies on its onset; however, self-reports of individuals seeking treatment suggest symptoms often started in their late teens or early 20s and may be chronic or intermittent.

Traumatic experiences have been identified as risk factors for later development of HVSB, including childhood sexual abuse (CSA), and particularly in women. Early substance use and impulse inhibition problems have also been proposed. HVSB may be related to a disposition to externalizing behaviors, potentially shared among antisocial personality disorder and SUD. Individuals with HVSB may be more likely to have family members with HVSB or addictive disorders. Despite these associations, most youth who experience CSA, early substance use, attention deficit hyperactivity disorder (ADHD), and disrupted family backgrounds do not develop HVSB.

Evidence for a correlation between variants in the dopamine transporter gene and number of sexual partners among men has been inconsistent. Links between dopamine availability and sexual behaviors are plausible but remain unproven. Neuroimaging studies have failed to find a consistent marker for HVSB or to find replicable similarities between HVSB and SUDs.

Psychiatric Comorbidity

Core features of HVSB such as impulsivity, obsessions, and compulsivity are shared with many psychiatric disorders. Impulsivity is seen in ADHD, bipolar disorders, SUDs, and some personality disorders. A high prevalence of psychiatric comorbidities is observed in community samples of individuals who defined their behavior as sexually compulsive. In one sample (N = 36), 39% met the criteria for lifetime mood disorders, 50% for lifetime anxiety disorders, and 64% for lifetime SUDs. The lack of longitudinal studies makes it difficult to determine whether PSBs precede or follow the Axis I diagnoses.

Some retrospective reports suggest associations between ADHD during childhood and later HVSB. Of seventy-two individuals seeking treatment for HVSB, 34% scored in the range of probable ADHD diagnosis; however, this may reflect the forensic population in which the study was done. In a small imaging study, men rated as sexually compulsive made significantly more errors than control participants on a measure of impaired inhibitory control.

One study found that 46% of a community-based sample of individuals reporting HVSB met the criteria for a personality disorder, predominantly Cluster C disorders. In a study of 403 adolescents seen in primary care settings, those rated as having three or more Axis II symptoms reported higher numbers of sexual partners, with the association being stronger in females than in males. These findings underscore difficulties in separating HVSB from personality disorders. Acting out sexually is a criterion for borderline personality disorder and may be seen in other Cluster B personality disorders, whereas Cluster C personality disorders may entail excessive self-criticism and guilt.

PARAPHILIAS AND PARAPHILIC DISORDERS
Definitions and Diagnosis

The *DSM-5* defines a paraphilia as "intense and persistent sexual interest other than sexual interest in genital stimulation or preparatory fondling with phenotypically normal, physically mature, consenting human partners." Noting that "a paraphilia by itself does not necessarily justify or require clinical intervention," the *DSM-5* further distinguishes a *paraphilic disorder* as "a paraphilia that is currently causing distress or impairment to the individual or a paraphilia whose satisfaction has entailed personal harm, or risk of harm, to others."

Eight specific paraphilic disorders are listed in the *DSM-5* as well as a category for *other specific paraphilic disorder*. The specific paraphilic disorders are listed because they are relatively common (compared to other paraphilic disorders), and satisfying them is likely to entail harm or criminal activity (eg, pedophilic disorder). The sexual disorders section of the *International Statistical Classification of Diseases and Related Health Problems* (11th revision) goes even further, recognizing that "specific patterns of sexual arousal that are merely relatively unusual, but are not associated with distress, dysfunction or harm to the individual or to others, are not mental disorders."

Distinguishing paraphilias and paraphilic disorders from crimes of a sexual nature has both clinical and legal ramifications. Although some persons with paraphilic disorders do commit sex crimes, most instances of rape, sexual assault of adolescent minors, and child molestation are committed by persons who do not have a paraphilic disorder. Unfounded worries about generalized sexual addiction feed into public support for lifelong registries of persons convicted of sex crimes, which are largely unsupported by research findings and can introduce unintended negative consequences to the individual and the community.

Etiology, Development, and Prevalence of Paraphilic Disorders

Most paraphilias manifest during adolescence, although the individual may not enact or acknowledge them to others at that time. The *DSM-5* adopts the grouping of paraphilias into two descriptive sets. Those with *anomalous activity preference* focus on atypical behaviors: sexual sadism and masochism, along with the *courtship disorders* (voyeurism, exhibitionism, frotteurism, and telephone scatologia—thought to be deviations from a psychological system whose normal function involves finding and wooing a potential sexual partner). Paraphilic disorders with *anomalous target preference*, on the other hand, are oriented toward targets other than adult humans: pedophilic disorder, fetishistic disorder, and transvestic disorder.

PEDOPHILIA AND SEX WITH MINORS

The paraphilias with the largest research base and most often coming to legal attention are those involving a predominant sexual attraction to children or adolescents. These should be distinguished from child molestation or CSA, most instances of which are not committed by persons with a predominant orientation toward minors. They should also be distinguished from sexual acts between younger and slightly older adolescents or young adults. The *DSM-5* characterizes *pedophilic disorder* as a recurrent, intense attraction to prepubescent children, generally younger than 13 years. An individual with pedophilic disorder must be at least 16 years of age and at least 5 years older than the child. The *DSM-5* further excludes "an individual in late adolescence in an ongoing sexual relationship with a 12 or 13 year old," recognizing that sexual exploration among adolescents does not reliably predict a lifelong, persistent attraction to children as sexual objects.

There is wide consensus that the prevalence of pedophilic disorder in the general public is unknown due to a lack of large-scale epidemiologic surveys, with estimates ranging from 0.5% to 5% of males.

The etiology of pedophilic disorder is poorly understood. Theories of developmental trauma or imprinting have been widely accepted, although most adult survivors of CSA do not have an attraction to children, and many persons with an attraction to minors were not themselves sexually abused. Poor impulse control, whether from ADHD or from a history of brain injuries, has been suggested as a mediating factor. Antisocial traits predict a greater likelihood of acting on paraphilic impulses and may be a mediating factor in paraphilic disorders involving sex with minors or nonconsenting partners.

COMPULSIVE SEX IN COMBINATION WITH SUBSTANCE USE

Sex and substance use combine some of the most powerfully reinforcing and potentially problematic behaviors known to humans. Since about the 1970s, we have seen an intersection of stimulants (cocaine and methamphetamines), dissociatives (ketamine), and "entactogens" or "empathogens" (eg, 3,4-methyl enedioxymethamphetamine, γ-hydroxybutyric acid) with sex, sometimes known as "partying" or "chemsex," particularly among men who have sex with men (MSM), although it also occurs in other groups. This combination can increase the risk of human immunodeficiency virus (HIV) and other sexually transmitted infections among vulnerable populations. Additionally, the association of sex with drug use and the ready availability of drugs within an individual's sexual networks can seriously impede efforts at treating SUDs. Researchers disagree whether it should be seen as primarily as an SUD, as PSB, or both.

The British Chemsex Study was one of the first quantitative publications on this topic. Of more than 1100 MSM respondents, around 20% reported engaging in compulsive sex in combination with substance use within the past year, and 10% within the past month. Although these numbers are concerning, it is impossible to extrapolate from these to prevalence numbers in the larger population.

Special Populations: Problematic Sexual Behaviors Among Lesbian, Gay, Bisexual, and Transgender Persons

We briefly address PSB among lesbian, gay, bisexual, and transgender persons and particularly among MSM in part because of the disproportionate amount of research and clinical attention paid to this population. These groups have historically been stigmatized, and their sexual behaviors often criminalized or pathologized. Consequently, there is a need to balance potential risks among lesbian, gay, bisexual, and transgender persons presenting with concerns for PSB. On the one hand, they may be at a higher risk for contracting HIV or being introduced by sexual partners to HVSB in the context of substance use. On the other hand, they may carry excessive shame and guilt about their sexual orientation and same-sex experiences; this may lead them to view relatively normal lesbian, gay, bisexual, and transgender experiences through a lens of pathology and may complicate efforts to access treatment for PSB, SUDs, mental health services, or general healthcare.

ASSESSMENT AND TREATMENT OF PROBLEMATIC SEXUAL BEHAVIORS

Assessment

Individuals presenting for an evaluation or treatment of PSB need a careful assessment to define the presenting problem. Did something precipitate the visit? Exactly what is the patient doing, at what frequency, and under what circumstances to define PSB? What is the gender and age of the partners involved with the individual? What is the development of the behavior—from childhood to present? What are exacerbating (ie, triggering) or alleviating factors?

In addition, carefully review how PSB has impacted areas of functioning: medical history (especially sexually transmitted infections); employment background and pattern; involvement with alcohol and drugs (including nicotine and cannabis) that may be used before, during, and after sexually compulsive behaviors; detailed history of legal problems (whether formally charged or convicted or not); quality of relationships with family, friends, and intimates (if any); and mental health functioning, including both diagnosable psychiatric conditions and subthreshold mood, anxiety, and cognitive disturbances. Regarding specific scales, Hook and colleagues provide a comprehensive review of 17 published instruments assessing PSB (see Suggested Readings).

It is important to establish whether there is victimization in the history, including sexual abuse, physical abuse, and head or other physical trauma. Some forms of compulsive sexual behavior (eg, child molestation) are legally reportable activities; others expose the patient to risk of arrest (eg, exhibitionism). Still others increase an individual's risk of infection or physical violence. All need to be empathically, but carefully, assessed in any extended evaluation.

Treatment Approaches

Treatment for individuals with PSB often occurs in the context of comorbid substance use or psychiatric disorders and in the absence of randomized controlled trials to guide best practice. Instead, the clinician is faced with a complex task of piecing together relevant findings from psychiatric literature, small trials, and observational reports to develop an evidence-informed, biopsychosocial approach for intervention. For individuals whose PSB has strong obsessive-compulsive characteristics, medications used to treat obsessive-compulsive disorder may relieve symptoms, particularly the selective serotonin reuptake inhibitors (SSRIs). As with SUDs, individuals presenting with PSB may have limited motivation for treatment, particularly if referred by a partner or mandated by law. Determining and enhancing motivation may be an important element of treatment.

Cognitive–Behavioral Therapy

Cognitive–behavioral therapy (CBT) is a general approach to treating addictive behavioral disorders that teaches patients the skills needed to achieve abstinence and to return to abstinence upon relapse. One generic CBT strategy involves identifying "triggers" (ie, persons, places, things, or internal experiences) that are specific to sexually compulsive behavior. Other skills common to CBT also are applicable, including distress tolerance (urge surfing), environmental manipulation (banning Internet access), diffusion techniques (mindfulness, meditation), and the like.

There are no randomized controlled trials of CBT for PSB generally. There is one randomized controlled trial of CBT-based HIV-prevention interventions for MSM, particularly those with PSB in the context of substance use. *Getting Off: A Behavioral Treatment Intervention for Gay and*

Bisexual Methamphetamine Users adapts the Matrix Model of manualized treatment for stimulant use disorders for clients who identify as gay and bisexual. It is effective at reducing both substance use and risky sexual behaviors. The client and counselor manuals are available for download at the Friends Community Center's website (see Suggested Readings).

Twelve-Step and Self-Help Groups

There are no controlled studies of the efficacy of 12-step self-help groups in the reduction of PSB, which is usually framed as "sexual addiction" or "sex and love addiction" in a 12-step context. As with 12-step programs for SUDs, the primary advantage is that the groups are convenient and widely available. Four 12-step approaches have been adapted to assist individuals with PSB: Sexaholics Anonymous, Sex Addicts Anonymous, Sex and Love Addicts Anonymous, and Sexual Compulsives Anonymous.

PHARMACOTHERAPY STRATEGIES
Selective Serotonin Reuptake Inhibitors

Empirically, about 60% of patients receiving SSRIs experience some form of treatment-emergent sexual dysfunction that involves all phases of a healthy sexual response. They include reductions in sexual desire, impaired arousal, and delayed or absent orgasm. Antidepressants may ameliorate dysphoric states that could predispose one toward PSB or result from its sudden cessation. In some penal systems that treat paraphilic disorders, in-custody persons are given high doses of SSRIs to produce dose-dependent sexual dysfunction as a side effect. One randomized, placebo-controlled trial of an SSRI (citalopram) and several small open-label trials of SSRIs have been published for treating PSB. They showed significant reductions in sexual drive, frequency of masturbation, and viewing of pornography compared to placebo. The effects of SSRIs on dampening libido and disrupting performance are general to all sexual functions, not just problematic ones. Patients may therefore be ambivalent about adherence.

Opioid Antagonists

Naltrexone is an opioid antagonist approved for treating alcohol and opioid use disorders. The putative mechanism of action for sexual compulsivity involves dampening the opioid–dopamine reward system. One open-label trial of high-dose naltrexone (150 to 200 mg per day) among adolescent sexual offenders was found to reduce PSB symptoms (eg, masturbating three or more times daily, reporting feelings of intrusive sexual thoughts or arousal, spending more than 30% of waking time thinking about sex) in 15 of the 21 subjects. A placebo-controlled trial of 30 MSM with high rates of methamphetamine use, binge drinking, and risky sexual behavior found that oral naltrexone 50 mg daily somewhat reduced all of these behaviors. Especially for nonparaphilic disorders, naltrexone may be a reasonable candidate for evaluation in clinical trials, but the lack of data makes it premature to consider its use in clinical situations.

Hormonal Therapies for Paraphilic Disorders

Because of public safety considerations, more drastic interventions are sometimes considered for paraphilic disorders and certain sadistic paraphilic disorders than for other forms of PSB. Although the evidence base is limited, a small number of open-label studies support the use of androgen-blocking medications, sometimes described as *chemical castration*, for men with paraphilic disorders involving children or violence against adults. Cyproterone acetate and triptorelin pamoate have approved indications in some European countries for paraphilic disorders. In the absence of randomized controlled trials, reviews of observational studies and open label trials show that these medications, as well as medroxyprogesterone acetate and luteinizing hormone–releasing hormone, reduce rates of reoffending when taken as prescribed for up to 1 year, particularly when implemented with CBT. When these men stop taking the medications, their likelihood to offend returns to baseline levels.

The World Federation of Societies of Biological Psychiatry has issued guidelines for the pharmacologic treatment of paraphilic disorders. Based on the (limited) available evidence, they suggest SSRIs at higher doses typical for obsessive-compulsive disorder, rated as Level C evidence, or "minimal research-based evidence to support this recommendation." Adding an antiandrogen agent is also suggested but with even less evidence (Level D).

SUMMARY

A number of types of compulsive or ego-dystonic sexual behavior may come to clinical attention, either at the initiative of the individual or their partner, or through involvement in the legal system. These include paraphilias and paraphilic disorders, concerns for HVSB, and the combination of compulsive sexual behavior with the use of drugs, particularly stimulants.

For persons referred to treatment in relation to crimes of a sexual nature, it is important to keep in mind that most individuals with paraphilias do not commit sexual crimes, and a majority of sexual crimes are likely committed by individuals who do not meet the criteria for a paraphilic disorder. Patients with paraphilic disorders whose satisfaction entails sexual acts of a nonconsensual nature or involving minor children may be candidates for hormone-blocking therapies, and may be most appropriately referred to specialist programs for further evaluation and treatment. The sexual orientation–like aspect of paraphilic disorders is highly resistant to change through any known therapies. Thus, treatment programs often aim at drive reduction through SSRI antidepressants or hormone-blocking agents for paraphilic disorders that may entail harm to others.

Although the concept of a general sexual addiction or hypersexual disorder has a long history, it has not been supported by rigorous studies, and has not yet produced evidence-based treatments. Research has been compromised by arbitrary cutoffs and a lack of consensus on definitions. Critics have noted frequent comorbidity of PSB with other psychiatric disorders, suggesting PSB may be an associated feature rather than an independent disorder. Many cases of self-diagnosed sexual addiction appear to be influenced by strongly negative attitudes toward sexuality or particular kinds of sexuality held by the individual or their partner.

Patients currently seek treatment for PSB, including paraphilias and HVSB, at rates that are sufficient to support healthy practices and a burgeoning residential recovery industry. Unfortunately, the evidence base for treatment remains poor. At minimum, there is evidence to support the use of SSRIs, with or without use of CBT. A comprehensive assessment is crucial to rule out comorbid psychiatric conditions, to be sure that a paraphilia or paraphilic disorder is not being missed or misinterpreted, and to evaluate psychosocial factors that may contribute to the behaviors or to the patient's discomfort with them.

ACKNOWLEDGMENTS

The authors wish to acknowledge support from the National Institute on Drug Abuse Grants P50 DA18185 and T32 DA026400. Matthew Brensilver, PhD, was coauthor on an earlier edition of this chapter.

REVIEW QUESTIONS

1. Which of the following best predicts a patient self-identifying as having pornography addiction?
   A. More than 60 minutes daily spent viewing pornography
   B. Endorsing negative social or religious attitudes about sex, pornography, or masturbation
   C. A history of childhood physical or sexual abuse
   D. Female gender

2. Which of the following statements about paraphilias are true? (Select all that apply.)
   A. Groping someone at a college party while intoxicated is evidence of frotteuristic disorder.
   B. The courtship disorder hypothesis proposes that voyeurism, exhibitionism, and some other paraphilias may be deviations in a psychological system whose function involves finding and wooing a potential sexual partner.
   C. Most sexual assaults are committed by persons with paraphilic rape fantasies.
   D. Merely having unusual sexual interests does not meet the criteria for a paraphilic disorder, unless they also cause distress or cause a person to act in a way that harms others.

3. Which of the following is an example of pedophilic disorder?
   A. A 37-year-old man with a history of dating adult women who gropes his 12-year-old stepdaughter while drunk
   B. A 28-year-old man with a long-standing attraction to prepubescent children and little interest in adult partners, who has started loitering at playgrounds
   C. A 17-year-old boy who is caught at school with a topless selfie from his 14-year-old girlfriend
   D. A 29-year-old woman who has sex with a young man she met at a bar, then finds out he is 17 years old and was using fake identification

ANSWERS

1. **B**
2. **B** and **D**
3. **B.** The case in **A** may be guilty of child molestation, but there is no evidence in the vignette of long-standing attraction to children. The cases in **C** and **D** could end up on a sex offender registry in some states, but there is no evidence here of pedophilic disorder.

SUGGESTED READINGS

Cantor JM, Klein C, Lykins A, et al. A treatment-oriented typology of self-identified hypersexuality referrals. *Arch Sex Behav.* 2013;42(5):883-893.

Grubbs JB, Exline JJ, Pargament KI, Hook JN, Carlisle RD. Transgression as addiction: religiosity and moral disapproval as predictors of perceived addiction to pornography. *Arch Sex Behav.* 2015;44(1):125-136.

Hook JN, Hook JP, Davis DE, Worthington EL Jr, Penberthy JK. Measuring sexual addiction and compulsivity: a critical review of instruments. *J Sex Marital Ther.* 2010; 36(3):227-260.

Reed GM, Drescher J, Krueger RB, et al. Disorders related to sexuality and gender identity in the ICD-11: revising the ICD-10 classification based on current scientific evidence, best clinical practices, and human rights considerations. *World Psychiatry.* 2016;15(3):205-221.

Shoptaw S, Reback CJ, Peck JA, et al. *Getting Off: A Behavioral Treatment Intervention for Gay and Bisexual Male Methamphetamine Users.* Los Angeles: Friends Research Institute, 2005.

Thibaut F, De La Barra F, Gordon H, et al. The World Federation of Societies of Biological Psychiatry (WFSBP) guidelines for the biological treatment of paraphilias. *World J Biol Psychiatry.* 2010;11(4):604-655.

47 Microprocessor-Based Disorders

Summary by Richard N. Rosenthal

Based on THE ASAM PRINCIPLES OF ADDICTION MEDICINE, 6th edition chapter by Richard N. Rosenthal, Zebulon Charles Taintor, and Jon E. Grant

Microprocessors are ubiquitous, serving as prosthetic brains, guides, knowledge sources, and calculators. Although they help us manage many aspects of our lives and provide much stimulation, they do not manage our time, our motivations, and our involvements. Some of us become dependent on the stimulation they provide, similar to addiction to substances, with significant negative life consequences

The Internet has six major uses that affect clinicians and their patients: (1) information on disease, diagnosis, treatments, and therapists; (2) support and self-help groups; (3) advice, diagnosis, and counseling where the only contact is over the Internet; (4) provision of addictive substances, both prescription and nonprescription; (5) platform for individual or group engagement in novel constructs such as social media and online gaming; and (6) opportunities for people to do things with intrinsic addiction vulnerability (eg, sex, gambling). Internet addiction, however, covers only part of the problems that people develop using devices built around microprocessors. These problems are due to the interaction of the novel technology and the people using it as opposed to intrinsic mental disorders such as depression and schizophrenia. Research on Internet addiction has burgeoned since the American Psychiatric Association announced that it would place Internet gaming disorder (IGD) into Section 3 (appendix) of the *Diagnostic and Statistical Manual of Mental Disorders*, 5th edition (*DSM-5*). Almost 70% of the 2135 articles listed after 1996 for Internet addiction on PubMed have been published since 2012, predominantly focused on IGD.

HISTORICAL PERSPECTIVE

The Internet was established in 1969 at the University of Southern California as a way of linking computers for national defense uses. Computers have always offered opportunities to impair functioning,

even before the Internet. For example, programmers had been described as so immersed in programming they failed to properly document their work. Problematic non–work-related Internet use arose quickly in the workplace after the Internet became functional in the business community. The first articles about Internet addiction appeared in the mid-1990s. Some portion of problematic microprocessor use may be more due to social adaptation to new technology than due to psychopathology. Internet social utilities such as social networks, commercial dating sites, special interest blogs, chats, and others have made forming new relationships with fellow online users a mainstream activity.

DIAGNOSTIC DILEMMAS

Addiction as used in popular media describes a much less serious phenomenon than what clinicians mean by "addiction." In considering whether microprocessors are a bona fide substrate for addictive processes, it is important to present some caveats:

- Using a computer or cell phone or playing videogames is normal, prosocial, and encouraged behavior.
- When people experience new and powerful tools, there is a learning curve to information acquisition, time management, and social behavior.
- Calling maladaptive microprocessor-related behavior a pathology rather than a bad habit may medicalize a social problem.

Important questions arise in the context of considering whether Internet addiction is a discrete disorder and whether it is an addiction or some other type of disorder. Debate has focused on whether Internet addiction is a separate and internally consistent disorder or a domain that contains several separate but related disorders supported through Internet-based activity, such as IGD. This distinction can be conceptualized as addiction *to* the Internet and addictions *on* the Internet. An analysis of treatment-seeking patients at a behavioral addictions clinic supports a range of different primary substrates such as gaming, chatting, or sexual content for those seeking treatment for pathologic Internet use. Recent attempts at classification have reframed Internet addiction as Internet use disorder, which as a behavioral addiction, might be eventually included in the substance-related disorders section of the *DSM-5* (like gambling disorder). Analogous to various specific substance use disorders (SUDs), this in turn might allow for specific use disorders such as Internet-gaming disorder, Internet-gambling disorder, Internet pornography–viewing disorder, etc.

Similar to drug-of-choice determinations among those with SUDs, it has been proposed that among those with specific instances of Internet use disorder, there will be a "first-choice use" of the genre of applications supported by the Internet, such as pornography/cybersex, gaming, gambling, or social networking.

Neuroimaging and Neuropsychological Correlates

Internet Addiction Disorder

Internet addiction disorder (IAD) was codified by Young in 1998 as an eight-item polythetic diagnostic set modeled on pathologic gambling. Neuroimaging research shows altered regional cerebral activity and structural changes generally consistent with studies of drug and other behavioral addictions. Individuals with IAD have increased glucose metabolism in the right orbitofrontal cortex, left caudate, and right insula and decreased metabolism in the bilateral postcentral gyrus, left precentral gyrus, and bilateral occipital regions. There is also decreased dorsal striatal D2 receptor availability in men, which is inversely correlated with IAD severity, consistent with a reward deficiency model for SUDs. Long-term IAD may lead to structural brain changes and altered function, but a causal relationship has not yet been established.

In sum, Internet addiction has been associated with structural and functional abnormalities in the orbitofrontal, dorsolateral prefrontal, anterior cingulate, and posterior cingulate cortices, regions that play crucial roles in salience attribution, inhibitory control, and decision-making.

Internet Gaming Disorder

Recent research has examined the specific version of IAD focusing on Internet gaming. Whether IGD should be regarded as a diagnostic disorder distinct from IAD awaits further understanding, but recent imaging studies have begun to paint a picture of a unique behavioral addiction. Men with high-severity IAD have greater activity in the anterior and posterior cingulate cortices, consistent with impaired inhibitory control and response inhibition, and Internet gamers with IAD have severity-associated abnormalities in the posterior cingulate cortex and thalamus.

The *DSM-5* workgroup had contemplated problematic Internet use as a compulsive–impulsive disorder in the group of impulse control disorders (ICD), and pathologic Internet use could be considered an ICD. Pathologic Internet use is modeled after pathologic gambling, a *DSM-IV* ICD, but gambling disorder has since been moved to the *DSM-5* substance-related and addiction disorders section. ICD hallmarks are repeated failure to resist impulses that are harmful to self or others and tension or arousal before and pleasure or relief during the act, followed by guilt or self-reproach. However, Internet addiction has addiction-specific symptoms, such as development of euphoria, craving, and tolerance in addition to ICD symptoms (Internet preoccupation, compulsive use, loss of control). Internet addiction has been narrowed in *DSM-5* to IGD and placed in the appendix, but the placement of gambling disorder in the substance-related disorders suggests other behavioral addictions may ultimately be validated for that group.

ASSESSMENT

Functional impairment is a good proxy for unhealthy and clinically relevant use of microprocessors. One can discuss the intensity and impact of use of microprocessor-containing devices and assign general risk categories based on the information provided. A simple screening cutoff can begin to establish whether use is normal or problematic:

- Normal use: A reasonable time spent accomplishing specific goals using microprocessors. High engagement does not necessarily mean pathology.
- Problem use: The use is causing clinically significant impairment. The patient repeatedly takes on undue risk, gets into legal problems, continues the use in spite of recurring social or interpersonal problems related to use, or the use interferes with fulfilling major role obligations.
- Use disorder: The patient experiences an inability to get along without it. Here, the problem is the level of impairment. As with SUDs, a person may have a false sense of being in control and "able to stop any time," when in fact they cannot.

Nervousness, aggression, agitation, insomnia, anorexia, tremulousness, and depression have been described after microprocessor deprivation, but microprocessor use withdrawal has not yet been documented sufficiently for inclusion into the *DSM*.

EPIDEMIOLOGY AND COMORBIDITY

The problem of understanding the prevalence of Internet addiction and related use disorders has its origin in the lack of internationally agreed upon standardized approaches to diagnosis, the multiplicity of instruments used to assess Internet-related psychopathology, and a deficit of large community-based studies. A meta-analysis of 80 studies of Internet addiction using the Internet Addiction Test (IAT) or the Young Internet Addiction Diagnostic Questionnaire generated a global base rate estimate of 6% but with regional differences such as 10.9% in the Middle East, 8% in North America, and 2.6% in Northern and Western Europe. In addition, a different systematic review found broad regional variations in Internet addiction prevalence rates such as 0.8% in Italy as compared to 26.7% in Hong Kong, attributable to differing assessments with different cutoff thresholds.

Given this, it is not surprising that the reported comorbidity of Internet-related disorders and other psychiatric disorders demonstrates a wide range of prevalence rates. However, compared to populations without IAD, mental disorder prevalence over all studies in persons with IADs is significantly increased. Despite different countries and age ranges, the prevalence rates of any personality disorder among those with Internet addiction are consistent at 27% to 30%. As with SUDs, there is an increased risk of co-occurring mental disorders including personality disorders, which if clinically unaddressed, could adversely affect treatment outcomes for IAD, IGD, and other Internet use disorders.

TREATMENT MODEL
Theory of Change

Motivation is key. If rewards are the issue, other rewards must be found. If obsessive–compulsive concerns are more important, efforts and medication are directed at developing different habits and thought patterns. Recovery is about learning to avoid triggers for impulsive Internet use, making use of social support for healthy reinforcers found in everyday life, and relearning how to use microprocessors in non-pathologic ways.

TREATMENT PLANNING
Evaluation–Diagnosis

Rating scales serve as diagnostic aids and can help patients realize the extent of their problems by offering objective data for feedback in motivational approaches. The 20-question IAT is best established and covers six factors: salience, excessive use, neglecting work, anticipation, lack of control, and neglecting social life on a 100-point scale with ranges of 20 to 49 indicating average online use, and 50 to 79 indicating occasional or frequent problem use. However, a meta-analysis of 11 studies reveals the IAT to be more reliable in college students compared to pre-college students and also has continent-dependent reliability in that Asian IAT samples are more reliable than European ones. Many new scales have been developed to improve and modernize the identification of Internet addiction since the publication of *DSM-5*, such as the 15-item Internet Disorder Scale.

Mortality

Murder and suicide have been reported (mostly in South Korea) after microprocessor deprivation. Usually, an adolescent kills the depriving parent or demonstrates through suicide that life is not possible without the microprocessor. IAT-identified Internet addiction has been significantly associated with depressive symptoms.

Morbidity

As more satisfying relationships are developed on the Internet, real-life social relationships get less time. Clinicians may rate these relationships less favorably, like drinking buddies of a person with an alcohol use disorder; therefore, clinicians must assess cyber relationships in detail and without bias. Identity fragmentation may occur if one's Internet persona is markedly different from one's real-life persona. Impairment can result from prolonged sitting in front of screens, with increased obesity and less exercise, but inactivity is preferable to accidents that occur while multitasking. The American College of Emergency Physicians issued an alert against "text walking" as the number of vehicle hits, falls, and running into trees, lamp posts, and other people has become noticeable in emergency rooms.

PRETREATMENT ISSUES
Motivation as Rationale for Choice of Treatment

Motivation prior to engagement in treatment may be scant or absent. Patients minimize, rationalize, or deny problems. A nonconfrontational discussion of impairment using the principles of motivational interviewing can help the patient gain perspective. The impact of the patient's microprocessor overuse are elicited and then fed back to assist the patient to use his or her native analytic capacity and values in determining that the overuse is actually problematic or impairing to help tip the decisional balance toward seeking help.

A departure from the abstinence-oriented approach of classic addiction treatment is therapeutic use of the Internet and microprocessors, aligned with moderation management concepts. Online support groups are thought to help, but there is no robust evidence of positive effects.

Treatment and Technique
Choice and Timing of Interventions
Similar to disorders of compulsive food intake, complete abstinence is not a feasible long-term treatment goal because use of microprocessors is unavoidable in today's world, and nonuse is associated with significant vocational and social disadvantage. Restricting microprocessor access by significant others in control may increase motivation or result in destructive anger; therefore, clinicians must expect to hear about and perhaps participate in decisions.

General and Stage-Specific Interventions
The general plan is reintroduction into the real world, which must be done in stages to ease transitions, replacing the rewards of the microprocessor abuse with more natural and socially appropriate reinforcers. Because a person's cognitive process maintains the IAD, appropriate psychotherapeutic strategies would include cognitive restructuring focused on the Internet applications of choice, behavioral exercises, and graded exposure therapy with increasing duration of offline activity.

RELEVANT TREATMENT RESEARCH
Compared to research on psychosocial treatments of SUDs, there is far less relevant treatment research on IADs because funding agencies have not yet recognized the problem as deserving much attention. A systematic review of 30 studies found overall research quality was impaired due to the disparities in the definition, diagnosis, and measurement of IGD; the lack of randomized controlled studies with proper blinding of data acquisition and analysis; and unavailability of recruitment dates, sample size justification, follow-up reports on changes in gaming or Internet

use, and effect sizes. Clearly, the research in this area is in need of standards for assessing and diagnosing, with better study design and execution.

Psychologically Based Treatments
As yet, there are no high-quality randomized controlled trials reported for psychosocial treatment of IAD as a stand-alone construct.

Pharmacotherapy and Psychologically Based Treatments
Pilot studies of pharmacotherapy for IADs have found success with escitalopram and with sustained-release bupropion. Treating comorbid psychiatric disorders may have utility as well. Methylphenidate treatment for attention deficit hyperactivity disorder (mean dose 30.5 mg per day) also reduced scores on hours of Internet use and the Internet Addiction Scale. However, if IAD follows suit with substance addictions, then the effective treatment of co-occurring mental disorders will generally have effect sizes insufficient as a stand-alone to treat the IAD.

However, one randomized trial of bupropion SR 300 mg daily in males with major depression and severe problem Internet gaming demonstrated significantly reduced severity of Internet addiction and mean online game playing time in addition to the expected reduction in depression severity. There remains no US Food and Drug Administration–approved pharmacotherapy for IAD.

KEY POINTS
1. As with other behavioral addictions, it remains to be demonstrated that Internet addiction is itself a discrete disorder, is inclusive of other microprocessor-related disorders, or is a substrate for other behavioral disorders.
2. Although there is high comorbidity with mood and anxiety disorders and attention deficit hyperactivity disorder, Internet addiction symptoms overlap but appear to be separate from those disorders.
3. Internet gaming disorder is included in the *DSM-5* in Section 3 (appendix).
4. Neuroimaging research shows altered regional cerebral activity and structural changes in patients with Internet addiction, which is generally consistent with studies of drug and other behavioral addictions.
5. Treatment should entail motivational interviewing engagement strategies and cognitive–behavioral therapy, with graded reintegration into the outside world and its healthier pleasures.

REVIEW QUESTIONS

1. Which of the following is *true*?
   A. Internet addiction disorder is a *DSM-5* disorder among the impulse control disorders.
   B. Internet sexual compulsive disorder is a *DSM-5* disorder among the impulse control disorders.
   C. Internet addiction disorder is a *DSM-5* disorder among the substance-related disorders.
   D. Internet gaming disorder is listed in the *DSM-5* appendix.
   E. Internet shopping disorder is listed in the *DSM-5* appendix.

2. Which of the following is *false* when approaching whether Internet addiction is a valid disorder?
   A. A monothetic approach requires that all criteria be met to make a diagnosis.
   B. A monothetic approach should have high sensitivity for true positives.
   C. High engagement in microprocessor use is pathognomonic.
   D. One must determine that Internet addiction is discrete, rather than a component of another disorder.
   E. High rates of pathologic Internet use found in online surveys may suffer from selection bias.

3. Which of the following is *true* regarding treatment of Internet addiction?
   A. Randomized controlled trials of naltrexone have demonstrated efficacy.

B. An abstinence-based approach to microprocessors is the most effective.
C. Treating comorbid attention deficit hyperactivity disorder with stimulants is sufficient to treat Internet addiction.
D. A motivational interviewing approach to treatment engagement with graded exposure and staged reintegration is clinically sensible.
E. Online self-help groups have demonstrated efficacy in multiple controlled studies.

ANSWERS

1. **D**
2. **C**
3. **D**

SUGGESTED READINGS

Brand M, Young KS, Laier C, Wölfling K, Potenza MN. Integrating psychological and neurobiological considerations regarding the development and maintenance of specific Internet-use disorders: an interaction of Person-Affect-Cognition-Execution (I-PACE) model. *Neurosci Biobehav Rev.* 2016;71:252-266.

Carli V, Durkee T, Wasserman D, et al. The association between pathological internet use and comorbid psychopathology: a systematic review. *Psychopathology.* 2013;46(1):1-13.

Griffiths M. Nicotine, tobacco, and addiction. *Nature.* 1996; 384(6604):18.

Winkler A, Dörsing B, Rief W, Shen Y, Glombiewski JA. Treatment of internet addiction: a meta-analysis. *Clin Psychol Rev.* 2013;33(2):317-329.

Zhu Y, Zhang H, Tian M. Molecular and functional imaging of internet addiction. *Biomed Res Int.* 2015;2015:378675.

48

Behavioral Syndromes to Consider as Forms of "Addiction"

Summary by Abigail J. Herron

| Based on THE ASAM PRINCIPLES OF ADDICTION MEDICINE, 6th edition chapter by Abigail J. Herron, Paul J. Rinaldi, and Petros Levounis

Three primary components have been described as the core elements of addiction: craving or compulsion, loss of control, and continued behavior despite associated negative consequences. Although the term *addiction* has been often used to exclusively describe impaired control over substance use, these core elements can also be seen in certain behaviors associated with short-term rewards that lead to persistent behavior despite adverse consequences. This shared feature of diminished control has given rise to the concept of *behavioral addictions*—syndromes similar to chemical addiction but with a behavior as the core of the disorder rather than a substance. Defining characteristics of these disorders include repetitive or compulsive engagement in a specific behavior despite adverse consequences, diminished control over the problematic behavior, and tension or an appetitive urge state prior to engagement in the behavior. Many of these disorders share features with substance use disorders (SUDs), whereas others do not. The shared characteristics of some behavioral disorders and SUDs have raised the question of whether they would more appropriately be classified as addictive disorders.

We include three of them here: compulsive buying disorder, excessive tanning, and kleptomania, which serve as specific examples of conditions that may merit reclassification as addictive disorders. We have chosen to include these disorders because they are activities that can be considered pleasurable, exciting, and naturally rewarding at normative levels, similar to substances of abuse.

COMPULSIVE BUYING DISORDER

Although compulsive buying disorder (CBD) is not specifically described in the *Diagnostic and Statistical Manual of Mental Disorders*, 5th edition

(*DSM-5*), diagnostic criteria have been proposed. These include being frequently preoccupied with buying or subject to irresistible, intrusive, and/or senseless impulses to buy; frequently buying unneeded items or more items than can be afforded; shopping for periods longer than intended; and experiencing adverse consequences, such as marked distress, impaired social or occupational functioning, and/or financial problems.

The estimated prevalence of CBD in the United States is approximately 5.8%, with estimates ranging from 1.8% to 8%. The usual age of onset for CBD appears to be in the late teens to early twenties. Most subjects identified are female, but studies have found that the prevalence of CBD between women and men was only slightly different.

Four phases have been identified in compulsive buying: anticipation, preparation, shopping, and spending. In the first phase, the person becomes preoccupied with either purchasing a specific item or with shopping in general. In the next phase, the person plans the purchase or shopping spree. This is followed by the actual shopping experience, during which many of those with CBD feel intense excitement. The actual purchase completes the cycle. Following the purchase, the person often experiences feelings of disappointment, shame, or guilt.

Neurobiological theories have focused on disturbed serotonergic, dopaminergic, or opioid neurotransmission. Some argue that CBD should be included in the nosologic classification as an addictive disorder. The reasoning is that some impulse control disorders share comorbidities, family histories, brain circuitry, and treatment responses to selective serotonin reuptake inhibitors (SSRIs) with SUDs. There is evidence that the brain circuitry in

SUDs—namely, the "reward system" of the brain—is involved in impulse control disorders.

There are no evidence-based treatments for CBD. Treatments have generally followed the same protocols as with other impulse control disorders—namely, cognitive–behavioral therapy (CBT) and pharmacotherapies. Pharmacotherapies have included the use of SSRIs, particularly fluoxetine and citalopram. There is some evidence of improvements with naltrexone, suggesting that opiate antagonists might play a role in CBD. Because the medication findings are mixed, no empirically supported treatment recommendations can be made. CBT has also been recommended and has been shown to yield significant improvements compared with a control group, and these improvements that were maintained during a 6-month follow-up.

EXCESSIVE TANNING

There is a subgroup of people for whom tanning is clearly excessive and seems to reflect frank psychopathology. Excessive tanning is not a discreet *DSM-5* diagnosis, nor is it mentioned as an example of a not otherwise specified impulse-control disorder. However, for this subgroup of people who tan excessively, their presentation, symptomatology, psychiatric comorbidity, consequences of behavior, and overall course of illness significantly resembles the trajectories of other behavioral addictions and SUDs. One small study even reported a group of regular sunbathers who exhibited symptoms similar to opioid withdrawal upon administration of naltrexone, an opioid antagonist.

Although most recent research has adopted the addiction paradigm in understanding excessive tanning, there are other psychiatric disorders that may also explain the manifestations of the illness. The following three disorders have been proposed as "possible underlying psychopathologies" for excessive tanning: obsessive-compulsive disorder (OCD), body dysmorphic disorder, and borderline personality disorder. At this time, limited research has been conducted to support or refute these explanations. Furthermore, an alternative formulation of the illness could suggest that excessive tanning may be a behavioral addiction that is often found to be comorbid with OCD, body dysmorphic disorder, and borderline personality disorder.

The lack of research in this area extends also to treatments. However, if we accept that excessive tanning is best appreciated as a behavioral addiction, then (1) addressing underlying or co-occurring psychiatric conditions and (2) providing CBT or motivational interviewing seem to be the most reasonable approach to treatment. A small study showed that young women who tan indoors very frequently markedly reduced their behavior following a motivational interviewing session delivered by a trained peer counselor. Interestingly, a comparison group that was given identical information but via the Internet with no person-to-person contact failed to show any significant difference from the control group.

A number of other psychosocial interventions have been tried in small samples of more normative populations, which have shown some promising results. Such interventions include showing patients ultraviolet photos of skin damage, showing patients "image norms of aspirational peers," approving of paleness, and providing feedback on the patient's suntanning behavioral patterns by a physician.

In addition to treatments, prevention has to play a major role in addressing the proposed illness, especially because there is little evidence of safe and effective therapeutic interventions. Current public heath efforts go beyond raising awareness of the risk of suntanning. State, federal, and international regulations are being considered and implemented to limit indoor tanning by imposing higher taxes and prohibiting minors from using such facilities.

KLEPTOMANIA

The *DSM-5* includes kleptomania in the category of disruptive, impulse-control, and conduct disorders, which also includes intermittent explosive disorder, conduct disorder, and pyromania. The *DSM-5* requires the following symptoms for a diagnosis of kleptomania:

- Recurrent failure to resist impulses to steal objects that are not needed for personal use or their monetary value
- Increasing sense of tension immediately before committing the theft
- Pleasure, gratification, or relief at the time of committing the theft
- Stealing that is not committed to express anger or vengeance and is no in response to delusion or a hallucination
- Stealing that is not better explained by conduct disorder, a manic episode, or antisocial personality disorder

Kleptomania is characterized by recurrent episodes of compulsive stealing. Often confused with shoplifting, it differs in that those with kleptomania do not steal for personal gain. They steal in response to an overwhelming urge that they are unable to resist.

The powerful urge causes feelings of anxiety, tension, or arousal. Stealing soothes these feelings. However, following this, there are often feelings of guilt, remorse, and fear. These feelings frequently serve as barriers to treatment seeking.

Kleptomania is a psychiatric disorder that is poorly understood and the subject of only a few empirical studies. Although the prevalence of the disorder in the general US population is unknown, it has been estimated at 6 per 1000 people.

Although kleptomania meets the criteria for impulse control disorder (inability to control one's impulse to steal and repeated expression of impulsive acts that lead to physical or financial damage), it shares many characteristics of OCD. There is evidence derived from studies of clinical characteristics, familial transmission, and treatment response that suggests that kleptomania may have subtypes that are more like OCD, addictive disorders, or mood disorders.

A correlational aspect linking kleptomania to OCD is seen in the biological perspective on OCD. Studies of the brain using magnetic resonance imaging showed that subjects with OCD had significantly less white matter than did normal control subjects, suggesting a widely distributed brain abnormality associated with OCD. OCD is considered a result of serotonin deficiency. The use of SSRIs has been used to treat both OCD and kleptomania and has been considered as demonstration of a link between the disorders.

However, prevalence rates between the two disorders do not show a strong relationship. Results of studies that examined the comorbidity of OCD in subjects with kleptomania have been inconsistent, with some showing a relatively high co-occurrence (45% to 60%), whereas others show low co-occurrent rates (0% to 6.5%). When rates of kleptomania have been examined in subjects with OCD, a similarly low co-occurrence was found (2.2% to 5.9%).

Kleptomania and SUDs have central qualities in common. These include recurring or compulsive participation in a behavior in spite of undesirable consequences; weakened control over the disturbing behavior; an overwhelming need or desire experienced before taking part in the problematic behavior; and a positive, pleasure-seeking condition throughout the act of the disturbing behavior. The anxiety, tension, or arousal that those with kleptomania experience and the relief that they feel upon stealing, followed by guilt or remorse, is consistent with opponent process descriptions and wanting-but-not-liking states described for SUDs. Similar to SUDs, a higher percentage of cases of kleptomania

have been noted in adolescents and young adults, with a smaller number of cases among older adults. Family history data also show a likely common genetic input to substance use and kleptomania. SUDs are more common in family members of persons with kleptomania than in the general population.

Treatment for kleptomania has many commonalities with SUD and OCD treatment. Treatment usually consists of a combination of therapies, including pharmacotherapy and talk therapy. Although there are no medications specifically approved for the treatment of kleptomania, the similarity and suggested biological dynamics of kleptomania and OCD and impulse control disorders led to the theory that similar groups of medications could be used for all of these conditions. Fluoxetine and other SSRIs have been widely used to treat kleptomania. Yet, there has not been strong evidence supporting the efficacy of SSRIs in treating the disorder. There has been some promising evidence supporting the use of mood stabilizers, antiseizure medications, and opioid antagonists, particularly naltrexone. Opioid receptor antagonists have been shown to lessen urge-related symptoms, which is a central part of impulse control disorders and substance dependence. In the past, psychoanalytic and dynamic approaches were used to treat kleptomania. Current practice usually includes CBT, which can include covert sensitization, exposure and response prevention, and imaginal desensitization.

SHARED FEATURES OF BEHAVIORAL AND CHEMICAL ADDICTIONS

Behavioral disorders resemble chemical addictions in a number of domains. Individuals with behavioral and chemical addictions demonstrate high levels of self-reported impulsivity and sensation seeking. They have similar natural histories, with increased prevalence in adolescents and young adults, chronic relapsing patterns, and the possibility of spontaneous recovery. Pathologic gambling, the most studied of the behavioral addictions, mirrors SUDs, with higher rates seen in men. A telescoping pattern is seen in women, with a later initiation of behavior but with a shortened period from initial behavior to addiction. Interpersonal conflicts are seen in both behavioral addictions and SUDs. The financial problems common to both can lead to illegal acts such as theft or forgery to offset the consequences of the behavior. Neurobiological and genetic parallels have also been shown between SUDs and impulse control disorders, with implications for the role of the dopamine and serotonin neurotransmitter systems.

In both types of addiction, behavior is often preceded by an urge or craving. Emotional dysregulation may contribute to cravings, and the resultant behavior can often decrease anxiety and lead to a positive mood or "high." Many individuals report a decrease in these positive effects over time, or a need to increase the intensity of their behavior in order to achieve the same effect, analogous to tolerance seen with substance use. In periods of abstinence from these behaviors, a dysphoric state may also be seen, analogous to withdrawal, although with no prominent medical symptoms, which does differ from withdrawal from substances. Although these behaviors are initially egosyntonic, they may become more egodystonic over time as the act becomes less pleasurable and more motivated by negative reinforcement.

CO-OCCURRENCE OF SUBSTANCE USE AND BEHAVIORAL ADDICTIONS

There is limited data from large national studies as to the co-occurrence of SUDs and behavioral disorders. Impulse control disorders have not been measured in most large-scale epidemiologic surveys, in part because validated instruments for the assessment of these disorders are largely lacking. Studies of clinical samples, however, suggest high rates of co-occurrence, most notably between pathologic gambling and SUDs. Clinical samples of other behavioral addictions suggest that co-occurrence of an SUD is common, with rates of SUDs between 22% and 50% in kleptomania, and approximately 60% in compulsive sexual behavior.

High comorbidity may suggest that these disorders are part of the same spectrum and should be classified together as addictive disorders. Yet, individuals with behavioral disorders have also been shown to have higher rates of other psychiatric disorders, including mood, anxiety, and personality disorders, which are not part of the addictive process. Comorbidity alone does not lend support for the classification of these disorders as addictive. This does highlight, however, that individuals with SUDs should be assessed for the presence of impulse control disorders.

DIAGNOSTIC CHALLENGES

Data about many of the impulse control disorders are lacking, and more evidence is needed to aid in the classification of these disorders. Empirically validated instruments to assess impulse control disorders would allow for the identification of behavioral disorders in large-scale epidemiologic studies, and

longitudinal assessments would be useful in mapping the temporal relationships between impulse control disorders and other psychiatric disorders and SUDs. Brief screening instruments would be helpful in the identification of impulse control disorders in both clinical and research populations.

Support for use of the term "addiction" rather than the term "dependence" has centered on confusion over different definitions of dependence. Physical dependence can occur following chronic administration of a drug, and features tolerance and withdrawal without the experience of the negative consequences of addiction. A change in terminology may allow the focus to shift from substance use and its adaptation-associated physical consequences to the harmful effects of addiction on multiple domains of functioning.

There are a number of advantages associated with categorizing certain impulse control disorders as addictive disorders. Rates of co-occurrence are high, there are common demographic and epidemiologic features, and there are parallels between presenting symptomology. Substance abuse treatment programs may be more likely to assess for the presence of impulse control disorders in their patient population than in general mental health or primary care settings. By expanding the scope of addiction to include these disorders, it may increase awareness, extend treatment for these conditions in the context of substance abuse treatment, and increase the availability of funding and research into these disorders.

Despite the advantages thus described, several disadvantages to reclassification exist. The primary rationale for the separate classification has been the lack of substance use with impulse control disorders, resulting in distinct consequences from use, particularly regarding the lack of significant physical sequelae from impulse control disorders. Additionally, categorizing impulse control disorders as addictive may increase stigmatization. Individuals without co-occurring chemical addiction may feel uncomfortable receiving treatment in a substance abuse treatment setting. Treatment programs that primarily treat substance abuse may not have a sufficient number of patients with impulse control disorders to offer groups dedicated to their treatment.

TREATMENT MODELS

Behavioral and chemical addictions can respond positively to the same treatments modalities. While research continues in this area, there are no currently approved medications for the treatment of behavioral addictions. Psychosocial therapies play many roles in the treatment of co-occurring chemical and behavioral addictions. They are used to directly target and reduce problem behaviors in both domains directly as well as indirectly through the rationale that reductions in one type of behavior are likely to lead to reduced symptom severity and reductions in another problematic behavior. Behavioral therapies can also be used to enhance treatment engagement and promote treatment adherence and can target other psychosocial problems that may occur.

Multiple psychosocial approaches have been employed in this treatment. Many treatments for behavioral addictions were originally developed for the treatment of SUDs, and psychosocial treatments for both types of disorders often employ a relapse prevention model, encouraging abstinence through identification of patterns of abuse, avoidance, or coping mechanisms for high-risk situations and lifestyle changes. CBT, motivational approaches, and 12-step approaches are mainstays of substance abuse treatment that have been successfully used in the treatment of a number of impulse control disorders, including pathologic gambling, compulsive sexual behavior, kleptomania, pathologic skin picking, and compulsive buying. CBT focuses on learning new skills and strategies to reduce negative thoughts and behaviors, helping individuals to identify patterns associated with ongoing substance use or other behaviors. Motivational approaches are brief interventions designed to produce internally motivated change in problematic behaviors. Contingency management, in which individuals receive incentives or rewards for demonstrating observable target behaviors (such as negative urine toxicology or treatment attendance), has been shown to be effective at reducing substance use and may be similarly effective when used for reducing other problematic behaviors.

Individuals with co-occurring disorders have also been shown to have poorer treatment outcomes, highlighting the need for effective treatment models to address co-occurring disorders. Integrated treatment, in which interventions and services are directed at both disorders by the same treatment team at the same time, is now recommended as the standard of care for SUDs and mental health disorders, and may also be the preferred model for co-occurring behavioral addiction and SUDs.

KEY POINTS

1. Evidence suggests parallels between chemical and behavioral addictions in many domains, including epidemiology, natural history, symptomology, and comorbidity.
2. Although controversy remains concerning the nomenclature, these shared features have treatment implications, with a number of behavioral disorders responding positively to modalities initially employed in the treatment of SUDs.
3. Evidence-based treatments are lacking in general, but the greatest support is for the use of psychosocial interventions such as CBT, relapse prevention therapy, motivational interviewing, and 12-step approaches.

REVIEW QUESTIONS

1. A 43-year-old woman with compulsive buying disorder is engaged in psychotherapy. Which of the following medications would be a reasonable addition to her treatment regimen?
   A. Disulfiram
   B. Acamprosate
   C. Naltrexone
   D. Naloxone
   E. Varenicline

2. Which of the following elements is *not* a shared feature of behavioral and chemical addictions?
   A. Chronic relapsing pattern
   B. Low levels of impulsivity
   C. Possibility of spontaneous relapse
   D. Increased prevalence in adolescents and young adults
   E. Telescoping pattern in women

3. Which of the following is recognized as a formal disorder in the *DSM-5* in the category of substance-related and addictive disorders?
   A. Kleptomania
   B. Internet gaming disorder
   C. Compulsive buying disorder
   D. Gambling disorder
   E. Excessive tanning

ANSWERS

1. **C.** There has been some evidence supporting the use of naltrexone, an opiate antagonist in the treatment of CBD. Disulfiram and acamprosate are used for alcohol use disorder. Naloxone is an opiate antagonist used in the treatment of opiate overdose. Varenicline is used for smoking cessation.
2. **B.** Individuals with behavioral and chemical addictions demonstrate high levels of self-reported impulsivity and sensation seeking.
3. **D.** Kleptomania is recognized as an impulse control disorder. Gambling is the only behavior included in the addictive disorders. The others are not recognized as formal disorders in the *DSM-5.*

SUGGESTED READINGS

Grant JE, Potenza MN. Compulsive aspects of impulse-control disorders. *Psychiatr Clin North Am.* 2006;29(2): 539-551. .

Grant JE, Potenza MN. Impulse control disorders: clinical characteristics and pharmacological management. *Ann Clin Psychiatry.* 2004;16(1):27-34.

Grant JE, Potenza MN, Weinstein A, Gorelick DA. Introduction to behavioral addictions. *Am J Drug Alcohol Abuse.* 2010;36(5):233-241.

Holden C. 'Behavioral' addictions: do they exist? *Science.* 2001; 294(5544):980-982.

Potenza MN. Should addictive disorders include non-substance-related conditions? *Addiction.* 2006;101(suppl 1):142-151.

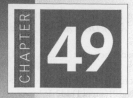

CHAPTER 49

Physician Health Programs and Addiction Among Physicians

Summary by Andrea Cole

> Based on THE ASAM PRINCIPLES OF ADDICTION MEDICINE, 6th edition chapter by Paul H. Earley

The available research about addiction among physicians and physician health programs (PHPs) is extensive and has been well-documented in several excellent overviews. Research on physician addiction elucidates the natural course of addiction in a highly regulated and monitored population. At the same time, physicians differ from the general population in terms of education, income, and regulatory oversight; therefore, conclusions about the efficacy of addiction treatment among physician-patients cannot simply be generalized to the population.

PREVALENCE

We have 20 years of debate about the prevalence of addiction among physicians. National studies show that in the general population, 3.8% of the population has a substance use disorder (SUD) at any given time. Prevalence studies among physicians vary depending on research methodology used. One study found a lifetime prevalence of an SUD at 7.9%. Physicians are less likely to smoke cigarettes than the general population, but some studies have found they are more likely to drink alcohol, use benzodiazepines, and use opioids unsupervised than the general population. Another view of unhealthy use of alcohol and drugs among physicians can be derived from complaints reviewed by state medical boards. One study shows 14% of board disciplinary actions were alcohol or drug related and another 11% were due to inappropriate prescribing practices, likely due to addiction. Alcohol and drug-related work impairment was the primary impetus for the formation of state PHPs in the United States and continues to account for the majority of physician impairment cases seen by most PHPs today.

CHARACTERISTICS OF ADDICTED PHYSICIANS

The median age for physicians to seek addiction treatment is 45 years. Although males account for the majority of physicians treated for addiction, the male-to-female ratio for physicians afflicted with addiction is smaller than in the nonphysician population. Rates of addiction by specialty have been relatively well-studied by methods including self-report surveys, analyses of participation in PHPs, and actions taken by medical boards. Psychiatry, emergency medicine, and anesthesiology are consistently overrepresented, that is, they present with substance use problems in greater numbers than would be expected if problems were evenly distributed in the physician population.

The problem of SUDs in anesthesiologists has been the focus of more research and debate than that which has occurred in other specialties. Postulated risk factors include ease of access to drugs, repeated exposure to subanesthetic levels of volatile compounds, and personalities that are not risk aversive. Whatever the risk factors, there is little question that the pattern of drug use reflects the unique access anesthesiologists have to high-potency agents with the potential to produce severe SUDs such as fentanyl and propofol. A particularly controversial question is whether anesthesia residents with SUDs involving these agents should be allowed to return to training given that lethal relapse is more common with these agents than with other substances.

DRUGS MISUSED

The most frequent problematic substance for physicians is alcohol, just as it is for the general population. In contrast, nicotine use disorders have declined in physicians over time and are currently lower than in the general population. Smoking status is an important consideration in prognosis for physicians in treatment for SUDs; those who smoke are at greater risk for relapse compared to other substance use.

Opioids are the second most common type of SUD in physicians presenting for addiction treatment. Although this finding has been stable over time, the type of opioids used has changed. Self-prescribing and diversion of medications intended for patients are not uncommon means of supply for physicians. SUDs caused by parenteral rather than oral opioids may be particularly severe and relatively quick to develop.

Other substances that are used by physicians include cocaine, amphetamines, and benzodiazepines. Cocaine use among physicians seems to have declined in recent years, along with the decline in the use of cocaine in medical practice. Physicians using amphetamines may have initially begun using due to attentional issues or the pressures of prolonged hours during residency, which then developed into an SUD. Psychiatrists report twice the rate of problematic use of benzodiazepines compared with other types of physicians and also report more self-prescription of benzodiazepines compared with other physicians, which may be why psychiatrists are overrepresented in addiction treatment programs for physicians.

Propofol is a sedative–hypnotic medication that presents unique problems for anesthesiologists, and its misuse outside of the medical professions is rare. Approximately 20% of anesthesia training programs report cases of propofol misuse by residents. The prevalence of propofol misuse has increased sharply in the past decade despite efforts within anesthesia training programs to provide training on the substantial dangers of self-administered propofol.

As among their nonphysician peers, the most commonly used illegal drug for residents is cannabis. Physicians from all specialties use cannabis, with those in emergency medicine, orthopedics, plastic surgery, anesthesiology, and psychiatry using more frequently. The legalization of marijuana in many US states has made central the question of whether those providing physician oversight should refer physicians who test positive for cannabis for further evaluation.

RISK FACTORS

The strongest predictor of SUDs in physicians is a family history of SUDs. Available data on medical student substance use trajectories are also consistent with findings in the general population: Regular alcohol and nicotine use also places one at greater risk for a subsequent SUD.

Although decades of research has failed to support the concept of an addictive personality, certain personality characteristics found in some physicians may place individuals at greater risk for SUDs. In particular, "sensation seeking" is correlated with recreational drug use among physicians in training. This personality characteristic may account for the finding in one study of a greater prevalence of illicit drug use in emergency medicine physicians compared with other specialties. The access of physicians to drugs with addictive potential is an important environmental risk factor for SUDs. Furthermore, trends in physician prescription drug use within classes of drugs have correlated with trends in availability and marketing of prescription drugs. Physicians' access to potent parenteral opioids and sedative–hypnotics may produce a severe SUD relatively quickly. A high degree of tolerance may develop to these drugs, correlating with dose escalation. Periods of abstinence result in loss of tolerance and raise the risk of fatal relapses.

ADDICTION COMORBIDITY

Thought and Mood Disorders

Although it is unclear whether physicians have higher rates of major depressive disorder than the general population, physicians do have higher rates of suicide than the general population. Physicians who complete suicide are more likely to have had SUDs and family histories of SUDs as well as other psychiatric disorders than those who do not complete suicide. Physicians have lower rates of schizophrenia and thought disorders than does the general population.

Pain

Physicians afflicted with pain are at greater risk for SUDs, particularly if prescribed long-term opioid medication. Self-prescription is not uncommon in this context, and this too raises the risk of an opioid use disorder. Physicians who have pain and addiction disorders pose regulatory challenges as to whether physicians in recovery who are prescribed opioid pain medication should be allowed to practice. More research is need in this area.

Post-Traumatic Stress Disorder

Post-traumatic stress disorder and alcohol use disorder are correlated, and the risk of alcohol-related relapse increases in the context of post-traumatic stress disorder triggers. Certain specialties such as emergency medicine and trauma surgery may result in more trauma exposure.

THEORIES OF ADDICTION AMONG PHYSICIANS

Family history of alcohol dependence in physicians is as high as 75%. Other reasons that physicians may be particularly vulnerable to addiction include: the stress of medical training, social isolation, history of parental deprivation, having a sense of omnipotence, and the need to appear self-sufficient and in control. The natural history of addiction in physicians is similar to that of nonphysicians. Typically, consequences of substance use are apparent in the personal lives of physicians before becoming evident in the work setting. For this reason, family members may prove more valuable in providing collateral history than work colleagues.

IDENTIFICATION, INTERVENTION, AND ASSESSMENT

Identification

Physicians present for assessment along a broad spectrum of symptom severity. Approaches that emphasize clinical intervention and support rather than discipline are more likely to encourage referral by colleagues and even self-referral. A variety of work-related behaviors may be clues to substance misuse, including irresponsible and unprofessional behavior, irregular work hours, changes in personal appearance, and signs consistent with intoxication or withdrawal.

Intervention

In interventions for physicians suspected of having an SUD, there are two safety considerations: the safety of patients treated by the physician under consideration and the health of the physician. If one accepts the definition of impairment provided by the Federation of State Medical Boards as an inability to practice with reasonable skill and safety due to illness, not all physicians with SUDs are impaired. For those who are impaired or likely impaired, the most prudent course is for the physician to stop practice until an assessment of fitness to practice is completed. Physicians should know the legal requirements in their respective states for reporting physician colleagues identified as impaired.

Most states have established a PHP that can provide assistance in intervention, refer for treatment if indicated, monitor the response to treatment, and advocate for permission to practice when necessary. As with reporting responsibilities for physicians, the roles, rights, and responsibilities of PHPs are often specified in state law. PHPs can serve as consultants to medical institutions or individual physicians when a possibly ill or impaired physician is identified.

Furthermore, state law often allows the PHP to evaluate such physicians and preserve the confidentiality of the findings to a far greater degree than institutions or colleagues as long as there is no potential for continued patient harm. The PHP can then become a "safe harbor" for evaluation and treatment and a more attractive option for a physician causing concern than a report to the licensing board.

Assessment

An assessment can be completed in the least intensive level of care that results in a comprehensive review of the physician as long as safety concerns are addressed. This comprehensive review requires not only a thorough diagnostic interview and medical evaluation, but also taking an extensive collateral history from individuals who have observed the physician at work, at home, and in social situations. The comprehensive review also requires the evaluator to contact clinicians who have treated the physician, and it requires a medical record review when pertinent. PHPs can direct a physician to a qualified evaluator or facility, discuss the results of the evaluation with the physician, and guide the physician to appropriate treatment resources when indicated.

TREATMENT

Clinical Considerations With Addicted Physicians as Patients

Treatment in a setting with fellow physicians promotes greater acceptance of the patient role and counterbalances the tendency to adopt the more comfortable role of providing medical advice to fellow patients. Physicians may excel in the didactic aspects of treatment while avoiding the emotional, interpersonal, and spiritual aspects of treatment. Furthermore, many physicians have developed the ability to distance themselves from the somatic and emotional pain inherent in a physician's work as a coping mechanism. Although this is often necessary and adaptive in a physician's professional role, it may impede the effectiveness of treatment.

Societal and regulatory expectations regarding acceptable outcomes for physicians treated for SUDs are an important influence on the treatment of physicians. Addiction medicine has recognized that addiction is often a persistent illness characterized by remission and relapse and has correctly come to measure treatment effectiveness by the results of treatment across multiple domains rather than solely through the lens of whether treatment recipients are abstinent. In contrast, complete abstinence is society's expectation in the case of physicians in recovery who are allowed to return to practice, and this expectation is enforced by licensing boards if resumption of drug use becomes evident.

Characteristics of the Treatment Setting

The challenges of engaging physicians in treatment, a perception that physicians benefit from intensive, multidisciplinary treatment, and public demands for safety if physicians with histories of addiction are allowed to practice have prompted the development of physician-specific, long-term residential addiction treatment programs. Although addiction treatment research has reported comparable outcomes for patients who receive intensive outpatient treatment, there are insufficient data to support the comparability of initial outpatient treatment for physicians. For physicians who are participants in physician health programs, treatment is accompanied by rigorous toxicology monitoring, which must meet forensic standards. Many PHPs also monitor performance at work and make sure concerns noted at the worksite are conveyed to clinicians providing treatment.

Many treatment settings and PHPs encourage involvement in 12-step programs and other peer support groups. There is an impressive body of research that meaningful involvement in Alcoholics Anonymous correlates with sobriety. Physician-specific groups can also be employed, with the goal of helping participants explore work triggers and address other issues they may face when returning to practice, such as how to respond to questions from peers. There is also a growing body of research supporting the use of pharmacologic agents in the treatment of addiction, and there are medications approved by the US Food and Drug Administration for the treatment of alcohol, opioid, and nicotine use disorders. Surveys have shown that just as with other types of patients, the use of these agents in physician patients has not been adopted to a significant extent.

Physician Health Programs

The importance of PHPs in promoting and supporting early intervention, appropriate treatment, and rigorous monitoring of the response to treatment cannot be overstated. Although the antecedents for PHPs can be traced to organizations such as International Doctors in Alcoholics Anonymous, which was founded in 1949, PHPs became organized when the American Medical Association convened its first conference on physician impairment in 1975, and state medical societies took on the charge to develop state committees on physician impairment. As of this writing, nearly every state has a PHP with a mission to restore physician health in a manner that does not endanger public health. All PHPs have agreements that specify what must be disclosed to state licensing boards and what may be kept confidential. Where confidentiality is allowed, it depends on the physician participant's cooperation with the treatment plan and record of abstinence as monitored by the PHP. The goal of PHPs is to maintain a therapeutic rather than disciplinary process whenever possible.

All PHPs monitor abstinence in its participants with SUDs. Programs typically use a toxicologic analysis of biologic matrices (especially urine) collected randomly with witnessed collection. The length of monitoring for SUDs of significant severity is typically 5 years. Given windows of detection for most addictive drugs, monitoring frequencies less than four times per month will not detect the resumption of sporadic drug use. Longer windows of detection can be examined via a hair analysis, which is typically performed four times per year. In addition to providing treatment and monitoring abstinence, PHPs also provide education on physician impairment, train on techniques to identify and report suspected impairment, and provide recovery support such as 12-step and therapeutic groups.

The treatment outcomes for participants in PHPs are among the best in addiction treatment. The largest study of PHP participants nationwide, published in 2008, demonstrated continuous abstinence in nearly 80% of PHP participants followed for 5 or more years. Among those who weren't continuously abstinent, nearly 75% had only one documented episode of drug use. These outstanding outcomes have given authority to PHPs when advocating for participants with licensing boards, specialty boards, and other regulatory entities.

CONTROVERSIES

Some public safety advocates have argued that physicians with SUDs should be reported to licensing boards regardless of whether there is evidence of impairment or patient harm as a consequence of addiction. Some argue further that such reports should be available to the general public in making decisions about where to seek care. In fact, beyond the important question of the rights of physicians to confidential treatment as patients, the possibility of confidential assessments and treatment is an important factor in colleagues referring colleagues and for physicians who use substances presenting themselves for PHP arranged evaluations. If all referrals resulted in disciplinary actions, fewer physicians would be referred, and the unintended consequence of less public safety could result. The structure of PHPs, in which confidentiality is maintained contingent on excellent performance as measured by rigorous, objective monitoring, strikes a good balance between privacy to facilitate treatment and public safety.

In nonphysician populations presenting for treatment of opioid use disorders, medication-assisted treatment has had a consistently beneficial effect on a variety of outcomes. In contrast, physicians in treatment supervised by PHPs have had excellent outcomes in the absence of medication-assisted treatment (with opioid agonists or antagonists). Concerns expressed about agonist medications include cognitive effects and the possibility that misuse of agonist medications may occur. The issue of *agonist medication becomes even more complex in* the case of physicians with persistent pain who have not experienced sufficient pain control without opioid agonist treatment.

Special concerns have been raised about the safety of anesthesiologists returning to practice after treatment for opioid use disorders given the risk of lethal relapse. Some have argued that the risk of relapse is too high given access to drugs inherent in the practice, and anesthesiologists with opioid use disorders should retrain for another specialty regardless of type of medication-assisted treatment. Others have argued that anesthesiologists should only be permitted to practice if long-acting naltrexone is mandated as a treatment component. Research to better inform these difficult decisions is sorely needed.

KEY POINTS

1. Physicians are less likely to use tobacco than the general population; however, some research indicates they are more likely to use alcohol and benzodiazepines than the general population.
2. Anesthesiology, emergency medicine, and psychiatry are specialties whose members are disproportionately represented in PHPs.
3. Opioid use disorder is particularly problematic for physicians given the speed with which addiction develops, the lethality of relapse, and the exposure to licensing actions as a consequence of impairment or diversion of drugs from patients to maintain the addiction.
4. Outcomes for physicians who participate in PHPs are among the best in addiction treatment.
5. To the degree that confidentiality encourages referral for treatment, it may better promote patient safety than would disciplinary approaches.

REVIEW QUESTIONS

1. Physicians are more likely to use which of the following as compared to the general population?
   A. Alcohol
   B. Benzodiazepines
   C. Tobacco
   D. Both A and B.

2. Which of the following is the strongest predictor of developing a substance use disorder in physicians?
   A. Family history of substance use disorder
   B. History of depression or anxiety
   C. Stress levels
   D. Type of specialty

3. Physician health programs typically provide:
   A. Case management to arrange for evaluations and subsequent treatment if indicated.
   B. A 5-year period in which fitness to practice is monitored from multiple perspectives including toxicology testing.
   C. Advocacy for participants in interactions with regulatory agencies.
   D. All of the above.

ANSWERS

1. **D.** Physicians are more likely than the general population to use alcohol and benzodiazepines. Physicians are less likely than the general population to use tobacco.
2. **A.** The strongest predictor of developing an SUD among physicians is a family history of SUDs. Other predictors include the personality characteristic of "sensation seeking" and having easy access to addictive drugs.
3. **D.** All of the functions listed are typical of physician health programs.

SUGGESTED READINGS

Brooks E, Gendel MH, Gundersen DC, et al. Physician health programmes and malpractice claims: reducing risk through monitoring. *Occup Med (Lond)*. 2013;63(4):274-280.

DesRoches CM, Rao SR, Fromson JA, et al. Physicians' perceptions, preparedness for reporting, and experiences related to impaired and incompetent colleagues. *JAMA*. 2010;304(2): 187-193.

DuPont RL, McLellan AT, White WL, Merlo LJ, Gold MS. Setting the standard for recovery: physicians' health programs. *J Subst Abuse Treat*. 2009;36(2):159-171.

Kaskutas LA. Alcoholics Anonymous effectiveness: faith meets science. *J Addict Dis*. 2009;28(2):145-157.

McLellan AT, Skipper GS, Campbell M, DuPont RL. Five year outcomes in a cohort study of physicians treated for substance use disorders in the United States. *BMJ*. 2008;337:a2038.

Oreskovich MR, Kaups KL, Balch CM, et al. Prevalence of alcohol disorders among American surgeons. *Arch Surg*. 2012; 147(2):168-174.

The California Diversion Program: A Cautionary Tale

Summary by Abigail J. Herron

Based on THE ASAM PRINCIPLES OF ADDICTION MEDICINE, 6th edition sidebar by
Paul H. Earley

In 1980, the California Board of Medical Quality Assurance opened a Diversion Program to assist physicians with alcohol and drug problems, "diverting" them from disciplinary action if they followed the requirements of the program. The participation of physicians who entered the program was not publicly disclosed, and audits were required as part of a standard oversight process by the state.

In 2003, the responsibility for these audits shifted from the state to a consumer group, the Center for Public Interest Law. The tone of the audits became more critical, alleging that several physicians had harmed patients. Press coverage regarding impaired physicians increased, including an example of a "diversion-protected" physician who used drugs, who in fact had been dropped from the Diversion Program for failure to comply with requirements. Much of the opposition to the program focused on the opinion that keeping the names of the physicians in the Diversion Program from the public was contrary to the public protection mission of the Medical Board of California. In 2007, as part of a required semiannual review of the program for renewal authorization, the Medical Board of California, under tremendous pressure from the Center for Public Interest Law, the media, and some legislators voted unanimously to deny renewal. The program was closed on June 30, 2008.

In response to a gaping hole in physician monitoring, local medical societies and hospital systems attempted to continue to provide such services, ultimately leading to the creation of a new 501(c)(3) organization, California Public Protection and Physician Health, which is focused on assisting in the re-creation of a full state-sanctioned physician health program to promote physician health. At the time of this writing, the Medical Board is writing regulations to govern the new organization.

This tale illustrates several key points. First, while the responsibility of physician health programs is the health and safety of all, they are sustained or destroyed by public opinion and politics. Second, physicians are safety-sensitive workers and are appropriately held to a higher standard. Effective treatment and monitoring decreases, but does not eliminate, public fear. Finally, the outcome of a few physicians can affect the entire organization, even after being ejected from the safe haven of a physician health program and turned over to disciplinary bodies.

Management of Intoxication and Withdrawal

50 Management of Intoxication and Withdrawal: General Principles

Summary by Tara M. Wright, Jeffrey S. Cluver, and Hugh Myrick

Based on THE ASAM PRINCIPLES OF ADDICTION MEDICINE, 6th edition chapter by Tara M. Wright, Jeffrey S. Cluver, and Hugh Myrick

INTOXICATION STATES

Intoxication is the result of being under the influence of, and responding to, the acute effects of alcohol or another drug. Intoxication states can range from euphoria or sedation to life-threatening emergencies when overdose occurs. It can mimic many psychiatric and medical conditions. Each substance has a set of signs and symptoms that are seen during intoxication. Identification and treatment of intoxication can lead to appropriate management of the withdrawal phenomenon and provide an avenue for entry into treatment.

Identification and Management of Intoxication

The identification of intoxication begins with the collection of patient data through a patient history, physical examination, and laboratory screening. Of immediate concern is life-threatening intoxication or overdose. Thus, the first priority is general supportive care and resuscitative actions. It is important to determine not only the severity of the substance ingestion but also the patient's level of consciousness, the substances involved, and any complicating medical disorders. Often, more than one substance is involved, and it is critical to know what substances have been ingested as well as how much of each substance. Questions regarding the quantity and frequency of substance use provide valuable information to the clinician. Discovering chronic patterns of substance use may aid in subsequent referral to addiction treatment.

Standardized questionnaires for self-administration by the patient or for use by the clinician are designed to elicit answers related to alcohol or substance use. Toxicology screens can provide valuable information regarding the type or types of substances used. They can aid in the differential diagnosis when atypical symptoms are present, particularly in cases where little clinical history is available. Urine is the most widely used specimen when screening for substances of abuse. Having knowledge of the sensitivities, specificities, and cross-reactivities of the particular urine drug test being used is of vital importance to the appropriate interpretation. In addition, one must have an understanding of the usual duration of detectability of particular substances. It is important to note that the rise in the use of synthetic or "designer" drugs can make identification of the causative substance(s) more difficult because these substances are frequently not detected by routine toxicology testing.

Testing for alcohol is most frequently accomplished by breathalyzer or blood alcohol levels; however, urine tests are also available that detect metabolites of alcohol. Laboratory assays that measure increases in liver enzymes—such as γ-glutamyltransferase, aspartate aminotransferase, and alanine aminotransferase—can be helpful in indicating possible heavy alcohol use. A biologic assay to monitor alcohol intake involves percent carbohydrate-deficient transferrin, a more sensitive and specific indicator of heavy alcohol consumption. The conjugated ethanol metabolites ethyl glucuronide and ethyl sulfate are other measures that can also be used to confirm or rule out recent drinking. They remain detectable in urine for several hours up to some days longer than ethanol, the time lag largely depending on the amount consumed. Another biomarker is serum-based phosphatidylethanol, which may be able to detect the presence of even a few days of heavy alcohol consumption for as long as 3 weeks after.

RECOGNIZING THE IMPACT OF EVER CHANGING DRUG TRENDS

Trends in substance use are ever changing as new drugs often burst on the scene rapidly. Because many of these drugs are synthetic and may not be detected in routine drug testing, it is imperative that the treating clinician keep abreast of recent substance use trends in their geographical area. To this end, the National Institute on Drug Abuse launched the National Drug Early Warning System in 2014 to create a national network to identify and monitor emerging drug problems.

WITHDRAWAL STATES

Substance withdrawal has been defined by the American Psychiatric Association as "the development of a substance-specific maladaptive behavioral change, usually with uncomfortable physiological and cognitive consequences, that is the result of a cessation of, or reduction in, heavy and prolonged substance use." The signs and symptoms of withdrawal usually are the opposite of a substance's direct pharmacologic effects. Substances in a given pharmacologic class produce similar withdrawal syndromes; however, the onset, duration, and intensity are variable, depending on the particular agent used, the duration of use, and the degree of neuroadaptation.

Evidence for the cessation of or reduction in use of a substance may be obtained by history or toxicology. The clinical picture must not be solely attributable to other medical conditions or a primary mental disorder. Withdrawal may, however, be superimposed on any medical condition or organic mental disorder. Therefore, a thorough physical examination is necessary, including appropriate laboratory analysis of basic organ functions.

Goals of Detoxification

Detoxification includes a set of interventions by which a substance an individual is physically dependent on is eliminated from the body. The American Society of Addiction Medicine (ASAM) lists three immediate goals for detoxification of alcohol and other substances: (1) "to provide a safe withdrawal from the drug(s) of dependence and enable the patient to become drug-free," (2) "to provide a withdrawal that is humane and thus protects the patient's dignity," and (3) "to prepare the patient for ongoing treatment of his or her dependence on alcohol or other drugs." Furthermore, it comprises three essential and sequential steps: evaluation, stabilization, and fostering patient readiness for and entry into treatment. It is important to distinguish detoxification from substance use disorder treatment. *Substance use disorder treatment/rehabilitation* involves a constellation of ongoing therapeutic services ultimately intended to promote recovery for patients with a substance use disorder. Detoxification may be the first step in this process.

Many risks are associated with substance use withdrawal, some of which are influenced by the setting in which detoxification occurs. For example, in persons who are severely physically dependent on alcohol, an abrupt, untreated cessation of drinking may result in marked hyperautonomic signs, seizures (which may be recurrent), withdrawal delirium, or even death. Other sedative–hypnotics also can produce life-threatening withdrawal syndromes. Withdrawal from opioids produces severe discomfort but generally is not life-threatening. A caring staff, a supportive environment, sensitivity to cultural issues, confidentiality, and the selection of appropriate detoxification medications are important components of a humane withdrawal experience. During detoxification, patients may form therapeutic relationships with treatment staff and other patients, providing an opportunity to explore alternatives to an alcohol- or drug-using lifestyle. Detoxification is therefore an opportunity to offer patients information and to motivate them for longer term treatment. Unfortunately, managed care organizations and other third-party payers often regard detoxification as separate from other phases of alcohol and other drug treatment, as though detoxification occurs in isolation from such treatment. In clinical practice, this separation should not exist; detoxification is but one component of a comprehensive treatment strategy.

General Principles of Management

There is a risk of serious adverse consequences for some patients who undergo withdrawal. A previous complicated withdrawal should alert the practitioner to the likely possibility of future complicated withdrawals. The kindling hypothesis has been well supported in alcohol research, such that past alcohol withdrawal seizures are a strong indicator of future alcohol withdrawal seizures. A widely used instrument in clinical and research settings for the initial assessment and ongoing monitoring of alcohol withdrawal is the Clinical Institute Withdrawal Assessment of Alcohol, Revised, a short test that rates the severity of withdrawal as observed by the clinician. In general, low scores (<8) suggest that pharmacotherapy may not be required, whereas high scores (>10) indicate a greater risk of alcohol withdrawal syndrome complications. Similarly, the Clinical Opiate Withdrawal Scale is a scale administered by the clinician to help determine the stage and severity of opioid withdrawal over time.

The duration of detoxification is not a clearly defined, discrete period. Because detoxification often requires a greater intensity of services than other types of treatment, there is a practical value in defining a period during which a person is "in detoxification." The detoxification period usually is defined as the time during which the patient receives detoxification medications, even though some signs and symptoms may persist for a much longer period. Another way of defining the detoxification period is by measuring the duration of withdrawal signs or symptoms. However, the duration of these symptoms may be difficult to determine in a correctly medicated patient because symptoms of withdrawal are largely suppressed by the medication.

Another problem in defining the duration of detoxification is the fact that many patients may have prolonged withdrawal signs or symptoms or protracted withdrawal syndrome. Symptoms may include disturbances of sleep, anxiety, irritability, mood instability, and craving. Despite advances in the literature elucidating the neurobiology of protracted withdrawal, appropriate pharmacologic management requires further exploration. The protracted withdrawal syndrome is hypothesized to be a period when individuals are at a heightened risk of relapse.

Pharmacologic Management

There are two general strategies for pharmacologic management of withdrawal: suppressing withdrawal through use of a cross-tolerant medication and reducing signs and symptoms of withdrawal through alteration of another neuropharmacologic process. Either or both may be used to manage withdrawal syndromes effectively. To suppress withdrawal with cross-tolerant medication, a longer acting medication typically is used to provide a milder, controlled withdrawal. Examples include the use of methadone for opioid detoxification and diazepam for alcohol detoxification. Medications that are not cross-tolerant are used to treat specific signs and symptoms of withdrawal (eg, the use of clonidine for opioid withdrawal).

Detoxification alone rarely constitutes adequate treatment. The provision of detoxification services

without continuing treatment at an appropriate level of care constitutes less than optimal use of limited resources. Maintaining abstinence can be a very difficult goal to achieve: It has been estimated that approximately 50% of patients with alcohol use disorder relapse within 3 months of detoxification. The appropriate level of care and content of treatment following detoxification must be clinically determined based on the patient's individual needs. ASAM's criteria are the most widely used and comprehensive set of guidelines used for determining the appropriate level of care for a patient within the continuum of addiction services. Using the criteria, levels of treatment are differentiated based on (1) degree of direct medical management provided; (2) degree of structure, safety, and security provided; and (3) degree of treatment intensity provided.

Detoxification Settings

The initial assessment should facilitate the selection of the appropriate level of care for detoxification. In determining the most appropriate setting, the practitioner should match the patient's clinical needs with the least restrictive and most cost-effective setting. Detoxification may take place in a variety of inpatient and outpatient settings. Multiple instruments have been designed to facilitate selection of an appropriate level of care. The ASAM Criteria contain detailed guidelines for matching patients to an appropriate intensity of services for detoxification. Both outpatient and inpatient settings can initiate recovery programs that may include referrals for problems such as medical, legal, psychiatric, and family issues.

Inpatient Detoxification

Inpatient detoxification is offered in medical hospitals, psychiatric hospitals, and medically managed residential treatment programs. It allows 24-hour supervision, observation, and support for patients who are intoxicated or experiencing withdrawal. The primary emphasis in this setting should be placed on ensuring that the patient is medically stable, assessing for adequate biopsychosocial stability, and linking the patient to appropriate inpatient and outpatient services once it is medically safe to do so. Inpatient detoxification provides the safest setting for the treatment of substance withdrawal because it ensures that patients will be carefully monitored and appropriately supported. Such monitoring is especially important if the patient is physically dependent on high doses of alcohol or other sedative–hypnotic drugs. In addition, inpatient detoxification separates the patient from substance-related social and environmental stimuli that might increase the risk of relapse.

Outpatient Detoxification

Outpatient detoxification usually is offered in community mental health and addiction centers, opioid treatment programs, and private clinics. Essential components to a successful outpatient detoxification include a positive and helpful social support network and regular accessibility to the treatment provider. Medical and nursing personnel involved must be readily available to evaluate and confirm that detoxification in the less supervised setting is safe. They must be able to interpret the signs and symptoms of alcohol and other drug intoxication and withdrawal, have knowledge of the appropriate treatment and monitoring of these conditions, and have the ability to facilitate the individual's entry into continued treatment as well as the ability to refer to a higher level of inpatient care if necessary.

Considerations in Selecting a Setting

The best detoxification setting for a given patient may be defined as the least restrictive and least expensive setting in which the goals of detoxification can be met. The treatment setting must be primarily based on a patient's clinical needs. Treatment providers should consider detoxification settings and patient matching within the context of a fundamental principle of high-quality patient care. The severity of the patient's withdrawal symptoms and the intensity of care required to ensure appropriate management of these symptoms are of primary importance. Pressures to achieve cost savings have a significant effect on the selection of treatment settings for detoxification. Many insurance companies, managed care organizations, and other payers have adopted stringent policies concerning reimbursement for alcohol and other drug detoxification services. These policies govern not only the setting in which the services are provided but also the maximum number and duration of detoxification episodes that are covered benefits. Such policies give insufficient weight to the variety of factors that affect the selection of a setting in which the patient has the greatest likelihood of achieving satisfactory detoxification. Some persons in need of detoxification, for example, may not be appropriate candidates for outpatient detoxification because of environmental impediments such as a spouse who is using alcohol or other drugs. Such a patient may be more appropriately detoxified in a residential setting such as a recovery house or other residential environment that is free of alcohol and other drug use.

Use of the ASAM Criteria

The ASAM Criteria are intended for use as a clinical tool for matching patients to appropriate levels of care. The criteria reflect a clinical consensus of adult and adolescent treatment specialists and incorporate the results of a comprehensive peer review by professionals in addiction treatment. They use six dimensions in the biopsychosocial assessment of individuals needing substance use services: (1) acute intoxication and/or withdrawal potential; (2) biomedical conditions and complications; (3) emotional, behavioral, or cognitive conditions and complications; (4) readiness to change; (5) relapse, continued use, or continued problem potential; and (6) recovery/living environment. Individual treatment plans are developed through the multidimensional assessment over five broad levels of treatment, which are based on the degree of direct medical management provided; the structure, safety, and security provided; and the intensity of treatment services provided. The five broad levels of care include early intervention, outpatient services, intensive outpatient/partial hospitalization services, residential/inpatient services, and medically managed intensive inpatient services. In between these broad levels are gradations in intensity of services.

Relapse

Many individuals undergo detoxification more than once, and some do so many times. When persons who are recently physically dependent return for repeat detoxification, it generally is with a more realistic expectation of what is needed to remain free from alcohol and other drugs. Compliance and relapse in addictive disease are comparable to rates of relapse in other illnesses, such as diabetes and hypertension. Therefore, patients with substance use disorders should be offered as many chances as they need for recovery. People with substance use disorders are at increased risk of relapse at certain points in their recovery, and relapse can occur at any time. The patient who relapse is an appropriate candidate for detoxification and continuing treatment, including relapse prevention education.

SPECIAL POPULATIONS

Although researchers have not yet thoroughly evaluated withdrawal strategies for certain populations, patients in several groups clearly require special consideration. These include adolescents; older adults; pregnant and nursing women; those who are HIV positive; patients with neurologic, cardiovascular, hepatic or renal, or other medical conditions; those with co-occurring chronic pain; and those with co-morbid psychiatric disorders.

KEY POINTS

1. A thorough patient history, physical examinations, laboratory screening, and gathering of collateral information are necessary in the management of both intoxication and withdrawal states.
2. Detoxification is essentially composed of three essential and sequential steps: evaluation, stabilization, and fostering patient readiness for and entry into treatment.
3. In determining whether to complete detoxification in an inpatient or outpatient setting, the patient's needs should always drive the selection of the most appropriate setting.
4. It is important to distinguish detoxification from substance abuse treatment. Substance abuse treatment/rehabilitation involves a constellation of ongoing therapeutic services ultimately intended to promote recovery. Detoxification may be the first step in this process.

REVIEW QUESTIONS

1. An elevation in which of the following laboratory assays is the most specific predictor of heavy drinking?
   A. Mean corpuscular volume
   B. Aspartate aminotransferase
   C. Percent carbohydrate-deficient transferrin
   D. Ethyl glucuronide
   E. Blood glucose

2. In an otherwise healthy adult, which of the following substances is *not* considered to have potentially life-threatening withdrawal symptoms?
   A. Alcohol
   B. Benzodiazepines
   C. Barbiturates
   D. Opioids
   E. Both A and B

3. Relative indications for inpatient detoxification from alcohol include all of the following *except*:
   A. younger age.
   B. past history of alcohol withdrawal seizures.
   C. pregnancy.
   D. comorbid acute medical or psychiatric illness.
   E. lack of stable housing.

ANSWERS

1. **C**
2. **D**
3. **A**

SUGGESTED READINGS

American Psychiatric Association. *Diagnostic and Statistical Manual of Mental Disorders*. 5th ed. Arlington, VA: American Psychiatric Association, 2013.

Mee-Lee D. *The ASAM Criteria: Treatment Criteria for Addictive, Substance-Related, and Co-Occurring Conditions.* 3rd ed. Rockville, MD: American Society of Addiction Medicine, 2013.

Substance Abuse and Mental Health Services Administration. *Detoxification and Substance Abuse Treatment (Treatment Improvement Protocol TIP 45).* Rockville, MD: Substance Abuse and Mental Health Services Administration, 2006.

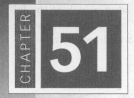

51 Management of Alcohol Intoxication and Withdrawal

Summary by Radha Sadacharan and Alan A. Wartenberg

Based on THE ASAM PRINCIPLES OF ADDICTION MEDICINE, 6th edition chapter by Alan A. Wartenberg

ALCOHOL INTOXICATION

Alcohol intoxication is defined by clinical manifestations of impairment that occur after alcohol consumption. At a blood alcohol concentration between 20 mg% and 99 mg%, loss of muscular coordination begins, and changes in mood, personality, and behavior occur. Although a level of 80 mg% is considered legal intoxication in the United States, many people may have significant impairment below that level.

As the blood alcohol concentration rises to the range of 100 mg% to 199 mg%, neurologic impairment occurs. Between 200 mg% and 299 mg%, obvious intoxication is present, except in persons with marked tolerance. Nausea and vomiting, as well as ataxia, may occur. As the level rises to 300 mg% to 399 mg%, hypothermia, along with severe dysarthria and amnesia, and stage I anesthesia is common. At blood alcohol levels between 400 mg% and 799 mg%, the onset of alcoholic coma occurs, depending largely on tolerance. Blood levels of alcohol between 600 mg% and 800 mg% are commonly fatal.

MANAGEMENT OF INTOXICATION

Even with very high blood alcohol levels, survival is probable if the respiratory and cardiovascular systems can be supported. Attention must be paid to the potential presence of nonbeverage alcohol (methyl alcohol, isopropyl alcohol, or ethylene glycol) as well as coingestion of other toxins (eg, opioids, benzodiazepines, tricyclic antidepressants) because these intoxications may present a similar clinical picture but require different management.

Medical treatment is supportive in the patient with alcohol intoxication. As with all patients with impaired consciousness, intravenous glucose should be given if rapid testing of blood glucose is not immediately available, after first giving 100 mg or more of intravenous thiamine. Alcohol is rapidly absorbed into the bloodstream; therefore, induction of emesis or gastric lavage is not indicated unless a substantial ingestion has occurred within a short time or when other drug ingestion is suspected.

The patient with acute intoxication may also exhibit some agitation as part of the intoxication syndrome, which is best managed nonpharmacologically. If needed, intramuscular administration of a rapid-onset, short-acting benzodiazepine, alone or in combination with a neuroleptic agent such as haloperidol, can be useful. There can be a potential synergistic response between the alcohol already in the patient's system and an exogenously administered sedative–hypnotic, so this approach should be used only as a last resort. There are no antidotes to alcohol that act like naloxone (an opioid antagonist) or flumazenil (a benzodiazepine/γ-aminobutyric acid [GABA] antagonist).

HANGOVER

A hangover is a constellation of unpleasant physical and mental symptoms that occur after heavy alcohol intake. Headache, malaise, diarrhea, nausea, and difficulty concentrating are the most common symptoms, often accompanied by sensitivity to light or sound, sweating, and anxiety. About 75% of individuals who drink to intoxication report experiencing a hangover at least some of the time. The pathophysiology of hangover is not completely understood. In part, it is believed to be the effect of the intermediate product of ethanol metabolism, acetaldehyde. Dehydration, electrolyte imbalance, sleep disruption, increased physical activity while intoxicated, hypoglycemia, and the many hormonal disruptions caused by alcohol may also play contributing roles.

Although many interventions have been tried to alleviate hangover symptoms, to date, none have clearly demonstrated effectiveness in rigorous investigations.

ALCOHOL WITHDRAWAL

In those with physiologic dependence on alcohol, the clinical manifestations of alcohol withdrawal begin 6 to 24 hours after the last drink, sometimes arising before the blood alcohol level has returned to zero. Early withdrawal signs and symptoms include anxiety, sleep disturbances, vivid dreams, anorexia, nausea, and headache. Physical signs include tachycardia, elevation of blood pressure, hyperactive reflexes, sweating, hyperthermia, and tremors. The severity of these symptoms varies, but in a majority, they are mild and transient, passing within 1 to 2 days. In more severe cases of withdrawal, these perceptual distortions or misperceptions may develop into frank hallucinations. It should be distinguished from that which is part of delirium tremens (DTs).

Withdrawal seizures usually begin within 8 to 24 hours after the patient's last drink and may occur before the blood alcohol level has returned to zero. Like hallucinosis, seizures can sometimes occur with minimal or absent other symptoms of withdrawal. Seizures peak 24 to 48 hours after the last drink. The risk of seizures appears to be, in part, genetically determined and is increased in patients with past withdrawal seizures or in those undergoing concurrent withdrawal from benzodiazepines or other sedative–hypnotic drugs. The association with seizure risk and repeated withdrawals has been described as a "kindling effect," which refers to animal studies demonstrating that repeated subcortical electrical stimulation is associated with increases in seizure susceptibility.

For up to 90% of patients, withdrawal does not progress beyond mild-to-moderate symptoms. In other patients, however, manifestations can include delirium. In the classic cases of withdrawal delirium, the manifestations steadily worsen and progress into a severe delirium accompanied by an autonomic storm: hence the term *delirium tremens*. DTs generally appear 72 to 96 hours after the last drink. In their classic presentation, DTs possess all the signs and symptoms of mild withdrawal, but in a much more pronounced form and with the development of marked tachycardia, tremors, diaphoresis, and fever. The patient develops global confusion and disorientation to place and time. Hallucinations are frequent, and marked psychomotor activity may develop. Severe disruption of the normal sleep–wake cycle also is common, with the possible absence of clear sleep for several days. The duration of the delirium is variable but averages 2 to 3 days. Historically, mortality in DTs was substantial. With the development

of effective therapy, including intensive care, death is now unusual.

Because alcohol withdrawal involves a constellation of nonspecific findings, efforts have been made to develop structured withdrawal severity assessment scales to objectively quantify the severity of withdrawal. The most extensively studied and best known is the Clinical Institute Withdrawal Assessment—Alcohol, or CIWA, and a shortened version known as the CIWA-A Revised (CIWA-Ar) (Table 51-1). The CIWA-Ar has well-documented reliability, reproducibility, and validity compared to ratings of withdrawal severity by experienced clinicians. In the case of the CIWA-Ar, a score ≤10 generally indicates mild withdrawal, a score of 11 to 15 indicates moderate withdrawal, and a score greater than 15 indicates severe withdrawal.

It is extremely important that staff responsible for patients' assessments be adequately trained in the utilization of the CIWA-Ar. The responsible clinician should be thoroughly familiar with the instrument and should train health professionals who will be monitoring the patients. Professionals using the CIWA-Ar need to understand that it is not a diagnostic instrument for alcohol withdrawal; the clinician must diagnose alcohol withdrawal based on the clinical setting. Confounding or exacerbating conditions, such as head trauma, central nervous system infections, other drug influences, and metabolic disturbances must be appropriately excluded.

Withdrawal scales can also contribute to appropriate triage of patients because it has been shown that high scores early in the course are predictive of the development of seizures and delirium. Marked autonomic hyperactivity, serum electrolyte abnormalities, and acute medical comorbidities, particularly infection and trauma, are associated with an increased risk of DTs or severe withdrawal.

The primary effect of alcohol on the central nervous system is as a depressant. Two neurotransmitter systems appear to play a central role in the development of alcohol withdrawal syndrome. Alcohol exerts its effects in part by enhancing the effect of GABA, a major inhibitory neurotransmitter. GABA mediates typical sedative–hypnotic effects such as sedation and a raised seizure threshold. Chronic alcohol intake leads to an adaptive suppression of GABA activity. A sudden relative deficiency in GABA neurotransmitter activity is produced with alcohol abstinence and is believed to contribute to the anxiety, increased psychomotor activity, and predisposition to seizures seen in withdrawal. Although alcohol enhances the effect of GABA, it inhibits the

TABLE 51-1	Clinical Effects of Alcohol
Blood Alcohol Level[a] (mg%)	**Clinical Manifestations**
20–99	Loss of muscular coordination Changes in mood, personality, and behavior
100–199	Neurologic impairment with prolonged reaction time, ataxia, incoordination, and mental impairment
200–299	Very obvious intoxication, except in those with marked tolerance Nausea, vomiting, marked ataxia
300–399	Hypothermia, severe dysarthria, amnesia, stage I anesthesia
400–799	Onset of alcoholic coma, with precise level depending on the degree of tolerance Progressive obtundation, decreases in respiration, blood pressure, and body temperature (hypothermia) Urinary incontinence or retention, reflexes markedly decreased or absent
600-800	Often fatal because of loss of airway-protective reflexes from airway obstruction by the flaccid tongue, from pulmonary aspiration of gastric contents, or from respiratory arrest from profound central nervous system obstruction

[a]Levels of 200–300 mg%, particularly when reached quickly ("chugging"), may result in coma, aspiration, and death in nontolerant individuals, particularly adolescents and young adults. In addition, presence of other depressant drugs, even in therapeutic doses (benzodiazepines, sedative–hypnotics, opioids), may result in respiratory depression, coma, and death at lower levels of alcohol.

sensitivity of the autonomic adrenergic systems, with a resulting upregulation with chronic alcohol intake. The discontinuation of alcohol leads to rebound overactivity of the brain and peripheral noradrenergic systems. Increased sympathetic autonomic activity contributes to tachycardia, hypertension, tremor, diaphoresis, and anxiety.

A second neurotransmitter, norepinephrine, also seems to be important in alcohol withdrawal presentations. Norepinephrine's metabolites are elevated in the body fluid during withdrawal; levels correlate with the sympathetic nervous system signs of withdrawal. Research has identified other neural effects of chronic alcohol intake, including effects on serotonergic systems, neuronal calcium channels, glutamate receptors, cyclic adenosine monophosphate systems, and the hypothalamic–pituitary–adrenal neuroendocrine axis; these too may play a role in withdrawal. Other recent studies suggest that the glutamatergic and N-methyl-D-aspartate dysregulation play a role in the development of central nervous system excitation as well, particularly seizures and delirium.

The role of genetics in alcohol withdrawal is a topic of active investigation. In animal models, the development of selectively bred strains demonstrates that severity of withdrawal and risk of seizures are strongly influenced by genotype. Investigations in humans have focused on genes regulating neurotransmitter systems. Several studies have found an association of the A9 allele, which affects central dopamine functions, with severity of alcohol withdrawal, alcohol withdrawal seizures, and DTs. To date, no relationship with genes involved in the serotonin, GABAergic, or endorphinergic systems have been found.

MANAGEMENT OF ALCOHOL WITHDRAWAL SYNDROMES

Pertinent laboratory tests generally include a complete blood count, electrolytes, magnesium levels, calcium levels, phosphate levels, liver enzymes, urine drug screen, pregnancy test (when appropriate), and breath or blood alcohol levels. Others, depending on suspected co-occurring conditions, may include chest x-ray, electrocardiogram, and tests for viral hepatitis, human immunodeficiency virus, or other infections. General management also involves maintaining adequate fluid balance and addressing nutritional and electrolyte deficiencies.

Supportive nonpharmacologic care is an important and useful element in the management of all patients undergoing withdrawal. Simple interventions such as reassurance, reality orientation, and general nursing care are effective.

Benzodiazepines are pharmacologically crosstolerant with alcohol and have the similar effect of enhancing the effect of GABA-induced sedation. It is believed that the provision of benzodiazepines alleviates the acute deficiency of GABA neurotransmitter activity that occurs with sudden cessation of alcohol use. Trials comparing different benzodiazepines indicate that all are similarly efficacious in reducing signs and symptoms of withdrawal and are more effective than placebo. However, longer-acting agents such as diazepam and chlordiazepoxide may be more effective at preventing seizures. Longer-acting agents also may contribute to an overall smoother withdrawal course, with a reduction in breakthrough or rebound symptoms. On the other hand, pharmacologic data and clinical experience suggest that longer-acting agents can pose a risk of excess sedation in some patients, including elderly persons and patients with hepatic synthetic dysfunction, and in patients with chronic pulmonary disease. In such patients, shorter-acting agents are preferable.

When a rapid control of symptoms is needed, medications with a faster onset offer an advantage. Given the evidence of equal efficacy, if a specific agent is available to a practitioner or program at a lower cost, cost is a legitimate factor to consider. The pharmacokinetics of different benzodiazepines should be taken into consideration depending on the clinical circumstances, including the age and health of the patient, and the stage and severity of withdrawal. Younger, healthier patients generally tolerate longer-acting drugs, which may produce a smoother course. Shorter-acting agents may be better tolerated in sicker patients, particularly those with hepatic insufficiency and/or pulmonary disease.

Drug latency may also be an issue when patients present with moderate-to-severe withdrawal because several commonly used drugs have longer periods between oral ingestion and peak levels, such as oxazepam (which takes 1.5 to 2 hours to peak) or chlordiazepoxide (1 to 2 hours), whereas diazepam may reach peak levels in 20 to 30 minutes.

Attention to tapering doses can be important when shorter-acting agents are used because tolerance to them can develop rapidly and withdrawal from them can lead to symptoms including seizures. Although physical dependence on benzodiazepines given therapeutically is a legitimate concern, it rarely occurs unless the benzodiazepine has been prescribed for 10 to 14 days, although shorter courses leading to withdrawal have been observed. Studies have indicated that nonbenzodiazepine sedative–hypnotics also are effective at reducing the signs and symptoms of withdrawal but have not been as extensively studied, and the size of studies with them is not adequate to confirm their effectiveness at reducing seizures and delirium.

Benzodiazepines have a greater margin of safety, with a lower risk of respiratory depression as well as overall lower misuse potential than the nonbenzodiazepine agents. Phenobarbital still is used by some programs because it has well-documented anticonvulsant activity, is inexpensive, and has low misuse liability. However, as with all barbiturates, oversedation is common. It is critically important to assess every patient for oversedation (sustained nystagmus, dysarthria, dysmetria, ataxia, mood lability, and depressed level of consciousness) prior to receiving additional doses and to withhold additional doses if such signs or symptoms are present.

In many studies examining the effectiveness of various medications for withdrawal, the medications were given in fixed amounts at scheduled times and were given for periods of 5 to 7 days. However, it has been shown that many patients can go through withdrawal with only minor symptoms even though they receive little or no medication. An alternative to giving medication on a fixed schedule is known as symptom-triggered therapy. In this approach, the patient is monitored through the use of a structured assessment scale and given medication only when symptoms cross a threshold of severity. Well-designed studies have demonstrated that this approach is as effective as fixed-dose therapy yet leads to the administration of significantly less medication and a significantly shorter duration of treatment.

Symptom-triggered therapy also facilitates the delivery of large amounts of medication quickly to patients with rapidly escalating withdrawal and thus reduces the risk of undertreatment that may arise with the use of fixed doses. Whenever fixed doses are given, it is very important that allowances be made to provide additional medication if the fixed dose should prove inadequate to control symptoms.

Loading dose therapy may also be considered, which involves monitoring the patient with CIWA-Ar scores until they reach a predetermined set point (generally, a score of 8 to 15) and then giving diazepam (10 to 20 mg), clorazepate (3.75 to 7.5 mg), or chlordiazepoxide (50 to 100 mg) on an hourly basis while evaluating the patient prior to each dose until symptoms diminish or signs of oversedation develop (eg, sustained nystagmus, ataxia, dysarthria, mood lability, or oversedation itself). The patient is then monitored for 2 to 3 hours without further medication. The average patient received three to five doses before reaching the end-point, and 80% of patients were adequately treated with a single episode of loading, whereas an additional 10% required a second loading dose regimen within the first 24 hours.

Treatment should allow for a degree of individualization so patients can receive large amounts of medication rapidly if needed. In all cases, medications should be administered by a route that has been shown to have reliable absorption. Therefore, benzodiazepines should be administered orally or, when necessary, intravenously. An exception is lorazepam, which has good intramuscular and sublingual absorption.

One technique is to use fixed-dose regimens that can be loosely based on the potential for mild, moderate, or severe withdrawal and then to order as-needed doses based on the development of an arbitrary CIWA-Ar score of 10 to 15. A major mistake is to continue tapering standing doses in patients who are receiving frequent as-needed doses. Another error is to give reduced doses to patients actively manifesting toxicity, when it is necessary to completely withhold doses of the drug until no signs of toxicity are present. Tapering should not begin until the patient is stable and CIWA-Ar scores are consistently below 10.

Carbamazepine has been widely used in Europe for alcohol withdrawal and has been shown to be equal in efficacy to benzodiazepines for patients with mild-to-moderate withdrawal. When compared with placebo, there is significantly less use of benzodiazepines for breakthrough symptoms. Carbamazepine does not potentiate the central nervous system respiratory depression caused by alcohol, does not inhibit learning, and has no addictive potential. One problem, however, is that rapid dose escalation is not well tolerated.

Although the evidence base is smaller, tapering doses of sodium valproate could be used in a similar fashion. Both medications may also be used as adjuncts to benzodiazepine-based regimens in patients who have past recurrent withdrawal seizures, who have prominent mood lability during withdrawal, or who have concurrent benzodiazepine withdrawal. However, studies of adequate size to assess the efficacy of these agents in preventing withdrawal seizures or delirium are not yet available. Patients treated with carbamazepine or sodium valproate should be monitored using withdrawal scales and receive benzodiazepines if severe withdrawal symptoms emerge. Both these agents have interactions with other drugs and have hepatic and/or hematologic toxicities and thus must be used carefully, if at all, in patients with certain comorbid medical disorders. Because they have not been shown to prevent withdrawal seizures and DTs, they should not be used as monotherapy without benzodiazepines in people at risk for such complications.

The routine use of phenytoin is no longer advocated as a method to prevent the occurrence of withdrawal seizures because it has been shown to be ineffective at preventing recurrent withdrawal seizures. Other anticonvulsants are the subject of active study and may be useful adjuncts in addition to benzodiazepine therapy.

β-Adrenergic–blocking agents as well as centrally acting α-adrenergic agonists also are effective at ameliorating symptoms in patients with mild-to-moderate withdrawal, primarily by reducing the autonomic nervous system manifestations of withdrawal. However, these agents do not have known anticonvulsant activity, and the studies to date have not been large enough to determine their effectiveness at reducing seizures or delirium. In addition, there is concern that the selective reduction in certain manifestations of withdrawal may mask the development of other significant withdrawal symptoms and may make it difficult to utilize withdrawal scales to guide treatment.

Neuroleptic agents, including the phenothiazines (eg, chlorpromazine, prochlorperazine) and the butyrophenones (haloperidol and droperidol), demonstrate some effectiveness at reducing the signs and symptoms of withdrawal and, for a time, were used extensively for that purpose. However, these agents are less effective than benzodiazepines in preventing delirium and may lead to an increase in the rate of seizures. They should not be used alone but always in conjunction with a benzodiazepine. There is limited published experience with the use of second-generation (or "atypical") antipsychotics.

Despite the relative lack of evidence of oral and intravenous alcohol for the management of alcohol withdrawal, several hospitals continue to use intravenous or oral alcohol in the management of alcohol withdrawal. Intravenous alcohol infusions require close monitoring because of the potential toxicity of alcohol. As a pharmacologic agent, ethyl alcohol has numerous adverse effects. Given the proven efficacy and safety of other agents, the use of oral or intravenous alcohol for alcohol detoxification is strongly discouraged. Indeed, the American Society of Addiction Medicine practice guidelines recommend against its use. However, the use of alcohol in the field to taper a patient down while awaiting access to medical management, such as in rural or military deployed settings where alcohol withdrawal medications are not immediately available, may be considered in rare situations.

Patients with alcohol use disorder are at risk for thiamine deficiency, which may lead to Wernicke disease and/or Korsakoff syndrome. Wernicke disease is an illness with acute onset characterized by the triad of mental disturbance, paralysis of eye movements, and ataxia. Mental status changes typically involve a global confusion and apathetic state, but in some patients, a relatively disproportionate disorder of retentive memory is apparent (Korsakoff syndrome). Wernicke–Korsakoff syndrome is a neurologic emergency that should be treated by the immediate intravenous administration of thiamine, with long-term thiamine and other B vitamin replacement. In patients with clinical evidence of thiamine deficiencies, such as memory issues, high-output heart failure (beriberi), or neuropathy, thiamine and multivitamin supplementation should be prolonged. The provision of intravenous glucose solutions may exhaust a patient's reserve of B vitamins, precipitating Wernicke disease. Therefore, intravenous glucose always should be accompanied by the administration of thiamine in the patient with alcohol use disorder. To reduce the risk of these sequelae, all patients presenting with alcohol withdrawal should receive thiamine at the time of initial presentation, followed by oral supplementation for several weeks. Because patients may also have other vitamin deficiencies, supplementation with B complex vitamins, including folic acid, is commonly employed.

It has also long been recognized that magnesium levels often are low during alcohol withdrawal. A closer study has found that magnesium levels usually are normal at admission but then drop later in withdrawal, before spontaneously returning to normal as symptoms subside. Providing supplemental oral magnesium to patients with a documented low magnesium level is without significant risk, but routine administration of magnesium for withdrawal is no longer recommended unless hypomagnesemia and hypokalemia are both present. In sicker and/or more debilitated patients, an evaluation of phosphorus stores, particularly after refeeding, should be considered, with repletion of those with hypophosphatemia.

The patient who presents after experiencing a withdrawal seizure raises several management issues. It is important to recognize that not all seizures in patients with alcohol use disorder are the result of withdrawal. All patients who present with their first seizure warrant a thorough neurologic examination and brain imaging, with lumbar puncture and electroencephalogram also appropriate in some cases. Patients who are known to have past withdrawal seizures and who present with a seizure that can be

attributed clearly to withdrawal may not require a full repeat evaluation. If the seizure was generalized, and if a careful neurologic examination reveals no evidence of focal deficits, there is no suspicion of meningitis, and there is no history of recent major head trauma, additional testing has an extremely low yield and may be safely omitted. There is a 6- to 12-hour period during which there is an increased risk of seizure. Withdrawal seizures often are multiple. For the patient who presents with a withdrawal seizure, rapid treatment is indicated to prevent further episodes.

Initial treatment should be followed by oral doses of longer-acting benzodiazepines over the ensuing 24 to 48 hours. Early studies indicated that a withdrawal seizure places the patient at increased risk for progression to DTs; therefore, close monitoring is warranted. The period of postictal "calm" or sedation may be followed by the development of delirium within 12 to 24 hours; therefore, adequate ongoing monitoring and treatment are necessary.

The patient who progresses to delirium raises many special management issues. The principles of successful treatment involve adequate sedation and meticulous supportive medical care. Careful management of fluids and electrolytes is important, given the patient's inability to manage his or her own intake and the presence of marked autonomic hyperactivity. Delirium often is encountered in patients admitted for acute medical problems whose alcohol dependence was not recognized and whose withdrawal was not adequately treated.

A high index of suspicion for the development of infection—whose presenting signs may be masked by the fever, tachycardia, and confusion of the underlying delirium—is essential, as is careful management of coexisting medical conditions. The use of cross-tolerant sedative–hypnotics has been shown to reduce mortality in DTs and is recommended. However, such medications have not been shown to reverse the delirium or reduce its duration. The goal is to sedate the patient to a point of light sleep or a calm but awake state. This will control the patient's agitation, thus preventing any potential harmful behaviors to the patient or staff and allowing staff to provide the necessary supportive medical care.

The use of intravenous benzodiazepines with rapid onset, such as diazepam, has been shown to provide more rapid control of the patient's symptoms. Due to the risk of respiratory depression, whenever this approach is used, providers should have equipment and personnel immediately available to provide respiratory support if needed.

Intravenous diazepam has both an "α" and a "β" half-life. The initial effect within 5 minutes is followed by a rapid uptake into lipid storage sites; this may result in late oversedation if several repeated boluses are used. Some clinicians prefer getting immediate control with intravenous diazepam and then (after two or three bolus doses) switching to intravenous lorazepam, which can maintain steady-state levels with bolus dosing without the high lipophilicity resulting in fat redistribution. Alternatively, midazolam can be used (1- to 2-mg boluses) to attain immediate control without a β half-life issue. Due to the first-pass hepatic metabolism of benzodiazepines, intravenous doses are equivalent to half the oral dose. Large doses of benzodiazepines may be needed to control the agitation of patients in DTs, with hundreds and even thousands of milligrams of diazepam or its equivalent used over the course of treatment. The practitioner should not hesitate to use whatever amounts are needed to control the agitation, while keeping in mind the possible accumulation of long-acting metabolites. In addition, intravenous preparations of both lorazepam and diazepam are stabilized with polyethylene or propylene glycol, and repeated high-dose use may result in both hyponatremia and metabolic acidosis.

For patients in whom withdrawal is not readily controlled with oral benzodiazepines and who are beginning to demonstrate signs of agitation, an intramuscular administration of a combination of lorazepam and an antipsychotic such as haloperidol is often effective at calming the patient, thus avoiding the need to use intravenous administration.

COMMON TREATMENT ISSUES

For patients with only mild withdrawal symptoms, no past seizures or DTs, and no concurrent significant medical or psychiatric conditions, management on an outpatient basis is reasonable. Such patients should have a responsible individual to monitor them and should be seen on a regular (daily if possible) basis until stabilized. Patients may be treated in an observation unit or admitted for a 1-day stay. If significant withdrawal does not develop and is easily controlled with little or no medication, patients can be discharged or transferred to an intensive outpatient rehabilitation program. Such programs achieve success rates comparable to inpatient/residential treatment for most patients. Patients who experience severe withdrawal symptoms, however, need continuous close monitoring and nursing support.

In medically or surgically hospitalized patients, withdrawal contributes to higher postoperative complications, mortality, and length of stay. Studies have shown that about 20% of patients admitted to the hospital have an alcohol use disorder, and the rate among those admitted for acute trauma or for conditions related to high alcohol intake, such as head and neck cancers, is even higher. Patients requiring more than small amounts of medication for withdrawal symptoms need an individualized assessment by clinicians experienced in the management of withdrawal.

Another event that frequently precipitates alcohol withdrawal is arrest and incarceration. In 1997, surveys showed that of 11 million individuals who were arrested, approximately 1.2 million had alcohol dependence. At the same time, only 28% of jail administrators reported that their institutions ever provided medically managed withdrawal programs for arrestees, despite the ruling of the US Supreme Court that failure to provide proper medical care amounts to a violation of the Eighth Amendment of the US Constitution. This situation has not changed significantly in the intervening years, so it is not surprising that inadequately treated alcohol withdrawal continues to contribute to deaths among newly arrested individuals. Healthcare professionals should remember this as they encounter patients referred from jails with possible withdrawal symptoms.

KEY POINTS

1. Alcohol intoxication is best managed with supportive care, with rare cases needing pharmacologic management for agitation.
2. The severity of alcohol withdrawal can vary greatly in individuals, from mild physical symptoms such as tachycardia and nausea to seizures or marked autonomic hyperactivity in the form of delirium tremens.
3. The use of CIWA-Ar, a validated tool for alcohol withdrawal severity rating, can guide treatment, for which benzodiazepines are the mainstay. Benzodiazepines significantly decrease the morbidity and mortality of alcohol withdrawal, withdrawal seizures, and delirium tremens. They may be administered for alcohol withdrawal in multiple treatment forms: utilizing a loading dose, a fixed schedule, or symptom triggered. Depending on comorbidities and age, fast-acting or longer-acting benzodiazepines may be preferable. Patients in alcohol withdrawal should also be treated with intravenous thiamine, with the goal of decreasing the incidence of Wernicke disease and Korsakoff syndrome.

REVIEW QUESTIONS

1. At what blood alcohol concentration do detectable impairments generally begin for nontolerant individuals?
   A. 50 mg%
   B. 150 mg%
   C. 250 mg%
   D. 350 mg%

2. Which of the following is *not* a common sign or symptom of alcohol withdrawal?
   A. Tachycardia
   B. Anxiety
   C. Hypotension
   D. Nausea

3. Which of the following neurotransmitters are primarily involved in the development of alcohol withdrawal?
   A. GABA and glycine
   B. GABA and glutamate
   C. Glutamate and dopamine
   D. Dopamine and serotonin

ANSWERS

1. **A**
2. **C**
3. **B**

SUGGESTED READINGS

Gershengorn HB. Not every drip needs a plumber. Continuous sedation for alcohol withdrawal syndrome may not require intubation. *Ann Am Thorac Soc.* 2016;13(2): 162-164.

Mayo-Smith MF. Pharmacological management of alcohol withdrawal. A meta-analysis and evidence-based practice guideline. American Society of Addiction Medicine Working Group on Pharmacological Management of Alcohol Withdrawal. *JAMA.* 1997;278(2):144-151.

Mayo-Smith MF, Beecher LH, Fischer TL, et al. Management of alcohol withdrawal delirium. An evidence-based practice guideline. *Arch Intern Med.* 2004;164(13):1405-1412.

Schuckit MA. Recognition and management of withdrawal delirium (delirium tremens). *N Engl J Med.* 2014;371(22): 2109-2113.

Wartenberg AA. Management of alcohol intoxication and withdrawal. In: Ries RK, Fiellin DA, Miller SC, Saitz R, eds. *The ASAM Principles of Addiction Medicine.* 6th ed. Philadelphia: Wolters Kluwer, 2018.

CHAPTER 52

Management of Sedative–Hypnotic Intoxication and Withdrawal

Summary by Jonathan M. Wai

Based on THE ASAM PRINCIPLES OF ADDICTION MEDICINE,
6th edition chapter by Steven J. Eickelberg, William E. Dickinson,
and Reham A. Attia

Sedative–hypnotics are a group of medications that are widely used to decrease anxiety and induce drowsiness to facilitate sleep. They are among the most widely prescribed medications in the Unites States and include benzodiazepines, barbiturates, "Z drugs," and carbamates. These medications are the second-most reported drug class causing emergency room visits, with opioids being the most reported.

SEDATIVE–HYPNOTIC INTOXICATION AND OVERDOSE

Clinical Picture

Benzodiazepines cause impaired motor activity and memory, even at low (therapeutic) doses. Mild-to-moderate toxicity presents with slurred speech, ataxia, and incoordination. Severe intoxication can induce stupor and coma. The older nonbenzodiazepine agents (eg, barbiturates) act directly on the γ-aminobutyric acid type A (GABA$_A$) receptor, unlike benzodiazepines, which increase the effect of GABA on the receptor by allosteric modulation. Because of this, and unlike benzodiazepines, barbiturates and the older agents can cause respiratory arrest and cardiac collapse at toxic levels. Benzodiazepines are rarely lethal when used alone but may become so when high doses are combined with alcohol, barbiturates, or opiates. Given the current high rates of benzodiazepine and opioid use in the United States, awareness of the potentiation of overdose possibility when combining these two medication classes is especially important. Older patients are especially vulnerable to the injurious effects of sedative–hypnotics.

Management

Management of sedative–hypnotic overdose is mostly supportive and should begin with a survey of the patient's airway, breathing, and circulation. Severe cases may require endotracheal intubation and continuous cardiac monitoring. Use of activated charcoal is not advised because of the increased risk of aspiration. Flumazenil, a benzodiazepine receptor antagonist, may be useful in reversing the effects of short-acting benzodiazepines after medical procedures but may not be widely used with benzodiazepine dependence due to the risk of seizures and cardiac arrhythmias from the acute withdrawal that is induced.

SEDATIVE–HYPNOTIC WITHDRAWAL

Overview

Chronic use of sedative–hypnotics can lead to physical and psychological dependence and withdrawal symptoms upon abrupt and sometimes tapered cessation of use. Withdrawal syndromes among all sedative–hypnotics share similar clinical characteristics. However, they may differ depending on the chronicity of the dependence and the rate of discontinuation.

The severity, onset, and duration of withdrawal depend on the pharmacologic factors of (1) medication dose, (2) duration of use, and (3) duration of medication action. In general, clinically significant withdrawal symptoms can occur within 4 to 6 months of low-dose sedative–hypnotic use or within 2 to 3 months of high-dose use.

Signs and Symptoms of Discontinuation

Frequent symptoms of withdrawal are anxiety, insomnia, restlessness, agitation, irritability, and muscle tension. Nausea, diaphoresis, lethargy, aches and pains, coryza, hyperacusis, blurred vision, nightmares, depression, hyperreflexia, and ataxia happen less frequently. Psychosis, seizures, confusion, paranoid delusions, hallucinations, and persistent

TABLE 52-1	Clinical Manifestations of Sedative–Hypnotic Withdrawal
Vital Signs	
• Tachycardia	
• Hypertension	
• Fever	
Central Nervous System	
• Agitation	
• Anxiety	
• Delirium	
• Hallucinations	
• Insomnia	
• Irritability	
• Nightmares	
• Sensory disturbances	
• Tremor	
Ears	
• Tinnitus	
Gastrointestinal	
• Anorexia	
• Diarrhea	
• Nausea	
High-Dose (Severe) Withdrawal	
• Seizures	
• Delirium	
• Death	

tinnitus are uncommon. There is considerable individual variation between patients who discontinue benzodiazepines. Table 52-1 provides a general summary of the spectrum of withdrawal signs and symptoms that may be experienced with varying severity up to 4 weeks with abstinence. Subjective symptoms may predominate without any objective findings.

Although the "Z drugs" (zolpidem, zopiclone, and eszopiclone) were first thought to be safer than the older agents because of selective binding to the α_1 subunit of the $GABA_A$ receptors, there are multiple case reports of severe withdrawal syndromes similar to benzodiazepine withdrawal after discontinuation.

Benzodiazepine Discontinuation

The signs and symptoms following benzodiazepine discontinuation can be described as falling under

one of four categories: (1) symptom recurrence or relapse, (2) rebound, (3) pseudowithdrawal, and (4) true withdrawal.

Symptom recurrence or relapse refers to the recurrence of symptoms, such as insomnia or anxiety, for which the benzodiazepine was initially intended to treat. Reemergence of symptoms is common after discontinuation and may occur with or without the prior existence of benzodiazepine dependence.

Rebound is characterized by the development of symptoms, within hours to days of medication discontinuation, which are qualitatively similar to the symptoms for which benzodiazepines were originally prescribed but of a higher intensity than before the medication treatment. These symptoms tend to be of short duration, which differentiates this syndrome from recurrence.

Pseudowithdrawal occurs when the expectations of withdrawal lead to the experience of abstinence symptoms in the absence of decreased medication dosages. Pseudowithdrawal symptoms may be influenced by expectations as reinforced by friends or media.

True withdrawal occurs when benzodiazepines are discontinued from an individual with physical dependence on the medication. It is marked by psychological and somatic signs and symptoms that can be suppressed by restarting the benzodiazepine or an equivalent cross-tolerant agent.

Prolonged Withdrawal/Postacute Withdrawal Syndrome

After prolonged benzodiazepine use, some patients may experience a prolonged withdrawal that may persist for weeks to months after discontinuation. This syndrome is irregular and unpredictable and without a linear pattern but often slowly abates over time in a waxing and waning pattern. Insomnia, perceptual disturbances, sensory hypersensitivities, and anxiety are common.

Role of the GABA–Benzodiazepine Receptor Complex

Tolerance and discontinuation syndromes are associated with receptor-level modulations. As tolerance to benzodiazepines develop, GABA receptors are downregulated and glutamate gated N-methyl-D-aspartate receptors are upregulated. If the sedative–hypnotic is rapidly decreased or stopped, there is a great imbalance as the downregulated GABA receptors are unable to overtake the upregulated glutamate receptors, resulting in withdrawal manifesting as central nervous system excitation.

Pharmacologic Characteristics Affecting Withdrawal

Benzodiazepine pharmacokinetics determine the time of onset of discontinuation symptoms. The elimination half-life of the drug determines the rate of decline of serum drug levels, which in turn correlates with the onset, duration, and severity of the withdrawal symptoms. Short-acting agents typically have withdrawal symptoms occurring within 24 hours after discontinuation, peaking in severity within 1 to 5 days and lasting from 7 to 21 days. Longer acting agents may have a withdrawal syndrome occurring after 5 days of cessation, peaking within 1 to 9 days, and lasting from 10 to 28 days. Short-acting benzodiazepines have more intense withdrawal syndromes than longer acting agents.

Higher doses and a longer duration of use increases the liability for increased withdrawal severity. Benzodiazepine use beyond 1 year predisposes patients to prolonged withdrawal sequelae, although such use minimally affects the severity of acute withdrawal.

Patients using short-acting, higher potency benzodiazepines (such as triazolam and alprazolam) develop tolerance more rapidly and also suffer from a more intense discontinuation syndrome that may require increased attention and medical monitoring.

Host Factors Affecting Withdrawal

Patients with increased psychiatric comorbidities are more likely to be physically dependent on benzodiazepines and experience withdrawal symptoms after discontinuation. Specifically, increased withdrawal symptoms have been associated with high initial anxiety or depression and decreased educational level. The reduction of fear and anxiety symptoms during withdrawal is the best predictor of a patient's success for achieving and maintaining abstinence.

Additional sedative–hypnotic, alcohol, opioid, and/or stimulant use contributes to a withdrawal syndrome of increased severity and a less predictable course. Because of the high comorbidity and increased risk of developing a use disorder, clinicians should be especially attentive to the presence of a comorbid alcohol use disorder or anxiety disorder when prescribing benzodiazepines. Heroin users as well as patients in methadone maintenance programs also have a high rate of comorbid benzodiazepine use.

A family history of alcohol use disorder is a risk factor for developing a sedative–hypnotic use disorder. Children of parents with alcohol use disorders have been shown to have mood changes associated with an increased risk of benzodiazepine dependence when administered a benzodiazepine in a controlled clinical setting.

In the acute medical setting, clinicians must be aware of conditions that are significantly influenced by adrenergic and psychological stress factors such as cardiac arrhythmias, asthma, systemic lupus erythematosus, and inflammatory bowel disease. The risk of exacerbating the acute medical condition must be weighed against the longer term benefit of benzodiazepine discontinuation. Patients with chronic medical conditions are more likely to experience a more severe withdrawal syndrome.

Older patients metabolize benzodiazepines at a significantly reduced rate. Younger age is generally associated with favorable withdrawal outcomes.

Sex has not been implicated as an influential factor in abrupt cessation of long-term, therapeutic drug use. However, women are prescribed benzodiazepines twice as often as men.

After a Roux-en-Y gastric bypass surgery, patients have reduced serum levels of phenobarbital and will require higher doses if using phenobarbital in a medically assisted withdrawal.

All classes of benzodiazepines (and phenobarbital) cross the placenta and are excreted in breast milk. Sedative–hypnotic discontinuation may be attempted with caution and regular monitoring in pregnancy. Neonatal benzodiazepine withdrawal syndrome can present as floppy infant syndrome or with tremors, irritability, hyperactivity, and cyanosis. Severe benzodiazepine withdrawal symptoms during pregnancy can place the fetus in distress, potentially causing miscarriage and may induce preterm labor.

PATIENT EVALUATION AND MANAGEMENT

Evaluating patients for benzodiazepine cessation and detoxification requires a combination of consultation and liaison; counseling; and clinical, diagnostic, and pharmacologic management skills. Clinicians should be flexible and able to tolerate ambiguities and variations in the course of withdrawal. A clinical evaluation and assessment of the patient should typically include the following steps:

Step 1: Determine the reason the patient is seeking evaluation and gather the appropriate collateral information necessary to best assess the clinical situation.

Step 2: Take a sedative–hypnotic use history, including dose, duration of use, substance used, and previous treatment interventions as well as discontinuation attempts/responses.

Step 3: Gather information on the history of alcohol and other drug use, including past treatment and withdrawal symptoms.

Step 4: Take a thorough psychiatric history, including previous diagnoses, hospitalizations, suicide attempts, and treatment. Be sure to ask if alcohol or drugs were used close to the time the diagnoses were made.

Step 5: Take a family history of substance use and psychiatric and medical illnesses.

Step 6: Gather the patient's medical history.

Step 7: Take a psychosocial history.

Step 8: Perform a physical and mental status exam.

Step 9: Conduct a urine drug screen for substances of abuse and check other laboratory values that are clinically indicated.

Step 10: Complete an individualized assessment focusing on factors that could influence the degree of withdrawal.

Step 11: Form a differential diagnosis.

Step 12: Determine the appropriate setting for treatment. Patients with polysubstance use should undergo withdrawal in an inpatient setting due to increased risk of sedation and overdose.

Step 13: Determine the most appropriate treatment method.

Step 14: Obtain informed consent.

Step 15: Begin the detoxification process. Be sure to monitor and adjust the treatment plan as needed.

Management

There are two main strategies for discontinuing sedative–hypnotics: minimal intervention and systematic discontinuation. Minimal intervention delivers simple advice to discontinue the benzodiazepine and is more effective for patients on low medication doses. Systematic discontinuation is useful for patients dependent on sedative–hypnotics. This can be done with either the tapering method or the substitution and tapering method. Patients with polysubstance use, high-dose sedative–hypnotic use, erratic behavior, unreliable substance use histories, and extensive mental health issues are better suited to discontinue sedative–hypnotic use in an inpatient facility with 24-hour medical monitoring.

Tapering

With the tapering method, the patient is slowly and gradually weaned from the medication using a fixed-dose schedule. Long-acting benzodiazepines are ideal for this method. The dose can be decreased weekly or every other week. The rate of discontinuation for patients who used benzodiazepines for the long term (>1 year) should not exceed 5-mg diazepam equivalents per week or 10% of the current (starting) dose per week, whichever is smaller. The first 50% of the taper is usually uncomplicated. For the final 25% to 35% of the taper, the reduction rate should be slowed to half of the previous dose reduction. Brief office visits should be scheduled at least weekly for a clinical assessment of the taper; physician input is an essential component. Patients unable to tolerate the taper should be considered for an alternative detoxification method or a higher level of care.

Substitution and Tapering

The substitution and taper method uses cross-tolerant long-acting benzodiazepines to substitute, at equipotent doses, for the sedative–hypnotics on which the patient is dependent. Chlordiazepoxide, clonazepam, and phenobarbital are the most commonly used substitution agents because there is negligible serum level variation between doses. Phenobarbital may be particularly useful in patients with high-dose dependence or with dependence with multiple substances. For an uncomplicated discontinuation of a short half-life benzodiazepine, substitution and tapering may be done in the outpatient setting. With this method, the equivalent dose of the cross-tolerant medication is calculated (Table 52-2) and administered in divided doses. As needed administration should only be given for the first 2 to 3 days for breakthrough withdrawal. Once the patient is stabilized on an adequate substitution dose, the taper is begun at a rate of 5 mg of diazepam equivalents or 10% of the starting dose per week. The taper is then slowed for the final 25% to 35%. The patient should be frequently monitored and given only the required amount of medication.

Phenobarbital Induction and Taper Protocol

Based on the Sedative–Hypnotic Tolerance Test, this method may be useful when the degree of dependence is difficult to determine and requires 24-hour medical monitoring. In this method, phenobarbital is dosed every 2 hours as needed for a Clinical Institute Withdrawal Assessment for Alcohol, revised (CIWA-Ar) score >15 for up to 48 hours, with doses held for signs of toxicity. After 48 hours, the 24-hour stabilizing dose is calculated and is tapered by 20% to 30% per day for the first half of the taper and then 10% every other day for the second half.

Anticonvulsants have been combined with phenobarbital tapers to manage benzodiazepine withdrawal;

TABLE 52-2 Sedative–Hypnotic Withdrawal Substitution Dose Conversions

Drug	Dose Equal to 30 mg of Phenobarbital
Benzodiazepines	
Alprazolam (Xanax)	0.5–1 mg
Chlordiazepoxide (Librium)	25 mg
Clonazepam (Klonopin)	1–2 mg
Clorazepate (Tranxene)	7.5 mg
Diazepam (Valium)	10 mg
Estazolam (Prosom)	1 mg
Flurazepam (Dalmane)	15 mg
Lorazepam (Ativan)	2 mg
Oxazepam (Serax)	10–15 mg
Quazepam (Doral)	15 mg
Temazepam (Restoril)	15 mg
Triazolam (Halcion)	0.25 mg
Barbiturates	
Pentobarbital (Nembutal)	100 mg
Secobarbital (Seconal)	100 mg
Butalbital (Fiorinal)	100 mg
Amobarbital (Amytal)	100 mg
Phenobarbital	30 mg
Nonbarbiturates–Nonbenzodiazepines	
Ethchlorvynol (Placidyl)	500 mg
Glutethimide (Doriden)	250 mg
Methyprylon (Noludar)	200 mg
Methaqualone (Quaalude)	300 mg
Meprobamate (Miltown)	1200 mg
Carisoprodol (Soma)	700 mg
Chloral hydrate (Noctec)	500 mg

however, this approach has fallen out of favor because of the adverse effects of anticonvulsants and the risk of medication interactions.

Adjunctive Withdrawal Management Measures

The anticonvulsants carbamazepine, sodium valproate, and gabapentin have all been found to be useful as adjunctive medications in managing benzodiazepine withdrawal. However, they have

the shortcomings of additional adverse effects, as mentioned previously. Propranolol can decrease the severity of withdrawal symptoms, although cannot be used alone for withdrawal, and can mask some of the symptoms that are used to determine substitution doses. Trazodone and mirtazapine are useful for decreasing anxiety and to improve sleep during withdrawal. Cognitive–behavioral therapy is useful for treating the underlying disorder for which the benzodiazepine was initiated for and may be particularly effective for patients with panic disorder.

Prolonged Benzodiazepine Withdrawal

Prolonged withdrawal may persist for weeks to months after medication discontinuation and has an irregular, unpredictable day-to-day course. Protracted symptoms may reflect long-term receptor site adaptations. Psychologically, patients with persistent withdrawal may have poor coping mechanisms and have a cognitive style that leads to apprehensiveness, body sensation amplification and mislabeling, and misinterpretation.

Management

An underlying psychiatric disorder should be ruled out before considering the diagnosis of prolonged withdrawal. Unlike an anxiety disorder, protracted withdrawal should diminish in symptoms and eventually resolve, albeit slowly and with a waxing and waning pattern. Propranolol can be useful in attenuating anxiety or tremors. Gabapentin can help with anxiety and insomnia. Sedating antidepressant medications may also be helpful in treating insomnia. Frequent follow-up visits for education, supportive psychotherapy, and reassurance are strongly advised.

COMMON TREATMENT ISSUES

Treatment is most often indicated for patients using multiple substances, on high doses, or with the diagnosis of a use disorder. Addiction treatment programs can be valuable to patients who are dependent on sedative–hypnotics. However, patients with problems from long-term therapeutic use of benzodiazepines should not be coerced to attend specialty programs designed to treat addiction because they may feel out of place. Careful prescribing is paramount to preventing iatrogenic benzodiazepine dependence. Clinicians must be responsible with the use of benzodiazepines and should frequently reevaluate the need in patients taking them.

KEY POINTS

1. Sedative–hypnotics inhibit central nervous system activity through their action at the GABA receptor.
2. Sedative–hypnotics should be prescribed cautiously and with careful attention to their effectiveness and the necessity of continuing the medication.
3. Proper recognition and management of sedative–hypnotic withdrawal is crucial to patient care and safety.

REVIEW QUESTIONS

1. Which is *not* one of the four categories of benzodiazepine discontinuation?
   A. Symptom recurrence
   B. Pseudowithdrawal
   C. Tolerance
   D. Rebound

2. What patient characteristics contribute to increased risk of morbidity and mortality when using sedative–hypnotics?
   A. Polysubstance use
   B. High-dose sedative–hypnotic use
   C. Extensive mental health issues
   D. All of the above.

3. When using the tapering method for people who use long term, how quickly should the dose be reduced?
   A. Immediately
   B. 10% reduction of initial dose per week
   C. 25% reduction of initial dose per week
   D. 10% reduction of initial dose per day

ANSWERS

1. **C.** The signs and symptoms following benzodiazepine discontinuation can be described as falling under one of four categories: symptom recurrence or relapse, rebound, pseudowithdrawal, and true withdrawal.
2. **D.** Patients with polysubstance use, high-dose sedative–hypnotic use, erratic behavior, unreliable substance use histories, and extensive mental health issues are better suited to discontinue sedative–hypnotic use in an inpatient facility with 24-hour medical monitoring.
3. **B.** The rate of discontinuation for patients who used benzodiazepines for the long-term (>1 year) should not exceed 5-mg diazepam equivalents per week or 10% of the current (starting) dose per week, whichever is smaller. The first 50% of the taper is usually uncomplicated. For the final 25% to 35% of the taper, the reduction rate should be slowed to half of the previous dose reduction.

SUGGESTED READINGS

American Psychiatric Association. *Diagnostic and Statistical Manual of Mental Disorders*. 5th ed. Washington, DC: American Psychiatric Association, 2013.

Galanter M, Kleber HD, Brady KT, eds. *The American Psychiatric Publishing Textbook of Substance Abuse Treatment. DSM-5 Edition*. Washington, DC: American Psychiatric Association, 2015.

Sadock BJ, Sadock VA, Ruiz P, eds. *Kaplan & Sadock's Comprehensive Textbook of Psychiatry*. 10th ed. Philadelphia: Wolters Kluwer, 2017.

Smith DE, Wesson DR. Benzodiazepine dependency syndromes. *J Psychoactive Drugs*. 1983;15(1-2):85-95.

Stahl SM. Anxiety disorders and anxiolytics. In: *Stahl's Essential Psychopharmacology: Neuroscientific Basis and Practical Applications*. 4th ed. Cambridge, UK: Cambridge University Press, 2013:397-403.

Management of Opioid Intoxication and Withdrawal

Summary by Kenneth L. Morford and Jeanette M. Tetrault

Based on THE ASAM PRINCIPLES OF ADDICTION MEDICINE,
6th edition chapter by Jeanette M. Tetrault and Patrick G. O'Connor

Opioids include substances that are derived directly from the opium poppy (such as morphine and codeine), the semisynthetic opioids (such as heroin), and the purely synthetic opioids (such as methadone and fentanyl). These compounds share several pharmacologic effects, including sedation, respiratory depression, and analgesia, and common clinical features of intoxication and withdrawal.

OPIOID INTOXICATION AND OVERDOSE

Although mild-to-moderate intoxication (characterized by euphoria or sedation) usually is not life threatening, severe intoxication or overdose is a medical emergency that causes many preventable deaths and thus requires immediate attention. As the prevalence of opioid use has increased in the United States, the incidence of opioid overdose has increased as well. Nonfatal opioid overdose is an additional cause of significant morbidity.

The pharmacologic actions responsible for opioid intoxication and overdose involve central nervous system (CNS) μ-, κ-, and δ-opioid receptors. Of primary concern in the management of overdose are interactions with μ receptors, which can lead to sedation and respiratory depression by direct suppression of respiratory centers in the brainstem and medulla. The level of tolerance to opioids can have a significant effect on an individual's risk of opioid overdose, and tolerance to respiratory depression may be slower than tolerance to euphoric effects. Patients who have undergone medically supervised withdrawal or those who have experienced intentional or unintentional abstinence from opioids for any reason (eg, incarceration) may be particularly susceptible to death from opioid overdose.

Physical examination of the patient with opioid intoxication may find CNS and respiratory depression as well as miosis and direct evidence of intravenous drug use, such as needle tracks or soft tissue infection. The opioid overdose syndrome, described as a triad of altered mental status, depressed respiration, and miotic pupils, has a sensitivity of 92% and a specificity of 76%. It is important to consider the differential diagnosis in patients presenting with symptoms of opioid intoxication, such as hypoglycemia, acidemia, or other fluid and electrolyte disorders or complications from end-stage liver disease. Intoxication from other substances should also be considered. Toxicology testing should be performed immediately in emergency settings. Opioid use and overdose may also be complicated by the effects of substances employed to "cut" substances purchased illicitly. Along with inert substances present to add bulk, active substances—including dextromethorphan, lidocaine, and scopolamine—may also be present.

In a case of suspected severe opioid intoxication resulting in overdose, general supportive management must be instituted simultaneously with the specific antidote, naloxone hydrochloride, a pure opioid antagonist, which can effectively reverse the CNS effects of opioid intoxication and overdose. Adult basic life support and adult advanced cardiac life support need to be available. The clinician needs to ensure that an adequate airway is established and that respiratory and cardiac function are appropriately assessed and managed. Adequate intravenous access is essential so that fluids and pharmacologic agents can be administered as needed. Finally, frequent monitoring of vital signs and cardiorespiratory status is required until it is clearly established that the opioid and any other intoxicating substances have been cleared from the patient's system. Additionally, the clinician must consider the half-life of the ingested substance as multiple doses of naloxone or an intravenous naloxone drip may need to be instituted in the case of ingestion of a long-acting opioid. When a patient presents to an emergency department with miosis and respiratory depression, pharmacologic therapy for opioid overdose should be instituted immediately. However, if the patient is breathing without assistance, specific pharmacotherapy should be withheld and the patient monitored. Naloxone can be given as an initial intravenous dose of 0.4 to 0.8 mg, which should quickly reverse neurologic and cardiorespiratory depression. The onset of action of intravenously administered naloxone, as manifested by antagonism of opioid overdose, is approximately 2 minutes. Although intravenous naloxone should work more rapidly than subcutaneous naloxone, it is also demonstrated that the subcutaneous route may be just as effective for managing patients before they arrive in the emergency department; additionally, the slower absorption time of the subcutaneous route may be compensated for by the delay in establishing adequate intravenous access. Intranasal naloxone, dosed at 2 mg, can be used effectively to reverse opioid overdose in both the prehospital and hospital settings.

Overdose with opioids that are more potent (such as fentanyl) or longer acting (such as methadone) may require higher doses of naloxone given over longer periods of time, as by ongoing naloxone infusion. In patients who do not respond to multiple or higher doses of naloxone, alternative causes of the failure to respond must be considered, including overdose with substances other than opioids. Of increasing concern are more potent opioids and opioid combinations, which may be less responsive to naloxone. These include carfentanil and U-47700 (also known as "gray death," which includes a dangerous combination of fentanyl, carfentanil, and heroin).

Pharmacologic management of acute opioid overdose may be the first step in engaging patients with a diagnosis of opioid use disorder into medical care and addiction treatment once the overdose event has resolved. Clinicians who manage patients with an opioid overdose should establish the need for ongoing addiction treatment as a major goal of patient management while caring for overdose-related complications. In the absence of acute medical or psychiatric issues, the patient can be discharged following the resolution of the symptoms of intoxication and establishment of follow-up referrals for addiction, medical, and psychiatric care.

OPIOID WITHDRAWAL

Opioid withdrawal syndrome is characterized by two phases, acute and chronic. In the initial acute opioid withdrawal phase, the patient typically experiences a range of symptoms for varying lengths of time (depending on the half-life of the opioid). Such symptoms include gastrointestinal distress such as diarrhea and vomiting, thermoregulation disturbances, insomnia, muscle and joint pain, and marked anxiety and dysphoria. Although these symptoms generally include no life-threatening complications unless there is an associated medical comorbidity (unlike alcohol withdrawal syndrome), the acute withdrawal syndrome causes marked discomfort, often prompting continuation of opioid use even in the absence of any opioid-associated euphoria.

In patients with chronic opioid use disorder presenting with acute withdrawal, medically supervised withdrawal or induction onto opioid agonist therapy is the first step of treatment. This period of altered physiologic function includes increased sedimentation rates; electroencephalogram changes; decreased blood pressure, heart rate, and body temperature; miosis; and a decreased sensitivity of the respiratory center to carbon dioxide, beginning about 6 weeks after withdrawal and persisting for 26 or more weeks and is often a precipitant to relapse to opioid use.

Methadone treatment, when prescribed at appropriate doses, provides a "narcotic blockade," which blocks the euphoric effect of exogenous opioids and stabilizes psychosocial functioning. In addition to biologic considerations, psychosocial concomitants of opioid use disorder also necessitate longer, more specialized adjunct treatments for these problems.

Several clinical tools are available to measure the severity of opioid withdrawal such as the Clinical Opiate Withdrawal Scale and the 10-, 13-, or 16-item Short Opioid Withdrawal Scales. Early findings may include abnormalities in vital signs, including tachycardia and hypertension. Bothersome CNS symptoms include restlessness, irritability, and insomnia. Opioid craving also occurs in proportion to the severity of physiologic withdrawal symptoms. Pupillary dilation can be marked. A variety of cutaneous and mucocutaneous symptoms (including lacrimation, rhinorrhea, and piloerection, also known as "gooseflesh") can occur as well. Patients frequently report yawning and sneezing. Gastrointestinal symptoms vary from anorexia to nausea, vomiting, and diarrhea as the withdrawal worsens.

As with the onset of the opioid withdrawal syndrome, the duration also varies with the half-life of the drug used and the duration of drug use. For example, meperidine withdrawal symptoms may peak within 8 to 12 hours and last only 4 to 5 days, whereas heroin withdrawal symptoms generally peak within 36 to 72 hours and may last for 7 to 14 days.

As in the management of opioid intoxication and overdose, management of the opioid withdrawal syndrome involves a combination of general supportive measures and specific pharmacologic therapies.

PHARMACOLOGIC THERAPIES FOR OPIOID WITHDRAWAL

Full Opioid Agonists

Slow Methadone Detoxification

It is important to distinguish between withdrawal from short-acting opioids such as heroin (plasma half-life of morphine, the main metabolite: 3 to 4 hours) and long-acting opioids such as methadone (plasma half-life: 13 to 47 hours). However, there is also considerable individual variation so that strong early opioid withdrawal symptoms from methadone are possible, as are delayed, severe symptoms due to heroin withdrawal. One treatment strategy employing this general principle is to stabilize patients with physiologic dependence on heroin with methadone and then gradually decrease the methadone dose over months rather than days. Initially, methadone may be given in 5- to 10-mg increments as needed as the physical signs of abstinence begin to appear, up to a total of 30 to 40 mg over the first 24 hours. In the ambulatory setting, this treatment strategy can only be employed by facilities licensed to prescribe methadone for the treatment of opioid use disorder. In the acute hospital setting, methadone can be used to treat opioid withdrawal without federal restriction. The protocol for slow methadone detoxification is similar to the strategy used for withdrawal from methadone maintenance treatment. After a stabilizing dose has been reached, methadone is tapered by 20% a day for inpatients, leading to a 1- to 2-week procedure. Alternatively, the dose is tapered by 5% per day for outpatients in a gradual cessation phase lasting as long as 6 months. Another recommendation is a dose-tapering rate of about 3% per week from methadone maintenance.

α₂-Adrenergic Agents

Clonidine Detoxification

It has been reported that clonidine ameliorates opioid withdrawal symptoms and that both morphine and clonidine blocks activation of the locus coeruleus, a major noradrenergic nucleus that shows increased activity during opioid withdrawal. Although opioids exert their effect through opiate receptors, clonidine activates α₂-adrenergic receptors. Consequently, clonidine does not possess the potential for creating the euphoria and physiologic dependence seen with opioids.

Clonidine was reported to reduce or eliminate most of the commonly reported withdrawal symptoms, including lacrimation, rhinorrhea, restlessness, muscle pain, joint pain, and gastrointestinal symptoms. However, symptoms such as lethargy and insomnia persisted. Sedation and dizziness from orthostatic hypotension were reported as the most significant side effects of clonidine. Although clonidine has been shown to be useful to decrease symptoms associated with the opioid withdrawal syndrome, its use for this purpose is considered off-label, and, because it is not an opioid agonist, many symptoms of opioid withdrawal remain untreated even though these symptoms can be ameliorated by a number of other adjunctive treatments (eg, nonsteroidal anti-inflammatory drugs, bismuth subsalicylate, pharmacotherapy for insomnia, dicyclomine).

For the treatment of opioid withdrawal, most protocols suggest 0.1 mg of clonidine every 4 to 6 hours as needed for withdrawal discomfort on the first day, followed by an increase in clonidine by 0.1 or 0.2 mg per day, to a maximum of 1.2 mg daily, with careful monitoring of blood pressure and withdrawal symptoms. The average maximum daily dose is roughly 0.8 mg. Toward the end of the detoxification period (days 5 to 7 in heroin detoxification), the clonidine dose is tapered by 0.1 to 0.2 mg daily to avoid rebound hypertension, headaches, and the reemergence of withdrawal symptoms. Clonidine can shorten the detoxification period from 20 days to 10 to 13 days, and success rates range from 36% to 80%.

Lofexidine, an analogue of clonidine that also is an agonist at the α₂-noradrenergic receptor, has shown promise as a detoxification agent. It generally is reported to be as effective as clonidine but more economical and with fewer side effects. This medication was approved for use by the U.S. Food and Drug Administration in May 2018.

Combined Clonidine and Naltrexone Treatment

This combination can be used only by experienced clinicians for rapid detoxification, although rapid detoxifications have limited efficacy and may be associated with severe morbidity and mortality. Naltrexone, at a 12.5 mg dose, is given the afternoon of the first day of withdrawal, after preloading with clonidine at 0.2 to 0.3 mg. Naltrexone is increased to 25 mg on the second day, 50 mg on the third day, and 100 mg on the fourth day. Clonidine is given at 0.1 to 0.3 mg three times per day, as needed, for the first 3 days and three times at 0.1 mg on the fourth day. About 75% of patients successfully completed detoxification and were discharged on maintenance doses of naltrexone. Some patients reported anxiety, restlessness, insomnia, joint pain, and muscle aches. Clonidine also caused hypotension but was well tolerated.

Buprenorphine Detoxification

Buprenorphine is a high-affinity, partial agonist at the μ-opioid receptor that is approved to be used for opioid use disorder. It has many advantages such as a ceiling effect, less misuse potential, and low toxicity. Its long duration of action diminishes withdrawal signs and symptoms on discontinuation. A review of 22 studies of over 1700 participants found that buprenorphine for opioid withdrawal was superior to clonidine and as effective as moderate doses of methadone for ameliorating withdrawal symptoms, treatment retention, and treatment completion.

Methadone-to-Buprenorphine Transfer

Some patients choose to transfer from methadone to buprenorphine for maintenance or detoxification. Buprenorphine can produce withdrawal discomfort among volunteers with physiologic dependence on opioids under certain conditions. Low buprenorphine doses may provide too little agonist effect (ie, insufficient relief from withdrawal syndrome) relative to the maintenance opioid (methadone). Alternatively, buprenorphine may directly precipitate withdrawal discomfort due to its partial μ-agonist properties leading to displacement of agonists. Among individuals maintained on the long-acting, full μ-opioid agonist methadone, the high-affinity partial μ-agonist buprenorphine is capable of abruptly reducing the extent of μ-opioid receptor stimulation. This would be expected to reduce opioid agonist effects or precipitate withdrawal symptoms.

The issue of transitioning patients from methadone to buprenorphine for the treatment of opioid withdrawal syndrome has been studied, and it is recommended that the dose of methadone be lowered for a successful detoxification. Those patients transferred on less than 30 mg reported significantly less withdrawal discomfort, and although withdrawal symptoms may occur during the buprenorphine induction, the intensity of the withdrawal symptoms may be lessened by the higher dose and frequency of buprenorphine administration.

Buprenorphine in Agonist-to-Antagonist Treatment

Opioid antagonists represent an alternative to opioid agonist treatment for patients with opioid use disorder. Opioid antagonists enhance relapse prevention and also protect patients from opioid overdose given its higher binding affinity than opioid agonists. Transitioning from opioids to extended-release naltrexone can be challenging. Buprenorphine might facilitate the transition from opioid agonists to antagonists in a three-step process: (1) buprenorphine

induction for individuals maintained on opioid agonists such as methadone, (2) buprenorphine-induced reduction in physical dependence, and (3) discontinuation of buprenorphine with eventual introduction of naltrexone.

In some situations, combination treatment may facilitate greater patient acceptance of agonist–antagonist switching. It is shown that the early use of naltrexone during detoxification in combination with benzodiazepines and clonidine facilitated naltrexone acceptance by patients and that the combination treatment may reduce the severity of withdrawal symptoms. The use of buprenorphine stabilization of opioid withdrawal symptoms before switching to naltrexone has the advantage of psychosocial stabilization during detoxification. This approach thus may represent a compromise between acute detoxification and long-term treatment of chronic opioid use disorder for highly motivated patients who have significant psychosocial support.

Other Agents

Agents other than opioid agonists and α-adrenergic agonists have been investigated to treat opioid withdrawal syndrome, such as memantine, gabapentin, and tramadol. These are found to be somewhat effective, but more research is needed for more widespread use. There is a very limited role for the use of anesthesia-assisted, ultrarapid opioid detoxification as it is riskier and no more successful than other methods.

As with the management of opioid overdose, medical detoxification is an important first step in the treatment of opioid use disorder. It must be made clear that detoxification alone, without plans for ongoing treatment, is not adequate to manage patients. In general, detoxification programs focus solely on one aspect of opioid use disorder and often lack appropriate linkages to ongoing treatment services. Therefore, this approach to the treatment of patients with opioid use disorder is not successful for most patients. The addition of psychosocial interventions to opioid agonist detoxification improves treatment retention, abstinence from opioids, and adherence to clinic visits. Opioid agonist treatment, on the other hand, is effective for the ongoing treatment of patients with opioid use disorder.

KEY POINTS

1. In opioid intoxication, general supportive management must be instituted simultaneously with the specific antidote, naloxone.
2. In cases of suspected opioid intoxication, the clinician needs to first ensure that an adequate

airway is established and that respiratory and cardiac functions are appropriately assessed.

3. Unlike opioid intoxication, opioid withdrawal syndrome generally includes no life-threatening complications; however, it causes marked discomfort, often prompting continuation of opioid use.

4. Methadone and buprenorphine detoxifications are the mainstay of pharmacologic interventions in the management of opioid withdrawal syndrome, with clonidine being a possible alternative.

REVIEW QUESTIONS

1. A patient calls to inquire about switching to buprenorphine maintenance from his methadone maintenance program. He says he is stable on 120 mg of methadone per day. What is the best recommendation?
   A. Make an appointment and switch to 32/8 mg of buprenorphine/naloxone 24 to 48 hours after his last methadone dose.
   B. Make an appointment for buprenorphine induction and tell him to stop methadone 48 hours in advance to get into the necessary withdrawal.
   C. Advise him to discuss with his program and consider slowly tapering down methadone to 30 mg daily with a period of 24 to 48 hours of abstinence prior to buprenorphine induction.
   D. Consider doing a crossover switch from methadone to buprenorphine by increasing the latter while decreasing methadone slowly.

2. A patient who is thought to be in opioid overdose does not respond to 0.8 mg IV naloxone. What is the best next step?
   A. Continue with supportive measures only and wait.
   B. Consider a second higher dose of naloxone.
   C. It must be solely due to intoxication from a different substance; give IV flumazenil, thiamine, and glucose and send an urgent blood toxicology test to find out.
   D. Try to give the dose subcutaneously.

3. A patient who has read about and met someone who had completed ultrarapid detoxification under anesthesia requests to get the procedure for his opioid use disorder. What is the best advice?
   A. Refer the patient to a program where it is conducted.
   B. Tell the patient that it is not a recommended protocol for detoxification and that he should

be on maintenance treatment. Refer him to a methadone maintenance treatment program or office-based buprenorphine provider.
   C. Educate him on the risks of such a procedure and inform him that it is not yet evidence based or recommended at this point. Explore other options with the patient.
   D. Make an appointment to do an office-based detoxification using naltrexone, clonidine, and other nonopioid supportive medications, as it will be similar to his request and without the risks of anesthesia.

4. Which of the following medications does *not* have a place in opioid detoxification?
   A. Methadone
   B. Buprenorphine
   C. Clonidine
   D. Naloxone

ANSWERS

1. **C.** It is recommended to switch to buprenorphine when the methadone dose is slowly lowered to 30 mg or less.
2. **B.** A second and higher dose should be administered in nonresponsive patients.
3. **C.** There is no consensus on the use of rapid detoxification under anesthesia, and there have been patients who had significant complications.
4. **D.** Although naloxone can be a part of buprenorphine/naloxone tablets, the purpose is not for detoxification, and naloxone can worsen withdrawal symptoms because it is an opioid antagonist.

SUGGESTED READINGS

Bickel WK, Amass L. Buprenorphine treatment of opioid dependence: a review. *Exp Clin Psychopharmacol.* 1995;3: 477-489.

Effective medical treatment for opiate addiction. National Consensus Development Panel on Effective Medical Treatment of Opiate Addiction. *JAMA.* 1998;280(22):1936-1943.

Margolin AKT. Opioid detoxification and maintenance with blocking agents. In: Miller NS, ed. *Comprehensive Handbook of Drug and Alcohol Addiction.* New York: Marcel Dekker, 1991:1127-1141.

O'Connor PG. Treating opioid dependence—new data and new opportunities. *N Engl J Med.* 2000;343(18): 1332-1334.

Substance Abuse and Mental Health Services Administration. *Medication-Assisted Treatment for Opioid Addiction in Opioid Treatment Programs. A Treatment Improvement Protocol TIP 43.* Rockville, MD: Substance Abuse and Mental Health Services Administration, 2008.

Management of Stimulant, Hallucinogen, Marijuana, Phencyclidine, and Club Drug Intoxication and Withdrawal

Summary by Jeffery N. Wilkins, Itai Danovitch, and David A. Gorelick

Based on THE ASAM PRINCIPLES OF ADDICTION MEDICINE, 6th edition chapter by Jeffery N. Wilkins, Itai Danovitch, and David A. Gorelick

Pharmacologic treatment of drug intoxication and withdrawal generally follows one of three approaches: increasing drug clearance, blocking the neuronal site at which the drug acts (eg, naloxone for opioid intoxication), and pharmacologically counteracting drug effects. The pharmacologic treatment of drug withdrawal generally follows one of two approaches: suppression by a longer-acting cross-tolerant medication (eg, buprenorphine for opioid withdrawal), and reducing the signs and symptoms of withdrawal by targeting key neurochemical or receptor systems (eg, the nonopioid clonidine to treat opioid withdrawal). A small number of the medications discussed in this chapter are approved by the US Food and Drug Administration for a substance use disorder indication, but the majority of medication uses described are experimental and awaiting controlled studies for validation.

Treatment of intoxication and withdrawal has increased in complexity: between 2009 and 2016, 793 new psychoactive substances were reported by 106 countries to the United Nations Office on Drugs and Crime. Many of these substances blur the traditional boundary between drug classes. For new psychoactive substances with mixed actions, consensus recommendations stress the importance of stabilizing vital signs and maintaining adequate ventilation and vascular access throughout the intoxication and withdrawal periods.

In this chapter, we present clinical recommendations drawn from published clinical guidelines for the treatment of intoxication and withdrawal in patients who may have taken stimulants, hallucinogens,

cannabinoids, club drugs, new psychoactive substances, or psychoactive herbs. The diagnostic criteria for specific drug intoxication and withdrawal syndromes can be found in the *Diagnostic and Statistical Manual of Mental Disorders*, 5th edition (*DSM-5*).

STIMULANTS

Stimulant Intoxication

Acute effects of stimulants principally are due to increased catecholamine neurotransmitter activity, mediated through the blockade of presynaptic neurotransmitter reuptake pumps (as by cocaine) and by presynaptic release of catecholamines (as by amphetamines). The resulting stimulation of brain reward circuits (corticomesolimbic dopamine circuit) mediates the desired (and addicting) psychologic effects of stimulants.

Treatment Approaches

Treatment approaches include the blockade of presynaptic catecholamine reuptake sites or postsynaptic receptors. Bupropion, aripiprazole, risperidone, topiramate, and modafinil block acute subjective effects in human laboratory experiments; combining escitalopram with modafinil does not enhance the efficacy of modafinil.

Additionally, another treatment includes decreasing the drug availability in the central nervous system by binding it peripherally with antidrug antibodies or by increasing its catabolism. For example, in phase I studies of treatment with a genetically enhanced bacterial cocaine esterase (intravenous) or butyrylcholinesterase (conjugated to albumin), cocaine availability was reduced by 90% within 2 minutes, and acute subjective and cardiovascular effects of an intravenous cocaine challenge were significantly reduced.

Stimulant Withdrawal

Abrupt cessation of stimulant use is associated with depression, anxiety, fatigue, difficulty concentrating, anergia, anhedonia, increased drug craving, increased appetite, hypersomnolence, and increased dreaming due to increased rapid eye movement sleep. Symptoms are usually mild and self-limited, resolving within 1 to 2 weeks. Hospitalization is rarely indicated and does not improve short-term outcome for stimulant addiction.

Medical Effects of Stimulant Withdrawal

The first week of stimulant withdrawal may be associated with myocardial ischemia.

Management of Stimulant Withdrawal

No medication has been consistently effective in controlled clinical trials, nor is any medication approved for this indication by any national regulatory authority. Symptoms are best treated supportively with rest, exercise, and a healthy diet. Short-acting benzodiazepines such as lorazepam are helpful for agitation or sleep disturbances. Severe or persistent depression (lasting more than 2 to 3 weeks) may require antidepressant treatment.

HALLUCINOGENS
Hallucinogen Intoxication

Hallucinogens fall primarily into two chemical groups: serotonin or tryptamine related (eg, lysergic acid diethylamide, psilocybin, or N,N-dimethyltryptamine), and phenylethylamine or amphetamine related (eg, 3,4,5-trimethoxyphenylethylamine [mescaline], 2,5-dimethoxy-4-methylamphetamine, or 3,4,5-trimethoxyamphetamine).

Note: 3,4-methylenedioxymethamphetamine (MDMA, "Ecstasy") has characteristics of both a hallucinogen and a stimulant and is considered separately.

Psychologic and Behavioral Effects of Hallucinogen Intoxication

Hallucinogens have in common the ability to dramatically change sensory perceptions. The subjective experience is influenced greatly by set and setting. Mood can vary from euphoria and feelings of spiritual insight to depression, anxiety, and terror.

Hallucinations are common. Reality testing usually remains intact.

Panic reactions are more common in those who have limited experience with hallucinogens or who ingest them unknowingly. Higher doses are associated with more intense experiences. Hallucinogens may trigger transient psychotic symptoms; however, development of a psychotic disorder is rare. People who use hallucinogens, unlike patients with schizophrenia, usually retain at least partial insight, and typically have visual rather than auditory perceptual disturbances. Hallucinogen ingestion may result in an acute toxic delirium.

Medical Effects of Hallucinogen Intoxication

Sympathomimetic effects are common, particularly pupillary dilation, hyperreflexia, piloerection, tachycardia, and increased blood pressure. Dry skin, increased muscle tone, agitation, and seizures are warning signs of a potential hyperthermic crisis. Complications that require treatment are rare in the absence of overdose.

Management of Hallucinogen Intoxication

After ensuring medical stability, the patient should be observed and placed in a quiet environment with minimal sensory stimulation. Physical restraints are contraindicated because they may exacerbate anxiety and increase the risk of rhabdomyolysis. The "talk-down" or reassurance technique may be helpful.

For patients who do not respond to reassurance alone, benzodiazepines such as lorazepam or diazepam are the medications of choice. If benzodiazepines are insufficient, a high-potency antipsychotic such as haloperidol may be needed. Phenothiazines should be avoided because they have been associated with poor outcomes and may exacerbate unsuspected anticholinergic poisoning.

Patients usually recover after several hours. Psychosis that does not resolve within 1 to 2 days suggests the ingestion of a longer-acting drug such as phencyclidine (PCP) or 2,5-dimethoxy-4-methylamphetamine. Symptoms persisting beyond a few days raise the possibility of a preexisting or concurrent psychiatric or neurologic condition.

Hallucinogen Withdrawal

There is no evidence to suggest a clinically significant hallucinogen withdrawal syndrome exists and no such diagnosis is included in the *DSM-5*. There is no role for medication in the treatment of hallucinogen withdrawal.

TABLE 54-1	Acute Psychological and Behavioral Effects of Intoxication With Lysergic Acid Diethylamide, Marijuana, Phencyclidine, and MDMA			
Effects	LSD	Marijuana	Phencyclidine	MDMA
"Abnormal" overall behavior and appearance	XX	X	XXX	X
Disoriented to person, place, time, or situation	XX	None	XX	None
Impaired memory	X	XX	XX	X
Inappropriate affect	XXX	X	XXX	XX
Depressed mood	XX	X	XX	X
Overly elated mood	XXX	XX	XX	XXX
Confused, disorganized thinking	XX	XX	XXX	X
Hallucinations	XXX	X	XXX	X
Delusions	X/XXX	XXX	XX	?
Bizarre behavior	XXX	X	XXX	?
Suicidal or danger to self	XX	XX	XX	?
Homicidal or danger to others	XX	X	XXX	X
Poor judgment	X/XXX	XXX	XXX	XX

Relative weighting: X, mild; XX, moderate; XXX, marked; /, common/rare; ?, insufficient research.
LSD, lysergic acid diethylamide; MDMA, 3,4-methylenedioxymethamphetamine.
Sources: Brust JC. Acute neurologic complications of drug and alcohol abuse. *Neurol Clin*. 1998;16(2):503-519; Frecska E, Luna LE. The adverse effects of hallucinogens from intramural perspective. *Neuropsychopharmacol Hung*. 2006;8(4): 189-200; Abraham HD, Aldridge AM, Gogia P. The psychopharmacology of hallucinogens. *Neuropsychopharmacology*. 1996;14(4):285-298.

MARIJUANA (CANNABIS)

Marijuana Intoxication

Desired psychological effects of marijuana intoxication include relaxation, euphoria, slowed time perception, altered sensory perception, and increased appetite. Undesired psychological effects include impaired concentration, anterograde amnesia, anxiety, panic attacks, paranoia, derealization/depersonalization, and psychosis (with visual rather than auditory hallucinations). Acute medical complications of LSD, marijuana, phencyclidine, and MDMA intoxication are listed in Table 54-1.

Marijuana Withdrawal

Marijuana withdrawal symptoms are reported by up to one third of persons who are frequent users, and may play an important role in relapse. This syndrome is recognized in the *DSM-5*. Withdrawal symptoms reduced (in clinical trials) with dronabinol (synthetic tetrahydrocannabinol), nabilone, nabiximols, and gabapentin.

DISSOCIATIVE ANESTHETICS

Dissociative Anesthetic Intoxication

PCP, ketamine, and dextromethorphan (DXM) are noncompetitive antagonists of the N-methyl-D-aspartate–glutamate excitatory amino acid neurotransmitter receptor. DXM is widely available as an ingredient in over 100 different over-the-counter cough and cold medicines. At the recommended antitussive dose of 15 to 30 mg every 6 to 8 hours, adverse reactions are rare. About 5% to 10% of those with white European ancestry are unable to demethylate DXM to dextrorphan. Such individuals are at an increased risk of toxicity from excess concentrations of DXM.

Dissociative Anesthetic Withdrawal

About one fourth of those who heavily use PCP report withdrawal symptoms, which includes depression, anxiety, irritability, hypersomnolence, diaphoresis, and tremor. DXM withdrawal has been associated with craving, dysphoria, and insomnia.

Prolonged Psychiatric Sequelae

Hallucinogens and dissociative anesthetics can trigger psychiatric sequelae that last beyond the period of acute intoxication, including anxiety, depression, or psychosis. The risk of a prolonged psychiatric reaction is increased with premorbid psychopathology, prior drug exposure, and a history of polydrug use. Treatment of prolonged anxiety or depression usually is psychosocial. Treatment of prolonged psychosis follows the guidelines for treatment of chronic functional psychosis.

"Flashbacks" are brief, self-limiting episodes in which perceptual abnormalities are unexpectedly reexperienced after acute intoxication has resolved. This condition is known as hallucinogen persisting perceptual disorder in the *DSM-5*. Flashbacks can occur with hallucinogens, MDMA, PCP, and marijuana. Flashbacks tend to decrease over time in frequency, duration, and intensity as long as no further drugs are taken.

There have been no clinical trials of pharmacologic treatment for hallucinogen persisting perceptual disorder. Repeated ketamine use produces cognitive deficits and depressed mood in the majority of active ketamine users; the degree of reversibility remains unclear.

INHALANTS
Inhalant Intoxication

Inhalants are a chemically heterogeneous group of volatile hydrocarbons found in glue, fuel, paint, aerosol propellant, and other products that can be inhaled for psychoactive effects. The initial euphoria or "rush" is followed by light-headedness, excitability, and perceptual changes. Higher doses may cause dizziness, slurred speech, and motor incoordination, followed by drowsiness and headache. There is no specific treatment.

Inhalant Withdrawal

Inhalant withdrawal is not a recognized clinical syndrome in the *DSM-5*. One study found that over 11% of patients evaluated for inhalant abuse reported withdrawal-like symptoms, including depressed mood, fatigue, anxiety, difficulty concentrating, tachycardia, diaphoresis, muscle trembling or twitching, increased tearing and nasal secretions, headache, nausea and vomiting, and craving for inhalants.

CLUB DRUGS

"Club drugs" are a pharmacologically heterogeneous group of drugs originally associated with a youth subculture that revolves around late-night dance parties known as "raves" or "trances." Common club drugs are MDMA ("Ecstasy"), an amphetamine analogue with stimulant and hallucinogenic properties, and γ-hydroxybutyric acid (GHB) and flunitrazepam ("roofies," "date rape pill"), both of which are central nervous system depressants.

MDMA

Effects of MDMA are those of a stimulant combined with a hallucinogen. MDMA often is taken concurrently with other drugs, such as LSD ("candyflipping"). DXM may be substituted for MDMA in street preparations. "Stacking" refers to taking multiple MDMA doses over a short period, often alternating with other drugs. There is no withdrawal syndrome that requires specific pharmacologic treatment.

MDMA INTOXICATION

MDMA is not detected by routine drug screens, which may be positive for amphetamines (products of MDMA metabolism). Gastric lavage with activated charcoal may be helpful within the first hour after ingestion. Induced emesis is not recommended.

Psychological and Behavioral Effects of MDMA Intoxication

Low-to-moderate oral doses of MDMA (50 to 150 mg) produce an intense initial effect ("coming on" or "rush") lasting 30 to 45 minutes, which includes increased wakefulness and energy, euphoria, increased sexual desire and satisfaction, heightened sensory perception, sociability, and increased empathy and sense of closeness to others, followed by several hours of less intense experience ("plateau"). Users start to "come down" 3 to 6 hours after ingestion.

Undesired effects with repeated use or higher doses include hyperactivity, fatigue, insomnia, anxiety, agitation, impaired decision-making, hallucinations, depersonalization/derealization, and bizarre or reckless behavior.

Initial treatment is the same as for hallucinogen intoxication: minimizing sensory stimulation with observation. Physical restraints are contraindicated. Severe or persisting symptoms may require benzodiazepines. Antipsychotics should be avoided.

γ-HYDROXYBUTYRATE

GHB ("liquid ecstasy") is a naturally occurring metabolite of the neurotransmitter γ-aminobutyric acid, approved for the treatment of narcolepsy. GHB is popular because of its reputed aphrodisiac, disinhibitory, and amnestic effects; short duration of action; absence of "hangover"; and nondetectability by standard drug screens. GHB is taken orally as a liquid, is rapidly absorbed from the gastrointestinal tract, and readily crosses the blood–brain barrier. Effects begin within 15 minutes of ingestion and last 2 to 4 hours. The blood elimination half-life is about 30 minutes, largely because of the rapid redistribution into other tissues.

γ-Hydroxybutyrate Intoxication

Signs and symptoms resemble those of a central nervous system depressant. GHB is not detected by routine drug toxicology assays, and there is no known antidote.

Psychological and Behavioral Effects of γ-Hydroxybutyrate Intoxication

At low doses, GHB produces relaxation, euphoria, sedation, disinhibition, sociability, and anterograde amnesia. Higher doses produce somnolence, confusion, and hallucinations. Unintended overdoses may occur because of the very steep dose-response curve of GHB and the great variability in potency of street preparations. Effects are prolonged and intensified when taken with other central nervous system depressants.

Medical Effects of γ-Hydroxybutyrate Intoxication

Low-to-moderate oral doses cause headache, dizziness, ataxia, hypotonia, and vomiting. Higher doses may cause incontinence, myoclonic movements, bradycardia, hypotension, hypothermia, generalized tonic-clonic seizures, and coma. Most patients recover completely within several hours with supportive care and do not require intubation. Death may result from respiratory depression.

γ-Hydroxybutyrate Withdrawal

Cessation of chronic GHB use leads to a discrete withdrawal syndrome resembling that of sedative–hypnotic withdrawal. Anxiety, restlessness, insomnia, tremor, nystagmus, tachycardia, and hypertension usually appear 2 to 12 hours after the last dose. Mild symptoms usually resolve gradually over 1 to 2 weeks. A more severe withdrawal may cause delirium with hallucinations, psychosis, agitation, and autonomic instability. Withdrawal can be managed with a long-acting benzodiazepine.

HERBS OF ABUSE

Many herbs contain psychoactive compounds with stimulant, anxiogenic, anxiolytic, hallucinogenic, euphoric, or dissociative effects. The perception that herbs are safer than illicit drugs, coupled with the absence of clearly established dosing parameters, contributes to their misuse. Routine toxicology screens do not detect many of these substances. An accurate diagnosis may rest on collateral information from family, friends, and first responders, in addition to a thorough clinical examination.

Herbs of Abuse Intoxication

Manifestations of the intoxication syndrome depend largely on the neurotransmitter systems that are activated. Hallucinogenic herbs achieve their psychotomimetic effects principally through activity at serotonergic or cholinergic receptors. Stimulating herbs generally augment the activity of norepinephrine or dopamine. Management of the intoxication syndromes generally follows that for the corresponding hallucinogen or stimulant intoxication.

Cathinone intoxication (whether induced by the khat plant or synthetic cathinones ["bath salts"]), may produce anorexia, insomnia/lack of fatigue, hyperactivity, excitation, euphoria, hyperthermia, increased respirations, mydriasis, arrhythmias, and hypertension.

Management of Psychological, Behavioral, and Medical Effects

Management is largely supportive (similar to amphetamine intoxication); symptoms are usually self-limited. Benzodiazepines are used for agitation, panic, or psychotic symptoms. Acetylcholinesterase inhibitors (eg, physostigmine) may reverse the effects of anticholinergic herbs (eg, jimsonweed).

Herbs of Abuse Withdrawal

Khat withdrawal may include irritability, fatigue, and rhinorrhea.

FLUNITRAZEPAM

Flunitrazepam is a potent, fast-acting benzodiazepine that is difficult to detect with routine toxicology screens because of the typically low concentration that is used. Flunitrazepam is illegal in the United States because of its association with date rape.

Flunitrazepam Intoxication

Flunitrazepam intoxication is characterized by sedation, disinhibition, anterograde amnesia, confusion, ataxia, bradycardia, hypotension, and respiratory depression. Treatment is supportive; activated charcoal and gastric lavage may be helpful. Severe respiratory depression or circulatory compromise can be treated with the benzodiazepine antagonist flumazenil. Flumazenil precipitates acute withdrawal in patients who are physically dependent on benzodiazepines and lowers their seizure threshold. Flumazenil has a short half-life, making repeated dosing necessary to avoid resedation.

Flunitrazepam Withdrawal

Withdrawal symptoms for flunitrazepam include anxiety, restlessness, tremors, headache, insomnia, and paresthesias. Treatment is similar to other benzodiazepines.

SEROTONIN SYNDROME

Serotonin syndrome includes a triad of highly variable signs and symptoms, typically consisting of:

- mental status changes (eg, anxiety, confusion, agitation, lethargy, delirium, coma),
- autonomic hyperactivity (eg, low-grade fever, tachycardia, diaphoresis, nausea, vomiting, diarrhea, dilated pupils, abdominal pain, hypertension, tachypnea), and
- neuromuscular abnormalities (eg, myoclonus, nystagmus, hyperreflexia, rigidity, trismus, tremor).

Patients with neuroleptic malignant syndrome, compared with serotonin syndrome, are more likely to present with extrapyramidal signs and autonomic instability and rarely present with the neuromuscular changes common in serotonin syndrome. Serotonin syndrome is most commonly seen after the ingestion of two or more serotonergic medications. Effective treatment requires early identification, immediate discontinuation of all serotonergic medications, supportive care (including intravenous hydration), and close monitoring.

KEY POINTS

1. Between 2009 and 2016, 106 countries reported 793 new psychoactive substances to the United Nations Office on Drugs and Crime.
2. The actions of many of these new psychoactive substances blur the boundary between stimulants and hallucinogens.
3. The risk for hallucinogen persisting perception disorder is increased when psychiatric comorbidity predates the initial hallucinogen intoxication.
4. It is important to rule out serotonin syndrome in the differential diagnosis of neuroleptic malignant syndrome.

REVIEW QUESTIONS

1. Which of the following statements does *not* apply to stimulants?
   A. Short-acting benzodiazepines such as lorazepam are helpful for agitation or sleep disturbance.
   B. Severe or persistent depression (>2 to 3 weeks) may require antidepressant treatment.
   C. Bupropion, aripiprazole, risperidone, topiramate, and modafinil block acute subjective effects in human laboratory experiments.

D. Modafinil is a medication approved by the US Food and Drug Administration for the treatment of stimulant use disorder.
   E. Myocardial infarction can occur in up to 6% of patients taking cocaine and up to 25% of patients taking methamphetamine.

2. Serotonin syndrome is commonly associated with which of the following?
   A. Mental status changes (eg, anxiety, confusion, agitation, lethargy, delirium, coma)
   B. Autonomic hyperactivity (eg, low-grade fever, tachycardia, diaphoresis, nausea, vomiting, diarrhea, dilated pupils, abdominal pain, hypertension, tachypnea)
   C. Neuromuscular abnormalities (eg, myoclonus, nystagmus, hyperreflexia, rigidity, trismus, tremor)
   D. All of the above.

3. Which of the following statements does not apply to intoxication with LSD, marijuana, phencyclidine, or MDMA?
   A. Impaired memory is associated with marijuana or phencyclidine intoxication.
   B. Hallucinations are commonly found in persons intoxicated with LSD or phencyclidine.
   C. Suicidal behavior is associated with LSD, marijuana, and phencyclidine intoxication.
   D. MDMA or LSD intoxication is not associated with overly elated mood.
   E. PCP intoxication is associated with the potential for harming others.

ANSWERS

1. **D**
2. **D**
3. **D**

SUGGESTED READINGS

Araújo AM, Carvalho F, Bastos Mde L, Guedes de Pinho P, Carvalho M. The hallucinogenic world of tryptamines: an updated review. *Arch Toxicol.* 2015;89(8):1151-1173.

Brezing CA, Levin FR. The current state of pharmacological treatments for cannabis use disorder and withdrawal. *Neuropsychopharmacol.* 2018;43(1):173-194.

Halpern JH, Lerner AG, Passie T. A review of hallucinogen persisting perception disorder (HPPD) and an exploratory study of subjects claiming symptoms of HPPD. In: Geyer MA, Ellenbroek BA, Marsden CA, Barnes TRE, Andersen SL, eds. *Current Topics in Behavioral Neurosciences.* Berlin/Heidelberg: Springer, 2016:1-28.

Liechti ME. Effects of MDMA on body temperature in humans. *Temperature (Austin).* 2014;1(3):192-200.

Wang RZ, Vashistha V, Kaur S, Houchens NW. Serotonin syndrome: preventing, recognizing, and treating it. *Cleve Clin J Med.* 2016;83(11):810-817.

Pharmacological Interventions and Other Somatic Therapies

Pharmacological Interventions for Alcohol Use Disorder

Summary by James Besante

Based on THE ASAM PRINCIPLES OF ADDICTION MEDICINE, 6th edition chapter by Hugh Myrick, Andrew J. Saxon, and Jerome H. Jaffe

Over the past three decades, several medications to treat alcohol use disorder have been developed and used by clinicians. The majority of these medications work by modifying the neurotransmitter systems that mediate alcohol reinforcement: endogenous opioids, catecholamines (eg, dopamine), serotonin (5-hydroxytryptamine [5-HT]), and excitatory amino acids (eg, glutamate). An alternative treatment strategy utilizes alcohol sensitizing agents, like disulfiram (Antabuse), which produce adverse effects when alcohol is consumed. The most commonly prescribed medications are discussed in this chapter. The latter part of the chapter also covers the treatment of co-occurring psychiatric symptoms and disorders in patients with alcohol use disorder.

MEDICATIONS USED TO REDUCE OR STOP ALCOHOL CONSUMPTION

Naltrexone

Naltrexone and, to a lesser extent, nalmefene—both of which are opioid antagonists with no intrinsic agonist properties—have been studied for the treatment of alcohol use disorder (AUD). Naltrexone was approved by the US Food and Drug Administration (FDA) for the treatment of opioid dependence in 1984 and for AUD in 1994. Nalmefene is approved in the United States as a parenteral formulation for the acute reversal of opioid effects (eg, after opioid overdose or analgesia).

The approval by the FDA of naltrexone for AUD was based on the results of two single-site studies, which showed it to be efficacious in the prevention of relapse to heavy drinking. In a 12-week trial in a sample of veterans with alcohol dependence, naltrexone was found to be well tolerated and to result in significantly less craving for alcohol and fewer drinking days than placebo. Among those who drank, naltrexone also limited the progression from initial sampling of alcohol to a relapse to heavy drinking, presumably because they experienced less euphoric effects from the alcohol consumed, suggesting that naltrexone blocked the endogenous opioid system's contribution to alcohol's "priming effect." Another study showed the medication to be well tolerated and superior to placebo in increasing the rate of abstinence and reducing the number of drinking days and relapse events. For patients who drank, those who received naltrexone and coping skills therapy were least likely to relapse to heavy drinking.

Naltrexone was shown to reduce craving for alcohol, alcohol's reinforcing properties, the experience of intoxication, and the chances of continued drinking following a slip. The literature on naltrexone treatment of AUD shows a clear advantage for naltrexone over placebo on a number of drinking outcomes, including relapse rates, time to relapse, percentage of drinking days, number of drinks per drinking days, and total consumption of alcohol during treatment. Naltrexone has also been shown to reduce the likelihood of heavy drinking, suggesting that it may be useful in patients who want to reduce their drinking to safe levels.

Because naltrexone only targets certain aspects of AUD (eg, reduced alcohol reinforcement, cue-induced craving), there has been an interest in combining it with medications that might influence other signs and symptoms of alcoholism. Symptoms often seen after alcohol cessation are difficulty sleeping, anxiety, irritability, decreased concentration, and depressed mood. This constellation of symptoms has been called protracted withdrawal. If not addressed, these symptoms are thought to lead to a relapse of alcohol use. The anticonvulsant gabapentin may help reduce these symptoms. As such, naltrexone has been evaluated in combination with gabapentin to determine if the combination was superior to naltrexone alone and/or placebo in decreasing alcohol use.

When gabapentin was combined with naltrexone, the combination group had a longer interval to heavy drinking than did the naltrexone-alone group, had fewer heavy drinking days than did the naltrexone-alone and placebo groups, and had fewer drinks per drinking day than did the naltrexone-alone and placebo groups. There was also some suggestion that the combination may work best in individuals who had previously experienced alcohol withdrawal.

Poor compliance with oral naltrexone has been shown to reduce the potential benefits of the medication. This has generated interest in the development and evaluation of long-acting injectable formulations of the medication, with the rationale that monthly administration would improve medication adherence and that parenteral administration would increase bioavailability by avoiding first-pass metabolism. Based on multiple studies that showed reduced rates of heavy drinking, greater likelihood of total abstinence, greater median time to a first drinking day, greater median time to a first heavy drinking day, lower median number of drinking days per month, and lower median heavy drinking days per month, the FDA approved long-acting naltrexone for monthly administration at a dosage of 380 mg per day.

The clinical use of naltrexone is relatively straightforward, despite the presence of a "boxed" warning on the label concerning hepatotoxicity. The medication should be prescribed at the time that psychosocial treatment is initiated. Because of adverse effects that could compound the adverse effects of alcohol withdrawal, the initiation of naltrexone therapy is probably best delayed until after the acute withdrawal period. Initial testing for liver enzyme abnormalities is warranted to avoid prescribing in the context of extreme elevations. Ongoing monitoring is required only if symptoms warrant it because the consistent effect of naltrexone in studies of AUD has been to decrease liver enzyme concentrations.

Oral naltrexone should be initially dosed at 25 mg per day to minimize adverse effects. The dosage can then be increased in 25-mg increments every 3 to 7 days to a maximum dosage of 150 mg per day using desire to drink or other symptoms that the patient identifies as reflective of risk of relapse to heavy drinking. It should be noted, however, that there is no clear evidence that a higher dosage is more efficacious than is the FDA-approved dosage of 50 mg per day. Nausea and other gastrointestinal symptoms are most common early in treatment as are neuropsychiatric symptoms (eg, headache, dizziness, lightheadedness, weakness) but are usually transient. Delaying or avoiding a dosage increase

can be used to address more persistent adverse events. In some patients, flulike symptoms occur, and the patient may not be willing to consider options other than discontinuation.

Long-acting naltrexone is only available as a 380-mg dose, which is administered as a deep intramuscular injection in the upper outer quadrant of the gluteal muscle of the buttock every 4 weeks. The medication is approved for use in patients who are abstinent from alcohol and who are also receiving psychosocial treatment. The precise length of the period of abstinence is not specified, and there is no evidence of any risk of consuming alcohol with naltrexone. Adverse effects with this formulation are similar to those of the oral medication, although pain and inflammation at the injection site may also occur. Local interventions, such as warm compresses, and nonsteroidal anti-inflammatory drugs can be used to treat such injection site reactions.

Acamprosate

Acamprosate is an amino acid derivative that increases γ-aminobutyric acid (GABA) neurotransmission and also has complex effects on excitatory amino acid neurotransmission, which is most likely the important therapeutic effect. It was first shown in a single-site study to be twice as effective as placebo at reducing relapse rates. Additionally, among patients who relapsed to drinking, acamprosate treatment was associated with less quantity and frequency of drinking than placebo, and it has been shown to reduce the risk of heavy drinking (ie, five or more drinks per day).

Acamprosate is FDA approved at a dosage of 1998 mg per day (two 333-mg capsules three times per day) in patient who are abstinent from alcohol and receiving psychosocial treatment. The most common adverse effects of the drug are generally mild and transient and may include gastrointestinal (eg, diarrhea, bloating) and dermatologic (eg, pruritus) complaints. In contrast to disulfiram and naltrexone, which are metabolized in the liver, acamprosate is excreted unmetabolized so that renal function is the rate-limiting factor in the drug's elimination. Renal function testing is warranted prior to initiation of the drug, particularly in individuals who have a history or are otherwise at risk of renal disease.

Baclofen

Baclofen, a GABAB receptor agonist, has been approved as an antispasmodic for more than 30 years and has recently been studied as a treatment for AUD, although it is not FDA approved for such treatment.

Patients treated with baclofen have been shown to be more likely to remain abstinent over a 1-month treatment period as well as having a greater number of cumulative abstinence days. There is, however, evidence of misuse, overdose, and other complications (eg, withdrawal reactions, including delirium) associated with baclofen, which underscores the need for more research on this medication before it can be recommended as a safe and efficacious treatment for AUD.

Anticonvulsants

Of growing interest is the use of anticonvulsants for the treatment of AUD, although currently, none are FDA approved for this indication. The efficacy of anticonvulsants for the treatment of AUD was initially demonstrated in placebo-controlled studies of carbamazepine, divalproex, and topiramate. Although these medications have different mechanisms of action, it is likely that these exert beneficial effects through their actions as glutamate antagonists and GABA agonists, helping to normalize the abnormal activity in these neurotransmitter systems seen following chronic heavy drinking.

Carbamazepine has been found to be superior to be placebo at increasing the time to the first heavy drinking day and at reducing drinks per drinking day and the number of consecutive heavy drinking days. Divalproex has been shown to reduce the risk of relapse to heavy drinking and to decrease irritability. Topiramate has been shown to significantly reduce drinks per day, drinks per drinking day, drinking days, heavy drinking days, and γ-glutamyl transpeptidase levels. The most common adverse effect of topiramate is numbness and tingling, with other common side effects including a change in the sense of taste, tiredness/sleepiness, fatigue, dizziness, loss of appetite, nausea, diarrhea, weight decrease, difficulty concentrating, and problems with memory and in word finding. Of clinical concern also are suicidal thoughts or actions, which have been reported uncommonly but at a frequency greater than that seen with placebo.

ALCOHOL-SENSITIZING AGENTS
Disulfiram

Alcohol-sensitizing agents alter the body's response to alcohol, making its ingestion unpleasant or toxic. Disulfiram (Antabuse) is the only alcohol-sensitizing medication approved in the United States for the treatment of AUD. It works by inhibiting the enzyme aldehyde dehydrogenase, which catalyzes the oxidation of acetaldehyde to acetic acid. The ingestion of alcohol while this enzyme is inhibited elevates blood acetaldehyde concentration, resulting in

the disulfiram–ethanol reaction (DER). Symptoms and signs of DER include warmness and flushing of the skin, increased heart rate, palpitations, decreased blood pressure, nausea, vomiting, shortness of breath, sweating, dizziness, blurred vision, and confusion. Most DERs are self-limited, lasting about 30 minutes. Severe DERs are associated with marked tachycardia or bradycardia, hypotension, and rarely, cardiovascular collapse, congestive heart failure, and convulsions. Severe reactions are usually associated with high doses of disulfiram ($>$500 mg per day).

Despite a lack of evidence demonstrating its efficacy in relapse prevention, disulfiram has long been used in the rehabilitation of patients with AUD. In the studies conducted, the difference in outcome between subjects receiving disulfiram and those given placebo has been modest. However, when compliance is ensured, these medications may be useful, and disulfiram may limit the severity of relapse when it occurs. There are no guidelines that can be offered to either identify patients for whom disulfiram is likely to benefit or match specific psychosocial interventions with particular patients to enhance compliance. In one large multicenter trial among patients who resumed drinking, those receiving 250 mg of disulfiram reported significantly fewer drinking days than did patients receiving lower doses or an inactive placebo. Thus, disulfiram may be helpful for reducing the frequency of drinking in patients who cannot remain abstinent and in those with whom special efforts are made to ensure compliance. Supervision of patients being treated with disulfiram may be an essential element in ensuring compliance and enhancing the beneficial effects of the medication.

Disulfiram is almost completely absorbed orally. Because it binds irreversibly to aldehyde dehydrogenase, renewed enzyme activity requires the synthesis of new enzyme so that the potential exists for a DER to occur 2 weeks from the last ingestion of disulfiram. Disulfiram commonly produces a variety of adverse effects, including drowsiness, lethargy, and fatigue. Although more serious adverse effects, such as optic neuritis, peripheral neuropathy, and hepatotoxicity occur rarely, patients should be monitored regularly for visual changes and neurologic symptoms and the medication discontinued if these appear. Further, liver enzymes should be monitored monthly during the first 3 months of treatment and quarterly thereafter to identify hepatotoxic effects. Psychiatric effects, such as psychosis or depression, are uncommon and probably occur only at higher dosages of the drug. These effects are mediated by disulfiram's inhibitory effect on enzymes involved in the metabolism of dopamine.

Due to the correlation between adverse effects and dosage, the daily dosage prescribed in the United States has been limited to 250 to 500 mg per day. However, efforts to titrate the dosage of disulfiram in relation to a challenge dose of ethanol have shown that some patients require in excess of 1 g per day of disulfiram to reach blood levels sufficient to produce a DER.

In deciding whether disulfiram should be used to treat AUD, patients should be made aware of the hazards of the medication, including the need to avoid over-the-counter preparations with alcohol and drugs that can interact with disulfiram and the potential for a DER to be precipitated by alcohol used in food preparation. Disulfiram is contraindicated in patients who do not have a goal of abstinence from alcohol and those who have not attained at least 48 hours of abstinence prior to the first administration of the drug. Given its potential to produce serious adverse effects when combined with alcohol, disulfiram cannot be recommended for use as part of a moderation approach to alcohol.

MEDICATIONS TO TREAT CO-OCCURRING PSYCHIATRIC SYMPTOMS OR DISORDERS IN PATIENTS WITH ALCOHOL USE DISORDER

Although most patients with AUDs report a reduction in mood or anxiety symptoms following acute withdrawal, for some, these symptoms may persist for months. Even among patients without substantial symptoms of alcohol withdrawal, low-level mood or anxiety symptoms may develop, a condition that has been called subacute withdrawal. In a substantial minority of these patients, these symptoms may reflect a diagnosable psychiatric disorder. Although medications are often prescribed during the postwithdrawal period in hopes of relieving these symptoms, there is no good evidence that the treatment of persistent or subacute withdrawal symptoms that do not meet diagnostic criteria for a co-occurring psychiatric disorder results in better outcomes in patients with AUD.

Many of the early studies of the efficacy of medications to treat mood disturbances targeted symptoms of depression and anxiety in unselected groups of patients with AUD after withdrawal. These and other methodologic limitations make the failure to demonstrate an advantage over control conditions through reductions in either psychiatric symptoms or drinking behavior difficult to interpret. Community studies have shown high rates of co-occurrence of psychiatric disorders in individuals with AUD, most commonly mood disorders, drug dependence, antisocial personality disorder, and anxiety disorder. Antidepressants, benzodiazepines and other anxiolytics, antipsychotics, and lithium have been used to treat anxiety and depression in the postwithdrawal state.

In patients with unipolar depression and AUD, several studies have shown a significant or near significant advantage for antidepressants over placebo at reducing symptoms of depression. However, most episodes of postwithdrawal depression will remit without specific treatment if abstinence from alcohol is maintained for a period of days or weeks. If depression persists after this period, treatment is warranted. Selective serotonin reuptake inhibitors and newer generation antidepressants have become the first-line treatment of depression because of their favorable side effect profile. However, they may exacerbate the tremor, anxiety, and insomnia often experienced by recently detoxified alcohol-dependent patients and may slightly increase the risk of gastrointestinal bleeding (particularly in combination with nonsteroidal anti-inflammatory drugs or aspirin).

Bipolar disorder co-occurs commonly with AUD. The presence of comorbid AUD is associated with an increased rate of mixed or dysphoric mania and rapid cycling, as well as greater bipolar symptom severity, suicidality, and aggression. However, controlled trials of medication to treat these comorbid disorders are difficult to conduct. A placebo-controlled trial of divalproex sodium in bipolar patients with *Diagnostic and Statistical Manual of Mental Disorder*, 4th edition (*DSM-IV*) alcohol dependence taking lithium showed that the drug significantly decreased the proportion of heavy drinking days, and manic and depressive symptoms improved equally in both groups.

Despite the risks that the use of benzodiazepines may create in patients with AUD beyond the period of acute withdrawal, judicious use of the drugs in this setting may be justified with close monitoring and supervision. Early relapse, which commonly disrupts alcohol rehabilitation, can result from protracted withdrawal-related symptoms such as anxiety, depression, and insomnia. To the extent that these symptoms can be suppressed by low doses of benzodiazepines, retention in treatment could be increased.

Buspirone, a nonbenzodiazepine anxiolytic, exerts its effects largely via its partial agonist activity at serotonergic autoreceptors. Although comparable to diazepam in the relief of anxiety and associated depression in outpatients with moderate-to-severe anxiety, buspirone is less sedating than diazepam, does not interact with alcohol to impair psycho-motor skills, and does not have abuse liability. This pharmacologic profile makes buspirone more suitable than benzodiazepines to treat anxiety symptoms among alcohol-dependent patients.

KEY POINTS

1. Naltrexone and nalmefene are opioidergic medications that have both been shown to directly reduce alcohol consumption. Only naltrexone is approved for use in the United States for alcohol use disorder. Naltrexone is also available as a monthly long-acting injection.
2. Acamprosate is an amino acid derivative that increases GABA neurotransmission and also has complex effects on glutamate neurotransmission, which is most likely responsible for its therapeutic effect. Acamprosate treatment has been shown to reduce relapse rates and is associated with less quantity and frequency of drinking, as well a reduction in heavy drinking.
3. Anticonvulsants such as topiramate and carbamazepine, as well as the antispasmodic baclofen, may be of limited use in patients with alcohol use disorder. However, none of these medications are FDA approved for this use, and further research is needed into the utility of these medications.
4. Patients often experience depressive symptoms, anxiety, and insomnia following acute alcohol withdrawal known as subacute withdrawal, which may persist for months. If a patient does not meet diagnostic criteria for a co-occurring psychiatric disorder, there is no strong evidence to support treating these symptoms.
5. Disulfiram is the only alcohol-sensitizing medication approved in the United States for the treatment of alcohol use disorder. It works by inhibiting the enzyme aldehyde dehydrogenase, and its ingestion elevates blood acetaldehyde concentration, resulting in DER.

REVIEW QUESTIONS

1. Oral naltrexone should be initially dosed at _____ to minimize adverse effects. The dosage can then be increased in 25-mg increments every 3 to 7 days to a maximum dosage of _____.

    A. 10 mg/day; 100 mg/day
    B. 10 mg/day; 150 mg/day

    C. 25 mg/day; 150 mg/day
    D. 25 mg/day; 380 mg/day
    E. 50 mg/day; 380 mg/day

2. Which of the following drugs is excreted unmetabolized, necessitating monitoring of renal function, particularly in individuals who have a history or are otherwise at risk of renal disease?

    A. Naltrexone
    B. Acamprosate
    C. Disulfiram
    D. Carbamazepine
    E. Diazepam

3. The most common adverse effect of topiramate is:

    A. nausea.
    B. numbness and tingling.
    C. sedation.
    D. memory deficits.
    E. muscle weakness.

4. Disulfiram works by inhibiting the enzyme _____, which leads to elevated serum levels of acetaldehyde and initiation of the disulfiram–ethanol reaction.

    A. methionine synthase
    B. glutathione S-transferase
    C. monoamine oxidase
    D. aldehyde dehydrogenase
    E. alcohol dehydrogenase

5. Symptoms of the disulfiram–ethanol reaction include all the following, *except*:

    A. increased heart rate.
    B. nausea.
    C. sedation.
    D. warmness and flushing.
    E. shortness of breath.

ANSWERS

1. **C**
2. **B**
3. **B**
4. **D**
5. **C**

SUGGESTED READINGS

Heilig M, Egli M. Pharmacological treatment of alcohol dependence: target symptoms and target mechanisms. *Pharmacol Ther*. 2006;111(3):855-876.

Petrakis IL. A rational approach to the pharmacotherapy of alcohol dependence. *J Clin Psychopharmacol*. 2006;26(suppl 1): S3-S12.

56 Pharmacological Interventions for Sedative–Hypnotic Use Disorder

Summary by Prameet Singh

Based on THE ASAM PRINCIPLES OF ADDICTION MEDICINE, 6th edition chapter by Jeffrey S. Cluver, Tara M. Wright, and Hugh Myrick

Although the sedative–hypnotic drug class includes benzodiazepines, barbiturates, carbamates, and "Z" drugs, this chapter focuses primarily on the first two categories. According to 2011 data from the Drug Abuse Warning Network, sedative–hypnotic anxiolytics were the second most frequently reported drug class to cause an emergency department visit (34%). Although the properties of benzodiazepines and barbiturates are similar, the relative safety and tolerability of benzodiazepines has led to their more widespread and lasting use. Medications in the benzodiazepine category all share a similar structure. Both barbiturates and benzodiazepines bind to the same receptor site on the γ-aminobutyric acid (GABA) receptor.

Other relatively new additions to this category of medications are the imidazopyridine derivatives (eg, zolpidem), zaleplon, and eszopiclone. These medications are chemically distinct from benzodiazepines but also bind to the GABA receptor at the ω subunit. It has been reported that the behavioral and subjective effects (including measures related to abuse potential) of the newer compounds are similar to those of the traditional benzodiazepines. Benzodiazepines and other sedative–hypnotics are often used in conjunction with other substances of abuse to enhance the effects of the other substances or to help an individual cope with unpleasant side effects of other drug use or withdrawal. Additionally, alone, or when used with other central nervous system (CNS) depressants, benzodiazepines and sedative–hypnotics can lead to respiratory depression, coma, and death.

PHARMACOLOGY

The effects of benzodiazepines and other sedative–hypnotics are mediated by their binding to the GABA receptor. When an agonist, such as a benzodiazepine or barbiturate, binds to the GABA receptor, the receptor opens its chloride channel, leading to an influx of chloride ions, which then decreases neuronal excitability. Clinically, this leads to the effects of decreased anxiety, increased sedation, muscle relaxation, and an elevated seizure threshold. The toxic effects of these compounds are caused by the excessive opening of chloride channels and can lead to respiratory depression, coma, and death. One essential difference between benzodiazepines and barbiturates is the mechanism by which they modify chloride ion influx at the GABA receptor. Barbiturates increase the duration that the chloride channel remains open, whereas benzodiazepines lead to an increased frequency of chloride channel opening. High doses of barbiturates lead to excessive activity of GABA at the $GABA_A$ receptor (which directly leads to respiratory depression), whereas high doses of benzodiazepines do not, causing the latter to be significantly safer in overdose. However, when taken in combination with other CNS depressants, such as opiates or alcohol, benzodiazepines can potentiate the action and thus contribute to death. Among the sedative–hypnotic agents, there are also important differences in the onset of activity, half-life of the medication, presence of active metabolites, and specificity of the clinical effects.

A compound with a high affinity for the GABA receptor that does not exert agonist or inverse agonist effects is flumazenil. Thus, it occupies the receptor without any intrinsic activity, operating thus as an agonist. This medication was developed and marketed to reverse the effects of benzodiazepines, including sedation and respiratory depression. It is ineffective in reversing effects of barbiturate overdose due to the site of action at the $GABA_A$ receptor.

DEFINITIONS

Physical dependence can be defined as an altered homeostasis at several levels of drug effect and activity. Discontinuation of the drug in this state leads to symptoms resulting from a disruption of this homeostasis. *Tolerance* can be defined as a decreased pharmacologic effect after repeated or prolonged exposure to the drug so that higher doses are needed to achieve the same initial clinical effects. Both physical dependence and tolerance are inevitable with prolonged and regular use of medications in the class of benzodiazepines and other sedative–hypnotics. Drug *misuse* generally refers to the inappropriate use of a medication such as the use of a higher dose than prescribed. The *Diagnostic and Statistical Manual of Mental Disorders*, 5th edition (*DSM-5*) criteria for a substance use disorder define a maladaptive pattern of substance use leading to clinically significant impairment or distress, defined by meeting multiple specified criteria within a 12-month period. Drugs with reinforcing properties, such as the ability to produce euphoria or other positive subjective experiences, are more likely to lead to a substance use disorder, although the development of physical dependence should not be equated with, or imply, the presence of a substance use disorder, although the two often coexist. Similarly, the misuse of a medication does not directly imply a substance use disorder, as may be the case in patients with severe anxiety disorders who do not achieve relief with their initially prescribed doses.

Issues of Abuse and Dependence

Benzodiazepines have largely replaced barbiturates and other sedative–hypnotics in clinical settings due to their preferred pharmacologic profile. Overall, there has been a trend toward decreased use of benzodiazepines and other sedative–hypnotics, but their use is still widespread. These medications are often initially prescribed for the treatment of anxiety disorders and insomnia, but their misuse often leads to euphoria and disinhibition, making them desirable as drugs of abuse.

There are notable differences among the compounds that correlate with the agents' onset of action. As is true of all drugs of abuse, the potential for misuse increases within the class based on the rapidity of onset of action. Lorazepam, alprazolam, and diazepam all appear to have a greater potential for abuse, based on their inherent lipophilic properties, and therefore, more rapid onset of action.

Misuse and abuse of benzodiazepines and sedative–hypnotics are commonly seen in individuals with other substance use disorders. In this context, sedative–hypnotics are often used to enhance the effects of other drugs and alleviate unpleasant side effects from use or withdrawal of other substances. Individuals seeking treatment for anxiety disorders, sleep disorders, and depression are at higher risk for developing sedative–hypnotic use disorder if they have a history of substance use disorders. A family history of substance use disorders also places an individual at higher risk for developing a sedative–hypnotic use disorder. The issue of alcohol use disorder warrants special caution because of the potential for dangerous interactions. The assumption that all individuals with an alcohol use disorder have a propensity for abusing benzodiazepines or becoming dependent has been challenged, but the risks of these medications should be carefully considered before prescribing them to this population. The American Psychiatric Association has published guidelines for benzodiazepine prescribing.

Interventions

In general, there are two clear indications for pharmacologic intervention in individuals who are taking benzodiazepines and other sedative–hypnotics and who meet the criteria for a use disorder. In a state of intoxication, a patient may require monitoring and even intervention to ensure a safe recovery. In patients experiencing acute withdrawal, pharmacologic management is often recommended because of the risk of serious consequences, including seizures and delirium tremens.

MANAGEMENT OF INTOXICATION AND WITHDRAWAL

The signs and symptoms of benzodiazepine and sedative–hypnotic intoxication are very similar to those of alcohol intoxication. Severe intoxication can lead to respiratory depression, coma, and death, especially with the barbiturates and other older, nonbenzodiazepine agents. The management of acute intoxication is mostly supportive, with special attention to airway management, because respiratory depression is the most likely cause of death in overdose. In overdose, it is also critical to know what other psychoactive agents (especially CNS depressants) may have been acutely or chronically ingested. Flumazenil can be used in the case of benzodiazepine intoxication and overdose, but its use is limited by the risk of precipitating withdrawal symptoms, including seizures, if it is not used with caution. Flumazenil can be considered in patients who have confirmed or suspected benzodiazepine toxicity and who have lost consciousness or are at risk of losing consciousness and who may require intubation. Flumazenil should be avoided in patients who have also recently ingested medications or substances that lower the seizure threshold, patients with known or suspected epilepsy, and patients who have developed physiologic dependence on benzodiazepines.

WITHDRAWAL

Withdrawal symptoms are most often seen in patients with physiologic dependence who abruptly discontinue taking benzodiazepines and other sedative–hypnotics. Individuals are likely to develop withdrawal symptoms when they have been taking high doses of sedative–hypnotics or if they have been taking low or moderate doses for a prolonged period. The severity of the withdrawal syndrome is a function of both the dose taken and the duration, with the latter often leading to protracted withdrawal syndromes. The withdrawal syndromes related to each of these patterns are disparate and require distinct management approaches. Although withdrawal symptoms are similar to those seen in alcohol withdrawal, the signs and symptoms of withdrawal manifest differently in each patient because of characteristics like age and overall state of health and the unique pharmacologic properties of each medication. The time to onset of withdrawal is a function of the half-life of the agent. Withdrawal from agents with short half-lives usually begins within 12 to 24 hours and reaches peak intensity within 1 to 3 days. With longer acting agents, withdrawal symptoms may begin later and not peak until 4 to 7 days after discontinuation. Symptoms may then continue for several more days or even weeks depending on the half-life of drug. Subjective symptoms can last for months and are often a precipitant to relapse.

Common physical manifestations include tachycardia, mild elevations in blood pressure, and diaphoresis. Anxiety, insomnia, restlessness, agitation, irritability, and muscle tension are frequent. Less frequent are nausea, diaphoresis, lethargy, aches and pains, hyperacusis, blurred vision, nightmares, depression, hyperreflexia, and ataxia. Psychosis, seizures, confusion, paranoid delusions, hallucinations, and persistent tinnitus are uncommon.

Another common occurrence during withdrawal is the reemergence of symptoms of anxiety and insomnia. Initially, these rebound symptoms are perceived to be more severe and intense than the original symptoms but within several weeks return to pretreatment levels.

MANAGEMENT
Benzodiazepine Taper

The withdrawal syndrome can be effectively treated by replacement with any cross-tolerant sedative–hypnotic and a gradual taper. Regardless of the misused sedative–hypnotic, long-acting benzodiazepines are the drug of choice, with consideration paid to liver function.

The approach with the most data to support its safety and efficacy is to initiate a taper that uses decreasing doses of the therapeutic agent over the course of 4 to 12 weeks. This is most often used in settings of long-term use and physical dependence, where there is not an urgent need to discontinue the current medication. In order for this strategy to be effective, the patient must be able to follow complex dosing regimens, adhere to regular follow-up appointments, and be free of other active substance use disorders. It is recommended that as lower doses are achieved, the dose reduction at each stage should be more modest, especially if short half-life drugs are being prescribed. More frequent dosing intervals can also be used in the later stages to help prevent the emergence of any withdrawal symptoms.

When tapering patients from medications with a short half-life, consideration should be given to converting to an equivalent dose of a longer acting agent and then gradually reducing the dose of the latter.

Anticonvulsants

Another strategy for the treatment of withdrawal is the use of carbamazepine. This anticonvulsant has been shown to be as effective as oxazepam in the treatment of alcohol withdrawal, and two open-label studies also demonstrated the effectiveness of this agent in the management of complicated benzodiazepine withdrawal. Based on the initial studies, the suggested dosing of carbamazepine is in the range of 200 mg three times a day for 7 to 10 days. Carbamazepine has the distinct advantage of having low abuse potential and limited cognitive side effects, especially during short-term use. Studies have also shown gabapentin and divalproex to be effective in the treatment of alcohol withdrawal in patients who experience mild-to-moderate symptoms.

Phenobarbital

A protocol has also been developed that utilizes phenobarbital during a medically supervised withdrawal, by converting patients from other sedative–hypnotics to equivalent phenobarbital doses. This practice is not commonly employed due to the decreased use of phenobarbital in clinical settings, but it does have evidence to support its safety and efficacy.

Flumazenil

The data on the use of flumazenil are limited and still emerging, but published reports and studies suggest that parenteral and subcutaneous flumazenil may be effective in the management of benzodiazepine withdrawal. Although flumazenil is generally thought of as a pure antagonist, it acts as a partial agonist with weak affinity at the benzodiazepine receptor site. Explanations for flumazenil's potential efficacy in the treatment of withdrawal symptoms include flumazenil-induced changes in receptor sensitivity and binding affinity, although the exact mechanism of action in ameliorating withdrawal symptoms is not clear. Factors that may limit the use of this strategy include the method of administration of the medication and the treatment setting (eg, an intravenous infusion would necessitate an appropriately monitored environment such as an inpatient unit).

Protracted Withdrawal Symptoms

One additional consideration is the treatment of residual symptoms of withdrawal in the days and weeks following the discontinuation of the medication used to manage the withdrawal. There are no definitive pharmacologic options for the treatment of protracted benzodiazepine withdrawal symptoms, and this is a subject that is in need of further investigation and understanding. Pharmacologic strategies with antihistamines, α-adrenergic agents, anticonvulsants, buspirone, and others have been described, but there is not an evidence base to support the use of a particular agent or strategy.

Treatment Setting

While discussing with the patient the pharmacologic strategy for the treatment of withdrawal, a decision must also be made regarding the setting in which the withdrawal will be treated. Although inpatient treatment is often optimal because of the close observation and controlled environment, this is often not feasible due to limited accessibility to inpatient resources and cost considerations and should therefore be limited to cases in which the patient is medically compromised or if there is a high risk of the patient developing severe symptoms, such as seizures. Medically supervised outpatient withdrawal is reasonable if the patient does not appear to be at risk for severe withdrawal, especially if the method of slowly reducing the sedative–hypnotic dose can be utilized. If outpatient management is undertaken, the patient should be given clear instructions and close follow-up appointments. It is preferable for the patient to have some level of supervision by friends or family, but this is not always possible. A written treatment contract with an agreed upon and relatively inflexible taper can be helpful. Urine drug screens and clinical and laboratory assessments for the use of alcohol or other misused agents should be utilized to monitor for complications that could arise from the concomitant use of other substances.

Postwithdrawal Treatment

Medically supervised withdrawal should not be seen as a definitive treatment in the case of sedative–hypnotic use disorder. This is the first step in the management of patients who often have other substance use disorders, anxiety and sleep disorders, and other co-occurring medical and psychiatric disorders. In the case of other substance use disorders, a treatment plan should include co-occurring medically supervised withdrawal from other substances and substance use disorder treatment in an appropriate setting. When treating patients with underlying anxiety and sleep disorders, other pharmacologic and psychotherapeutic treatments—particularly, cognitive–behavioral therapy—should be initiated to counter any reemerging symptoms that may be experienced following withdrawal, which may help to reduce the risk of relapse.

KEY POINTS

1. Due to their inherent pharmacologic properties, use of benzodiazepines and other sedative–hypnotic medications can lead to clinically significant and dangerous intoxication and withdrawal states.
2. The withdrawal syndrome is a function of both dosage and duration of use, with the latter being just as important and a predictor of a protracted withdrawal syndrome.
3. Management of severe intoxication includes supportive medical care in an appropriate setting and the judicious use of flumazenil.
4. Selecting a strategy for the management of withdrawal states must include consideration of the dose and length of time that the medication has been used, the pharmacologic properties of the medication(s) being discontinued, as well as comorbid substance use and other psychiatric conditions. Outpatient pharmacologic interventions are likely to work if accompanied by psychosocial treatments, including cognitive–behavioral therapy and a treatment contract.

REVIEW QUESTIONS

1. The sedative–hypnotic withdrawal syndrome is influenced by:
   A. the doses used.
   B. the duration of use.
   C. a history of seizures.
   D. a history of overdoses.
   E. the dose used and duration.

2. Which of the following strategies has the most evidence to support its efficacy in the management of benzodiazepine withdrawal?
   A. Alcohol drip
   B. Benzodiazepine taper
   C. Carbamazepine taper
   D. Flumazenil infusion
   E. Phenobarbital taper

3. What is the preferred treatment setting for patients being treated for benzodiazepine withdrawal?
   A. Depends on the treatment
   B. Inpatient
   C. Intensive outpatient
   D. Outpatient
   E. Partial hospital

ANSWERS

1. **E.** The withdrawal syndrome is a function of the dose used as well as the duration with the latter being as if not more important in the overall course

2. **B.** When possible, a prolonged taper of a benzodiazepine is a preferred management strategy. This strategy cannot always be safely employed, especially in cases of benzodiazepine use disorder, abrupt discontinuation, and concurrent substance use involving other CNS depressants.

3. **A.** The treatment will dictate the treatment setting. A prolonged taper can be completed in an outpatient setting if the patient has appropriate social support and can keep frequent appointments, whereas a patient at high risk for a complicated withdrawal course (eg, history of seizures, concurrent use of alcohol or other sedatives, medically compromised) should be treated in an inpatient setting.

SUGGESTED READINGS

American Psychiatric Association. *Benzodiazepine Dependence, Toxicity, and Abuse.* Washington, DC: American Psychiatric Publishing, 1990.

Baandrup L, Ebdrup BH, Rasmussen JØ, et al. Pharmacological interventions for benzodiazepine discontinuation in chronic benzodiazepine users. *Cochrane Database Syst Rev.* 2018; (3):CD011481.

O'Brien CP. Benzodiazepine use, abuse, and dependence. *J Clin Psychiatry.* 2005;66(suppl 2):28-33.

Substance Abuse and Mental Health Services Administration. *Detoxification and Substance Abuse Treatment. Treatment Improvement Protocol (TIP) Series, No. 45.* Rockville, MD: Substance Abuse and Mental Health Services Administration, 2006. DHHS Pub. No. (SMA) 13-4131.

Welsh JW, Tretyak V, McHugh RK, Weiss RD, Bogunovic O. Review: adjunctive pharmacologic approaches for benzodiazepine tapers. *Drug Alcohol Depend.* 2018;189:96-107.

CHAPTER 57

Pharmacological and Psychosocial Treatment for Opioid Use Disorder

Summary by David Kan

Based on THE ASAM PRINCIPLES OF ADDICTION MEDICINE, 6th edition chapter by David Kan, Joan E. Zweben, Susan M. Stine, Thomas R. Kosten, Elinore F. McCance-Katz, and John J. McCarthy

Pharmacologic interventions for opioid use disorder (OUD) continue to expand. Detoxification is of limited long-term efficacy. Opioid agonist therapy (OAT) has the best data supporting improved outcomes in overdose prevention, relapse prevention, and treatment retention.

OVERVIEW OF PHARMACOLOGIC INTERVENTIONS

Opioid Antagonists

Naloxone is short acting (half-life [$t_{1/2}$] = 30 to 80 minutes) and intranasally or parenterally administered to counter the life-threatening depression of the central nervous and respiratory systems caused by opioid overdose. It is also combined with buprenorphine in the medication as a treatment for both medically assisted withdrawal and long-term, office-based OAT. In this formulation, naloxone serves to reduce the medication's abuse potential.

In comparison to naloxone, *naltrexone* has a prolonged duration of action due to its longer half-life (mean $t_{1/2}$ = 4 hours), active metabolite (6β-naltrexol, mean $t_{1/2}$ = 13 hours), and greater affinity for the κ-opioid receptor. Clinical studies indicate that 50 mg of naltrexone will block the pharmacologic effects of 25 mg of intravenous heroin for up to 24 hours. Naltrexone is available in pill form as well as a 28- to 30-day injectable formulation.

Opioid Full and Partial Agonists

Methadone is an orally active, long-acting synthetic opioid that reduces nonprescribed opioid use, withdrawal symptoms, and drug craving. A stable dose of methadone ranging from 80 to 120 mg per day, usually higher than what is required for pain management, produces a tolerance to the effects of exogenous opioid compounds, such as intravenously administered heroin or oral pain medications (eg, oxycodone, hydrocodone, hydromorphone), while also blocking the euphoric effects of these substances. This phenomenon is referred to as *agonist blockade*.

Levomethadyl acetate (LAAM) is structurally similar to methadone but with a longer half-life and active metabolites norLAAM and dinorLAAM. It is approved by the US Food and Drug Administration (FDA) for opioid maintenance treatment but is no longer marketed due to its association with cardiac arrhythmias (torsade de pointes).

Buprenorphine is a high-affinity μ-opioid partial agonist and κ-opioid antagonist that received FDA approval as pharmacotherapy for OUD in October 2002. Its safety profile is considered favorable due to a "ceiling effect" on respiratory suppression originating from its partial agonist properties. Buprenorphine is available in office-based practice. Because of its partial agonist property and higher affinity to μ-opioid receptors than other full agonists, buprenorphine has the potential to precipitate withdrawal symptoms. This is one of the factors to consider when patients with opioid dependency are inducted onto buprenorphine or during the transfer from long-acting opioid agonists to buprenorphine.

Nonopioid Agonists: α-Adrenergic Agents

Both *clonidine* and *lofexidine* are antihypertensives used to treat autonomic symptoms during opioid withdrawal. With opioid abstinence, the loss of opioid suppression of the locus coeruleus system leads to increased adrenergic activity. Both clonidine and lofexidine, centrally acting α_2-adrenergic presynaptic receptor agonists, decrease adrenergic neurotransmission through feedback inhibition. The use of clonidine has been hampered by side effects of sedation and hypotension. Lofexidine was recently approved by the FDA for medically supervised withdrawal from opioids. Lofexidine is associated with lower rates of hypotension than is clonidine.

ABSTINENCE SYNDROMES AND MEDICALLY SUPERVISED WITHDRAWAL

The opioid abstinence syndrome is characterized by two phases: acute withdrawal, lasting 5 to 14 days, followed by a protracted abstinence (PA) syndrome lasting months or longer (discussed in the following text). The acute withdrawal syndrome consists of a distinctive constellation of symptoms, including gastrointestinal distress, disturbances in thermal regulation, dilated pupils, insomnia, muscle and joint aches, marked anxiety, and dysphoria. Although these symptoms generally include no life-threatening complications, acute withdrawal causes marked discomfort, often prompting continuation of opioid use.

Opioid Agonists and Partial Agonists

Based on the principle of cross-tolerance, opioid-based medically supervised withdrawal is the replacement of the misused opioid(s) with another opioid, typically one with a longer half-life, and then slowly tapered.

Methadone is commonly used and can be administered once daily. Initial dosages of methadone start in the range of 15 to 30 mg per day. Additional methadone may be given as necessary based on clinical findings. Importantly, a simple conversion of short-acting prescription opioids into an equivalent dosage of methadone can lead to overdose due to incomplete cross-tolerance and methadone accumulation over the first several days of dosing. In general, any methadone dose above 40 mg daily should involve careful and gradual increases over at least several days. In an acute setting, the starting dosage should be maintained through the second or third day after the peak level is attained, and then the methadone can be slowly tapered by approximately 10% to 15% per day. Longer term medical supervision is available through federally licensed opioid treatment programs.

Buprenorphine has been studied as a treatment for opioid withdrawal. It has several advantages, including long duration of action due to its slow dissociation from μ-opioid receptors, milder withdrawal signs and symptoms, and an enhanced safety profile stemming from its partial agonist properties. Such qualities may permit accelerated withdrawal without significant distress. The optimal dose of buprenorphine has not yet been determined; studies have used various protocols ranging from several days to weeks with dosages ranging from 2 to 8 mg daily.

Medically supervised withdrawal is associated with increased risk of overdose death in return to opioid use. Long-term OAT is considered the current standard of care.

Nonopioid Medication Treatments

The α-adrenergic agents are widely used to treat symptoms of noradrenergic hyperactivity during medically supervised withdrawal, particularly in treatment settings where controlled substances may be unavailable or unsuitable for use.

A regimen of *clonidine* 0.1 to 0.2 mg every 4 hours, up to 1.2 mg per 24 hours, has been used with careful monitoring of blood pressure. Given clonidine's limited effectiveness in managing subjective withdrawal symptoms, adjuvant therapy (nonsteroidal anti-inflammatory drugs for myalgia and bone pain, medications for insomnia, antiemetics, and antidiarrheal medications) may be needed.

In clinical trials, *lofexidine* demonstrated fewer side effects than did clonidine, particularly hypotension. Lofexidine is typically initiated at 0.54 mg every 5 to 6 hours up to a total dose of 2.88 mg per day. Doses required to effectively manage withdrawal symptoms, however, vary for each patient depending on amount, frequency, and duration of opioid use. Other side effects include insomnia, dry mucous membranes, sedation, and dizziness.

Rapid and Ultrarapid Opioid Detoxification

Most opioid and nonopioid approaches to medically supervised withdrawal require a prolonged time frame of a week or more. In contrast, "rapid" and "ultrarapid" opioid withdrawal protocols attempt to complete withdrawal in shorter periods, ranging from as little as 2 or 3 days to 8 days. These "rapid" protocols use an opioid antagonist to cause an accelerated withdrawal response along with additional medications (eg, clonidine and sedation) to minimize acute withdrawal symptoms. The proposed risk of minimizing relapse has not been borne out in clinical experience. These methods have not been in widespread use. Ultrarapid methods use anesthetic sedation and complete the procedure in several hours, but it is not recommended due to the risks of general anesthesia as well as the risk of overdose after opioid tolerance is lost.

LONG-TERM TREATMENTS FOR OPIOID USE DISORDER

In patients with a history of OUD, studies found that certain physiologic functions, including temperature, sleep, respiration rate, weight, basal metabolic rate, blood pressure, hematocrit, sensitivity of the respiratory center to carbon dioxide, sedimentation rate, and electroencephalograph patterns, take months to return to normal. Clinically, these symptoms are less characterized and are termed PA. Although the concept of PA has been controversial, it remains a useful model for scientific hypothesis testing and development of new therapeutic approaches.

Naltrexone Maintenance Treatment

Clinically, oral naltrexone is initiated after withdrawal from opioids, at least a 5- to 7-day opioid-free period for short-acting opioids and a 7- to 10-day period for long-acting agents. The initial dose of naltrexone used generally is 25 mg on the first day, followed by 50 mg daily or an equivalent of 350 mg weekly, divided into three doses (100, 100, and 150 mg). Common side effects are nausea and vomiting. The most serious (but quite rare) potential side effect of naltrexone is liver toxicity, which seems to be dose dependent and reversible.

Naltrexone has proven to be effective in highly motivated subsamples of patients with opioid use disorder. However, in other populations, medication adherence remains problematic and is associated with poor retention in treatment. Long-acting injectable (LAI) naltrexone was approved by the FDA to treat opioid dependence in 2010. A significantly lower rate of patients can be successfully inducted into LAI naltrexone compared with buprenorphine. LAI naltrexone had higher rates of opioid relapse mostly occurring earlier in treatment. LAI naltrexone was not inferior to buprenorphine once patients were stabilized on treatment with both medications.

Ongoing Methadone Treatment

The rationale for long-term methadone maintenance is to relieve the PA syndrome, block euphoric effects from misused opioids, and enhance psychosocial stabilization during recovery. Side effects include constipation, drowsiness, decreased sexual interest, sleep apnea, hypogonadism in men, and risk of prolonged QT syndrome. Maintenance treatment generally requires 60 mg or more of methadone per day; doses less than 60 mg per day appear to be inadequate for most patients and are associated with poorer treatment outcomes. The duration of methadone maintenance treatment is best seen in terms of years rather than months. For many patients, 5 to 10 years—or even a lifetime—of methadone administration may be required.

Factors affecting methadone's pharmacologic effectiveness include the presence of chronic diseases, medications interacting with methadone, and altered physiologic states, especially pregnancy. Methadone dosage likely needs to be adjusted when CYP450 3A4 inhibitors (cimetidine, certain antiretroviral agents), enhancers (rifampin, phenytoin, carbamazepine), or drugs competing with methadone for metabolism (ethanol, disulfiram) are used concomitantly.

Early treatment termination, illicit use of non-opioid substances, and diversion of take-home doses to the illicit market remain significant issues for most opioid treatment programs. Several interventions, including behavioral approaches and medications, assist in the reduction of concurrent substance use.

Ongoing Buprenorphine Treatment

Buprenorphine is administered through sublingual route due to its high first-pass effects. It has the ability to block subjective responses to doses of morphine up to 120 mg, and 8 mg of buprenorphine has comparable effectiveness to 60 mg of methadone. There are multiple formulations, the "mono" tablet, containing only buprenorphine, and a tablet, film, or bioerodible mucoadhesive containing buprenorphine and naloxone in approximately a 4:1 ratio designed to discourage illicit diversion and injection use. The recommended therapeutic dose of buprenorphine/naloxone is 16 mg/4 mg to 24 mg/8 mg. Transdermal formulations are approved for pain. Depot formulations of buprenorphine have recently been FDA approved.

Office-based treatment of OUD with sublingual formulations of buprenorphine/naloxone has demonstrated safety and effectiveness in reducing opioid use and craving with significant improvements over time in psychosocial functioning.

Buprenorphine can produce withdrawal discomfort among individuals with opioid dependency, due to either insufficient substitution of the full agonist or the rapid displacement of opioid agonist by the higher affinity compound and blockade of the μ-opioid receptors. It is important to avoid buprenorphine-precipitated withdrawal, which is usually sudden and more severe and uncomfortable than is a naturally occurring withdrawal. In general, after physical assessment to rule out acute, life-threatening conditions, treatment with buprenorphine should begin when there are no signs of opioid intoxication or sedation and signs of opioid withdrawal. The FDA has recommended patients receive buprenorphine even if they are misusing benzodiazepines or sedatives because the risk of nonprescribed opioid use outweighs the risk of buprenorphine in these patients. The typical first dose of buprenorphine is 4 mg, and patients should be monitored for 30 to 60 minutes to assess for acute adverse effects. Another 4 to 8 mg for a maximum first-day dose of 12 mg of buprenorphine can be given if withdrawal symptoms persist 2 to 4 hours after the first dosing. The first day's dose should be followed by dosage increases over subsequent days until withdrawal symptoms are suppressed within about 2 hours after taking the medication and lasting until the next day's dosing. In-home buprenorphine inductions have been demonstrated to be safe and effective

SPECIAL ISSUES IN MAINTENANCE TREATMENT
Opioid Agonist Treatment During Pregnancy

Opioid misuse during pregnancy and its associated environmental and medical factors lead to adverse consequences including high rates of infection, premature delivery, and low birth weight. Ongoing treatment with methadone has been the recommended standard of care based on longer duration of maternal drug abstinence, increased obstetrical care adherence, avoidance of associated risk behaviors, reduction in fetal illicit drug exposure, and improved neonatal outcomes observed in pregnant women receiving methadone treatment. All opioid use is associated with neonatal abstinence syndrome (NAS), which can be treated without damaging consequences. Pregnant women should receive appropriate methadone doses to treat OUD. A rooming-in model of care where the mother and fetus are not separated and where the mother is an active part of NAS management has been shown to reduce NAS symptoms and length of hospitalization. Usually, the dose required during pregnancy and frequency of dosing, particularly in the third trimester, is higher than are nonpregnant doses. Based on available data, buprenorphine may represent an alternative to methadone for the treatment of opioid dependence during pregnancy. It may carry the advantage of reducing the severity of NAS. Of note, the mono buprenorphine formulation should be used to minimize impact on the fetus.

Interactions of Opioid Agonist and HIV Pharmacotherapy

Opioid agonist treatment has multiple beneficial effects on clinical status in patients with HIV infection, primarily as a result of improving adherence to treatment and decreasing risky behaviors. Both methadone and buprenorphine treatments are compatible with highly active antiretroviral therapy (HAART) for HIV. The complexity of multiple-agent antiretroviral treatment complicates the use of methadone owing to pharmacokinetic interactions. Methadone is primarily metabolized by liver enzymes CYP450 3A4. When medications that inhibit or induce the activity of CYP450 3A4 are started or discontinued, the dose of methadone may need to be adjusted accordingly. Several HAART drugs compete with methadone for metabolizing enzymes, thus requiring methadone dose changes during concomitant treatment for HIV.

To date, drug interactions between buprenorphine/naloxone and HAART show a more promising profile than that of methadone. There are no current recommendations on buprenorphine dose change or antiretroviral dose change when used together.

Methadone-to-Buprenorphine Transfer

Some patients will be transferred from methadone to buprenorphine for maintenance or medically supervised withdrawal due to its more favorable safety profile, subjectively milder withdrawal, easier completion of taper, and decreased stigma. It is also accessible over a wider geographic area due to its availability in office-based primary care settings and may be more appropriate as an early intervention strategy for those with less physical dependence or short dependence histories. However, if the patient is stable on methadone, careful scrutiny of the factors motivating the transfer request is required.

Transferring patients from a longer acting agonist such as methadone to buprenorphine may be challenging due to withdrawal discomfort, attrition, or return to drug use. A number of small clinical studies show that a methadone-to-buprenorphine transfer is feasible over a range of starting methadone doses up to 60 mg per day. Two important factors to consider are the methadone dose before the transfer and the interval between the last methadone dose and the initiation of buprenorphine. Recommendations from the Center for Substance Abuse Treatment (*TIP 40: Clinical Guidelines for the Use of Buprenorphine in the Treatment of Opioid Addiction*) for patients taking methadone are to taper methadone to 30 mg or less per day for 1 week or more before initiating buprenorphine. Induction should not begin until at least 24 hours after the last dose of methadone and should start at 2 mg of the monotherapy formulation. If signs or symptoms of withdrawal are seen after the first dose, a second dose of 2 mg should be administered and repeated, if necessary, to a maximum of 8 mg buprenorphine on day 1. More recently, a Physician Clinical Support System guidance offered similar recommendations except that these use a lower starting dose (20 or 30 mg of methadone), *objective signs on Clinical Opioid Withdrawal Scale* to quantify withdrawal, and a higher dose of buprenorphine up to 32 mg on day 1. If withdrawal is precipitated, management with ancillary medications is advised. Patients on moderate-to-high doses of methadone (>60 to 100 mg) are still possible to transfer directly from methadone to buprenorphine/naloxone but with greater discomfort and risk of return to use.

Buprenorphine in Agonist-to-Antagonist Treatment

Buprenorphine has been used in several studies as a transitional agent between agonists and antagonists. Combination drug treatment may facilitate greater patient acceptance of agonist–antagonist switching due to the substitution of agonist effects and reduction of physical dependence from full agonists. It also improves stabilization of patients with opioid dependency before switching to naltrexone, allowing engagement in psychosocial aspects of treatment. Stabilization would be followed by rapid transition to naltrexone, using clonidine to relieve any withdrawal symptoms caused by discontinuation of buprenorphine.

KEY POINTS

1. Methadone and buprenorphine are commonly used opioid agonists for medically supervised withdrawal. Clonidine and lofexidine, α_2-adrenergic agonists, are useful for symptomatic management for withdrawal especially when controlled substances are not available. Low-dose naltrexone, an opioid antagonist, is used during withdrawal to facilitate rapid resolution

of symptoms and early transition into antagonist therapy.
2. Methadone and buprenorphine are effective long-term opioid maintenance therapies. Buprenorphine is available through office-based treatment with easier access; however, it may not be sufficient to maintain patients with high-level physical dependence. Methadone programs are usually more restrictive but with the advantages of timely psychosocial intervention and contingency management.
3. Methadone or buprenorphine is recommended for patients with opioid dependency during pregnancy, with better maternal and fetal outcomes.
4. For patients who are HIV positive and maintained on methadone, the dosage of either methadone or HAART medications may need adjustment. Buprenorphine has fewer drug interactions; however, decreased HAART adherence in office-based settings may be a concern.

REVIEW QUESTIONS

1. Which of the following statements is *false* regarding buprenorphine/naloxone?
   A. Naloxone is added to reduce injection use potential of buprenorphine because it will precipitate withdrawal when used intravenously but not sublingually.
   B. Buprenorphine can be administered three times a week because of its long half-life.
   C. Buprenorphine has higher affinity to μ-opioid receptors than full agonists; thus, it can precipitate withdrawal in patients with opioid dependency.
   D. When used in medically supervised withdrawal, buprenorphine could have a faster completion due to its partial agonist property.
   E. None of the above

2. Which of the following statements is *false* regarding opioid agonist therapy?
   A. The average range of effective methadone doses is 20 to 40 mg per day.
   B. Buprenorphine has a ceiling effect, which means with doses greater than 32 mg, it will not cause additional respiratory suppression. This is due to its partial agonist property.
   C. Some patients may need to be on opioid agonist therapy for a long time, even for the rest of their lives, because OUD is a chronic biologic disease with altered brain structure and function. Currently, there is no curative medication available.

D. Naltrexone is a μ-antagonist with complete blockade of μ-opioid receptors and is less likely to be tolerated than buprenorphine.

3. Which of the following is the reason that the opioid antagonist naloxone can be coadministered with buprenorphine sublingually with no adverse effect?

A. Low dose of naloxone used
B. Development of tolerance to naloxone
C. Poor sublingual absorption of naloxone
D. Low affinity of naloxone for opioid receptors
E. Significant first-pass metabolism of naloxone

ANSWERS

1. **E**
2. **A**
3. **C**

SUGGESTED READINGS

Substance Abuse and Mental Health Services Administration (SAMHSA): *TIP 63: Medications for Opioid Use Disorder – Full Document (Including Executive Summary and Parts 1-5)*. https://store.samhsa.gov/product/TIP-63-Medications-for-Opioid-Use-Disorder-Full-Document-Including-Executive-Summary-and-Parts-1-5-/SMA18-5063FULLDOC.

CHAPTER 58

Special Issues in Office-Based Opioid Treatment

Summary by Andrew J. Saxon

Based on THE ASAM PRINCIPLES OF ADDICTION MEDICINE, 6th edition chapter by Andrew J. Saxon

EPIDEMIOLOGIC AND REGULATORY ISSUES

Most individuals with opioid use disorder (OUD) cannot access adequate treatment services. In 2014, 357,293 individuals entered treatment for heroin-related OUD, but only 28.3% received medication treatment.

Similarly, 132,387 entered treatment for prescription-related OUD, but only 20.7% received medication treatment. These data reflect a circumstance that has been prevalent throughout the past 100 years. However, these data do not reflect individuals receiving office-based opioid treatment, which is making medication treatment more widely available.

Like today, thousands of untreated individuals who are dependent on opioids also worried society in the early part of the 20th century. Although controversy raged then as it does now about how best to handle individuals with OUD, many experts of that generation already had recognized the high likelihood that patients with OUD would resume opioid use after enforced withdrawal. Physicians in many areas of the country thus viewed opioid addiction as a medical disorder; they advocated and practiced the ongoing prescribing of opioids from their offices as a form of harm reduction.

In 1919, the US Supreme Court ruled that the Harrison Act disallowed such prescribing to individuals with OUD for "maintenance" purposes. The decision was largely based on a small number of reports of inappropriate prescribing and increasing concern (from doctors, regulators, and the public) about the safety of and wisdom in prescribing opioids to individuals with OUD. This decision effectively ended the first era of office-based treatment for opioid addiction.

Thus, from the 1920s onward, physicians were actively discouraged from treating heroin-addicted individuals and, indeed, medical school curricula provided no training to physicians in this regard.

Convicted violators of federal narcotics laws caused an overload in the federal penal system, so Congress established federal narcotics hospitals at Lexington, Kentucky, and Fort Worth, Texas, in the 1930s. Despite high recidivism rates, these isolated facilities remained the only treatment option for individuals with OUD until the advent of methadone maintenance 30 years later.

The divergence between mainstream medicine and opioid addiction treatment has had some unfortunate consequences. Licensed opioid agonist treatment programs often lack the resources to provide comprehensive medical care, with the result that comorbid medical disorders may be unattended, delaying care and driving up its ultimate cost. Similarly, a high prevalence of co-occurring psychiatric disorders, particularly mood and anxiety disorders, is seen among patients with OUD, and licensed programs typically cannot provide the treatment these conditions require.

Many potential patients who need and desire opioid agonist treatment and who are willing to enroll in licensed programs cannot overcome the barriers to entry. One state, Wyoming, does not offer any such licensed opioid agonist treatment. In other states, licensed clinics, by virtue of economic necessity and neighborhood acceptance, tend to be sited primarily in urban locations. Even within larger metropolitan areas, specific neighborhoods or communities can bar licensed clinics.

Inadequate treatment capacity creates another barrier for potential patients who do live in reasonable proximity to a licensed clinic: Many clinics have waiting lists that discourage potential patients from even attempting entry.

Many more potential patients lack the financial resources to pay for their treatment. In several states, Medicaid does not cover the cost of treatment in federally licensed clinics. Medicare does not cover this service at all.

Finally, the very nature of licensed opioid agonist treatment clinics, with the potential to be recognized and stigmatized by passersby, waiting lines for medication administration, rigid attendance policies, and lack of privacy, deters some potential patients.

However, three important developments have now altered the landscape.

1. Since March 2000, licensed opioid agonist treatment programs can apply for exceptions so that stable, long-term patients can enter methadone medical maintenance and have visits to obtain medication less frequently than once per week.
2. The Drug Addiction Treatment Act, passed in 2000, allows qualified physicians and (with rule changes in 2016) qualified nurse practitioners and physician assistants to prescribe certain opioid agonist medication in office-based settings.
3. In October 2002, the US Food and Drug Administration approved buprenorphine and buprenorphine/naloxone for the treatment of opioid dependence (now called opioid use disorder). These medications were placed in Schedule III and are available for use in office-based opioid treatment.

RESEARCH ISSUES
Research Related to Stable, Long-Term Patients in Office-Based Practices

The available research regarding patients on methadone maintenance who have achieved some measure of stability shows that most can transfer successfully to office-based care. In addition, in virtually all cases, patients who fail in an office-based treatment because of substance relapse or rule violations can be returned from office-based care to licensed opioid treatment clinic care to receive intensified counseling and monitoring without undue harm. The controlled studies also suggest that relapse or other problems in previously stable patients in office-based practice occur at rates no greater than those of similarly stable patients who remain in licensed opioid treatment clinic care.

Research Related to Patients Entering Directly Into Office-Based Practices

In Scotland, most patients who receive methadone have it prescribed in general practitioners' offices and ingest it in community pharmacies. England also has had a policy since the 1980s of encouraging individuals with OUD to get methadone maintenance treatment (MMT) through office-based treatment by general practitioners. General practitioners in France can prescribe up to 28 days' supply of take-home medications and a maximum daily buprenorphine dose of 16 mg. Thousands of patients per year have received buprenorphine in this office-based paradigm.

Multiple studies of direct office entry for opioid maintenance treatment have been conducted in the United States since the 1990s. All of these early evaluations of direct entry to office-based treatment for opioid addiction support its viability as a treatment option and show its acceptance by patients, physicians, and pharmacists. Treatment retention in these office-based investigations did not fall markedly below—nor did illicit opiate use rise strikingly above—rates reported in recent clinic-based investigations of opioid agonist treatment.

Recent work indicates that although many patients initiated on an office-based treatment with buprenorphine leave treatment too soon, patients who remain in office-based treatments over a period of years reduce their illicit opioid use to negligible amounts. In addition, other studies have shown that adding intensive counseling such as cognitive–behavioral therapy to physician management alone for patients in office-based buprenorphine programs did not improve outcomes. Thus, high-quality physician management, as described, is a very potent intervention for these patients when provided in conjunction with buprenorphine treatment.

CLINICAL ISSUES

The patient assessment and the appropriate selection of patients for transfer from clinic-based to office-based care are key elements of a comprehensive paradigm. Studies suggest that more episodes of MMT and longer time in treatment are associated with a greater likelihood of a good outcome after transfer to office-based care.

Hair testing studies suggest that many of the patients who relapse after transfer to office-based care had intermittent ongoing use while still in methadone clinic care and that this ongoing use was missed because of infrequent urine toxicology testing. Because hair testing is not routinely available, an alternative might be to obtain weekly or more frequent urine screens for some period before the anticipated transfer of any apparently stable patient from a licensed clinic to office-based care.

How thoroughly one would assess and how stringently one would screen patients for potential transfer to office-based care may depend on how much illicit substance use is to be tolerated in the office-based setting. Safety concerns would dictate that patients who are using illicit drugs should not have any take-home methadone to minimize the potential for overdose.

Patients who use illicit drugs may pose a greater risk of diverting methadone to raise cash to buy drugs. Nevertheless, the controlled studies indicate that substance use did not differ on the basis of treatment in office-based versus standard clinic care.

Office-based practitioners vary in their ability to tolerate and manage relapse. Some may feel very uncomfortable and immediately wish to transfer the patient back to licensed clinic care, whereas others may prefer to intensify services in other ways.

A monitoring plan that would be practical in an office-based setting would involve the following:

1. Monthly nonrandom urine specimens at the time of scheduled office visits
2. A few unscheduled callbacks per year, with medication checks and provision of random urine specimens
3. A very quick callback after any positive urine specimen to obtain a repeat specimen within a few days

Psychosocial interventions form another potentially valuable element of office-based treatment for transferred patients. Such interventions would be brief and might be minimal or unnecessary for highly stable, long-term patients.

In the context of an office visit, it would be desirable for the physician to ask about the patient's drug and alcohol use and cravings, how the patient is doing at work and/or with family or childcare responsibilities and financial and housing circumstances, about psychiatric and medical status, and about the use of leisure time.

The majority of patients who now enter office-based treatment for OUD do so directly and not in transfer from licensed opioid treatment programs. To a great extent, patient selection for direct entry into office-based treatment must rely on the specific areas of expertise and clinical skills of the treating provider.

With a thorough assessment, including a complete history and physical examination, the physician should ascertain whether he or she can comfortably manage—either by direct care and/or by adequate referral networks—the combination of substance use problems, general medical problems, psychiatric problems, and life crises likely to arise in the treatment of each patient. Providers should

exercise caution and refer patients who are not good candidates for their practice setting to licensed treatment programs or to other office-based providers who have the expertise to handle such patients.

No solid scientific data are available to guide precise techniques or monitoring schedules. Urine toxicology testing and periodic medication callbacks, coupled with regular clinical evaluation, likely will continue to serve as the mainstays of monitoring. For newly entering patients, tight control of medication dispensing, when practical, likely will enhance the patient's progress toward stability.

Buprenorphine and buprenorphine/naloxone are the only agonist medications approved for the treatment of patients directly entering office-based care in the United States. Although daily observation of medication ingestion would not be practical in most office-based settings, buprenorphine can be administered effectively three times a week, a schedule that probably is feasible in some office-based settings and/or their affiliated community pharmacies.

Indicators of ensuing clinical stability include the following:

1. Compliant behavior
2. Regular, timely attendance at scheduled office visits
3. Successful compliance with medication callbacks
4. Negative urine toxicology tests
5. Productive use of time
6. Supportive interpersonal relationships
7. Absence of criminal justice involvement

Careful pharmacotherapy of newly entering patients can contribute to their stability. Providers should frequently inquire about symptoms such as rhinorrhea, lacrimation, chills, nausea, diarrhea, muscle aches, and insomnia and assess whether these symptoms could be related to opioid withdrawal. They should query patients about thoughts of drug use or cravings. If such symptoms are occurring, an increase in the medication dose should be given serious consideration. Similarly, physicians should ask about possible side effects (such as constipation, excess sedation, or lowered libido) that may suggest the need for a reduction in dose.

The potential for medication diversion plays into decisions about medication dose and frequency of dispensing. Diversion by a patient undermines and endangers the patient's efforts toward achieving a stable recovery from OUD.

Possible signs of diversion include failing a medication callback, a request for early refills, a sudden unexplained increase in disposable income, a sudden request for a dose increase in a previously stable patient without an apparent explanation for instability, or a urine specimen negative for the presence of buprenorphine and its metabolite, nor-buprenorphine.

Diversion can be prevented at the outset by using a provider-initiated written treatment agreement detailing consequences of diversion, which could include loss of take-home medication privileges, more frequent medication callbacks, or ultimately discontinuation of treatment for repeated episodes of diversion. Repeated episodes of diversion clearly indicate that office-based treatment is not an appropriate setting and consideration for transfer to a more structured, licensed program may be required.

Psychosocial treatments may be even more important to some patients who are newly entering office-based treatment programs than to stable patients who already have received regular counseling at a licensed program. Studies of various intensities of psychosocial services in licensed methadone programs do offer some illumination on this point: Patients who receive minimal psychosocial services do not fare as well as do those who receive moderate or high levels of services; however, the higher cost of more intensive services may nullify any slight advantage they hold over moderate services. Some recent studies of patients newly entering buprenorphine/naloxone treatment programs showed no advantage in treatment outcomes with the addition of extra counseling added to physician visits compared to physician visits alone. So, for many patients, basic counseling provided by the provider during visits to prescribe medication may be sufficient.

At present, physicians are eligible to practice office-based treatment of opioid addiction with the completion of 8 hours of formal training. In states where it is permitted, nurse practitioners and physician assistants are eligible to practice office-based treatment upon completion of 24 hours of formal training. Expert consensus suggests that appropriate training should consist of most of the following topics:

1. Overview of opioid dependence and rationale for agonist treatment
2. Legislation permitting office-based treatment with general opioid pharmacology
3. General opioid pharmacology
4. Pharmacology of buprenorphine and buprenorphine/naloxone
5. Efficacy and safety of buprenorphine
6. Clinical use of buprenorphine including induction, stabilization, and withdrawal

7. Patient assessment and selection
8. Office management, including treatment agreements, urine testing, record keeping, and confidentiality
9. Co-occurring psychiatric and medical disorders
10. Psychosocial treatments
11. Special populations including adolescents, pregnant women, and patients with pain

KEY POINTS

1. A high demand exists for medication treatment for opioid use disorders.
2. This demand can be addressed in part through office-based opioid treatment.
3. In the United States, buprenorphine and buprenorphine/naloxone are the two medications approved and available for office-based opioid treatment.
4. With required training, a bit of experience, and use of straightforward monitoring techniques physicians, nurse practitioners, and physician assistants can successfully treat opioid use disorder in their offices with these medications.

REVIEW QUESTIONS

1. A patient with opioid addiction was inducted on buprenorphine/naloxone, and the dosage was increased to 16 mg/4 mg within 1 week to manage withdrawal symptoms. The patient returns to the office for an evaluation, provides a urine specimen positive for opiates, and admits to injecting heroin again a few times because he was not sleeping well. Which of the following is the most reasonable immediate response?
   A. Increase the amount of medication prescribed with longer intervals between office visits.
   B. Increase the dosage of buprenorphine/naloxone.
   C. Discontinue buprenorphine/naloxone.
   D. Refer for increased counseling.
   E. Stop urine toxicology testing altogether to save resources.

2. Which of the following is an opioid withdrawal symptom suggesting that a patient on methadone or buprenorphine/naloxone in office-based treatment program may need an increase in medication dosage?
   A. Drowsiness
   B. Constipation
   C. Chills
   D. Headache
   E. Urinary hesitancy

3. Which of the following procedures serves as both a deterrent to and a way to detect medication diversion from office-based treatment?
   A. A written treatment agreement
   B. Surveillance cameras
   C. Body search
   D. Medication callback
   E. Keeping the medication dose low

ANSWERS

1. **B.** The patient is still having withdrawal symptoms (insomnia) and needs a higher dosage to relieve the symptoms.
2. **C.** The other listed symptoms are all side effects of opioids.
3. **D.** A written agreement would deter but not detect diversion. Surveillance cameras and a body search would be impractical and unpleasant for patients in a healthcare setting. Keeping the dose low could contribute to instability.

SUGGESTED READINGS

Carroll KM, Weiss RD. The role of behavioral interventions in buprenorphine maintenance treatment: a review. *Am J Psychiatry.* 2017;174(8):738-747.

Fiellin DA, Moore BA, Sullivan LE, et al. Long-term treatment with buprenorphine/naloxone in primary care: results at 2-5 years. *Am J Addict.* 2008;17(2):116-120.

Fudala PJ, Bridge TP, Herbert S, et al. Office-based treatment of opiate addiction with a sublingual-tablet formulation of buprenorphine and naloxone. *N Engl J Med.* 2003;349(10): 949-958.

King VL, Kidorf MS, Stoller KB, et al. A 12-month controlled trial of methadone medical maintenance integrated into an adaptive treatment model. *J Subst Abuse Treat.* 2006;31(4): 385-393.

Salsitz EA, Joseph H, Frank B, et al. Methadone medical maintenance (MMM): treating chronic opioid dependence in private medical practice—a summary report (1983-1998). *Mount Sinai J Med.* 2000;67(5-6):388-397.

Concerning Veterans and Office-Based Treatment of Opioid Use Disorder

Summary by Tim K. Brennan

Based on THE ASAM PRINCIPLES OF ADDICTION MEDICINE, 6th edition sidebar by Tim K. Brennan

Office-based treatment with buprenorphine has seen a rapid uptake for veterans with an opioid use disorder who are treated by the Department of Veterans Affairs (VA). In 2004, there were 300 patients receiving buprenorphine at the VA. By 2010, there were 6147 patients receiving buprenorphine, and in 2016, there were 12,525 patients. Unfortunately, these 12,525 patients only represent 20.9% of the total number of veterans receiving care for opioid use disorder at the VA. Another 6.8% of veterans receive treatment with naltrexone. This means approximately 72% of veterans receiving opioid use disorder treatment at the VA are not receiving buprenorphine or naltrexone. Although some of these veterans may be on methadone maintenance treatment, one wonders how many of them would prefer the ease of being on buprenorphine instead. Of course, this treatment gap is not unique to the VA, and there remains a clear nationwide need for more incentives for widespread implementation of buprenorphine prescribing.

Pharmacological Treatment of Stimulant Use Disorders

Summary by David A. Gorelick

Based on THE ASAM PRINCIPLES OF ADDICTION MEDICINE, 6th edition chapter by David A. Gorelick

Stimulants such as cocaine and amphetamines are the second most widely used illegal drugs in the United States, surpassed only by cannabis.

There is no US Food and Drug Administration (FDA)-approved pharmacotherapy for stimulant use disorder. As such, all of the medications referenced in this chapter are being used in an "off-label" capacity.

COCAINE USE DISORDER

Goals of Treatment

The behavioral mechanisms by which medication achieves treatment goals are poorly understood and can vary across patients and medications.

Currently available medications are considered to act by one or more of three mechanisms:

1. Reducing or eliminating the positive reinforcement from taking a cocaine dose
2. Reducing or eliminating a subjective state (such as "craving") that predisposes a person to taking cocaine
3. Reducing or eliminating negative reinforcement from taking a cocaine dose (as by reducing withdrawal-associated dysphoria)

Medication does not address other mechanisms such as making cocaine-taking aversive and increasing the positive reinforcement obtained from non–cocaine-taking behaviors. The latter is crucial to successful treatment because it ensures that other behaviors are reinforced to replace cocaine taking as it is extinguished. However, such medications do not exist and, as a result, this mechanism is engaged by psychosocial interventions that address issues such as vocational rehabilitation, the patient's social network, and use of leisure time.

Medication is almost never used without some psychosocial treatment component.

The type, intensity, and duration of psychosocial treatment that should accompany pharmacologic treatment are questions with little data to guide clinical decision making.

Pharmacologic Mechanisms

Four pharmacologic approaches are potentially useful in the treatment of cocaine use disorder:

1. Substitution treatment with a cross-tolerant stimulant (analogous to methadone or buprenorphine maintenance treatment for opioid use disorder)
2. Treatment with an antagonist medication that blocks the binding of cocaine at its site of action
3. Treatment with a medication that functionally antagonizes the effects of cocaine (as by reducing the reinforcing effects of or craving for cocaine)
4. Alteration of cocaine pharmacokinetics so that less drug reaches or remains at its site(s) of action in the brain

No medication currently is approved by the FDA or any other national health authority for the treatment of cocaine use disorder, chiefly because no medication has met the scientifically rigorous standard of consistent, statistically significant efficacy in replicated, controlled clinical trials.

Cocaine's positively reinforcing effects derive from its blockade of the dopamine reuptake pump, causing presynaptically released dopamine to remain in the synapse and enhancing dopaminergic neurotransmission.

Cocaine's local anesthetic effects are believed to contribute to cocaine-induced kindling, the phenomenon by which previous exposure to cocaine sensitizes the individual so that later exposure to low doses produces an enhanced response.

CHOICE OF MEDICATION

Antidepressants

A systematic review and meta-analysis of 28 published clinical trials found that antidepressants as a class (including tricyclics, selective serotonin reuptake inhibitors, serotonin-norepinephrine uptake inhibitors, and the monoamine oxidase inhibitor selegiline) were no more effective than placebo in terms of dropout from treatment or number of weeks of continuous cocaine abstinence. However, there was some variation in efficacy across types of antidepressants.

Heterocyclic Antidepressants

Tricyclic and other heterocyclic antidepressants are the most widely used and best studied class of medications for the treatment of cocaine use disorder.

A systematic review and meta-analysis of 18 published clinical trials (17 with desipramine, 1 with imipramine) found no advantage over placebo for dropout rates but a significant advantage in proportion of participants achieving at least 3 weeks of continuous abstinence. This advantage over placebo disappeared when the analysis was limited to the three studies that involved participants with moderate-to-severe cocaine use disorder, suggesting that the therapeutic effect is not very robust.

Patients with depression and without antisocial personality disorder may respond best to **desipramine**. Patients dually dependent on cocaine and opioids may do better on **desipramine** if their opioid use disorder is treated with **buprenorphine** rather than methadone, or if they receive contingency management.

No unexpected or medically serious side effects have been reported in published clinical trials of heterocyclic antidepressants. However, patients who relapse to cocaine use while still on antidepressant medications could, in theory, be at increased risk of cardiovascular side effects. Both cocaine and the tricyclics have quinidine-like membrane effects that, when superimposed, could lead to cardiac arrhythmias.

Selective Serotonin Reuptake Inhibitors

A systematic review and meta-analysis of eight published clinical trials (five with fluoxetine, one each with citalopram, paroxetine, and sertraline) found no significant advantage over placebo in dropout rates or craving for cocaine.

Monoamine Oxidase Inhibitors

Selegiline, marketed in the transdermal form for treatment of depression, is fairly selective for monoamine oxidase type B (the predominant type in the brain) at recommended doses (10 mg per day for parkinsonism, 12 mg per day for depression). A recent multisite controlled clinical trial using **selegiline** administered via a skin patch (**selegiline** transdermal system) found no evidence for efficacy in cocaine use disorder.

Dopamine Agonists (Antiparkinson Agents)

A systematic review and meta-analysis of 24 published clinical trials that evaluated direct dopamine receptor agonists (bromocriptine, pergolide, pramipexole, cabergoline, hydergine), the indirect dopamine agonist amantadine, and the amino acid dopamine precursor L-dopa together as a class found no evidence of efficacy compared to placebo.

Disulfiram can be considered a functional dopamine agonist because it blocks the conversion of dopamine to norepinephrine by the enzyme dopamine β-hydroxylase, thereby increasing dopamine concentrations. Several of the dozen published controlled clinical trials found disulfiram (250 mg per day) more effective than placebo. Some of this heterogeneity in treatment response may be due to genetic factors, such as activity of the enzyme dopamine β-hydroxylase and allelic variation in the dopamine D2 and α1A-adrenergic receptors.

Stimulants

A systematic review and meta-analysis of 14 published clinical trials found that stimulants as a class (including dexamphetamine, mixed amphetamine salts, methamphetamine, lisdexamfetamine, methylphenidate, modafinil, and mazindol) were significantly better than placebo in promoting at least 3 weeks of sustained abstinence but did not increase proportion of cocaine-free urine samples among those who did not achieve sustained abstinence or improve study retention. Among specific stimulants, only dexamphetamine (three studies) and mixed amphetamine salts (one study) were significantly better than placebo in promoting at least 3 weeks of sustained abstinence. None of these studies reported significant adverse effects, suggesting that stimulant substitution treatment might be safe in patients who use cocaine.

Antipsychotics

The older (first generation) antipsychotics, which are potent dopamine receptor antagonists (chiefly

D2 [postsynaptic] subtype), do not significantly alter cocaine craving or use. A systematic review and meta-analysis of 14 published clinical trials found that the newer (second generation) antipsychotics as a class (aripiprazole, olanzapine, quetiapine, risperidone) reduced study dropout, but did not significantly reduce the proportion of subjects achieving at least 3 weeks of continuous abstinence or the number of participants using cocaine during treatment.

Caution should be exercised when prescribing any antipsychotic to cocaine users because of their potential vulnerability to neuroleptic malignant syndrome. Cocaine or amphetamine users may also be at elevated risk of antipsychotic-induced movement disorders.

Anticonvulsants

A systematic review and meta-analysis of 20 published clinical trials found that anticonvulsants as a class (carbamazepine, gabapentin, lamotrigine, phenytoin, tiagabine, topiramate, and vigabatrin) had no significant effect on dropout rate, cocaine use, or cocaine craving. A separate meta-analysis including only the two topiramate trials found a significant benefit for topiramate over placebo. A recent controlled clinical trial (not included in either meta-analysis) also found topiramate (maximum dose 200 mg daily) performed significantly better than placebo for increasing cocaine-negative urine samples and reducing self-reported cocaine use for amount; mean reduction −0.78 times per week for frequency but only during the first 4 weeks of the 12-week trial.

Nutritional Supplements and Herbal Products

Nutritional Supplements

There is no evidence from controlled clinical trials that the use of amino acid mixtures, either alone or with other nutritional supplements (vitamins and minerals) or of various herbal and plant-derived products, has any efficacy in the treatment of substance use disorders.

Calcium Channel Blockers

There is no evidence for the efficacy of calcium channel blockers (such as amlodipine) in the treatment of cocaine addiction.

Other Physical Treatments

Meta-analyses of nine published studies found no significant benefit of active acupuncture over sham treatment for the treatment of drug withdrawal (including cocaine), including studies using acupuncture of the outer ear at the five standard locations recommended by the National Acupuncture Detoxification Association.

AMPHETAMINE USE DISORDER

As with cocaine use disorder, controlled clinical trials find that most medications do not show efficacy for the treatment of amphetamine use disorder. The most promising approaches to date are agonist substitution with stimulants and blockade of μ-opioid receptors.

Three of five controlled clinical trials with D-amphetamine (one using a sustained-release formulation) found a significant reduction in amphetamine or methamphetamine use compared with placebo as did one controlled clinical trial with slow-release methylphenidate (54 mg daily).

The μ-opioid receptor antagonist naltrexone, marketed for the treatment of alcohol and opioid use disorder, significantly reduced amphetamine use in controlled clinical trials in both oral and subcutaneous implant formulations. It is still considered "off label" for use in amphetamine use disorder.

SPECIAL TREATMENT SITUATIONS
Mixed Use Disorders
Opioid Use Disorder

Concurrent opioid use disorder is a common clinical problem among patients with cocaine use disorder. Three different pharmacologic approaches have been used for the treatment of such patients with dual cocaine and opioid use disorders:

1. Adjustment of methadone dose
2. Maintenance with another opioid medication
3. Addition of medication targeting the cocaine dependence

Higher methadone doses (usually 60 mg or more daily) generally are associated with less opioid use by patients in methadone maintenance. This relationship also holds in general for cocaine use among patients in methadone maintenance programs, although exceptions have been reported. Increasing the methadone dose as a contingency in response to cocaine use can be effective at reducing such use (and more so than decreasing the methadone dose in response to a cocaine-positive urine sample).

Buprenorphine is a partial opioid agonist (μ-receptor agonist/κ-receptor antagonist) used for the agonist substitution treatment of opioid use disorder. Some (but not all) studies in patients with both opioid and cocaine use disorder suggest that cocaine use (as well as opioid use) is reduced at higher buprenorphine doses (16 to 32 mg daily).

Alcohol Use Disorder

Alcohol use disorder is common in patients with cocaine use disorder, with comorbidity rates of up to 90% and is associated with poorer treatment outcomes. Possible mechanisms include the following:

1. Production of the toxic psychoactive metabolite cocaethylene
2. Stimulation of cocaine craving by alcohol
3. Alteration of medication metabolism by the hepatic effects of alcohol

Psychiatric Comorbidities

Patients with cocaine use disorder have high rates of psychiatric comorbidity (ie, psychiatric diagnoses other than another substance use disorder), with rates as high as 65% for lifetime disorders and 50% for current disorders.

The most common comorbid disorders are major depression, bipolar spectrum, phobias, and posttraumatic stress disorder.

Personality disorders are common among treatment-seeking individuals who are cocaine-dependent, with rates in this population as high as 69%. The most common of these is antisocial personality disorder.

Depression

Desipramine, **imipramine**, and **bupropion** have usually, but not always, been found effective, whereas selective serotonin reuptake inhibitors (eg, **fluoxetine**) are usually not effective.

Bipolar Disorder

Case series and open-label trials suggest that "mood-stabilizing" anticonvulsants such as **valproate**, **divalproex**, **lamotrigine**, and **carbamazepine** are more effective than lithium at reducing cocaine use in dually diagnosed patients. Combining **lithium** with an anticonvulsant may be helpful in treatment-resistant patients.

Second-generation antipsychotics have generated mixed results in patients with cocaine use disorder.

Attention Deficit Hyperactivity Disorder

Up to one fourth of adults with cocaine use disorder have either adult attention deficit hyperactivity disorder (ADHD) or a history of childhood ADHD. Clinical trials generally show efficacy in reducing cocaine use for the commonly used ADHD medications dextroamphetamine (up to 60 mg per day), methamphetamine (15 mg per day), and bupropion (up to 100 mg three times a day), but not for methylphenidate or atomoxetine.

Schizophrenia

Although schizophrenia is not a common comorbid psychiatric disorder among individuals with cocaine use disorder, cocaine use is common among treatment-seeking patients with schizophrenia.

First-generation (so-called "typical") antipsychotics, at doses that are effective in the treatment of schizophrenia, do not significantly alter cocaine craving or use.

Several case series and open-label trials suggest that the second-generation (so-called "atypical") antipsychotics, including clozapine, olanzapine, quetiapine, risperidone, and aripiprazole, may be more effective at reducing cocaine and other drug use among patients with schizophrenia, but this has not been confirmed in several controlled clinical trials.

Gender-Specific Issues

Women tend to be excluded from or underrepresented in many clinical trials of cocaine use disorder pharmacotherapy, in part because of concern, embodied in former FDA regulations, over the risk to the fetus and neonate should a female participant become pregnant. In the absence of directly relevant and systematically collected data, caution should be used when prescribing medications to pregnant women with stimulant use disorder and to those with pregnancy potential, keeping in mind both the risks of medication and the risks of continued stimulant use. Tricyclic antidepressants, bupropion, and buprenorphine appear to have little potential for morphologic teratogenicity or disruption of pregnancy, although there are little or no data on behavioral teratogenicity.

Amantadine is associated with pregnancy complications, lithium with cardiac malformations and neonatal toxicity, anticonvulsants with increased risk of congenital malformations, and antipsychotics with nonspecific congenital anomalies and neonatal withdrawal.

Disulfiram and naltrexone may generate different treatment responses in men versus women. The reasons for such gender differences are poorly understood but may include differences in medication pharmacokinetics, hormonal interactions, or subjects' psychological and/or socioeconomic status.

Age

Although adolescents constitute a substantial minority of heavy cocaine users, they have been largely excluded from clinical trials of cocaine pharmacotherapies because of legal and informed consent considerations.

KEY POINTS

1. There are no FDA-approved pharmacotherapies for cocaine use disorder.
2. There are no FDA-approved pharmacotherapies for amphetamine use disorder.
3. Some medications are used in an "off-label" capacity as clinicians await the results of clinical trials.

REVIEW QUESTIONS

1. Which of the following is *not* a common pharmacologic approach to the treatment of stimulant use disorder?
   A. Functionally antagonize effects of the stimulant.
   B. Create an aversive contingency for taking the stimulant.
   C. Substitute with a cross-tolerant stimulant.
   D. Block stimulant binding to its site of action.

2. Which of the following antidepressants has evidence from more than one controlled clinical trial for efficacy in treating cocaine use disorder?
   A. Desipramine
   B. Sertraline
   C. Selegiline
   D. Phenelzine

3. Which of the following medications can be considered a functional dopamine agonist?
   A. Olanzapine
   B. Carbamazepine
   C. Amlodipine
   D. Disulfiram

ANSWERS

1. **B**
2. **A**
3. **D**

SUGGESTED READINGS

Castells X, Cunill R, Pérez-Mañá C, Vidal X, Capellà D. Psychostimulant drugs for cocaine dependence. *Cochrane Database Syst Rev.* 2016;(9):CD007380.

Gorelick DA. Pharmacokinetic strategies for treatment of drug overdose and addiction. *Future Med Chem.* 2012;4(2):227-243.

Indave BI, Minozzi S, Pani PP, Amato L. Antipsychotic medications for cocaine dependence. *Cochrane Database Syst Rev.* 2016;(3):CD006306.

Mills EJ, Wu P, Gagnier J, Ebbert JO. Efficacy of acupuncture for cocaine dependence: a systematic review & meta-analysis. *Harm Reduction J.* 2005;2(1):4.

Minozzi S, Amato L, Pani PP, et al. Dopamine agonists for the treatment of cocaine dependence. *Cochrane Database Syst Rev.* 2015;(5):CD003352.

Minozzi S, Cinquini M, Amato L, et al. Anticonvulsants for cocaine dependence. *Cochrane Database Syst Rev.* 2015;(4):CD006754.

60

Pharmacological Interventions for Tobacco Use Disorder

Summary by Jon O. Ebbert, J. Taylor Hays, David D. McFadden, Ryan T. Hurt, and Richard D. Hurt

Based on THE ASAM PRINCIPLES OF ADDICTION MEDICINE, 6th edition chapter by Jon O. Ebbert, J. Taylor Hays, David D. McFadden, Ryan T. Hurt, and Richard D. Hurt

Each year, 480,000 Americans die of tobacco-related diseases. The epidemic of tobacco-caused diseases has spread throughout the world, and globally, about 6 million people die annually of tobacco-related diseases; by 2030, the annual rate is expected to rise to 8 million tobacco-related deaths.

In this chapter, we review the neurobiologic basis for tobacco use disorder, discuss available pharmacotherapeutic strategies, and provide guidance for the optimal use of pharmacotherapy in a clinical setting.

NEUROBIOLOGY OF TOBACCO USE DISORDER

The neurobiology of tobacco use disorder provides both a rationale for pharmacotherapy and a framework for understanding why medications sometimes fail. Nicotine has multiple and complex effects on the central nervous system. The binding of nicotine to nicotinic acetylcholine receptors (nAChRs) results in conformational changes of the receptors. This stimulation of nAChRs results in the release of dopamine, norepinephrine, glutamate, vasopressin, serotonin, γ-aminobutyric acid, β-endorphins, and other neurotransmitters. In the mesolimbic system, or "reward center," nicotine causes the release of dopamine, creating positive reinforcing effects and serving as a critical mediator of addiction.

Our understanding of the neurobiology of tobacco use disorder places several important facts regarding pharmacotherapeutic interventions into context: (1) rapid delivery of nicotine by conventional tobacco cigarettes facilitates the development of tobacco use disorder, (2) nicotine replacement therapy (NRT) products approved by the US Food and Drug Administration (FDA) to treat tobacco use disorder are relatively inefficient mechanisms for

nicotine delivery, and (3) nonnicotine medications have mechanisms of action and targets that allow them to be used in combination with NRT.

NICOTINE REPLACEMENT THERAPY

The FDA has approved five nicotine replacement products for the treatment of tobacco use disorder: nicotine gum, nicotine patches, nicotine nasal spray, a nicotine vapor inhaler, and nicotine lozenges. NRT comes in two main types: short-acting NRT (gum, lozenge, nasal spray, and inhaler) and longer-acting NRT (nicotine patch). If NRT is selected for treatment, combination therapy with a nicotine patch and a short-acting NRT is usually preferred over monotherapy with a short-acting NRT product.

Nicotine Gum

Nicotine gum is available in over-the-counter 2- and 4-mg doses and is effective as monotherapy or in combination with other forms of NRT.

Nicotine Lozenge

Nicotine lozenges are available in 2-mg and 4-mg over-the-counter doses. As with the other short-acting NRT products, lozenges are most often used in combination with other NRT products and nonnicotine pharmacotherapies.

Nicotine Nasal Spray

Nicotine nasal spray requires a prescription in the United States, delivers nicotine directly to the nasal mucosa, and is effective for achieving abstinence as monotherapy. The nasal spray device delivers nicotine more rapidly than other forms of NRT and reduces withdrawal symptoms quickly.

Nicotine Inhaler

The nicotine vapor inhaler, which is also a prescription product in the United States, is effective for increasing abstinence as monotherapy but only with extensive use (greater than six cartridges per day).

Nicotine Patch

Nicotine patches are available in over-the-counter doses of 7 mg, 14 mg, and 21 mg. In almost every randomized clinical trial performed to date, nicotine patch therapy has been demonstrated to be effective compared with placebo, usually with a doubling of the abstinence rate. Use of high doses of nicotine patch therapy (>21 mg per day) is appropriate for patients who previously failed standard-dose patch therapy (≤21 mg per day) or for individuals who experience nicotine withdrawal symptoms with standard-dose patch therapy. Patients who smoke more heavily will be significantly underdosed with standard-dose patch therapy. High-dose nicotine patch therapy has been shown to be safe and well tolerated in patients who smoke more than 20 cigarettes per day. The nicotine patch dose can be estimated based on the number of cigarettes smoked per day (Table 60-1).

Side effects of nicotine patch therapy are relatively mild and include localized skin reactions at the patch site. Topical corticosteroid therapy may be helpful in controlling these local symptoms. Rotation of the patches to different sites of the skin helps to reduce the frequency of this side effect. Vivid dreams can occur with nicotine patch therapy. Patches can be left on at night if individuals wake up with significant tobacco cravings and a strong desire to smoke. However, if patches keep patients awake, they can be taken off at night and a new one can be applied the next morning.

TABLE 60-1 Recommended Initial Dosing of Nicotine Patch Therapy Based on the Number of Cigarettes Smoked Daily

Cigarettes Smoked per Day	Patch Dose (mg/d)[a]
<10	7–14
10–20	14–21
21–40	21–42
>40	≥42

[a]Nicotine patches are available in the following doses: 7 mg, 14 mg, and 21 mg.

NONNICOTINE MEDICATIONS
Bupropion Sustained Release

Bupropion is a monocyclic antidepressant that inhibits the reuptake of both norepinephrine and dopamine. Bupropion is hypothesized to be effective for patients through its dopaminergic activity on the pleasure and reward pathways in the mesolimbic system and nucleus accumbens. Bupropion also has an antagonist effect on nAChRs.

Bupropion sustained release (SR) is the formulation approved by the FDA for the treatment of tobacco use disorder. Bupropion SR 300 mg per day attenuates weight gain during treatment among patients who are continuously abstinent from smoking. Treatment with bupropion SR should be initiated 1 week before the tobacco quit date at an initial dose of 150 mg per day for 3 days and then increased to 150 mg twice daily. The usual length of treatment is 6 to 12 weeks, but bupropion SR can be safely used longer. As with other antidepressants, this medication is associated with a small risk of seizures (0.1%). Therefore, bupropion SR is contraindicated for those who have a history of seizures, serious head trauma with skull fracture, or a prolonged loss of consciousness; an eating disorder (ie, anorexia nervosa or bulimia); or in those with concomitant use of medications that lower the seizure threshold. The most common adverse effects of bupropion SR are insomnia and dry mouth. If individuals experience insomnia, taking bupropion SR once per day may be as effective and will decrease the insomnia.

Varenicline

Varenicline selectively binds to the $\alpha_4\beta_2$ nAChRs, where it both blocks nicotine from binding to the receptor (antagonist effect) and stimulates receptor-mediated activity (agonist effect), leading to the release of dopamine. Varenicline has been shown to reduce cravings and nicotine withdrawal symptoms. Varenicline is not metabolized and is excreted virtually unchanged in the urine with a serum half-life of 17 hours.

Seminal clinical trials have demonstrated varenicline to be more effective than placebo or bupropion SR for achieving abstinence, with end-of-treatment continuous smoking abstinence rates (ie, no smoking since the target quit date) of 44% for varenicline, 30% for bupropion SR, and 18% for placebo (odds ratio of 3.85 for varenicline compared to placebo). The end-of-treatment 7-day point prevalence smoking abstinence rates (ie, no smoking, not even a "puff," in the last 7 days) were approximately

50% for varenicline, 35% for bupropion SR, and 20% for placebo. An additional 12 weeks of varenicline (24 weeks total) was effective at maintaining abstinence in patients who had stopped smoking after 12 weeks of open-label varenicline treatment; in this study, 70% of patients receiving varenicline were continuously abstinent from weeks 13 to 24 compared with 50% assigned to placebo ($p < 0.001$). A Cochrane meta-analysis concluded that varenicline is superior to bupropion and single forms of NRT but comparable to multiple forms of NRT taken simultaneously (eg, nicotine patch and nicotine nasal spray).

Varenicline has been studied in patients with chronic obstructive pulmonary disease and patients with stable coronary heart disease with impressive end-of-treatment smoking abstinence rates (odds ratios of 8 and 6, respectively, compared to placebo). In a randomized, placebo-controlled trial of patients with schizophrenia or schizoaffective disorder, varenicline was efficacious (end-of-treatment smoking abstinence 19% versus 5% for placebo) with no evidence of exacerbation of psychiatric symptoms. Among patients with schizophrenia and bipolar disease who attained initial abstinence with varenicline, maintenance of abstinence with varenicline significantly improved outcomes after 1 year of treatment and was not associated with adverse psychiatric effects.

Treatment with varenicline should be initiated 1 to 5 weeks before the patient's stop date at a dose of 0.5 mg daily for 3 days, with an increase to 0.5 mg twice per day for the subsequent 4 days, and a second increase to 1 mg twice per day for the duration of therapy. The initial course of treatment is 12 weeks, but clinical trials suggest that continuing varenicline for a total of 24 weeks increases abstinence rates. The long-term safety of varenicline has been evaluated in a 52-week placebo-controlled trial. In this study, 37% of patients who used cigarettes who were treated with varenicline were abstinent, compared with 8% in the placebo group. Available data suggest that varenicline is as effective in those with light physical dependence (eg, 5 to 10 cigarettes per day) as it is in those with heavier physical dependence.

The most frequent adverse effect of varenicline is nausea, which is reported by approximately 30% of the participants. The nausea is most often mild to moderate, and study participants infrequently discontinue therapy due to nausea (<3%).

In February 2008, the FDA issued a public health advisory because of postmarketing surveillance reports of suicidal thoughts and aggressive or erratic behavior in people who had taken varenicline. However, a reanalysis of 17 clinical trials conducted with varenicline revealed no evidence that varenicline is associated with adverse psychiatric events. Additionally, meta-analyses have not observed a link between varenicline and risk of suicide or attempted suicide, suicidal ideation, depression, or death. A large clinical trial randomly assigned 8144 participants with and without psychiatric histories to varenicline, bupropion, nicotine patch, or placebo and observed no significant increase in neuropsychiatric adverse events, including suicide, attributable to varenicline or bupropion relative to nicotine patch or placebo. The FDA has removed the black box warning regarding serious neuropsychiatric events associated with the use of varenicline.

In 2011, a meta-analysis of 14 randomized clinical trials was published suggesting a small percentage point increase (0.24%) in serious cardiovascular events in patients receiving varenicline versus placebo. The FDA issued a warning of the potential association with cardiovascular events along with the caveat that the risk of using varenicline must be weighed against the risks of smoking. Meta-analyses have not found an increased risk of cardiovascular disease events. The only trial for which the cardiovascular status was adjudicated by an independent event committee demonstrated no significant difference in serious cardiovascular events with varenicline compared to placebo. A nationwide historical cohort in Denmark with 17,926 patients receiving varenicline and 17,926 patients receiving bupropion observed no increased risk of cardiovascular events with varenicline compared with bupropion.

The FDA also issued a warning on the risk of seizures with varenicline. Case studies of seizures have been published, but, to date, no comprehensive assessment of a link between varenicline and seizures has been published in the peer-reviewed literature. A warning was also issued regarding the possibility that varenicline changes the response to ingested alcohol. Intriguingly, varenicline has been associated with reduced alcohol consumption and cravings.

COMBINATION PHARMACOTHERAPY

Combination pharmacotherapy has been shown to increase treatment efficacy. Adding a short-acting NRT to the nicotine patch is superior to the nicotine patch alone. Nicotine lozenges in combination with standard-dose nicotine patches are more effective than other combinations. Combining bupropion with the nicotine inhaler provides a better

TABLE 60-2	Combining Long-Acting and Short-Acting Pharmacotherapy
Long-Acting (pick 1 or 2)	**Short-Acting (add 1 or 2)**
Nicotine patch	Nicotine gum
Bupropion	Nicotine inhaler
Varenicline	Nicotine lozenge
	Nicotine nasal spray

treatment effect than either alone, and triple therapy using bupropion, the nicotine inhaler, and the nicotine patch doubles the smoking abstinence rate compared to monotherapy with the nicotine patch. A meta-analysis has suggested that combining varenicline with NRT is superior to varenicline as monotherapy.

Bupropion SR and varenicline have different mechanisms of action and do not interact with each other. Data from one large, randomized, placebo-controlled clinical trial suggests that in patients who smoked more heavily ($\geq$20 cigarettes per day), the combination of varenicline and bupropion increases smoking abstinence outcomes compared to monotherapy with varenicline.

When developing treatment plans in the clinical setting, a reasonable starting point is to combine a long-acting medication (eg, nicotine patch, bupropion, and/or varenicline) with one or more short-acting NRTs (eg, nicotine gum, lozenge, inhaler, or nasal spray) for withdrawal symptom control (Table 60-2).

Cigarette Smoking Reduction

Almost one-half of current cigarette smokers report a preference to achieve smoking abstinence via tapering down the number of cigarettes smoked daily until ultimately stopping completely rather than stopping abruptly. Among cigarette smoking patients not prepared to set a quit date, NRT decreases the number of cigarettes smoked and increases smoking abstinence. Varenicline has also been demonstrated to increase smoking abstinence rates significantly more than placebo among patients willing to reduce their smoking rate before quitting.

GENETICS AND ACHIEVING SMOKING ABSTINENCE

Genetic variation within the *CHRNA5-A3-B4* gene cluster encoding nicotinic receptor subunits has been associated with success in achieving short-term smoking abstinence among patients seeking treatment. A meta-analysis concluded that *CHRNA5* genetic variation predicted delayed abstinence and an earlier age of lung cancer diagnosis. Variation in nicotine metabolism may also affect treatment outcomes. Nicotine is metabolized by the liver mixed-function oxidase system cytochrome P450 2A6 (CYP2A6). NRT may be more effective among individuals with fast rather than slow CYP2A6 nicotine metabolism.

ELECTRONIC NICOTINE DELIVERY SYSTEMS

Electronic nicotine delivery systems (ENDS) consist of battery-powered atomizers producing nicotine vapor, which then cools either in the mouthpiece of the device or in the user's mouth to form an aerosol. The liquid placed into the device, commonly referred to as "e-juice," is composed of humectants (eg, propylene glycol, vegetable glycerin), flavoring agents, and nicotine. A Cochrane systematic review concluded that weak evidence exists that ENDS containing nicotine help patients achieve tobacco abstinence in the long term compared with placebo ENDS and that ENDS have similar efficacy to nicotine patches. The long-term health consequences of ENDS remain unknown.

TREATMENT OF SMOKELESS TOBACCO USE

Smokeless tobacco is tobacco consumed orally and not burned. A Cochrane systematic review has shown that varenicline and the nicotine lozenge are effective pharmacotherapies for increasing long-term ($\geq$6 months) smokeless tobacco abstinence rates.

POSTCESSATION WEIGHT GAIN

Many individuals smoke cigarettes to control body weight. Among 4000 female smokers calling a telephone tobacco quitline, more than 50% of women of normal weight (body mass index: 18.5–24.9 kg/m^2) and more than 80% of women who are obese (body mass index: >30 kg/m^2) expressed concern about postcessation weight gain. Despite the effectiveness of pharmacotherapy in smoking abstinence, currently available medications have only minor favorable effects on postcessation weight gain. Weight gain is mildly attenuated relative to placebo at the end of 12 weeks of treatment with varenicline (−0.41 kg), NRT (−0.45 kg), and bupropion (−1.12 kg).

CLINICAL DECISIONS ABOUT PHARMACOTHERAPY

Adding pharmacotherapy to a behavioral intervention doubles smoking abstinence rates, and "real-world" studies suggest a tripling effect of combining pharmacotherapy and behavioral interventions compared to using neither. Tailoring or individualizing dosing for patients is critical to the success of pharmacotherapy. Relapse and remission characterize tobacco use disorder, and recent estimates suggest that patients may make 30 or more quit attempts before achieving lasting smoking abstinence. The patient's past experiences and preferences must be an integral part of the clinical decision-making process. We present a menu to the smoker (see Table 60-2) and discuss the rationale for pharmacotherapy along with expected effects and side effects.

Duration of Pharmacotherapy

Longer use of pharmacotherapy is useful in selected patients to maintain smoking abstinence. The optimal length of pharmacotherapy has not been established for any of the available medications. Bupropion administered for approximately 12 months to patients abstinent from smoking at the end of a short course of pharmacotherapy showed mixed results. Prolonged nicotine patch therapy (5 months) combined with nicotine nasal spray for 1 year also seems to prevent smoking relapse. Long-term smoking abstinence outcomes are better after 24 weeks of treatment than after 12 weeks for both nicotine patch therapy and varenicline.

Tapering of Pharmacotherapy

Varenicline and bupropion do not need to be tapered, and a Cochrane review observed no significant differences in adverse symptoms between abrupt discontinuation or gradual tapering of the nicotine patch.

CONCLUSIONS

Untreated tobacco use disorder results in the deaths of over 60% of patients who currently smoke from tobacco-caused illnesses. Pharmacotherapy plays an essential role in treating tobacco use disorder. Nicotine replacement therapy, varenicline, and bupropion form the foundation of clinical pharmacologic treatment strategy. Relapse to tobacco use requires treatment intensification, which should include combination pharmacotherapy. People who use smokeless tobacco benefit from varenicline and the nicotine lozenge. The risk-benefit ratio for ENDS presently remains unknown, and incorporation of these products into clinical treatment in the United States remains controversial.

KEY POINTS

1. Pharmacotherapy is a cornerstone in the comprehensive treatment of tobacco dependence.
2. First-line medications available for the treatment of tobacco dependence include nicotine replacement therapy, bupropion, and varenicline.
3. Combination pharmacotherapy with multiple forms of nicotine replacement therapy and/or nonnicotine pharmacotherapy increase tobacco abstinence rates compared to single-agent therapy.

REVIEW QUESTIONS

1. The neurotransmitter involved with the reinforcing effects of nicotine is:
   A. serotonin.
   B. norepinephrine.
   C. γ-aminobutyric acid.
   D. dopamine.
   E. glutamate.

2. Varenicline binds to which receptor?
   A. Acetylcholine
   B. Dopamine
   C. Adrenergic
   D. Glutamate
   E. Opioid

3. Which of the following has been demonstrated to increase long-term smoking abstinence rates in people who use smokeless tobacco?
   A. Bupropion SR
   B. Varenicline
   C. Nicotine lozenges
   D. Nicotine patch
   E. Both B and C.
   F. None of the above.

ANSWERS

1. **D.** Dopamine is involved with the reinforcing effects of nicotine. Nicotine can lead to the release of these other neurotransmitters, but dopamine is the one implicated in reinforcement.
2. **A.** Varenicline binds specifically to the $\alpha_4\beta_2$ nicotine acetylcholine receptor. Although nicotine binds to nicotine receptors throughout the body, varenicline binds specifically to this receptor, which is a major nicotine receptor in the central nervous system.
3. **E.** A Cochrane systematic review concluded that varenicline and nicotine lozenges increase long-term (>6 months) tobacco abstinence compared to placebo. Bupropion SR and the nicotine patch have not been demonstrated to increase long-term tobacco abstinence rates.

61 Pharmacological Interventions for Other Drugs and Multiple Drug Use Disorders

Summary by Jeffery N. Wilkins, Mark Hrymoc, and David A. Gorelick

Based on THE ASAM PRINCIPLES OF ADDICTION MEDICINE, 6th edition chapter by Jeffery N. Wilkins, Mark Hrymoc, and David A. Gorelick

Pharmacologic treatment of addiction (substance use disorder in *Diagnostic and Statistical Manual of Mental Disorders*, 5th edition [*DSM-5*] terms) follows at least five different strategies, including the use of agonists (including partial agonists), or the use of antagonists at the site(s) of action (receptors) for the drug, medications that alter reinforcement or drug craving, medications that increase drug metabolism or decrease crossing of the blood–brain barrier, and medications that produce aversive conditions for drug taking (eg, disulfiram for alcohol). In almost all cases, the pharmacologic treatments discussed in this chapter are experimental and are not approved by the US Food and Drug Administration (FDA).

CANNABIS (MARIJUANA)

There is no recognized or proven role for pharmacotherapy in the treatment of cannabis use disorder.

Two medications showed efficacy in single controlled clinical trials. Anticonvulsant gabapentin in adults with cannabis use disorder led to significant increases in cannabinoid-negative urine samples. Glutamate modulator *N*-acetylcysteine in cannabis-dependent adolescents led to significant increases in cannabinoid-negative urine samples; however, no significant benefit was discovered for adults in a controlled clinical trial.

In addition, in a placebo-controlled trial, the anxiolytic buspirone significantly reduced marijuana use in adults with marijuana dependence per *DSM-IV* (now termed moderate-to-severe cannabis use disorder in the *DSM-5*) but only in those who completed the study. In a controlled clinical trial, oral dronabinol (synthetic Δ9-tetrahydrocannabinol [THC], the chief psychoactive constituent of cannabis) had

no significant effect on cannabis use in adults with marijuana dependence, although it did significantly reduce cannabis withdrawal symptoms.

ANABOLIC STEROIDS

There is no established medication for the treatment of anabolic steroid abuse. Approximately 2.9 to 4 million US residents aged 13 to 50 years have used anabolic steroids, with 1 million classified as having anabolic steroid use disorder. Two pharmacologic treatment approaches have been suggested: hormonal treatments to restore hypothalamic–pituitary–gonadal dysfunction caused by the use of steroids and medications to relieve specific psychiatric symptoms associated with steroid withdrawal.

Hormonal treatments can be implemented with tapering doses of a long-acting steroid such as testosterone enanthate. This approach could be considered analogous to treating heroin withdrawal with a long-acting opiate such as methadone.

The second approach uses standard psychotropic medications to target the depression, irritability, and aggression often associated with anabolic steroid use, although these symptoms often resolve without medication. Anabolic steroid–associated depression is most often treated with selective serotonin reuptake inhibitor (SSRI) antidepressants; two placebo-controlled trials and two open-label trials suggest that SSRIs may also be effective in the treatment of the commonly co-occurring body dysmorphic disorder. Low-dose neuroleptics, both phenothiazines and second generation (eg, risperidone), have reportedly been effective for managing anabolic steroid–induced psychosis, hostility, and agitation.

PHENCYCLIDINE AND KETAMINE

Phencyclidine (PCP) and ketamine are both *N*-methyl-D-aspartate (NMDA) receptor antagonists but have different legal status in the United States. PCP is no longer legally available, whereas ketamine, a synthetic analogue of PCP, is legally available as an anesthetic, although subject to misuse.

There is little systematic experience with the pharmacologic treatment of PCP and ketamine addiction. Desipramine and the anxiolytic buspirone have significantly improved psychological symptoms such as depression in small outpatient controlled clinical trials of persons using PCP, but neither medication significantly reduced PCP use when compared with a double-blind placebo.

INHALANTS

Inhalants are a heterogeneous group of volatile abused substances that include adhesives, aerosols, solvents, anesthetics (including nitrous oxide), gasoline, cleaning agents, and nitrites. Many people who use inhalants who enter treatment have co-occurring psychiatric and addictive disorders, typically involving alcohol and marijuana, which can complicate treatment.

The mainstay of treatment is psychosocial, including techniques such as cognitive–behavioral therapy, multisystem and family therapy, 12-step facilitation, and motivational enhancement.

TOBACCO (NICOTINE) WITH OTHER DRUGS

Among US adults with current tobacco use disorder, 8.2% have a current (nonalcohol) drug use disorder, an odds ratio of 3.2 for having a drug use disorder compared with those without a tobacco use disorder. Conversely, 52.4% of those with a current drug use disorder have a tobacco use disorder. Comorbidity rates may exceed 70% among patients in treatment.

Most studies find that smoking cessation treatment does not adversely influence the outcome of treatment for other substance use disorders. Limited evidence suggests that individuals with multiple substance use disorders (eg, alcohol, stimulants, cannabis) may respond better to the combination of nicotine replacement therapy and bupropion than to either treatment alone.

Tobacco and Alcohol

Among adults with moderate-to-severe tobacco use disorder, 22.8% have an alcohol use disorder (odds ratio, 4.4). Conversely, among adults with an alcohol use disorder, 34.5% have a tobacco use disorder.

Tobacco-related diseases are a greater cause of morbidity and mortality in patients with alcohol use disorders than are alcohol-related medical conditions, highlighting the importance of smoking cessation treatment for this population.

Cigarette smokers with a current alcohol use disorder (but not those in remission) tend to have a more severe form of tobacco use disorder and may need more intensive treatment, including higher doses of medication. Most, but not all, studies suggest that tobacco and alcohol use disorders can be successfully treated at the same time without adversely affecting outcome.

Naltrexone is an FDA-approved treatment for both alcohol and opioid use disorders, with some evidence for efficacy in the treatment of tobacco use disorder. In one recent controlled trial, naltrexone reduced both heavy drinking and smoking in those who drank socially and are not addicted. Naltrexone significantly improved prolonged abstinence quit rates in heavy drinkers but not in moderate-to-light or nondrinking smokers.

Based on limited evidence, nicotine-replacement therapy in the form of nicotine patches may be more effective than naltrexone at reducing cigarette smoking in patients with moderate-to-severe alcohol use disorder. More research is needed to determine whether adding nicotine replacement therapy to a higher dose of naltrexone in tobacco smokers with alcohol use disorder will significantly reduce smoking.

In addition, topiramate has been shown to reduce alcohol use and cigarette smoking.

Varenicline, which is also approved by the FDA for smoking cessation, also significantly increased smoking abstinence in smokers with moderate-to-severe alcohol use disorder.

Tobacco and Opioids

More than three fourths of individuals with moderate-to-severe opioid use disorder smoke cigarettes, including patients in methadone maintenance treatment (MMT). Opioid drugs, including methadone, may acutely increase cigarette smoking.

Limited evidence suggests that nicotine replacement therapy, with or without bupropion, can be effective for smoking cessation in patients on methadone maintenance. Treatment outcomes are improved with concurrent psychosocial treatment, including motivational interviewing.

Nicotine and Cocaine

Cigarette smoking is associated with poorer short-term outcomes of outpatient treatment for moderate-to-severe cocaine use disorder but not for concurrent opioid use disorder, suggesting the importance of offering smoking cessation treatment to patients with cocaine use disorder.

OPIOIDS WITH OTHER DRUGS
Opioids and Alcohol

Heavy drinking or alcohol use disorder occur in one third or more of those with opioid use disorder, including those in MMT, and is associated with poor treatment outcomes. Conversely, cessation of illicit opioid use and retention in MMT are positively correlated with a reduction in concurrent alcohol and/or cocaine misuse and the absence of the psychosocial complications associated with such misuse. There does not appear to be a strong association between methadone dose and alcohol use.

Buprenorphine reduces alcohol intake in animal studies but shows inconsistent effects in human clinical trials. Disulfiram, at typical doses used to treat alcohol use disorder, can be effective in the treatment of patients with comorbid opioid use disorder when coordinated with careful medication monitoring and incentives for compliance, as found in MMT programs.

Strong preclinical evidence suggests that medications that alter (especially decrease) glutamatergic neurotransmission might successfully treat co-occurring substance use disorders. Candidate medications include acamprosate, N-acetylcysteine, D-cycloserine, gabapentin, lamotrigine, memantine, modafinil, and topiramate, although most act at multiple receptor systems.

Opioids and Cocaine

Cocaine use is common among those with an opioid addiction and is associated with greater opioid use, even among those in MMT. A popular pattern involves simultaneous use of the two drugs ("speed balling"), which is said to provide a qualitatively better subjective experience ("high") than either drug alone.

For patients already in MMT, increasing the methadone dose (usually to >60 mg per day) can reduce both opioid and cocaine use. High doses of methadone maintenance are more effective at achieving sustained heroin abstinence but have no effect on cocaine abstinence. At equivalent doses, methadone is more efficacious than buprenorphine in promoting cocaine abstinence and heroin abstinence.

Although one meta-analysis did not demonstrate a direct association between high doses of methadone and decreased cocaine use, some studies have demonstrated decreased cocaine use in patients receiving higher doses of methadone maintenance,

likely due to a two-step process whereby high-dose methadone maintenance first reduces heroin use, which subsequently leads to decreased cocaine use. Contingency management targeting cocaine abstinence may improve cocaine abstinence in patients on MMT. The literature regarding adjunctive medication, including dopamine agonists, in MMT patients is inconclusive and often negative.

Varenicline reduces tobacco smoking but has no impact on cocaine use in methadone-maintained patients with cocaine use disorder who also smoked cigarettes.

Buprenorphine, equivalent to 16 to 32 mg per day as sublingual tablet, reduces both cocaine and opioid use in patients with both use disorders, although lower doses do not.

A clinical trial using injectable, sustained-release naltrexone in individuals with heroin use disorder found a dose-dependent effect on the percentage of urine samples negative for opioids, cocaine, and amphetamines.

HALLUCINOGENS

Hallucinogens include compounds that influence serotonergic neurotransmission, such as lysergic acid diethylamide, psilocybin, and N,N-dimethyltryptamine, and those that influence catecholaminergic neurotransmission (such as mescaline and amphetamine analogues like 3,4-methylenedioxymethamphetamine).

At present, no pharmacologic treatment is available for the treatment of hallucinogen use disorder. Single doses of the SSRI antidepressant citalopram or the $5\text{-HT}_{2A/C}$ receptor antagonist ketanserin attenuated many of the acute psychologic effects of 3,4-methylenedioxmethamphetamine in human experimental studies. The mainstay of treatment remains psychosocial intervention, which can require residential treatment in patients with severe personality disorganization.

Prolonged psychotic reactions appear to occur chiefly in individuals who have preexisting psychiatric disorders; these can be difficult to distinguish from hallucinogen-induced precipitation or exacerbation of a preexisting psychotic disorder such as schizophrenia. Low doses of a high-potency neuroleptic have been recommended.

Lysergic acid diethylamide use has been associated with perceptual abnormalities, such as illusions, distortions, and hallucinations that persist or recur intermittently for long periods (up to years) after the last use. When these abnormalities occur after a period of normal perceptual functioning, they are termed flashbacks.

Case reports suggest that naltrexone, clonidine, or benzodiazepines can be helpful in the treatment of both persisting perceptual abnormalities and flashbacks, whereas antipsychotics (eg, haloperidol, risperidone) have been reported to worsen the condition. SSRIs do not represent an optimal initial therapeutic choice because both harms and benefits have been reported.

KEY POINTS

1. Although agonist treatments for withdrawal symptoms and substance use disorders are effective for opioid and/or tobacco use disorders, they are effective only for cannabis withdrawal but not for cannabis use disorder.
2. Varenicline treatment significantly reduces heavy drinking and increases smoking abstinence in men but not in women. This demonstrates the importance of taking gender into account when treating comorbid substance use disorders.
3. The opioid antagonist naltrexone and the opioid partial agonist buprenorphine are effective in treating comorbid tobacco and alcohol use disorders and comorbid stimulant (eg, cocaine) and opioid use disorders, respectively.
4. Effective pharmacologic treatment of anabolic steroid, PCP, ketamine, inhalant, or hallucinogen use is largely limited to managing substance-induced depression, anxiety, agitation, and psychosis.
5. One third of patients on buprenorphine or methadone maintenance treatment for opioid use disorder also have at-risk alcohol use or alcohol use disorders, resulting in poor physical and mental health as well as treatment noncompliance, social deterioration, and increased mortality.

REVIEW QUESTIONS

1. Which of the following represents a class of medications for the pharmacologic treatment of substance use disorder?
   A. Receptor agonists (including partial agonists), or receptor antagonists
   B. Medications that alter reinforcement or drug craving
   C. Medications that increase drug metabolism or decrease blood–brain barrier crossings
   D. Medications that create an aversive contingency for drug taking (eg, disulfiram)
   E. All of the above.

2. Which of the following statements is *incorrect* regarding pharmacotherapy controlled clinical trials of cannabis use disorder?
   A. The anticonvulsant gabapentin reduced marijuana use in adults.
   B. The glutamate modulator *N*-acetylcysteine reduced cannabis use in adolescents.
   C. The glutamate modulator *N*-acetylcysteine reduced cannabis use in adults.
   D. The anxiolytic buspirone was effective at reducing marijuana use in adults who completed the study.
   E. Synthetic Δ9-tetrahydrocannabinol (dronabinol) significantly reduced marijuana withdrawal symptoms but had no effect on cannabis/marijuana use.

3. Which of the following treatments is considered most effective at reducing cocaine use by patients in methadone maintenance treatment?
   A. Higher dose of methadone
   B. Desipramine
   C. Bupropion
   D. Citalopram
   E. Buprenorphine

ANSWERS

1. **E.** All 4 classes of medication listed in A through D are actively used in the treatment of substance use disorders.
2. **C.** *N*-acetylcysteine has been demonstrated to reduce cannabis use in adolescents, a subsequent study found no efficacy in adults.
3. **A.** Patients on methadone maintenance with cocaine use disorders are less likely to use cocaine if they are on a high dose of methadone than on a low dose.

SUGGESTED READINGS

Brezing CA, Levin FR. The current state of pharmacological treatments for cannabis use disorder and withdrawal. *Neuropsychopharmacology*. 2018;43(1):173-194.

Compton W. The need to incorporate smoking cessation into behavioral health treatment. *Am J Addict*. 2018;27(1):42-43.

Fridberg DJ, Cao D, Grant JE, King AC. Naltrexone improves quit rates, attenuates smoking urge, and reduces alcohol use in heavy drinking smokers attempting to quit smoking. *Alcohol Clin Exp Res*. 2014;38(10):2622-2629.

O'Malley SS, Zweben A, Fucito LM, et al. Effect of varenicline combined with management on alcohol use disorder with comorbid cigarette smoking: a randomized clinical trial. *JAMA Psychiatry*. 2018;75(2):129-138.

Soyka M. Alcohol use disorders in opioid maintenance therapy: prevalence, clinical correlates and treatment. *Eur Addict Res*. 2015;21(2):78-87.

62 Neuromodulation for Addiction-Related Disorders

Summary by David A. Gorelick

Based on THE ASAM PRINCIPLES OF ADDICTION MEDICINE,
6th edition chapter by David A. Gorelick

Brain neuromodulation uses noninvasive electromagnetic or electrical methods to transiently alter neuronal firing in the brain. The most studied and widely used method of neuromodulation is transcranial magnetic stimulation (TMS), which is not approved by the US Food and Drug Administration (FDA) for the treatment of substance use disorders because of the limited number of controlled clinical trials. TMS is approved by the FDA for the treatment of depression.

TMS uses wire coils placed on the scalp to project a fluctuating magnetic field into the brain. Because brain tissue is a conductive medium, this fluctuating magnetic field generates electrical currents in the brain. These electrical currents influence neuronal firing. The configuration of the coil determines the brain region(s) targeted by the magnetic field and the depth of penetration. The most commonly used figure-8 coils penetrate about 2 to 3 cm into the cortical surface; so-called H or deep coils may penetrate 5 to 6 cm.

The majority of sham-controlled human laboratory (phase I) studies (usually one or two sessions) find that high-frequency repetitive TMS (rTMS) targeted at the prefrontal cortex or dorsolateral prefrontal cortex (DLPFC) significantly reduces self-reported cravings for tobacco, alcohol, cocaine, methamphetamine, or heroin for several hours. rTMS targeted at the DLPFC was effective at reducing cigarette smoking in several small, short-term phase II controlled clinical trials, using either low-frequency or high-frequency pulses, figure-8 or deep coils, alone or combined with a nicotine patch and in patients with schizophrenia. Of two small phase II controlled clinical trials for cocaine use disorder, one found high-frequency rTMS targeted to the left DLPFC effective at reducing cocaine use, whereas the second, using a deep coil to target the bilateral prefrontal cortex, did not. We are not aware of any outpatient controlled clinical trials evaluating rTMS as treatment for other substance use disorders.

When administered in accordance with international consensus safety guidelines relating to patient/subject selection and pulse intensity and frequency, rTMS has an excellent record of short-term safety and tolerability, for both the treatment of depression and in studies of substance use disorders. Common adverse effects include transient scalp and face discomfort and paresthesia and headache. The only serious adverse effect is seizure, which is very rare. The few reported cases were in individuals taking concomitant medications known to lower the seizure threshold or who were experiencing substance withdrawal.

The mechanism of action of rTMS for reducing substance craving and use remains unclear. It may involve both modulation of neurotransmitter activity (such as dopamine and glutamate) and of neuronal firing in brain circuits, such as the frontal cortex–striatal circuit, that mediates substance craving and seeking behavior. The latter mechanism may explain the efficacy of rTMS targeting the DLPFC.

A less well-studied method of brain neuromodulation is transcranial direct current stimulation. Transcranial direct current stimulation involves passing very low amplitude (typically 0.5 to 2 mA) direct electrical current into the brain by placing two large electrodes at different spots on the scalp. The mechanism of action is not well understood but may involve subthreshold depolarization (increasing excitability) of neurons near the anode electrode and hyperpolarization (decreasing excitability) near the cathode electrode. Several human laboratory studies found that transcranial direct current stimulation significantly reduced cravings for tobacco, alcohol, cocaine, heroin, and cannabis.

KEY POINTS

1. Brain neuromodulation uses noninvasive electromagnetic or electrical methods to transiently alter neuronal firing in the brain.

2. The most studied and widely used method of neuromodulation is TMS, which is not approved by the FDA for the treatment of substance use disorders because of the limited number of controlled clinical trials.

3. Several studies have shown a reduction in cravings for substances following neuromodulation, and it remains an area of active study.

REVIEW QUESTIONS

1. TMS uses what form of electromagnetic energy to alter neuronal firing?
   A. X-rays
   B. Fluctuating magnetic fields
   C. Stable magnetic fields
   D. Alternating electrical current
   E. Direct electrical current

2. The most common serious adverse effect from TMS is:
   A. paralysis.
   B. headache.
   C. stroke.
   D. seizure.
   E. muscle twitching.

ANSWERS

1. **B**
2. **D**

SUGGESTED READINGS

Rossi S, Hallett M, Rossini PM, Pascual-Leone A. Safety, ethical considerations, and application guidelines for the use of transcranial magnetic stimulation in clinical practice and research. *Clin Neurophysiol.* 2009;120(12):2008-2039.

Salling MC, Martinez D. Brain stimulation in addiction. *Neuropsychopharmacology.* 2016;41(12):2798-2809.

Spagnolo PA, Goldman D. Neuromodulation interventions for addictive disorders: challenges, promise, and roadmap for future research. *Brain.* 2017;140(5):1183-1203.

Tendler A, Barnea Ygael N, Roth Y, Zangen A. Deep transcranial magnetic stimulation (dTMS)–beyond depression. *Expert Rev Med Devices.* 2016;13(10):987-1000.

Psychologically Based Interventions

63 Enhancing Motivation to Change

Summary by James O. Prochaska and Janice M. Prochaska

Based on THE ASAM PRINCIPLES OF ADDICTION MEDICINE,
6th edition chapter by James O. Prochaska

What motivates people to take action? The answer to this key question depends on what type of action is to be taken. What moves people to start therapy? What motivates them to continue therapy? What moves people to progress in therapy or to continue to progress after therapy?

Answers to these questions can provide better alternatives to one of the field's most pressing concerns: What types of therapeutic interventions would have the greatest effect on the entire population at risk for or experiencing addictive disorders?

What motivates people to change? The answer to this question depends in part on where they start. What motivates people to begin thinking about change can be different from what motivates them to begin preparing to take action. Once people are prepared, different forces can move them to take action. Once action is taken, what motivates people to maintain that action? Conversely, what causes people to regress or relapse to their addictive behaviors?

THE STAGES OF CHANGE

Change is a process that unfolds over time through a series of stages: precontemplation, contemplation, preparation, action, maintenance, and termination. Precontemplation is a stage in which the individual does not intend to take action in the foreseeable future (usually measured as the next 6 months). Individuals may be at this stage because they are uninformed or underinformed about the consequences of a given behavior. Or individuals may have tried to change a number of times and become demoralized about their ability to do so.

Individuals in both categories tend to avoid reading, talking, or thinking about their high-risk behaviors. In other theories, such individuals are characterized as "resistant," "unmotivated," or "not ready" for therapy or health promotion programs. In fact, traditional treatment programs were not ready for such individuals and were not motivated to match their needs.

Individuals who are in the precontemplation stage typically underestimate the benefits of change and overestimate its costs but are unaware that they are making such mistakes. If they are not conscious of making such mistakes, it is difficult for them to change. As a result, many remain in the precontemplation stage for years, with considerable resulting harm to their bodies, themselves, and others.

A common belief is that people with addictive disorders must "hit bottom" before they are motivated to change. So family, friends, and physicians wait helplessly for a crisis to occur. When individuals show the first signs of a serious physical illness, such as cancer or cardiovascular disease, those around them usually become mobilized to help them seek an early intervention. Evidence shows that early interventions often are lifesaving, and so it would not be acceptable to wait for such a patient to "hit bottom."

Contemplation is a stage in which individuals intend to take action within the ensuing 6 months. Such persons are more aware of the benefits of changing, but also are acutely aware of the costs. When addicted persons begin to seriously contemplate giving up favorite substances, their awareness of the costs of changing can increase. There is no free change. This balance between the costs and benefits of change can produce profound ambivalence, which may reflect a type of love–hate relationship with an addictive substance and thus can keep an individual stuck at the contemplation stage for long periods of time. This phenomenon often is characterized as "chronic contemplation" or "behavioral procrastination." Such individuals are not ready for traditional action-oriented programs.

Preparation is a stage in which individuals intend to take action in the immediate future (usually measured as the ensuing month). Such persons typically have taken some significant action within the preceding year. They generally have a plan of action, such as participating in a recovery group, consulting a counselor, talking to a physician, buying a self-help book, or relying on a self-change approach. It is these individuals who should be recruited for action-oriented treatment programs.

Action is a stage in which individuals have made specific, overt modifications in their lifestyle within the preceding 6 months. Because action is observable, behavior change often has been equated with action. But in the transtheoretical model, action is only one of six stages. In this model, not all modifications of behavior count as action. An individual must attain a criterion that scientists and professionals agree is sufficient to reduce the risk of disease. In smoking, for example, only total abstinence counts. With alcohol use disorders, many believe that only total abstinence can be effective, whereas others accept controlled drinking as an effective action.

Maintenance is a stage in which individuals are working to prevent relapse but do not need to apply change processes as frequently as one would in the action stage. Such persons are less tempted to relapse and are increasingly confident that they can sustain the changes made. Temptation and self-efficacy data suggest that maintenance lasts from 6 months to about 5 years.

One of the common reasons for early relapse is that individuals are not well prepared for the prolonged effort needed to progress to maintenance. Many persons think the worst will be over in a few weeks or a few months. If, as a result, they ease up on their efforts too early, they are at great risk of relapse. To prepare such individuals for what is to come, they should be encouraged to think of overcoming an addiction as running a marathon rather than a sprint. They may have wanted to enter the Boston Marathon, but they know they would not succeed without preparation and so would not enter the race. With some preparation, they might compete for several miles but still would fail to finish the race. Only those who are well prepared could maintain their efforts mile after mile. Using the Boston Marathon metaphor, people know they have to be well prepared if they are to survive Heartbreak Hill, which runners encounter at about mile 20. What is the behavioral equivalent of Heartbreak Hill? The best evidence available suggests that most relapses occur at times of emotional distress. It is in the presence of depression, anxiety, anger, boredom, loneliness, stress, and distress that humans are at their emotional and psychological weak point.

How does the average person cope with troubling times? He or she drinks more, eats more, smokes more, and takes more substances to cope with distress. It is not surprising, therefore, that persons struggling to overcome addictive disorders will be at greatest risk of relapse when they face distress without their substance of choice. Although emotional distress cannot be prevented, relapse can be prevented if patients have been prepared to cope with distress without falling back on addictive substances.

If so many Americans rely on oral consumptive behavior as a way to manage their emotions, what is the healthiest oral behavior they could use? Talking with others about one's distress is a means of seeking support that can help prevent relapse. Another healthy alternative is exercise. Physical activity helps manage moods, stress, and distress. Also, 60 minutes per week of exercise can provide a recovering person with more than 70 health and mental health benefits. Thus, exercise should be prescribed to all sedentary patients with addictions. A third healthy alternative is some form of deep relaxation, such as meditation, yoga, prayer, massage, or deep muscle relaxation. Letting the stress and distress drift away from one's muscles and one's mind helps the patient move forward at the most tempting of times.

Helping patient populations to not smoke, eat healthy, exercise, and effectively manage stress have recently been recommended by three federal agencies that have major responsibilities for substance use disorders and mental illness. The Substance Abuse and Mental Health Services Administration, the National Institutes of Health, and the Center for Medicare & Medicaid Innovation have independently concluded that those health risk behaviors are major causes of chronic diseases, disabilities, and premature deaths in almost all populations. But populations with severe mental illness and substance use disorders die an average of 10 years earlier. The New Recovery Advocacy Movement believes that any commitment to enhance health can be motivators that can begin the recovery process. Therefore this Movement also recommends holistic health care.

Termination is a stage at which individuals have zero temptation and 100% self-efficacy. No matter whether they are depressed, anxious, bored, lonely, angry, or stressed, such persons are certain they will not return to their old unhealthy habits as a method of coping. It is as if they never acquired the habit in the first place. In a study of former smokers and people with alcohol use disorders, fewer than 20% of each group had reached the stage of no temptation and total self-efficacy. The New Recovery Advocacy Movement also recognizes that many people want to be recovered so that they can dedicate their time and resources to enhancing other aspects of their health and well-being. Although the ideal is to be cured or totally recovered, it is important to recognize that for many patients, a more realistic expectation is a lifetime of maintenance.

USING THE STAGES OF CHANGE MODEL TO MOTIVATE PATIENTS

The stages of change model can be applied to identify ways to motivate individuals more.

Recruitment

Too few studies have paid attention to the fact that professional treatment programs recruit or reach too few persons with addictions. Across all diagnoses in the *Diagnostic and Statistical Manual of Mental Disorders,* 5th edition, fewer than 25% of persons with addictive disorders enter professional treatment in their lifetimes. With smoking, the deadliest of addictions, fewer than 10% ever participate in a professional treatment program.

Given that addictive disorders are among the costliest of contemporary conditions, it is crucial to motivate many more persons to participate in appropriate treatment. These conditions are costly to the addicted individuals, their families and friends, employers, communities, and healthcare systems. Health professionals no longer can treat addictive disorders just on a case basis; instead, they must develop programs that can reach addicted persons on a population basis.

How can more people with addictive disorders be motivated to seek the appropriate help? By changing both paradigms and practices. There are two paradigms that need to be changed. The first is an action-oriented paradigm that construes behavior change as an event that can occur quickly, immediately, discretely, and dramatically. Treatment programs that are designed to have patients immediately quit abusing substances are implicitly or explicitly designed for the portion of the population in the preparation stage.

The problem is that with most unhealthy behaviors, fewer than 20% of the affected population is prepared to take action. Among smokers in the United States, for example, about 40% are in the precontemplation stage, 40% are in the contemplation stage, and 20% are in the preparation stage. Among college students with an alcohol use disorder, about 85% are in the precontemplation stage, 10% are in the contemplation stage, and 5% are in the preparation stage. When only action-oriented interventions are offered, less than 20% of the at-risk population

are being recruited. To meet the needs of the entire addicted population, interventions must meet the needs of the 40% in the precontemplation stage and the 40% in the contemplation stage.

A treatment program for addicted gamblers in Windsor, Ontario, used creative communications to let their prospective population know that wherever they are at, the program can work with them. This program had generous support of 2% of earnings from local casinos, but they were not reaching many people. So, on the back of city buses, they placed ads with a traffic light logo: red light (not ready), yellow light (getting ready), and green light (ready). Not only did they dramatically increase their recruitment, some clients would take pride in saying, "Hey, there goes my bus!"

The second paradigm change that is required is movement from a passive–reactive approach to a proactive approach. Most professionals have been trained to be passive–reactive: to passively wait for patients to seek their services and then to react. The problem with this approach is that most persons with addictive disorders never seek such services. The passive–reactive paradigm is designed to serve populations with acute conditions. The pain, distress, or discomfort of such conditions can motivate patients to seek the services of health professionals. But the major killers today are chronic lifestyle disorders such as the addictions. To treat the addictions seriously, professionals must learn how to reach out to entire populations and offer them stage-matched treatments.

Principles and Processes of Change

To help motivate patients to progress from one stage to the next, it is necessary to know the six principles and processes of change that can produce such progress.

Principle 1: The benefits for changing must increase if patients are to progress beyond precontemplation.

A technique that can be used in population-based programs involves asking a patient in the precontemplation stage to describe all the benefits of a change such as quitting smoking or starting to exercise. Most persons can list four or five. The therapist can let the patient know that there are eight to ten times that number and challenge the patient to double or triple the list for the next meeting. If the patient's list of benefits of exercise begins to indicate many more motives, such as a healthier heart, healthier lungs, more energy, healthier immune system, better moods, less stress, better sex life, and enhanced self-esteem, he or she will be more motivated to begin to seriously contemplate such a change.

Principle 2: The "cons" of changing must decrease if patients are to progress from contemplation to action. In 12 studies of 12 different behaviors, research has found that the perceived costs of changing were lower in the action than in the contemplation stage.

Principle 3: The relative weight assigned to benefits and costs must cross over before a patient will be prepared to take action.

Principle 4: The strong principle of progress holds that to progress from precontemplation to effective action, the rewards for changing must increase by one standard deviation.

Principle 5: The weak principle of progress holds that to progress from contemplation to effective action, the perceived costs of changing must decrease by one-half standard deviation.

Principle 6: It is important to match particular processes of change with specific stages of change. Table 63-1 presents the empirical integration found between processes and stages of change. Guided by this integration, the following processes would be applied to patients in various stages of change:

- Consciousness raising (get the facts) involves increased awareness of the causes, consequences, and responses to a particular problem. Interventions that can increase awareness include observations, confrontations, interpretations, feedback, and education. Some techniques, such as confrontation, pose considerable risk in terms of retention and are not recommended as highly as motivational enhancement methods such as personal feedback about the current and long-term consequences of continuing the addictive behavior. Increasing the costs of not changing is the corollary of raising the rewards for changing. Therefore, consciousness raising should be designed to increase the perceived rewards for changing.

- Dramatic relief (pay attention to feelings) involves emotional arousal about one's current behavior and the relief that can come from changing. Fear, inspiration, guilt, and hope are some of the emotions that can move individuals to contemplate changing. Psychodrama, role-playing, grieving, and personal testimonies are examples of techniques that can move people emotionally. It should be noted that earlier literature on behavior change concluded that interventions such as education and fear arousal did not motivate behavior change. Unfortunately, many interventions were evaluated in terms of their ability to move people to immediate action. However, processes such as consciousness raising and dramatic relief are intended to move people to the contemplation rather than the action stage. Therefore, their effectiveness should be assessed according to whether they lead to the expected progress.

- Environmental reevaluation (notice your effect on others) combines both affective and

TABLE 63-1 Principles and Processes of Change That Mediate Progression Between the Stages of Change

Precontemplation	Contemplation	Preparation	Action	Maintenance
Consciousness raising				
Dramatic relief				
Environmental reevaluation				
	Social liberation			
	Self-reevaluation			
		Self-liberation		
			Reinforcement management	
			Helping relationships	
Pros of changing increasing			Counter conditioning	
	Cons of changing decreasing		Stimulus control	
		Self-efficacy increasing		

Source: In Ries RK, Miller SC, Fiellin DA, Saitz R, eds. *The ASAM Principles of Addiction Medicine*. 6th ed. Philadelphia: Wolters Kluwer, 2019.

cognitive assessments of how an addiction affects one's social environment and how changing would affect that environment. Empathy training, values clarification, and family or network interventions can facilitate such a reevaluation.

■ Self-reevaluation (create a new self-image) combines both cognitive and affective assessments of an image of one's self free from addiction. Imagery, healthier role models, and values clarification are techniques that can move individuals in this type of intervention. Clinically, patients first look back and reevaluate how they have lived as addicted individuals. As they progress into the preparation stage, they begin to develop a focus on the future as they imagine how life could be if they were free of addiction.

■ Self-liberation (make a commitment) involves both the belief that one can change and the commitment and recommitment to act on that belief. Techniques that can enhance such willpower include public rather than private commitments. Motivational research also suggests that individuals who have only one choice are not as motivated as those who have two choices. Three choices are even better, but four choices do not seem to enhance motivation. Wherever possible, then, patients should be given three of the best choices for applying each process. With smoking cessation, for example, there are at least three good choices: quitting "cold turkey," using nicotine replacement therapy, and using nicotine fading. Asking clients to choose which alternative they believe would be most effective for them and which they would be most committed to can enhance their motivation and their self-liberation.

■ Counterconditioning (use substitutes) requires the learning of healthier behaviors that can substitute for addictive behaviors. Counterconditioning techniques tend to be quite specific to a particular behavior. They include desensitization, assertion, and cognitive counters to irrational self-statements that can elicit distress.

■ Reinforcement management (use rewards) involves the systematic use of reinforcements and punishments for taking steps in a particular direction. Because successful self-changers rely much more on reinforcement than punishment, it is useful to emphasize reinforcements for progressing rather than punishments for

regressing. Contingency contracts, overt and covert reinforcements, and group recognition are methods of increasing reinforcement and incentives that increase the probability that healthier responses will be repeated. To prepare patients for the longer term, they should be taught to rely more on self-reinforcements than on social reinforcements. Clinical experience shows that many patients expect much more reinforcement and recognition from others than they actually receive. Relatives and friends may take action for granted. Average acquaintances typically generate only a few positive consequences early in the action stage. Self-reinforcements obviously are much more under self-control and can be given more quickly and consistently when temptations to lapse or relapse are resisted.

■ Stimulus control (manage your environment) involves modifying the environment to increase cues that prompt healthy responses and decrease cues that lead to relapse. Avoidance, environmental reengineering (such as removing addictive substances and paraphernalia), and attending self-help groups can provide stimuli that elicit healthy responses and reduce the risk of relapse.

■ Helping relationships (get support) combine caring, openness, trust, and acceptance as well as support for changing. Rapport building, a therapeutic alliance, counselor calls, buddy systems, sponsors, and self-help groups can be excellent resources for social support. If patients become dependent on such support to maintain change, the support will need to be carefully faded, lest termination of therapy becomes a condition for relapse.

■ Social liberation (notice the public effort) is the process by which changes in society increase the options and opportunities to have healthier and happier lives freer from addiction. Social networks provide the ability to participate in positive interactions free from the pressures to rely on substance use.

KEY POINTS

1. Behavior change is a process that unfolds over time through a sequence of stages: precontemplation, contemplation, preparation, action, and maintenance.

2. Behavior change initiatives can motivate change by enhancing the understanding of the pros and diminishing the value of the cons.

3. Most at-risk populations are not prepared for action and will not be served by traditional action-oriented programs. Helping individuals set realistic goals, like progressing to the next stage, will facilitate the change process.
4. Specific principles and processes of change need to be emphasized at specific stages for progress to occur.

REVIEW QUESTIONS

1. In the transtheoretical model, success includes:
   A. increasing the pros of changing.
   B. increasing self-efficacy.
   C. movement to the next stage of change.
   D. all of the above.

2. Which process of change would you most likely use to help someone move from the precontemplation stage to the contemplation stage?
   A. Consciousness raising (get the facts)
   B. Stimulus control (manage your environment)
   C. Counterconditioning (use substitutes)
   D. Reinforcement management (use rewards)

3. Which process or principle of change would you most likely use to help someone move from the preparation stage to the action stage?
   A. Dramatic relief (pay attention to feelings)
   B. Self-liberation (make a commitment)
   C. Increasing the pros
   D. Reinforcement management (use rewards)

ANSWERS

1. **D**
2. **A**
3. **B**

SUGGESTED READINGS

DiClemente CC. *Addiction and Change: How Addiction Develops and Addicted People Recover.* 2nd ed. New York: Guilford Press, 2018.

Mauriello LM, Johnson SS, Prochaska JM. Meeting patients where they are at: using a stage approach to facilitate engagement. In: O'Donohue W, James L, Snipes C, eds. *Practical Strategies and Tools to Promote Treatment Engagement.* New York: Springer Publishing, 2017:25-44.

Prochaska JO. Enhancing motivation to change. In Ries RK, Miller SC, Fiellin DA, Saitz R, eds. *The ASAM Principles of Addiction Medicine.* 6th ed. Philadelphia: Wolters Kluwer, 2019.

Prochaska JO, Prochaska JM. *Changing to Thrive: Using the Stages of Change to Overcome the Top Threats to Your Health and Happiness.* Center City, MN: Hazelden Publishing, 2016.

Van Marter D, Levesque D, de Auguiar E, Castle P, Mauriello L. Promoting responsible drinking among employed adults through a mobile health intervention: outcomes of a randomized effectiveness trial. Poster presented at: American Public Health Association Annual Meeting; November 7, 2017; Atlanta, GA.

Group Therapies

Summary by Dennis C. Daley and Antoine Douaihy

Based on THE ASAM PRINCIPLES OF ADDICTION MEDICINE,
6th edition chapter by Dennis C. Daley, Antoine Douaihy,
Roger D. Weiss, and Delinda E. Mercer

Group therapies are used widely in the treatment of substance use disorders (SUDs) and co-occurring psychiatric disorders. These are often the main form of treatment used. We use the term *group therapy* to refer to milieu therapy, psychoeducational recovery, coping skills, family therapy, and therapy groups including motivational interviewing (MI) groups. Groups may address early recovery issues such as initiating abstinence and engaging the patient in a recovery process, anger management, behavior change, relapse prevention, and co-occurring psychiatric disorders. It can also address treatment engagement and participation. Groups also are widely used in the treatment of specific populations such as women, persons in the criminal justice system, those with co-occurring psychiatric disorders, and families.

GOALS OF GROUP THERAPIES

The long-term goals of treatment are to help the individual with the SUD to achieve and maintain abstinence and improve his or her quality of life. Short-term goals are to evaluate and reduce substance use, increase motivation to change, address problems caused or worsened by the SUD, and improve functioning. Groups help patients achieve these goals by creating a milieu in which members can bond with each other, thus reducing the stigma associated with SUDs and the humiliation of having lost control of one's own behavior. The specific ways in which groups can help achieve this include providing education on SUDs, recovery, and relapse; resolving ambivalence and enhancing motivation to change; evoking hope and optimism for change; providing an opportunity to give and receive feedback from peers; teaching recovery skills to manage the SUD; addressing problems resulting from the SUD; providing a context in which the group member can identify with others and give and receive support; creating an experience in which feelings, thoughts, and conflicts can be freely expressed; preparing the patient for involvement in long-term recovery; and facilitating the

patient's interest in mutual support programs. Patients can be oriented to group programs so they understand the goals and structure of groups, potential benefits, and what is expected from their participation. Practitioners can describe the types and formats of the groups offered, and how these differ from Alcoholics Anonymous, Narcotics Anonymous, or other recovery meetings in the community.

TYPES OF GROUP THERAPIES

Many of the problems or issues addressed in different models of group treatment are similar. The specific issues or problems addressed depend on the treatment model and number of sessions offered. Groups usually fall into one of the following categories:

- Milieu groups: These are offered in residential programs and involve a review of the day's schedule, goals for group members, and a review of learning at the end of the day.
- Psychoeducational recovery groups: These provide information about SUDs and recovery topics such as cravings, social pressures to use, boredom or other negative emotions, social support, sober relationships, relapse, and family issues in addiction.
- Coping skill groups: These teach problem-solving methods, stress management, or relapse prevention strategies to help patients learn skills to manage the challenges of recovery.
- Therapy or counseling groups: Participants identify problems, conflicts, or struggles to explore during the session. Members give and receive feedback from one another. MI groups can improve recognition of ambivalence, support autonomy, strengthen commitment to change, and facilitate engagement and participation in treatment. MI combination groups combine elements of MI with elements of other counseling approaches, such as cognitive–behavioral therapy.
- Specialized groups: These can be based on the needs and interests of a specific group of individuals.

FORMAT OF GROUP SESSIONS AND INTERVENTIONS OF LEADERS

Group sessions usually last 60 to 90 minutes. Groups can be limited to a specific number of sessions in which all participants start the group together, or be open-ended, so that new patients can be added to the group. Group leaders may use any of the following intervention strategies:

- Educational presentations in which members are provided information about substances, symptoms, causes and effects of SUDs, treatments for SUDs, recovery, relapse, family issues, medical or psychiatric illnesses, and other issues specific to the group members
- Brief, real-life stories to illustrate an issue or point discussed
- Guest presenters, including professionals to speak on a specific topic, or individuals in recovery to share their personal stories
- Videotapes, DVDs, or audiotapes to provide information and show recovery in action
- Workbooks, journals, or worksheets in which clients share answers to questions about their SUDs or recovery or specific issues discussed by the group
- Visual handouts to provide information and stimulate discussion such as a diagram of the brain and areas affected by substance use and addiction
- PowerPoint slides to show visual examples of the effects of substances or SUDs or recovery
- Behavioral assignments related to the group topic reviewed in structured recovery sessions
- Role plays to address interpersonal problems, to practice dealing with pressure to engage in substance use, or to help a group member learn to ask another person for help or support
- Monodramas to externalize a problem, conflict, or recovery issue such as a member creating a dialogue between his "healthy, recovering self" and his "unhealthy, addicted self"
- Creative media (arts, crafts, media) or other healthy lifestyle strategies and activities based on "mind–body focusing" (eg, meditation, guided relaxation, yoga, exercise) that aid in recovery and help improve health and the quality of life

Recovery Group Sessions

Each session focuses on a topic relevant to recovery. It begins with a check-in (10 to 20 minutes), in which patients briefly report any substance use, strong cravings, or "close calls." This is followed by a discussion of the topic for the session (40 to 60 minutes).

Each session provides materials from a workbook or other handout with information about the topic and questions for members to relate the material to their lives. During discussions, patients are encouraged to ask questions, share experiences, and identify strategies to manage the issue discussed. The sessions end with a brief review of patients' plans for the coming week (10 to 15 minutes). Patients may also discuss mutual support meetings and other steps they would take in their recovery.

Problem-Solving (Therapy) Groups

Problem-solving therapy groups meet weekly for 90 minutes for 12 or more sessions. The goals are to help patients identify, prioritize, and discuss problems in recovery and to identify strategies to manage these. Patients give and receive support and feedback from each other. After the check-in period, participants are asked to identify a problem or recovery issue for discussion. Often, more than one member identifies a similar problem or issue. Common issues discussed include struggles with motivation to change or remain abstinent; obsessions, compulsions, or close calls to use; lapses or relapses; boredom, anxiety, anger, depression, or other negative emotions; concerns with mutual support programs, a 12-step program, or a sponsor; interpersonal problems and conflicts; social pressures to use substances; financial, job, and lifestyle problems; other addictions; and religion and spirituality. At the end of each session, patients state their plans for the coming week in terms of meetings or other steps to aid their recovery or resolve a problem.

Group Process Issues

Counselors can attend to the group process to keep the group focused and productive. This requires engaging quiet members in discussions and facilitating their self-disclosure and limiting or redirecting members who talk too much and dominate discussions, listen poorly, or use the group session for individual therapy.

Family Psychoeducational Workshop

A family psychoeducational workshop aims to educate the family, provide support, help reduce the family's burden, increase helpful behaviors, decrease unhelpful behaviors, and provide hope. The family psychoeducational workshop is semistructured involving multiple families and members with SUDs present. Families share their questions, concerns, and feelings during the meeting. They learn about symptoms, causes and effects of SUDs, treatment, relapse, and helpful recovery resources for the affected member and families. These can last several hours or all day.

Motivational Interviewing Groups

MI groups are defined as groups that use the MI spirit, processes, and technical skills to increase motivation for change and foster healthy interactions among group members. MI groups more commonly combine MI and other therapeutic interventions such as cognitive–behavioral therapy groups. MI groups are different from educational groups because they focus more on group interactions. MI groups increase self-efficacy and readiness to change. They also facilitate outpatient treatment engagement, attendance, and completion. Increasing participation in aftercare is an outcome of MI groups.

RESEARCH ON GROUP THERAPIES

Controlled trials of group interventions are limited, and many studies report results from "programs" that involve multiple components (eg, individual plus group, multiple types of group treatments, group plus other services). Sobell and Sobell found only five studies that compared the same intervention in both an individual and group format. All five studies found both types of treatment to be effective, but none showed a significant difference in outcomes of patients receiving individual versus group treatment, suggesting that group therapy is as effective as individual treatment.

Weiss et al. reviewed 24 prospective treatment outcome studies comparing group therapy with one or more treatment conditions. The results of the studies were mixed, varying on the nature of the research design, the population studied, and the format of treatment (content, intensity, and length). The findings showed three important patterns: additional specialized group therapy can enhance the effectiveness of "treatment as usual," no differences were found between group and individual modalities, and no single type of group therapy demonstrated any consistent superiority in efficacy. The content of the group did not make a difference. The authors concluded that the most notable finding of that study was the paucity of research on this topic. More recently, positive evidence about MI groups is emerging across pilot and clinical trials. The findings from these trials are consistent across studies and demonstrated that MI groups can reduce drinking frequency and quantity. The evidence supporting MI groups in other areas is limited. However, researchers and clinicians agree on the importance of group therapies, and groups remain one of the principal modalities of treatment in most SUD treatment programs.

Although evidence suggests that group treatments are effective for SUDs, limitations to the research conducted on group treatments arise from two sources: variations in content and differences in process. Difficulties in designing and evaluating group treatment make it more challenging to conduct studies of group therapy. Also, dropout rates are higher among clients in groups compared to in individual therapy.

ADHERENCE TO GROUP SESSIONS AND TREATMENT DROPOUT

Most randomized clinical trials show significant reductions in drug use, improved health, and reduced social pathology. Patients who comply with sessions and attend a sufficient number of sessions show better outcomes than do those who drop out prematurely. Two problems in the treatment of SUDs are poor adherence with session attendance and early termination. The reasons patients cite most commonly for early drop out are time problems, an actual relapse or the desire to use, not finding the group helpful, wanting a different treatment (eg, individual therapy), improvement in the SUD, lack of interest in treatment, or the need for hospitalization.

THE NEED FOR PHYSICIAN INPUT AND SUPPORT

Physicians can provide input into group program development and support and facilitate patients' participation in groups. They can suggest specific topics for recovery groups and/or conduct a group. Some treatment programs use physicians to present groups on topics such as medical aspects of addiction, medications, or addiction and the brain. Physicians can educate, encourage, and motivate patients to participate in treatment groups as part of their overall treatment program. The physician can discuss the patient's group participation to identify and resolve any barriers related to continued participation, to understand the reasons for poor adherence or early dropout, and to help the patient reengage in group. The physician can also collaborate with group therapists about patients' clinical status or problems with adherence.

CONCLUSIONS

Group therapies play a critical role in the treatment of SUDs and should be supported by all clinicians. Different group therapies can be used depending on a given patient's progress in relation to the stages of change and the treatment context. A combination of group and individual treatment is optimal. Staff training and ongoing supervision can enhance the effectiveness of group therapies. Due to the nature of more severe forms of addiction to opioids or alcohol, patients who participate in group therapies often benefit from medications in addition to therapy. Group therapies can encourage attendance at mutual support programs, provide education, increase readiness to change, increase treatment engagement and participation, and explore experiences and resistances. Therapy groups are designed to explore psychological, personal, and interpersonal issues in a safe environment in which self-disclosure, self-awareness, and self-change are encouraged and valued. Group leaders can utilize recovery materials and creative ways to facilitate behavior change and teach coping skills and strategies.

KEY POINTS

1. Different group therapies can be used depending on a given patient's progress in relation to the stages of change and the treatment context.
2. Due to the nature of more severe forms of addiction to opioids or alcohol, patients who participate in group therapies often benefit from medications in addition to group therapy.
3. Group therapies can encourage attendance at mutual support programs, provide education, increase readiness to change, increase treatment engagement and participation, and explore experiences and resistances.

REVIEW QUESTIONS

1. Which of the following statements is *true* about a problem-solving therapy group?
   A. The group leader presents a recovery topic with specific objectives and points for discussion.
   B. Group participants complete written workbook or journal assignments on a topic assigned between group sessions so that they come prepared to the session.
   C. Group members identify and discuss personal problems or issues specific to their current situations.
   D. Family members are included so that they can learn ways to confront the patient who relapses after a period of recovery.

2. Which of the following best describes Sobell and Sobell's findings regarding the research literature that compared five studies of cognitive–behavioral individual and group therapies?
   A. All five studies found both types of treatment to be equally effective.
   B. Group therapy was superior to individual therapy in all but one study.
   C. Nearly 65% of patients dropped out of group treatment in the first month.
   D. Patients prefer Alcoholics Anonymous or Narcotics Anonymous mutual support groups to professional treatment groups.

3. Which of the following was *not* identified as a reason patients dropped out of group therapy before completing treatment?
   A. The patient had time problems.
   B. The patient relapsed.
   C. The patient did not find group therapy helpful.
   D. The patient did not like the group therapist, especially if he or she was not in recovery from an addiction.
   E. The patient needed to be hospitalized.

ANSWERS

1. **C**
2. **A**
3. **D**

SUGGESTED READINGS

Daley DC, Douaihy A. *Group Treatments for Addiction: Counseling Strategies for Recovery and Therapy Groups.* Murrysville, PA: Daley Publications, 2011.

Daley DC, Douaihy A. *Relapse Prevention Counseling: Clinical Strategies to Guide Addiction Recovery and Reduce Relapse.* Eau Claire, WI: PESI Publishing & Media, 2015.

Daley DC, Marlatt GA. *Overcoming Your Drug or Alcohol Problem: Therapist Guide.* New York: Oxford University Press, 2006.

Sobell LC, Sobell MB. *Group Therapy for Substance Use Disorders: A Motivational Cognitive-Behavioral Approach.* New York: Guilford Press, 2011.

Velasquez MM, Maurer GG, Crouch C, DiClemente CC. *Group Treatment for Substance Abuse: A Stages-of-Change Therapy Manual, 2e.* New York: Guilford Press, 2012.

Weiss RD, Jaffee WB, DeMeril VP, Cogley CB. Group therapy for substance use disorders: What do we know? *Harvard Review of Psychiatry.* 2004;12(6):339-350.

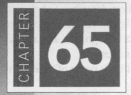

CHAPTER 65

Individual Treatment

Summary by Harshit Sharma

Based on THE ASAM PRINCIPLES OF ADDICTION MEDICINE,
6th edition chapter by Deborah L. Haller and Edward V. Nunes

HISTORY OF PSYCHOTHERAPY FOR SUBSTANCE USE DISORDERS

The first theory-based psychotherapy (psychoanalysis), founded in the late 19th century by Sigmund Freud, was limited in treating substance use disorders (SUDs) because it (1) failed to address overt symptoms like substance use, (2) aroused anxiety and painful affects in vulnerable individuals provoking return to use, and (3) provided limited support or direction for change as therapists were expected to maintain "neutrality." Alcoholics Anonymous (AA), a self-help program, emerged in 1935. In contrast to psychoanalysis, AA focused on alcohol use as the problem behavior and abstinence as the goal. The first therapeutic community to rehabilitate individuals with SUD through a residential program was established in 1958.

It was not until the 1960s that provisions for substance use counseling were included in legislation to fund community mental health centers. When insurance began paying for it, the number of patients with SUDs accessing treatment saw a dramatic rise. However, the interventions were poorly defined and delivered mostly by counselors whose primary credential was their own recovery. This era also saw the emergence of evidence-based psychotherapies. In addition, discovery of the brain reward system helped establish a biological basis for SUDs.

In the 1980s, substance use researchers began to adapt and test therapies originally developed to treat diseases such as depression and anxiety. Among these, cognitive–behavioral therapy emerged as a forerunner of therapies for SUD including cognitive–behavioral relapse prevention, coping skills therapies, and the community reinforcement approach (CRA). Contingency management (CM) grew out of applications of classical behavioral theory and principles of reinforcement. Motivational interviewing (MI) evolved from social psychological theories of interpersonal influence and social learning.

DEVELOPMENT OF PSYCHOTHERAPIES FOR SUBSTANCE USE DISORDERS: THE TECHNOLOGY MODEL

The technology model consists of (1) developing new (or adapting existing) interventions for populations with SUDs, (2) specifying a process for determining the efficacy of interventions, (3) creating a network of treatment programs in which promising interventions may be tested, (4) disseminating positive research findings in a user-friendly format, (5) training clinicians to deliver interventions with fidelity, and (6) providing technical assistance to clinicians and programs to facilitate adoption of these interventions in a timely manner. The National Institute on Drug Abuse launched the Behavioral Therapies Development Program, the objectives of which included development, pilot testing, and standardization of novel and adapted interventions for SUDs, divided into three distinct stages (I, II, and III), similar to the phases of medication development. Stage I serves to answer key questions including: (1) Is the treatment tolerable and feasible? (2) Is the therapy replicable? (3) Does the therapy show promise of effectiveness, based on clinical outcomes from preliminary and pilot studies?

As a result of this initiative, a large cohort of stage I projects were funded, several of which developed into therapies that have proven effective, advancing through stage II and III trials. Stage II represents formal efficacy testing and identifying mechanisms of action of psychotherapies. An intervention that produces a statistically and clinically significant beneficial effect is considered appropriate to advance to stage III testing. The goal of stage III research is to evaluate the generalizability and ease of implementation of treatments. Once determined to be effective, the treatments are implemented and disseminated throughout the larger community.

COMMON ELEMENTS OF EFFECTIVE PSYCHOTHERAPIES

Examination of psychotherapies developed to treat SUDs suggests a set of common elements that include the following.

Focusing Directly on Substance Use

All of the effective behavioral and psychotherapeutic approaches for SUDs maintain a focus on controlling and ameliorating substance use.

Enhancing Motivation to Reduce/ Stop Substance Use and Adhere to a Treatment Plan

Opposing desires (to both use and quit) create a state of ambivalence, which is typical of patients seeking treatment for SUDs. This manifests as efforts to reduce substance use, punctuated by cravings, return to use, and/or fluctuating engagement with treatment. Patients need help to resolve the ambivalence in favor of quitting.

Coping Skills to Avoid Substance Use and Change Lifestyle

Whether patients are struggling to achieve initial abstinence, prevent a return to use, or effect other lifestyle changes to improve their prospects for a long-term recovery, they need to be taught skills and strategies to achieve these ends.

Changing Reinforcement Contingencies

Addictive substances function as reinforcers, becoming increasingly salient and predominant as the SUD progresses. As a patient's behavior increasingly falls under the control of the substance, more time is spent seeking it out and using it, while normal or healthy sources of reinforcement (eg, family, friends, work) are displaced. Thus, an effort to reconnect a patient with their former sources of healthy reinforcement may help to combat the reinforcement value of substances, resulting in a reduction in use. To reduce the likelihood of return to use, patients need to reclaim positive reinforcers and rebuild their lives.

Managing Painful Effects

To avoid negative occurrences such as return to use, patients need to learn to recognize, label, and tolerate painful effects as part of the recovery process from SUD. For example, approaches such as SE therapy and MI encourage the expression of feelings; cognitive behavioral approaches teach skills for tolerating and managing strong effects.

Improving Interpersonal Functioning and Social Support

Individuals with SUDs often have damaged or lost contact with positive social networks. Any remaining relationships often revolve around others who are also in recovery or actively using substances (eg, "drug buddies"). The absence of positive social support can interfere with efforts to recover from SUDs.

Fostering the Treatment Alliance

A treatment alliance refers to the collaborative relationship that develops between the patient and therapist. The alliance is composed of three components—that is, shared goals, tasks, and emotional bonds—and accounts for as much as 15% of the variance in treatment outcomes. A treatment alliance is a common mediator of effectiveness of treatments across a wide range of therapies and disorders. It affects retention, completion, and outcomes among patients with SUDs.

OVERVIEW OF EVIDENCE-BASED PSYCHOTHERAPIES FOR SUBSTANCE USE DISORDERS

Motivational Interviewing and Motivational Enhancement Therapy

MI is a way of approaching and talking to patients that is designed to increase their commitment to reducing or stopping substance use and taking the steps necessary to do so. MI is founded on guiding principles, called the "spirit" of MI—namely, collaboration, evocation, and respect for the autonomy of the patient. The most recent formulation of MI also includes acceptance of the patient for who they are and empathy as an essential stance of the therapist. By expressing genuine curiosity and openness to the patient's experience and values, the clinician builds and communicates empathy. However, MI is not simply an empathic, exploratory interview. It is strategic, seeking to guide the patient toward change. MI prescribes a group of interviewing skills, which include open questions, reflections, affirmations, summarizations, and avoidance of statements that run counter to MI principles (eg, confrontation, argumentation, unsolicited advice). MI therapists are trained to recognize, elicit, and respond to "change talk." Change talk consists of statements by the patient that reflect one or more of desire, ability, reasons, need, and commitment to change their substance use behavior. MI approaches have been shown to be effective in multiple randomized trials; the evidence seems strongest for nicotine and alcohol use disorders, though less consistent for other SUDs.

Brief Advice

Any encounter between a clinician and a patient represents an opportunity for therapeutic effect. Although not a formal psychotherapy, brief advice has been shown to be beneficial in influencing patients to reduce substance use. In some respects, it may seem to be the polar opposite of MI. However, brief advice can be incorporated into the MI paradigm by asking permission before giving advice. This maintains the collaborative nature of the interaction and respects the patient's autonomy.

Supportive–Expressive Therapy

Supportive–expressive (SE) therapy is a time-limited approach, adapted for use with both cocaine and opioid use disorders. It represents an effort to apply psychoanalytic and psychodynamic principles in a systematic way to manage SUDs. SE has two main components. The first employs supportive techniques to assist patients in feeling comfortable discussing their feelings and life experiences, while addressing the role that the substance has played with regard to problematic feelings and behaviors. The second component involves the use of expressive techniques to help the patient understand and work through relationship issues. Clinical trials testing the effectiveness of SE among patients with SUDs have generated mixed results, with some evidence of efficacy in cocaine and opioid use disorders.

Cognitive–Behavioral Approaches: Relapse Prevention and Coping Skills Therapies

Cognitive–behavioral relapse prevention therapy and related approaches are founded on functional analysis, where the sequences of thoughts, feelings, behaviors, and circumstances that lead to substance use for a given patient are reviewed and understood. The therapist then introduces coping skills to promote the unlearning of these maladaptive patterns and to substitute more adaptive patterns that will oppose and prevent substance use. This is a structured, time-limited (8 to 12 weeks), and goal-oriented treatment, which can be flexibly adapted for a variety of individual obstacles, skill deficits, settings, and formats. Through role plays and practice, patients are taught skills including

drug refusal, decisional delay, and talking oneself through cravings. Relapse prevention and coping skills therapies have extensive evidence from clinical trials supporting efficacy in treatment of nicotine, alcohol, and cocaine use disorders.

Community Reinforcement Approach

CRA is a cognitive–behavioral approach that places greater emphasis on examining the reinforcers in a patient's life and helps the patient to reengage and reconnect with healthy sources of reinforcement (eg, family, friends, work, recreation). The theory is that this will interfere with and replace drug-seeking behaviors, which are under the control of reinforcement by the substance. CRA often is combined with contingency management in which voucher-based rewards are used to enhance abstinence. These two approaches seem synergistic because the vouchers provide concrete rewards within the therapy, whereas the CRA attempts to foster rewards within the patient's life outside of therapy.

Contingency Management

CM seeks to directly harness the principles of reinforcement and behavior modification by making concrete rewards or punishments contingent upon some key target behavior. The target behavior usually is abstinence from substance use as confirmed by urine testing, but other targets such as attendance also can be reinforced. The basic principle is that contingent rewards or punishments will help reduce the likelihood of substance use and help patients achieve and sustain abstinence. CM has been applied effectively for substances such as cocaine, heroin, and cannabis where use over the last several days can be readily detected in urine. The use of CM for alcohol use disorder is limited by its quick washout, resulting in false-negative breath tests. Recently, ethyl glucuronide, a longer lasting metabolite of alcohol, has been used successfully as the basis for a CM intervention for alcohol use disorder. Principles of learning suggest that positive reinforcement tends to produce behaviors that are more durable and generalizable beyond the immediate context. Hence, many of the most successful CM treatments have worked with rewards, often where the magnitude of the reward increases with each consecutive negative urine; this procedure is intended to shape prolonged periods of abstinence. Among psychotherapeutic and behavioral treatments for SUDs, CM has shown the most consistent and strongest evidence of efficacy compared to control conditions, at least during treatment. Response tends to be bimodal, however; around half the patients rapidly achieve abstinence, whereas the remainder achieve little or no abstinence. Also, the impact tends to wear off, at least partially, when the treatment ends, with some patients returning to use.

Individual Drug Counseling

Individual drug counseling (IDC) was one of the first science-based treatments for SUDs. The IDC approach includes assessing the patient's status prior to initiating treatment and recommends use of the Addiction Severity Index and a urine toxicology to ascertain abstinence. The phases of treatment in IDC include (1) treatment initiation (targeting denial and ambivalence); (2) early abstinence, which focuses on advice for minimizing return to use, dealing with cravings and high-risk situations (similar to cognitive–behavioral approaches) and 12-step meeting attendance; (3) maintaining abstinence by addressing the potential for return to use, dealing with relationships while in recovery, living a drug-free lifestyle, encouraging spirituality, and dealing with character defects; (4) advanced recovery; (5) dealing with specific problems, including return to use; (6) counselor characteristics and training; and (7) counselor supervision. IDC incorporates the essential elements of the 12-step approach, while also addressing the important issue of intervention fidelity, thus allowing it to be compared with other evidence-based interventions for SUDs. Study results show that high-quality substance use counseling delivered by trained clinicians, 12-step meeting attendance, and a commitment to abstinence can make for an effective therapy.

Twelve-Step Facilitation

Twelve-step facilitation (TSF) is characterized as a guided approach to "facilitating" early recovery and is intended to give clinicians a tool to help their patients engage productively in AA or other 12-step groups. The therapy focuses on two general goals: acceptance of the need for abstinence and surrender, which includes a willingness to engage in the TSF as a means to achieving sobriety. The act of surrender to the "group conscience" involves acknowledging that 12-step programs have helped millions of people to achieve and sustain sobriety and that the best chance at recovery comes through following the 12-step path. TSF counselors assess patients' substance use, advocate for abstinence, explain basic 12-step concepts, and actively support and facilitate involvement in AA or Narcotics Anonymous. TSF has been studied to produce long-term abstinence in patients with alcohol use disorder and has recently shown some promise in patients with stimulant use disorder.

Medical Management

Medical management interventions originally were developed to provide clinicians who were treating patients in pharmacotherapy trials with a standard, well-specified set of goals and talking points to cover during clinic visits. Typically, clinicians are asked to systematically address symptoms, side effects, and medication adherence and to troubleshoot any problems in an empathic, supportive, and nonjudgmental manner. Medical management interventions focus on medication adherence, monitoring side effects, and troubleshooting problems with adherence. In addition, they also focus on abstinence as a goal and address problems in achieving or sustaining abstinence, sometimes recommending 12-step participation.

DIFFERENTIAL THERAPEUTICS: HOW TO MATCH PATIENTS WITH THERAPIES

Choosing the best treatment for a given patient remains more art than science. In the absence of strong indicators for matching patients to specific substance use treatments, a sensible approach is to make a best guess as to where to start and then be prepared to switch interventions if the initial effort fails. Unfortunately, clinicians (and treatment programs) tend to offer just one or only a few predominant treatment methods in a "one-size-fits-all" approach. Many clinicians have not been formally schooled in the evidence-based approaches described in this chapter; accordingly, they may be at a loss as to what to do next when their "go to" intervention fails to produce the desired results. Clinicians must be prepared to deliver alternative interventions themselves or else refer their patients to other therapists who have a larger repertoire of treatment options.

VIRTUAL THERAPY AND COMPUTER-DELIVERED TECHNOLOGY-BASED INTERVENTIONS

Over the past decade, technology has played an increasingly important role in the treatment of SUDs. A large proportion of patients with SUDs do not seek out or otherwise engage in treatment due to various barriers. Technology-assisted interventions can help to overcome these barriers (like low motivation to change, stigma, high cost, and/or limited availability of services) by making treatment more accessible. Patients who are not yet ready to seek out treatment may still be willing to complete a screening tool anonymously through the Web, including those that provide feedback and/or advice to change. If an intervention, such as a cognitive–behavioral intervention, can be delivered through a computer, or an app on a phone, then clinicians at a treatment program can prescribe the intervention and monitor patient participation. However, many interventions and apps, although developed and marketed, do not have adequate empirical evidence yet to support their efficacy and lack funding to support their growth.

TECHNOLOGY TRANSFER: HOW TO TRAIN CLINICIANS TO DELIVER EVIDENCE-BASED PSYCHOTHERAPIES

Although a number of effective treatments for SUDs are available, these are not widely used in the community-based treatment system. Technology transfer refers to the process of taking a new technology (like evidence-based psychotherapy in this case) and getting it into widespread use in the community. A fundamental precept of technology transfer is that clinicians need encouragement, feedback, and supervision in order to learn and successfully use new psychotherapeutic skills. Clinical trials among physicians have repeatedly shown that traditional methods of introducing new treatments (journal articles, lectures, and didactic symposia or workshops) may increase knowledge but do not get physicians to actually practice the new methods. Studies of methods for training community-based clinicians in MI have tended to confirm the lack of effectiveness of didactic workshops alone. These findings suggest that efforts to disseminate new psychotherapies for SUD into the treatment community should shift focus away from didactic exercises to feedback and clinical supervision. Treatment programs should be encouraged to set aside time for clinical supervision intended to introduce, build, and maintain new clinical skills.

KEY POINTS

1. The behavioral therapies development process has three distinct stages: (1) materials development (including manual and rating forms) and pilot testing, (2) efficacy testing in highly selected samples with expert therapists, and (3) effectiveness testing in typical patients (real-world settings) and typical therapists.
2. For clinics to successfully implement these interventions, staff requires didactic training, clinical supervision, and feedback.
3. Effective individual interventions include dynamic, motivational, and multiple behavioral interventions.

DEDICATION

This chapter is dedicated to the memory of the late Dr. Bruce Rounsaville, our friend and colleague and the previous author of this chapter.

REVIEW QUESTIONS

1. Which of the following is a key component of the technology model?
   A. Developing/adapting interventions and targeting and training clinicians to deliver them with fidelity
   B. Determining the efficacy of the interventions
   C. Conducting effectiveness studies in real-world treatment settings
   D. All of the above.

2. Which of the following is not a significant element of efficacious treatments for the substance use disorders?
   A. Building an alliance, enhancing motivation to change, and managing painful affects
   B. Understanding unconscious motivations and defenses
   C. Focusing directly on substance use and changing reinforcement contingencies
   D. Teaching coping skills, improving functioning, and enhancing social support

3. True or False: In cognitive–behavioral relapse prevention and related approaches, the therapist introduces coping skills to promote the unlearning of maladaptive patterns and to substitute more adaptive patterns that will oppose and prevent substance use.

ANSWERS

1. **D**
2. **B**
3. **True**

SUGGESTED READINGS

Bien TH, Miller WR, Tonigan JS. Brief interventions for alcohol problems: a review. *Addiction*. 1993;88(3):315-335.

Carroll KM. *A Cognitive-Behavioral Approach: Treating Cocaine Addiction. Therapy Manuals for Drug Addiction. Manual 1*. Rockville, MD: National Institute on Drug Abuse, 1998.

Mark D, Luborsky L. *A Manual for the Use of Supportive-Expressive Psychotherapy in the Treatment of Cocaine Abuse*. Philadelphia: University of Pennsylvania, 1992.

Mercer DE, Woody GE. *Individual Drug Counseling. Therapy Manuals for Drug Addiction Series. Manual 3*. Rockville, MD: National Institute on Drug Abuse, 1999.

Miller WR, Rollnick S. *Motivational Interviewing: Helping People Change*. 3rd ed. New York: Guilford Press, 2013.

66 Contingency Management and the Community Reinforcement Approach

Summary by Sarah H. Heil, Christopher A. Arger, Danielle R. Davis, and Stephen T. Higgins

> Based on THE ASAM PRINCIPLES OF ADDICTION MEDICINE, 6th edition chapter by Sarah H. Heil, Danielle R. Davis, Christopher A. Arger, and Stephen T. Higgins

Contingency management (CM) interventions and community reinforcement approach (CRA) therapy for treating substance use disorders (SUDs) are based on the conceptual framework of learning and conditioning theory. Especially fundamental to these treatment approaches is operant conditioning, which is the study of how systematically applied environmental consequences increase (reinforce) or decrease (punish) the frequency and patterning of voluntary behavior. In this model, drug use is considered a normal, learned behavior that falls along a continuum ranging from little use and few problems to excessive use and many untoward effects. The same principles of learning and conditioning are assumed to operate across this continuum.

This conceptual framework has played a significant role in the development of the field of behavioral economics, which underscores how unhealthy behaviors can be conceptualized in terms of behavioral choice wherein less healthy options are repeatedly chosen over more healthy alternatives. One of the decision-making processes that behavioral economics research has demonstrated as integral to understanding these suboptimal choice patterns is delay discounting, in which greater preference is shown for more immediate, smaller magnitude reinforcement (eg, smoking a cigarette) over more delayed, larger magnitude reinforcement (eg, better health). CM and CRA interventions are designed to reorganize the patient's environment to systematically increase reinforcement obtained while abstinent from drug use and to reduce or eliminate reinforcement obtained through drug use and associated activities.

TREATMENT MODEL

In this treatment model, reinforcement derived from drug use and the associated lifestyle is deemed to have monopolized the behavioral repertoire of the patient. Primary emphasis is placed on decreasing drug use by systematically increasing the availability and frequency of alternative reinforcing activities either through relatively contrived sources of reinforcement as in CM interventions or more naturalistic sources as in CRA therapy. Additionally, arranging the environment so that aversive events or the loss of reinforcing events (ie, punishment procedures) occur as a consequence of drug use can also decrease drug use. By *contrived*, we mean a set of contingencies that are put in place explicitly and exclusively for therapeutic purposes (eg, earning vouchers exchangeable for retail items contingent on cocaine-negative urine toxicology results). By *naturalistic*, we mean a set of contingencies that are already operating in the natural environment for nontherapeutic purposes but can be used to support the therapeutic process (eg, teaching a spouse to deliver praise when a patient avoids bars and to withhold praise or express disapproval for going to bars).

Some treatments are designed to deliver contrived consequences during the initial treatment period, with a transition to more naturalistic sources later in treatment. The rationale for that sequence is that the lifestyle of the patient is often so disrupted upon treatment entry that it is largely devoid of effective alternative sources of reinforcement that can compete with the reinforcement derived from drug use. Contrived sources of alternative reinforcement delivered through CM are designed to promote initial abstinence, thereby allowing time for therapists and patients to work toward reestablishing more naturalistic alternatives (eg, job, stable family life, participation in self-help and other social groups that reinforce abstinence).

TREATMENT PLANNING

Detailed information is collected on drug use, treatment readiness, psychiatric functioning, employment/vocational status, recreational interests, current social supports, family and social problems, and legal issues. A practical needs assessment questionnaire is also used to determine whether the patient has any pressing needs or crises that may interfere with initial treatment engagement (eg, housing, legal, transportation, childcare).

PRETREATMENT ISSUES
Selection and Preparation of Patients

There is no patient with SUDs for whom CM or CRA is contraindicated. With CM, it is quite common to have patients sign a written contract stipulating all aspects of the CM arrangement to avoid any confusion about the contingencies.

Therapist Characteristics

To implement CRA effectively, therapists need to be directive but also flexible. Particularly in the early stages of treatment, therapists try to work around patient schedules and generally make participation in treatment convenient to the patient. Within ethical boundaries, therapists must be committed to doing what it takes to facilitate lifestyle changes on the part of patients. Therapists often accompany patients to appointments or job interviews. They initiate recreational activities with patients and schedule sessions at different times of day to accomplish specific goals. They have patients make phone calls from their office. They search newspapers and online postings for job possibilities or ideas for healthy recreational activities in which patients might be able to participate.

TREATMENT TECHNIQUE

The basic elements of CM and CRA interventions are described using the CRA + Vouchers treatment for cocaine use disorder for illustration purposes.

Contingency Management

The CM component of the CRA + Vouchers treatment involves vouchers exchangeable for retail items that are earned contingent on negative results in thrice-weekly urine toxicology testing. In our studies, the first negative specimen earns a voucher worth $2.50. The value of each subsequent consecutive negative specimen increases by $1.25. A bonus is provided for every three consecutive negative specimens. The intent of the escalating magnitude of reinforcement and bonuses is to reinforce continuous abstinence. A positive specimen or failure to submit a scheduled specimen resets the value of vouchers back to the initial value. This reset feature is designed to punish relapse to use after a period of sustained abstinence, with the intensity of the punishment tied directly to the length of sustained abstinence that was broken. In order to provide patients with a reason to continue abstaining from drug use after a reset, submission of five consecutive negative specimens after a positive specimen returns the value of the voucher back to where it was prior to the reset.

Community Reinforcement Approach

The CRA component of the CRA + Vouchers treatment has seven elements:

1. Patients are taught how to recognize antecedents and consequences of their drug use and to use this information to put together self-management plans to decrease the chances of future cocaine use.
2. Patients are also assisted with systematically developing a new social network that will support a healthier lifestyle and with getting involved in recreational activities that do not involve drug use.
3. Various other forms of individualized skill training are provided to patients, usually to address some specific skill deficit that may directly or indirectly influence their risk for future drug use.
4. Unemployed patients are offered employment assistance.
5. Patients with romantic partners who do not use drugs are offered behavioral couples therapy, which is an intervention designed to teach couples positive communication skills and how to negotiate reciprocal contracts for desired changes in each other's behavior.
6. All patients receive HIV/AIDS education.
7. Pharmacotherapy is offered to all patients who meet criteria.

EMPIRICAL SUPPORT
Community Reinforcement Approach + Vouchers Intervention

The CRA + Vouchers intervention garnered significant interest when it was introduced in the 1990s because of its efficacy with cocaine use disorder. At a time when most clinical trials investigating treatments for cocaine use disorder were consistently producing negative outcomes, a series of controlled trials examining this approach produced reliably positive outcomes. Subsequent trials dismantled the CRA + Vouchers intervention to examine the contribution of each component. These studies demonstrated the importance of the contingency and of voucher magnitude in the CM portion of the intervention and provided evidence that CRA contributed in numerous ways to the positive outcomes observed. Additional trials examined the CRA + Vouchers treatment with other SUDs, using different modalities, and in other settings, demonstrating the generality of the intervention across drug classes, formats, and to communities outside the United States.

Developing Contingency Management as a Treatment for Illicit Substance Use Disorders

Up to this point, the emphasis has been on the combination treatment of CRA + Vouchers. However, prior to the introduction of CM in the form of vouchers, there was strong empirical data in the literature on CM for the treatment of SUDs using other forms of reinforcement. That work was almost exclusively conducted with patients enrolled in methadone treatment for opioid use disorder. Although methadone is effective at eliminating the use of illicit opioids, a subset of patients continue using other nonopioid drugs. A commonly used reinforcer in this area of CM is the medication take-home privilege, where an extra daily dose of opioid medication is dispensed to the patient for ingestion at home on the following day, thereby granting the patient a break from the routine of having to travel to the clinic to ingest the medication under staff supervision.

Subsequent to these seminal studies, research on CM for SUDs has developed in many exciting directions. A recent PubMed search of "contingency management" involving SUDs returned more than 500 publications. In the following sections, we briefly summarize some of the current trends in the evolving CM literature.

Extending Contingency Management to Special Populations

Special populations appears to be an area where CM is finding a niche, perhaps because CM has been demonstrated to be among the most effective treatments at promoting abstinence in these populations. One of the best examples of this is the use of voucher-based reinforcement of abstinence among pregnant cigarette smokers. A series of clinical trials have systematically replicated the efficacy of vouchers delivered contingent on smoking abstinence, with some also documenting significant increases in fetal growth and improved birth outcomes. One of these trials also demonstrated that vouchers increased abstinence above control levels when implemented by obstetrical staff in a large urban hospital working with community tobacco interventionists. Another reported the first econometric analysis of this approach, showing vouchers to be highly cost effective.

Extending Contingency Management into Community Clinics

In addition to one of the studies noted in the prior section, a number of other studies have demonstrated that CM interventions implemented by clinical rather than research staff can be effective. It is also anticipated that some of the novel technologies being integrated into CM interventions, like using videos recorded on and submitted via cell phone to objectively monitor abstinence, will also facilitate the integration of CM into routine care in community clinics. In another effort to increase uptake of the voucher-based CM approach by community clinics, a variation known as prize-based CM was developed. In this procedure, rather than reinforce each occurrence of the target response, patients earned the opportunity to draw from a bowl that contained vouchers of varying value, including many that are of zero value but offer verbal praise, some that are of relatively low monetary value, still fewer of moderate value, and a very few worth high monetary value. Studies have demonstrated this approach to be efficacious for increasing cocaine and other drug abstinence in drug-free and methadone community clinics.

Investigating Longer Term Outcomes of Contingency Management

There is often observed a weakening in the magnitude of treatment effects when comparing overall effects when incentives are in place versus after their discontinuation. Some studies have expressly focused on promoting better longer term outcomes by seeking to build on correlational data, suggesting that one key to fostering longer term abstinence is increasing during-treatment abstinence, whereas others have focused on voucher-based maintenance therapy. Important to underscore is that this need for greater focus on promoting and sustaining longer term behavior change is a priority and a challenge for CM. Also important to note, however, is that the need for greater focus on sustaining behavior change is not unique to CM and extends to all behavioral, psychosocial, and pharmacologic interventions for SUDs and other chronic conditions where behavior is a proximal cause.

Developing Community Reinforcement Approach as a Treatment for Alcohol Use Disorder

CRA was developed and most extensively researched in the treatment of alcohol use disorder. In the initial study, CRA was designed to rearrange and improve the quality of the reinforcers obtained by patients through their vocational, family, social, and recreational activities. Patients treated with CRA demonstrated marked reductions in time spent drinking and superior outcomes on a number of other measures.

After publication of the seminal study, CRA was subsequently expanded to include additional components, including disulfiram therapy with monitoring by a significant other to ensure medication compliance, counseling directed at crises resolution, a "buddy" system in which individuals in the participant's neighborhood volunteered to be available to give assistance with practical issues and a switch from individual to group counseling to reduce cost. This revised intervention proved superior to standard care in terms of percent of time spent drinking, unemployed, away from family, and institutionalized. Another study completed as part of the original CRA series examined the effects of adding a social club, designed to have the social atmosphere of a tavern but without alcohol, to a standard regimen of outpatient counseling. Greater improvements were observed in terms of alcohol consumed as well as in ratings of behavioral impairment and time spent in heavy-drinking situations in the social club group as compared to the control group. Since these initial studies, research on CRA has continued and, like CM, has been adapted for use with special populations. Next, we briefly review some of these efforts.

Extending the Community Reinforcement Approach to Special Populations

Adolescents
The first study with adolescents involved individuals randomly assigned to CRA or supportive counseling. The CRA intervention had three major components: stimulus control, urge control, and social control/contracting. Abstinence from drug use was significantly higher as compared to the supportive counseling condition. School attendance, employment, family relationships, and depression symptoms were also better in the CRA condition as compared to the supportive counseling condition. Additional evidence supporting the efficacy of CRA with adolescents has been sufficiently positive to warrant a large-scale dissemination effort throughout the United States.

The Homeless
The efficacy of CRA has been examined in adults with alcohol use disorder and youth living on the street. In studies with adults, those treated with CRA showed greater improvement on measures of drinking over a 1-year period. In the study with homeless youth, substance use and depression scores decreased more among a larger proportion of those treated with CRA than usual care, whereas measures of social stability increased more among those treated with CRA versus usual care.

Significant Others
CRA has also been adapted for use with significant others of treatment-resistant patients with alcohol use disorder, an approach that has come to be referred to as community reinforcement and family training. The intervention includes education about alcohol problems, information and discussion of the positive consequences of not drinking, assistance with involving the patient with alcohol use disorder in healthy activities, increasing the involvement of the significant other in social and recreational activities, training on how to respond to drinking episodes (including dangerous situations), and how to recommend treatment entry to the family member with alcohol use disorder. A series of controlled trials have consistently supported the efficacy of this approach in getting unmotivated individuals with alcohol use disorders and individuals with illicit drug use disorders to enter treatment.

KEY POINTS

1. CM and CRA treatments are designed to reorganize the patient's environment to reduce/eliminate reinforcement obtained through drug use and to increase reinforcement obtained while abstinent.
2. Each component of CM and CRA contributes significantly to the positive outcomes associated with the combined intervention.
3. The evidence supporting the efficacy of CM and CRA is quite robust.

ACKNOWLEDGMENTS

Preparation of this work was supported by R01 HD075669, R01 HD078332, R01 DA036670, P20 GM103644, and T32 DA07242 from the National Institutes of Health.

REVIEW QUESTIONS

1. From the operant conceptual framework, treatments for substance use disorders should:
   A. target drug use and addiction as a brain disease.
   B. increase reinforcement for abstinence.
   C. arrange for the loss of reinforcers following drug use.
   D. both B and C.

2. CM and CRA treatment approaches have been tested and are efficacious with all of the following populations *except*:
   A. pregnant cigarette smokers.
   B. people who consume edible marijuana products.
   C. adolescents with substance use disorders.
   D. homeless patients with alcohol use disorder.

3. Which of the following is *false* regarding the CM/CRA model?
   A. Drug use is considered a normal learned behavior.

B. A family history of alcoholism is *not* necessary to develop a substance use disorder.
C. Substance use disorders result as a secondary consequence of primary psychiatric problems.
D. Consequences related to drug use fall along a spectrum of a few problems to many problems.

ANSWERS

1. **D**
2. **B**
3. **C**

SUGGESTED READINGS

Budney AJ, Higgins ST. *The Community Reinforcement Plus Vouchers Approach. Therapy Manuals for Drug Addiction. Manual 2.* Rockville, MD: National Institute on Drug Abuse, 1998.

Godley SH, Meyers RJ, Smith JE, et al. *The Adolescent Community Reinforcement Approach for Adolescent Cannabis Users. Cannabis Youth Treatment (CYT) Series. Volume 4.* Rockville, MD: Center for Substance Abuse Treatment, Substance Abuse and Mental Health Services Administration, 2001. DHHS Pub. No. (SMA) 07-3864.

Higgins ST, Silverman K, Heil SH, eds. *Contingency Management in Substance Abuse Treatment.* New York: Guilford Press, 2008.

Mazur JE. *Learning and Behavior.* 8th ed. New York, NY: Routledge, 2017.

Meyers RJ, Smith JE. *Clinical Guide to Alcohol Treatment: The Community Reinforcement Approach.* New York: Guildford Press, 1995.

67 Behavioral Interventions for Nicotine/Tobacco Use Disorder

Summary by Erika Litvin Bloom, Christopher W. Kahler, Adam M. Leventhal, and Richard A. Brown

Based on THE ASAM PRINCIPLES OF ADDICTION MEDICINE, 6th edition chapter by Erika Litvin Bloom, Christopher W. Kahler, Adam M. Leventhal, and Richard A. Brown

RELEVANCE FOR SUBSTANCE USE DISORDER TREATMENT

The majority of patients in treatment for a non-nicotine substance use disorder (SUD) also smoke cigarettes, and about 50% to 80% of these patients who smoke indicate an interest in or desire to quit smoking. Studies have found that inclusion of nicotine/tobacco use disorder (NTUD) treatment in the context of other SUD treatment programs does not reduce long-term treatment completion. Furthermore, most studies have found that NTUD interventions initiated during other SUD treatment do not harm treatment outcomes and may even be associated with better substance use outcomes. In addition, other recent studies have found that patients who quit smoking on their own following other SUD treatment have significantly better substance use outcomes compared to those who continue smoking.

Nevertheless, patients may be unaware of this data and express a preference for delaying NTUD treatment until after finishing an SUD treatment, out of concern that stopping nicotine/tobacco use will jeopardize their sobriety from other substances. We recommend that all patients in SUD treatment who use nicotine/tobacco be informed of these research outcomes to address concerns about interference with treatment for their other SUDs; be provided at least a brief NTUD intervention, including offering pharmacologic aids; and be encouraged to quit smoking as soon as possible. Referral to state-sponsored telephone "quitlines" is also recommended. Such direct advice to quit smoking from a clinician may be at least as effective, if not more effective, than more extensive motivational interventions. Interventions with this population can generally mirror those used with all patients who smoke, which are reviewed in the following sections. The use of pharmacotherapy may be especially important given that patients with other SUDs tend to smoke more cigarettes per day than do those without other SUDs.

The prevalence of electronic cigarette (e-cigarette) use has increased dramatically in recent years. Many individuals report that they have used e-cigarettes as treatment for NTUD (ie, they have stopped smoking cigarettes and have switched to e-cigarettes). However, the long-term safety and efficacy of e-cigarettes has not yet been determined. These devices have not been approved by the US Food and Drug Administration for NTUD treatment.

TREATMENT PLANNING

- *Ask* patients whether they smoke cigarettes: All patients should be asked whether or not they have ever smoked, when they last smoked a cigarette, and the typical number of cigarettes they currently smoke per day.
- *Advise* all patients to quit: Patients report that physician advice to quit smoking is often an important factor in their deciding to make a quit attempt, and trials have found that brief advice (<3 minutes) by a clinician to quit smoking increases the odds of abstinence by about 30%.
- *Assess* willingness to make a quit attempt: Patients present with differing levels of motivation for quitting smoking, and interventions should be based on a patient's readiness to change.
- *Assist* patients in making a quit attempt, as described in the following sections.
- *Arrange* follow-up contacts to help prevent relapse.

TREATMENT AND TECHNIQUE
Preparing for Quitting

We recommend a "preparation" period before quitting smoking, the length of which can vary according to program needs. There are three key objectives for this period: (1) patients' motivations to quit and commitment to the program should be clarified and reinforced, (2) patients should self-monitor their daily smoking behavior to begin to learn about their smoking triggers, and (3) a target quit day should be clearly established to allow patients the time to "mentally prepare" and develop coping strategies for quitting smoking.

Motivating Patients to Quit Smoking

Patients who smoke may be ambivalent about the prospect of quitting. This may be especially true for those who have failed in prior quit attempts. Acknowledging this ambivalence without directly challenging patients can help diffuse some of its power to undermine their commitment. A useful and effective method for exploring readiness to change is to have patients rate on a numeric scale (eg, from 0 to 10) the importance they place on quitting smoking and the confidence they have in successfully quitting. After a patient has provided these ratings, a clinician can inquire further about factors influencing each rating. For example, a clinician might ask, "What made you give a rating of 4 to the importance of quitting rather than a 0?" In this way, the patient is prompted to generate reasons to quit smoking on his or her own. Similarly, exploring confidence ratings can reveal roadblocks that may prevent more motivated patients from taking action and can help identify potential strategies for overcoming these roadblocks.

The challenge is to move patients from general acceptance of potential negative consequences (eg, "smoking is dangerous to health") to personalized acceptance (eg, "smoking is dangerous to *my* health"). For patients who have low importance ratings, personalized information and feedback can raise awareness of the ways in which smoking is affecting their health. Feedback can take several forms, including evidence of the effects of smoking on the patient's current physical symptoms (eg, "smoker's cough") and laboratory findings, impact of smoking on disease states, and relationship between smoking and risk. Feedback about the deleterious effects of continued smoking should be paired with feedback about the benefits of cessation. After each piece of information, clinicians should elicit patients' reactions, answer their questions, and then empathize with and validate their concerns before providing new information. It can also be helpful to have patients write down their specific reasons for both quitting and continuing smoking, because the latter can help patients identify likely barriers to quitting.

For patients who place higher levels of importance on quitting but are not taking action because of a lack of confidence, clinicians can emphasize that it may take several quit attempts before they are finally successful. It is also useful to explore reasons for continued smoking and barriers to quitting so that potential solutions for overcoming barriers can be discussed. Given that the majority of patients who smoke are not willing to quit immediately, it is important that clinicians have modest expectations of whether their patients will make a quit attempt. Patients who are chronically stuck may benefit from encouragement to take small steps toward action, such as cutting down the number of cigarettes they smoke, delaying their first cigarette of the day, or trying to quit for just 24 hours. The goal of intervention with a patient who is not committed is to move him or her closer to change. Follow-up visits can allow for continued monitoring of readiness and for repeated interventions to enhance motivation and facilitate quitting.

Self-Monitoring of Smoking Behavior

Keeping a written or electronic record of cigarettes smoked can help increase knowledge about the factors cueing and maintaining smoking behavior. Self-monitoring also interrupts the automatic smoking habit and encourages patients to think about every cigarette they smoke and why they smoke it. Often, this procedure reduces the number of cigarettes smoked per day. An assessment of mood at the time of each cigarette also can be useful. The situational notations allow patients to identify antecedents that trigger their smoking.

Patients may find self-monitoring of their smoking behavior inconvenient. It is important that clinicians present the rationale for self-monitoring clearly and follow through at all sessions by reviewing the self-monitoring information with patients to highlight its relevance in their quitting efforts.

Choosing a Quit Date

Central to the quit plan is setting a quit date, ideally within 2 weeks. Setting this date allows patients to plan for quitting and to obtain the necessary support, which may include the following:

- Telling their family and friends about their quit date
- Making sure that all tobacco products and associated cues, such as ashtrays and cigarette lighters, have been removed
- For those who drink alcohol, avoiding drinking alcohol as much as possible while quitting (alcohol

use is involved in about one fourth of all relapses to smoking)

■ Thinking about potential triggers for smoking and considering situations in which relapse might be likely to occur

■ Reading self-help materials that are available through numerous agencies

■ Accessing state-funded "quitlines," which offer from three to six sessions of proactive counseling

■ Pharmacotherapies, including nicotine replacement therapies (gum, inhaler, nasal spray, lozenge, and patch), varenicline, and bupropion SR

Patients should be advised to smoke their last cigarette on the night before their quit date so that they wake up a nonsmoker.

Providers should schedule a specific time to connect immediately with the patient after the quit day to reinforce successes and troubleshoot difficulties in cessation efforts. Follow-up contacts also provide an opportunity to work with patients who have relapsed to smoking. Clinicians can help patients view a relapse as a learning experience that is part of the normal process of quitting and encourage patients to continue their efforts to quit.

CESSATION STAGE INTERVENTIONS

Self-management (sometimes termed *self-control* or *stimulus control*) procedures are a critical component of behavioral smoking interventions. Self-management procedures refer to strategies intended to rearrange environmental cues that "trigger" smoking or to alter the consequences of smoking. Using their smoking records, patients develop a list of trigger situations. They then begin to intervene in these situations to break up the smoking behavior chain (ie, situation, urge, smoke) by using one of three general strategies:

■ *Avoid* the trigger situation: foregoing a coffee break at work with other people who smoke, leaving the table after dinner, and avoiding social situations involving alcohol.

■ *Alter* or change the trigger situation: drinking tea or juice in the morning instead of coffee, watching television in a nonsmoking room, and putting cigarettes in the trunk of the car before driving.

■ Use an *alternative* or substitute in place of the cigarette, often in conjunction with avoiding or altering trigger situations or in situations that cannot be avoided or altered: chewing gum, sugarless candy, or cut-up vegetables; toothpicks; relaxation techniques in stressful situations; or activities such as needlework that can keep the hands busy.

Patients should choose strategies that they think will work for them and then try out different approaches, rejecting those that are not useful until they have successfully managed all or most trigger situations without smoking.

Positive social support can be a source of motivation for quitting and has been shown to increase abstinence. It can also provide positive reinforcement for maintaining abstinence and act as a buffer against stressful life events that might precipitate a relapse. Social support outside of treatment might include making specific requests to friends and family members about steps they can take to support the patient's abstinence efforts.

Because the majority of patients who smoke who initially quit resume smoking within several months of treatment termination, maintenance is a critical issue for smoking cessation programs. The most commonly used behavioral maintenance strategies are based on the relapse prevention model. Preliminary evidence suggests that extending behavioral treatment and pharmacotherapy may improve cessation outcomes.

Relapse prevention theory proposes that the ability to cope with "high-risk" situations for relapse determines an individual's probability of maintaining abstinence. High-risk situations often involve at least one of the following elements: negative moods, positive moods, social situations involving alcohol, and being in the presence of those who smoke. To help patients identify high-risk situations, a clinician can ask, "If you were to slip and smoke a cigarette after quit day, in what situation would it be?" For each high-risk situation, patients can develop a set of strategies for managing the situation without smoking. They should be reminded that these high-risk situations are similar to the trigger situations they have previously addressed and that they can apply similar self-management strategies (ie, avoid, alter, or use an alternative) as well as other problem-solving skills.

When patients experience a slip, they often progress to further smoking and full relapse. In the event that a slip happens, a few steps can be taken to regain abstinence. First, a slip is an important time for clinicians to assess motivation or commitment to quitting. Has motivation changed or is the patient ambivalent about quitting? Does the patient support the goal of quitting completely or does he or she believe that occasional cigarettes are unlikely to be harmful? If motivation is flagging, then use of the motivational interventions described previously is appropriate. If motivation remains high, then it is important for the clinician and the patient to review the circumstances of the slip to better determine why it happened. The lessons learned from the slip are reviewed, and plans for avoiding similar slips in the future can then be made.

A negative addiction such as smoking can be replaced with a "positive addiction" by increasing participation in activities that are incompatible with smoking and are a source of pleasure. Patients are encouraged to set aside time as often as possible (ideally, on a daily basis) for this purpose. It is in this context that we strongly encourage patients to engage in some type of regular physical exercise. Exercise may also be a good alternative to dieting for individuals who are concerned about gaining weight after quitting smoking.

SPECIAL POPULATIONS

Alcohol consumption is the third leading cause of death in the United States, and excessive drinking results in numerous well-documented physical and mental health problems. The combined effects of excessive drinking and smoking are enormous.

A recent clinical trial found that incorporating a brief alcohol intervention into NTUD treatment for people who drank heavily but who were not alcohol dependent led to significantly lower levels of drinking and increased the odds of smoking abstinence. Steps for a brief alcohol intervention include assessing alcohol use and problems, providing clear advice to reduce drinking for those who are drinking excessively, assessing readiness to change drinking patterns, and helping patients set safer drinking goals and make plans for achieving those goals. It is also important to educate patients that any alcohol use, and especially heavy drinking, can greatly increase the odds of a smoking relapse.

Patients with psychiatric comorbidities are twice as likely to smoke as individuals without psychiatric comorbidities. Psychotic disorders, mood disorders, anxiety disorders, and attention deficit hyperactivity disorder are among the most common psychiatric diseases among people who smoke. Certain clinical characteristics of patients with psychiatric comorbidities and contextual factors present only in psychiatric settings should be taken into account when applying behavioral treatments for smoking.

Patients with psychiatric comorbidities with NTUD are more likely to have sociodemographic risk factors that could lead to poorer smoking outcomes, including being divorced or separated, disabled, uninsured, and having fewer years of education. Those who smoke also have more comorbid

psychiatric disorders, lower global functioning, and poorer psychiatric treatment compliance relative to patients with a psychiatric disease who do not smoke. Thus, patients who smoke in the psychiatric setting may be encountering the most severe and complex psychosocial problems of any population. Despite these challenges, severity and chronicity of psychiatric disease do not predict whether patients who are depressed are willing to accept a combined behavioral–pharmacologic nicotine-dependent treatment program, nor does severity predict current motivation to quit smoking.

Another clinical characteristic that may differ in patients with a psychiatric disease who smoke is nicotine withdrawal severity. Evidence suggests that patients with anxiety, depression, and eating disorder symptoms are more likely to experience greater nicotine withdrawal symptoms when discontinuing nicotine/tobacco use, which in turn suggests that these patients may potentially benefit from an assessment and treatment to buffer the effects of nicotine withdrawal. Despite the risk of more severe withdrawal in the short term, patients should be informed that there is increasing evidence that nicotine/tobacco abstinence does not worsen, and may even improve, psychiatric functioning over the long term. These patients also are more likely to experience cognitive problems because disorders such as major depression and psychosis often present with disturbances in memory, concentration, and thinking. Nonetheless, studies have demonstrated that skill building and motivational enhancement techniques can be applied to these patients, including those with active psychotic disorders, although modifications should be made to meet the needs of this population.

KEY POINTS

1. A simple set of procedures for working in healthcare settings with patients who smoke is to follow the five As of intervention: *ask* patients whether they use nicotine/tobacco, *advise* nicotine/tobacco abstinence, *assess* willingness to quit, *assist* in quitting, and *arrange* follow-ups to prevent relapse.
2. Key elements of behavioral intervention for NTUD include exploring and increasing motivation and readiness to quit, self-monitoring of smoking behavior, choosing a quit date, managing triggers using self-management strategies (avoid, alter, alternative), obtaining social support, identifying and coping with high-risk situations for relapse, managing slips, and making lifestyle changes such as engaging in regular physical exercise.

3. An NTUD intervention initiated during the treatment for other SUDs does not harm treatment outcomes and may even be associated with better drinking and other substance use outcomes; therefore, all patients SUD treatment who smoke should be provided at least a brief NTUD intervention, including offering pharmacologic aid, with encouragement to quit smoking as soon as possible.

4. Patients with psychiatric comorbidities are more likely to have sociodemographic risk factors that could lead to poorer smoking outcomes and may experience greater nicotine withdrawal upon quitting; nonetheless, studies have demonstrated that skill building and motivational enhancement techniques can be applied to psychiatric patients.

REVIEW QUESTIONS

1. The five As is a model for brief smoking cessation intervention in healthcare settings. Which of the following is the correct order of the steps?
   A. Ask, advise, assess, assist, arrange
   B. Ask, assist, advise, assess, arrange
   C. Ask, arrange, advise, assist, assess
   D. Arrange, assist, assess, advise, ask

2. Which of the following is *not* a recommended technique for increasing a patient's readiness to quit?
   A. Provide feedback about the deleterious effects of continued smoking that is paired with feedback about the beneficial effects of nicotine/tobacco abstinence.
   B. Ask patients to write down specific, self-relevant reasons for wanting to stop smoking and also wanting to continue to smoking.

C. Use double-sided reflective statements to highlight both sides of ambivalence.
D. Directly challenge patients' ambivalence about quitting.

3. Which of the following is *not* one of the primary self-management strategies that are a critical component of behavioral interventions for nicotine/tobacco use disorder?
   A. Avoiding trigger situations
   B. Keeping a written record of cigarettes smoked
   C. Altering, or changing, trigger situations
   D. Using alternatives, or substitutes, in place of cigarettes

ANSWERS

1. **A**
2. **D**
3. **B**

SUGGESTED READINGS

Abrams DB, Niaura R, Brown RA, et al, eds. *The Tobacco Dependence Treatment Handbook: A Guide to Best Practices.* New York: Guilford Press, 2003.

Babb S, Malarcher A, Schauer G, Asman K, Jamal A. Quitting smoking among adults—United States, 2000–2015. *MMWR Morb Mortal Wkly Rep.* 2017;65(52):1457-1464.

Fiore MC, Jaén CR, Baker TB, et al. *Treating Tobacco Use and Dependence: 2008 Update. Clinical Practice Guideline.* Rockville, MD: US Department of Health and Human Services, Public Health Service, 2008.

Kalman D, Kim S, DiGirolamo G, Smelson D, Ziedonis D. Addressing tobacco use disorder in smokers in early remission from alcohol dependence: the case for integrating smoking cessation services in substance use disorder treatment programs. *Clin Psychol Rev.* 2010;30(10):12-24.

Marlatt GA, Donovan DM, eds. *Relapse Prevention: Maintenance Strategies in the Treatment of Addictive Behaviors.* 2nd ed. New York: Guilford Press, 2005:92-129.

Network Therapy

Summary by Dmitry Ostrovsky

Based on THE ASAM PRINCIPLES OF ADDICTION MEDICINE,
6th edition chapter by Marc Galanter and Helen Dermatis

Traditional psychotherapeutic approaches in substance use disorders (SUDs) are marred by high dropout rates and relapse. Network therapy utilizes people close to the patient to aid in the prevention of relapse and dropout. Traditional psychotherapy does not reliably identify conditioned reinforcing factors of drug-seeking behaviors due to the often unconscious nature of such factors. Thus, it is often difficult to alter the stimulus-response sequence, when neither the patient nor the therapist is aware that a conditioned sequence is taking place.

THE NETWORK THERAPY TECHNIQUE

The network approach is useful for (1) patients who experience a "loss of control," meaning they cannot limit consumption to a reasonable and predictable level, and (2) patients who have consistently demonstrated relapse. Network therapy is not for patients who can learn to set limits or for those with unusual destabilizing circumstances such as homelessness or psychosis. In those cases, inpatient detoxification or long-term residential treatment may be more useful.

Key Elements

The first key element is the cognitive–behavioral therapy (CBT) approach. Emphasis is placed on triggers to relapse and behavioral techniques for avoiding them while exploring underlying psychodynamic issues. Second, recruiting the patient's social network is integral. This includes peer support in Alcoholics Anonymous (AA) as well as involvement of family (particularly spouses) and friends, which has been shown to be effective at enhancing the outcomes of therapy. Last, the utilization of community reinforcement resources provides even more robust results. The role of "primary care therapist" is one who directly coordinates and monitors network members' roles, as well as combines psychotherapeutic and self-help aspects. The therapist is responsible for the overall management of circumstances inside and outside the office.

COGNITIVE–BEHAVIORAL THERAPY AND SOCIAL SUPPORT
Cognitive–Behavioral Therapy

The CBT format is useful for many SUDs. CBT is goal directed and focuses on current circumstances in the patient's life. Patients begin each session with a recounting of recent events directly relevant to their addiction and recovery, followed by active interactions between the therapist, the patient, and the network members. CBT emphasizes psychoeducation in the context of relapse prevention so that patients and network members are taught to anticipate triggers to substance use. Guided recall is used with the patient and network members to recognize a sequence of triggers that may not initially be apparent but will emerge over the course of exploration.

Social Support

It has been found that the size of the supportive social network in the person's life and the number of members who were abstainers or recovering from SUDs had a positive effect on sobriety.

Contrast With Other Approaches

Interpersonal models posit that SUDs reflect relational problems. Network therapy (NT) assumes that even if interpersonal issues are resolved, SUDs may continue. However, if abstinence is achieved, NT assumes that interpersonal relationships will often subsequently improve. However, NT does bear relation to relapse prevention treatment. Both focus on trigger anticipation, mitigation, or prevention. NT is also similar to couple's therapy in that the spouse is encouraged to support abstinence behaviors. However, in NT, the main goal remains maintaining abstinence.

Initial Encounter: Starting a Social Network

The patient will be asked to bring his or her spouse or a close friend to the first session, who will assist in history taking and implementing a viable treatment plan. Patients with SUDs will usually present with initial denial and/or rationalization of their addiction. The network member will be invaluable in cutting through denial. Some patients insist on attending the first meeting alone, and this is often associated with the desire to continue substance use and fear of an independent alliance forming between the therapist and network member. Although one can delay for one or two sessions, it should be unambiguously stated early on that effective treatment can only be undertaken on the basis of a therapeutic alliance that includes the support of significant others.

The therapist should ensure the provision of necessary social supports to achieve the goals that are agreed upon. First, the therapist should be available for phone consultation and should indicate that the patient should call if problems arise. This makes the therapist's commitment clear and sets the tone for a "team effort." This also undercuts the patient's sense of "being on one's own" as a cause for relapse when problems do arise. The patient should also develop a support network that can handle the majority of day-to-day problems, which should leave the therapist to respond to occasional difficult questions. If problems in management arise in the period between initial sessions, the first few sessions may be scheduled at intervals as frequent as 1 to 3 days. Frequent appointments should always be initially scheduled if a pharmacologic detoxification is indicated, so the patient will not manage more than a few days of medication at a time.

It is essential to forge the network into a working group to provide interappointment support for the patient. Contacts between network members generally include phone calls, dinner arrangements, and social encounters that should be preplanned during the joint session. Encounters should occur at times when alcohol or drug use is likely to occur. Make it clear to network members that after the patient is stabilized, little unusual effort apart from infrequent meetings with the patient and therapist will be required in the long term.

Defining the Network's Membership

This process is undertaken with active collaboration of the patient and therapist. The therapist must carefully promote the choice of appropriate network members by strategically considering the interactions that may take place among network members. Balance between network members is important to consider. For example, do not choose

the patient's current partner to be in network with an ex-partner.

Defining the Network's Task

The therapist's relationship to the network is that of a task-oriented team leader as opposed to a family therapist oriented toward insight. Competing and alternative goals should be suppressed or prevented from interfering with the primary goal of maintaining abstinence. Network members are not scrutinized as in traditional family therapy to prevent the development of competing goals for the network's meetings and to support the members' continued involvement without an assault on their psychological defenses. Their constructive behavior should be commended and appreciation for their contribution to therapy should be acknowledged.

The Use of Alcoholics Anonymous

Self-help modalities (eg, AA, Narcotics Anonymous) should be used whenever possible. The therapist should mobilize the support network to encourage the patient's involvement with AA for a reasonable trial (eg, at least two meetings per week for 1 month). Patients in AA sometimes experience a conversion, wherein they adopt the group ethos and express a deep commitment to abstinence. When conversion occurs, the therapist can take a more passive role in monitoring the patient's abstinence and AA involvement but should still monitor the patients' commitment to AA.

Use of Pharmacotherapy in the Network Format

Pharmacotherapy can be employed for use in network therapy. For example, if disulfiram is used, the recommendations for the network include the following: (1) have the patient take the medication every morning in front of a network member, (2) have the patient take the pill so a network member can observe swallowing, (3) have the observer record the time of day in an administration list, (4) have the observer bring the list to office at each network session, and (5) have the observer inform the therapist of any missed doses. At the outset, see the patient with their group on a weekly basis for the first month. Unstable cases may require more frequent contacts with the network. As the patient stabilizes, taper sessions to biweekly and then monthly intervals as needed. Network sessions should be held every 3 months for the duration of individual therapy. There should be bilateral communication between network members and the therapist regarding potential relapse.

Adapting Individual Therapy to the Network Treatment

The patient may feel deprived of attention unless individual therapy is framed as an opportunity for further growth following a period of network-ensured abstinence. For insight-oriented therapy, the clarification of unconscious motivations is a primary objective. For supportive therapy, bolstering established constructive defenses is primary. For individual therapy in NT, the primary objectives include addressing exposure to cues/triggers that might precipitate substance use and establishing a stable social context and an appropriate social environment that is conducive to abstinence with minimal disruption of life circumstances. Disruptions in the place of residence, friendships, and employment should be specifically addressed. After these priorities are considered, the patient's unresolved psychological conflicts may be examined and take a more prominent role in therapy. As treatment progresses and the patient remains stable, the context of treatment will begin to resemble a more traditional psychotherapeutic context.

RESEARCH ON NETWORK THERAPY TREATMENT

Network therapy is included under the American Psychiatric Association's *Practice Guidelines for the Treatment of Patients With Substance Use Disorders* as an approach for facilitating treatment plan adherence. The Substance Abuse and Mental Health Services Administration includes a description of NT in its National Registry of Evidence-based Program and Practices, and NT is listed as one of its treatment improvement protocols (TIP 39: Substance Abuse Treatment and Family Therapy). To date, five studies, each addressing the technique's validation from a different perspective, have demonstrated NT's effectiveness in treatment and in training.

Treatment by Psychiatry Residents

A large psychiatric residency program developed and implemented an NT training sequence for patients dependent on cocaine treated by residents. A training manual was developed as a guide and tool for ensuring uniformity of practice. Videotaped NT sessions were used to illustrate typical therapy situations. An NT rating scale was developed and evaluated for its reliability in distinguishing between NT and systemic family therapy for addiction. It was then used by clinical supervisors as a didactic aid to monitor therapist adherence to the study treatment manual. PGY-3 (third year of training) psychiatry residents were taught to apply the NT approach and worked with a sample of 47 patients with cocaine addiction. Of these patients, 77% established networks. Out of 17 patients who completed the 24-week regimen, 15 produced urine that was negative for cocaine in their last three toxicologies. However, only a minority (4 out of 18) of those who attended the first week, but did not complete the full course, met this outcome. Overall, the inexperienced residents achieved results similar to those reported for experienced professionals.

Treatment by Addiction Counselors

Another study was conducted in a community-based addictions clinic using the same NT training sequence that was used for the psychiatry residents described previously. A cohort of 10 patients with cocaine dependence were treated with a format that included NT as well as the clinic's usual package of modalities and 12-step–oriented treatment regimens. Twenty patients with cocaine dependence received the standard clinic treatment and were used as controls. It was found that in the NT group, 88% of 107 urinalyses were negative and the mean retention in treatment was 13.9 weeks, whereas in the control group, 66% of 82 urinalyses were negative and the mean retention in treatment was 10.7 weeks. The results show positive effects of NT on abstinence and treatment adherence as well as demonstrate its feasibility in a community-based setting.

Adaptations of Network Therapy Treatment

NT has been combined with relapse prevention and a voucher reinforcement system in the treatment of patients with opioid dependence undergoing naltrexone therapy during a 6-month course. The network incorporated one significant other for each patient, who monitored adherence to naltrexone. They found that patients who were on methadone at baseline had higher rates of treatment retention than those on heroin at baseline. In both cohorts, higher rates of treatment retention were noted in patients who had a network component.

PRINCIPLES OF NETWORK TREATMENT
Start a Network as Soon as Possible

It is important to see the patient as soon as possible because the window of opportunity for openness to treatment is generally brief. If the person is married, engage the spouse early on (preferably during the first phone call), explain that addiction is a family problem, and enlist the spouse in ensuring that the patient arrives to the first office visit with at least 1 day of sobriety.

During the initial interview, build a strong case for the grave consequences of the patient's addiction before they can introduce their system of denial. This prevents the spouse from having to contradict the patient during the initial meeting. Make clear that the patient needs to be abstinent starting immediately. For patients with alcohol use disorders, consider starting disulfiram treatment as soon as possible and have the patient continue taking it under network member supervision. Start arranging for a network at the first session. From the very first meeting, consider how to ensure sobriety until the next meeting and plan that with the network (eg, daily AA attendance, planned activities).

Manage the Network With Care

Include people who are trusted and close to the patient. Avoid members with substance abuse problems as well as superiors or subordinates at work. Create a network that is also balanced generationally. The mood for the meetings should be trusting and free of recrimination. Avoid letting members feel guilty or angry at meetings and explain issues in terms of problems presented by the addiction. Do not examine members' psychological motives. Set a directive tone and give explicit instructions to support and ensure abstinence by meeting as frequently as necessary to ensure abstinence before tapering meetings as needed. Finally, do not work on family relations or focus on network members' personal issues.

Keep the Network's Agenda Focused
Maintaining Abstinence

At the outset of each session, the patient and network should report on any patient exposure to alcohol or drugs. The patient and network should be educated on the nature of relapse and on how to sustain abstinence. Cues to conditioned drug seeking should be examined.

Supporting the Network's Integrity

Network members should attend network meeting sessions. However, they may also be asked to undertake other supportive activities with the patient. The patient is expected to ensure that network members keep meeting appointments and stay involved with treatment. The therapist aids the patient in ensuring network membership stability, sets meeting times, and summons the network for emergencies such as relapse.

Securing Future Behavior

The therapist should utilize all modalities available to ensure the patient's stability, including a stable and drug-free residence; avoidance of friends who abuse substances; attendance at 12-step meetings; medications such as disulfiram, naltrexone, buprenorphine etc.; observed urinalysis; ancillary psychiatric care; as well as mutually acceptable written contingency contracts.

KEY POINTS

1. Network therapy utilizes people close to the patient to aid in the prevention of relapse and dropout.
2. It has been found that the size of the supportive social network in the person's life and the number of members who were abstainers or recovering from substance use disorders had a positive effect on sobriety.
3. Self-help modalities (eg, AA, Narcotics Anonymous) should be used whenever possible in NT.

REVIEW QUESTIONS

1. When would be the most appropriate time to engage a spouse in a network for a patient with alcohol use disorder?
   A. Whenever the patient feels it is appropriate
   B. Preferably during the first phone call, before the first meeting
   C. During the first meeting with the patient
   D. After the first meeting with the patient

2. What is something that is *not* included as a component of network therapy?
   A. Avoidance of traditional group psychotherapeutic interventions between patient and network
   B. Including people who are trusted and close to the patient
   C. Flexibility in setting the goals of treatment (eg, abstinence vs. harm reduction)
   D. Using the network to aid in ensuring sobriety between meetings

3. Which of the following is *not* a component of network management?
   A. Creating a network that is balanced generationally
   B. Avoiding personality conflicts
   C. Avoiding members with substance abuse problems
   D. Letting the patient independently choose who will be in the network

ANSWERS

1. **B**
2. **C**
3. **D**

SUGGESTED READINGS

Galanter M, Dermatis H, Glickman L, et al. Network therapy: decreased secondary opioid use during buprenorphine maintenance. *J Subst Abuse Treat.* 2004;26(4): 313-318.

Galanter M, Keller DS, Dermatis H. Using the Internet for clinical training: a course on network therapy. *Psychiatr Serv.* 1997;48(8):999-1000, 1008.

Glazer SS, Galanter M, Megwinoff O, Dermatis H, Keller DS. The role of therapeutic alliance in network therapy: a family and peer support-based treatment for cocaine abuse. *Subst Abuse.* 2003;24(2):93-100.

Meyers RJ, Miller WR, Smith JE, Tonigan JS. A randomized trial of two methods for engaging treatment-refusing drug users through concerned significant others. *J Consult Clin Psychol.* 2002;70(5):1182-1185.

Therapeutic Communities and Modified Therapeutic Communities for Co-Occurring Mental and Substance Use Disorders

Summary by George De Leon and Stanley Sacks

Based on THE ASAM PRINCIPLES OF ADDICTION MEDICINE, 6th edition chapter by George De Leon and Stanley Sacks

Drug-free residential programs for substance use disorders appeared a decade later than did therapeutic communities (TCs) in psychiatric hospitals, first pioneered by Maxwell Jones and others in the United Kingdom. The term *therapeutic community* evolved in these hospital settings, although the two models arose independently. TCs for substance use disorders emerged in the 1960s as a self-help alternative to existing conventional treatments.

TRADITIONAL THERAPEUTIC COMMUNITIES

Traditional TCs are similar to each other in structure, staffing pattern, perspective, and treatment regimen, although they differ in size (30 to several hundred beds in a facility) and client demography. Staffs are composed of TC-trained clinicians, with and without recovery experiences, and other human service professionals who provide medical, mental health, vocational, educational, family counseling, fiscal, administrative, and legal services. The recommended planned duration of stay in long-term TCs has gradually decreased over the years from 15 to 24 months to 9 to 12 months.

The Therapeutic Community Perspective

The TC perspective or theory shapes its program model and unique approach: community as method. The perspective consists of four interrelated views: (1) view of the substance use disorder, (2) view of the individual, (3) view of the recovery process, and (4) view of healthy living.

View of the Disorder

Substance use disorder is viewed as a disorder of the whole person, affecting some or all areas of functioning. Cognitive and behavioral problems are evident, as are mood disturbances. Thinking may be unrealistic or disorganized; values are confused, nonexistent, or antisocial. Frequently, there are deficits in verbal, reading, writing, and marketable skills. Moral or even spiritual issues, whether expressed in existential or psychological terms, are apparent. Thus, the individual suffers from an internal problem, not from the drug itself. Substance use is a symptom, not the essence of the disorder.

View of the Person

In TCs, individuals are distinguished in terms of psychological dysfunction and social deficits rather than according to drug use patterns. In many TC residents, vocational and educational problems are marked; middle-class, mainstream values are either missing or not sought. Usually, these residents emerge from a socially disadvantaged sector. In the sociodemographic research literature, people who use substances generally demonstrate poor employment and educational histories among those who enter publically funded treatment, particularly TCs. Their TC experience is better termed *habilitation*, ie, development of a socially productive and conventional lifestyle for the first time. Among residents from more advantaged backgrounds, the term *rehabilitation* is more suitable, which emphasizes a return to a lifestyle previously lived, known, and perhaps rejected.

Regardless of differences in social background, drug preference, or psychological problems, however, most individuals admitted to TCs share clinical characteristics that reflect immaturity and antisocial dimensions. Whether they are antecedents or consequences, these characteristics are commonly observed to correlate with serious substance involvement. More importantly, a positive change in these characteristics is considered to be essential for stable recovery.

View of Recovery

In the TC perspective, recovery involves a change in lifestyle as well as in social and personal identity. Thus, the primary psychological goal of treatment is to change the negative patterns of behavior, thinking, and feeling; the main social goal is to develop the skills, attitudes, and values of a responsible drug-free lifestyle. Stable recovery, however, depends on a successful integration of these social and psychological goals. Behavioral change is unstable without insight, and insight is insufficient without felt experience. Several key assumptions underlie the recovery process in the TC.

View of Healthy Living

TCs adhere to certain precepts, values, and a social perspective that guide and reinforce recovery. For example, there are community sanctions to address antisocial behaviors and attitudes such as the negative values of the street, jails, or negative peers and irresponsible or exploitative sexual conduct. Positive values are emphasized as being essential to social learning and personal growth. These values include truth and honesty (in word and deed), a work ethic, self-reliance, earned rewards and achievement, personal accountability, responsible concern (being one's brother's or sister's keeper), social manners, and community involvement. The precepts of healthy living are constantly reinforced in various formal and informal ways (eg, signs, seminars, in groups, community meetings).

The Therapeutic Community Approach: Community as Method

The TC approach can be summarized in the phrase "community as method." Theoretical writings offer a definition of "community as method" as "the purposive use of the community to teach individuals to use the community to change themselves."

The fundamental assumption underlying community as method is that individuals obtain maximum therapeutic and educational impact when they engage in and learn to use all of the diverse elements of the community as the tools for self-change. Thus, "community as method" means that the community itself provides a *context* for social learning. Its membership establishes *expectations* or standards of participation in the community. It continually *assesses* how individuals are meeting these expectations and *responds* to them with strategies that promote continued participation. The diverse elements and activities of the community can be organized in terms of the program stages, the TC program model, and specific methods that facilitate the process of change.

The Therapeutic Community Program Model

The TC program model is its social and psychological environment. Each component of the environment reflects an understanding of the TC perspective, and each is used to transmit community teachings and to promote affiliation and self-change.

Therapeutic Community Methods

In the TC, all activities both planned (eg, groups, meetings) and unplanned (eg, interpersonal, social interactions) facilitate recovery and healthy living. However, planned activities are viewed as interventions or methods, designed to impact both individuals and the general community in specific ways.

Therapeutic/Educative Activities

Therapeutic/educative activities consist of various group processes and individual counseling. They increase communication and interpersonal skills, bring about an examination of behavior and attitudes, and offer instruction in alternative modes of behavior. The main groups include encounters, probes, and tutorials. These differ somewhat in format and objectives, but all have the common goal of fostering trust, personal disclosure, intimacy, and peer solidarity to facilitate therapeutic change.

Community and Clinical Management Elements

Community and clinical management elements maintain the physical and psychological safety of the environment and ensure that resident life is orderly and productive. They protect the community as a whole and strengthen it as a context for social learning. The main elements are staff managed and include privileges, disciplinary sanctions, surveillance, and urine testing.

The Program Stages and Phases

Recovery in the TC is a developmental process, one that occurs in a social learning setting. The developmental process itself can be understood as a passage through stages of learning. The learning that occurs at each stage facilitates change at the next, and each change reflects movement toward the goals of recovery. Three major program stages characterize change in long-term residential TCs: orientation/induction, primary treatment, and reentry.

Stage 1: Orientation/Induction (0 to 60 Days)

The main goal of stage 1 is to provide new residents with a formal orientation to the TC. The aim of orientation in the initial phase of residence is for the individual to be assimilated into the community through full participation and involvement in all of its activities. Formal seminars and informal peer instruction focus on dissemination of information and instruction concerning program philosophy, rules, house regulations, and community expectations as to participation in the program meetings and group activities.

Stage 2: Primary Treatment (2 to 12 Months)

The stage of primary treatment consists of three subphases that roughly correlate with time in the program (2 to 4, 5 to 8, and 9 to 12 months). The daily therapeutic–educational regimen of meetings, groups, job assignments, and peer and staff counseling remains the same throughout the year of primary treatment. However, progress is reflected at the end of each phase in terms of explicit behavioral indicators (eg, resident "sets an example" by month 8) and more broadly in terms of three interrelated dimensions of change: community status (role model), development or maturity, and overall psychological adjustment. Staff informally assesses progress in this stage and throughout with input from peers and, in recent years, with clinical scales.

Stage 3: Reentry (13 to 24 Months)

Reentry is the stage at which the individual must strengthen skills for autonomous decision making and the capacity for self-management and must rely less on rational authorities or a well-formed peer network. The main objective of the early reentry phase (13 to 18 months) is to prepare for separation from the TC. Particular emphasis is placed on life-skills seminars that provide training for living outside the community. Plans are developed for long-term psychological, educational, housing, and vocational objectives. Clients may be attending school or holding full-time jobs, either within or outside the TC while still living in the facility.

The objective of the later reentry phase (18 to 24 months) is successful separation from the TC.

Clients have a "live-out" status; they hold full-time jobs or attend school full time, and they maintain their own households, usually with live-out peers. They may participate in Alcoholics Anonymous or Narcotics Anonymous or attend family or individual therapy sessions. Contact with the TC is gradually reduced to weekly telephone calls and monthly visits with a primary counselor.

Research: The Effectiveness of Traditional Therapeutic Communities

Over the past five decades, a considerable scientific knowledge base has developed from follow-up studies on thousands of individuals treated in TCs worldwide. Overall, the weight of the research evidence from multiple sources (multiprogram field effectiveness studies, single program controlled studies, meta-analytic statistical surveys, and cost–benefit studies) is compelling in supporting the hypothesis that the TC is an effective and cost-effective treatment for certain subgroups of people with substance use disorders, particularly those who present with serious co-occurring social and psychological problems.

MODIFIED THERAPEUTIC COMMUNITY FOR PERSONS WITH CO-OCCURRING MENTAL AND SUBSTANCE USE DISORDERS

Over time, TCs adapted to changing needs and populations, different settings, and advances in research and practice. In the early and mid-1990s, the modified TC (MTC) was developed from the theoretical framework of the traditional TC model, as detailed in the definitive text, *The Therapeutic Community: Theory, Model, and Method*, adapted to treat individuals with co-occurring disorders. The use of MTC in this report is intended "to capture those adaptations of the TC model designed to serve substance-using individuals with co-occurring mental disorders, most of which were serious (ie, schizophrenia and other psychotic disorders, bipolar disorders and major depression) mental disorders."

Description of the Modified Therapeutic Community Program

Modifications

The MTC model retains yet reshapes most of the central elements, structure, and processes of the traditional TC to accommodate the many needs that accompany co-occurring disorders, particularly psychiatric symptoms, cognitive deficits, and reduced level of functioning. Three key alterations were made in designing the MTC program for persons with co-occurring disorders: (1) increased flexibility, (2) decreased intensity, and (3) greater individualization. Other adaptations in the MTC for co-occurring disorders include more flexibility in program activities, shorter duration of various activities, less confrontation and intensity of interpersonal interaction, greater emphasis on orientation and instruction in programming and planning, fewer sanctions and greater opportunities for corrective learning experiences, more explicit affirmation for achievements, greater sensitivity to individual differences, and greater responsiveness to the special developmental needs of the clients (Table 69-1).

TABLE 69-1	Residential Interventions
Community Enhancement	
Morning Meetings	to increase motivation for the day's activities and to create a positive family atmosphere
Concept Seminars	to review the concept of the day
General Interest Seminars	to provide information in areas of general interest (eg, current events)
Program-Related Seminars	to address issues of particular relevance (eg, homelessness, HIV prevention, psychotropic medication)
Orientation Seminars	to orient new members and to introduce all new activities
Evening Meetings	to review house business for the day, to outline plans for the next day, and to monitor the emotional tone of the house
General Meetings	to provide a public review of critical events
Therapeutic/Educative	
Individual Counseling	to incorporate both traditional mental health and unique modified TC goals and methods
Psychoeducational Classes	are predominant, in a format to facilitate learning among persons with co-occurring disorders and to include topics such as entitlements/money management, positive relationship skills training, triple trouble group, and feelings management
Conflict Resolution Groups	are modified encounter groups designed specifically for persons with co-occurring disorders
Gender-Specific Groups	to combine features of "discussion groups" and therapy groups focusing on gender-based issues
Community & Clinical Management	
Policies	to form a system of rules and regulations to maintain the physical and psychological safety of the environment, ensuring that resident life is orderly and productive, strengthening the community as a context for social learning
Social Learning Consequence	to prescribe a set of required behaviors as a response to unacceptable behavior, designed to enhance individual and community learning by transforming negative events into learning opportunities
Vocational	
Peer Work Hierarchy	a rotating assignment of residents to jobs necessary for the day-to-day functioning of the facility, serving to diversify and develop clients' work skills and experience
World of Work	a psychoeducational class providing instruction in applications and interviews, time and attendance, relationships with others at work, employers' expectations, discipline, promotion, etc.
Recovery & World of Work	a psychoeducational class that addresses issues of mental illness, addiction, etc. in a work context

TC, therapeutic communities.
Adapted from Sacks et al., 1999.

Interventions

All program activities and interactions, singly and in combination, are designed to produce change. Although each intervention has specific individual functions, all share community and therapeutic and educational purposes.

Outcomes

A series of studies in homeless, criminal justice, and aftercare settings demonstrated better outcomes for MTCs compared to controls on measures of substance abuse, mental health, crime, employment, and housing. MTCs have been listed on the National Registry of Effective Programs and Practice since 2008.

The Medically Integrated Therapeutic Community

The Affordable Care Act furnished an opportunity for the continued adaptation and growth of the MTC model, which is ideally suited for alterations to support integration with primary care services. The rationale for such an approach is based on the fact that the conceptual framework of the MTC (and the TC) endorses a view of "whole person" treatment that is compatible with holistic, person-centered medicine, and the model has been modified in the past to suit special populations, retaining core TC principles while adding interventions to accommodate particular services.

KEY POINTS

1. The TC approach can be summarized with the phrase "community as method."
2. The TC program model is its social and psychological environment wherein each component of the environment reflects an understanding of the TC perspective and each is used to transmit community teachings and to promote affiliation and self-change.
3. The weight of the research evidence from multiple sources is compelling in supporting the hypothesis that the TC is an effective and cost-effective treatment for certain subgroups of people with substance use disorders, particularly those who present with serious co-occurring social and psychological problems.

REVIEW QUESTIONS

1. Which statement best summarizes the TC approach?
   A. Community as method
   B. The use of encounter groups
   C. Peers serve as role models
   D. Residents progress through program stages and phases

2. MTCs for persons with co-occurring substance use:
   A. do not rely on the community.
   B. have three key alterations: increased flexibility, decreased intensity, and greater individualization.
   C. have more frequent encounter groups.
   D. are a type of aftercare program.

3. Which statement best summarizes the status of TC research?
   A. There is a need for larger samples.
   B. It is too anecdotal.
   C. The results are equivocal.
   D. There exists a substantial empirical base.

ANSWERS

1. **A**
2. **B**
3. **D**

SUGGESTED READINGS

De Leon G. Is the therapeutic community an evidence-based treatment? What the evidence says. *Int J Ther Communities.* 2010;31(2):104-128.

De Leon G. *The Therapeutic Community: Theory, Model, and Method.* New York: Springer, 2000.

Sacks S, Banks S, McKendrick K, Sacks JY. Modified therapeutic community for co-occurring disorders: a summary of four studies. *J Subst Abuse Treat.* 2008;34(1):112-122.

Substance Abuse and Mental Health Services Administration. *Substance Abuse Treatment for Persons With Co-Occurring Disorders. A Treatment Improvement Protocol (TIP) Series, No. 42.* Rockville, MD: Substance Abuse and Mental Health Services Administration, 2005. DHHS Pub. No. (SMA) 05-3992.

Vanderplasschen W, Colpaert K, Autrique M, et al. Therapeutic communities for addictions: a review of their effectiveness from a recovery-oriented perspective. *ScientificWorldJournal.* 2013;2013:427817.

CHAPTER 70

Aversion Therapies

Summary by P. Joseph Frawley

Based on THE ASAM PRINCIPLES OF ADDICTION MEDICINE,
6th edition chapter by P. Joseph Frawley, Matthew Owen Howard,
Ralph L. Elkins, and Kalyan Dandala

AVERSION THERAPY AS PART OF A MULTIMODALITY TREATMENT PROGRAM

Patients with substance use disorders have been conditioned by their drug of choice. Studies have shown that patients with alcohol use disorder increase the number of swallows and amount of salivation in response to the sight of alcohol, as compared to controls without alcohol use disorder. Studies of patients with nicotine use disorder seeking to quit show that those who are least likely to quit have a much larger conditioned drop in pulse (presumably to compensate for the increase in pulse rate caused by smoking) when presented with a cigarette. Patients with cocaine use disorder experience progressively steeper drops in skin temperature and increased galvanic skin response (a sign of arousal) when viewing progressively more intense and explicit pictures of cocaine use. These responses can be shown to decay in strength as time away from the drug increases.

The presence of these phenomena suggests that one of the consequences of addiction is that the body becomes conditioned to drink or use drugs in the presence of certain stimuli. This may contribute to the sensation of physical craving experienced by substance use disorders.

Aversion therapy, or counterconditioning, is a powerful tool in the treatment of alcohol and other drug addiction. Its goal is to reduce or eliminate the "hedonic memory" or craving for a drug and to simultaneously develop a distaste and avoidance response to the substance. Unlike punishments, which often are delayed in time from the use episode, aversion therapy relies on the immediate association of the sight, smell, taste, and act of using the substance with an unpleasant or "aversive" experience. Also, with punishment, it is the individual who receives the negative consequences, whereas in aversion therapy, it is the behavior—the negative consequence is only paired with the act of using a drug. This has a very important benefit to self-esteem. While the patient is engaging in positive recovery activities, he or she is receiving immediate positive support for a new way of behaving and thinking. It is only when the patient is engaging in an old behavior—alcohol or drug use—that he or she experiences immediate and consistent discomfort. Hence, self-esteem is rebuilt by separating the drug from the self.

The development of an aversion can be very specific; for example, inadequate treatment can occur when aversion is developed only to one type of alcoholic beverage. Also, repetition is an essential part of training and conditioning; adequate trials are needed to develop an aversion and to maintain and reinforce it to prevent extinction.

Contrary to popular belief, disulfiram is not a classic aversion treatment. In aversion therapy for alcohol addiction, alcohol is not absorbed into the system. With disulfiram, alcohol must be absorbed and metabolism begun for it to produce its toxic effect. Aversion relies on safe but uncomfortable experiences that can be repeated, whereas disulfiram plus alcohol induces a profoundly toxic reaction. For this reason, patients given disulfiram are not given alcohol at the same time that they are prescribed disulfiram; as a result, they have not actually experienced a disulfiram reaction. Thus, disulfiram does not change the way the addict feels about alcohol. He or she may fear the consequence of drinking, just as he or she fears being arrested for drinking and driving; nevertheless, he or she still retains the euphoric recall of past episodes of drinking alcohol, hence the craving for the alcohol itself. Aversion works to eliminate or reduce euphoric recall by recording new negative experiences with the drug.

USES OF AVERSION THERAPY
Aversion Therapy for Alcohol Use Disorder
Nausea Aversion

Studies in rats suggest that humans and other organisms may be biologically predisposed to form long-lasting conditioned aversions to consumables such as alcohol and foodstuffs, the consumption of which is followed by nausea and vomiting.

The usual treatment session involves having the patient take nothing except clear liquids by mouth for 6 hours prior to treatment in order to reduce the likelihood of aspiration. After receiving a full explanation of the treatment procedure, the patient is taken to the treatment room, which has shelves containing all types of alcoholic beverages along the walls, as well as cutouts of various liquor ads on the walls: The intent is to have the majority of the patient's visual stimuli associated with visual cues for drinking. The patient receives an oral dose of emetine and is given water and electrolytes to provide a volume of easily vomited material. Shortly before the expected onset of nausea, the nurse administering the treatment pours a drink of the patient's preferred alcoholic beverage. The patient is instructed to smell the beverage, take a small mouthful, swish it around in the mouth to get the full flavor of it, and then to spit it out into the basin. This ensures that the patient has well-defined visual, olfactory, and gustatory sensations associated with the preferred beverage prior to the onset of the nausea. The nausea and vomiting ensue shortly thereafter, and the "sniff, swish, and spit" procedure described previously is altered to "sniff, swish, and swallow," with the swallowed alcoholic beverage being returned shortly as emesis so that no significant amount of alcohol is retained to be absorbed. After a session, the patient is returned to the hospital room, where another drink of alcoholic beverage is given containing an oral dose of emetine and tartar emetic, which induces a slower acting residual nausea lasting up to 3 hours. The average patient receives five treatment sessions, which are given every other day over a 10-day period. In the private sector, Smith and Frawley compared 249 inpatients receiving aversion therapy as part of a multimodality treatment program with 249 inpatients from a large (>9000 patients) treatment registry of patients receiving multimodality treatment but without aversion therapy. All were matched on 17 baseline characteristics. Of the patients receiving aversion therapy, 84.7% had total abstinence from alcohol at 6 months, compared with 72.2% in the control group ($p < 0.01$); at 1 year, 79% of those treated with aversion had maintained abstinence versus 67% of those without such treatment ($p < 0.05$). The daily drinkers group showed the greatest benefit from aversion therapy (84% vs. 67%, $p < 0.001$).

Faradic Aversion

The faradic aversion treatment paradigm consists of pairing an aversive level of electrostimulation with the sight, smell, and taste of alcoholic beverages. At the direction of the therapist (forced choice trial), the patient reaches for a bottle of alcoholic beverage, pours some of it in a glass, and tastes it without swallowing. Electrostimulus onset occurs randomly throughout the entire behavior continuum, from reaching for the bottle through tasting the alcoholic beverage. The number of electrostimuli with each trial varies. An additional 10 free choice trials are designed so that the patient is negatively reinforced, with removal of the aversive stimulus if he or she selects a nonalcoholic choice such as fruit juice. The patient is instructed not to swallow any alcohol at any time throughout the faradic session, and this behavior is closely monitored by the therapist.

Covert Sensitization

Conditioned nausea responses can be trained in some patients with alcohol use disorder through the use of imagination and verbal suggestion without the use of an emetic drug. In covert sensitization, patients are helped to imagine personally relevant drinking scenes that emphasize the motivational, sensory, and behavioral precursors and concomitants of alcohol ingestion. The drinking scenes then are paired repeatedly with verbally induced nausea. Most cooperative participants can learn to experience genuine and intense nausea reactions by focusing on the therapist's noxious verbal suggestions; these suggestions prompt recipients to remember and recreate prior feelings and thoughts that have been prominent in their former nausea experiences. Such verbally induced nausea is designated *demand nausea*. Repeated presentations of the drinking scenes (the conditioned stimulus) followed by episodes of verbally induced demand nausea (the unconditioned stimulus) can, over extended conditioning trials, produce conditioned aversions to alcohol in many of the participants. The goal of treatment is for a patient's demand nausea to transition to conditioned nausea, an automatic consequence of the patient's focusing on a drinking scene without any attempted therapist or self-induction of nausea.

In one study of 52 patients, 33 were able to develop verbally induced nausea after imagined drinking scenes; of these, 23 were able to develop conditioned nausea to either the desire for alcohol or other alcohol-related physical stimuli. Those who developed conditioned nausea had an average of 13.74 months of total abstinence as compared to 4.52 months for those who failed to progress beyond the demand nausea stage.

Effect of Aversion on Craving for Alcohol

The *Diagnostic and Statistical Manual of Mental Disorders*, 5th edition (*DSM-5*) now includes craving as a diagnostic criterion, which then can be used for determining substance use disorder severity. The changes in autonomic response to the presentation of alcohol or drug stimuli mentioned previously demonstrate some physiologic correlates of craving. There has been shown an association between the strength of autonomic markers in aversion therapy and abstinence from alcohol. Patients who had reported loss of all urges to drink after aversion therapy had a 1-year abstinence of 89%, those who reported loss of only uncontrollable urges had an abstinence rate of 56.8%, and those who still had urges after treatment reported abstinence rates of 6.3% at 1 year (Table 70-1). In the current treatment protocol for patients in aversion treatment, nurses use a Likert scale that ranges from −5 for high craving to +5 for strong aversion based on the observed physical and emotional reaction the patient has to seeing, smelling, and tasting their favorite drinks. There is a progression from craving to aversion over the course of the treatment. Functional magnetic resonance imaging (fMRI) studies done before and after aversion therapy for alcohol have shown a pronounced reduction in cue-induced brain activation in the occipital cortex after aversion treatment.

TABLE 70-1	Percent Abstinence From Alcohol During Specified Follow-Up Periods		
Follow-Up Period	Aversion (%)	Match (%)	p Value x^2, 1 df
0–6 mo	85	72	0.01
0–12 mo	79	67	0.05

df, degree of freedom.
Adapted from Smith JW, Frawley PJ, Polissar NL. Six- and twelve-month abstinence rates in inpatients with alcohol use disorder treated with either faradic aversion or chemical aversion compared with matched inpatients from a treatment registry. *J Addict Dis.* 1997;16(1):5-24.

Aversion Therapy in Tobacco/Nicotine Use Disorder

A review of modern smoking cessation treatments concluded that programs that use rapid smoking aversion or satiation had superior outcomes. Rapid smoking involves smoking cigarettes with inhalations every 6 seconds; although nicotine is taken into the system during rapid smoking, the aversion developed to smoking is adequate to prevent relapse. Sessions last an average of 15 minutes, during which the subject smokes an average of 5 cigarettes. The treatment sessions are usually daily for 5 days with a tapering frequency of booster treatments after that. When compared to the physical effects of normally paced smoking, clients undergoing rapid smoking experience increased burning in the lungs, palpitations, facial flush, headache, and feeling faint or weak. The best results have been reported by programs in which aversion was combined with several other modalities, including relapse prevention, relaxation training, written exercises, contract management, booster sessions of aversion, and group support. A study of patients with cardiopulmonary disease who underwent satiation treatment found no myocardial ischemia or significant arrhythmia in this group; five patients with ischemic changes on the treadmill did not experience the changes during the satiation treatment.

Faradic aversion has also been used for smoking cessation: Each time a patient brings a cigarette toward his or her lips, a mild electrical stimulus is administered automatically by a 9-V battery. With faradic aversion, the smoke is not inhaled but merely puffed; inhaling may lead to early relapse because of maintenance of the nicotine dependence. One advantage of this form of treatment is that less medically sophisticated staff can supervise the administration of the treatment.

In both forms of treatment, patients personally administer the aversive agent to themselves, while the therapist serves as a coach.

Aversion Therapy for Marijuana Use Disorder

In clinical practice, aversion therapy for marijuana uses faradic aversion. The protocol for faradic aversion is similar to that of the treatment for alcohol, except that it uses a variety of bongs, drug paraphernalia, and visual imagery. An artificial marijuana substitute and marijuana aroma are used in treatment. A 1-year abstinence rate of 84% was reported after 5 days of treatment, combined with three weekly group sessions on self-management techniques.

Aversion Therapy for Stimulant (Cocaine/Amphetamine) Use Disorder

In a study of the use of chemical aversion for the treatment of cocaine use disorder, an artificial cocaine substitute called Articaine was developed from tetracaine, mannitol, and quinine. Patients snorted this substance and paired it with nausea induced by emetine. Of those so treated, 56% were continuously abstinent and 78% currently abstinent for the prior 30 days at 6 months after treatment; at 18 months, 38% were continuously abstinent and 75% currently abstinent. For those treated for both alcohol and cocaine use, 70% were continuously and currently abstinent from cocaine at 6 months, and 50% were continuously abstinent and 80% currently abstinent at 18 months after treatment.

A well-designed experimental evaluation of aversion therapy treatments for cocaine use disorder enlisted volunteer participants from the Augusta VA Medical Center Substance Abuse Treatment Program. The abstinence rate at 6 months' posttreatment follow-up was reported as 57.9% for participants who had received emetic therapy, significantly exceeding the 26.5% 6-month abstinence finding for control group participants. Covert sensitization also produced a significant therapeutic benefit, but its effect did not extend beyond 3 months posttreatment. A result unique to participants who received emetic therapy was a total loss of cravings for cocaine by the end of treatment.

Aversion Therapy for Opioid Use Disorder (Heroin and Prescription Opioids)

One study employed a unique approach to aversion therapy by pairing aversive stimuli with cognitive images of heroin use. Patients were asked to verbalize only after they had conjured up a strong mental image. In the second part of the treatment, patients were asked to conjure up images of socially appropriate behavior, including employment, education, or nondrug entertainment. Latency to verbalization was measured: At baseline, patients could rapidly conjure up positive thoughts about heroin use but had significant delays in conjuring up thoughts about rewarding nondrug activities. Subjects were in a halfway house for heroin use disorder and received group therapy in conjunction with relaxation therapy, along with aversion treatment. A faradic stimulator was used; once patients had conjured up drug images, faradic aversion was applied. At other times, patients were given 15 seconds to conjure up images

of nondrug, socially appropriate behavior to prevent aversion from being applied. With this training in an average of 15 sessions, latency for drug-related images increased, whereas that for socially appropriate images decreased. Of the 50 patients in the trial, 30 completed the treatment, and at 24 months, 80% of these were reported to be drug free. Since 2012, a new approach to aversion therapy for heroin has been developed. This heroin treatment combines hypnotically guided covert sensitization with the program's well-established medical (emetic) counterconditioning. Seven heroin counterconditioning sessions are provided within the traditional 10-day inpatient multimodal treatment format that is used for alcohol and other drug dependencies. The first three sessions provide training in hypnotically induced nausea followed by four sessions where emetine is added to enhance the nausea.

A novel treatment for prescription opioid use disorder has been developed at the Schick Shadel Hospital. This treatment capitalizes on the use of naltrexone to negate the psychotropic effects of prescription opioids. Recipients who are dependent on prescription opioids first are detoxified; they then are started on a daily naltrexone regimen that begins in the morning of the first treatment day. The recipients then use prescription opioids in their customary manner during emetic therapy sessions. The treatment has been well received and is being requested by an increasing number of patients.

USE OF REINFORCEMENT (BOOSTER) AVERSION TREATMENTS

Researchers followed up at 1 year on 437 of 600 patients treated with chemical and faradic aversion for alcohol, marijuana, or cocaine. The 1-year complete abstinence rate for alcohol for those who did not return for any reinforcements was 29.4%; for one booster aversion treatment, the abstinence rate was 50.5%; for two booster aversions, the abstinence rate was 68.5%; and for more than two aversions, the abstinence rate was 80%.

USE OF SUPPORT PROGRAMS AND 12-STEP MEETINGS AFTER RECEIVING AVERSION THERAPY

Follow-up studies found that those who used some form of support group after aversion treatment did better than those who did not use such support, with an additive effect of the use of reinforcement (booster) aversion treatments and support and/ or 12-step meetings after completion of a hospital aversion program. Total abstinence was associated with use of support groups after treatment, but for those with urges to drink, increased support use was negatively associated with abstinence. A similar pattern was found for patients going to Schick Shadel Hospital–sponsored support groups.

SAFETY OF AVERSION THERAPY

Faradic aversion has virtually no unsafe side effects and has been found to be safe for patients with pacemakers and pregnant women (because the current only travels between two electrodes on the arm). To be eligible for chemical aversion therapy, patients must be free of medical contraindications such as esophageal varices, serious coronary artery disease, or active gastrointestinal pathology. There was no increased incidence of medical utilization or hospitalization in the 6 months after treatment in a group treated with aversion therapy, as compared to matched controls treated without aversion.

The contraindications to covert sensitization are similar to those for chemical aversion; however, with this therapy, emesis can be prevented in most cases. The drawback to covert aversion therapy is that the induction of nausea or other aversive state is not as predictable as with medication and requires more patient preparation.

AVERSION THERAPY AS PART OF ESTABLISHED CARE FOR SUBSTANCE USE DISORDERS

Selecting the appropriate treatment for a particular patient involves the patient having full informed consent. The practitioner needs to counsel the patient about the risks of continuing the addiction and the risks, benefits, and expected outcomes of various methods of treatment. Studies of patients who voluntarily received aversion therapy do not show higher rates of leaving against medical advice than is found in patients in Minnesota Model programs. Patients seeking aversion therapy in clinical settings complete treatment at the same rate as patients seeking alternative established treatments.

Aversion therapy has been recognized by both governmental and private agencies as appropriate treatment for patients with addictive disease.

NEED FOR FURTHER RESEARCH

A study of emetic therapy for cocaine use disorder, funded by the National Institute on Drug Abuse, demonstrated that recipients not only lost their cravings for cocaine but also developed strong active revulsions for the placebo cocaine materials and for cocaine-related cues. However, the revulsions were not measurable by the 0 to 10 cravings scale that was used in the study. Future studies should incorporate bidirectional scales that measure maximum craving at one extreme and maximum revulsion at the other extreme with a neutral zero-craving midscale region.

Future research should better characterize the physiologic changes that coincide with the transition from cue-induced cravings to cue-induced revulsion within a course of emetic aversion treatments. The dynamically expanding field of brain imaging research is likely to provide the greatest near-term advancements in our basic understanding and possible clinical applications of cue-induced brain changes that occur during the emetic therapy–induced transition from cocaine cravings to revulsions. Recent studies have reported activations of specific brain regions during cue-induced cravings for cocaine. Reliable changes in brain activation patterns may be revealed by comparing the initial episodes of cue-induced cravings that typify the beginning of treatment with those that accompany the late-treatment cue-induced revulsions of successfully conditioned participants. The landmark positron emission tomography scan findings obtained from human volunteers with cocaine addictions have shown that dopamine in the dorsal striatum is involved in cocaine craving and addiction. The dorsal striatum is a region that has been implicated in habit learning and in action initiation. The dorsal striatum is therefore a high-interest area for studies of possible transitions from cravings to revulsions. Cue-induced craving to revulsion changes are also likely to be found in brain regions that include the amygdala, the nucleus accumbens, the dorsal anterior cingulate cortex, the ventral anterior cingulate cortex, and the frontal cortex. An obvious clinical application of such information would be to assess the strength of the attained aversion at the end of treatment. Additionally, the findings could support propitious individually tailored timings of booster treatments.

fMRI also may be well suited to studies of emetic therapy–induced changes of cue-induced cravings to revulsions. The fMRI technology, unlike positron emission tomography scan technology, does not involve the injection of radioactive compounds. Therefore, it can be safely used during repeated measures of the same participants across different time periods.

A variety of researchers have reported that some patients do not seem to develop aversions, leading researchers to develop and study lines of selectively bred taste aversion–prone and taste aversion–resistant rats. Such studies give promise to one day be able to identify biologic indices to separate conditionable and nonconditionable potential emetic therapy recipients. Additionally, studies of the two lines may support the development of pharmacologic or nutritional interventions to increase the nausea-based conditionability of taste aversion–resistant patients with substance use disorders.

KEY POINTS

1. Aversion therapy has its best outcomes with daily drinkers compared to periodic drinkers.
2. Aversion therapy involves retraining the emotional memory through repetitive negative immediate associations with the substance.
3. Aversion therapy can be a part of a multimodal treatment program.
4. Aversion therapy has been successfully applied to multiple types of substance use disorders.

REVIEW QUESTIONS

1. Which of the following is *false* regarding disulfiram therapy when compared to aversion therapy?
   A. Disulfiram reactions are not expected to be repeated, whereas aversion therapy utilizes repetition.
   B. For both disulfiram therapy and aversion therapy to work, alcohol must be absorbed into the bloodstream.
   C. Disulfiram does not directly affect the hedonic memory of alcohol, whereas aversion therapy does.
   D. Disulfiram therapy requires a regular decision to take the medication, whereas aversion therapy is administered in a controlled setting for distinct periods of time.

2. Which of the following is not a key component of the development of an aversion?
   A. Pairing the sight, smell, and taste of the alcohol or other drug with a negative stimulus
   B. Repetition of negative pairing with the alcohol or other drug
   C. Awareness of negative consequences of alcohol or other drug use in at least three major areas of life
   D. The use of a negative unconditioned stimulus that is paired with the conditioned stimulus

3. Which of the following is a specific goal of aversion therapy?
   A. Learning new coping skills
   B. Losing the hedonic memory for a drug or alcohol
   C. Improved communication skills
   D. Changing people, places, and activities associated with the use of alcohol or other drugs

ANSWERS

1. **B**
2. **C**
3. **B**

SUGGESTED READINGS

Hall RG, Sachs DP, Hall SM, Benowitz NL. Two-year efficacy and safety of rapid smoking therapy in patients with cardiac and pulmonary disease. *J Consult Clin Psychol.* 1984;52(4):574-581.

Howard MO. Pharmacological aversion treatment of alcohol dependence. I. Production and prediction of conditioned alcohol aversion. *Am J Drug Alcohol Abuse.* 2001;27(3): 561-585.

Smith JW. Long term outcome of clients treated in a commercial stop smoking program. *J Subst Abuse.* 1988;5(1): 33-36.

Smith JW, Frawley PJ, Polissar L. Six- and twelve-month abstinence rates in inpatient alcoholics treated with aversion therapy compared with matched inpatients from a treatment registry. *Alcohol Clin Exp Res.* 1991;15(5):862-870.

CHAPTER **71**

Family Involvement in Addiction, Treatment, and Recovery

Summary by Kathleen A. Gross and Maritza E. Lagos

Based on THE ASAM PRINCIPLES OF ADDICTION MEDICINE, 6th edition chapter by Kathleen A. Gross, Maritza E. Lagos, Elmira Yessengaliyeva, Matthew M. LaCasse, and Michael R. Liepman (deceased)

DEFINITION OF TERMS

An individual's "family" may consist of parents and siblings (*family of origin*), spouse and children (*family of procreation*), or all relatives and unrelated key individuals (*significant others*) who play important family roles (*extended family*). A *family with a member with addiction* has one or more members who are addicted and may become a *recovering family* with treatment and recovery support but not a *recovered family* because addiction is a chronic disorder.

Codependence refers to the harmful overinvolvement with others that both *enables* active addiction to continue and reduces the well-being of the codependent individual. A *supportive enabler* rescues others from the consequences of addictive behavior, while diminishing his or her own resources and self-esteem. The *hostile enabler* demonstrates disrespect, anger, and aggression, exacerbating the patient's guilt and shame. Codependency recovery groups, including Al-Anon, Nar-Anon, and Adult Children of Alcoholics/Dysfunctional Families, teach individuals how to stop enabling and encourage them to pursue recovery for themselves, remaining supportive of efforts toward treatment and recovery but allowing the patient to take responsibility for the consequences of his or her own addictive behavior.

THE IMPORTANCE OF FAMILY IN ADDICTION

Many providers are unaware of the ways in which addiction impacts the family, or conversely, how the family impacts addiction. Understanding this relationship is vital to the recognition and successful resolution of many addiction and recovery issues. Addiction disorders are common, and they correlate overwhelmingly with familial genetic and environmental factors.

They also contribute to morbidity and mortality among *all* family members, including those who do not have a substance use disorder (SUD). Relatives and significant others often play important roles in perpetuating addiction disorders, but they also can actively discourage substance abuse, assist in making a diagnosis of addiction, encourage treatment, and support ongoing recovery.

FAMILY CONSEQUENCES OF ADDICTION

Families can be harmed by the consequences of SUD in ways that include realignment of priorities, deterioration of values, emergence of illness and disability, escalation of violence, confrontation with avoidable early losses, and precipitation of addiction among other family members. Adult drug and alcohol intake, responses to substance use and abuse by others, and ways of coping with consequences are observed by children and shape their attitudes and behaviors. A child's exposure to drinking, smoking, and drug use in the home provides behavioral role modeling, suggests tacit approval, and may increase ease of access, all of which encourage early experimentation and increase the risk of addiction, especially in homes where use of alcohol and drugs do not always correspond to community legal, cultural, or health-related norms.

Traumatic injury and illness due to the psychological and physiologic effects of drugs and alcohol may result in hospitalization, permanent disability, or death. Family members also may be injured in motor vehicle accidents, house fires, domestic violence, or other incidents. Interpersonal verbal, physical, and sexual violence may erupt. Loss of a parent, child, or sibling also may occur as a consequence of institutionalization; running away from home; adolescent pregnancy, or premature marriage, divorce, or separation. Other family structural changes may result as various members distance themselves from the increasingly dysfunctional family.

FAMILY ADJUSTMENT TO ADDICTION AND RECOVERY

The early onset, gradual progression, and intermittent, chronic nature of addiction disorders may lead families to accept addictive behaviors as a fact of life, especially when addiction is a multigenerational problem. Family members often exhibit self-defeating behaviors based on distorted versions of certain normal defense mechanisms, such as *classic denial, minimization, projection,* and *rationalization.* As a chronic disease, addiction insidiously alters family "rules, roles, and customs/rituals." Most families that suffer from the disease of addiction demonstrate characteristic interpersonal interaction patterns, including the following "rules": (1) *Don't talk* (avoid discussion of dysfunctional family events); (2) *don't feel* (suppress all true emotions); and (3) *don't trust* (be proactive in preventing disappointment). Following these rules may have short-term protective benefits for individuals, but they discourage healthy, intimate, nurturing relationships within and outside the family. Family members also may take on stereotyped "roles" such as *enabler, hero, scapegoat, lost child,* and *mascot.* These roles are internalized in childhood and persist into adulthood, although individuals may change roles over time.

THE PHYSICIAN'S ROLE

Use of the family version of the CAGE questionnaire (f-CAGE) markedly improves screening sensitivity and specificity. Another tool, the Family Drinking Survey, is a more extensive inquiry into the family effects of alcohol and drug use. The Risk Inventory for Substance Abuse–Affected Families specifically assesses impairment in performing parental functions. In many cases, despite awareness of the negative effects of substance abuse, the patient and some family members may have the perception that substance use also makes their lives better in some ways. By recognizing the role the substance plays in modulating how families interact, the physician can better understand resistance to treatment and recovery.

The physician may support families in confronting and motivating a family member to seek needed treatment. Motivational interviewing techniques may be persuasive, but if resistance is met, inclusion of family members is indicated. If the patient is extremely defensive, family members may be referred to a family therapist who is trained in treating addiction.

FAMILY THERAPY FOR ADDICTION

When compared with individual-oriented care, family-oriented treatment approaches have been shown to result in superior rates of treatment engagement, treatment retention, positive treatment outcomes, and aftercare participation. Several approaches have been tailored to the unique needs of specific groups of patients with SUDs.

Adults

Behavioral couples therapy, the most extensively researched family approach, has strong empirical evidence of its efficacy. It can be used in a variety of formats, is cost-effective, and benefits both the couple and their children; there is, however, some evidence that those diagnosed with antisocial personality disorder or those experiencing intimate partner violence may have better outcomes with individual approaches.

Adolescents

Adolescents exposed to unstructured group therapy approaches tend to imitate one another's pathologic attitudes and behaviors and often do poorly. In contrast, family therapy specifically improves treatment outcomes in terms of drug use, association with antisocial peers, and acting-out behavior. Several family-based approaches have been studied. The Behaviour Exchange Systems Training program supports parents in coping with their adolescent's substance use; it has demonstrated parental reductions in symptoms of impaired mental health and increases in satisfaction and assertive parenting behaviors. Prosocial family therapy is a preventive intervention for juvenile offenders. It integrates specific parental training with nonspecific family therapy based on a theoretical model of risk-protection factors. Brief strategic family therapy targets drug use behavior and other associated behaviors, such as oppositional defiance, underachievement, aggression, delinquency, and risky sexual behaviors. Multidimensional family therapy uses both individual and family sessions to address various family issues, including expectancies about intoxicant use, parental addiction, and the prevention of family relapse. Multisystemic therapy and the Youth Support Project were developed specifically for juvenile offenders. Multisystemic therapy empowers parents and other caregivers to influence delinquent youth and support them in taking progressively more responsibility for their own behavior. Youth Support Project was developed especially for families at high risk for and difficult to enroll and retain in addiction treatment.

Older Adults

Given the demographic changes occurring in the United States, older adults will account for a larger segment of adults experiencing SUDs. Older adults may have well-established SUDs, relapse after long-term abstinence, or experience addiction for the first time as they face retirement, loss of family and friends, isolation, chronic illness, and other challenges. They may surround themselves with enablers or other substance abusers, or they may live in secretive isolation, hiding their shame from others. Age-appropriate screening tools such as the Michigan Alcoholic Screening Test, Geriatric Version may be used to improve detection. If available, family input is very helpful for assessing the extent of functional impairment, in monitoring adherence, and in facilitating entry into treatment, if needed.

Military Personnel and Veterans

Those who have served in the military are at particularly high risk for addiction. Under constant stress, exposed to danger, and away from home and family, they may develop maladaptive coping strategies, including abuse of intoxicants. This type of behavior is often part of the combat culture, but many other unique issues may contribute and complicate the presentation and treatment. For example, although effective treatments for posttraumatic stress disorder exist, many veterans isolate themselves and rely on intoxicants to suppress anxiety. Their addiction treatment also must address their posttraumatic stress disorder, and involvement of the partner is critical. Multifamily therapy groups can be helpful in addressing some of these issues, allowing men and women to find peers who understand them by virtue of their common experiences. Here, again, family involvement is very helpful and likely to improve outcomes.

Pregnant Women

About 15% of pregnancies are complicated by substance abuse. Although women may attempt to stop using drugs and alcohol once the pregnancy is discovered, pre-pregnancy patterns of substance use may nevertheless be continued well into the period of greatest teratogenic risk, the first trimester. Relatives, although concerned, may continue to enable, and the woman herself may experience ambivalence about substance use during pregnancy. Involving the family may be helpful in detecting and treating addiction in pregnant and postpartum women. When abstinence is established early in pregnancy, the family may become less concerned; however, recovery efforts should be strongly encouraged and supported throughout the pregnancy. Family involvement in

Al-Anon and the implementation of family-oriented psychoeducation and treatment can reduce the likelihood of ongoing family enabling.

KEY POINTS

1. A patient's family significantly influences addiction progression, treatment, and recovery.
2. Family members themselves may need treatment for the maladaptive coping behaviors that have emerged.
3. Family treatment not only improves the well-being of all family members but also supports the recovery of the involved family member.
4. Families may unintentionally undermine the recovery process of change if their own treatment needs are not addressed.
5. In addition to standard couples and family addiction therapies, specialized treatment options are available for the families of adolescent children, elderly adults, pregnant women, active duty military personnel, and veterans with SUDs.

REVIEW QUESTIONS

1. Family involvement in the treatment for SUDs:
   A. increases the likelihood that the patient will seek treatment.
   B. increases the likelihood that the patient will complete treatment.
   C. increases the likelihood that the patient will maintain recovery.
   D. All of the above.
   E. None of the above.

2. Family members of a person suffering from a SUD may:
   A. provoke guilt and shame felt by the person suffering from SUD.
   B. provide encouragement to recover.
   C. offer excuses to relapse.
   D. interfere with treatment and recovery.
   E. All of the above.

3. Which of the following is a useful screening tool to use in a family where someone may have alcohol use disorder?
   A. COWS
   B. DAST
   C. AUDIT-C
   D. f-CAGE

ANSWERS

1. **D**
2. **E**
3. **D**

SUGGESTED READINGS

Baird MA. Care of family members and other affected persons. In: Fleming MF, Barry KL, eds. *Addictive Disorders.* St. Louis: Mosby Year Book, 1992;195-210.

Dembo R, Cervenka KA, Hunter B, et al. Engaging high risk families in community based intervention services. *Aggress Violent Behav.* 1999;4(1):41-58.

Dube SR, Felitti VJ, Dong M, Giles WH, Anda RF. The impact of adverse childhood experiences on health problems: evidence from four birth cohorts dating back to 1900. *Prev Med.* 2003;37(3):268-277.

Frank SH, Graham AV, Zyzanski SJ, White S. Use of the Family CAGE in screening for alcohol problems in primary care. *Arch Fam Med.* 1992;1(2):209-216.

McGann KP. Self-reported illnesses in family members of alcoholics. *Fam Med.* 1990;22(2):103-106.

Steinglass P. Family systems and motivational interviewing: a systemic-motivational model for treatment of alcohol and other drug problems. *Alcohol Treat Q.* 2008; 26(1-2):9-29.

72 Twelve-Step Facilitation Approaches

Summary by Tim K. Brennan

Based on THE ASAM PRINCIPLES OF ADDICTION MEDICINE,
6th edition chapter by Kathleen M. Carroll

HISTORY

Twelve-step–based treatment has been around for many decades in the United States and around the world and has served to form the foundation of many well-known treatment programs. Today, facilities and treatment networks may refer to themselves as "12-step based" or "12-step informed." Although the specifics may differ, the central tenant of these 12 step–based programs is abstinence from all psychoactive substances and self-help meeting attendance. Twelve-step facilitation (TSF), which is different than 12-step–based treatment, was started in 1992 in order to provide individual, manual-guided treatment to patients over the course of 12 to 24 weeks. One can conceive of TSF as a formalized treatment approach to the 12 steps.

THE 12 STEPS

The twelve steps of Alcoholics Anonymous are as follows:

Step 1: We admitted we were powerless over alcohol—that our lives had become unmanageable.

Step 2: Came to believe that a Power greater than ourselves could restore us to sanity.

Step 3: Made a decision to turn our will and our lives over to the care of God *as we understood Him.*

Step 4: Made a searching and fearless moral inventory of ourselves.

Step 5: Admitted to God, to ourselves, and to another human being the exact nature of our wrongs.

Step 6: Were entirely ready to have God remove all these defects of character.

Step 7: Humbly asked Him to remove our shortcomings.

Step 8: Made a list of all persons we had harmed, and became willing to make amends to them all.

Step 9: Made direct amends to such people wherever possible, except when to do so would injure them or others.

Step 10: Continued to take personal inventory and when we were wrong promptly admitted it.

Step 11: Sought through prayer and meditation to improve our conscious contact with God *as we understood Him*, praying only for knowledge of His will for us and the power to carry that out.

Step 12: Having had a spiritual awakening as the result of these steps, we tried to carry this message to alcoholics, and to practice these principles in all our affairs.

TWELVE-STEP FACILITATION OVERVIEW

The TSF manual was created by a multidisciplinary group of people and designed to be used in a large research protocol. Specifically, the core topics of TSF are assessment and overview, acceptance, surrender, and getting active. Assessment is self-explanatory and includes a thorough alcohol and substance use history, wherein the patient identifies both positive and negative consequences of their drug and alcohol use. Overview education is provided about the various 12 steps and explanation regarding the concept of addiction. Acceptance involves working with the patient so that they might realize that addiction is a chronic, progressive disease over which they have no control and the concept that their life has become unmanageable as a result. Further, acceptance includes the idea that their willpower alone is insufficient to combat the problem. Surrender involves giving oneself over to a "higher power," accepting the fellowship and social support of other recovering people, and following the plan laid out in the 12-step program. Active involvement is the attendance and close personal involvement in 12-step programs. Importantly, TSF does not portend to describe a causal theory regarding the patient's substance use disorder. The emphasis is on acceptance of a loss of control and the importance of fellowship with the 12 steps to enter into recovery.

TREATMENT MODEL OF 12-STEP FACILITATION

TSF can be adapted to different individuals and contains guidelines on conducting sessions with involved friends or family members. The TSF sessions follow a consistent format and begin with a review of the previous week's attendance at various 12-step–based self-help programs. The patient keeps a recovery journal in which they describe their reactions to any 12-step–based programming or literature such as Alcoholics Anonymous' *Big Book*. These reactions are then discussed with the TSF therapist.

The therapist introduces a new "recovery topic" each week and devotes that session to exploring the relevant topic. For example, the therapist might explore discrepancies between the patient's stated goals and their completed actions. They might help the patient identify "people, places, and things" that may trigger relapse to substance use as well as protective "people, places, and things" that might help promote abstinence. Tasks are assigned at the conclusion of the session, wherein the patient receives homework assignments regarding meeting attendance and selected readings.

THEORY OF CHANGE

Change in TSF is based on the belief that building a meaningful relationship with the 12-step traditions can promote change within a patient. The theories of change in the 12-step traditions themselves evolved historically via practice as opposed to an academic theory that was first postulated by a social or behavioral scientist. There are some overlapping similarities between the change principles of the 12-step traditions and more formalized cognitive–behavioral therapies. TSF is inherently practical and pragmatic, so emphasis is based on doing "whatever works" in order to avoid substance use.

TREATMENT PLANNING AND EVALUATION IN 12-STEP FACILITATION

The first few sessions of TSF are devoted to obtaining an extremely thorough drug and alcohol use history. Emphasis is placed on the various time periods in the patient's life during which they used drugs and alcohol. Five-year increments are the typical unit of measure during the evaluation, with particular attention paid to the most recent year. As the frequency of substance use is revealed, the therapist will attempt to highlight the loss of control for the patient.

The TSF therapist explores both the positive and negative consequences of substance use with the patient. Many patients will reveal that their initial substance use was largely positive and perhaps served to ameliorate certain ongoing emotional or social distress or psychiatric symptoms such as low mood or anxiety. As negative consequences are revealed, the therapist will highlight them as evidence of the "unmanageability" that is referenced in the first step. Patients will be asked about their attempts at limiting substance use or abstinence as negative effects began to pile up in their life. Various domains are explored with the patient, including physical health, legal history, social environment (eg, friends, romantic history), sexual health, psychological health, and financial stressors. During the evaluation period, the TSF therapist will ask the patient to discuss their overall impression of their substance use history. For some patients, this may be the first time that they have visualized their entire substance use history at one time. The TSF therapist will guide the patient toward the logical conclusion that they are suffering from an addiction and have lost control of their substance use.

Once the diagnosis is established and understood by the patient, the TSF therapist can begin emphasizing the 12-step–based tradition of recovery. An emphasis is placed on the success that people have had in 12-step–based treatment. A plan is developed for the patient to begin attending meetings as assigned. The TSF sessions themselves are conversational in nature but fundamentally structured. Many TSF therapists may begin their session by asking the patient "how has your last week of recovery gone?" Specific details need to be related on a week-to-week basis to encourage active participation in recovery.

INDICATIONS FOR 12-STEP FACILITATION TREATMENT

TSF therapy is intended for patients with severe drug and alcohol use disorders. TSF is not intended for patients "at risk" for developing a substance use disorder. There are no established contraindications to TSF treatment, although patients who do not agree with the 12-step concept are obviously not good candidates for treatment.

PRETREATMENT ISSUES
Motivation

TSF views motivation as being related to patient denial about their substance use disorder. Fundamentally, recovery is an active process, and so the TSF therapist will attempt to engage the patient's interest in a commitment to the 12 steps. The relationship between the TSF therapist and the patient is not adversarial, nor is it one of threat or coercion. The TSF therapist is instructed to remain nonjudgmental and educational toward the patient. Issues related to motivation and denial are addressed in a direct and empathetic way.

Therapist Characteristics

TSF was designed to be used by therapists with a postgraduate education (master's level) or at least substantial experience in and commitment to the 12-step traditions. Important skills in a therapist include active listening, empathy, constructive problem solving, and appropriate ability to give direct but nonadversarial feedback. Obviously, a familiarity with the 12 steps themselves and openness to their success is fundamental. A TSF therapist needs to know exactly where the 12-step meetings are and what they entail.

RESEARCH

Historically, 12-step–based recovery programs have had very little exposure or interest in participating in formalized research. Because these programs are fundamentally anonymous and typically occur outside the typical healthcare infrastructure, there was little need to participate in research. Their "success" was essentially implied by the many millions of people who engaged in 12-step–based programs. Recently, there have been some research studies that examine the evidence for manualized 12-step–based treatment.

TSF has been studied compared to cognitive–behavioral therapy and motivational enhancement therapy, and results showed that there was no statistical difference in effectiveness between the three modalities. However, TSF has been associated with higher rates of self-help participation, which itself has been associated with better substance use outcomes.

KEY POINTS

1. TSF is professionally delivered and involves a manual-guided approach to participation in the 12 steps.
2. TSF is intended for patients with severe drug and alcohol use disorders and not for those "at risk" of developing a substance use disorder.
3. Research regarding the effectiveness of TSF and 12-step programs in general is relatively new and remains ongoing.

REVIEW QUESTIONS

1. Which of the following is *true* regarding TSF?
   A. TSF was designed by the founders of Alcoholics Anonymous.
   B. TSF therapists must be in recovery themselves to participate in TSF.
   C. TSF is covered by Medicaid but not by Medicare.
   D. TSF involves a nonconfrontational approach.

2. What is the typical length of TSF?
   A. 6 weeks
   B. 12 to 24 weeks
   C. 6 months
   D. 1 year

3. Which of the following statements is *true* regarding research into TSF effectiveness?
   A. TSF has been proven to be less efficacious than cognitive–behavioral therapy or motivational enhancement therapy.
   B. TSF has been proven to be equally efficacious to cognitive–behavioral therapy and motivational enhancement therapy.
   C. TSF has never been studied in comparison to cognitive–behavioral therapy and motivational enhancement therapy.
   D. TSF has been proven to be more efficacious than motivational enhancement therapy, but less efficacious than cognitive–behavioral therapy.

ANSWERS

1. **D**
2. **B**
3. **B**

SUGGESTED READINGS

Ferri M, Amato L, Davoli M. Alcoholics Anonymous and other 12-step programmes for alcohol dependence. *Cochrane Database Syst Rev.* 2006;(3):CD005032.

Humphreys K. *Circles of Recovery: Self-Help Organizations for Addictions.* Cambridge, United Kingdom: Cambridge University Press, 2004.

Humphreys K. The trials of Alcoholics Anonymous. *Addiction.* 2006;101(5):617-618.

National Institute on Drug Abuse. *Principles of Drug Addiction Treatment: A Research-Based Guide.* 3rd ed. Bethesda, MD: National Institute on Drug Abuse, 2018. https://www.drugabuse.gov/publications/principles-drug-addiction-treatment-research-based-guide-third-edition. Updated January 2018. Accessed September 14, 2018.

Nowinski J, Baker S, Carroll K. *Twelve Step Facilitation Therapy Manual: A Clinical Research Guide for Therapists Treating Individuals with Alcohol Abuse and Dependence.* Rockville, MD: National Institute on Alcohol Abuse and Alcoholism, 1999. NIH Publication No. 94-3722.

 Relapse Prevention: Clinical Models and Intervention Strategies

Summary by Antoine Douaihy, Dennis C. Daley, G. Alan Marlatt, and Dennis M. Donovan

> Based on THE ASAM PRINCIPLES OF ADDICTION MEDICINE, 6th edition chapter by Antoine Douaihy, Dennis C. Daley, G. Alan Marlatt, and Dennis M. Donovan

Substance use disorder (SUD) is a highly prevalent public health issue with serious personal and societal consequences. SUDs are often associated with a wide range of medical problems, co-occurring with other psychiatric disorders, and implicated in significant social and economic consequences. SUDs are psychiatric disorders defined by the American Psychiatric Association in the *Diagnostic and Statistical Manual of Mental Disorders,* 5th edition, and chronic health disorders with similar rates of relapse or exacerbation as other chronic medical conditions, such as congestive heart failure, asthma, and diabetes mellitus. Few adults with SUDs seek and obtain treatment, and the majority of these people experience relapse within 12 months. Longitudinal studies show that the treatment of SUDs is associated with major reductions in substance use, related problems, and societal costs. Although most people with an SUD eventually abstain or manage to control their use without professional help, many suffer from a long-lasting chronic condition and cycle through episodes of lapse, relapse, treatment reentry, and recovery. High rates of relapse have led many researchers to conceptualize addiction as a "chronic relapsing illness" and understand relapse prevention (RP) as an iterative process of change rather than as a full inoculation against relapse. Numerous approaches and models have been suggested to explain the relapse process. Focusing on the complexity of the relapse process helps us better understand the challenges of the change process and identify RP interventions that may enhance recovery and reduce relapse risk. Healthcare practitioners need to be careful about the context of using the term *relapse,* which could have potential negative connotations and implies fault on the part of the person.

LAPSE, RELAPSE, AND RECOVERY

The definitions of the terms *relapse* and *relapse prevention* have evolved over the years. The lack of consensus regarding the conceptualization of relapse has made it difficult to assess treatment outcomes and different estimates of relapse rates. Relapse has been described as a discrete phenomenon and as a process of behavior change. Relapse denotes meaning that goes beyond the dichotomous outcome. Marlatt has identified a *lapse* as the initial episode of use of a substance after a period of abstinence, a *relapse* as a continued use after the initial slip (ie, "a breakdown or setback in the person's attempt to change or modify any target behavior"), and a *prolapse* as a behavior that is consistent with getting back on track in the direction of positive behavior change.

The definition of relapse has a significant impact on the conceptual and clinical approach to assessment. The ways in which practitioners quantify and qualify relapse determine how they will respond to an individual's behaviors associated with the relapse. If a person is involved in a treatment program that identifies *any drinking* behavior, such as one drink after a period of abstinence as a relapse, it is more probable for him or her to engage in heavier drinking behaviors, which is explained by the phenomenon of the "abstinence violation effect" (eg, self-blame and loss of perceived control that individuals often experience after the violation of self-imposed rules). However, if the same person is receiving treatment in a program that does not convey that this behavior (ie, one drink) is a relapse, it is more probable for that person to have an increased awareness of his or her reactions to drinking and may be less vulnerable to the abstinence violation effect. Lapse and relapse may also be defined according to the individual's goals for change. If abstinence is a goal, then a drink may be considered as a lapse, but if the individual maintains harm reduction goals, then a lapse may be defined as a harmful consequence of drinking behavior.

Recovery in the context of SUDs refers to a long-term process in which there is change not only in the use of substances but also in personal and social aspects of a person's life. The road to recovery remains anything but linear and smooth, and the outcome anything but predictable. Domains of change during the recovery process can include physical, psychological, spiritual, behavioral, interpersonal, sociocultural, familial, and/or financial. Recovery tasks and areas of clinical focus are contingent on the stage or phase of recovery the individuals are in as well as what they want and desire to change. Although some individuals achieve full recovery, others only achieve partial recovery. The latter group is at risk for multiple relapses over time, yet still can benefit from the cumulative effects of multiple treatments.

Recovering from an SUD involves gaining information, increasing self-awareness, developing skills for "sober" living, and following a program of change. The program of change may incorporate psychotherapy, pharmacotherapy, case management, peer support, participation in mutual support programs including 12-step programs like Alcoholics Anonymous or Narcotics Anonymous, and self-management approaches. As recovery progresses, individuals may rely more on themselves after initially using their support system, with the goal of improving their overall quality of life. RP aims to help sustain their recovery by gaining information on relapse warning signs and risk factors and learning specific strategies to manage these signs and risk factors.

EFFECTIVENESS AND EFFICACY OF RELAPSE PREVENTION

Based on systematic reviews and large-scale treatment outcome studies, the RP model continues to be an influential cognitive–behavioral approach framework that can inform both theoretical and clinical approaches to understanding and facilitating behavior change in SUDs. Despite several limitations to studies on RP, the literature generally favors the efficacy and effectiveness of RP and shows that RP strategies, especially as a component of a multimodal treatment approach, enhance the recovery of individuals with SUDs and is particularly well suited for implementation in continuing care contexts.

DETERMINANTS OF RELAPSE

In this section, we highlight select findings that are relevant to the main tenets of the RP model.

Intrapersonal Determinants

Self-Efficacy

Self-efficacy refers to a person's beliefs in their capability to organize and carry out specific courses of action to attain some goal or situation-specific task. These beliefs have great influence on self-regulation and the quality of human functioning because they shape the goals individuals set for themselves. This construct is intimately related to the individual's coping abilities and reflects the degree of confidence about successfully managing a high-risk situation. The person's personal belief in their ability to control use of a substance is a reliable predictor of lapses immediately after treatment and over long-term outcomes. Self-efficacy is a predictor of outcomes across all types of addictions, including gambling, smoking, and drug use; low levels of self-efficacy are predictive of relapse, whereas high levels are predictive of a lower relapse risk.

Outcome Expectancies

A factor enhancing the likelihood of relapse is the set of cognitive expectancies that the individual develops about the expected outcomes associated with the addictive behavior. These are known as outcome expectancies. Outcome expectancies are central to the RP model and have been studied extensively in the domain of alcohol use. Underlying motives for engaging in addictive behaviors include both a desire to change one's mood and to increase sociability. Individuals who developed an addiction typically have developed a set of expectancies that anticipate positive outcomes from engaging in the behavior, serving as a source of motivation to engage in it. Such outcome expectancies are shaped by an individual's past direct and indirect experiences with the behaviors related to the addiction, including vicarious learning through the modeling they see early on displayed by parents and later on by peers.

Motivation

An important element in determining the likelihood of relapse is the individual's commitment to or motivation for self-improvement. The motivation may relate to the relapse process in two distinct ways: the motivation for positive behavior change and the motivation to engage in the problematic behavior. Motivation is judged with regard to a particular action or outcome. The most common motivation obstacle to seeking help early on is ambivalence. An ambivalence toward change is highly related to self-efficacy and outcome expectancies. Thus, it is important to assess commitment and motivation to change and understand that motivation for change is composed of multiple dimensions that are modestly intercorrelated. Interventions designed to enhance commitment to change, such as motivational interviewing, should be a component of any RP approach.

Coping

Based on the cognitive–behavioral model of relapse, the most critical predictor of relapse is the individual's ability to utilize adequate coping strategies in dealing with high-risk situations. What predicts sustained sobriety is the individual's capacity for dealing with life's challenges, particularly with coping strategies that exclude avoidance. Coping has been shown to be a critical predictor of substance use treatment outcomes and is often the strongest predictor of behavioral lapses in the moment. Despite findings that coping can prevent lapses, there is limited evidence to show that skills-based interventions lead to improved coping.

Negative Emotional States

Many studies report a strong link between negative affect and relapse to substance use if the patient does not use active coping strategies to manage the mood or emotion. Thus, practitioners should incorporate strategies to decrease and manage negative emotional states such as anxiety, anger, boredom, depression, loneliness, or guilt and shame as a part of the RP approach. Again, it is not the emotional state that determines if a relapse occurs but the use of coping strategies to manage this state. Because physical and psychological withdrawal symptoms can predict relapse, addressing them early in treatment has the potential to reduce the risk of lapse. Because co-occurring anxiety or mood disorders are common among individuals in treatment for SUDs, aggressively treating these disorders is warranted as a part of a comprehensive RP approach.

Interpersonal Determinants

Functional social support or the level of emotional support is highly predictive of long-term abstinence across several addictive disorders. The social support network size, the perceived quality of social support, and the level of support from people who do not use substances have also been shown to predict relapse.

Clinical Relapse Prevention Interventions to Reduce Lapse and Relapse Risk

The literature emphasizes individualizing RP strategies, taking into account the individual's level of motivation, severity of substance use, ego functioning,

and sociocultural environment. These RP interventions can be provided in individual or group sessions. They aim to facilitate the acquisition and practice of coping skills and to encourage behavioral change.

Strategy 1: Help Individuals Understand Relapse as a Process and Event and Learn to Identify Warning Signs

Attitudinal, emotional, cognitive, and behavioral changes may occur days, weeks, and even longer before resuming the use of substances. Warning signs can be obvious, such as reducing or stopping Alcoholics Anonymous or Narcotics Anonymous meetings or counseling without discussing it with a therapist or a sponsor. Relapse can also be conceptualized as links in a relapse chain—each link represents a warning sign or high-risk situation. Reviewing with the individual the relapse history and relapse calendar (ie, use of a daily inventory that helps identify high-risk situations, relapse warning signs, or significant life events that could lead to a relapse) is essential. The practitioner can ask the individual to review any relapse experience in detail to learn the connections between thoughts, feelings, events, or situations and a return to substance use.

Strategy 2: Help Individuals Identify Their High-Risk Situations and Develop Effective Cognitive and Behavioral Coping

The need to recognize and manage high-risk factors or situations is an essential component of RP. High-risk factors involve intrapersonal and interpersonal situations in which the person feels vulnerable to substance use. Relapse is more likely to occur as the result of a lack of coping skills than the high-risk situation itself, so the practitioner should assess the person's coping style to identify targets for an intervention. A person heading for a relapse usually makes several minidecisions over time, each of which brings him or her closer to creating a high-risk situation or giving in to the decision to use a substance. These choices are called "apparently irrelevant decisions," and they need to be identified and addressed with individuals to decrease lapse risk.

In Marlatt's cognitive–behavioral relapse model, for example, in addition to teaching individuals "specific" RP skills to deal with high-risk factors, the practitioner could teach "global" approaches such as problem-solving or skills-training strategies (such as behavioral rehearsal, covert modeling, and assertiveness training), cognitive reframing (such as coping imagery and reframing reactions to lapse/relapse), and lifestyle interventions (such as mindfulness, exercise, and relaxation).

Strategy 3: Help Individuals Enhance Their Communication Skills and Interpersonal Relationships and Develop a Recovery Social Network

Positive family and social supports generally enhance recovery for the person with an SUD. Families and concerned significant others are more likely to support the recovery of their loved one struggling with an SUD if they are engaged in treatment and have an opportunity to ask questions, share their concerns and experiences, learn practical coping strategies, and learn behaviors to avoid. This opportunity is more likely to occur if the family member with the SUD understands the effect of it on the family and concerned significant others and makes amends for some of its adverse effects. Individuals can be encouraged to get active in mutual support programs (eg, 12-step programs) and use the "tools" of the program (eg, meetings, sponsor, 12 steps, slogans, recovery literature). Linking them with specific mutual support programs or introducing them to a "buddy" or person already active in a program or a peer navigator who can attend meetings with them are some ways to enhance their recovery network. Some individuals may need help asking for help or support from others.

Strategy 4: Help Individuals Reduce, Identify, and Manage Negative Emotional States

Negative affective states, such as depression and anxiety, or negative feelings, such as boredom or anger, are factors in a substantial number of relapses when individuals do not use coping skills to manage them. Helping individuals become aware of their moods and emotions or feelings, understand the connection between thoughts and emotions, and changing how they think can help them manage these without resorting to substance use. Individuals may also benefit from changing behaviors relevant to a specific emotional state. Examples include engaging in exercise or pleasant activities to reduce depression, challenging anxious thoughts, taking up a new hobby or activity to reduce boredom, or making amends to a loved one hurt by the addiction to reduce feelings of guilt. Finally, if there is concern about an anxiety or a mood disorder, facilitating an evaluation and/or treatment are important interventions.

Strategy 5: Help Individuals Identify and Manage Cravings and Cues That Precede Cravings

A strong desire or craving for a substance can be triggered by exposure to environmental or internal cues associated with prior use. Cues such as the sight or smell of the substance can trigger cravings that are evidenced in increased thoughts of using and physiologic changes (eg, anxiety). The practitioner can provide information about cues and how they trigger cravings for alcohol or other drugs. Monitoring and recording cravings, associated thoughts, and outcomes in a daily log or journal can help individuals become more vigilant and prepare them to cope when they occur. Cognitive interventions include changing thoughts about the craving or desire to use, challenging euphoric recall, talking oneself through the craving, thinking beyond the high by identifying negative consequences of using (immediate and delayed) and positive benefits of not using, using 12-step recovery slogans, and delaying the decision to use. Behavioral interventions include avoiding, leaving, or changing situations that trigger or worsen a craving; redirecting activities or becoming involved in pleasant activities; obtaining help or support from others by admitting and talking about cravings and hearing how others have survived them; and considering anticraving medications.

Strategy 6: Help Individuals Identify and Challenge Cognitive Distortions

Marlatt's RP model observed that "the patient's cognitive errors and distortions may increase the probability that an initial slip will develop into a total relapse." Twelve-step programs refer to these patterns as "stinking thinking" and suggest that individuals need to alter their thinking if they are to remain substance free. Teaching them to identify their negative thinking patterns or cognitive errors and to evaluate how these affect recovery and relapse is one strategy. Individuals can be taught to use counterthoughts to challenge their thinking errors or specific negative thoughts. For example, "I'll die if I don't get a drink" can be changed to "Even though I have a strong desire to drink at this time, I can put it off for a few hours. I know it will go away and I don't have to drink."

Strategy 7: Help Individuals Work Toward a More Balanced Lifestyle

Individuals can benefit from global changes to restore or achieve balance in their lives. Development of a healthy lifestyle may reduce stress that makes the patient more vulnerable to relapse. A person's lifestyle can be assessed by evaluating patterns of daily activities, sources of stress, daily hassles and uplifts, the balance between "wants" (ie, activities engaged in for pleasure or self-fulfillment) and "shoulds" (ie, external demands), health, exercise and relaxation patterns, interpersonal activities, and religious beliefs. Working with the person to develop positive habits or substitute indulgences (such as jogging, meditation, mindfulness-based activities, relaxation, exercise, hobbies, or creative tasks) for an addictive disorder can help balance their lifestyles.

Strategy 8: Consider the Use of Medications in Combination With Psychosocial Treatments

There are medications used for their anticraving effects and other benefits available for each of the major classes of addictive substances such as alcohol, opioids, and tobacco. The best use of medications may be in combination with one another and *with psychosocial interventions. Individuals with SUDs receiving psychosocial treatments and/or mutual support programs should be offered medication options.*

Strategy 9: Facilitate the Transition Between Levels of Care for Individuals Completing Residential or Hospital-Based Inpatient Treatment Programs or Structured Partial Hospital or Intensive Outpatient Programs

Interventions used to enhance treatment entry and adherence that also lower the risk of relapse include providing a single session of motivational therapy before discharge from residential or intensive treatment, using telephone or mail reminders of initial treatment appointments, and providing reinforcers (rewards or incentives) for appropriate participation in treatment activities or for providing negative urine tests. Individuals who return to the hospital, to residential treatment, or to other higher levels of care should be "linked" to the next level when possible (ie, meet or talk with a staff member from the receiving clinic or program).

Strategy 10: Incorporate Strategies to Improve Adherence to Treatment and Medications

Many clinical and systems strategies can improve adherence to treatment among individuals with SUDs, psychiatric illnesses, or co-occurring disorders. Incorporating these strategies (eg, motivational incentives) into treatment setting operations or integrating these (eg, motivational interviewing) into the therapy can help improve adherence and thus reduce relapse risk.

CONCLUSIONS

Relapse is a major challenge in the treatment of SUDs. The dynamic model of relapse acknowledges the complexity and unpredictable nature of substance use behavior after the commitment to abstinence or a harm reduction goal. Clinical RP strategies can be used throughout the continuum of care and can be integrated with other treatment modalities such as motivational interviewing, case management, peer support, pharmacotherapy, spirituality, mindfulness meditation, 12-step mutual support groups, and family-based interventions.

KEY POINTS

1. Lapse and relapse are common during and after treatment for substance use disorders.
2. Many factors, intrapersonal and interpersonal, contribute to relapse.
3. Relapse prevention interventions can be adapted to individual and group sessions and incorporated into the treatment of substance use disorders.
4. Medications for substance use disorders are an essential component of relapse prevention.

REVIEW QUESTIONS

1. Marlatt defined lapse as the initial episode of substance use after a period of abstinence. Which of the following is *true* of a lapse?
   A. Once a person with opioid use disorder lapses to alcohol or any drug use, they end up in a full-blown relapse to opioid addiction.
   B. An individual with alcohol use disorder is considered moving from lapse to relapse after 1 week or more of daily excessive drinking.
   C. A lapse does not always end in a relapse because the person may stop it quickly.
   D. In abstinence-based outpatient treatment programs, a lapse usually leads to the person getting discharged for showing low motivation to change.

2. Which of the following examples are *not* "intrapersonal" determinants of relapse? Select all that apply.
   A. Celebrate.
   B. A woman in recovery from intravenous opioid addiction who has been abstinent for 8 months receives a flu shot and unexpectedly feels a strong craving for heroin.
   C. A young man in recovery with several months being free of alcohol or drugs feels restless

and bored with his life and starts to think about "needing some action," which drugs can provide.

D. A woman in recovery from cocaine addiction randomly runs into her old dealer who offers to give her cocaine until payday.

3. Which of the following statements are *true* with regard to the high-risk factor of "social pressure to use substances"? Select all that apply.

A. Social pressures can be direct (the person is offered substances) or indirect (the person is in a situation in which substances are being used by others).

B. Avoiding all "high-risk" people, places, and events is the only way to cope with social pressure to use substances.

C. Being around social drinkers is no threat to an individual with an alcohol use disorder who is in recovery because these individuals do not usually drink to excess.

D. It is not the social pressure situation itself but the person's use of coping skills that ultimately determines if social pressure leads to substance use.

ANSWERS

1. **C.** Although some practitioners and individuals in recovery believe that any substance use is a relapse, many can quickly stop the initial lapse from leading to a full-blown relapse. This can occur after a single use of a substance (eg, a few drinks, joint, pills) or after a brief binge drinking episode.

2. **A and D.** "Intrapersonal" determinants related more to internal factors (thoughts, feelings, motivation, craving, expectancies) and can occur in any situation or context, even those that do not involve any social interaction. "Interpersonal" determinants refer to people (dealers, others who get high or use in front of the person in recovery), places, events, and situations (bars, parties, places associated with using) in which the recovering individual feels direct or indirect pressure to engage in substance use.

3. **A and D.** Numerous direct and indirect social pressures can impact a person's relapse; therefore, awareness of these is an important part of recovery. Because there are so many social pressures (eg, a family event, a wedding), it is impossible for a person in recovery to avoid them all. Learning and using coping skills will determine if a person in recovery relapses or refuses to give in to social pressures.

SUGGESTED READINGS

Daley DC, Douaihy A. *Relapse Prevention Counseling: Strategies to Aid Recovery From Addiction and Reduce Relapse Risk*. Murrysville, PA: Daley Publications, 2011.

Daley DC, Maccarelli L. Relapse prevention. In: Douaihy A, Daley D, eds. *Substance Use Disorders: Pittsburgh Pocket Psychiatry*. New York: Oxford University Press, 2014:247-268.

Donovan D, Witkiewitz K. Relapse prevention: from radical idea to common practice. *Addict Res Theory*. 2012;20(3):204-217.

Hendershot CS, Witkiewitz K, George WH, Marlatt GA. Relapse prevention for addictive behaviors. *Subst Abuse Treat Prev Policy*. 2011;6:17.

Marlatt GA, Donovan DM. *Relapse Prevention: Maintenance Strategies in the Treatment of Addictive Behaviors*. 2nd ed. New York: Guilford Press, 2005.

74

Digital Health Interventions for Substance Use Disorders: The State of the Science

Summary by Lisa A. Marsch and Jacob T. Borodovsky

| Based on THE ASAM PRINCIPLES OF ADDICTION MEDICINE, 6th edition chapter by Lisa A. Marsch and Jacob T. Borodovsky

Advances in digital technologies—including Web/mobile devices, cloud computing, and data analytics—have created unprecedented opportunities to assess and modify health behavior and health outcomes. In this new area of science, referred to as "digital health," digital therapeutic devices and platforms provide interactive and self-directed behavior therapy as well as tools to help individuals replace self-defeating patterns of behavior (eg, substance use) with healthier behavioral repertoires.

Digital therapeutics can be available 24/7 and thus allow for "on-demand," ubiquitous access to therapeutic support, thereby creating unprecedented models of intervention delivery and reducing barriers to accessing care. Because most choices about health (such as whether to take prescribed medications or follow other medical advice, what to eat and drink, where and when to exercise, and whether to smoke) are made during everyday activities, harnessing mobile devices to understand and influence these choices in real time constitutes one of the most promising opportunities for improving health outcomes in the United States.

Digital therapeutics may be particularly transformative in the field of substance use disorder (SUD) treatment for a number of reasons. First, most individuals currently receiving SUD treatment still spend the majority of their time outside of the treatment facility. Digital technologies can extend the reach and the impact of the treatment system by offering anytime/anywhere resources—literally "in one's pocket"—and at times when patients may be at greatest need (eg, at risk for relapse). Additionally, a significant portion of care offered in SUD treatment settings is not science based and thus may not have the maximal therapeutic impact. Digital therapeutics allow for the widespread delivery of science-based resources and tools, with fidelity to best practices. Further, SUD is a chronic relapsing disorder, and digital therapeutics can offer

ongoing access to recovery support resources in a manner that can be personalized to an individual's needs, stage of recovery, and clinical trajectory over time. Finally, the vast majority of individuals with a diagnosable SUD do not receive treatment for their disorder. This treatment gap is due, in part, to factors such as the stigma associated with many models of SUD care, limited access to care in many contexts (eg, rural settings, health insurance coverage, cost), and lack of clinical staff. With regard to the last point, even if the SUD clinician workforce were to be dramatically expanded, it could never be sufficiently scalable to meet the full needs of the population or to offer anytime/anywhere care. Digital therapeutics can help create science-based, scalable solutions to meet SUD needs at a population level.

This chapter provides an overview of the state of the science of applying digital health interventions to SUDs. We summarize the peer-reviewed literature focused on the development and evaluation of digital (ie, computer-, smartphone-, and Web-based) therapeutics for SUDs evaluated in a variety of adult populations (age ≥18 years). We first summarize the peer-reviewed literature concerning the evaluation of SUD-specific digital therapeutics (eg, alcohol- or cannabis-only interventions). We then summarize the literature on therapeutics evaluated for a diverse array of populations with SUDs. This heterogeneity includes both (1) samples with different primary SUDs across individuals and (2) samples with individuals diagnosed with multiple co-occurring SUDs.

DIGITAL THERAPEUTICS FOR SPECIFIC SUBSTANCE USE DISORDERS

Alcohol

Digital therapeutic interventions for hazardous alcohol use and for alcohol use disorder have a large body of literature underlying their evidence base. Those interventions guided by behavioral therapy techniques such as self-monitoring, goal setting, and goal-related feedback along with action planning have been deemed to be particularly effective. Notable alcohol-specific digital therapeutic interventions include Check Your Drinking, Health-Call, Alcohol–Comprehensive Health Enhancement Support System, and Location-Based Monitoring and Intervention for Alcohol Use Disorders. These interventions are delivered via computer or mobile phones and utilize several evidence-based therapeutic strategies such as personalized normative feedback, self-determination and relapse prevention theories, motivational enhancement therapy, and the community reinforcement approach. The content of these interventions is usually divided into several distinct modules, each of which addresses different but interrelated therapeutic targets (eg, stress management, craving coping mechanisms, refusal skills). Often, the way in which therapy is delivered as well as the content of the therapy become increasingly tailored and personalized to a particular patient (eg, specific triggers, unique treatment goals, peer support networks) by utilizing the information that an individual provides when completing intervention modules. Additionally, the data collected over time can be provided to counselors who can integrate this information into their treatment plans. Randomized controlled trials (RCTs) and observational studies have generally demonstrated that these interventions can produce significant changes in drinking behaviors such as greater reductions in the number of heavy drinking days, the number of drinks per week, or the number of drinks per day compared to treatment-as-usual control groups.

Cannabis

Several digital health interventions have also been specifically developed for addressing the clinical patterns and consequences of cannabis use disorder (CUD). The digital intervention for CUD summarized in this review include Quit the Shit, Can Reduce, and Reduce Your Use. Digital therapeutics for CUD are often computer- or Web-based programs that are either self-directed and automated or include interactions with live counselors via Web-based chat functions. Similar to digital interventions for alcohol, interventions for CUD generally use some combination of manualized clinical protocols for evidence-based therapies such as motivational enhancement therapy, motivational interviewing, cognitive–behavioral therapy (CBT),

or contingency management. Further, digital interventions for CUD (similar to those developed for alcohol) contain multiple psychotherapeutic modules that provide patients with opportunities to set goals; engage in cognitive restructuring; and develop self-awareness, coping strategies, and problem-solving skills to prevent relapse. Daily diaries are also a notable component of digital interventions for CUD. Individuals are asked to keep track of relevant clinical events such as cravings, cannabis consumption events, and volume of cannabis consumed. Such information can be used by patients or their clinicians to track progress and provide automated or clinician-delivered personalized feedback. In general, mobile- or smartphone-based interventions for CUD (as opposed to computer based) have not yet progressed to the same level of sophistication as those developed for alcohol use disorders. Results from RCTs and observational studies have generally demonstrated that these interventions produce similar or better treatment retention, cannabis use reduction (eg, number of days cannabis was used, number of joints used per day), cannabis abstinence, or overall reductions in clinical severity of CUD compared to control groups (eg, waitlist controls, treatment as usual).

Cocaine

Cocaine-specific digital health interventions are rare in the published scientific literature, but they do exist. One example is Snow Control, a 6-week Web-based self-help program for cocaine use grounded in CBT, motivational interviewing, and self-control theories. This intervention draws on paradigms similar to those utilized by alcohol- and cannabis-specific interventions. Results from an RCT demonstrated greater retention in the Snow Control group than in the psychoeducation control group but showed no differences in cocaine abstinence or reduced cocaine use.

DIGITAL THERAPEUTICS FOR DIVERSE SAMPLES WITH SUBSTANCE USE DISORDERS

Other types of digital health interventions have been developed to address a broader range of SUDs than those discussed previously. We reviewed data for four such digital health interventions: Self-help Alcohol and Other Drug Use and Depression, Computer-Based Training for Cognitive–Behavioral Therapy, Breaking Free Online, and the most extensively tested intervention for SUDs, the Therapeutic Education System.

Researchers have evaluated the effectiveness of these interventions by testing them in real-world community treatment centers responsible for the care of heterogeneous substance use populations (eg, alcohol, opioids, cocaine, cannabis). These interventions can be delivered on either desktop computers or mobile platforms and are usually self-directed (ie, patients are capable of receiving therapeutic content from the intervention without instruction or guidance from clinic staff). They can be used in conjunction with traditional in-person therapy (ie, as an additional supplement to treatment as usual) or can be employed in a stand-alone fashion to replace clinician interaction.

Importantly, digital health interventions designed to address heterogeneous SUDs utilize many of the same evidence-based psychotherapeutic principles as the substance-specific interventions discussed previously. They contain multiple modules grounded in CBT, motivational interviewing, and contingency management. These therapeutic approaches are translated into interactive videos and graphics that provide patients with opportunities to identify personal patterns of drug use and enhance their coping, refusal, and problem-solving skills. Homework assignments are often used to reinforce those skills. The content of these interventions may also address several domains of life problems (eg, relationships, finances, work/school, housing) and help patients take steps toward resolving conflicts in these domains. Results from RCTs and observational evaluations have generally demonstrated that compared to treatment-as-usual control groups, those who receive these interventions experience better outcomes such as lower dropout rates, higher rates of abstinence, longer periods of continuous abstinence, or greater reductions in the frequency of substance use (ie, number of days used or number of times used per day).

CONCLUSIONS AND FUTURE OPPORTUNITIES

The pattern of results observed in the scientific literature to date indicates that digital interventions improve clinical outcomes among patients with SUDs and have the potential to substantially increase the scope of SUD care. Indeed, in several trials, digital therapeutics produced clinical outcomes that were as good as, or better than, outcomes produced in models of clinician-delivered care. However, there are still several areas of research that will be necessary to explore in order to tap the full potential of digital therapeutics for SUDs. One critical area for expanded research is in the study of mechanisms by which digital therapeutics promote behavior change, including changes in SUDs. "Mechanisms" refer to intervention-induced changes in psychological, behavioral, and/or biological factors, which, in turn, are then responsible for health behavior changes. Understanding how these tools can lead to changes in substance-taking behaviors will help determine the conditions under which research results are or are not replicable.

An additional and vital area of research is to identify improved strategies for engaging individuals in the use of digital therapeutics for SUDs. Even the best interventions cannot elicit behavior change if patients do not actually use them. There is a tremendous opportunity to understand individual trajectories of use of digital interventions over time to better understand the optimal patterns of use and how individuals' clinical needs may change.

This is also a time of great opportunity to evaluate how to best scale-up access to science-based digital therapeutics in real-world settings. A research agenda that balances scientific rigor (eg, developing maximally *potent* interventions) with relevance (eg, developing maximally *implementable* digital health tools) may enable entirely new models for offering personalized, useful resources for SUD treatment to individuals anytime and anywhere. This approach could expand the ability of healthcare providers to both track and influence the health behavior of patients. Additionally, healthcare systems may consider digitally driven business models that provide accessible, engaging, scalable, and cost-effective methods for promoting translational science to the population level.

Although much of the work on digital health and SUDs has focused on Web and mobile digital therapeutics, there is a tremendous opportunity to embrace the full spectrum of digital health tools to produce the most impactful therapeutic resources for SUDs. This may include an expanded agenda focused on the role of passive sensing technologies on smartphones or wearable sensors to infer information about an individual's behavior, health, and environment and then prompt the delivery of real-time and adaptive SUD interventions. This may also include the use of social media (used by over 2.5 billion people), to enable a deeper understanding of both individual and population-level trends in health behavior and market demands in the health space (including SUDs) and/or offer social media–based interventions for behavior change. Additionally, this may include expanded clinical application of the increasingly sophisticated data analytic methodologies becoming possible due to the rich data afforded via mobile data collection, passive sensing, and social media. For example, innovative approaches to predictive modeling, such as the rapidly advancing field of machine learning, allow for the creation of systems that learn from data instead of simply following preprogrammed instructions. Together, these emerging trends enable an entirely new offering of tools for collecting rich data about individuals' behavior, health, and environment; provide personalized interventions and resources based on individuals' needs and preferences; and enable dynamic computational models to predict and characterize individuals' changing needs and health trajectories over time.

Finally, an increased focus on digital health ethics is sorely needed. As research and development in digital health ventures into uncharted territory—in which information is obtained about individuals in entirely new ways in their homes, in their social interactions, and as they navigate through their daily lives—numerous privacy and ethical considerations arise, particularly when addressing sensitive topics such as SUDs. These include questions such as who owns the data? When, where, and with whom are data shared? How do patients, clinicians, payers, governmental, and industry stakeholders develop best practices for digital health in the space of public health? Moreover, how do we engineer digital health technology to be secure, respect individual privacy, and be usable by a broad array of end users without technological expertise? A systematic research agenda focused on the intersection of privacy and ethics in digital health for SUDs is essential as digital technologies are increasingly transforming the health sector. Collectively, these activities can lead to entirely new models for delivering scalable, sustainable, science-based care for SUDs.

KEY POINTS

1. Technology-based interventions offer viable solutions to implementation- and utilization-related problems that affect standard substance use disorder treatment models.
2. Technology-based interventions for substance use disorders can yield clinical outcomes that are as good as, or better than, in-person interventions.
3. When evaluating technology-based interventions for substance use disorders, the emphasis should remain on determining the psychotherapeutic mechanisms that are primarily responsible for driving behavioral changes.

REVIEW QUESTIONS

1. Which type of psychotherapy is *not* usually incorporated into the design of digital health interventions for substance use disorders?
   A. Motivational interviewing
   B. Cognitive–behavioral therapy
   C. Psychoanalysis
   D. Contingency management

2. True or False: Digital therapeutic interventions for substance use disorders can generate outcomes (eg, abstinence, retention) similar to or better than traditional in-person therapy.

3. True or False: Ethical concerns regarding use of digital therapeutics for substance use disorders have largely been resolved.

ANSWERS

1. **C.** Motivational interviewing, cognitive–behavioral therapy, and contingency management are all evidence-based psychotherapeutic models that have been incorporated into digital health technologies for SUDs.
2. **True.** A body of scientific literature documenting the results from randomized controlled trials demonstrates that technology-based interventions and in-person interventions yield similar outcomes. Some data also suggest that technology-based interventions achieve outcomes superior to those achieved by in-person interventions.
3. **False.** The use of technology-based interventions for substance use disorders is a relatively new area of clinical science, and many new ethical concerns (eg, data privacy, protection, data ownership) have arisen as a result of this new area of research. These concerns have yet to be completely resolved.

SUGGESTED READINGS

Campbell AN, Nunes EV, Matthews AG, et al. Internet-delivered treatment for substance abuse: a multisite randomized controlled trial. *Am J Psychiatry*. 2014;171(6):683-690.

Kaner EF, Beyer FR, Garnett C, et al. Personalised digital interventions for reducing hazardous and harmful alcohol consumption in community-dwelling populations. *Cochrane Database Syst Rev*. 2017;9:CD011479.

Marsch LA, Gustafson DH. The role of technology in health care innovation: a commentary. *J Dual Diagn*. 2013;9(1):101-103.

Nahum-Shani I, Smith SN, Spring BJ, et al. Just-in-time adaptive interventions (JITAIs) in mobile health: key components and design principles for ongoing health behavior support. *Ann Behav Med*. 2018;52(6):446-462.

Ramsey A, Lord S, Torrey J, Marsch L, Lardiere M. Paving the way to successful implementation: identifying key barriers to use of technology-based therapeutic tools for behavioral health care. *J Behav Health Serv Res*. 2016;43(1):54-70.

Medical Management Techniques and Collaborative Care: Integrating Behavioral with Pharmacological Interventions in Addiction Treatment

Summary by Richard N. Rosenthal

> Based on THE ASAM PRINCIPLES OF ADDICTION MEDICINE,
> 6th edition chapter by Richard N. Rosenthal, Richard K. Ries,
> and Joan E. Zweben

OVERVIEW OF ISSUES AND APPROACHES
Clinical Skills Any Clinician Should Use

Because the outcome of substance use disorder (SUD) treatment has been related to the time spent in treatment, techniques that maximize treatment engagement and retention promote better outcomes. One technique likely to sustain engagement and retention in treatment is to facilitate the therapeutic alliance through psychological support. Psychological support is among the most necessary components of management of patients with addiction, especially those with more severe dependence, so clinicians should specifically support the development of a therapeutic alliance with the patient. Alliance building is a core tactical technique of supportive therapy that uses straightforward approaches accessible to clinicians who may not have had any formal psychotherapy training and includes expression of interest, expression of empathy, expression of understanding, and repairing a misalliance.

For patients who may lack insight that their substance use is problematic, motivational enhancement strategies (described in the following sections) are beneficial. The therapist identifies the patient's readiness to change and makes reflective statements matched to his or her current stage to elicit intrinsic motivation.

Misalliances occur in all human relationships, including addiction treatment. However, when patients with SUDs get frustrated or resentful about the treatment, they frequently drop out of treatment, change to another provider, relapse, or enact elements of each. The clinician's willingness to entertain a patient's grievances, whether factual or a misconstruction, is a powerful interpersonal reinforcer for patients who may have little experience with a nonjudgmental person willing to listen. Trust is a factor associated with a lower risk of substance use in detoxified patients with SUDs in primary care.

Motivational interviewing (MI) is an evidence-based technique for interacting with patients to enhance better communication, engagement, and motivation to change. It encourages internally driven change through a collaborative effort that elicits, using clinical feedback, the patient's own recovery-oriented thoughts and feelings (intrinsic motivation), and promotes and supports the patient's sense of autonomy. In addition to the standard supportive stance, the motivational interviewer further explores the patient's feelings and comments and, more specifically, "rolls with the resistance." This moves the patient's "decisional balance" toward treatment engagement and reducing substance use.

Behavioral Therapies in the Context of Detoxification

The rates of relapse after detoxification are quite high. Only 20% to 50% of patients receive postdetoxification treatment for substance dependence, yet engagement in follow-up treatment increases the time to a second detoxification admission. Psychosocial treatments in addition to detoxification demonstrate beneficial effects on treatment completion, use of opiates, follow-up abstinence, and compliance with clinic visits. With outpatient detoxification and longer durations compared to inpatient detoxification, MI with boosters to support continued motivation for treatment engagement plus some form of contingency management is a sensible approach to treatment. Contingency management–provided incentives do not have to be monetary rewards but can be anything that the patients value, offering an opportunity for clinicians' or patients' creativity.

Medication Adherence

Medications do not work unless one takes them. Better adherence can improve the efficacy of pharmacologic interventions for SUDs, so behavioral interventions for medication adherence are sensible. Some factors that adversely affect patients' adherence to a medication regimen are co-occurring mental disorders, medication side effects, long waiting times, and inadequate understanding of the proposed treatment. Providing information, counseling, reminders, self-monitoring, reinforcement, family therapy, additional supervision or attention, and higher convenience of care are interventions that are modestly effective at increasing long-term medication adherence. Network therapy enlists others in the patient's support team to help optimize the patient's medication adherence. Network therapy for patients dependent on opioids on 16 mg per day Suboxone demonstrated higher abstinence rates compared to medication management in an 18-week randomized controlled trial.

Medical Management

Medical management is composed of several psychosocial interventions that were integrated for use in the Project COMBINE study. The medical management intervention is semistructured and brief in both duration (about nine sessions) and length of sessions (about 20 minutes), making it suitable for delivery in a primary care environment. The National Institute on Alcohol Abuse and Alcoholism's *Medical Management Treatment Manual* is a very clinically useful, evidence-based practice manual available to clinicians who combine medications and psychosocial interventions in typical office visits. Targeted feedback of medical information and individualized advice motivates the patient toward medication adherence and reducing harmful substance use, educates the patient about the need for medication, and offers referrals to support groups such as Alcoholics Anonymous.

Strategies to Integrate Medication Treatment and Behavioral Therapies

To date, there is not much empirical data to support the beneficial effects of treatment matching. No singular treatment is a "slam dunk," so it is necessary to have a variety of strategies and barriers in place to assist a person struggling with addiction craving and to prevent relapse. Both external and internal structures can be brought to bear in this process and that combination of different interventions, whether psychosocial or pharmacologic, may have *convergent* or *complementary* effects on the inhibition of relapse. Considering adjunctive treatments to pharmacotherapies for SUDs, the empirically supported and well-operationalized behavioral therapies have a range of possible targets such as enhancing medication adherence, reducing attrition, addressing co-occurring problems, promoting abstinence, and targeting specific weaknesses of the pharmacologic agent.

Pharmacotherapies for alcohol dependence biologically enhance mechanisms of either external or internal control. Disulfiram, as an aversive agent, supports external control. Conversely, medications that affect the endogenous reward system, like the neuromodulator acamprosate or reward inhibitors like naltrexone, can be considered enhancers of mechanisms of internal control. So, in constructing a combination medication and psychosocial intervention for substance dependence, one aligns psychosocial interventions that either augment the control impact of the medication or offer a complementary control locus.

Using Matching Data to Facilitate Integration

A convergent strategy uses 12-step facilitation (TSF) to reduce social support for drinking behavior through linking with the proabstinence social support found in Alcoholics Anonymous. In Project MATCH, patients with alcohol dependence with social networks supportive of continued drinking had better short-term outcomes if they were assigned to TSF. Among Project MATCH subjects with low self-efficacy, those receiving cognitive–behavioral therapy (CBT) drank far less frequently than did those receiving motivational enhancement therapy (MET). Across Project MATCH therapies (CBT, MET, and TSF), patients with alcohol dependence ($N = 141$) treated in a more confrontational and directive therapy who tended to resist relinquishing control had worse drinking outcomes than did those with less reluctance, especially in the MET group.

Other Strategies

Combination strategies can target the SUD and, in addition, attempt to treat co-occurring mental or medical disorders. It is clear that both disorders need to be targeted independently, although there may be convergent effects in treating the co-occurring disorder (COD). In addition, some interventions for mental disorders can have adverse impact on SUDs. Patients with type A alcohol use disorder (later onset) may respond positively to selective serotonin reuptake inhibitor treatment compared to placebo with reductions in drinking, but patients with type B (early onset, prior to age 25 years) alcohol use disorder may actually do worse (see Pettinatti et al under "Suggested Readings"; concept from Babor et al.).

Principles for Care Integration

Research data are needed to demonstrate whether convergent or complementary strategies have more robust effects. In the spirit of constructing multiple obstacles to relapse, clinical practice engages strategies that may be both convergent and complementary. Individual patient characteristics such as genetics, addiction severity, comorbidity, and drug of choice will likely influence the optimal combination of medications and psychosocial interventions. Use a stage-wise approach to recovery to help guide the choice of an appropriate mix of medication and therapy, with the clinician determining the important tasks for a particular stage in treatment.

For example, in establishing abstinence, several acute issues typically need to be dealt with, including negative mood states and craving, conditioned cues, access to substances, and immersion in contexts supportive of substance use. One can pick treatments based on the impact in those domains:

■ Reducing social isolation and offering social support for sobriety with mutual self-help groups and TSF, behavioral couples therapy, or network therapy
■ Supporting treatment engagement with MI

■ Supporting cognitive and coping skills functioning in early recovery with CBT/relapse prevention and/or improving baseline cognitive deficits with appropriate medications
■ Reducing alcohol craving with naltrexone and opioid craving with buprenorphine or methadone
■ Supporting self-efficacy and resilience for craving and negative states with CBT
■ Reducing substance use with contingency management and supporting alcohol abstinence with disulfiram or acamprosate

COLLABORATIVE CARE WITH COUNSELORS AND PSYCHOTHERAPISTS

Addiction treatment practitioners differ widely in their attitudes, preparation, and skills; however, many states have moved to license professional counselors with standardized training and credentials who will represent the predominant form of addiction counseling. Addiction treatment personnel also vary in the degree to which they are accustomed to working with physicians and other medical personnel. Understanding the background and orientation of specific staff can enhance communication and teamwork.

Counselors

Historically, therapeutic communities, developed in the 1960s, relied on recovering noncredentialed staff. Today, nonlicensed, recovering counselors work in short-term Minnesota Model "chemical dependency" inpatient programs, as peer counselors in COD and community-based addiction programs, and predominate in 12-step–oriented therapeutic communities. Some counselors obtain graduate degrees and licenses, building the cadre of professionals in recovery. Some counselors have little training, whereas others have completed comprehensive credentialing or certification programs that may require 200 to 300 hours of coursework plus supervised field placement experience. Many programs have a 12-step perspective exclusive of important evidence-based approaches, including US Food and Drug–approved addiction medications, but the current emphasis on offering evidence-based approaches exerts increasing influence on these certificate programs.

At their best, counselors present powerful role models as peers, a contribution deeply valued by addicted patients. Whereas some have superb skills, others may have rigid, non–patient-centered concepts of recovery and have difficulty tolerating the ambiguities of complex clinical populations, such as COD patients who may need extended time or harm reduction approaches on the path toward abstinence.

Licensed Providers

Licensed professionals, both in recovery and not, work in addiction treatment settings. Most have basic clinical skills, but their competence in treating addicted patients may vary greatly. Graduate schools of nursing, psychology, medicine, and social work typically do not integrate sufficient training in the assessment and treatment of addiction into their core curricula.

Clinical experience may tell little about qualifications. In many free-standing drug treatment centers, the failure of the patient to adhere to the strict rules leading to dropout or premature discharge is explained as "he hasn't reached his bottom," when the reality is that the patient may have an untreated COD that impairs his or her abilities to participate in groups, speak coherently, or control affect and impulse. In selecting appropriate therapists for referral, physicians should look for evidence of recent systematic training, either through conferences or coursework.

Tensions can occur between staff who treat and staff who do not treat patients who are recovering and between those with and without professional training and licenses. Clinicians who use addiction treatment concepts such as "enabling" and "codependency" to disapprove of or to discredit colleagues who take certain positions discourage appropriate forms of helping and foster premature therapy termination. Because a patient's time in treatment correlates with positive outcomes in many treatment outcome studies, engaging and retaining patients in treatment is paramount.

Terminating patients for manifesting symptoms of their psychiatric or addictive disorder is simply bad treatment. Physicians can be the voice of reason, preventing premature termination of therapy, while avoiding colluding with patient behaviors that have a negative impact on their treatment, others' treatment, or on the recovery environment.

Physicians in leadership roles should establish weekly in-service sessions on both basic and specialized topics. A multidisciplinary team can develop a shared language and can become knowledgeable about integrating the treatment of addictive, psychiatric, and medical disorders. Securing continuing education credits for each of the staff's disciplines enhances participation and commitment to a high-quality training sequence.

Collaboration With Psychotherapists in the Community

The programmatic approach to addiction treatment typically is highly structured with multiple behavioral expectations, so psychodynamically oriented therapists may have difficulty incorporating behavioral commitments because their treatment style tends to be more patient and process driven. Therapists with a more directive orientation such as CBT and MI or with a supportive orientation may adapt more easily to working with an addiction medicine physician.

Addiction treatment often includes breath and urine testing if resources permit—psychotherapists without addiction training rarely arrange testing and may consider it invasive and abhorrent. These differences pose an adaptive challenge to the physician who is arranging for treatment of patients with a COD.

Pharmacotherapy Support and Collaborating to Achieve Treatment Adherence

Recovering patients who require medications have clinical needs that have historically been out of the scope of practice for addiction treatment programs, and programs have slowly incorporated on-site treatment of or referral for pharmacotherapy for either addiction or other mental disorders. Pharmacotherapy in addiction treatment is increasingly being utilized, especially with the support of professional counseling organizations and nationally known private recovery systems.

Adherence to treatment recommendations is critical to a patient's successful treatment. Behavioral strategies frequently yield poor results for patients because the actual obstacles to adherence were never identified. Thus, physicians should help counselors and psychotherapists explore these issues with patients during treatment.

Many recovering patients define recovery as living a comfortable and responsible lifestyle without the use of psychoactive drugs, so they may have complex feelings and attitudes toward medications that need to be understood and addressed. The patient with substance dependence who at one time consumed illicit substances may reject pharmacotherapy, horrified at the idea of "putting something foreign in my body" or "relying on drugs." For some, medication undermines the sense of mastery that promotes sobriety, whereas for others, it provides maintenance while recovery concepts are internalized and mastered. Clinicians should handle this issue carefully and individually.

In addition, some disorders require psychiatric medications for appropriate treatment, such as antipsychotic agents for schizophrenia or mood stabilizers for bipolar disorder, without which the risk for relapse to substance use is increased. Family members or 12-step program participants may criticize the patient or pressure them to discontinue use of the medication, generating conflict that undermines treatment. Because physicians often lack the time to deal with such issues, patients should be specifically delegated to other treatment team members who may need additional training on how to handle medication issues. Family psychoeducation about addiction and co-occurring psychiatric disorders can be helpful in aligning family members to the treatment team and the goals of treatment. Educating therapists about medications usually yields multiple benefits as well. Empathic, reflective listening combined with appropriate information can also improve medication adherence significantly.

Medication adherence can be monitored through refill requests because treatment-adherent patients typically initiate contact with their physicians for refills before running out of medicine. Prescribing for an extended period deprives the physician of this feedback. In most states, prescribers of controlled substances must check a prescription monitoring program database to ensure the patient is not obtaining the same or similar medications elsewhere.

Communication with other treatment staff is essential when noncompliance is suspected. Discontinuation of psychotropic medication and the reemergence of distressing psychiatric symptoms in patients with COD often precedes relapse to substances or indicates its recurrence.

Physicians need to communicate to nonphysician therapists what to expect and what might constitute warning signs of impending problems when prescribing medications for withdrawal phenomena. Physicians should provide guidance to therapists when patients who do not abstain skip prescribed medication because they fear their interaction with drugs and alcohol. Therapists are in a good position to detect developing problems and initiate communication with the physician or clinician responsible for coordinating care.

The physician should discuss with the patient and other members of the treatment team the indications for discontinuing medications and the process by which such discontinuation should occur. Progress should be reviewed by the patient with program staff, a private therapist, or the prescribing physician before discontinuing medication. Both the patient

and the nonphysician therapist should be educated by the physician about the dangers of psychiatric and addiction relapse that attend such a decision.

KEY POINTS

1. Treatment techniques that maximize a patient's engagement and retention promote better outcomes.
2. Clinicians should support the development of a therapeutic alliance with the patient.
3. Medical management techniques provide feedback of medical information and individualized advice that encourages medication adherence and a reduction in harmful substance use.
4. The best approaches to relapse prevention place as many barriers as practical of differing content and strategies in the way of relapse opportunities, strategies that can be convergent or complementary.
5. The physician should be an important leader of the multidisciplinary addiction treatment team that can provide medical knowledge, evidence-based methods, and administrative support for needed clinical integration.

REVIEW QUESTIONS

1. Which of the following is true?
   A. When a patient gets angry due to a misinterpretation, the clinician should quickly get him to understand why he has a wrong understanding in order to maintain the therapeutic alliance.
   B. Using clinical feedback, motivational interviewing elicits the patient's own recovery-oriented thoughts and feelings.
   C. Exploration of the patient's beliefs and ambivalence about alcohol dependence and the nature of treatment has no positive impact on medication adherence.
   D. Most of the evidence-based behavioral therapies for addiction focus on abstinence.
   E. Medical management is an easy and successful intervention because the content is independent of the patient.

2. Which of the following is true?
   A. Complementary addiction treatment strategies focus on the same therapeutic target in the same way.
   B. Placing multiple obstacles that increase the patient's effort needed for relapse behavior is a poor recovery strategy because it diverts the patient's focus away from abstinence.

C. Treatment outcomes for alcohol dependence are always augmented by selective serotonin reuptake inhibitor treatment.

D. Treatment with naltrexone to reduce alcohol craving paired with cue extinction therapy for alcohol craving is an example of a convergent strategy.

E. Twelve-step facilitation is not helpful if a patient's social network supports continued drinking, especially when compared to MET or CBT.

3. Which of the following is true?

A. Therapists with a directive style tend to align with an addiction medicine physician more easily than do those with a psychodynamic orientation and process-oriented style.

B. Psychosocial treatments in addition to detoxi-fication demonstrate beneficial effects on treatment completion, use of opioids, follow-up abstinence, and compliance with clinic visits.

C. Enlisting a patient's supportive significant others can assist them in medication adherence.

D. Therapists are usually well trained about addictions, so physicians have little role in educating them about medications for treating SUDs.

E. A, B, and C

ANSWERS

1. **B**
2. **D**
3. **E**

SUGGESTED READINGS

Babor TF, Hofmann M, DelBoca FK, et al. Types of alcoholics, I. Evidence for an empirically derived typology based on indicators of vulnerability and severity. *Arch Gen Psychiatry.* 1992;49(8):599-608.

Carroll KM, Kosten TR, Rounsaville BJ. Choosing a behavioral therapy platform for pharmacotherapy of substance users. *Drug Alcohol Depend.* 2004;75(2):123-134.

Center for Substance Abuse Treatment. *Managing Depressive Symptoms in Substance Abuse Clients During Early Recovery. Treatment Improvement Protocol (TIP) Series 48.* Rockville, MD: Substance Abuse and Mental Health Services Administration, 2008. DHHS Publication No. (SMA) 08-4353.

Dutra L, Stathopoulou G, Basden SL, et al. A meta-analytic review of psychosocial interventions for substance use disorders. *Am J Psychiatry.* 2008;165(2):179-187.

Haynes RB, Ackloo E, Sahota N, et al. Interventions for enhancing medication adherence. *Cochrane Database Syst Rev.* 2008;(2):CD000011.

Pettinati HM, Weiss RD, Dundon W, et al. A structured approach to medical management: a psychosocial intervention to support pharmacotherapy in the treatment of alcohol dependence. *J Stud Alcohol Suppl.* 2005;(suppl 15):170-178.

Powers MB, Vedel E, Emmelkamp PM. Behavioral couples therapy (BCT) for alcohol and drug use disorders: a meta-analysis. *Clin Psychol Rev.* 2008;28(6):952-962.

Rosenthal RN. Basic treatment techniques for persons with mental disorders and co-occurring substance use disorders. In: McQuistion HL, Sowers WE, Ranz JM, Feldman JM, eds. *Handbook of Community Psychiatry.* New York: Springer, 2012:257-273.

Substance Abuse and Mental Health Services Administration. *Substance Abuse Treatment for Persons With Co-Occurring Disorders. Treatment Improvement Protocol (TIP) Series, No. 42.* Rockville, MD: Substance Abuse and Mental Health Services Administration, 2005. DHHS Publication No. (SMA) 13-3992.

Mutual Help, Twelve-Step, and Other Recovery Programs

76 Twelve-Step Programs in Addiction Recovery

Summary by Edgar P. Nace

Based on THE ASAM PRINCIPLES OF ADDICTION MEDICINE, 6th edition chapter by Edgar P. Nace

This chapter describes the structure and usefulness of 12-step programs. Emphasis is placed on Alcoholics Anonymous (AA) because it is the progenitor of all subsequent 12-step programs.

ALCOHOLICS ANONYMOUS

AA is a fellowship of men and women who offer their hope, strength, and experience to anyone desiring to not drink. Meetings are held at various times throughout the day and evening. There are speaker meetings, step discussion meetings, women's meetings, and other formats. Participation is anonymous, there is no cost, and questions are not asked of newcomers. Participants are not told what to do but learn what worked for experienced members.

AA has a single purpose: "to carry its message to the alcoholic who still suffers." In 2010, AA membership exceeded 2 million, and there were 115,770 groups registered. AA does not engage in fund-raising or lobbying; it endorses no causes and does not promote itself. It is interested in the person with alcohol use disorder, not alcoholism per se. AA will decline outside contributions and does not provide treatment or educational services. Personal anonymity is a guiding principle.

AA refers to itself as a fellowship. A fellowship is a "mutual association of persons on equal and friendly terms; a mutual sharing, as of experience, activity, or interest." There are no dues, but a collection is commonly taken at meetings to ensure that AA remains self-supporting and not dependent on outside funds. There are no age or educational requirements. All are welcome based on a desire to stop drinking. Admitting that one is an "alcoholic" is not necessary, nor will AA attempt to proffer a diagnosis on an attendee. It is left to each participant to decide whether he or she is an "alcoholic" as per AA.

AA meetings may be open or closed. Closed meetings are for those who consider themselves as an "alcoholic" per AA (or, in the medical field, as a

person with an alcohol use disorder) or are questioning whether they might have this disease. Open meetings are for anyone interested in attending a meeting. For example, when medical students are required to attend an AA meeting as part of their training in psychiatry, they attend an open meeting. If a person with alcohol use disorder did not wish to be seen at an AA meeting except by other people with this disease, he or she would attend only closed meetings.

A meeting is usually 1 hour in duration and may be followed by informal socializing. A "speakers" meeting will consist of a member telling her story—emphasizing "what it was like" (the drinking experience), "what happened" (the process of recognizing the consequences of drinking and doing something about it), and "what it is like now" (how life has changed since beginning recovery from alcoholism). Step meetings focus on one of the 12 steps in a discussion format. (See Alcoholics Anonymous under Suggested Readings for a list of the 12 steps). Discussion meetings are those where a topic is picked (eg, gratitude) and the group shares thoughts and experiences of the same.

It is not unusual to hear persons say that as they struggle to get comfortable with AA, they hear the same thing over and over again, that one person talks too much, or that they can't identify with those in the meeting (eg, "I've never been in jail," "I'm better educated"). With time, such individuals may see that they do have a common bond with those who are different from them in terms of life experiences as they recognize that they all share the struggle to not drink. A good attitude toward meetings was expressed by a recovered alcoholic counselor who, when asked, "Hey, how was the meeting last night," would respond, "It was great; I didn't drink the whole time I was there."

New members to AA, as well as members who have relapsed or been without a sponsor for a prolonged period of time, are encouraged to ask for a sponsor. The sponsor offers a helping hand and serves as a mentor. He or she guides the person being sponsored in understanding the 12 steps and typically goes over each step with the person being sponsored.

Predecessors to Alcoholics Anonymous

June 10, 1935, is the founding date of Alcoholics Anonymous. That date is the last day that Dr. Bob Smith took a drink—a beer to steady his nerves before surgery. Dr. Bob and Bill Wilson had met in Bob's hometown of Akron, Ohio, in May 1935, and became the cofounders of AA. Their unplanned yet fateful meeting would spur the formation of the most successful self-help movement known.

Nearly 100 years before the founding of AA, the Washingtonian Total Abstinence Society was formed in 1840 in Baltimore, Maryland. After hearing a lecture on temperance, six members of a drinking club (all men), decided to quit the club and form the Washingtonian society. They initially held private meetings, met nightly because they had been drinking nightly, and invited local people with this disease of alcoholism to attend. Later, they held public meetings as interest in their society was growing, assessed dues, and formed committees to recruit others struggling with alcohol. In 1841, a branch for women was formed—the Martha Washington Society.

The Washingtonians grew rapidly but did not develop a central organization. They became divided over the issue of alcohol prohibition and began to fade away by the end of the decade. AA is similar in that mutual self-help, personal shared commitment, and a religious/spiritual foundation are utilized.

Following on the heels of the Washingtonians was the Independent Order of Good Templars, founded in 1851. A pledge of abstinence was required, and expulsion could be expected if the pledge wasn't kept. Many other fraternal temperance societies and reform clubs formed during the 19th century and emphasized anonymity, a principle later adopted by AA.

The Oxford Group, also now out of existence, was a direct predecessor of Alcoholics Anonymous. The Oxford Group considered spiritual growth as the solution to many of mankind's problems. "Four absolutes"—absolute honesty, absolute purity, absolute unselfishness, and absolute love—as well as the "five Cs"—confidence, confession, conviction, conversion, and continuance—were necessary for spiritual change to occur.

Founded in the early 1900s, the Oxford Group strove to recapture the fervor of first century AD Christianity. The group was not founded to specifically help people with alcohol use disorder, but under the leadership of Episcopal priest Rev. Sam Shoemaker, it became active with such people in New York City.

Roland H., who was from a wealthy Connecticut family, had suffered from a chronically active alcohol use disorder and had exhausted his family's financial resources. Using his experience with the Oxford Group, Roland H. encountered an old friend Edwin Thatcher (also known as Ebby) who, in 1934, was about to be committed to a state institution. Ebby responded to Roland H.'s outreach and got sober attending Oxford Group meetings. Ebby was also a lifelong friend of Bill Wilson and spoke to Bill about his recovery through faith. Ebby and others from the Oxford Group persisted in meeting with Bill and he also eventually attended Oxford Group meetings.

It must be apparent now to anyone familiar with AA that a nascent process of one person with alcohol use disorder reaching out to another was in effect.

Bill eventually checked himself in to Towns Hospital where he had been detoxified several times in the past. William D. Silkworth was a neurologist who took care of Bill and who had a reputation for helping people with alcohol use disorder—an estimated 50,000 over the course of his medical career. During this hospital stay, Bill Wilson was depressed and resistant to the notion of a "higher power." Bill described that during his stay in Towns Hospital, he had cried out in despair, experienced the room lit up with a white light, and felt ecstatic. He asked Dr. Silkworth if this was the effect of brain damage, and Silkworth reassured him that it wasn't.

Bill then began to share his drinking experiences with others with this same disease after the Oxford Group meetings and began to sense that one person talking to another in a nonjudgmental manner was the tool or dynamic that helped him stay alcohol free. Over the next 6 months, Bill fervently told his story to other people with alcohol use disorder. He stayed sober, but they didn't.

In spite of being discouraged by these initial efforts, while on a business trip to Akron, Ohio, Bill recognized he was craving alcohol and found a minister's phone number in a hotel directory. The call led him to Henrietta Seiberling, a member of the local Oxford Group and the daughter-in-law of the president of Goodyear Tire. Although she did not have alcoholism herself, Henrietta had been trying to help a local surgeon who was in her Oxford Group and invited Bill to her house the next day to meet Dr. Bob Smith.

Bill knew he wasn't going to take a drink, and thanked Bob for hearing him out. Bob, while listening to Bill, would say "Yes, that's like me, that's just like me." Bill remained sober thereafter, but Bob went to a medical convention in Atlantic City and returned to home intoxicated. With Bill's help and the help of Dr. Bob's wife, Bob acquired lasting sobriety on June 10, 1935. That date is considered the founding of Alcoholics Anonymous.

The identity of AA gradually took shape beginning in the late 1930s. AA was able to form its identity by 1939 when the book *Alcoholics Anonymous* was written by Bill Wilson. That book remains the bible of AA, and every member is encouraged to read it. However, its reviews when first published were discouraging: "no scientific merit or interest."

There were about 100 members when AA officially adopted the name Alcoholics Anonymous in 1939. When Dr. Bob Smith, cofounder of AA, died in 1950, there were about 90,000 members.

Today, the number exceeds 2 million worldwide, with over half its members in the United States.

Other 12-Step Programs

Narcotics Anonymous

Narcotics Anonymous (NA) is the second largest 12-step program focused on substance use disorders. NA grew out of AA in Los Angeles in the late 1940s and follows the format of AA, with 12 steps and 12 traditions. NA substituted the word "addiction" for "alcohol" and removed drug-specific references. NA is open to all people with substance use disorders without regard to the type of drug or combination of drugs.

NA published *Narcotics Anonymous* in 1983 and NA literature states, "NA is a nonprofit fellowship or society of men and women for whom drugs had become a major problem. We . . . meet regularly to help each other stay clean . . . . We are not interested in what or how much you used but only in what you want to do about your problem and how we can help."

Cocaine Anonymous

Cocaine Anonymous began in Los Angeles in 1982. Cocaine Anonymous is adapted from the AA program and follows the 12-step model. It is open to all individuals who want to stop using cocaine as well as all other addictive substances.

Marijuana Anonymous

Marijuana Anonymous was founded in June 1989 and is based on the 12-step program of AA. Marijuana Anonymous is for those who experience marijuana as controlling their lives. Their website states, "We lose interest in all else; our dreams go up in smoke. Ours is a progressive illness often leading us

to addiction to other drugs, including alcohol. Our lives, our thinking, and our desires center around marijuana-scoring it, dealing it, and finding ways to stay high."

Gamblers Anonymous

Gambling disorder was included in the *Diagnostic and Statistical Manual of Mental Disorders*, 5th edition. It is part of the "Substance-Related and Addictive Disorders" section as a nonsubstance–related disorder. Decades before gambling disorder became an official diagnosis, those inflicted by gambling addiction found a way to organize their own self-help organization, called Gamblers Anonymous. As with substance use disorders, a 12-step approach is seen as helpful to those with gambling addiction. Gamblers Anonymous was founded in Los Angeles in 1957.

Al-Anon and Alateen

Al-Anon is an international fellowship of friends or relatives of people with alcohol use disorder who have been impacted by another's drinking. They share their experiences, strength, and hope and follow their own 12-step format. Al-Anon is not family or group therapy and does not provide counseling in any formal sense. Alateen grew out of Al-Anon and is for teenagers aged 13 to 17 years, although the age range may vary by group. Alateen meetings are sponsored by Al-Anon members; adults do not attend except for a few Al-Anon sponsors.

Al-Anon was founded in 1951 by Lois Wilson, the wife of AA cofounder Bill Wilson. She realized that much of her life had been directed toward helping Bill get sober and felt the need to develop her own spiritual life as a loved one of someone with a drinking disorder.

Al-Anon meetings focus not on the drinker but rather on the family member or friend of a drinker who tolerates abuse, or indulges in excessive caretaking, and who may have developed low self-esteem because they thought they could help the person with alcohol use disorder stop or control alcohol use. Al-Anon members learn that they didn't cause the alcoholism and can't cure it or control it but are affected by it and, therefore, need help for themselves.

SMART Recovery

In 1985, Rational Recovery was founded; it was the forerunner to what is now SMART Recovery. Rational Recovery's first meeting took place in a hospital in Cambridge, Massachusetts, in 1990. In 1994, the board of Rational Recovery Self Help, Inc., voted to change the name to SMART Recovery (Self-Management and Recovery Training).

SMART Recovery offers tools and techniques to implement its four-point program: (1) building and maintaining motivation; (2) coping with urges; (3) managing thoughts, feelings, and behaviors; and (4) living a balanced life.

Reliance on self-empowerment is emphasized, rather than a commitment to a spiritual orientation, although each participant is encouraged to use what is found helpful.

Women for Sobriety

Women for Sobriety, founded in 1976, is an abstinence-based program. Although physical recovery is claimed to be the same for both sexes, Women for Sobriety asserts that the psychological recovery is different for women. As part of the recovery, a 13-point program of affirmations is utilized daily in order to remove negative thinking and to develop a sense of self. The organization claims to have a worldwide presence and states that hundreds of meetings are held daily.

Physician Facilitation of 12-Step Participation

Physicians and other clinicians would do well to inform patients of the existence, format, and benefits of participating in a 12-step or other self-help program. This obligation is based on empirical evidence that AA participation (and, by extension, the use of other 12-step programs) and engagement and commitment to AA are consistent predictors of positive outcomes for patients. Even attendance at AA (apart from "commitment") produces modest yet positive results.

Practical Information and Advice for Your Patients

1. Offer a brief explanation of 12-step programs. For example, they are a fellowship of men and women who offer their hope, strength, and experience to anyone desiring not to drink or do drugs. There is no cost, the meetings are at various times throughout the day or evening, participation is anonymous, questions are not asked of newcomers, and there are different formats (eg, women's meetings, speaker meetings, step discussion meetings).
2. Try to discern whether your treatment approach and advice to the patient are in synchrony with what he or she is learning in the 12-step program. If you find contradictions or conflict between your treatment approach and what the patient is reporting from AA, try to resolve and explain any possible differences.

3. Counter objections. Fear of stigma is common, but as one gains sobriety, respect usually replaces negative associations such as stigma. Another objection is inability to identify with others in the program (eg, "I've never been in jail"). Finding a group that one feels comfortable with makes sense, but emphasis should be put on seeing the commonalities of the addiction experience that cuts across personal experience and socioeconomic differences.

Outcome Studies

Support for encouraging membership in AA (and by extension other 12-step programs) is found in several large studies. Project MATCH compared patients with alcohol use disorder randomly assigned to cognitive–behavioral therapy, motivational treatment, and 12-step facilitation. Twelve-step facilitation is a professionally led group therapy, which points patients to 12-step participation. In the outpatient arm of this study, patients in 12-step programs had significantly higher rates of abstinence at 1-year and 3-year follow-ups. AA participation for those in the other treatment arms, CBT and MT, also predicted abstinence. A large Veterans Administration study found that at 1 year and at 18 months, those whose aftercare was only AA or another 12-step program had abstinence rates twice those who did not attend any 12-step program. The rate of abstinence for the 12-step participants was approximately 45%, whereas for the nonparticipants, it was just under 25%. See Chapter 77 for more details.

Why Are 12-Step Programs Effective?

No one answer or variable is known to explain why any individuals benefit from 12-step participation. There are, however, several dynamics that may account for or explain, at least in part, why benefits ensue.

- Group cohesiveness: A sense of belonging leads to continued engagement, which facilitates sustained abstinence.
- Improved self-governance: Acceptance of supportive, caring interactions with others provides a counterbalance to the drive to drink through a "borrowing" of self-governance from the group. A sense of oneself as an autonomous being capable of taking charge of one's life, yet in need, interdependently, of relationships with others develops.
- Self-awareness: The participant begins to understand motivations and feelings that led to substance use and that they are not unique in regard

to how feelings, moods, and frustrations were managed in the past.

■ Spirituality: Twelve-step programs emphasize spirituality over any specific religious creed. Reference to God occurs throughout the 12 steps and the 12 traditions, but an emphasis is put on each individual's understanding of a "higher power." But how is spirituality manifested in the context of a 12-step program? Spirituality may be experienced as a release from the compulsion to use substances. This "release" may occur slowly or, in some instances, suddenly and is experienced as having been "given" rather than achieved. From a decrease in the compulsion to use substances emerges a feeling of gratitude, which promotes thankfulness for what one has rather than what one doesn't have. Humility is part of spirituality and accompanies an acceptance of being "powerless" over alcohol or drugs.

KEY POINTS

1. Understanding 12-step programs, as well as programs that are not 12-step based, will allow physicians as well as clinicians to confidently recommend these programs to patients in need.
2. Referral requires no variables to be considered beyond the desire to be free from alcohol or drug use. No cost is incurred by the patient beyond the expenditure of time. Age, gender, ethnicity, education, or status will not limit the potential utility of active participation.
3. Resistance to and objections about 12-step programs can be expected. A calm, encouraging stance will usually overcome patients' initial fears or concerns. Participation in a 12-step program does not conflict with or replace other clinical interventions such as medicine, psychotherapy, or commitment to a religious preference.

REVIEW QUESTIONS

1. The primary purpose of Alcoholics Anonymous is to:
   A. provide group counseling to the person with an alcohol use disorder.
   B. carry its message to the person with an alcohol use disorder who still suffers.

   C. educate the person with an alcohol use disorder about the harms of drinking.
   D. indoctrinate the concept of spirituality in new members.

2. The founding of Alcoholics Anonymous was most directly influenced by:
   A. the Oxford Group.
   B. the American Psychiatric Association.
   C. the Catholic Church.
   D. Dr. William Silkworth.

3. Which of the following is the primary criterion for going to Alcoholics Anonymous?
   A. Agreeing to tell your story
   B. Accepting that you are a person with an alcohol use disorder
   C. Agreeing to sign a pledge not to drink
   D. Having a desire not to drink

4. Physicians should know that AA:
   A. will not allow members to take medicines.
   B. will inform the doctor that his/her patient is attending.
   C. provides detoxification services.
   D. has no opinion about medications or medical issues.

ANSWERS

1. **B**
2. **A**
3. **D**
4. **D**

SUGGESTED READINGS

Alcoholics Anonymous. *Twelve Steps and Twelve Traditions.* New York: Alcoholics Anonymous World Services, 1978.

Kurtz E. *Not-God: A History of Alcoholics Anonymous.* Center City, MN: Hazelden Pittman Archives Press, 1979.

Matching alcoholism treatment to client heterogeneity: Project MATCH posttreatment drinking outcomes. *J Stud Alcohol.* 1997;58(1):7-29.

Thomsen R. *Bill W. The Absorbing and Deeply Moving Life Story of Bill Wilson, Co-Founder of Alcoholics Anonymous.* New York: Harper & Row, 1975.

White WL. *Slaying the Dragon: The History of Addiction Treatment and Recovery in America.* Bloomington, IL: Chestnut Health Systems/Lighthouse Institute, 1998.

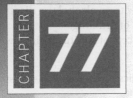
77 Recent Research into Twelve-Step Programs

Summary by Barbara S. McCrady

▐ Based on THE ASAM PRINCIPLES OF ADDICTION MEDICINE,
6th edition chapter by Barbara S. McCrady

Alcoholics Anonymous (AA) is ubiquitous, both in the United States and around the world. Worldwide, there are an estimated 109,872 groups and 1,962,499 members. The formal structure of AA is similar across nations, although there is some variability in emphasis on different parts of the AA program, and differences in the demography of membership are apparent, depending on the cultural context in which AA occurs. Although most addiction professionals have some familiarity with AA and other self-help groups based on 12-step principles, professionals' scientific knowledge about AA often is more limited. The past 25 years have witnessed an explosion of research on AA and on treatments designed to facilitate involvement in AA, with close to 400 articles appearing since 2002. Despite earlier skepticism about the possibility of conducting research on AA, researchers have used a range of methodologies, including ethnographic methods, epidemiologic studies, longitudinal studies of treatment-seeking and non–treatment-seeking populations, controlled clinical trials, and meta-analyses, to develop a body of new research about AA that has some coherence, confirms some previous findings and beliefs, and challenges others. This chapter provides a selective review of earlier research on AA and a more comprehensive review from 2002 through 2017.

UTILIZATION OF ALCOHOLICS ANONYMOUS

AA members enter the program by a number of routes, including self-referral or referral by family or friends, referral from treatment centers, or through coercion from the legal system, employers, or the social welfare system. A variety of research methods have illuminated patterns of utilization of AA. First, population surveys provide information on the utilization of AA in both the general and in populations

with alcohol problems. In general populations, AA attendance among respondents with a history of alcohol dependence as defined by the *Diagnostic and Statistical Manual of Mental Disorders*, 4th edition (*DSM-IV*) ranges from approximately 20% to 25%. However, surveys of those seeking assistance for an alcohol use disorder (AUD) find that 80% to 90% report having attended a 12-step program, including about 12% who attended only a 12-step program and about 67% who attended both formal treatment and a 12-step program.

Data derived from a number of different methodologies converge in suggesting clearly different patterns of involvement with AA. Three patterns are most common: individuals who initially are actively involved with AA but taper off over time, individuals with a steady level of involvement over time, and individuals who have a more variable or less engaged type of involvement. Data also suggest that consistent involvement is associated with better outcomes.

FACTORS ASSOCIATED WITH SUCCESSFUL AFFILIATION WITH ALCOHOLICS ANONYMOUS

Despite the AA's membership diversity, research shows that certain factors are associated with more successful affiliation with AA. However, it should be emphasized that research to identify characteristics of those more likely to affiliate with AA does not imply that individuals without those characteristics will not affiliate. Over time, a body of single studies has accrued a wide range of characteristics found to be predictive of affiliation with AA, including male gender, more serious alcohol problems, greater commitment to abstinence, more social support to stop drinking, less support from and more stress in marriage/intimate relationships, fewer psychological problems such as depression or poor self-esteem, use of a more avoidant style for coping with problems, and having a greater desire to find meaning in life.

The personal characteristic of spirituality, religiosity, or purpose in life has been examined in a series of studies. Professionals and the public alike believe that individuals who are more religious will be more successful in AA because of the intrinsically spiritual nature of the recovery program. Research has found that professionals are less likely to refer patients to AA who engage in lower levels of religious behaviors and that religious involvement predicts greater AA engagement, but research also has found that regardless of initial level of spirituality or religiosity, individuals who become involved with AA increase their own religious and spiritual beliefs and practices.

Thus, data generally support the view of AA as a program that attracts a diverse membership but that those with more severe drinking problems and those with a greater commitment to change are more likely to affiliate with AA. Patient religiosity affects clinicians' referrals to AA, and patients with agnostic and atheist beliefs may attend fewer meetings, but patients who go to AA increase their religiosity regardless of their initial beliefs. Patients with comorbid psychiatric disorders also affiliate with AA, although those with social anxiety or a diagnosis of schizophrenia are somewhat less likely to attend.

ALCOHOLICS ANONYMOUS AND POPULATION SUBGROUPS

Two contrasting views of AA lead to different predictions about AA and different population subgroups. One perspective suggests that AA is a program of recovery for persons with AUD and that the common experience of alcoholism should supersede superficial individual differences. Because AA groups are autonomous, individual meetings may take on the character of the predominant population in attendance, allowing for meetings that are comfortable for persons of different backgrounds. In the United States, "special interest" groups for certain subpopulations divided by gender, sexual orientation, age, or ethnicity are very common. An alternative perspective is that because AA was developed by educated, middle-aged, white, Christian, heterosexual males, its relevance to less educated, young or older persons, persons of color, non-Christians, gays and lesbians, or women is suspect. AA's own triennial surveys have found an increase in the proportion of women in AA from about 22% in 1968 to about 38%, leveling off starting in 1989. The average age

of AA members responding to AA's triennial survey has increased to about 50 years, and the triennial survey data reveal a broad diversity among the membership in age and occupational status but limited racial/ethnic diversity.

Women may perceive more barriers to utilizing AA, particularly in terms of access, child care, and a sense of stigma about their AUD, but there is little evidence of gender differences in actual help seeking from or affiliation with AA. Women may use AA differently from men, as they attend more meetings but are less likely to have a sponsor. Women also are more likely than men to call other AA members for help, to have experienced a spiritual awakening, and to have read AA literature. There also may be aspects of AA that make it less appealing to women, including a perception that AA is too punitive and focused on shame and guilt; disagreement with program principles related to powerlessness, surrender, and reliance on a higher power; and a perception that AA is male dominated.

AA membership has an underrepresentation of members in American racial/ethnic minorities, with membership including only 3% Hispanics, 4% Blacks, 1% American Indian, and 1% Asians.

There is some hesitancy about involving adolescents in AA because of their developmental status and concern that adolescent AUD is, in some cases, an age-limited phenomenon. However, several studies have suggested a strong association between AA and Narcotics Anonymous involvement and abstinence in adolescents with more severe AUD, similar to that found in adults. Research to date has focused on adolescents in inpatient treatment programs, arguably the population with the most severe problems. In this population, 44% participated in AA after discharge and were more likely to attend AA meetings that had more same aged peers.

Recent research also supports understanding of those with coexisting psychiatric disorders in AA. Specifically, participation in AA and other 12-step programs has been found to be associated with positive substance use outcomes for individuals with coexisting psychiatric disorders. In addition, patients with coexisting psychiatric disorders show increases in self-efficacy, and the social support received in 12-step groups with a dual focus on recovery and psychiatric disorders mediates the relationship between group involvement and positive outcomes. Importantly, although there is a perception that AA members do not support the use of psychiatric medications, surveys of AA members found that the majority of members support the use of such medications.

Thus, it appears that individuals from minority groups have a mixed experience in AA, not only seeing particular value in the support for sobriety but also having a different set of experiences with AA, some of which are somewhat negative.

THE EFFECTIVENESS OF ALCOHOLICS ANONYMOUS

Answering the apparently simple question "Does AA work?" is a challenge. One approach is to look at the success of AA as an organization: The broad dissemination of the program around the world and the large membership suggest that AA has been enormously successful at attracting persons to AA as a program of recovery. The AA triennial surveys also point to the substantial proportion of abstaining, long-term members. More difficult questions, however, have less clear-cut answers: "How effective is *AA in comparison* to treatments for alcohol use disorder?" "Is AA involvement *necessary* to the successful resolution of alcohol problems?" "Does AA *lead to* better outcomes or is it simply a correlate?" "What are the most effective strategies to *engage* individuals with AA?" Research to answer these questions has used several different methodologies: (1) randomized clinical trials (RCTs) comparing AA or treatments designed to involve individuals in AA with different forms of AUD treatment, (2) naturalistic studies of treatments designed to engage individuals with AA, (3) studies examining the unique contribution of AA to the prediction of outcomes in clinical and nonclinical samples, and (4) studies of effective approaches to engaging patients in AA.

RCTs in which persons are randomly assigned to different treatment conditions are considered the most rigorous experimental tests of therapeutic effectiveness. Only three RCTs directly comparing AA alone to different forms of treatment have been reported in the research literature, and no RCT has been reported since 1991. Each of the three RCTs has serious methodologic problems and all used populations mandated to treatment, so it is inappropriate to draw specific conclusions about the effectiveness of AA from these studies.

AA and 12-step–oriented treatments have close conceptual links in their adherence to the classic disease concept of AUD, emphasis on abstinence, the importance of AA involvement, and working through the 12 steps. Differences between AA and 12-step–oriented treatment programs are substantial, however, and the two should not be equated.

Several important RCTs of treatments based on 12-step principles have been reported over the past several years. In contrast to RCTs, which typically include strict experimental controls to maximize internal validity, naturalistic study designs evaluate existing treatment programs and patient populations. Experimental controls are lacking, but the inclusion of a broader sample and the evaluation of extant treatments provide information complementary to that obtained from RCTs. A large study of male veterans being treated for AUD in 15 different Veterans Administration medical centers found that patients who participated in 12-step–oriented treatment were about 1.5 times more likely to be abstinent than patients whose treatment was cognitive–behavioral in orientation. In the year after treatment, patients from the 12-step–oriented programs attended significantly more self-help groups than patients from the cognitive–behavioral programs and had significantly fewer outpatient visits and inpatient treatment days; subsequent costs of treatment were 64% higher for patients who had not participated in a 12-step–oriented treatment unit.

Many studies have examined the contribution of AA attendance and involvement to the successful resolution of a drinking problem. One of the most consistent and robust findings is that there is a positive correlation between AA attendance and drinking outcomes. Finally, the literature on methods to engage individuals with AA is limited, but findings suggest that methods for engagement may need to vary depending on the individual's past experience with the program and that simple, directive methods can be effective.

In sum, the research literature suggests that involvement with AA is clearly associated with positive outcomes and that AA involvement leads to positive outcomes, rather than simply being a correlate. Data simply do not exist to determine whether AA itself is *more effective* than different approaches to recovery, but an accumulating body of literature suggests that treatment programs (inpatient and outpatient) based on 12-step principles may be more successful in effecting total abstinence over time and may be more cost-effective than other treatment models.

MECHANISMS OF CHANGE IN ALCOHOLICS ANONYMOUS

With empirical evidence that AA is beneficial for many individuals with AUDs, investigators are now seeking to understand why AA is beneficial.

This line of research necessarily involves three integrated aims, and it is important to keep them distinct. First, investigators are seeking to identify the active ingredients of AA that mobilize behavior change. Such catalysts may not only include prescribed behaviors such as sponsorship, reading core AA literature, and AA step work but may also include less formal or more subtle processes, such as frequency and nature of social support offered through AA participation. Second, actual active ingredients must produce changes that enhance the probability of successfully changing behavior; active ingredients in and of themselves are not explanations for behavior change. And third, mobilized changes in an individual must predict later reductions in drinking.

AA-related benefit occurs because of a tapestry of social interactions, prescribed behaviors, and mobilized psychological processes. There is strong evidence that social support for abstinence in 12-step programs is an important element accounting for a 12-step–related benefit, but evidence also indicates that the nature and temporal benefits associated with such support are complex and are only beginning to be understood. Likewise, consistent support is found for the benefit of two AA-prescribed behaviors: AA meeting attendance and engagement in the AA program by having and being an AA sponsor. Because sponsorship is a vital prerequisite for working the 12 steps, an important outstanding question is whether sponsorship per se predicts positive outcome or, alternatively, whether being guided through the 12 steps by a sponsor accounts for the AA-related benefit. Changes in spirituality or religious/spiritual practices appear to be an important mechanism by which AA exerts a positive impact of outcomes. Contrary to conventional wisdom, cognitive shifts that appear to account for AA-related benefit are not AA specific. Although changes in many beliefs and values occur among AA-exposed individuals, such changes do not seem to have a direct and definitive effect explaining reduced drinking.

FUTURE DIRECTIONS

Research on AA has become increasingly sophisticated over the past 25 years, and a body of accrued knowledge provides a richer and more articulated research-based picture of AA than was available previously. However, there are important research and conceptual issues not well addressed in the current body of literature.

KEY POINTS

1. AA is ubiquitous in the United States, and AA involvement typically is recommended by primary care physicians as well as treatment programs for persons with AUD.
2. An accumulating research base provides a more nuanced understanding of the characteristics of individuals most and least likely to affiliate with AA, barriers to affiliation, and patterns of utilization over time.
3. Knowledge about the effectiveness of AA does not come from gold standard, RCTs, but results from studies utilizing several different research methodologies that converge on a conclusion that involvement with AA, for those who affiliate, leads to better long-term drinking outcomes.
4. Active ingredients in AA include attendance, working the steps in the program, and having a sponsor.
5. Mechanisms by which AA is efficacious include increases in self-efficacy, social support, and spirituality.

REVIEW QUESTIONS

1. What does research suggest as the program ingredient that contributes *the most* to an AA member's success?
   A. Reading the Big Book
   B. Going to meetings
   C. Getting a sponsor
   D. Learning how to avoid people, places, and things

2. Among those listed, what characteristic is *most* common among individuals who affiliate with AA?
   A. Having mild alcohol dependence
   B. Being from racial or ethnic minority groups
   C. Being atheist
   D. Being female

3. Which statement is *true* regarding AA?
   A. AA is only open to those who consider themselves religious or spiritual.
   B. Those who are not religious or spiritual are more likely to become religious or spiritual after participating in AA.
   C. People who are religious tend to benefit least from AA compared to those that are not.
   D. AA is limited to Christians only.

ANSWERS

1. **C**
2. **D**
3. **B**

SUGGESTED READINGS

Matching alcoholism treatments to client heterogeneity: Project MATCH posttreatment drinking outcomes. *J Stud Alcohol.* 1997;58(1):7-29.

Moos RH, Moos BS. Participation in treatment and Alcoholics Anonymous: a 16-year follow-up of initially untreated individuals. *J Clin Psych.* 2006;62(6):735-750.

Tonigan JS, Rynes KN, McCrady BS. Spirituality as a change mechanism in 12-step programs: A replication, extension, and refinement. *Subst Use Misuse.* 2013;48(12): 1161-1173.

Ullman SE, Najdowski CJ, Adams EB. Women, Alcoholics Anonymous, and related mutual aid groups: review and recommendations for research. *Alcohol Treat Q.* 2012;30(4):443-486.

Witbrodt J, Kaskutas, L, Bond J, Delucchi K. Does sponsorship improve outcomes above Alcoholics Anonymous attendance? A latent class growth curve analysis. *Addiction.* 2012;107(2):301-311.

Spirituality in the Recovery Process

Summary by Sonya Lazarevic

Based on THE ASAM PRINCIPLES OF ADDICTION MEDICINE,
6th edition chapter by Marc Galanter

WHAT IS SPIRITUALITY?

Spirituality consists of the nonmaterial issues that give a person meaning and purpose in life; these can be found in not only in a person's religious orientation but can also be seen in his or her ethnic heritage, altruism, humanism, or naturalism. The issue of spirituality is prominent within contemporary culture, as evidenced in a probability sampling of American adults, among whom 95% of respondents replied positively when asked if they believe in "God or a universal spirit." Responses to a follow-up survey suggest that this belief affects the daily lives of the majority (51%) of those sampled, who indicated that they had talked to someone about God or some aspect of their faith or spirituality within the previous 24 hours.

Understanding the Phenomenon

Spirituality can be classified among *latent constructs* like personality, culture, and cognition. These are not observed directly but inferred from observations of their component dimensions. Such constructs are typically multidimensional and understood from the vantage point of more than one discipline. The presence of formal doctrine may be considered associated more with religion than with spirituality.

Alcoholics Anonymous as a Spiritual Recovery Movement

Spirituality parallels recovery from addiction in the way that attitudes are transformed in intensely zealous groups and the way that the denial of illness and the self-defeating behaviors of people with substance use disorders may be reversed through induction into 12-step groups such as Alcoholics Anonymous (AA). Members of the lay public may conclude that certain healthcare issues are inadequately addressed by the medical community and then coalesce to implement a response to this perceived deficit to form a spiritual recovery movement premised on achieving remission based on beliefs independent of evidence-based medicine. Such movements may ascribe their effectiveness to higher metaphysical or nonmaterial forces and claim to offer relief from illness.

AA can be considered a highly successful example of a spiritual recovery movement, which have three primary characteristics. These movements (1) claim to provide relief from disease, (2) operate outside the modalities of established empirical medicine, and (3) ascribe their effectiveness to higher metaphysical powers. The appeal of such movements in the contemporary period is due in part to the fact that many physicians tend not to discuss the spiritual concerns of their patients.

People who are highly distressed over the consequences of their addiction are therefore candidates to respond to the strong ideological orientation of AA toward recovery and are operantly reinforced by the relief produced by affiliation with the group's ideology and behavioral norms, all related to abstinence and a spiritually grounded lifestyle. Significantly, AA generates distress in its members by pressing them to give up their addictive behaviors, but the distress associated with this conflict is relieved if they sustain affiliation and cleave to the group.

Spirituality as a Psychological Construct

Two empirically grounded perspectives have played a material role in framing how we conceptualize recovery:

1. Derived from a model of psychopathology based on the work of Emil Kraepelin, which categorizes diseases diagnosed on the basis of explicit and discrete symptoms. This approach is evident in the development of criteria for substance use disorders employed in the *Diagnostic and Statistical Manual of Mental Disorders* (*DSM*).

Remission can take place with the resolution of the specific symptoms.

2. Derived from behavioral psychology, whose model of stimulus–response sequences has led to the ordering of experience around discrete phenomena that can be observed by a researcher or clinician. Here, recovery can also be defined in terms of observable, measurable responses to substance use, lending credence to recovery as a process defined in behavioral terms.

A third perspective is defined on the basis of the patient's reports of his or her own subjective experience. Research would typically rely on self-report scales, such as those that can be facilitated by the development of instruments like the Life Engagement Test, the General Well-Being Schedule, or the Spiritual Self-Rating Scale.

Spirituality and Religious Experience

The relative role of spiritual experience in the 12-step recovery process has been investigated from a variety of perspectives, generally in relation to patients' experiences in AA. Kelly et al. reviewed studies that applied tests to ascertain how AA achieves beneficial outcomes and found little support for a role of AA's specific spiritual mechanisms. In fact, with regard to religiosity, Tonigan et al. found that although atheists were less likely to attend AA meetings, those who did join derived equal benefit as did spiritually focused individuals.

Spiritually Grounded Recovery in Alcoholics Anonymous

The AA "program of recovery" is mentioned in numerous places in the Big Book, *Alcoholics Anonymous*, and is associated there with terms such as "spiritual experience" and "spiritual awakening" and with working AA's 12 steps. Four of the steps include the word "God," which is qualified "as we understood Him." Some clarity is lent to this latter phrase in the Big Book where it is pointed out that "with few exceptions, our members find that they have tapped an unsuspected inner resource, which they presently identify with their own conception of a Power greater than themselves." Flexibility on the issue of theistic belief is also made clear in one chapter that addresses any person with alcohol use disorder "who feels he is an atheist or agnostic," encouraging their membership as well.

A spiritually grounded definition of recovery can be useful as well. Such a concept relates to the importance of nondemographic subject factors,

originally proposed as "quality of life" issues, among which spirituality can be considered. In this context, a series of suitable criteria for "diagnosing" addiction could be developed. These could then be used to assess the spiritual aspect of recovery associated with the 12-step experience. Resolution of these issues could be considered as important to the spiritual aspect of recovery from addiction. A series of criteria could include:

- loss of sense of purpose due to excessive substance use,
- a feeling of inadequate social support because of one's addiction,
- continued use of a substance while experiencing moral qualms over its consumption, and
- loss of the will to resist temptation when the substance is available.

Another aspect of the *DSM* format can be considered as well. The manual stipulates "course specifiers" of remission such as "on agonist therapy" and "in a controlled environment." It could be added "fully engaged in a program of Twelve-Step recovery," which would be equally explanatory to many clinicians.

But are spiritually grounded criteria measurable? In recent years, methodologies have been developed and validated that could be used to assess outcomes based on such subjectively experienced criteria. They employ a systematic approach to measurement and can be used to describe spiritually related states.

A. Affective state:
   i. A sense of well-being, measured by the General Well-Being Schedule or the Subjective Happiness Scale
   ii. Contentment with one's life circumstances, measured by the Satisfaction with Life Scale
   iii. Positive affect, assessed with the Positive and Negative Affect Schedule
   iv. Feelings of support, employing a scale for Perceived Social Support
B. Existential variables: meaningfulness in one's life, assessed by the Purpose in Life Test
C. Flow as measured by Experience Sampling or the Flow Scale
D. Spirituality as measured by the Spirituality Self-Rating Scale
E. Personality assessment: The Classification of Strengths
F. AA involvement: measures affiliation and commitment to the AA fellowship

Alcoholics Anonymous in the Professional Context

The spiritually oriented 12-step approach has been integrated into professional treatment in some settings where it serves as the overriding philosophy of an entire program or, in others, where it is but one aspect of a multimodal eclectic approach. The Minnesota Model for treatment, typically located in an isolated institutional setting, is characterized by an intensive inpatient stay during which a primary goal of treatment is to acculturate patients to acceptance of the philosophy of AA and to continue with AA attendance after discharge. Although a variety of exercises are included during the stay, this approach has been criticized as overly dogmatic because of its sole reliance on the 12-step approach. A more eclectic option is illustrated in the integration of 12-step groups into a general psychiatric facility for the treatment of patients dually diagnosed for major mental illness and substance abuse.

In summary, spirituality is a matter of personal meaning that is widely accepted. It is also central to the recovery process from addiction for many AA members. The fellowship of AA, in fact, can be considered a movement developed in relation to people's spiritual needs. Although spirituality is subjectively experienced, it can be assessed systematically in given individuals by employing currently available empirical techniques. By such means, an important aspect of addiction recovery can be defined and studied.

KEY POINTS

1. The phenomenon of spirituality is multidimensional.
2. Spirituality is prominent in American culture.
3. AA may be considered a spiritual recovery movement.
4. Spirituality parallels recovery from addiction.

REVIEW QUESTIONS

1. Recovery framework is derived from a:
   A. behavioral model.
   B. disease model.
   C. spiritual model.
   D. subjective experience of the person with addiction.

2. A probability sampling of American adults suggests about what percent of US adults believe in "God or a universal spirit"?
   A. 70%
   B. 80%
   C. 85%
   D. 95%

3. Examples of spiritually grounded measurable criteria to describe spiritually related states include all of the following *except*:
   A. existential variables.
   B. flow.
   C. AA involvement.
   D. exercise.
   E. personality assessments.

ANSWERS

1. **C**
2. **D**
3. **D**

SUGGESTED READINGS

Alcoholics Anonymous World Services. *Alcoholics Anonymous: The Story of How Many Thousands of Men and Women Have Recovered from Alcoholism*. New York: Alcoholics Anonymous Publishing, 1955.

Campbell A, Converse PE, Rogers WL. *The Quality of American Life*. New York: Russell Sage Foundation, 1976.

Galanter M, Dermatis H, Bunt G, et al. Assessment of spirituality and its relevance to addiction treatment. *J Subst Abuse Treat*. 2007;33:257-264.

Kelly JF, Magill M, Stout RL. How do people recover from alcohol dependence? A systematic review of the research on mechanisms of behavior change in Alcoholics Anonymous. *Addict Res Theory*. 2009;17:236-259.

Kraeplin E. *Clinical Psychiatry: A Textbook for Students and Physicians*. New York: Macmillan, 1902.

Tonigan JS, Miller WR, Schermer C. Atheists, agnostics and Alcoholics Anonymous. *J Stud Alcohol*. 2002;63:534-541.

Medical Disorders and Complications of Addiction

79

Medical and Surgical Complications of Addiction

Summary by Karsten Lunze

> Based on THE ASAM PRINCIPLES OF ADDICTION MEDICINE, 6th edition chapter by Richard Saitz

MEDICAL HISTORY

In addition to the usual history taking and a thorough alcohol and substance use assessment probing typical past withdrawal symptoms, questions should address past hospitalizations and any medical conditions that might be related to substance use, which might not be volunteered by the patient without direct questioning. Screening for depression and anxiety, assessment of sexual practices, intention to conceive a child, and behavior that might lead to injury (including being alert for signs of violence) are particularly important.

Physical Examination

The physical examination may be complete or, where appropriate, may focus on body systems related to any reported symptoms or clinical observations.

Tests

Reasonable, inexpensive tests that all patients should undergo at least once include a complete blood count, glucose, liver enzymes, cholesterol, serum creatinine, and urinalysis (to assess for the presence of asymptomatic renal disease). Of particular importance in those who heavily drink is identifying hypertriglyceridemia, which is associated with and can be a cause of pancreatitis. Persons with alcohol use disorders or human immunodeficiency virus (HIV) sometimes present with unsuspected anemia or pancytopenia.

Sexually Transmitted Diseases

The US Preventive Services Task Force (USPSTF) recommends that all pregnant women, all people aged 15 to 65 years, and any others at high risk (ie, men who have sex with men, people who inject drugs, those with other sexually transmitted diseases) be tested for HIV. Persons with substance use disorders who have been sexually active or who inject drugs should be screened routinely for sexually transmitted diseases, including syphilis

and chlamydia. The serologic test for syphilis (rapid plasma reagin or venereal disease research laboratory test) frequently is falsely positive in people who use injection drugs and should be confirmed by direct treponemal tests.

For preexposure prophylaxis for the prevention of HIV infection among those without an HIV infection, a once-daily pill of tenofovir and emtricitabine is recommended for sexually active men who have sex with men, heterosexually active men and women who are at a substantial risk of HIV, for persons who inject drugs, and HIV-discordant couples.

Other Infectious Diseases

Persons with alcohol and other substance use disorders who are likely to be infected should be screened for tuberculosis. If screening is positive, a radiograph should be performed. Provided the radiograph is not consistent with active tuberculosis, prophylactic pharmacotherapy should be considered regardless of age.

To screen for chronic hepatitis and cirrhosis, test patients who use injection drugs, those with heavy alcohol use, and persons with multiple sexual partners or who engage in high-risk sexual activity for international normalized ratio, bilirubin, aspartate amino transferase (AST) and alanine amino transferase (ALT), albumin, and arterial pressure levels.

If any of the first three tests are abnormal, test for hepatitis B (surface antigen and core antibody) and hepatitis C antibodies. Previously vaccinated individuals should have the antisurface hepatitis B antibody levels determined to assess current immunoprotection. Consider testing for immunity to hepatitis A in people who inject drugs, those who practice anal intercourse, and those who are not from endemic areas.

Cancer Screening and Testing for Other Conditions

The USPSTF recommends annual screening for lung cancer with low-dose computed tomography in adults aged 55 to 80 years who have a 30 pack-year smoking history and who currently smoke (or have within the past 15 years), provided life expectancy is not limited and they would be willing to have curative lung surgery.

Biennial mammography should be offered to women aged 50 to 74 years, given a possible small decrease in breast cancer mortality. Screening prior to age 50 years should be individualized based on patient preferences and values after discussing risks and benefits because almost half of the women screened will suffer a false positive and the consequences of further testing to clarify the diagnosis. A family history of breast cancer can indicate the need for earlier testing or referral to a specialist for genetic testing. Those who smoke are at a higher risk of cervical cancer; thus, cervical cytology (Pap smears) should be performed as recommended by the USPSTF.

Men between the ages of 65 and 75 years who ever smoked should have abdominal aortic aneurysm screening with ultrasonography once. Prostate cancer screening remains controversial. The USPSTF recommends against the use of the prostate-specific antigen test for prostate cancer screening because many men are harmed by it and few, if any, derive benefit.

Colorectal cancer screening should be done as recommended by the USPSTF. Currently recommended approaches include yearly fecal occult blood testing, flexible sigmoidoscopy every 5 years, and both procedures or a colonoscopy every 10 years. Positive occult blood testing or sigmoidoscopy should be followed by an examination of the complete colon.

Adults older than 65 years should receive thyroid function testing and vision and hearing screening. Persons with substance use disorders can have poor diets, inadequate calcium intake, little sun exposure, and minimal intake of milk products; therefore, bone mineral density testing and screening for vitamin D deficiency with a 25-hydroxyvitamin D should be considered.

Preventive Counseling

In addition to specific counseling related to addiction, preventive health counseling for these patients should include healthy dietary habits, safe sexual practices and contraception, gun safety, seat belt and helmet use, use of designated drivers, and safe lifting to prevent low back injury. Additionally, those who inject drugs should be educated about sterile injection practices. Patients should be encouraged to engage in regular primary and preventive healthcare with a primary care physician in addition to their addiction specialty care, and mental healthcare should be offered when appropriate.

Naloxone for Overdose Reversal

People with opioid use disorder and their significant others should be prescribed intranasal (or intramuscular) naloxone to prevent an overdose and should be educated regarding how to use the medication and how to call for emergency services.

Preventive Medication to Reduce Cardiovascular Risk

The potential benefit of a reduction in cardiovascular risk should be weighed against the potential harm of an increase in risk for gastrointestinal hemorrhage (in older people, those with gastrointestinal pain, ulcers, nonsteroidal anti-inflammatory drug use, liver disease, or alcoholic gastritis). Clinical conditions associated with substance use disorders such as end-stage liver disease and alcoholic gastritis would also increase the risk. The USPSTF recommends aspirin for the prevention of heart disease and colorectal cancer in "adults aged 50 to 59 years who have a 10% or greater 10-year cardiovascular risk, are not at increased risk for bleeding, have a life expectancy of at least 10 years, and are willing to take low-dose aspirin daily for at least 10 years." More information and links to resources to calculate cardiovascular risks can be found at http://my.americanheart.org/cvriskcalculator.

Folate and Other Vitamins and Minerals

Because folate deficiency is common in patients with alcohol use disorders, women of childbearing age should take 400 to 800 µg daily to prevent fetal neural tube defects. Recommend a daily multivitamin for people with alcohol use disorders and those with deficient diets because they are at risk of thiamine, vitamin D, pyridoxine, niacin, riboflavin, zinc, and folic acid deficiency. In people with alcohol use disorders, encourage eating foods with a high magnesium content (such as peanuts) or a magnesium supplement to prevent magnesium deficiency.

Osteoporosis

Risks for osteoporosis are higher in people with alcohol use disorders and other persons with an addiction. All adults with insufficient intake should be supplemented for calcium and vitamin D, with dosing adjusted for age and gender.

CARE DURING HOSPITALIZATION
Withdrawal

In patients with a history of moderate-to-severe alcohol use disorder and recent regular heavy use, withdrawal symptoms should be anticipated. Opiate and other drug withdrawal should be identified and managed pharmacologically, both for the patient's comfort and to prevent complications of the medical disorder for which the patient was hospitalized. For inpatient methadone administration to treat opioid dependence, see https://professional.heart.org/professional/Guidelines Statements/ASCVDRiskCalculator/UCM_457698 _ASCVD-Risk-Calculator.jsp. Buprenorphine is a reasonable alternative, as is the provision of clonidine together along with other supportive medications such as ibuprofen, diphenoxylate, dicyclomine, and diphenhydramine or promethazine. At hospital admission, when deciding on the best treatment for the patient, the patient's disposition at discharge should be anticipated. If the patient plans to abstain from the substance at hospital discharge, the opioid can be tapered off if symptoms allow. Coordination of care to the outpatient setting is key to ensure a smooth transition.

Pain

Patients with addictive disorders, including those on opioid agonist treatment, usually are very tolerant to the substance they use. Therefore, pain control can be achieved only with substantially higher doses of opioids. Once a dose is determined, pain medications should be given on a regular schedule rather than as needed to avoid making the patient demand medication to relieve uncontrolled symptoms.

MEDICAL CONSEQUENCES OF ALCOHOL, TOBACCO, AND OTHER DRUG USE
Alcohol
Cardiovascular Consequences

Hypertension can occur as a transient symptom of withdrawal and can become chronic. Chronic heavy drinking can lead to alcoholic cardiomyopathy and congestive heart failure, along with its potential complications. Treatment consists of alcohol abstinence and standard therapy for congestive heart failure.

Rhythm disturbances, particularly supraventricular tachyarrhythmias, can occur as a consequence of alcohol use or withdrawal. Referred to as "holiday heart" when following excessive alcohol consumption, these usually resolve spontaneously or after treatment for withdrawal (with benzodiazepines and β-blockers) and abstinence.

Liver and Gastrointestinal Consequences

In alcoholic hepatitis, concentrations of AST is usually higher than ALT. A higher ALT concentration suggests another or a concomitant etiology, such as hepatitis C. Although steatohepatitis is best diagnosed by a liver biopsy, clinically, it is often diagnosed when a serology for hepatitis B and C is negative, the abnormality persists with abstinence, and an ultrasound examination is consistent with the diagnosis. Classic alcoholic hepatitis presents with fever, leukocytosis, right upper quadrant pain and tenderness, and elevations of the AST concentration out of proportion to ALT elevations. Management consists of abstinence from alcohol as well as supportive care, with attention to fluid and electrolyte balance, vitamin K for coagulopathy, clotting factor replacement when there is active bleeding and coagulopathy, and attention to volume and mental status.

Cirrhosis, and associated hypoalbuminemia, coagulopathy, and hyperbilirubinemia, can develop in those with chronic alcohol use either as a consequence of hepatitis C, recurrent alcoholic hepatitis, or chronic use of more than two to three standard drinks per day (although it is more common in heavy alcohol use). Hepatocellular carcinoma can occur, particularly when a hepatitis C infection is present. Surgical treatment may be hampered by complications of cirrhosis, which include hepatic encephalopathy, esophageal or gastric variceal bleeding, ascites and spontaneous bacterial peritonitis, volume overload and edema, and hepatorenal syndrome. End-stage liver disease of many etiologies can be addressed with liver transplantation.

Alcohol is directly toxic to the gastric mucosa and can lead to asymptomatic or symptomatic gastritis. Vomiting can lead to a Mallory-Weiss tear and hematemesis. Alcohol can lead to stomatitis, esophagitis, pancreatitis, duodenitis, esophageal cancer, and gastric cancer. An endoscopy is warranted for persistent reflux symptoms or epigastric pain, particularly if weight loss is present or if patients are 40 years or older.

In people with alcohol use disorder, amylase is often elevated because of chronic parotitis, rather than due to pancreatitis. Epigastric pain might be indicative of pancreatitis, a potentially lethal complication of alcohol use, for which an abdominal computed tomography scan is the most sensitive and specific test. Severity can range from mild epigastric symptoms to a mortal condition complicated by acidosis, adult respiratory distress syndrome, and hypovolemia. Standard therapy for acute pancreatitis (volume repletion, nothing by mouth, and parental opiate pain control) should be instituted early.

Renal and Metabolic Consequences

Hepatic disease can lead to renal consequences, which manifest as nephrotic syndrome and glomerulonephritis from chronic hepatitis C and hepatorenal syndrome in severe cirrhosis. Acute renal failure can occur from rhabdomyolysis after alcohol intoxication or seizure or from volume depletion from vomiting, diarrhea, and diuresis.

People with heavy alcohol use who present for acute medical care should be evaluated for fluid and electrolyte abnormalities. Medical management should focus on volume repletion at least until the patient no longer manifests postural changes in blood pressure and heart rate and until excess losses are not continuing, and correction of metabolic acidosis and alkalosis.

Hyperglycemia or hypoglycemia can be seen in people with alcohol use disorders as a result of pancreatic insufficiency or in end-stage cirrhosis.

Pulmonary Consequences

Alcohol intoxication can lead to respiratory depression and aspiration, which may result in a chemical or infectious pneumonia. Tachypnea can be the result of pulmonary infection, respiratory alkalosis of liver disease, alcohol withdrawal, or compensation for a metabolic acidosis.

Neurologic Consequences

Alcohol intoxication can lead to head trauma, and signs and symptoms of intracranial hemorrhage—particularly subdural hematoma—can be confused with intoxication. In addition, heavy drinking increases the risk for ischemic and hemorrhagic strokes. Imaging of the brain is indicated when there are signs of significant head trauma and abnormal mental status, when focal neurologic deficits are present, or when neurologic symptoms do not resolve with declining alcohol levels. Alcohol can lower the seizure threshold in epileptics, and seizures may be the presenting sign of an intracranial hemorrhage.

Acute cognitive impairment caused by a thiamine deficiency, or Wernicke-Korsakoff syndrome, presents with confusion, ataxia, or nystagmus. Parenteral thiamine, 100 mg administered before glucose, is the initial treatment. Chronically, Wernicke-Korsakoff syndrome can develop into Korsakoff syndrome, a memory impairment disorder classically characterized by confabulation. More commonly, chronic alcohol use disorder is associated with nonspecific dementia. Alcoholic cerebellar dysfunction results in ataxia and incoordination and is often irreversible.

People with alcohol use disorder can suffer from peripheral neuropathy, usually from vitamin deficiency, pressure on a nerve, or ethanol toxicity. It presents as sensory disturbance, including burning, pain, and numbness in a stocking-glove distribution.

Alcohol withdrawal symptoms (eg, diaphoresis, tremor) begin 6 to 48 hours after the last drink. Many patients can be managed as outpatients, provided there are few symptoms and no comorbidities. Benzodiazepines are the only medications proven to ameliorate symptoms of withdrawal, to decrease the risk of seizures and delirium, and to speed the achievement of a calm but awake state in patients experiencing delirium. Pharmacotherapy is indicated for asymptomatic patients at risk for complications (ie, with comorbidities or past seizures) and for those with significant symptoms (use tools such as the Clinical Institute Withdrawal Assessment for Alcohol scale). Seizures, when they occur, almost always resolve spontaneously. Seizures can recur and generally do so within 6 hours of the first seizure. Benzodiazepines prevent further seizures and progression to delirium tremens. Delirium should be managed in a setting where frequent and intensive monitoring is possible because of the risk of death from the condition and its treatment. Other medications to be used as adjunctive therapies include β-blockers for tachycardia, clonidine for hypertension, and haloperidol for psychosis or agitation, when these signs and symptoms fail to respond to benzodiazepines.

Infectious Diseases

Among people with alcohol use disorder, immune defenses are impaired through various mechanisms, including undernutrition, splenic dysfunction, leukopenia, impaired granulocyte function, as well as suppression of the gag reflex during intoxication and overdose. Fever in people with alcohol use disorders cannot be attributed to a minor viral syndrome or withdrawal. Other causes must be reasonably excluded. Pneumonia is more common in people with alcohol use disorders and is associated with increased mortality risk. Tuberculosis must be considered in this population, particularly in the presence of symptoms consistent with the diagnosis. Meningitis in people with alcohol use disorders has a broader etiology than in the general population. Brain abscess can result from poor dentition, leading to transient bacteremia and local infection, for example, in a preexisting subdural hematoma. In patients with cirrhosis and ascites, spontaneous bacterial peritonitis can occur with minimal or absent abdominal tenderness. Diagnosis is made by paracentesis. Spontaneous bacterial empyema can occur when pleural effusion is present. Sexually transmitted diseases, including HIV, are more common in people who drink heavily than in the general population, in part because sexual risk-taking behavior and potential sexual abuse are more common. In people with HIV, *Pneumocystis carinii* pneumonia and other opportunistic infections must be considered when pneumonia is diagnosed.

Trauma

Trauma, including physical and sexual abuse, can lead to unfavorable addiction treatment outcomes. Providers should be attuned to the high rates of injury (both past trauma and the risk of future injury) when counseling people with alcohol use disorders.

Alcohol can interfere with balance and coordination as well as judgment, thus predisposing the patient to injury. Heavy episodic drinking poses a particular risk of injury and accidents. Because these patients often present to emergency departments and trauma centers, these facilities should routinely screen for alcohol problems and should refer patients with alcohol-related disorders for treatment.

Injury can be a motivating factor for discontinuing alcohol use or a focus of counseling to prevent future injuries.

Endocrinologic Consequences

Alcohol causes sexual dysfunction and hypogonadism in men, both through direct effects on the testes and through secondary effects in chronic liver disease, in which gynecomastia may be seen. In women, alcohol delays menopause and is associated with menstrual disorder and decreased fertility. Alcohol increases high-density lipoprotein but also serum triglycerides, which can lead to heart disease, hepatic steatosis, and pancreatitis. Moderate drinking can decrease the incidence of diabetes mellitus, but more than three drinks a day increases the risk.

Fetal, Neonatal, and Infant Consequences

Even low amounts of alcohol consumed during pregnancy can lead to developmental disabilities and neurobehavioral deficits in the offspring. Fetal alcohol syndrome involves craniofacial abnormalities, growth retardation, and neurologic abnormalities, which persists throughout life. Because no safe amount of alcohol during pregnancy has been identified and there is no treatment for the effects of alcohol on the fetus, abstinence is mandatory during pregnancy.

Hematologic Consequences

In addition to the iron deficiency anemia that can result from gastrointestinal hemorrhage or chronic blood loss, people with alcohol use disorders can develop pancytopenia (leukopenia, thrombocytopenia, and anemia) from alcohol's direct toxic effects on the bone marrow or splenic sequestration as manifested in the splenomegaly associated with cirrhosis and portal hypertension. There may be leukopenia or an impaired quantitative and qualitative white blood cell response to infection. Megaloblastic anemia may be as a result of folate deficiency. If there is iron deficiency lowering the mean corpuscular volume and hemolytic anemias related to liver disease with reticulocytosis or megaloblastic processes simultaneously increasing it, the mean corpuscular volume may be noncontributory in differentiating the cause of anemia; the red cell distribution width should be elevated in this situation.

The treatment for bone marrow suppression is abstinence. For iron deficiency, it is identification of the cause and iron replacement. For folate deficiency, treatment consists in folate replacement (after testing for concomitant vitamin B_{12} deficiency and treating it as needed). Coagulopathy usually is a result of chronic liver disease, although a trial of vitamin K replacement is warranted at least once.

Oncologic Risks

Alcohol is a risk factor for several malignancies including of the lip, oral cavity, pharynx, larynx, esophagus, stomach, breast, liver, intrahepatic bile ducts, prostate, and colon. The risk is particularly increased with concurrent tobacco use. Even moderate levels of alcohol use may increase the risk of certain cancers. For example, the risk of breast cancer increases with the consumption of one to two standard drinks per day.

Musculoskeletal Consequences

Intoxication to the point of overdose may result in the individual remaining in one position for prolonged periods of time, which can lead to compression nerve palsies, rhabdomyolysis, and compartment syndrome. Surgical consultation is required for the latter.

Hyperuricemia and gout are more common in alcohol use disorders. Treatment is with colchicine, using caution in renal or hepatic insufficiency, or indomethacin, using caution in the presence of gastritis or renal insufficiency. A brief course of corticosteroids and a single injection of adrenocorticotropic hormone may be safer choices for persons with alcohol use disorders. Chronic treatment in the setting of renal disease, tophaceous gout, or polyarticular gout should be with allopurinol or probenecid.

Excessive regular alcohol use or heavy episodic drinking increases the risk of skeletal fractures through a higher risk of trauma or alcohol-related osteopenia or both. Heavy alcohol use can lead to osteonecrosis of the bone, such as that at the femoral head.

Vitamin Deficiencies

Malabsorption and poor dietary intake can lead to deficiencies of thiamine, pyridoxine, niacin, riboflavin, vitamin D, zinc, and fat-soluble vitamins when there is malabsorption because of pancreatic disease. Vitamin replacement is safe and should be done empirically.

Consequences in the Perioperative Patient

Heavy alcohol consumption is a risk factor for postoperative complications. In the perioperative period, withdrawal is a concern, and both withdrawal and postoperative pain must be managed appropriately. Attempting to achieve abstinence prior to elective surgery has been shown to reduce morbidity.

Sleep

Although alcohol can help people fall asleep, it also can be stimulating and lead to disrupted sleep and daytime fatigue. Alcohol increases the risk of obstructive sleep apnea and worsens the disease (because of its depressant effects on respiration and relaxation of the upper airway) and can increase the risk of periodic limb movements of sleep. Treatment should include attention to sleep hygiene and pharmacotherapy with drugs with a low or no risk of dependence (eg, trazodone).

Tobacco

Tobacco use is the leading cause of preventable illness and premature death. Its adverse health effects range from cosmetic damage to severe illness as outlined in the following section.

Smoking increases the risks of myocardial infarction and sudden death due to poorer control of hypertension and atherosclerosis. It can precipitate angina by facilitating vasospasm and hypercoagulability and can precipitate dysrhythmia. Those who smoke are at a higher risk of cerebrovascular and peripheral vascular diseases. Smoking is also the leading cause of both chronic obstructive pulmonary disease and bronchogenic carcinoma. It leads to pulmonary hypertension, interstitial lung disease, and pneumothorax. The decline in lung function and mortality risks of both diagnoses can be decreased with smoking cessation. In addition, smoking is associated with cancer of the oral cavity,

larynx, esophagus, bladder, kidney, pancreas, stomach, and cervix. These risks decrease promptly after smoking cessation.

Smoking causes gastric and duodenal ulcers and can exacerbate gastroesophageal reflux disease. Smoking cessation, in addition to pharmacotherapy, is usually necessary for effective treatment. It has hypercoagulable effects and is a risk factor for deep vein thrombosis. Tobacco use is known to increase the risk of Graves disease (hyperthyroidism) and hypothyroidism, increase insulin resistance and the risk of diabetes, and decrease estrogen in both genders and is associated with decreased bone mineral density, osteoporosis, and fractures. In men, it is one of the leading causes of erectile dysfunction and decreases sperm number and function. Tobacco use during pregnancy causes low birth weight, spontaneous abortion, and perinatal mortality and may increase the risk of sudden infant death syndrome and neurodevelopmental impairment.

Consequences in the Perioperative Patient

Smoking increases the risk of postoperative pneumonia, atelectasis, reactive airways exacerbations, and respiratory failure. If possible, smoking cessation at least 2 months before elective surgery is advisable.

Cessation and Treatment of Withdrawal

Nicotine replacement—bupropion or varenicline, if appropriate—should be provided for medically ill patients who are hospitalized because nicotine withdrawal and craving can complicate treatment for other medical illnesses. Nicotine replacement can precipitate myocardial ischemia, but the alternative, smoking a cigarette, also can do so. Therefore, in general, even those who smoke who have coronary artery disease can use nicotine replacement, unless they are experiencing unstable angina or a myocardial infarction.

Opiates, Cocaine, and Other Drugs

Medical, surgical, and other complications of drugs are related to their route of administration (unsafe injection, inhalation) and to their organ effects, particularly their effects on the brain.

Injection Drug Use

Intravenous drug use is a major risk factor for HIV and hepatitis C infections. Tetanus can develop in nonimmune individuals. False-positive screening tests for syphilis often are found in people who inject drugs; therefore, treponemal specific tests are needed to determine the diagnosis.

Due to unsafe injections, skin and soft tissue infections are common in people who use injected drugs. Commonly caused by staphylococci and streptococci, local epidemiology and practices can point to other, unusual causative pathogens (eg, *Pseudomonas aeruginosa, Serratia* species) and polymicrobial infections from the use of saliva to prepare the injection. Cellulitis and minor infections can usually be treated with penicillin, cephalosporins, or macrolides. Abscesses need additional surgical drainage. Soft tissue infections become life threatening if fasciitis results in significant local ischemia (as with cocaine injection). Intravenous injection can result in septic thrombophlebitis, arterial injection with embolus and digital ischemia, and infections or venous valvular damage in the extremities, marked by leg ulcers, edema, and a propensity to develop deep vein thrombosis.

One of the most serious infectious consequences of injection drug use is bacterial endocarditis. Thus, in an injection drug user, fever even in the absence of cardiac murmurs and other typical signs of subacute bacterial endocarditis needs to be worked up (blood culture, eventual empiric antibiotic treatment). Mycotic aneurysms; endophthalmitis; congestive heart failure; brain, spleen, or myocardial abscesses and emboli; renal failure from interstitial nephritis; pulmonary septic emboli with effusions; stroke; and heart block can complicate the course. Injection drug users can also develop septic arthritis in unusual locations (sternoclavicular or sacroiliac joints), spinal epidural or vertebral infections, osteomyelitis, or meningitis.

In addition to infectious complications, the injection of drugs can lead to pulmonary and hepatic talc granulomatosis from injected crushed tablets containing talc, pulmonary hypertension from granulomatous disease or drug-related vasoconstriction, needle embolization, pneumothorax or hemothorax from injections into large central veins gone awry, and pulmonary emphysema related or unrelated to talc granulomatosis.

A common renal complication related specifically to injection drug use is nephropathy, primarily because of HIV infection. Amyloidosis and nephrotic syndrome can occur because of chronic skin infections. A hepatitis C infection can lead to glomerulonephritis. The coagulopathy that results from liver and kidney disease in injection drug users can lead to neurologic complications, particularly hemorrhagic stroke. Cerebral infarction can result from the injection of crushed tablets and even from a melted suppository (intravenously and via inadvertent intra-arterial injection).

Inhalation of Drugs

The inhalation of drugs has effects related to the size of the particles: Larger particles affect the airways, whereas smaller ones affect the alveoli. In addition to the granulomatous complications previously listed, chronic bronchitis from inhaled smoke; bronchospasm; barotrauma with resultant pneumothorax or pneumomediastinum from prolonged breath holding or stimulant use; hemoptysis from airway irritation; and emphysema from inhaled tobacco, marijuana, or opiates can occur. Freebasing can lead to upper airway and facial burns.

Withdrawal

Although withdrawal is not fatal in an otherwise healthy person, in the acutely ill or hospitalized patient, withdrawal should be treated with the aim of symptomatic relief and to prevent hyperadrenergic states that complicate treatment of the acute medical problem (eg, coronary syndromes).

Neurologic Consequences

Seizures can occur as a result of sedative withdrawal, stimulant use, or proconvulsant metabolites (meperidine). Similarly, a hemorrhagic stroke can occur with the use of methamphetamines, phenylpropanolamine, lysergic acid diethylamide, and phencyclidine from hypertension, vasculitis, or other vascular mechanisms. Cocaine use can lead to both hemorrhagic and ischemic strokes. Anabolic steroids can cause a stroke by promoting hypercoagulability. Although classic syndromes of dementia have not been described for people who use drugs other than alcohol, chronic cognitive deficits can be seen in those who use cocaine, sedatives (barbiturate), and toluene. Neuropathy (including plexopathies and Guillain-Barré syndrome) may be caused by heroin use, compression neuropathy caused by any drug, quadriplegia in those who sniff glue, and combined systems degeneration from vitamin B_{12} deficiency induced by nitrous oxide use. Parkinsonism can develop from the use of a meperidine analogue, MPTP (1-methyl-4-phenyl-1,2,3,6-tetrahydropyridine).

Gastrointestinal Consequences

In addition to hepatitis C, which is almost universal in those who use injection drugs, cocaine itself can cause hepatic necrosis, probably because of ischemia. Ecstasy and phencyclidine use has been reported to cause liver failure. Androgenic steroids can cause hepatic toxicity. Anticholinergic and opiate abuse will cause constipation. "Body packing" (ie, transporting cocaine, heroin, or other drugs in bags that are swallowed) can lead to mechanical obstruction of the intestines. A rupture can lead to overdose.

Hematologic Consequences

Amyl nitrate, isobutyl nitrate, and other "poppers" can cause methemoglobinemia.

Cardiovascular Consequences

In addition to causing endocarditis and myocardial abscess, drugs can directly affect the cardiovascular system. Cocaine can cause severe hypertension, cardiomyopathy, cardiac dysrhythmias, angina, myocardial infarction, sudden death, and stroke. Chest pain often occurs during or after cocaine use, but most persons evaluated in emergency departments with chest pain and cocaine use do not have a myocardial infarction. Nonetheless, heart attacks do occur and are thought to be related to coronary vasospasm, in situ thrombosis, or the accelerated development of atherosclerosis. Other stimulants can also produce cardiac complications. Anabolic steroids can lead to coronary artery disease as well as cardiomyopathy. Drugs with anticholinergic effects (eg, muscle relaxants, antihistamines, antidepressants) cause tachycardia and dysrhythmias in intoxication or overdose. Inhalants (eg, volatile fluorocarbons) can cause dysrhythmias.

Renal and Metabolic Consequences

Any drug that leads to sedation with intoxication or overdose can lead to muscle compression and rhabdomyolysis and, thus, to acute renal failure. Rhabdomyolysis can also be seen with amphetamine, cocaine, and phencyclidine use. Cocaine can lead to accelerated hypertension and renal failure, hypertensive nephrosclerosis, thrombotic microangiopathy, and renal infarction. Amphetamines can result in a drug-related polyarteritis nodosa. Ecstasy use can lead to hyponatremia when users drink excess water to prevent the hypovolemia associated with its use. Toluene inhalation can lead to metabolic acidosis.

Injury

Although much of the literature focuses on alcohol as a risk factor for injury, cocaine and other drugs also have been associated with an increased risk of motor vehicle crashes and other violent injuries, including fatal shootings.

Oncologic Risks

Although the magnitude of risk remains unclear, marijuana, when smoked, can lead to squamous cell carcinoma of the oral cavity and to lung cancer.

Pulmonary Consequences

Drugs that produce sedation with use or overdose can lead to respiratory depression and death. Atelectasis can develop, as can aspiration and chemical pneumonitis. Opiate use can lead to bronchospasm, as a result of its stimulation of histamine release, and pulmonary edema in the setting of overdose. The pulmonary consequences of sedatives are limited primarily to respiratory depression and arrest from overdose; worsening of sleep-disordered breathing; as well as tachypnea, hyperventilation, and respiratory alkalosis from withdrawal syndromes.

Marijuana use can lead to obstructive lung disease and fungal infection from contamination. Cocaine use can lead to nasal septal perforation, sinusitis, epiglottitis, upper airway obstruction, and hemoptysis, primarily from irritant and vasoconstrictive effects. Cocaine use can lead to pulmonary hemorrhages, edema, hypertension, emphysema, interstitial fibrosis, and hypersensitivity pneumonitis. The treatment for most of these diseases is withdrawal of the cocaine and supportive care, although corticosteroids and bronchodilators are warranted in some cases. Pulmonary hypertension and edema can result from use of stimulants (specifically amphetamines).

Inhalants can lead to methemoglobinemia, tracheobronchitis, asphyxiation, and hypersensitivity pneumonitis. Nitrous oxide can cause respiratory depression and hypoxemia. Anabolic steroids can induce prothrombotic states and can lead to pulmonary embolism.

Endocrinologic Consequences

Most drugs of abuse can affect a variety of hormone levels. Opiates can impair gonadotropin release, which may lead to impaired sperm motility in men, and women may have menstrual and ovulatory irregularities. Cocaine is a risk factor for the more frequent occurrence of diabetic ketoacidosis, in part because of its adrenergic effects. Barbiturate use can lead to osteomalacia from vitamin D deficiency. Clinical metabolic consequences have been clearly linked to use of anabolic steroids. Women develop androgenization, and lipids are adversely affected.

Consequences in the Perioperative Patient

As with other substances, attention to and treatment of withdrawal symptoms can avert the development of tachycardia and hypertension, which may complicate interpreting assessments and operative and anesthetic treatments. The anesthesiologist must be informed of any recent drug use because of potential interactions between β-blockers and cocaine and because of the potentiation of sedative and anesthetic drugs. Finally, anesthesia and pain management generally require much higher doses than usual in the patient with an opiate dependency. Nutritional issues often require attention in addicted persons undergoing surgery because wound healing may be impaired.

Sleep

Many persons with addictive disorders experience sleep disturbances because of drug effects, lifestyles, or comorbid psychiatric conditions. The often desired effect of drugs on sleep (stimulants and nicotine suppress sleep, opioids induce sleep) can contribute to their use for self-medication. Therefore, the management of sleep disorders, particularly insomnia, is difficult but important in persons with an addiction. Attention to sleep hygiene (ie, a quiet location, using the bed only for sleep and sex, eliminating napping) and judicious use of drugs less likely to lead to misuse, such as trazodone, are the best approaches.

Fetal, Neonatal, and Infant Consequences

No clear teratogenic effects of opiates are known, but opiate exposure in utero can lead to neonatal abstinence syndrome, which manifests primarily with seizures. Benzodiazepines have been associated with cleft lip and palate, although studies may have been confounded by alcohol use. Toluene and other inhalants use can cause an embryopathy, preterm labor, and intrauterine growth retardation. Dextroamphetamine and cocaine are associated with teratogenesis. Cocaine use during pregnancy can induce neonatal irritability and can also cause behavioral and learning disorders.

KEY POINTS

1. Care for patients with an addiction needs to address both their medical and surgical needs and those related to substance use.
2. When caring for patients with an addiction, keep in mind that unhealthy substance use can affect virtually any organ system in the body.
3. Preventive care should be targeted to the patient's background and follow current guidelines.

ACKNOWLEDGMENTS

Karsten Lunze is supported in part by the National Institute on Drug Abuse (K99DA041245 and R00 DA041245).

REVIEW QUESTIONS

1. In patients with opiate use disorder:
   A. pain management often is a challenge during medical hospitalization because opioids would worsen the addiction.
   B. controlling pain with opioids is not necessary because their pain receptors are not responsive due to their opioid use.
   C. pain should be addressed and may require higher doses of opioids administered on a regular schedule.

2. True or False: Medical and surgical complications among patients with substance use disorders or unhealthy alcohol use can only be treated by addiction specialists.

3. Medical and surgical complications of addiction may be:
   A. the consequence of drug-specific organ effects.
   B. related to the methods of administration, such as inhalation, injection, or ingestion.
   C. caused by drug contaminants or the vehicles for drugs used.
   D. due to the behavioral habits associated with substance use.
   E. all of the above.

ANSWERS

1. C
2. **False**
3. E

SUGGESTED READINGS

Douaihy AB, Kelly TM, Sullivan C. Medications for substance use disorders. *Soc Work Public Health*. 2013;28(3-4):264-278.

Gordon AJ, Bertholet N, McNeely J, et al. 2013 Update in addiction medicine for the generalist. *Addict Sci Clin Pract*. 2013;8:18.

Saitz R. Clinical practice. Unhealthy alcohol use. *N Engl J Med*. 2005;352(6):596-607.

World Health Organization. *Guidelines for the Psychosocially Assisted Pharmacological Treatment of Opioid Dependence*. Geneva: World Health Organization, 2009.

Cardiovascular Consequences of Alcohol and Other Drug Use

Summary by Steven Pfau and Samit Shah

Based on THE ASAM PRINCIPLES OF ADDICTION MEDICINE,
6th edition chapter by Steven Pfau and Samit Shah

Diseases of the heart and blood vessels account for substantial medical morbidity and mortality worldwide and affect a staggering proportion of the population. Lifetime risk for coronary heart disease alone at age 40 years approaches 50% for men and 33% for women in the United States. Although use of some substances may rarely precipitate uncommon cardiovascular conditions—cocaine use causing aortic dissection, for example—much more importantly, substance use may contribute to the pathogenesis of very common cardiovascular conditions. The most common cardiovascular diseases in Western society—hypertension, coronary artery disease (CAD), atrial fibrillation, heart failure, and stroke—have important associations with the use of alcohol, nicotine, and illicit substances. As a general practitioner, a specialist in addiction medicine, or a cardiovascular specialist, it is important to understand the implications of these relationships, as it is likely that treatment of a common cardiac condition (eg, hypertension) will require recognizing and addressing risky substance use or a co-occurring substance use disorder (eg, alcohol). Here, we review these very frequent associations and the relationship of substance use to the development and clinical manifestations of heart disease.

ALCOHOL

Clinical heart disease related to alcohol use is an old observation, familiar to physicians for over a century, and the term *alcoholic heart disease* was first used in 1902. There is significant evidence that alcohol use adversely impacts cardiovascular health, and recent data suggests that alcohol use independently increases the risk of developing the most common cardiovascular conditions such as atrial fibrillation, myocardial infarction (MI), and congestive heart failure, with a similar effect to more commonly

recognized cardiovascular risk factors such as obesity and hypertension. The manifestations of alcohol-related heart disease depend in large part on the amount of alcohol ingested and the time period of exposure. For definitions used in this discussion, drinking no more than 3 standard (14 g) drinks in a day or 7 drinks a week for women (and those older than 65 years) and drinking no more than 4 drinks in a day or 14 drinks a week for men is considered low-risk drinking.

Alcoholic Cardiomyopathy

Chronic heavy alcohol consumption can result in a clinical picture characterized by four-chamber cardiac enlargement, loss of left ventricular systolic function, and the development of typical symptoms of congestive heart failure: dyspnea on exertion, orthopnea, and nocturnal dyspnea. In Western societies, alcohol-related cardiomyopathy is second only to ischemia as a cause of dilated cardiomyopathies. Worldwide, as many as one third to one half of cases of dilated cardiomyopathy may be attributable to alcohol use. The likelihood of developing clinical cardiomyopathy correlates with mean daily alcohol intake and the duration of drinking. Asymptomatic left ventricular dysfunction is present in as many as one third of patients with alcohol use disorder. The signs and symptoms of alcoholic cardiomyopathy are not unique, and the history is primary in establishing the diagnosis. Chronic and prolonged alcohol use, usually 80 to 90 g of alcohol daily for at least 5 years, is of primary importance. The prognosis in alcoholic cardiomyopathy is strongly correlated with continued use of alcohol. When detected early and treated aggressively with alcohol abstinence and standard medical therapy for dilated cardiomyopathies and congestive symptoms, the prognosis may be better than in other dilated cardiomyopathies.

This may be explained in large part by improvement in left ventricular function with abstinence. However, with continued alcohol use, the prognosis is as poor or worse than in other nonischemic dilated cardiomyopathies. Without complete abstinence, the 4-year mortality approaches 50%. Therefore, treatment should focus on abstinence, with other standard medical therapies for heart failure: loop diuretics, angiotensin-converting enzyme inhibitors, β-blockers, and spironolactone.

Coronary Artery Disease and Stroke

There is a complex relationship between alcohol and the incidence of coronary artery disease as diagnosed by noninvasive or invasive testing, a clinical event such as MI, or mortality from coronary disease. Low-to-moderate alcohol consumption appears to be largely protective when compared to those patients who abstain from alcohol. In patients with established coronary heart disease, both cardiovascular mortality and all-cause mortality are lower with low-to-moderate alcohol intake, with the dose response curve indicating a possible benefit between 5 and 26 g/dL. The evidence for the beneficial effect of alcohol at low consumption levels has been debated, particularly because the epidemiologic data suffer, in addition to the potential bias of self-reporting of alcohol intake, the likely influence of uncontrolled confounding (low use being associated with more physical activity, higher income, positive health behaviors) and lack any long-term randomized controlled trials. The epidemiologic evidence for increasing CAD risk with heavy alcohol use has also been consistent, leading to the so-called J-shaped curve of alcohol-related cardiovascular risk. Consumption of low-risk amounts of alcohol is also associated with a lower risk of stroke, although the data are less robust than that for CAD. At any level of consumption, alcohol is associated with a lower risk of ischemic stroke and a higher risk of hemorrhagic stroke and may be explained by those antithrombotic properties of alcohol that may be protective from CAD. The increased risk of stroke with heavy alcohol use is consistent across many studies, with an increased relative risk of total, ischemic, and hemorrhagic stroke of approximately 1.6. A retrospective cohort analysis of the Swedish Twin Registry over 43 years showed that two drinks of alcohol per day before the age of 60 years increased the risk of stroke by 34% compared to lighter drinking. Heavy alcohol intake shortened the time to stroke by 5 years and was more significant a risk factor for stroke than hypertension or diabetes mellitus in patients younger than age 75 years.

Heart Failure

Patients with chronic congestive heart failure may be particularly susceptible to the cardiotoxic effects of alcohol. Regardless of any ambiguity with "low-to-moderate" risk drinking, heavy alcohol consumption (greater than six drinks per day) is strongly associated with an increased risk of developing clinically evident heart failure and heart failure–related mortality in adults. The 2013 American College of Cardiology Foundation/American Heart Association Guideline for the Management of Heart Failure lists excessive alcohol consumption as a common factor that may precipitate decompensated congestive heart failure, and the recommendation is to counsel patients appropriately.

Hypertension

Alcohol use, especially in excess, is associated with hypertension, and alcohol may be responsible for as much as 16% of the global burden of hypertensive disease. Regular consumption of more than two drinks a day is associated with increased blood pressure, and the degree of blood pressure increase is dose dependent. The elevation in blood pressure is accompanied by the expected rise in hypertension-related cardiovascular morbidity and mortality. Alcohol can be an important factor in hypertension that is refractory to standard therapy, which may be 10% to 15% of patients with hypertension, and there is an increased risk of cardiovascular complications when compared to medication-responsive hypertension. Reduction of alcohol consumption is associated with significant decreases in blood pressure in patients with hypertension. In patients being treated for hypertension, alcohol consumption should be limited to two drinks per day or less.

Atrial Fibrillation and Other Arrhythmias

Atrial fibrillation is the most common clinical arrhythmia in adults, with a lifetime risk of one in four for men and women older than 40 years. The prevalence varies from 1% in patients younger than 60 years to 17.8% in patients older than 85 years. Alcohol use has also been associated with an increased risk for the development of atrial fibrillation. *Holiday heart* is a term that has historically been applied to atrial fibrillation that occurs after binge drinking and typically implies the absence of other heart disease. Because of early structural abnormalities that occur in the heart with chronic heavy alcohol use, the occurrence of atrial fibrillation in those patients with a history of heavy alcohol use must be considered as a potential harbinger of significant heart disease. Atrial fibrillation in the setting of alcohol use disorder must be evaluated in the same manner as new-onset atrial fibrillation occurring in any other context: a full history and physical exam; 12-lead electrocardiogram; echocardiogram; and blood tests for kidney, thyroid, and liver function. In addition to atrial fibrillation, heavy alcohol consumption has also been linked to ventricular arrhythmias. An analysis of a large national database of 7600 inpatients with alcoholic cardiomyopathy showed that 33% suffered an arrhythmia, with atrial fibrillation occurring in 22% of patients, ventricular tachycardia in 10%, atrial flutter in 5%, and ventricular fibrillation in 2%. Thus, the proarrhythmic effects of alcohol ingestion are common and can be life-threatening in susceptible patients.

CIGARETTE SMOKING AND TOBACCO USE

Cigarette smoke is a complex mixture of chemicals, including nicotine, many of which have been closely associated with a direct role in coronary atherosclerosis and its clinical manifestations. It is estimated that 15.1% of the US adult population were active smokers in 2015 (>35 million people). The importance of cigarette smoking as a risk factor for atherosclerotic vascular disease cannot be overemphasized. Cigarette smoking has been identified as an important risk factor for virtually every clinical manifestation of atherosclerosis, including the presence and progression of CAD, carotid artery disease, peripheral vascular disease including abdominal aortic aneurysm, thoracic aortic plaque burden, ischemic stroke, and particularly the incidence of acute MI. Notably, children who are raised in homes where one or both parents are smokers are at substantially elevated risk of developing carotid atherosclerotic plaque later in life, suggesting that the irreversible cardiovascular effects of cigarette smoke occur even with secondhand exposure. Every individual regularly exposed to cigarette smoke should be considered as high risk for cardiovascular disease. In a given individual, smoking cessation is associated with a rapid decline in the risk for acute MI, approaching the level of a nonsmoker after 2 to 3 years. Mandatory smoking prohibition programs have repeatedly been associated with decreased hospitalization rates after an acute MI. Stopping smoking has also been shown to reduce to the risk

of congestive heart failure and cardiovascular death. However, people who are former heavy smokers (>32 pack-years) remain at elevated risk of cardiovascular events but at comparatively lower risk than people who continue to smoke.

Electronic Cigarettes

Electronic cigarettes (e-cigarettes) are classified by the US Food and Drug Administration as "electronic nicotine delivery systems." The highest rate of e-cigarette use is among people who are current and former smokers with relatively low rates of use among nonsmokers. However, up to 20% to 30% of middle and high school students who have reported using e-cigarettes have never tried conventional cigarettes, suggesting that e-cigarettes may increasingly be the initial exposure to nicotine in young people. From a cardiovascular perspective, the most concerning constituents of e-cigarette vapor are nicotine, carbonyls, and particulates. The amount of nicotine delivered in each "puff" from an e-cigarette is highly variable and depends on characteristics of each device. It is generally estimated that it would take 30 puffs from an e-cigarette to deliver the 1 mg of nicotine that is typically delivered from a conventional cigarette. The cardiovascular effect of nicotine exposure from e-cigarettes is therefore lower than that of conventional cigarettes (as the latter is accompanied by thousands of other combustion-generated chemicals). People who are former smokers as well as patients with known cardiovascular disease who are maintained on therapeutic doses of non–e-cigarette nicotine-replacement therapy have not been shown to have adverse outcomes.

COCAINE

The "recreational" use of cocaine has been associated with a wide variety of cardiovascular complications. Cocaine is the illicit drug most likely to precipitate an emergency room visit, responsible for 57% of recreational substance–related emergency room visits. Many of these visits are for complaints of chest pain; this is particularly important because cocaine is the most common illicit drug used by individuals older than 50 years. In addition to chest pain, other conditions such as acute MI, aortic dissection, stroke, heart failure, and sudden cardiac death have all been associated with acute and chronic cocaine use. In the coronary arteries of human subjects, cocaine use results in vasoconstriction, platelet aggregation, and endothelial dysfunction, all of which are effects that may be accentuated by the presence of atherosclerosis and cigarette smoking.

In general, presentation with cardiovascular symptoms occurs early after cocaine use, with a markedly elevated risk of cocaine-related MI within the first 24 hours. Cocaine-related chest pain is the most frequent cardiovascular presentation associated with cocaine use. However, the incidence of acute MI in this group of patients is relatively low, with reports ranging from 0.7% to 6%. Observation with serial measurement of troponin is the best compromise of cost and sensitivity when evaluating this group of patients. When MI in the context of cocaine use does occur, the treatment approach may differ from non–cocaine-associated MI. Dual antiplatelet therapy with aspirin and P2Y12 platelet receptor inhibitors is considered beneficial, and most experts agree with following standardized treatment algorithms for antiplatelet regimens. β-Adrenergic receptor blockers are a class of medications that have demonstrated reduced mortality in a large number of clinical trials when administered in the setting of acute MI. In the setting of cocaine use, there is a theoretical possibility of β-blockers precipitating arterial vasoconstriction by unopposed cocaine-induced alpha-receptor stimulation. However, two studies have shown that the effect of β-blocker administration to patients did not meaningfully affect hemodynamic or clinical outcomes. In fact, people who had received β-blockers had lower blood pressure and lower rates of MI, and in one study, there was a trend toward decreased postdischarge mortality when compared to subjects who did not receive them. Still, the most recent American Heart Association/American College of Cardiology practice guidelines to address cocaine-related chest pain/acute coronary syndrome do not endorse β-blockers in early management and give a class IIIC recommendation to the use of β-blockers in patients with acute coronary syndromes and active cocaine use.

Other important presentations of cocaine-related cardiovascular disease include aortic dissection and stroke. The proportion of aortic dissection that is related to cocaine varies depending on the population studied, ranging from 0.5% to 37%. Cocaine-related dissection tends to occur more frequently in young subjects with hypertension. Both ischemic stroke and intracerebral hemorrhage related to cocaine use have been reported with approximately equal frequency. Hemorrhage appears to be more frequent in individuals with ongoing use, whereas ischemic stroke and transient ischemic attack are more common in patients who are remote cocaine users. Most strokes occur within 6 to 24 hours of using cocaine and individuals who smoke crack cocaine are at an increased risk of stroke compared to those with intranasal use.

OPIOIDS

From a strictly cardiovascular perspective, opioids have significant medicinal value. The hemodynamic effects of lowering heart rate and blood pressure as well as decreasing preload, combined with their analgesic and anxiolytic properties, have made morphine a cornerstone of the treatment of acute coronary syndromes. Opioids have not been associated with any direct toxic effects on myocytes or other components of the heart. The primary risks of opioid use from a cardiovascular point of view are those associated with method of administration, namely, intravenous injection. It is estimated that as many as 21 million people worldwide injected drugs in 2007, indicating a very large number of people at risk. It is difficult to estimate the incidence of injection-related endocarditis, but the number of hospitalizations for this diagnosis is rising in the United States. The demographics of infectious endocarditis related to injection drug use are changing, and there have been significant increases in endocarditis-related hospital admissions in young people between the ages of 15 and 34 years old, with the greatest impact on Caucasian women. Infectious endocarditis in someone who has used an injection drug is characterized by several distinguishing features. First, it is much more common for the right heart valves, especially the tricuspid valve, to be involved. As much as 75% of endocarditis in individuals with injection drug use involves the right heart valves, but left-sided endocarditis in those who use drugs may be associated with a worse prognosis. Second, polymicrobial infections and endocarditis due to fungal pathogens are much more common in those who use injection drugs. Polymicrobial endocarditis is much more likely to require valve surgery and carries a higher mortality than single-organism infections. Fungal endocarditis mortality ranges from 37% to 80%, even with aggressive surgical and medical therapy. Finally, because patients with opioid use disorder have a high likelihood of continued use if left untreated, recurrent endocarditis is common. A recurrence of endocarditis after valve replacement surgery carries a particularly ominous prognosis.

AMPHETAMINES

Amphetamines are a group of synthetic compounds used both medicinally and recreationally. Phenylpropanolamine is an amphetamine frequently used as an appetite suppressant and nasal decongestant. Other derivatives are used only recreationally and include mephedrone/methylenedioxypyrovalerone (MDPV or "bath salts"); 3,4-methylenedioxymethamphetamine (MDMA or "ecstasy"); and methyldiethanolamine (MDEA or "Eve"). Amphetamines produce a dose-dependent elevation of blood pressure and an increase in heart rate, and the most common presentation in patients seen in the emergency room after recent amphetamine use is tachycardia and hypertension. Amphetamine-related stimulants are associated with acute MI and may be associated with a worse prognosis in those who present with acute coronary syndromes. Amphetamines may cause myocardial ischemia by several mechanisms, including focal or diffuse vasospasm, increased myocardial demand on preexisting coronary disease, and increased platelet reactivity. Similarly, ischemic and hemorrhagic stroke have been associated with amphetamine use. Phenylpropanolamine, a common ingredient in appetite suppressants, was removed from over-the-counter sale by the US Food and Drug Administration because of a strong association with an increased risk for hemorrhagic stroke, especially in young women. Some amphetamine derivatives developed as appetite suppressants (such as fenfluramine) are strong serotonin receptor (especially the $5-HT_{2B}$ receptor) agonists and were removed from the market after evidence linking them to the development of a specific form of valvular heart disease previously associated with serotonin-secreting carcinoid tumors; similar lesions have been described in recreational amphetamine use. Cardiomyopathy is perhaps the most commonly associated heart disease in acute and with chronic amphetamine use. As many as 5% of all patients presenting to emergency rooms in the United States with decompensated heart failure may have chronic stimulant use.

CANNABIS AND SYNTHETIC MARIJUANA

Observational data suggest a temporal relationship between the smoking of marijuana and the onset of acute MI and a worsened outcome of MI. In patients with known coronary artery disease, marijuana use has been shown to decrease myocardial oxygen delivery, increase myocardial oxygen demand, and decrease the time to develop angina during exercise. However, population-based studies have found no increased risk of cardiovascular mortality associated with marijuana use. Marijuana use has also been temporally associated with stroke in adult users as well as children, with a 17% increase

in risk of acute ischemic stroke in young adults after marijuana use. The mechanism of cerebrovascular events is potentially due to cerebral vasospasm and transient intracranial arterial stenosis. The vasoactive effect of marijuana has been suggested in the coronary arteries as well, as there are documented reports of slow contrast flow on coronary angiograms of patients who have suffered ventricular arrhythmias after using marijuana.

Synthetic cannabinoids known by the street names "K2," "Spice," and "Black Mamba" are "designer drug" compounds that are synthesized to have higher binding affinity to the CB1 cannabinoid receptor than the $\Delta9$-tetrahydrocannabinol found in naturally grown marijuana. Recreational use has been increasing, and in 2012, there were 28,531 emergency department visits for synthetic cannabinoid use, and over 40% of patients reported adverse cardiovascular effects. There have been multiple reports of myocardial ischemia by electrocardiographic changes or serum biomarkers in children and adults who have used synthetic cannabinoids. Notably, case reports of ischemic stroke in individuals with synthetic marijuana use have demonstrated acute thrombotic occlusion in the intracranial vessels, suggestive of thromboembolic events. The underlying mechanism for these clinical syndromes remains unclear, but synthetic cannabinoids have been associated with significant cardiovascular morbidity and clinicians should remain vigilant when treating patients who are at risk for using these substances.

CONCLUSION

In summary, both short-term and chronic use of common addictive substances have myriad effects on the circulatory system. The development and progression of several cardiac diseases are related to exposure to these substances, and addiction is strongly linked to poor outcomes in terms of cardiovascular health. Alcohol, nicotine, and marijuana are the most frequently encountered substances and are often used by patients with some of the most common medical conditions, including hypertension, dyslipidemia, and coronary artery disease. In addition, the use of less common substances such as opioids, amphetamines, and novel synthetic compounds exposes patients without a preexisting disease to catastrophic cardiovascular illnesses. As a result, the cardiovascular effects of addictive substances will be encountered by pediatric and adult general practitioners, addiction medicine clinicians, and specialists in nearly every field.

KEY POINTS

1. Use of illicit substances, tobacco use, and heavy alcohol use are all strongly associated with the development of common cardiovascular conditions such as hypertension, coronary artery disease, congestive heart failure, atrial fibrillation, and stroke.

2. Heavy alcohol use, tobacco use, cocaine, methamphetamines, and marijuana have all been directly implicated in deleterious cardiovascular effects, whereas opioids are primarily detrimental to cardiovascular health when administered intravenously due to a risk of endocarditis.

3. Alcohol-related cardiomyopathy and the elevated risk of coronary artery disease in the setting of tobacco use may be reversed by cessation of substance use, but ongoing use after the onset of cardiovascular disease is associated with a very poor prognosis.

REVIEW QUESTIONS

1. The most common cause of dilated cardiomyopathy in the United States is:
   A. methamphetamine use.
   B. alcohol use.
   C. ischemic heart disease.
   D. tobacco use.
   E. history of cocaine use.

2. Use of marijuana or synthetic cannabinoids like "K2" has been most strongly associated with:
   A. myocardial infarction.
   B. atrial fibrillation.
   C. congestive heart failure.
   D. stroke.
   E. diabetes mellitus.

3. There may be a "J-shaped" association between alcohol use and coronary artery disease and stroke. People who consume low-to-moderate amounts may have a reduced risk of cardiovascular events compared to the general population and those who are consume heavy amounts are at increased risk. Which of the following is at the upper limit

of daily consumption to be considered "moderate" intake for a man?
   A. 14 g, or approximately one standard drink
   B. 26 g, or approximately two standard drinks
   C. 40 g, or approximately three standard drinks
   D. 55 g, or approximately four standard drinks
   E. 90 g, or approximately six standard drinks

ANSWERS

1. **C.** Alcohol use is the second most common cause of dilated cardiomyopathy in the United States. Even in patients with a known history of alcohol use disorder, the evaluation for a new diagnosis of cardiomyopathy should involve an assessment for ischemic heart disease because alcohol may worsen hypertension and precipitate the onset of coronary artery disease.

2. **D.** Marijuana use has been implicated in the development of ischemic stroke secondary to intracranial vasospasm or altered cerebrovascular reactivity in the setting of cannabinoid exposure. There does not appear to be a significant effect on coronary artery disease aside from the known risk of chronic inhaled smoke exposure.

3. **B.** This is equivalent to approximately two standard drinks according to the National Institute on Alcohol Abuse and Alcoholism. An analysis of the Physicians Health Study cohort found that there may be reduced cardiovascular mortality in people who drink up to two drinks per day.

SUGGESTED READINGS

Fernández-Solà J. Cardiovascular risks and benefits of moderate and heavy alcohol consumption. *Nat Rev Cardiol.* 2015;12(10):576-587.

Grana R, Benowitz N, Glantz SA. E-cigarettes: a scientific review. *Circulation.* 2014;129(19):1972-1986.

Havakuk O, Rezkalla SH, Kloner RA. The cardiovascular effects of cocaine. *J Am Coll Cardiol.* 2017;70(1):101-113.

Pacher P, Steffens S, Haskó G, Schindler TH, Kunos G. Cardiovascular effects of marijuana and synthetic cannabinoids: the good, the bad, and the ugly. *Nat Rev Cardiol.* 2018;15(3):151-166.

Wurcel AG, Anderson JE, Chui KK, et al. Increasing infectious endocarditis admissions among young people who inject drugs. *Open Forum Infect Dis.* 2016;3(3):ofw157.

Liver Disorders Related to Alcohol and Other Drug Use

Summary by Paul S. Haber and Chris Tremonti

> Based on THE ASAM PRINCIPLES OF ADDICTION MEDICINE,
> 6th edition chapter by Paul S. Haber and Carl H. Freyer

The liver is commonly affected by regular or heavy alcohol or illicit drug use. This may be the result of direct toxicity, metabolic or immunologic damage initiated by drug use, or infections acquired through drug use. This chapter describes the more common examples (Table 81-1), emphasizing clinical manifestations, diagnosis, and management.

ALCOHOL-RELATED LIVER DISEASE

Alcohol-related liver disease (ALD) is a significant cause of mortality, with almost 20,000 deaths in the United States alone in 2014. Although the level of consumption is the key risk, other factors contribute to the development of ALD.

Risk Factors

- *Amount of alcohol consumed:* Population studies across Europe conclude that the greater the population level of alcohol consumption, the higher the prevalence and mortality of ALD. The risk of ALD rises continuously without a clear threshold, but most cases of ALD are associated with sustained heavy drinking, >50 g daily for several years in men, and >30 g daily for women. Even in those with intakes at these levels, only 10% develop cirrhosis. It is not seen with one-off binges.
- *Sex:* Studies suggest women are at greater risk for ALD owing to their size, body composition, and faster metabolism of alcohol. Women have reduced levels of gastric alcohol dehydrogenase, leading to increased bioavailability of alcohol, and sex hormones also appear to regulate hepatic enzymes of alcohol metabolism. Typically, women will have a higher blood alcohol level even if they consume the same amount as men.
- *Genetic factors:* There is substantial heritability in the development of alcohol use disorder, with twin studies showing approximately 50% heritability. Polymorphism of the enzymes involved

in alcohol metabolism (alcohol dehydrogenase, aldehyde dehydrogenase, and cytochrome P450 2E1) have consistently been associated with alcohol use disorders.

- *Cofactors for alcoholic liver disease*
  - *Obesity and nonalcoholic fatty liver disease:* There is both experimental and clinical evidence of an alcohol–obesity interaction in the liver. Alcohol-fed rats develop more severe liver disease if given a high fat diet. In patients who have a history of heavy alcohol consumption, a high body mass index has been associated with increased steatosis, as well as being a risk factor for the development of alcoholic hepatitis and cirrhosis.
  - *Chronic viral hepatitis:* Chronic viral hepatitis—in particular, hepatitis C—is more common in patients with alcohol use disorder, possibly due to increased prevalence of injectable drug use. Patients with a chronic hepatitis infection are also more at risk of developing fibrosis with prolonged heavy alcohol use, again particularly in patients with hepatitis C, but also in those with hepatitis B.
  - *Ingestion of hepatotoxins:* Chronic alcohol consumption can lead to increased risk of hepatotoxicity from a number of other drugs, including acetaminophen, industrial solvents, anesthetic gases, isoniazid, phenylbutazone, and illicit drugs, such as cocaine. Furthermore, patients with ALD are at a higher risk of hepatic injury secondary to acetaminophen ingestion, which can be seen even with consumption of as little as 4 g per day. That said, acute alcohol use appears to be protective in cases of acetaminophen poisoning.
- *Nutrition:* ALD is universally associated with nutritional impairment, which can both accelerate progression of the disease and also be a marker for severity of the disease. Patients with ALD can

TABLE 81-1	Associations Between Drugs and Liver Disease
Hepatic drug toxicity	• Alcohol • MDMA • Cocaine • Phencyclidine • Androgenic steroids
Toxic interactions with other drugs	• Alcohol plus MDMA • Alcohol plus cocaine • Alcohol plus acetaminophen
Systemic effect of drugs leading to liver injury	• Hyper- and hypothermia • Shock • Rhabdomyolysis
Infectious complications	• Viral hepatitis: A to D, particularly B and C • Bacteria: subacute bacterial endocarditis, septicemia
Coinjected material	• Talc (hepatic granulomas) • Lead (by-product of meth-amphetamine synthesis)
Unrelated to drugs	• Fatty liver • Focal liver diseases

MDMA, 3,4-methylenedioxymethamphetamine.

also lose regulation of vitamins including zinc and vitamin A, potentially leading to further liver damage. Protein deficiency can cause fatty liver disease, further adding to the burden of the malnourished ALD patient.

Pathogenesis of Alcohol-Related Liver Disease

The pathogenesis of ALD is multifactorial. Ethanol metabolism within the liver leads to the generation of hepatotoxic metabolites. Oxidative stress with subsequent inflammation and liver injury are recognized. This, in association with endotoxin-mediated activation of cytokine production by several cell populations within and beyond the liver, leads to activation of hepatic stellate cells and progressive fibrogenesis.

Clinical Features

ALD has three main clinicopathologic entities that often overlap and coexist in patients:

■ *Alcoholic fatty liver or steatosis* is typically asymptomatic, although patients may have anorexia, nausea, or right upper quadrant pain. The liver can be enlarged, evenly massive, but there are no signs of chronic liver disease. It can be seen in either short- or long-term heavy alcohol use but is reversible with a period of abstinence.

■ *Alcoholic hepatitis* presents with the classic symptoms and signs of hepatitis—jaundice, anorexia, fever, and right upper quadrant pain—in conjunction with heavy alcohol use. The liver is typically enlarged and tender. In more severe cases, patients may present with signs and symptoms of hepatic failure, including confusion from hepatic encephalopathy. Severe cases have a short-term mortality of around 50%. Patients with alcoholic hepatitis will have moderately elevated aspartate aminotransferase (AST) and alanine aminotransferase (ALT), with an AST:ALT ratio of 2:1. Serum bilirubin, γ-glutamyltransferase, international normalized ratio, and neutrophils will also be elevated, and the latter warrants investigation for concomitant infection. The severity of alcoholic hepatitis is usually assessed using the Maddrey Discriminant Function or the Model for End-Stage Liver Disease score; high scores predict mortality. Recovery may take many months even after abstinence has been achieved.

■ *Alcoholic cirrhosis* often presents with the complications of liver failure: portal hypertension, ascites, and variceal bleeding. Patients may also experience anorexia, weight loss, nausea, malaise, and disturbed sleep–wake cycles, the latter of which is due to hepatic encephalopathy. The clinical examination can be a treasure trove for any budding physician and can include palmar erythema, spider naevi, caput medusa, and gynecomastia. In decompensated disease, there may be jaundice, encephalopathy with or without asterixis, petechial hemorrhage, or ecchymoses and ascites. Clinicians should be mindful to look for asterixis, but it may be absent in both mild and the most severe stages of encephalopathy. Patients with alcoholic cirrhosis are at risk for hepatocellular carcinoma, and 6-monthly screening by imaging is recommended.

Diagnosis and Assessment of Severity of Alcohol-Related Liver Disease

The diagnosis of ALD requires the presence of one of the aforementioned clinical pictures combined with a history of prolonged heavy alcohol ingestion. Blood tests should include liver tests, including tests of function: bilirubin, albumin, and international normalized ratio. An ALT higher than AST or levels >500 IU/L should prompt an investigation for other causes of liver injury. The treating clinician should be vigilant to other contributors to chronic liver disease, such as drug ingestion, viral hepatitis B and C, human immunodeficiency virus (HIV), and iron overload. A full blood count may reveal thrombocytopenia secondary to portal hypertension as well as macrocytic anemia in severe cases. Other causes for liver disease should only be considered with a compatible history or when there is failure to improve with abstinence.

Imaging is not necessary to establish the diagnosis, but it can help assess severity and complications. Transient elastography (FibroScan) employs noninvasive ultrasound technology to estimate the degree of liver fibrosis and is now used routinely. Patients with cirrhosis also require an endoscopy to assess for varices.

Liver biopsies have a number of constraints, including sampling error and potential for bleeding, and is now limited to patients with a complex disease process, confounding factors in the history, or those being assessed for a transplant.

Treatment of Alcoholic Liver Disease
Treatment of Causative Factors

Abstinence from alcohol remains the mainstay treatment of ALD. Abstinence improves both survival and degree of steatosis, even in the setting of cirrhosis. Patients should be advised to stop drinking entirely. Repeat blood tests at 6 weeks should show an improvement in the patient's biochemistry, and failure to see this should prompt a thorough review of the patient's abstinence or an investigation into other causes. Although cirrhosis is irreversible, the patient's liver function may improve with resolution of decompensation. Many patients report feeling greatly improved across domains of health and vitality. Patients should also be monitored closely for possible psychological complications due to the risk of suicide.

Treatment should include a comprehensive treatment of alcohol use disorder as described elsewhere in this volume. The severity of liver disease and concurrent comorbidities influences the choice of medication. Naltrexone can be used safely in early ALD with judicious monitoring of liver function. Disulfiram, which interferes with alcohol metabolism, can also be used in compensated noncirrhotic liver disease but not in advanced liver disease because of the risk of fatal hepatotoxicity. Acamprosate has the best safety profile and has been used safely in Child–Pugh scores of A and B. Baclofen is safe in liver disease, but the efficacy is limited and this drug may be abused or taken in overdose. Topiramate may be effective in experienced hands but is not established in advanced liver disease.

Managing Acute Alcoholic Hepatitis

Abstinence, nutritional support, and treatment of alcohol withdrawal remain the mainstays of treatment for acute alcoholic hepatitis. Many clinicians have avoided steroids in the past because of the risk of infection; however, the American Association for the Study of Liver Disease currently recommends a trial of prednisolone 40 mg daily in patients with severe hepatitis, with continuation beyond 7 days based on a favorable Lille score. The effectiveness of pentoxifylline was not confirmed by a large UK trial and conflicting results have been reported using N-acetylcysteine.

Treatment of Alcohol-Induced Cirrhosis

Abstinence from alcohol is the only treatment that can alter the course of alcohol-induced cirrhosis. The management of cirrhotic complications is no different than other cirrhotic liver diseases, and will not be covered here. Liver transplantation remains an option, despite unpopular public opinion; 5-year survival rates are comparable to non–alcohol-related liver transplants. An evaluation should confirm patients have been alcohol free for at least 6 months, with adequate family and support network, and no other major substance use or mental health issues. Up to half of patients will return to drinking posttransplant, with a third of these patients developing alcohol-related harms.

VIRAL HEPATITIS
Hepatitis B Virus
Epidemiology, Transmission, and Outcome

Around 240 million people worldwide are chronically infected with hepatitis B virus (HBV). Sexual exposure and intravenous drug use are the most common causes of spread in the Western world, and the longer the duration of intravenous drug use, the greater the risk of exposure. Horizontal transmission is less common in developed countries. Those infected as adults have clearance rates of around 90% to 95%, whereas 90% of those infected by vertical transmission remain infected for life.

Clinical Features and Diagnosis

Acute hepatitis B is often subclinical. Patients may experience a transient prodrome of fever and arthralgias, followed by an acute illness of anorexia, nausea, vomiting, and jaundice. Chronic hepatitis B is associated with progressive hepatic fibrosis but is not typically symptomatic. Chronic hepatitis B, however, is more aggressive than hepatitis C, and 40% of males and 15% of females with perinatally acquired chronic HBV will eventually die of liver failure or cirrhosis.

Serologic testing should be done in all at-risk patients and in those with suggestive symptoms. The presence of HBsAg (the hepatitis B surface antigen) implies an active current infection, whereas anti-HBs (hepatitis B antibodies) suggests clearance. The presence of hepatitis B core antibodies (anti-HBc) confirms a previous infection, and its absence in those with surface antibodies indicates past immunization. All at-risk patients should be offered immunization.

Treatment

A chronic hepatitis B infection may be characterized by four phases: immune tolerance, immune clearance, immune control, and immune escape. Antiviral treatment is indicated in immune clearance and immune escape phases when ALT is abnormal and HBV DNA is raised or for those with clinical evidence of liver disease. The goals are to suppress HBV DNA, surface antigens, and HBe antigens. First-line treatments currently include tenofovir, entecavir, and pegylated interferon. Patients with cirrhosis and those at higher risk of hepatocellular carcinoma (particularly men aged 40 years and older) should also be screened with 6-monthly abdominal imaging.

Hepatitis C Virus

Epidemiology

An estimated 71 million people worldwide are infected with hepatitis C virus (HCV). Transmission is blood-borne and, in the Western world, this is mostly via injection drug use. The incidence varies but is approximately 20% for each year of injection drug use. Vertical transmission occurs in around 5% of mothers with HCV; comorbid HIV increases the risk twofold. Breastfeeding, provided there is no cracking of the nipple, is safe. Guidelines recommend testing at-risk infants at 18 months, after clearance of maternal HCV antibody. Although the screening of blood products has virtually eliminated transmission via blood donation, healthcare workers remain at risk from needlestick injuries. Transmission rates from an HCV RNA–positive needlestick injury range from 0% to 7%. Tattooing and intranasal use of cocaine are also associated with HCV transmission. Sexual transmission, however, is uncommon, with one study showing transmission among monogamous couples as low as 1 in 190,000 sexual encounters. Unlike hepatitis B, spontaneous clearance of acute HCV is low and estimated at 30% to 40% of infected patients.

Clinical Features and Diagnosis

Acute HCV infection is typically subclinical but may result in a mild hepatitis, which suggests a better immune response and higher chance of spontaneous clearance. Chronic HCV infection is also asymptomatic if there are no signs of chronic liver disease. Around 15% of patients will develop cirrhosis after 20 years of infection. The main risk factors are duration of chronic infection, age 40 years and older at the time of infection, alcohol consumption, and HIV/hepatitis B coinfection. Chronic hepatitis C also has a number of extrahepatic manifestations, including mixed cryoglobulinemia, renal disease (membranoproliferative or membranous glomerulonephritis), autoimmune thyroid disease, diabetes mellitus, and leukocytoclastic vasculitis.

At-risk patients should be screened with HCV antibodies, and if positive, be tested for HCV RNA. A positive RNA test suggests active infection, and such patients should be tested for viral load and genotyping. A positive antibody test with a negative RNA test suggests clearance of infection, but RNA testing should be repeated in 3 to 6 months for confirmation. Patients should also be assessed for the presence of hepatitis by reviewing liver function tests and fibrosis with transient elastography or another noninvasive marker.

Treatment

The development of highly efficacious and well-tolerated oral direct-acting antivirals (DAAs) has revolutionized the treatment of chronic hepatitis C, and treatment should now be considered for all patients. The World Health Organization has set a goal of HCV elimination by 2030, but few countries are on track to achieve this. The goal of DAA treatment is sustained virologic response, defined as HCV RNA clearance 12 weeks after treatment completion. This is considered a cure. Patients without cirrhosis experience resolution of fibrosis, and patients with cirrhosis can see a partial reversal of fibrosis. Once daily treatment is now available for all genotypes using a single tablet with a combination of antivirals. For retreatment in rare cases of treatment failure, the choice of DAAs depends on previous treatment, genotype, viral load, presence of cirrhosis, and resistance-associated variants. Local guidelines should be consulted because of the rapidly changing scene in HCV treatment.

Although pharmacologic treatment is now highly effective, access for many patients is limited because of stigmatization, incarceration, and social marginalization, and clinicians should be mindful of these issues. Holistic treatments should also include immunization against hepatitis A and B in at-risk patients, as well as counseling on concurrent alcohol use because these accelerate fibrosis in HCV. Treatment serves as an effective prevention strategy by reducing the infected pool and reducing further transmission. Accordingly, patients who are still injecting should be offered antiviral treatment in addition to harm reduction strategies. All patients with HCV and cirrhosis require 6-monthly screenings for HCC. Sadly, many patients still progress to advanced cirrhosis requiring transplantation, which should be considered in patients with a Model for End-Stage Liver Disease score >15. These patients should still receive DAA because HCV recurrence posttransplant is almost 100%, but caution is required on the choice of regime in decompensated patients.

Hepatitis D Virus

Hepatitis D cannot replicate without coinfection with hepatitis B because it requires HBsAg to allow entry to the hepatocyte. Coinfection with hepatitis B can be seen in patients who inject. Testing should be considered in patients with cleared hepatitis B infections that relapse and is diagnosed by rising titers of HDV immunoglobulin G or immunoglobulin M antibodies. Treatment is directed at the hepatitis B infection.

Hepatic Toxicity Associated With Other Drug Use

Both cocaine and 3,4-methylenedioxymethamphetamine (MDMA; "Ecstasy") have been associated with hepatitis and fulminant liver failure. Unexplained liver test abnormalities, particularly in young adults with hepatomegaly, should prompt inquiry into illicit drug use and a urinary drug screen. A negative drug screen may reflect a delay in presentation. Although cocaine-related hepatic injury is uncommon, it can cause fulminant hepatic failure. Typically, this is seen with systemic heat shock–like features of cocaine toxicity such as hyperthermia, rhabdomyolysis, hypoxia, and hypotension. Cocaine, a potent vasoconstrictor, is thought to cause hepatitis by ischemia. Patients will have severely deranged ALT and AST levels and liver failure.

MDMA can cause two syndromes, the first of which is similar to that of cocaine hepatitis, presenting with severe liver injury shortly after ingestion. The second syndrome presents days to weeks after ingestion with jaundice and pruritus, and may proceed to fulminant liver failure. In both cocaine and MDMA hepatitis, other differentials, including hepatitis B and C, need to be excluded before making the diagnosis. Meticulous supportive care should be employed, with rigorous rehydration and active cooling measures. Newer synthetic stimulants (eg, cathinones), phencyclidines, as well as khat, have also been linked to similar syndromes.

Benzodiazepines, opioids, and cannabis are generally considered nonhepatotoxic.

KEY POINTS

1. Hepatitis C can now be readily cured by physicians without a referral to specialists. Elimination of this infection is now a feasible goal.
2. Alcohol liver disease is still growing in prevalence and has become the most prevalent form of severe liver disease. The level of consumption is still the key determinant.
3. Abstinence remains the mainstay of treatment for alcohol liver disease.
4. Cocaine and other stimulants cause liver injury rarely, but it can be life-threatening.
5. Hepatitis C is easily treatable with direct-acting antivirals, even in patients with ongoing substance use and/or advanced liver disease.

REVIEW QUESTIONS

1. Mr. JB is a 36-year-old man who migrated to the United States from Thailand 5 years ago. He presents to the clinic with results of a routine hepatitis screen organized by his family doctor. He has no significant past medical history and takes no regular medications. He lives with his partner and three children. He drinks four standard drinks a day, has a 20-pack-year smoking history, and denies any intravenous or illicit drug use. He is currently unemployed. On examination, he has no peripheral signs of chronic liver disease, and his liver is not palpable.

   His test results are as follows:

   Complete blood count is within normal limits.
   Liver function tests are within normal limits.
   HBsAg positive, anti-HBs negative, anti-HBc positive, HBeAg negative, and anti-HBe positive
   HBV DNA: 2000 IU/mL
   Abdominal ultrasound shows normal liver span and texture with no evidence of portal hypertension.

Which one of the following statements is *not* correct?

A. He has evidence of chronic hepatitis B infection and should commence treatment. You refer him to a liver specialist.

B. He is currently in the immune control phase of chronic hepatitis B infection. You recommend yearly liver function tests and hepatitis B serologic testing. You refer him to a liver specialist for follow-up.

C. You recommend that his family also be screened for hepatitis B.

D. You discuss his alcohol intake and suggest he consider reducing the weekly intake, with two alcohol-free days a week.

E. You encourage him to consider stop smoking tobacco.

2. A 45-year-old woman presents to the clinic because she noticed that her eyes are yellow. Her body mass index is 30 and she has a history of type 2 diabetes mellitus, hypertension, and dyslipidemia. Her medications are metformin, an angiotensin-converting enzyme inhibitor, and a statin. She drinks five standard drinks a day on a week day, and more on the weekend, and has done so for the past 20 years. She is a lifelong nonsmoker and denies any illicit drug use, including intravenous drugs.

On examination, she is jaundiced, has palmar erythema, scleral icterus, and multiple spider naevi on her chest. Her abdomen is not distended, and there is no evidence of hepato/splenomegaly or ascites.

Her tests results are as follows:

Complete blood count: Hb102 (macrocytosis), white cell count: 4.0, platelets: 109

Electrolytes are within normal range.

Liver function tests:

Bilirubin: 3 mg

γ-Glutamyltransferase: 430

Alkaline phosphatase level: 110

AST: 75

ALT: 40

Albumin: 34 g/L

International normalized ratio: 1.3

Abdominal ultrasound shows evidence of cirrhosis and portal hypertension.

Which of the following statements about her diagnosis and management are correct? Select all that apply.

A. She has nonalcoholic fatty liver disease.

B. She has evidence of significant and severe liver damage.

C. She should be advised to cease alcohol altogether.

D. Her low platelets are solely due to bone marrow suppression.

E. Her liver tests reflect a degree of alcohol-related hepatitis.

F. She should immediately commence prednisolone.

G. Macrocytosis in alcohol-related liver disease is multifactorial.

ANSWERS

1. **A**
2. **B, C, E,** and **G**

SUGGESTED READINGS

Grebely J, Dore GJ. Treatment of HCV in persons who inject drugs: treatment as prevention. *Clin Liver Dis.* 2017;9(4):77-80.

Hirnschall G. Towards the elimination of hepatitis B and C by 2030: the draft WHO Global Hepatitis Strategy, 2016-2021 and global elimination targets. Presented at: World Hepatitis Summit 2015; September 2-4, 2015; Glasgow, Scotland. http://www.worldhepatitissummit.org/docs/default-source/default-document-library/2015/resources/towards-elimination-dr-gottfried-hirnschall.pdf?sfvrsn=6. Accessed November 8, 2018.

Leggio L, Lee MR. Treatment of alcohol use disorder in patients with alcoholic liver disease. *Am J Med.* 2017;130(2):124-134.

Louvet A, Mathurin P. Alcoholic liver disease: mechanisms of injury and targeted treatment. *Nat Rev Gastroenterol Hepatol.* 2015;12(4):231-242.

Thompson AJ. Australian recommendations for the management of hepatitis C virus infection: a consensus statement. *Med J Aust.* 2016;204(7):268-272.

82 Renal and Metabolic Disorders Related to Alcohol and Other Drug Use

Summary by Catreena Al Marj and Laith Al-Rabadi

Based on THE ASAM PRINCIPLES OF ADDICTION MEDICINE, 6th edition chapter by Laith Al-Rabadi, Catreena Al Marj, Girish Singhania, A. Ahsan Ejaz, and Stanley D. Crittenden

The renal complications of drugs of abuse encompass the spectrum of tubular, glomerular, interstitial, and vascular kidney diseases as well as many adverse pathophysiologic and metabolic consequences. The causal links are apparent in some cases such as human immunodeficiency virus (HIV) nephropathy, hepatitis C–associated glomerular disease, or subcutaneous injection drug-related amyloidosis. However, with other diseases such as accelerated hypertension or subtypes of focal and segmental focal glomerulosclerosis, the relationship, even if strongly suspected, has not been proven definitively. Many harmful effects of drug use are related to infectious agents inoculated during drug use or acquired owing to high-risk behavior exposures or via direct pharmacologic effects of drugs. For example, repeated bouts of intense vasoconstriction associated with cocaine use cause harmful renal and metabolic effects.

OVERVIEW OF NEPHROLOGY AND RENAL CLINICAL SYNDROMES

Injury to the kidney results in a multiplicity of signs and symptoms. Acute tubular necrosis attributed to volume depletion and rhabdomyolysis remain the most common form of acute kidney injuries seen in alcohol and other drugs like heroin, cocaine, amphetamines, methadone, and lysergic acid diethylamide. In addition, proteinuria caused by altered permeability of capillary walls, hematuria caused by rupture of capillary walls, and azotemia (elevated serum blood urea nitrogen and creatinine) caused by impaired filtration of nitrogenous wastes can also occur. These manifestations ultimately lead to oliguria (reduced urine production <500 mL per day), edema caused by decreased renal clearance of salt and water, and hypertension caused by fluid retention and disturbed renal hormonal homeostasis.

The nature and severity of disease in a given patient are dictated by the nature and severity of the underlying renal injury.

ALCOHOL

Patients who are dependent on alcohol may present with severe anion gap acidosis following a binge drinking episode, even if ethanol is no longer detectable in the serum. Ketoacidosis is induced by poor dietary intake, especially a lack of carbohydrates, and the inhibition of gluconeogenesis and acceleration of lipolysis by alcohol. The urine test results can be weakly positive or negative for ketones because, in many patients, β-hydroxybutyrate comprises most of the ketonuria. Standard tablets or dipsticks use the nitroprusside reaction, which are positive when acetone or acetoacetate is present but are negative with β-hydroxybutyrate. Therefore, a specific serum β-hydroxybutyrate should be requested.

Altered mental status and coma induced by alcohol intake can lead to immobilization and ischemic compression of muscles, causing rhabdomyolysis and subsequent acute kidney failure. Other acid–base disturbances include non–anion gap acidosis secondary to diarrhea and, occasionally, renal tubular acidosis. Decreased serum potassium levels often are seen in connection with gastrointestinal losses and secondary hyperaldosteronism. Correction of this electrolyte abnormality is important because hypokalemia can accelerate or worsen hepatic encephalopathy, in part through the enhancement of ammoniagenesis. In addition, hypokalemia (along with hypophosphatemia) increases the risk for rhabdomyolysis. The correction of hypomagnesemia is critical to allow for the repair of any renal potassium wasting.

One of the most frequent electrolyte abnormalities among people with an alcohol use disorder is hypomagnesemia. Hypomagnesemia is due to a combination of poor nutrition and gastrointestinal losses coupled with direct renal tubular alcohol toxicity, which decreases renal magnesium reabsorption. Severe hypomagnesemia should be treated with a slow intravenous infusion, whereas oral replacement can be used for therapy of milder forms of hypomagnesemia.

Hypophosphatemia often is seen in alcoholism and may contribute to rhabdomyolysis and encephalopathy.

Hepatorenal Syndrome

Chronic alcohol ingestion can lead to hepatorenal syndrome (HRS) if fulminant liver failure or cirrhosis occurs. This syndrome is thought to reflect a state of profound renal vasoconstriction and splanchnic vasodilatation associated with severely impaired liver function, often with other systemic signs of liver failure (eg, portal hypertension, esophageal varies, ascites). HRS is a diagnosis of exclusion. A slow rise in serum creatinine and oliguria, accompanied by low urinary sodium concentration (usually <10 mEq/L) are characteristics of HRS. In this instance, the urinary sediment may not be helpful because it is well known that bilirubin pigmented casts, which are indistinguishable from the "muddy brown" casts seen in acute tubular necrosis, can be found in patients with jaundice even when they have apparently normal renal function. In addition, because malnutrition and decreased muscle mass are the almost universal in these patients, the serum creatinine may be within normal limits or minimally elevated, and the blood urea nitrogen may be normal or low, whereas the glomerular filtration rate is actually markedly reduced.

HRS can develop following episodes of gastrointestinal bleeding, diuresis, or spontaneous bacterial peritonitis; however, many patients have no specific inciting event. Death is likely unless the patient is rescued by liver transplantation. However, recent studies have shown improvement in renal function and longer survival through the use of albumin, vasoconstrictor sympathomimetic agents (midodrine or terlipressin), and/or a somatostatin analogue (octreotide).

Toxic Alcohols

The ingestion of toxic alcohols—methanol, ethylene glycol, and isopropyl alcohol—is occasionally seen in patients who are dependent on alcohol who has ingested a toxic alcohol as a substitute for ethanol. The metabolic products of these alcohols (facilitated by the enzyme alcohol dehydrogenase) are severely toxic and produce organ damage and anion gap acidosis from the nonvolatile organic acids produced.

The presence of an osmolal gap (ie, the difference between the calculated and measured serum osmolality >15) should raise suspicion of toxic alcohol ingestion when no other reason for this gap is apparent, such as ethanol or mannitol use.

Calculated osmolality $= 2 \times$ (sodium mmol/L) + (glucose mg/dL) / 18 + (blood urea nitrogen mg/dL) / 2.8 + (ethanol / 3.7)

In cases of ethylene glycol ingestion, the presence of calcium oxalate crystals in the urine is highly suggestive but not diagnostic.

Fomepizole, an intravenous medication that competitively inhibits alcohol dehydrogenase more than ethanol, is a very effective treatment and safer than an ethanol infusion. As long as kidney function is maintained, the alcohol will be removed by renal excretion. With severe intoxication, hemodialysis is used to efficiently remove the alcohol and the toxic products and is useful in the treatment of the concurrent metabolic acidosis. Failure to recognize and promptly treat these alcohol intoxications can lead to multiple organ system damage and failure to the brain, liver, and kidneys, and for methanol, to blindness.

OPIOIDS

There is a high rate of viral, bacterial, and fungal contamination associated with intravenous drug use. These infections include HIV, hepatitis B and C viruses, and local pyogenic abscesses and systemic endocarditis with staphylococcal or streptococcal bacterial infections.

Nephrotic Syndromes Associated With Opioid Misuse

HIV-associated nephropathy (HIVAN) refers to the presence of a kidney disease developing in association with an HIV infection. HIVAN presents as nephrotic syndrome with progressive renal failure. African American race, low CD4 counts, and positive family history of renal disease are risk factors for the development of HIVAN. The typical patient with HIVAN presents with nephrotic-range proteinuria. The most common histologic finding is a form of focal and segmental glomerular sclerosis with collapse of the glomerular tufts, also named *collapsing focal and segmental glomerulosclerosis* (FSGS).

Ultrasound reveals normal-sized or enlarged kidneys that are hyperechoic. Renal insufficiency appears very early in the disease and is typically rapidly progressive, leading to end-stage renal disease in a matter of weeks or months. Use of angiotensin-converting enzyme inhibitors appears to decrease the magnitude of proteinuria and postpone progression, as drugs of this class do in other nephrotic syndrome diseases. The most recently identified gene protein apolipoprotein L1 (ApoL1) has been implicated in the African American predisposition to HIVAN. It seems that these mutations may also be contributed to higher rates of focal and segmental glomerulosclerosis and hypertensive end-stage renal disease in patients of African descent.

All patients presenting with nephrotic syndrome of unknown etiology should be tested for hepatitis B and C virus infections. The association between hepatitis B and membranous nephropathy is well established. It is important to diagnose this cause of membranous nephropathy because immunosuppressive treatment—often used in the idiopathic form of nephrotic syndrome—actually may enhance ongoing hepatitis B viral replication and is contraindicated. Antiviral therapy targeted at hepatitis B virus replication may prove beneficial. The most common presentation of renal disease in patients with hepatitis C is a combination of nephritic and nephrotic syndromes.

Heroin-associated nephropathy (HAN) is a form of focal and segmental glomerulosclerosis that was, at one point, the predominant cause of end-stage kidney disease in African Americans. Heroin-associated nephropathy more or less disappeared with the surge of AIDS in African Americans, and the incidence of HIVAN markedly increased. Investigators hypothesized that the availability of contaminant-free heroin may account for the disappearance of heroin-associated nephropathy.

Nephritic–Nephrotic Syndromes Associated With Opioid Misuse

In addition to significant proteinuria, the presence of hematuria, hypertension, and variable degrees of renal insufficiency in the setting of past or present injecting drug use should raise the suspicion of hepatitis C virus–related glomerular disease. The most common pattern of injury in patients with a hepatitis C infection is membranoproliferative glomerulonephritis with or without cryoglobulinemia. Less commonly, membranous nephropathy or fibrillary glomerulonephritis and immunotactoid glomerulopathy may be encountered. In cases with associated essential mixed cryoglobulinemia, serum cryoglobulins are detected. In addition, palpable purpura, arthralgias, peripheral neuropathy, and nonspecific systemic complaints may be present.

The emergence of the new direct-acting antivirals for the treatment of hepatitis C has offered the opportunity to reach sustained viral response rates exceeding 90%. Multiple all-oral interferon-free regimens based on various combinations of direct-acting antivirals were approved by the US Food and Drug Administration. Combined antiviral therapy and immunosuppression (cyclophosphamide or rituximab with steroids) may be the treatment of choice for patients with severe renal disease.

Nephritic Syndromes Associated With Opioid Misuse

The presence of a nephritic urinary sediment (proteinuria, hematuria, and often red blood cell casts), variable degrees of hypertension, and renal insufficiency in the setting of injecting drug use should raise the suspicion of immune complex–mediated postinfectious glomerulonephritis. In this circumstance, bacterial sepsis, pyogenic abscesses, and acute bacterial endocarditis are commonplace. The most frequent pathogen is *Staphylococcus aureus*. Less often, *Streptococcus viridans*, gram-negative rods, or *Candida* species are isolated. The complication of renal septic emboli is characterized by persistent fevers, gross or microscopic hematuria (occasionally accompanied by flank pain), and signs of embolization to other organs (including the brain and lungs).

COCAINE

Cocaine is an alkaloid extracted from a shrub plant (*Erythroxylum coca*). It has an estimated half-life of 30 to 90 minutes, with 80% to 90% of cocaine being metabolized. The remainder is excreted unchanged in the urine, where its metabolites can be detected for approximately 48 hours. A wide spectrum of renal complications can occur with both acute and chronic uses.

Cocaine-Related Vasculitis

Several case series have described vasculitic syndrome in the setting of cocaine use. This entity has recently been attributed to levamisole. Approximately 70% of illicit cocaine consumed in the United States was contaminated with levamisole. Levamisole is added to cocaine because it potentiates its stimulant effects. Levamisole-induced syndrome has a characteristic clinical presentation. Skin lesions are distinctive vasculopathic purpura, typically involving the ears, the nose, cheeks, and extremities. Renal manifestation is not very common. Patients usually present with hematuria, proteinuria, and worsening renal function. A kidney biopsy, if performed, shows necrotic crescentic lesions with or without immune complex formation. The spectrum of autoantibody findings is interesting. Perinuclear antineutrophil antibodies are almost always found in high titers (86% to 100%), and cytoplasmic antineutrophil antibodies are present in about 50% of the cases. Moreover, antiphospholipid antibodies and antinuclear antibodies are also often present. The ideal treatment for levamisole-induced vasculitis is not known. Nearly all cases resolve upon the cessation of cocaine use.

Acute Kidney Injury and Rhabdomyolysis Associated With Cocaine Use

Rhabdomyolysis is a common cause of acute renal failure associated with cocaine abuse. The presentation in the emergency department of a young adult with a history of illicit drug use (especially cocaine), who is agitated, confused, combative, and hyperthermic and who has a urinalysis highly suggestive of this disease (ie, brownish-red urine positive for blood but without red blood cells on microscopy), is a common scenario. In addition, blood testing usually reveals a markedly elevated serum creatine kinase level.

Drugs associated with rhabdomyolysis include cocaine, phencyclidine, methamphetamines, 3,4-methylenedioxymethamphetamine (MDMA, ecstasy), heroin, and alcohol. The presence of volume depletion, hypotension, acidosis, and hypoxemia increases the likelihood of acute tubular necrosis and rhabdomyolysis.

CLUB DRUGS

The amphetamine-type drug MDMA is also known as *ecstasy*. MDMA is rapidly absorbed, reaching plasma peak levels in approximately 2 hours. It is metabolized by the liver and excreted by the kidneys. Toxicity is mostly idiosyncratic and not related to overdose. Hence, first-time users tend to have more serious complications. Clinical manifestations associated with MDMA toxicity include hyponatremia, rhabdomyolysis, acute hyperthermia, and cardiac and neurologic injuries. MDMA induces its effect by releasing serotonin, dopamine, and norepinephrine into the central nervous system

and inhibiting reuptake of these neurotransmitters. Moreover, MDMA leads to the release of arginine vasopressin, which explains its ability to cause hyponatremia, the most common renal complication of MDMA. Hyponatremia with MDMA is at least partially dilutional, given excessive water or other hypotonic beverage intake. However, the excessive release of arginine vasopressin seems to be a major factor in impairing free water excretion. Cerebral edema can occur because of the acute fall in serum sodium leading to devastating complications such as mental status changes, seizures, and possibly coma and brainstem herniation, resulting in death. Acute kidney injuries have been described in several case reports. However, it is rare and mostly associated with nontraumatic rhabdomyolysis in the setting of hyperthermia, extreme exertion, and volume depletion. MDMA has also been reported to produce accelerated hypertension and acute kidney injury due to its marked sympathomimetic effects (much like cocaine). Therapy for acute ecstasy-induced adverse events is mostly supportive care and includes aggressive cooling, intravenous fluids, and correction of electrolytes. Severe symptomatic hyponatremia is a medical emergency, and treatment includes 100 to 200 mL of 3% saline administered as soon as possible with the goal of increasing the serum sodium concentration by 3 to 5 mEq/L, which should acutely lower intracranial pressure and improve symptoms.

"Bath salt" crystals may contain designer drugs that are derivatives of pyrrolidinopropiophenone (such as 3,4-methylenedioxypyrrovalerone) or mephedrone. These substances may promote severe renal arteriolar vasoconstriction in a manner similar to cocaine, thereby producing renal hypoperfusion and renal ischemia, resulting in acute tubular necrosis. Rhabdomyolysis also may promote kidney injury in the setting of "bath salt" intoxication. Finally, hyperuricemia can be found with acute "bath salt" intoxication. This raises the possibility of acute uric acid deposition and nephropathy contributing to the development of acute kidney injury.

INHALANTS

An unusual cause of metabolic acidosis and hypokalemia that is encountered more often in teenagers involves toluene intoxication from glue sniffing. Distal renal tubular acidosis has been described in this setting. However, the principal mechanism producing the acidosis seems to involve the increased manufacture of hippuric acid derived from toluene metabolism.

TOBACCO USE AND RENAL DISEASE

Tobacco use appears to have a deleterious effect on renal function. Cigarette smoking is related to proteinuria, accelerated atherosclerotic vascular disease, and ischemic nephropathy. In addition, increased risk of progression to renal insufficiency related to tobacco smoking has been documented in patients with diabetes mellitus and severe essential hypertension. Accelerated atherosclerotic vascular disease related to cigarette smoking is well known to contribute to the development and progression of ischemic nephropathy. Moreover, an increased risk of sustained proteinuria and poorer prognosis of renal disease have been ascribed to tobacco smoking. Idiopathic nodular glomerulosclerosis is a progressive vasculopathic lesion linked to hypertension and cigarette smoking. It is an enigmatic condition that resembles nodular diabetic nephropathy but occurs in nondiabetic patients with tobacco use and hypertension.

CANNABINOIDS

A recent report reveals that heavy marijuana consumption may be the cause of a serious illness called cannabinoid hyperemesis syndrome. There have been few case reports of acute renal failure secondary to cannabinoid hyperemesis syndrome. The unique combination of intractable vomiting and constant hot showers seems to put patients with cannabinoid hyperemesis syndrome at significant risk of severe volume depletion and prerenal failure. Patients present with abdominal pain and intractable vomiting.

Synthetic cannabinoids—a group of compounds with cannabis- or marijuana-like effects—have become more popular among young populations as recreational drugs. Synthetic cannabinoids (SCs), originally developed for research and drug development, produce effects similar to those of cannabis (ie, effects due to Δ-9-tetrahydrocannabinol [THC]). SCs are not detected by routine urine drug screenings, which make them appealing to people who may undergo random urine toxicology testing.

Acute renal injury related to the use of SCs has not become recognized until recently. Most patients present with emesis, abdominal pain, or flank pain. Urine microscopy findings were variable. Ultrasound findings range from normal to increased echogenicity. Acute tubular necrosis is the most common histologic finding. Interstitial nephritis was also present in a few cases. The pathogenesis remains elusive. Volume depletion due to nausea and vomiting causing acute tubular necrosis is one possible etiology. The potential direct nephrotoxic effects of SCs or the additives has been suggested and supported by some studies.

CONCLUSIONS

Renal disease is seen frequently in people who use alcohol, tobacco, and other drugs. As described throughout this chapter, the use of drugs both causes and exacerbates a wide spectrum of kidney diseases. The relationships between drug use and renal diseases range from causality associated with known harmful exposures believed to lead to nephrologic manifestations to the peculiar challenges of managing patients with drug-related problems and need for renal replacement therapy, which requires treatment adherence, disease insight, and self-management. In patients with injection drug use, clinicians must also consider the potential for infectious complications and complicated decision making around dialysis catheter central access.

Renal and metabolic consequences of illicit substance use are common, may be quite serious, and sometimes are difficult to diagnose and manage. Alcohol, tobacco, and other drug use must be considered in the differential diagnosis of any patient with an unexplained renal pathology. Careful collaboration between nephrology, primary care, and addiction specialists can ensure safe and effective treatment of patients with substance use disorders and acute or chronic kidney disease.

KEY POINTS

1. Patients who are dependent on alcohol may present with multiple electrolyte abnormalities. Correction of these imbalances will decrease the risk for hepatic encephalopathy and rhabdomyolysis.
2. In patients who misuse opioids, the spectrum of glomerular pathology can include nephrotic syndrome, nephritic syndrome, and nephrotic–nephritic syndrome.
3. Renal complications can occur with acute and chronic use of cocaine and include vasculitis, hypertension, rhabdomyolysis, and glomerular forms of renal injury.
4. Tobacco use is related to proteinuria, accelerated atherosclerotic vascular disease, and ischemic nephropathy. Idiopathic nodular glomerulosclerosis is a progressive vasculopathic lesion linked to hypertension and cigarette smoking.
5. Acute renal injury related to the use of SCs has not become recognized until recently.

Acute tubular necrosis is the most common histologic finding.

6. Clinical manifestations associated with MDMA toxicity include hyponatremia, rhabdomyolysis, acute hyperthermia, and cardiac and neurologic injuries.

REVIEW QUESTIONS

1. Nephrotic syndrome is characterized by:
   A. proteinuria >3.5 g per day.
   B. proteinuria <3.5 g per day.
   C. hematuria.
   D. red blood cell casts.

2. Failure to recognize alcohol intoxication can lead to multiple organ system damage and failure. Intoxication with which of the following can also cause blindness if not promptly treated?
   A. Ethylene glycol
   B. Isopropyl alcohol
   C. Methanol
   D. Ethanol

3. A 22-year-old Caucasian male with a known history of illicit drug use presents to the emergency department in an agitated, confused, and combative state. He is also found to be hyperthermic.

A urinalysis shows brownish-red urine that is positive for blood but without red blood cells on microscopy. The most likely diagnosis for this patient is:
   A. urinary tract infection.
   B. rhabdomyolysis.
   C. malignant hyperthermia.
   D. viral myositis.

ANSWERS

1. **A**
2. **C**
3. **B**

SUGGESTED READINGS

Akkina SK, Ricardo AC, Patel A, et al. Illicit drug use, hypertension, and chronic kidney disease in the US adult population. *Transl Res.* 2012;160(6):391-398.

Buettner M, Toennes SW, Buettner S, et al. Nephropathy in illicit drug abusers: a postmortem analysis. *Am J Kidney Dis.* 2014;63(6):945-953.

Cooper C, Bilbao JE, Said S, et al. Serum amyloid A renal amyloidosis in a chronic subcutaneous ("skin popping") heroin user. *J Nephropathol.* 2013;2(3):196-200.

Singh VP, Singh N, Jaggi AS. A review on renal toxicity profile of common abusive drugs. *Korean J Physiol Pharmacol.* 2013;17(4):347-357.

83 Gastrointestinal Disorders Related to Alcohol and Other Drug Use

Summary by Paul S. Haber and Chris Tremonti

Based on THE ASAM PRINCIPLES OF ADDICTION MEDICINE, 6th edition chapter by Paul S. Haber and Praveen Gounder

This chapter describes gastrointestinal (GI) effects of alcohol and drugs. Disorders of the liver are covered in Chapter 81.

GASTROINTESTINAL PROBLEMS RELATED TO ALCOHOL

Alcohol use can affect any part of the GI system from mouth to colon, but (setting aside the liver) alcoholic pancreatitis is the major clinical concern.

The Parotid Glands and Oral Cavity

Alcohol use disorder can lead to sialosis, a painless symmetrical enlargement of the parotid glands. Patients often have poor dental hygiene and oral mucosal health, characterized by glossitis and stomatitis. It is unclear whether this is due to changes in salivary flow, poor nutrition, or the direct effects of alcohol. Alcohol is a known risk factor for the development of oral cancers, which is compounded by tobacco use.

The Esophagus

Acute alcohol consumption relaxes the lower esophageal sphincter and can lead to reflux episodes. However, the link between long-term alcohol use and gastroesophageal reflux disease appears much weaker and requires high amounts of consumption. Mallory-Weiss syndrome, a condition in which tears in the gastric mucosa at the cardioesophageal junction leads to hematemesis, is commonly seen in patients vomiting and retching following alcohol binges.

The Stomach

Gastritis—inflammation of the gastric mucosa—can be seen with exposure of the stomach to 20% alcohol. However, alcohol gastritis can be a difficult entity to define because of confounding factors that may be causing inflammation, in particular, *Helicobacter pylori* infection. *H. pylori* eradication may prove more effective in patients with "alcohol gastritis" than abstinence. There is a relationship between alcohol and peptic ulcer disease. Gastric hemorrhage, erosive lesions and ulceration are also commonly seen in people admitted for alcohol use disorder.

The Pancreas

Acute Pancreatitis

Acute pancreatitis refers to an acute inflammatory process of the pancreas. Alcohol remains the most common cause of acute pancreatitis in males and second most common in females after gallstones. Clinical severity ranges from mild and self-limited to severe, with local and systemic complications, organ failure, and potentially death.

Risk Factors and Pathogenesis

Several mechanisms have been postulated as to why alcohol causes pancreatic injury. Extrahepatic metabolism of alcohol in the pancreas leads to the production of reactive oxygen species and other toxic metabolites, including nonoxidative alcohol metabolites. These lead to premature activation of pancreatic enzymes and in turn to autodigestion. Tobacco appears to be a cofactor for developing alcoholic pancreatitis.

Clinical Features, Investigations, and Diagnosis

Patients typically present with pain in the upper abdomen that radiates through to the back and is exacerbated by eating. The diagnosis of pancreatitis requires two of three criteria: (1) abdominal pain consistent with pancreatitis (persistent, severe epigastric pain of acute onset, often radiating to the back), (2) serum lipase (or amylase) levels three times the upper limit of normal, and (3) computed tomography (or, less commonly, magnetic resonance imaging or transabdominal ultrasound) findings characteristic of pancreatitis. Clinically acute pancreatitis is also associated with acute phase changes on blood tests.

Regardless of alcohol history, gallstone pancreatitis must be excluded by ultrasound examination. Patients with gallstone pancreatitis require urgent endoscopic retrograde cholangiopancreatography with endoscopic sphincterotomy if there is biliary sepsis, biliary obstruction, or worsening or persistent jaundice. Note that patients on methadone and other opioids can develop dilated common bile ducts without gallstones.

Chronic Pancreatitis

Chronic pancreatitis features chronic inflammation, glandular atrophy, and fibrosis. Patients typically present with pain accompanied by either exocrine insufficiency, endocrine insufficiency, or both. This can manifest as steatorrhoea, weight loss, deficiency of fat-soluble vitamins, or diabetes mellitus. Fecal elastase-1 may be a useful screening test.

Risk Factors and Pathogenesis

Chronic excessive alcohol intake accounts for three quarters of cases of chronic pancreatitis, but it remains unclear why some patients are more affected than others. Several genetic factors, including differences in alcohol dehydrogenase, have been studied. Recurrent episodes of acute pancreatitis can lead to chronic pancreatitis, and use of tobacco can also accelerate this process.

Clinical Features

Patients typically present with pain accompanied by either exocrine insufficiency, endocrine insufficiency, or both. Fecal elastase-1 may be a useful screening test.

Treatment

Complete abstinence from alcohol is essential to minimize progression of the disease, and this may help to control pain. Analgesia management is complex. Opioids should not be withheld if nonopioid medications are insufficient, but clinicians must be wary of potential substance misuse. Antidepressants and pregabalin may also be effective at providing pain relief but again are at risk of misuse. Recent studies have shown some role for antioxidants in older patients and those with alcohol-related pancreatitis. Randomized trials have also shown some analgesic benefit with early endoscopic or surgical intervention.

The Small Intestine

Patients who drink excessively often develop both acute and chronic diarrhea secondary to altered motility and poor nutrition. Acute alcohol intake can also cause increased gut permeability, leading to abnormal absorption of luminal content and leakage of mucosal contents (such as albumin). Patients commonly develop folate deficiency, which also causes intestinal injury and further exacerbates malabsorption and diarrhea.

The Colon

Alcohol can cause nonulcerative inflammatory changes in the human colonic epithelium that are reversible with abstinence.

Alcohol and Gastrointestinal Cancer

Alcohol use is a recognized risk factor for several GI neoplasms, including tumors of the tongue, mouth, pharynx, larynx, esophagus, stomach, pancreas, colon, and liver. Surprisingly, the risk is even increased with small daily amounts of alcohol intake, which is within the guidelines of many Western countries. That said, alcohol is typically a "cocarcinogen," which worsens the exposure to other carcinogens, rather than being a complete carcinogen itself. For example, alcohol is a known risk factor for hepatocellular carcinoma, but it is unclear if it is a direct hepatic carcinogen independent of the development of cirrhosis from alcoholic liver disease. Nonetheless, the risk appears to be dose related and is exacerbated by tobacco. Concurrent use of alcohol and tobacco confers an almost 40-fold risk for esophageal and oropharyngeal cancers.

GASTROINTESTINAL SYMPTOMS ASSOCIATED WITH OPIOIDS

Opioids, including heroin, are known to reduce bowel function through the blockade of propulsive peristalsis, inhibition of secretion of intestinal fluids, and increased fluid absorption, even at low doses. Because of this, most patients using opioids will experience symptoms of reduced GI motility, such as constipation, bloating, early satiety, and pain. Narcotic bowel syndrome is now a recognized phenomenon with significant pain secondary to ileus and opioid-induced hyperalgesia. The degree of GI symptoms will vary depending on the opioid used and its route of administration. Bowel symptoms usually respond to increased fluid intake and fiber supplementation to correct for poor dietary intake.

Laxatives are not often required, but osmotic agents such as lactulose are the laxatives of choice. Both methylnaltrexone and alvimopan, peripherally acting opioid-receptor antagonists, are available for opioid-induced constipation, but their use is not widespread.

LAXATIVE MISUSE AND GASTROINTESTINAL SYMPTOMS

Unexplained chronic diarrhea can be caused by surreptitious laxative misuse. It can be associated with bulimia or seen in older patients as a form of Munchausen syndrome. The diagnosis rests on identification of laxatives by stool alkalinization, osmolality studies, or a bag search in the hospital.

MISUSE OF ANTICHOLINERGICS AND GASTROINTESTINAL SYMPTOMS

Misuse of anticholinergic drugs such as amitriptyline and other tricyclic depressants can lead to constipation, abdominal pain, and dry mouth.

EFFECTS OF TOBACCO ON GASTROINTESTINAL FUNCTION

The Upper Gastrointestinal Tract

Tobacco smoking is linked to exacerbations of reflux symptoms. Nicotine lowers esophageal sphincter pressure and causes reflux in response to straining during coughing and deep breathing. Smoking cessation is recommended for the treatment of reflux, although cessation alone does not usually resolve the symptoms. There is also a dose-related link between tobacco and peptic ulcer disease because tobacco increases the risk of peptic ulcer complications and ulcer-related mortality and delays ulcer healing. Patients who smoke tobacco also have a threefold increased risk of pancreatic cancer. The evidence is less clear cut for pancreatitis, but it still seems appropriate to advise patients that quitting smoking will reduce the risk of recurrence.

The Lower Gastrointestinal Tract

Inflammatory Bowel Disease

A curious relationship exists between tobacco smoking and inflammatory bowel disease. Smoking has consistently been shown to increase the risk of Crohn's disease but decrease the risk of ulcerative colitis. The severity of ulcerative colitis has been shown to worsen in patients who stop smoking. Smoking may also increase the risk of recurrence of Crohn's disease. Tobacco smoke appears to interfere with epithelial integrity and immune responses to pathogenic bacteria, but research in this area is ongoing.

Nicotine may have therapeutic potential for ulcerative colitis. Nicotine influences immune cellular function, increases mucin production, relaxes colonic smooth muscle, increases endogenous glucocorticoids, and influences rectal blood flow and intestinal permeability. Nicotine-based therapy has been explored using strategies including topical colonic administration of nicotine that avoids exposure to tobacco smoke. A Cochrane review of transdermal nicotine patches for the treatment of mild-to-moderate ulcerative colitis suggested that these agents can improve ulcerative colitis compared to placebo but have significant adverse events and have not been shown to be more effective than other treatments.

Gastrointestinal Malignancy

Tobacco smoking has been strongly linked to cancers of the upper aerodigestive tract and pancreas as discussed previously. The link between smoking and stomach cancer is weaker but is present in most studies.

GASTROINTESTINAL PROBLEMS ASSOCIATED WITH PSYCHOSTIMULANTS (COCAINE AND AMPHETAMINES)

Cocaine may lead to ischemic injury to the gut, leading to intestinal perforation, infarction, or ischemic colitis. Young people subjected to prolonged hypotension or hypoxia after an opioid overdose may develop ischemic infarction to the gut. These uncommon injuries typically present with abdominal pain and peritonitis but may be occult in a critically ill and unconscious person.

GASTROINTESTINAL PROBLEMS ASSOCIATED WITH CANNABIS

Cannabinoid receptors are widely expressed throughout both the upper and lower GI tract and are also expressed on hepatic stellate cells. Consequently, cannabinoids may influence a range of GI functions in health and disease. Nausea and vomiting are side effects of many chemotherapeutics and reduce the quality of life of patients with diabetes, cancer, and HIV and AIDS. Cannabis and other cannabinoids appear to be effective antiemetics. Dronabinol has been approved by the US Food and Drug Administration for refractory chemotherapy-induced nausea and vomiting, and other cannabinoid regimens are under study. The antiemetic effect has been demonstrated in an animal model and is related to the expression of CB1 receptors in the dorsal vagal nucleus.

Paradoxically, cannabis has also been linked to a series of cases with hyperemesis. This syndrome is now well recognized, although the mechanism is not understood. Cannabis hyperemesis syndrome should be considered in the differential diagnosis of patients with intractable vomiting and/or compulsive hot water bathing. Cessation of cannabis, as confirmed by a negative urine drug screen for cannabinoids, led to the cessation of the cyclical vomiting illness and a return to regular cannabis use heralded a return of the hyperemesis weeks to months later. Several pharmacologic approaches have been tried including benzodiazepines, haloperidol, and capsaicin, but evidence is limited to case reports. Capsaicin activates the transient receptor potential vanilloid-1 receptor as does heat, suggesting a link with relief from hot showers. Capsaicin cream (typically 0.025% to 0.075% applied to the abdomen or back) is increasingly being used in the emergency department setting, notwithstanding the absence of controlled trials, as it may allow safe discharge from the hospital, although side effects include heat and burning at the application site.

"BODY PACKING" AND GASTROINTESTINAL CONCERNS

Persons smuggling illicit drugs may ingest packages containing large amounts of cocaine, heroin, or other drugs, aiming to retrieve them after reaching their destination. This is referred to as body packing, cocaine packing, or body stuffing syndrome. Multiple packages made from latex condoms, wax, or plastic bags are used and may also be placed into the rectum or vagina. Hospitals close to international airports may encounter these cases, and some have developed a management policy for this challenging problem. These patients may present with life-threatening symptoms of intoxication, including seizures and cardiorespiratory collapse, as well as mechanical obstruction from the ingested drug packets. Lethal drug absorption through rubber condoms may occur without rupture.

Clinical monitoring comprises frequent clinical and neurologic assessments and daily abdominal examinations to detect complications of acute drug intoxication, bowel obstruction, or perforation. The patient should be kept in the hospital until all drug packages have cleared due to the risk of life-threatening overdose if a rupture occurs. Plain abdominal x-rays are helpful and can be repeated daily until the gut is cleared, typically in 3 to 6 days. Dilute contrast has been reported to assist in the identification of the packages. In some cases, computed tomography is required. Symptomatic cases may require early surgery. With the sophisticated packaging now commonly used by drug smugglers, an endoscopy may be safe when performed in a highly controlled setting, especially when a packet is available to test its strength against the snare. Asymptomatic patients are candidates for endoscopy if whole bowel irrigation has failed or is otherwise contraindicated.

KEY POINTS

1. Alcohol remains a leading cause of acute pancreatitis, which ranges in severity from mild and self-limiting to severe with organ failure and death.
2. Alcohol is responsible for over three quarters of cases of chronic pancreatitis, which can lead to complex pain management problems as well as exocrine and endocrine insufficiency.
3. Tobacco smoking is related to both gastroesophageal reflux disease and peptic ulcer disease.
4. Cannabis is being extensively researched for use in nausea; however, it may also be a cause of cannabis hyperemesis syndrome.
5. Both tobacco smoking and alcohol are risk factors for a number of GI malignancies.

REVIEW QUESTIONS

1. Which of the following is not a cause of constipation?
   A. Morphine
   B. Advanced age
   C. Dehydration
   D. Colorectal cancer
   E. Male gender

2. Which of the following cancers is not associated with alcohol use?
   A. Primary brain cancer
   B. Mouth cancer
   C. Stomach cancer
   D. Pancreatic cancer
   E. Esophagus cancer

3. A 32-year-old female with severe opioid dependence is now stable on methadone maintenance treatment but complains of troublesome constipation. The most appropriate management would be:
   A. detoxification from methadone.
   B. reduce methadone dose until constipation improves.

C. decreased fluid intake.
D. regular laxative use.
E. switch to buprenorphine.

ANSWERS

1. **E**
2. **A**
3. **D**

SUGGESTED READINGS

Kleeff J, Whitcomb DC, Shimosegawa T, et al. Chronic pancreatitis. *Nat Rev Dis Primers.* 2017;3:17060.

National Cancer Institute. Alcohol and cancer risk. https://www.cancer.gov/about-cancer/causes-prevention/risk/alcohol/alcohol-fact-sheet. Reviewed June 24, 2013. Accessed March 15, 2018.

Ness-Jensen E, Lagergren J. Tobacco smoking, alcohol consumption and gastro-oesophageal reflux disease. *Best Pract Res Clin Gastroenterol.* 2017;31(5):501-508.

84

CHAPTER

Respiratory Tract Disorders and Selected Critical Care Considerations Related to Alcohol and Other Drug Use

Summary by Joseph Lurio

> Based on THE ASAM PRINCIPLES OF ADDICTION MEDICINE, 6th edition chapter by Drew A. Harris, Jason J. Heavner, and Kathleen M. Akgün

The respiratory tract is a unique interface between the body and the environment—the lungs contain the largest surface area of the body that is exposed to the external environment. A variety of addictive drugs present acute and chronic insults to the respiratory system and can overwhelm the capacity for recovery. Inhalation, injection, or ingestion of addictive drugs can have adverse effects within the airways, lung parenchyma, and pulmonary vascular bed. Respiratory complications also may arise indirectly from the effects of drugs on the central nervous system (CNS), cardiovascular system, and immune system.

RESPIRATORY FUNCTION

The respiratory tract contains and excludes foreign materials, provides an interface for immune sampling of antigens, and provides a large surface area for absorption of inhaled substances and drugs. The respiratory tract also detoxifies and metabolizes proteins, drugs, and other potentially injurious substances. Drugs of abuse can derange these critical, interrelated functions of the respiratory tract and lungs. Because respiration is under extensive neural control in the CNS, it is susceptible to the effects of CNS depressants and stimulants. Addictive drugs may affect the lung through direct local inflammation, increased susceptibility to infections, airway reactivity, impairment of pulmonary vascular integrity, acute lung injury, structural injury, and derangements of gas exchange. Polysubstance use is associated with a variety of injuries, making it difficult to ascribe a particular respiratory complication to a single agent. Coexisting pulmonary pathology may worsen the acute and chronic physiologic effects of an addictive drug on the lungs.

COMMON PULMONARY COMPLICATIONS

Respiratory Depression

With the exception of nicotine, cocaine, and amphetamines/stimulants, all of the drugs discussed in this chapter inhibit respiration, causing respiratory depression or respiratory failure. Besides hypoventilation, gag and cough reflexes may be depressed, resulting in aspiration pneumonitis.

Atelectasis

In patients with respiratory depression, shallow respirations result in decreased functional residual capacity, which contributes to airway closure in dependent regions of the lung during expiration. Ineffective cough and aspirated oral and gastric secretions, with loss of surfactant, contribute to the development of atelectasis. Unventilated areas distal to closed airways maintain perfusion, resulting in shunting and subsequent hypoxemia.

Aspiration Syndromes

The risk of aspirating oropharyngeal or gastric contents into the lower respiratory tract increases with decreasing levels of consciousness. The common aspiration syndromes include aspiration pneumonitis, aspiration pneumonia, airway obstruction, and diffuse aspiration bronchiolitis.

Respiratory Infections

Chronic users of addictive drugs are susceptible to a variety of respiratory infections. Persons who use drugs are at risk of direct infection from injecting, inhaling, or snorting substances contaminated with pathogens. The types of respiratory infections in people who use drugs include sinusitis, acute bronchitis, community-acquired and aspiration pneumonias, septic emboli, fungal infection, and mycobacterial infections.

Respiratory Complications of Contaminants

Illicit drugs vary greatly in purity. Adulterants—pharmacologically active substances used to increase quantities of the drug of interest or enhance drug delivery—are frequently identified in illicit drugs. Commonly used adulterants include mannitol and other sugars, cellulose, and talc, as well as other drugs such as phenobarbital, fentanyl, methaqualone, caffeine, procaine, noscapine, and levamisole. Additionally, drugs can be contaminated with manufacturing by-products such as lead, aluminum, and glass. The lungs act as a filter, trapping inhaled or injected foreign substances, which may incite local inflammatory or fibrotic responses. *Bacillus* and *Clostridium* species have been found to be the most common microbiologic contaminants of intravenous drugs, whereas *Aspergillus* contamination of marijuana (both illicit and medicinal) has been reported, causing pneumonitis in immunocompromised individuals.

Respiratory Complications of Injected Drugs

Opiates, stimulants, and combinations thereof are commonly injected into the veins. The resulting pulmonary complications may be acute or chronic. Acute problems are likely to be severe, including respiratory failure and acute pulmonary edema. Chronic pulmonary problems include the development of interstitial and bullous lung disease, endovascular and respiratory infections, pulmonary hypertension, tuberculosis, and cancer. Talc granulomatosis can develop when talc (magnesium silicate) is used as a filler in medications such as buprenorphine, oxycodone, and methylphenidate. A syndrome similar to sarcoidosis may result, with insidious onset of granulomatous interstitial fibrosis. Dyspnea, particularly with exertion, and cough are the most common symptoms.

Pulmonary Hypertension

People who use intravenous drugs may develop chronic pulmonary hypertension from multiple mechanisms, including chronic hypoxemia related to interstitial lung disease and vasoconstriction; pulmonary embolization of particulate matter from crushed tablets used for injection; pulmonary arterial thrombosis at sites of foreign body granulomatosis; thromboembolic disease; and pulmonary arterial hypertension from the drug itself (eg, cocaine) or from an adulterant.

Septic Thromboemboli and Drug or Needle Embolization

Septic pulmonary embolism is a common pulmonary complication among those who use intravenous drugs and may result from tricuspid endocarditis or from infected injection site thrombophlebitis. Occasionally, needles may break off inadvertently during injection, or entire needles may embolize if left in place after injection.

Other Complications of Injected Drugs

Pneumothorax, empyema, mycotic aneurysms of the pulmonary vasculature, hemothorax, and bullous emphysema may also develop in those who use intravenous drugs.

Respiratory Complications of Inhaled Drugs

Inhalation of talc or other fibrogenic substances may lead to the development of granulomatous inflammation or fibrosis. Smoke consists of gas and particulate phases, including carbon monoxide, oxidants, aldehydes, alcohols, nitrosamines, benzene derivatives, and other inorganic and organic substances, many of which cause mucosal injury and inflammation. Inhaled drugs may also cause chronic bronchitis, emphysema, bronchospasm, hemoptysis, and asphyxiation. Barotrauma can result from maneuvers to increase drug delivery by hyperinflating the lung (ie, "shotgunning").

TOBACCO AND NICOTINE

Within the lung, smoking has profound effects, altering the immunologic and structural milieu. Cigarette smoke contains more than 4500 components, which are associated with a high rate of lung cancer, chronic obstructive pulmonary disease, bronchitis, and airway reactivity. Smoking is also associated with acute and chronic lower respiratory tract infections (bronchitis and pneumonia) and obstructive and restrictive lung diseases. People who smoke have a more rapid decline in forced expiratory volume in 1 second than do those who do not smoke, which may lead to symptoms such as dyspnea on exertion and fatigue. Chronic airflow obstruction is common and, when associated with persistent hypoxemia, may lead to pulmonary hypertension, cor pulmonale, and right heart failure. Smoking may also cause interstitial lung disease. Finally, smoking can cause spontaneous pneumothorax, hemoptysis, hypersensitivity pneumonitis, and lipoid pneumonia.

MARIJUANA

Smoking marijuana results in inhaling three times more tar than in cigarettes, causing a fivefold higher carboxyhemoglobin level in the blood than cigarettes. Although earlier studies have conflicting results, more recent data suggest that long-term marijuana use is associated with an increased risk of lung cancer. Heavy marijuana use is also associated with laryngeal cancer. People who smoke marijuana may suffer some of the same complications as those who smoke tobacco, including chronic obstructive pulmonary disease and bullous emphysema. Pathogens such as *Aspergillus* can contaminate marijuana (including medical grade batches), potentially resulting in pulmonary infection as well as hypersensitivity pneumonitis.

COCAINE

Cocaine crosses the blood–brain barrier and stimulates the CNS where, in addition to the well-known effects on the limbic system, it can increase the respiratory rate. Approximately 20% to 30% of the inhaled dose actually reaches the lung. Freebasing is the practice of using volatile solvents to convert cocaine from a salt to a base and to remove adulterants. This potentially incendiary chemical process can lead to extensive cutaneous and inhalational burns. Use of volatile solvents has largely been supplanted by freebase obtained by treating cocaine hydrochloride with bicarbonate of soda ($NaHCO_3$). The final freebase product is highly potent and has a rapid onset of action and, therefore, is more likely to induce pulmonary, cardiac, neurologic, and other complications. Smoked cocaine may induce lung injury through vasoconstriction, by impairing the integrity of the pulmonary capillary bed, and by effects on the pulmonary vasculature (ie, "crack lung"). Barotrauma is common with crack cocaine inhalation and is associated with prolonged and forceful deep inhalation. A variety of upper airway complications are associated with inhaled cocaine, including mucosal irritation or inflammation, resulting in perforation of the nasal septum, sinusitis, and epiglottitis. Cocaine inhalation, but not injection, causes measurable and clinically significant bronchospasm in asthmatic as well nonasthmatic, nonatopic individuals. Cocaine can also cause alveolar hemorrhage. Additionally, 70% of cocaine in the United States is contaminated with levamisole—an anthelmintic agent. Levamisole-contaminated cocaine is

associated with an antineutrophil cytoplasmic antibody-mediated vasculitis. Finally, cocaine can cause both noncardiogenic and cardiogenic pulmonary edema, drug-induced pulmonary artery vasoconstriction and subsequent pulmonary infarction, and "crack lung"—a self-limited eosinophilic hypersensitivity pneumonitis.

AMPHETAMINES AND OTHER STIMULANTS

Effects of amphetamines are predominantly cardiovascular and neurologic. Amphetamines were used in the early part of the last century to treat respiratory illness because of their sympathomimetic effects and can induce some bronchodilation and vasoconstriction. Amphetamines have adverse effects on the immune system, including a decrease in CD4 T-helper cells and an increase in immunosuppressive cytokines. Such changes may adversely affect the delayed hypersensitivity response to microbial pathogens. Extreme agitation and hyperthermia during amphetamine intoxication may result in rhabdomyolysis and severe metabolic acidosis, which is associated with an increased respiratory drive. A direct central effect also may increase respiratory drive. Pneumomediastinum, subcutaneous emphysema, and retropharyngeal emphysema have been reported with the use of inhaled 3,4-methylenedioxymethamphetamine (ie, "ecstasy"). Finally, amphetamines can cause noncardiogenic pulmonary edemas and pulmonary hypertension.

CAFFEINE

Caffeine, a phosphodiesterase inhibitor and an adenosine and benzodiazepine receptor antagonist that raises intracellular cyclic adenosine monophosphate, has pulmonary effects that are similar to theophylline, including smooth muscle relaxation and mild bronchodilator properties. Caffeine may also falsely elevate the serum theophylline level. Pulmonary complications are rare and usually are associated with a large overdose or unintentional ingestion by children. Respiratory alkalosis, chest pain, seizures, aspiration, respiratory failure, and pulmonary edema associated with cardiac arrhythmias may occur.

OPIOIDS

Opioids have their most dramatic effects on the respiratory system by acting on the CNS. Opioids binding to μ_2 receptors cause a reduction in responsiveness to carbon dioxide and depresses the pontine and medullary centers that regulate respiratory automaticity and cough. Opioids may induce respiratory complications indirectly through the CNS and also have effects on airways, pulmonary vasculature, and the immune system. Opioids induce histamine release from mast cells, which may lead to pulmonary vein constriction, increased pulmonary capillary permeability and pulmonary edema, and bronchoconstriction. In addition, chronic opioid use is associated with increased rates of central and obstructive sleep apnea. Finally, intranasal heroin has been reported to cause hypersensitivity pneumonitis.

ALCOHOL

Alcohol ingestion may cause acute intoxication accompanied by respiratory depression and common pulmonary complications including atelectasis, hypoxemia, respiratory failure, respiratory acidosis, aspiration pneumonia, and acute respiratory distress syndrome (ARDS). Alcohol may cause metabolic acidosis from alcoholic ketoacidosis, with resultant compensatory respiratory alkalosis. The consumption of other toxic alcohols, including isopropanol, ethylene glycol, and methanol, continues to be a public health issue. Patients presenting with alcohol intoxication and high anion gap metabolic acidosis should be evaluated for the presence of an unexplained osmolar gap, which increases the concern for a coingestion. Among patients with cirrhosis, chronic respiratory alkalosis is common, even in the absence of metabolic acidosis. This condition may be due to the respiratory stimulant effect of poorly cleared progesterone and estradiol on the CNS. Patients with asthma may experience a worsening of asthma symptoms after the consumption of alcohol, particularly those who are histamine sensitive. Additionally, alcohol use is associated with adult-onset asthma.

Cirrhosis with ascites may lead to pleural effusions. Massive ascites, with or without hepatic hydrothorax, may restrict diaphragmatic and pulmonary excursion, leading to rapid shallow breathing, dyspnea, atelectasis, and hypoxemia in severe cases. Hepatopulmonary syndrome affects 15% to 30% of patients with cirrhosis and consists of portal hypertension, intrapulmonary microvascular vasodilatation, and an increased alveolar–arterial oxygen gradient with hypoxemia in patients with cirrhosis. A liver transplant reverses hepatopulmonary syndrome. Alcohol also causes pulmonary arterial hypertension, although the pathogenesis of this complication is not clear. Individuals who chronically abuse alcohol are twice as likely to develop ARDS and to die from ARDS once it develops. Chronic alcohol abusers with sepsis are more likely to develop ARDS and are at increased risk for transfusion-related acute lung injury.

SEDATIVE–HYPNOTICS

Sedative–hypnotic drugs may exert significant respiratory depressant effects when abused or when mixed with alcohol and opiates. Benzodiazepines, barbiturates, γ-hydroxybutyrate, and zolpidem bind γ-aminobutyric acid receptors, which normally function as targets for inhibitory neurotransmitters and promote sedation, hypnosis, anxiolysis, anterograde amnesia, and anticonvulsant activity. Adverse respiratory effects are mainly related to respiratory depression from overdose. Benzodiazepines can worsen sleep-disordered breathing by decreasing the tone of the upper airway muscles, resulting in increased obstructive events. Increased central apneas and reduced ventilatory response to carbon dioxide also lead to worse nocturnal hypoxemia.

VOLATILE SUBSTANCES

The abuse of inhalants is highly prevalent throughout the world (although overall use is decreasing), particularly among teenagers. Volatile substances are aromatic and include short-chain hydrocarbons, such as toluene, gasoline, butane, butyl and amyl nitrites, and organofluorines, which are found in adhesives, paints, paint thinners, dry cleaning fluids, refrigerants, and propellants. When sniffed or vigorously inhaled within a hermetic container ("huffed"), these are readily absorbed in the lungs. Intoxicating or euphoric as well as dysphoric effects follow within seconds. Pulmonary complications include severe respiratory depression, barotrauma (pneumomediastinum), persistent cough, noncardiogenic pulmonary edema, and asphyxiation. Butyl and isobutyl nitrites may cause methemoglobinemia, which manifests as cyanosis with low oxygen saturation of hemoglobin but with normal partial pressure of oxygen. CO-oximetry will specifically measure methemoglobin levels. Intravenous methylene blue may be administered for treatment. Metabolic acidosis may occur, with compensatory respiratory alkalosis resulting from distal renal tubular acidosis or from increased anion gap acidosis. Nitrates and other inhalants may be directly irritating to the airway mucosa, which can cause chronic cough. Finally, people who use inhalants may develop asphyxiation from plastic bag suffocation, respiratory depression, displacement of oxygen in the inspired air, and acute noncardiogenic pulmonary edema.

NITROUS OXIDE

Nitrous oxide is a widely used inhalational anesthetic–analgesic agent, which also is used in a variety of commercial products (such as a propellant for whipped cream chargers). Pulmonary complications include pneumomediastinum, respiratory depression, and hypoxemia because of displacement of oxygen, leading to asphyxiation. Treatment is supportive, including supplemental oxygen and respiratory support.

ANABOLIC STEROIDS

Anabolic steroids induce a prothrombotic state and may cause pulmonary embolism, strokes, and other forms of thrombosis. Other respiratory complications are less common but may occur after a stroke and include atelectasis, pneumonia, aspiration, neurogenic pulmonary edema, and sleep-disordered breathing.

KEY POINTS

1. A variety of addictive drugs present acute and chronic insults to the respiratory system and can overwhelm the capacity for recovery.
2. Inhalation, injection, or ingestion of addictive drugs can have adverse effects within the airways, lung parenchyma, and pulmonary vascular bed.
3. With the exception of nicotine, cocaine, and amphetamines/stimulants, all of the drugs discussed in this chapter inhibit respiration, causing respiratory depression or respiratory failure.

REVIEW QUESTIONS

1. Which of the following is a common side effect of amphetamine intoxication?
   A. Increased respiratory rate
   B. Decreased respiratory rate
   C. Hypoxemia
   D. Respiratory acidosis
   E. None of the above.

2. Which of the following substances is *most* harmful to the respiratory system?
   A. Cocaine
   B. Sedative–hypnotics
   C. Tobacco
   D. Cannabis
   E. Amphetamines

3. Which of the following substances is a frequent contaminant of cocaine?
   A. Thimerosal
   B. Levamisole
   C. Methimazole
   D. Clotrimazole

ANSWERS

1. **A**
2. **C**
3. **B**

SUGGESTED READINGS

Brugman S, Irvin C. Lung structure and function. In: Mitchell RS, Petty T, Schwartz M, eds. *Synopsis of Clinical Pulmonary Disease.* 4th ed. St. Louis, MO: Mosby, 1998:1-17.

Global Initiative for Asthma. Global strategy for asthma management and prevention. Updated 2018. https://ginasthma.org/2018-gina-report-global-strategy-for-asthma-management-and-prevention/. Accessed November 20, 2018.

Global Initiative for Chronic Obstructive Lung Disease. Global strategy for the diagnosis, management, and prevention of chronic obstructive pulmonary disease. 2018 report. https://goldcopd.org/wp-content/uploads/2017/11/GOLD-2018-v6.0-FINAL-revised-20-Nov_WMS.pdf. Accessed November 20, 2018.

West JB. *Respiratory Physiology: The Essentials.* 8th ed. Baltimore: Lippincott Williams & Wilkins, 2008.

Wilson KC, Saukkonen JJ. Acute respiratory failure from abused substances. *J Intensive Care Med.* 2004;19(4):183-193.

Neurological Disorders Related to Alcohol and Other Drug Use

Summary by Emmanuelle A.D. Schindler and Jason J. Sico

Based on THE ASAM PRINCIPLES OF ADDICTION MEDICINE, 6th edition chapter by Emmanuelle A.D. Schindler, Monica M. Diaz, Brian C. Mac Grory, Brian B. Koo, Darren C. Volpe, Hamada Hamid Altalib, Huned S. Patwa, and Jason J. Sico

Alcohol and many drugs of abuse may affect different levels of the neuraxis, including the brain, spinal cord, peripheral nervous system, and muscles. Effects may be both acute and chronic.

TRAUMA AND TRAUMATIC BRAIN INJURY

When trauma occurs, acute intoxication may be partly responsible and may mask the extent of neurologic injury. In traumatic brain injury (TBI), contusions, intracranial hemorrhage, and/or extracranial hematomas can occur. Surgical intervention(s) may be complicated among those who chronically use alcohol who have platelet and clotting factor dysfunction. A TBI can acutely cause changes in mentation as well as a postconcussion syndrome, which includes vertigo, nausea, vomiting, headaches, photophobia, phonophobia, and difficulties with vision. Longer term TBIs may cause chronic headaches, epilepsy, aberrations in sleep, and neurobehavioral and neurocognitive changes. Spinal cord injuries (eg, contusion, transection, vascular compromise) most commonly occur in the cervical region. Symptoms may include weakness in the arms and/or legs, sensory loss in the extremities or perianal region, and genitourinary and bowel dysfunction. Trauma may also cause injury to a peripheral nerve or nerves, plexus, or individual nerve root. For patients who may have been immobile for an extended period (which may occur with drug use), compartment syndrome must be considered.

HEADACHE
Alcohol and Other Sedative–Hypnotics

The common "hangover" headache involves multiple systems: vascular, inflammatory, and endocrine.

Headaches that arise from alcohol withdrawal likely stem from cerebrovascular dysfunction and pain hypersensitivity. Those with alcoholic cirrhosis are at risk for intracranial hemorrhage, which can either present as a focal or holocranial headache. Frequent use of butalbital-containing medications is highly correlated with chronification of headaches. Benzodiazepines may offer an indirect benefit by addressing comorbid anxiety, insomnia, somatoform symptoms, or neck pain.

Caffeine

Caffeine has reasonable efficacy in headache treatment and is standard treatment for headaches acquired after dural puncture. When consumption becomes chronic, headaches can occur due to withdrawal.

Cocaine, Amphetamines, and Methylenedioxymethamphetamine

Cocaine-induced headaches can occur immediately, in delayed fashion (hours), or in times of withdrawal. Patients report using cocaine as an abortive for migraine or cluster headache attacks. In general, stimulant drugs can cause intracranial hemorrhage or vasculopathy, which present with headache.

Heroin and Opioids

Heroin intoxication or withdrawal can produce headaches. Concerning patterns of dependence and addiction can emerge when opioids are used on an outpatient basis for headache management. As an exception, it is widely accepted to use opioids in patients with cancer-related head and face pain.

Other Substances

Headache prevalence is positively correlated with both active and passive cigarette smoking. Patients with cluster headache are stereotypically heavy smokers, although smoking habits largely do not affect the disorder. The effect of relaxation induced by cannabis may play into its reported efficacy in treating headaches. In regular users, the withdrawal from cannabinoid products can result in rebound headaches. The use of nabilone, a synthetic cannabinoid, has demonstrated efficacy in one trial for the treatment refractory medication overuse headaches. Hallucinogens, such as lysergic acid diethylamide (LSD) and psilocybin, can induce headaches of different types. There are anecdotal reports of lasting therapeutic effects with limited exposure to hallucinogens in both migraine and cluster headaches. Ketamine has been shown to reduce the duration and/or severity of migraine auras.

NEUROBEHAVIORAL AND COGNITIVE DISORDERS

Alcohol and Other Sedative–Hypnotics

Wernicke encephalopathy, caused by a thiamine deficiency, involves neurobehavioral symptoms, abnormal eye movements, and ataxia. Without the administration of intravenous thiamine, there is a progression to coma and death. With early thiamine treatment, recovery can be complete, but if delayed, patients may develop Korsakoff syndrome, an irreversible condition characterized by impaired memory, retrograde amnesia, and confabulation. Pellagra is caused by nicotinic acid deficiency and results in dermatitis, gastroenteritis, and neurobehavioral/cognitive symptoms. With prompt nicotinic acid replacement, recovery can occur over hours or days, but pellagra is fatal if untreated. Marchiafava–Bignami disease is a rare alcohol-related condition involving demyelination and necrosis of the corpus callosum, presenting predominantly with psychiatric symptoms, and which may end fatally if untreated. Alcohol-related dementia refers to progressive global cognitive decline that is gradual in onset. Neuropsychological testing shows cognitive impairment in 50% to 70% of people who drink heavily. Barbiturates and benzodiazepines can produce mental clouding or paradoxical hyperactivity in older adults. Long-term benzodiazepine treatment leads to cognitive dysfunction.

Cocaine, Amphetamines, and Methylenedioxymethamphetamine

Cocaine acutely causes hyperalertness, psychomotor agitation, pressured speech, sense of well-being, and elation. Chronic cocaine users have significant impairments in executive function, attention span, and memory; this cognitive dysfunction may stem from widespread microvascular lesions. Acutely, amphetamine-based stimulants cause effects similar to cocaine; chronically, they damage dopaminergic and serotonergic nerve terminals, which impacts mood, attention, memory, and learning.

Cannabis and Synthetic Cannabinoids

Acute effects of cannabis include a sense of well-being, mild euphoria, and relaxation, although dysphoria, depression, or a delusional syndrome may rarely occur. Deficits in attention, memory, and sense of time may also be seen. Chronic cannabis use has been associated with broad neuropsychological impairments.

Heroin and Opioids

Opioids cause a sense of relaxation and a state of euphoria. Heroin users demonstrate visual memory impairment and impulsive and risky decision making. Prescription opioid dependence also impairs decision making and strategic planning.

Other Substances

Hallucinogens (eg, LSD, psilocybin) produce profound changes in perception, mood, and cognition acutely, although panic attacks and psychotic reactions (in susceptible individuals) may also occur. Hallucinogens alone have not been found to cause permanent cognitive alteration. Acutely, phencyclidine produces schizophrenia-like symptoms, and permanent neuropsychiatric change has been claimed. Toluene, found in many solvents, paints, and glues, is associated with white matter lesions and can result in dementia as well as pyramidal, cerebellar, and oculomotor signs. Inhalation of gasoline containing tetraethyl lead can result in lead encephalopathy.

SEIZURES

Alcohol and Other Sedative–Hypnotic Agents

Most alcohol-related seizures are due either to withdrawal or neurologic injury comorbid with chronic alcoholism, such as TBI or infection. In chronic users, withdrawal seizures occur 6 to 48 hours after the last drink. Alcohol withdrawal seizures are typically generalized tonic–clonic (grand mal) seizures, with up to 10% resulting in status epilepticus. Most alcohol-related seizures occur singly or in brief clusters, and thus, treatment with an anticonvulsant (other than benzodiazepines) is not advised.

Seizures in people with benzodiazepine and barbiturate use disorders occur most often as a withdrawal phenomenon.

Cocaine, Amphetamines, and Methylenedioxymethamphetamine

New-onset seizures from cocaine most often follow intravenous administration of cocaine hydrochloride or smoking of alkaloidal "crack." Seizures occur immediately or within a few hours of administration; delayed seizures might be related to the proconvulsant cocaine metabolite, benzoylecgonine. Seizures with amphetamine-like psychostimulants usually occur concurrently with associated signs of agitation, psychosis, fever, hypertension, and cardiac arrhythmia. Hyponatremia resulting from excessive fluid intake is most commonly associated with methylenedioxymethamphetamine-related seizures.

Heroin and Opioids

Heroin is an independent risk factor for a first-time seizure. Anecdotal reports of opioid medication toxicity leading to seizure have been described with fentanyl, pentazocine, and propoxyphene. Meperidine readily causes seizures and myoclonus through the proconvulsant properties of its metabolite, normeperidine.

Other Substances

Cannabidiol is approved for adjunctive therapy in two medically refractory seizure disorders—Dravet and Lennox-Gastaut syndromes. Phencyclidine at high doses can cause seizures and myoclonus; such cases are accompanied by other signs of overdose, such as marked hyperthermia, myoglobinuria, respiratory depression, and hypertension. Seizures are not expected with hallucinogens but can occur at very high doses. Seizures accompanied by hallucinations are features that point to intoxication with inhalants as opposed to hallucinogens or alcohol. Seizures may also accompany severe anticholinergic poisoning.

STROKE

Tobacco and Nicotine

Cigarette smoking increases the risk of every type of stroke. Smoking leads to accelerated atherosclerosis, acute and chronic elevations in blood pressure, elevated fibrinogen levels, arterial wall damage, platelet dysfunction, and inhibition of prostacyclin formation. Smokeless tobacco has also been demonstrated to increase the risk of acute ischemic stroke.

Alcohol

Heavy alcohol use increases the relative risk of stroke, whereas light-to-moderate consumption may be protective. Alcohol use is associated with several factors that contribute to stroke, including cardiovascular, endocrine, and hematologic functions.

Cocaine, Amphetamines, and Methylenedioxymethamphetamine

Stroke associated with cocaine use has a tendency to occur in the first 6 hours after use of the drug and is more common when smoked. Cocaine's relationship with strokes is largely related to its vasoconstrictive and prothrombotic properties. Similar to cocaine, amphetamine-like drugs increase sympathetic tone and are associated with strokes.

Opioids and Cannabinoids

Ischemic and hemorrhagic strokes have been described in the setting of heroin use and may occur in the absence of other risk factors. Most cases of cannabis-related strokes occur shortly after exposure. Cannabis has been associated with cardiac arrhythmias, systemic hypotension, impaired cerebral autoregulation, and intracranial vasculopathy and vasospasm.

Other Substances

Ischemic strokes have been reported up to several days after use of LSD, which can cause vasoconstriction in systemic and cerebral arteries. Cerebral infarction, intracerebral and subarachnoid hemorrhage, and hypertensive encephalopathy have followed the use of phencyclidine, which can cause systemic hypertension lasting hours or days. Stroke has also been reported in users of anabolic–androgenic steroids without any concomitant risk factors.

NEUROMUSCULAR (NERVE, MUSCLE, AND SPINAL CORD) DISORDERS

Alcohol

Acute alcohol myopathy presents with myalgias, weakness, and elevation of creatine kinase. Chronic, heavy alcohol use is associated with a painless, progressive proximal weakness; cardiomyopathy; and peripheral neuropathy (motor, sensory, and/or autonomic).

Heroin and Opioids

Intravenous use of heroin has been associated with neuropathies attributed to compression, muscle edema, and immune mechanisms (eg, Guillain-Barré syndrome). Myopathy and acute transverse myelitis have also been seen in individuals who use heroin.

Inhalants

n-Hexane exposure can lead to "glue-sniffer's neuropathy," a severe sensorimotor polyneuropathy that can evolve to an incompletely reversible quadriplegia. Nitrous oxide use can result in a myelopathy similar to that caused by vitamin B_{12} deficiency.

Other Substances

Rhabdomyolysis has been reported after the use of cocaine, amphetamines, heroin, phencyclidine, marijuana, and LSD. Cocaine has rarely been associated with mononeuritis multiplex from presumed vascular insult.

MOVEMENT DISORDERS
Alcohol

An alcohol-induced cerebellar tremor is an intentional tremor that is worse when touching distant objects and typically manifests gradually with long-standing alcohol use. In alcoholic liver failure, asterixis ("negative myoclonus") involves jerking movements resulting from transient loss of muscle tone when maintaining a posture. Alcohol withdrawal tremor is coarse, irregular, and seen best distally in the hands. It occurs acutely during the first 1 to 2 days following abstinence and is responsive to benzodiazepines, baclofen, and β-blockers. Transient parkinsonian symptoms, choreiform movements, and dyskinesias have also been reported in alcohol withdrawal after chronic use. Alcohol can improve the symptoms of an essential tremor and autosomal dominantly inherited myoclonus-dystonia.

Cocaine, Amphetamines, and Methylenedioxymethamphetamine

Cocaine and amphetamine-like drugs may result in a number of de novo hyperkinetic movement disorders as well as an exacerbation of preexisting conditions. Repeated exposure to cocaine depletes dopamine, the clinical correlate to depression and parkinsonism.

Heroin and Opioids

Opioid intoxication and withdrawal states have been associated with myoclonus, which is responsive to benzodiazepine therapy. When heroin pyrolysate is heated on an aluminum base and inhaled ("chasing the dragon"), a cerebral and cerebellar spongiform leukoencephalopathy can develop, presenting with various neurologic symptoms, including choreoathetoid movements, parkinsonism, quadriparesis, dementia, and death. A toxic by-product of opioid production, 1-methyl-4-phenyl-1,2,3,6-tetrahydropyridine, can lead to acute levodopa-responsive parkinsonism.

Cannabis

With cannabis use, several case reports describe a transient amelioration of symptoms in various movement disorders, such as Huntington disease and Tourette syndrome, although clinical trials have failed to demonstrate significant clinical improvement.

NEUROLOGIC COMPLICATIONS OF INFECTIOUS DISEASES

Neurologic complications of HIV involve opportunistic central nervous system (CNS) infection (eg, toxoplasmosis, cryptococcal meningitis/cryptococcomas, progressive multifocal leukoencephalopathy), malignancies (eg, primary CNS lymphoma), stroke, peripheral neuropathy, and HIV–associated neurocognitive disorder. Parenteral drug use also subjects patients to an array of local and systemic infections with neurologic consequences. Endocarditis can lead to meningitis, cerebral infarction, diffuse vasculitis, cerebral or spinal abscess, or subarachnoid hemorrhage. Infectious hepatitis can cause encephalopathy or precipitate a hemorrhage due to deranged clotting. Vertebral osteomyelitis can cause radiculopathy or spinal cord compression.

Coexisting intoxication, withdrawal, and nutritional and metabolic anomalies must not detract from the consideration of a CNS infection. *Clostridium tetanus* spores can migrate from the skin to the CNS, leading to tetanus, manifesting with trismus (lockjaw), opisthotonos, risus sardonicus (facial muscle spasms leading to a sardonic smile), and dysautonomia. Botulism begins at injection sites and in the nasal sinuses and presents with bilateral symmetric cranial neuropathies and symmetrical descending weakness of the upper extremities without sensory deficits. Malaria transmission has been reported with intravenous drug use in endemic areas. Cerebral malaria causes cerebral edema leading to elevated intracranial pressure, encephalopathy, seizures, and possibly coma and death. A *Candida* CNS infection is uncommon but can occur in intravenous drug users with neutropenia. Endophthalmitis, cerebral abscesses, vascular thrombosis, and subarachnoid hemorrhages from a ruptured mycotic aneurysm can occur.

High-risk sexual behavior associated with intravenous drug use increases the risk for syphilis. Neurosyphilis is divided into early (meningitis, cranial neuropathies, strokes, gummas) and late (tables dorsalis, dementia) stages. Human T-cell lymphotropic virus type I/II is a retrovirus that can be transmitted intravenously and sexually and causes a chronic and progressive spinal disease characterized by hyperreflexia, spasticity, clonus, lower extremity weakness, and a neurogenic bladder and/or bowel.

KEY POINTS

1. Alcohol and other substances can cause acute and chronic manifestations with intoxication, longstanding use, or withdrawal states anywhere along the neuraxis.
2. Alcohol and illicit substances can affect several parts of the nervous system simultaneously; this is especially true in patients who are acutely intoxicated.
3. In younger persons with neurologic dysfunction, including new-onset stroke, seizure, or movement disorders, history and laboratory investigations should include use of alcohol and illicit substances.

REVIEW QUESTIONS

1. Which of the following substances is *least* associated with new-onset seizures?
   A. LSD
   B. Cocaine
   C. Marijuana
   D. Alcohol

2. A patient admitted for alcohol withdrawal has tenderness over the temple without neck stiffness. There is no papilledema. A magnetic resonance imaging scan shows a stable, chronic subdural hematoma without evidence of brain contusion. What is the etiology of this patient's headache?
   A. Subdural hematoma
   B. Subarachnoid hemorrhage
   C. Postconcussive syndrome
   D. Increased intracranial pressure
   E. Carotid dissection

3. A patient with severe alcohol use disorder sees you for weakness and myalgias. On examination, he has moderate symmetric weakness of the proximal muscles in the arms and legs with normal tone. Sensation to pinprick is mildly decreased in the feet; he has no spinal sensory level to pinprick. Creatinine kinase is elevated at 1,050 U/L. What is the most likely cause of his weakness?
   A. Alcohol myopathy
   B. Cervical radiculopathy
   C. Compressive neuropathy
   D. Right parietal lobe stroke

4. Concerns of dependence and addiction limit the use of opioids in the treatment of headache *except* for which condition?
   A. Migraine headaches
   B. Cluster headaches
   C. Tension-type headaches
   D. Headaches secondary to cerebral metastatic disease

ANSWERS

1. **C**
2. **C**
3. **A**
4. **D**

SUGGESTED READINGS

Brust J. *Neurological Aspects of Substance Abuse*. 2nd ed. Boston: Butterworth- Heinemann, 2004.

Brust JCM. Stroke and substance abuse. In: Mohr JP, Wolf PA, Grotta JC, et al, eds. *Stroke: Pathophysiology, Diagnosis, and Management*. 5th ed. Philadelphia: Elsevier Saunders, 2011:790-813.

Martin PR, Adinoff B, Weingartner H, Mukherjee AB, Eckardt MJ. Alcoholic organic brain disease: nosology and pathophysiologic mechanisms. *Prog Neuropsychopharmacol Biol Psychiatry*. 1986;10(2):147-164.

Mukamal KJ, Kuller LH, Fitzpatrick AL, et al. Prospective study of alcohol consumption and risk of dementia in older adults. *JAMA*. 2003;289(11):1405–1413.

Silver JM, McAllister TW, Yudofsky SC, eds. *Textbook of Traumatic Brain Injury*. 2nd ed. Washington, DC: American Psychiatric Publishing, 2011.

Human Immunodeficiency Virus, Tuberculosis, and Other Infectious Diseases Related to Alcohol and Other Drug Use

Summary by Carol A. Sulis and Simeon D. Kimmel

Based on THE ASAM PRINCIPLES OF ADDICTION MEDICINE, 6th edition chapter by Carol A. Sulis and Simeon D. Kimmel

Acute infections account for 60% of hospital admissions among people who inject drugs (PWID) in the United States each year and complicate a substantial proportion of admissions among other drug users. Cellulitis, cutaneous abscesses, endocarditis, hepatitis, pneumonia, and tuberculosis have been common problems for decades; AIDS and infection with type II human T-cell lymphotropic virus are more recent problems.

HOST DEFENSES

Among PWID, infection and colonization with resistant organisms follow a breach of skin and mucosal barriers. Repeated injection of nonsterile materials leads to a polyclonal elevation of immunoglobulin that can cause diagnostic confusion in PWID who develop autoantibodies such as rheumatoid factor or who have a biologic false-positive test for syphilis or hepatitis C. People who smoke have defective mucociliary function and are predisposed to sinopulmonary infections caused by encapsulated organisms such as *Streptococcus pneumoniae* or *Klebsiella pneumoniae*. Various immunomodulatory effects of alcohol have been postulated but not proven and are influenced by the type and amount of alcohol ingested, genetic factors, and other comorbidities.

SKIN AND SOFT TISSUE INFECTIONS

Skin and soft tissue infections are common among PWID. The type of infection (cellulitis, abscess, or ulcer), location and severity, and causative organisms usually are related to the duration and site of injection and local epidemiology. *Staphylococcus aureus* and streptococci are the organisms most often seen.

Since 1999, there has been a dramatic increase in the incidence of methicillin-resistant *S. aureus* infections. Risk factors for acquisition include use of alcohol, methamphetamines, and injection drugs. The mainstay of therapy is incision and drainage of abscesses, judicious use of appropriate antibiotics, and meticulous hygiene.

PWID who mix their drugs with saliva or who lick their needles before injecting may develop polymicrobial infections with viridans streptococci, *Haemophilus* spp., *Eikenella corrodens*, and oral anaerobes. Repeated injection of vasoactive opiates can cause ischemic necrosis at the injection site, rendering the damaged areas susceptible to superinfection. Both inhalation and injection of cocaine cause vasospasm with resulting areas of tissue necrosis serving as a nidus for infection. Streptococcal infection in areas of cocaine-induced tissue ischemia can cause large necrotic ulcers with extensive tissue loss.

GINGIVITIS

Acute necrotizing ulcerative gingivitis (trench mouth, Vincent angina) is characterized by severe pain, gingival necrosis, and bleeding. Patients have fever, malaise, and fetid breath. Development of acute necrotizing ulcerative gingivitis appears to be associated with smoking, stress, immunosuppression, and poor oral hygiene. Treatment may include use of antiseptic mouthwash, systemic antibiotics such as penicillin or clindamycin, or débridement.

ENDOCARDITIS

Infective endocarditis (IE) is the most common cardiac complication of injection drug use. Most cases of IE in PWID occur in structurally normal valves, and more than 50% is caused by *S. aureus*, of which variable proportions are methicillin resistant. The resulting lesion, called a vegetation, is composed of layers of platelets and fibrin covering clumps of relatively sequestered microorganisms. Most vegetations are located on heart valves but can occur on any endothelial surface. The sustained bacteremia that characterizes IE occurs when microorganisms are released as the vegetation fragments. The size of the vegetation is related to the type of pathogen. Underlying alcohol use disorder is identified as a risk factor in 40% of episodes of pneumococcal endocarditis, and concurrent meningitis is present in 70% of this subgroup of patients.

Clinical features include fever accompanied by a panoply of cardiac abnormalities (murmur, conduction delay, congestive heart failure, and valvular dysfunction), complications from emboli or from metastatic seeding of other structures during bacteremia (causing meningitis, brain abscess, osteomyelitis, or splenic abscess), and a wide spectrum of immune complex–mediated phenomena (arthritis, glomerulonephritis, aseptic meningitis, Osler nodes, Roth spots, splinter hemorrhages, and other manifestations of vasculitis). The most reliable clues are the presence of embolic phenomena and visualization of vegetations on echocardiography. Empiric therapy should be targeted to the most likely pathogens and adjusted once blood culture results become available. Initial therapy with an antistaphylococcal antibiotic is appropriate for most PWID; use of vancomycin should be considered in areas with a high prevalence of methicillin-resistant *S. aureus* or penicillin-resistant pneumococcus. Most patients require a minimum of 4 weeks of intravenous antibiotics. Left-sided endocarditis is associated with a worse prognosis, as is infection with gram-negative bacilli or fungi. Heart failure is the leading cause of death. After cure, patients remain at a substantially increased risk of reinfection, and injection drug use is the most common risk factor. Concurrent treatment of addiction with methadone, buprenorphine, or naltrexone may improve adherence to the initial antibiotic regimen and reduce the risk of reinfection. Patients should follow American Heart Association guidelines and be given prophylactic antibiotics when undergoing certain invasive dental procedures.

NONCARDIAC VASCULAR INFECTIONS

Direct injury to blood vessels during injection drug use and vasospasm from cocaine use are associated with endothelial injury and thrombus formation. Bacterial seeding of the thrombus can cause septic thrombophlebitis. The predominant pathogen is *S. aureus*; however, gram-negative bacilli (especially *Pseudomonas aeruginosa*) are reported with increased frequency in PWID. Management of septic thrombophlebitis generally includes both intravenous antibiotics and short-term anticoagulation.

RESPIRATORY INFECTIONS

Cigarette smoke disrupts mucociliary function and macrophage activation. Alteration in the level of consciousness accompanied by a depressed gag reflex compromises airway protection and permits aspiration of oropharyngeal flora. Alcohol use disorder is associated with oropharyngeal colonization with enteric gram-negative bacilli and abnormal phagocyte function. Injection drug use is associated with a large number of insults, including drug-induced bronchospasm, pulmonary edema, and the development of various types of foreign-body granuloma from contaminants in injected materials. Pneumonia, both aspiration and community acquired, is present in up to one third of PWID evaluated for fever and complicates a variable percentage of admissions for treatment of alcohol withdrawal or cocaine intoxication. Lung abscesses can complicate aspiration pneumonia, necrotizing bacterial pneumonia, or septic emboli.

Four to 6% of the US population has a latent tuberculosis infection. PWID and people with alcohol use disorder have an increased incidence of reactivation tuberculosis. Infection is spread by the aerosolization of acid-fast bacilli in respiratory secretions. Directly observed therapy is strongly encouraged when nonadherence is anticipated and is preferred for patients with risk factors such as homelessness or addictive disorders. Rifampin can reduce methadone levels, and patients often require adjustment of their maintenance dose. Patients with underlying hepatitis or who use hepatotoxins such as alcohol have an increased risk of developing hepatitis when using isoniazid, rifampin, or pyrazinamide and should be monitored

HEPATIC AND GASTROINTESTINAL INFECTIONS

Hepatic cirrhosis results from an irreversible injury to the hepatic parenchyma and is most often caused by alcohol use disorder or viral hepatitis. Infection is the leading cause of death in patients with cirrhosis. Gram-negative enteric bacilli such as *Escherichia coli* and *K. pneumoniae* and encapsulated respiratory pathogens such as *S. pneumoniae* are the most frequent causes of infection in these patients; however, severe infections with many other organisms have been described. Spontaneous bacterial peritonitis is a common and potentially fatal infectious complication in patients with cirrhosis and ascites. Pathogenesis involves translocation of bacteria from the gut to mesenteric lymph nodes and is associated with deficiencies in humoral response and phagocytic function.

NERVOUS SYSTEM INFECTIONS

Manifestations of central nervous system infections are easily missed if symptoms are mistakenly attributed to intoxication or withdrawal. Delirium, acute confusional states, encephalopathy, or coma may accompany overdose, intoxication, infection, or a large number of noninfectious etiologies. Clinical features should guide diagnostic strategies, with management based on lumbar puncture and neuroradiologic imaging results. Endocarditis is the most common cause of central nervous system symptoms in PWID and can cause meningitis (aseptic or purulent), brain abscesses from septic emboli, or hemorrhage from a mycotic aneurysm rupture.

Contamination of skin ulcers with spores of *Clostridium* spp. can cause neurologic symptoms from the elaboration of neurotoxins. Wound botulism is caused by contamination of injection sites or skin ulcers with *Clostridium botulinum*. Toxin causes a descending, symmetric, flaccid paralysis. Over the past 15 years, there has been a dramatic increase in reported cases among people who injected black tar heroin—the dark, gummy substance derived from crude preparations of opium that may be contaminated by spore-containing adulterants such as dirt.

HIV AND AIDS

Among US adults with known risk factors who were diagnosed with HIV in 2015, 6% reported injection drug use and another 3% reported sex with a PWID. This is a 48% decrease in HIV diagnosis among PWID compared with 2008. However, increasing rates of injection drug use, riskier injection practices, and riskier sexual practices while using drugs threaten these gains. A primary HIV infection should be considered in any patient with a history of potential exposure and compatible symptoms. Various guidelines describe when to begin antiretroviral therapy, what drugs to initiate, when and how to change therapy, and appropriate laboratory monitoring and screening tests. Additional guidelines provide disease-specific recommendations for the use of primary or secondary prophylaxis for the prevention of opportunistic infections. Immunizations for hepatitis A and B, influenza, and pneumococcus should be administered as needed.

Drug–drug or drug–food interactions can profoundly affect the absorption and efficacy of certain medications. For example, methadone levels can be significantly decreased when given with certain protease inhibitors (ritonavir, nelfinavir, or lopinavir) and nonnucleoside reverse transcriptase inhibitors (efavirenz, etravirine), and often require an increase in methadone maintenance dosage. Use of maintenance methadone can have variable effects. Methadone decreases the level of some nucleoside reverse transcriptase inhibitors (abacavir), requiring an increase in antiretroviral dosage, and increases the level of others (zidovudine), requiring a decreased dosage. Atazanavir may cause an increase in buprenorphine levels and result in sedation or mental status changes, although this is less likely if used with a boosted protease inhibitor. In contrast, limited data suggest that buprenorphine needs no dosage adjustment and is less likely to be associated with adverse events when given with active antiretroviral regimens that include efavirenz or an integrase inhibitor. Overdoses due to interactions between 3,4-methylenedioxymethamphetamine (MDMA, ecstasy) or γ-hydroxybutyrate and protease inhibitors have been reported.

SEXUALLY TRANSMITTED DISEASES

Although the prevalence of sexually transmitted diseases is higher in people who use drugs, the presentation, diagnosis, and management of most sexually transmitted diseases are not profoundly influenced by drug use. One exception is that the diagnosis and treatment of syphilis in PWID may be confounded by an increased prevalence of biologic false-positive nontreponemal screening tests such as venereal disease research laboratory or rapid plasma reagin tests for syphilis.

KEY POINTS

1. Infectious complications in people who use drugs are more frequent, more difficult to diagnose, and more challenging to treat than similar infections in people who do not use drugs.
2. IE is the most common cardiac complication of injection drug use.
3. PWID and people with alcohol use disorder have an increased incidence of reactivation tuberculosis. Smoking can increase transmission.

REVIEW QUESTIONS

1. A 24-year-old patient who uses injecting drugs presents with chills and fever. On exam, he is hypotensive and tachycardic and has a 4/6 systolic ejection murmur. What is the most likely diagnosis?
   A. Endocarditis
   B. Toxic shock from a group A beta-hemolytic streptococcal infection
   C. Spontaneous bacterial peritonitis
   D. Anthrax

2. A 45-year-old homeless patient with alcohol use disorder is admitted with 3 months of fever, night sweats, bloody cough, and 20-pound weight loss. What should you do first?
   A. Place the patient in airborne infection isolation and obtain a chest x-ray.
   B. Obtain a tuberculin skin test or interferon γ release assay.
   C. Obtain 3 sputum acid-fast bacilli smears.
   D. Treat with antibiotics.
   E. Test for HIV.

3. A 60-year-old patient with newly diagnosed HIV is brought in with fever and confusion. He was started on antiretroviral therapy 2 weeks prior. What should you do first?
   A. Perform a lumbar puncture.
   B. Stop any antiretroviral drugs that could be causing confusion.
   C. Check CD4 and viral load.
   D. Perform a head computed tomography scan.
   E. Give steroids.

ANSWERS

1. **A**
2. **A**
3. **D**

SUGGESTED READINGS

Darouiche RO. Spinal epidural abscess. *N Engl J Med.* 2006;355(19):2012-2020.

Levine D, Brown P, eds. Infections of intravenous drug abusers. *Infect Dis Clin North Am.* 2002;16:535-792.

Li JS, Sexton DJ, Mick N, et al. Proposed modifications to the Duke Criteria for the diagnosis of infective endocarditis. *Clin Infect Dis.* 2000;30(4):633-638.

Rao N, Ziran BH, Lipsky BA. Treating osteomyelitis: antibiotics and surgery. *Plast Reconstr Surg.* 2011;127 (suppl 1):177S-187S.

Wilson W, Taubert KA, Gewitz M, et al. Prevention of infective endocarditis: guidelines from the American Heart Association: a guideline from the American Heart Association Rheumatic Fever, Endocarditis, and Kawasaki Disease Committee, Council on Cardiovascular Disease in the Young, and the Council on Clinical Cardiology, Council on Cardiovascular Surgery and Anesthesia, and the Quality of Care and Outcomes Research Interdisciplinary Working Group. *Circulation.* 2007;116(15):1736-1754.

87 Sleep Disorders Related to Alcohol and Other Drug Use

Summary by Sanford Auerbach and Yelena Gorfinkel Pyatkevich

Based on THE ASAM PRINCIPLES OF ADDICTION MEDICINE,
6th edition chapter by Sanford Auerbach and
Yelena Gorfinkel Pyatkevich

OVERVIEW OF SLEEP

Sleep is essential for normal human function. Wakefulness (lack of sleepiness), vigilance, and performance on monotonous tasks deteriorate after a single sleepless night. "Sleep need" is difficult to define but usually is accepted as the amount of sleep required for optimal function during wakeful periods. Sleep need varies in individuals from 3 to 10 hours of sleep over a 24-hour period. Self-reports of sleep time often are subject to both overestimates and underestimates. It is clear that objective measures of sleep and sleepiness are critical to the study of sleep and the effects of alcohol on sleep. The nocturnal polysomnogram (PSG) is the standard method of determining the presence and stage of sleep. Similarly, the multiple sleep latency test is a standard and accepted measure of daytime sleepiness; it employs a PSG while a patient is allowed to take naps on five separate occasions throughout a day.

Sleep Architecture

Sleep is a dynamic process, featuring fluctuations in brain wave activity, muscle tone, eye movement, and autonomic activity. It consists of two discrete states: rapid eye movement (REM) and non–rapid eye movement (NREM) sleep. Each can be defined in physiologic terms by using the elements of the PSG: electroencephalogram, electrooculogram, and electromyogram.

Sleep Rhythms

The components of sleep do not occur randomly throughout the course of the night. In fact, a clear pattern emerges from the ultradian or short rhythms of sleep. The "light" stages of NREM are seen first. These are followed by a transition to slow-wave sleep (SWS), followed by lighter stages of NREM again, and then REM sleep. Typically, there are three to four NREM–REM cycles, each

lasting 90 to 120 minutes. More importantly, sleep–wake rhythms follow a circadian or approximately 24-hour biologic pattern. The sleep–wake cycle is considered a circadian rhythm that is tightly synchronized with circadian variations in core body temperature. Although individuals may have different periodicities in their clocks ("larks" and "owls"), there are many factors that maintain or influence these rhythms. Although activity levels, social cues, mealtimes, and other external scheduling factors play some role, the most powerful zeitgeber ("time-giver"; ie, environmental circadian time cues) has proved to be exogenous light.

DISORDERS OF SLEEP
Restless Legs Syndrome

Restless legs syndrome (RLS) is estimated to be present in 5% to 15% of the general population. It affects both sexes and has been described in both children and adults. The usual presentation includes an urge to move, usually accompanied by uncomfortable sensations. Symptoms tend to be worse when the individual is inactive, especially in the evening when preparing for sleep. Movement may relieve the symptoms for a brief period of time. Uremia, anemia, iron deficiency, and neuropathies have been implicated in many so-called secondary cases. RLS may also be aggravated or triggered by the use of several medications, including antidepressants, lithium carbonate, neuroleptics, and caffeine. The most commonly used medications are dopaminergic drugs (ropinirole, pramipexole, rotigotine) and calcium channel α 2-δ ligands (gabapentin, pregabalin, gabapentin enacarbil). Success has also been demonstrated with benzodiazepines, other anticonvulsants, opioids, and others such as clonidine. Opioids are of particular interest. Some patients report that they began to use opioids on a regular basis when they received them for an unrelated disorder and realized that they were able to sleep for the first time in years.

Obstructive Sleep Apnea

Obstructive sleep apnea (OSA) is a common syndrome characterized by repetitive episodes of sleep-related upper airway obstructions, which usually are associated with oxygen desaturation. It is a treatable disorder that accounts for many of the cases of excessive somnolence and insomnia encountered in most sleep centers. Common risk factors include obesity, sedative use, alcohol consumption, diabetes, stroke, and age. Disrupted sleep can certainly contribute to daytime sleepiness with impairments of alertness, concentration, mood, and behavior. There are several cardiopulmonary consequences, including arrhythmia, systemic arterial hypertension, and polycythemia. These changes can become chronic.

Central Sleep Apnea

Central sleep apnea is a disorder characterized by recurrent episodes of apnea during sleep resulting from a temporary loss of ventilatory effort. Central sleep apnea may be associated with desaturations and arousals, as in OSA. A pattern of sleep-related, irregular respirations known as ataxic breathing, or Biot respirations, has been associated with chronic opioid therapy with risk seemingly dose related.

Insomnia

Insomnia refers to a pattern of disrupted sleep (eg, delayed sleep onset, frequent arousals, early awakening) in an individual given sufficient opportunity to sleep that is associated with a pattern of daytime distress and symptoms. The requirement of daytime symptoms distinguishes the insomniac from the individual with an insufficient sleep disorder. Most recently, it was suggested that insomnia should be considered a comorbid disorder. This represents a shift from the thinking that insomnia is a symptom.

Extrinsic Factors

Several extrinsic factors affect sleep, including exercise, sleep environment, medications, and drug effects. Exercise has been long recognized as a factor promoting sound sleep. Environmental stimuli, such as room temperature and light, often are factors in the initiation and maintenance of sleep. Meals around bedtime may also play a role in proper sleep.

Medical and psychiatric factors and certain medical conditions contribute directly to specific sleep disorders such as OSA or RLS. However, other disorders simply lead to problems with the wake–sleep transition at sleep onset or at other times through the night, including the most vulnerable time in the circadian cycle. The role of psychiatric disorders always should be considered in the assessment of sleep disorders. Sleep disruption is not uncommon in any person with a comorbid psychiatric syndrome, but most of the attention has been directed toward the relationship between affective disorders and sleep. Insomnia is the prominent feature, although hypersomnia may be seen in depression, especially in bipolar depression. Similarly, during manic episodes, one may see periods of sleeplessness, with an apparent reduction in sleep need.

ALCOHOL AND SLEEP

Effect of Alcohol on Sleep in the Individual Without Alcohol Dependence

Alcohol probably is the sleep-promoting agent that is most widely used by the general public. Despite this wide use, alcohol can actually be mildly stimulating. Because alcohol is rapidly metabolized, the direct effect of evening alcohol consumption usually is during the sleep cycle. As predicted by the hypnotic effect, sleep latency is shortened and there is an increase in the amount of NREM sleep and SWS that occurs at the expense of REM sleep, which is suppressed during the acute phase. As the effects of the alcohol dissipate, there is a rebound effect, in which sleep becomes lighter and more easily disrupted. REM increases, with an associated increase in dreams and nightmares. There is an increase in sympathetic arousals, with tachycardia and sweating. After adjusting for blood alcohol levels, these effects may be more prominent on women than men. As alcohol consumption continues, the hypnotic effects may diminish, but the late sleep disruption persists. Ultimately, the net effect is a feeling of fatigue during the individual's waking hours. It would seem that the hypnotic effects of alcohol should be related to direct effects of alcohol on the central nervous system. Unfortunately, this explanation does not account for the observation that sleepiness can be observed after the alcohol is no longer detectable. Although it is customary to advise patients with sleep difficulties to avoid late-evening alcohol, there is evidence that even early-evening alcohol consumption may disrupt sleep in the last half of the night. Similarly, alcohol administered early in the day has been shown to have a negative effect on multiple sleep latency tests and tests of divided attention, even when given later in the day when alcohol levels are undetectable. Finally, the hypnotic effects seem to be enhanced in the previously sleep-deprived individual. In particular, low-dose alcohol administered after a night of reduced sleep is associated with reduced performance on a driving simulator.

Effect of Alcohol on Sleep in the Individual With Alcohol Dependence

It is not uncommon for persons with alcohol dependence to report some combination of insomnia, hypersomnia, circadian rhythm disorders, or parasomnias (abnormal sleep-related behaviors). Various studies of patients with alcohol dependence have demonstrated increased sleep latencies, decreased sleep efficiencies, and decreased total sleep, with reductions in both REM and SWS. As the dependence continues, patients often report that they no longer are able to initiate sleep without a drink. After a time, the usual rhythms of sleep become quite disrupted.

Sleep in Alcohol Withdrawal

The alcohol withdrawal syndrome frequently is marked by severe insomnia and sleep fragmentation. The reduction of SWS during this period has been related to a loss of restful sleep and feelings of daytime fatigue. The rebound of REM sleep has been regarded as a component of the pathophysiology of hallucinations encountered in the withdrawal syndrome. In fact, sleep during withdrawal may consist simply of fragments of REM sleep. It is of some interest that the rebound of SWS does not appear to occur. Nightmares and vivid dreams are not uncommon features of alcohol withdrawal and probably reflect the observed REM "pressure." It has been speculated that the rebound of REM encountered in acute withdrawal states such as delirium tremens may account for much of the associated clinical symptomatology. The increase in muscle activity also has suggested a possible relationship with REM sleep behavior disorder (dream-enacting behaviors in sleep).

Sleep During Alcohol Recovery

In the patient with alcohol dependence, sleep is not immediately recovered with abstinence; in fact, it may require months or even years. In the first 2 to 3 weeks of recovery, increased sleep latency may be seen, accompanied by increased sleep fragmentation and reduced total sleep time. There may be a decrease in SWS and an increase in REM density; such an increased density of REMs suggests an apparent rebound effect. The effects on REM may be exaggerated in patients with secondary depression, who also may exhibit a shortened REM latency

(duration of onset of REM after sleep onset) and a greater percentage of sleep time spent in REM sleep. A recovering person with alcoholism who begins to drink again will experience an increase in SWS, with an increase in total sleep time and reduction in fragmentation. This response, which involves a perceived immediate improvement in sleep, is thought to contribute to relapse, even though continued alcohol use inevitably leads to further sleep disruption.

SPECIFIC SLEEP DISORDERS ASSOCIATED WITH ALCOHOLISM

Patients with alcohol dependence appear to be at increased risk of developing OSA, especially if they snore. Alcohol has been shown to increase the frequency and duration of obstructive events in patients with established OSA. Alcohol has been related to a loss of restful sleep and feelings of daytime fatigue. The rebound of REM sleep has been regarded as a component of the pathophysiology of hallucinations encountered in the withdrawal syndrome. In fact, sleep during withdrawal may consist simply of fragments of REM sleep. It is of some interest that the rebound of SWS does not appear to occur. Nightmares and vivid dreams are not uncommon features of alcohol withdrawal and probably reflect the observed REM "pressure." It has been speculated that the rebound of REM encountered in acute withdrawal states such as delirium tremens may account for much of the associated clinical symptomatology. The increase in muscle activity also has suggested a possible relationship with REM sleep behavior disorder (dream-enacting behaviors in sleep).

Sleep During Alcohol Recovery

In the alcohol-dependent patient, sleep is not immediately recovered with abstinence; in fact, it may require months or even years. In the first 2 to 3 weeks of recovery, increased sleep latency may be seen, accompanied by increased sleep fragmentation and reduced total sleep time. There may be a decrease in SWS and an increase in REM density; such an increased density of REMs suggests an apparent rebound effect. The effects on REM may be exaggerated in patients with secondary depression, who also may exhibit a shortened REM latency (duration of onset of REM after sleep onset) and a greater percentage of sleep time spent in REM sleep. A recovering person with alcoholism who begins to drink again will experience an increase in SWS, with an increase in total sleep time and a reduction in fragmentation.

This response, which involves a perceived immediate improvement in sleep, is thought to contribute to relapse, even though continued alcohol use inevitably leads to further sleep disruption.

SPECIFIC SLEEP DISORDERS ASSOCIATED WITH ALCOHOLISM

Patients with alcohol dependence appear to be at increased risk of developing OSA, especially if they snore. Alcohol has been shown to increase the frequency and duration of obstructive events in patients with established OSA. Alcohol administration to asymptomatic men has been associated with increased episodes of desaturation, as well as an increase in frequency and duration of hypopneas and apneas. Moreover, the depressant effects of alcohol can decrease the likelihood of arousal from an obstructive event, thus prolonging the duration of each respiratory event. There is also an increase in snoring, as well as interruption in normal nocturnal respiration. These changes in airflow resistance are sufficient to cause OSA in those who consume moderate to-high doses of alcohol in the evening, even if they do not otherwise have OSA.

OTHER DRUGS AND SLEEP
Stimulants

The commonly used stimulants include the amphetamine-type (methylphenidate, dextroamphetamine, etc.) and the nonamphetamine-type (modafinil and armodafinil) stimulants. Cocaine also has a similar effect on sleep. It is widely accepted that a primary effect of stimulants is to prolong sleep latency and reduce total sleep time. Stimulants have a specific inhibitory effect on REM sleep so that there is a prolonged REM latency with a reduction in total REM throughout the sleep period. Presumably, this effect is attributable to the dopaminergic stimulation of the arousal system, although serotonergic systems also may be involved. When used episodically, these agents contribute to periods of sleeplessness that can last for days, but these usually are followed by a rebound hypersomnia. Tolerance to this effect can develop with continued use, even in those who take these agents for medical disorders such as narcolepsy or attention deficit hyperactivity disorder. After a period of persistent, chronic use, withdrawal of stimulants often leads to initial insomnia, which may persist with a decrease in sleep efficiency, increased periods of nocturnal wakefulness, increased amounts of REM sleep with a shortened REM latency, and increased stage 1 NREM sleep.

MDMA (Ecstasy)

Ecstasy ((±)3,4-methylenedioxymethamphetamine [MDMA]) is a psychostimulant and a synthetic derivative of amphetamine with both stimulant and hallucinogenic properties. Chronic use is associated with a significant decrease in serotonergic activity and also serves as a releaser and reuptake inhibitor of monoamines, including dopamine and norepinephrine. Acute MDMA administration disrupts sleep and REM sleep, specifically, without producing daytime sleepiness. Compared with control subjects, recreational MDMA users showed evidence of hyperarousal and impaired REM function. Sleep is usually disrupted for 48 hours following ingestion with additional REM suppression. Chronic use has also been associated with further sleep disturbance.

Opioids

The primary effect on sleep of acute administration of opioids to normal subjects or abstinent users is to shorten sleep latency and reduce total sleep time, sleep efficiency, REM sleep, and SWS. Chronic use, however, usually leads to tolerance to some of these effects. Even the longer acting opioids, such as methadone, contribute to insomnia, with disruption of sleep architecture and increased arousals accompanying chronic administration. Opioids play a role in the treatment and management of specific sleep disorders, such as RLS and sleep disorders secondary to pain syndromes. On the other hand, opioid use has been implicated as a cause of central sleep apnea.

Nicotine

When compared with nonsmokers, smokers experience an increase in sleep latency and an increase in arousals with resulting poorer sleep maintenance and a relative increase in sleep apneas and leg movements. A possible biphasic response is that low doses promote sleep and higher doses disrupt sleep. Unlike most of the other agents discussed in this chapter, nicotine can increase rather than decrease REM. Withdrawal from nicotine is associated with sleep disruption and increased daytime sleepiness. Smoking and nicotine may be associated with other sleep disorders. Some researchers speculate that in addition to the direct effect of nicotine on sleep mechanisms and architecture, tobacco and the irritation it causes to the upper airway may contribute to OSA. There also appears to be an association with bruxism. Although nicotine has been implicated as an aggravating factor in RLS, there are rare cases where it seemed to be palliative. Some of the effect of nicotine on RLS has also been attributed to the enhanced metabolism of agents such as ropinirole that are commonly used in the treatment of RLS.

Caffeine

The effects of caffeine overlap those of the stimulants. Caffeine has a long history of use to combat fatigue and sleepiness in normal individuals and to improve performance in shift workers, and it can trigger insomnia in experimental conditions as well. Unlike many other stimulants, caffeine appears to exert its effect by blocking adenosine receptors (primarily A1 and A2A) on neurons and glial cells of all brain areas. Caffeine, through antagonism of adenosine receptors, affects brain functions such as sleep, cognition, learning, and memory. The half-life of caffeine ranges from 3 to 7 hours, with effects persisting for as long as 8 to 14 hours. Thus, the effects of late-morning caffeine intake may continue into the evening. There is considerable variability in individual responses to caffeine. Caffeine often is used in combination with alcohol, and together, these can lead to even further aggravation of insomnia. Although alcohol has hypnotic properties, its half-life is much shorter than that of caffeine and its major effects disappear within a few hours. At that point, the rebound effect of alcohol withdrawal and the persistent stimulatory effect of caffeine jointly contribute to further sleep disruption. Although few formal studies of caffeine withdrawal and its effects on sleep have been conducted, it has been noted that within 18 to 24 hours, some patients develop headache, fatigue, irritability, sleepiness, and flulike symptoms.

Marijuana

Cannabis sativa contains over 70 different cannabinoids including Δ9-tetrahydrocannabinol and cannabidiol. Some of the hypnotic effects have been attributed to the ability of cannabinoids to modulate spontaneous neuronal activity and evoke inhibition of the locus coeruleus noradrenergic neurons. In a study of chronic marijuana users, abstinence from tetrahydrocannabinol increased ratings of anxiety, depression, and irritability and decreased the reported quantity and quality of sleep. It was suggested that these abstinence symptoms may contribute to continued use. Abstinence has been associated with a decrease in total sleep time, sleep efficiency, and REM sleep with an increase in waking after sleep onset and periodic limb movements in sleep. Findings such as these have emphasized the importance of addressing the treatment of addiction in people who use marijuana heavily. The hypnotic effect of marijuana may be a bit oversimplified. Although tetrahydrocannabinol has been usually implicated and its hypnotic properties described, it appears that another major constituent of marijuana, cannabidiol, may actually induce alertness. It appears that this alerting system may be modulated by the cannabidiol impact on dopaminergic release and activation of neurons in the hypothalamus and dorsal raphe nucleus. In addition, there have been a few studies that have looked specifically at the impact of marijuana on sleep architecture. It seems that the acute administration leads to a decrease in REM sleep and an increase in SWS. Abstinence seems to lead to a rebound effect with a decrease in REM latency and an increase in the relative amount of REM sleep and SWS. With long-term administration (>7 days), some tolerance probably develops to the SWS effects but not to the REM sleep effects. Finally, some studies have suggested that cannabinoids may be useful in the treatment of insomnia and RLS and may also lead to an improvement in the frequency of obstructive sleep-related breathing effects.

Benzodiazepines

Benzodiazepines and the related drugs (zolpidem, zopiclone, eszopiclone) are often referred to collectively as benzodiazepine-receptor agonists. They bind to the γ-aminobutyric acid (GABA$_A$) alpha subunits resulting in sedative, hypnotic, anticonvulsant, muscle relaxant, and anxiolytic properties and, of course, corresponding side effects. Their primary effect is to reduce sleep latency, increase total sleep time, and reduce nocturnal arousals. Benzodiazepines have only a minimal effect on REM sleep. With acute and chronic use, there can be an increase in spindle activity, and there is a decrease in the amount of SWS. The related agents, zolpidem and zaleplon, have similar effects, although it is thought that these have less effect on SWS. The traditional view has been that the sleep-promoting effects are lost within 2 to 3 weeks of use. Recent reviews, however, suggest that the development of tolerance to the hypnotic effects of benzodiazepines is quite variable and that drug effects may persist for extended periods of time. Benzodiazepine use is associated with the potential for physical dependence. Typical symptoms of withdrawal, which result secondary to an abrupt discontinuation, include agitation, anxiety, dysphoria, rebound insomnia, diarrhea, tachycardia, delirium, and seizures.

Gabapentin

Gabapentin was initially introduced as an antiepileptic drug but has been commonly used for certain types of pain and as a hypnotic. It is also commonly used in the treatment of alcohol and other drug use disorders and withdrawal. A number of cases, however, have described substance use disorder associated with gabapentin, all in patients with a prior substance use disorder. Some report euphoric effects similar but weaker to cocaine when combined with quetiapine. Some people with opioid use disorders use gabapentin to potentiate the desired opioid effects. Withdrawal from gabapentin has also been described and includes agitation, confusion and disorientation, diaphoresis, tremor, tachycardia, hypertension, and insomnia. Gabapentin improves wake after sleep onset and increases total sleep time. These results are both from objective PSG results and from subjective patient questionnaires. In addition, subjective questionnaires also indicated an improvement in overall sleep quality. Adverse side effects include headaches, dizziness, and gastrointestinal disturbances. Overall, it is a second-line therapy for insomnia unless the patient has comorbid RLS and/or chronic neuropathic pain.

Clonidine

Clonidine is a nonselective α_2 adrenergic agonist that has been used to help with sleep initiation and maintenance, especially in the pediatric population. Although it is commonly used among people with substance use disorders to help with both alcohol and opioid withdrawal, it is also a drug that is misused. Clonidine works at the level of the prefrontal cortex, mediating inattentiveness, hyperactivity, and impulsivity. At the level of the thalamus, its actions are associated with sedation. At the level of the locus coeruleus, it is associated with hypotensive and sedative effects. As a consequence, it is commonly used to treat patients with attention deficit hyperactivity disorder and children with neurodevelopmental disorders. Clonidine has also been successful in reducing the central nervous system noradrenergic activity and helping in symptoms of posttraumatic stress disorder. Clonidine has been used extensively to aid in symptoms of opioid withdrawal by reducing the sympathetic overactivity like tachycardia, hypertension, seating, flashes, and restlessness as well as insomnia. Unfortunately, there is evidence of an increase in the misuse of clonidine. Explanations for clonidine misuse might be related to the medication's ability to potentiate opioid analgesia. Other thoughts include clonidine's ability to reduce core withdrawal symptoms, to dampen other adverse effects of other drugs, or to self-medicate comorbid undiagnosed psychopathology.

KEY POINTS

1. Assessments of sleep disturbances should include a careful sleep history, looking at the amount of sleep obtained, timing of sleep, co-occurring medical and psychiatric disorders, evidence of intrinsic sleep disorders such as OSA or RLS, and extrinsic factors (ie, sleep environment).

2. Occasionally, additional diagnostic studies are required. A PSG should be considered if OSA or narcolepsy is suspected or for evaluating parasomnia (abnormal sleep-related behavior). A multiple sleep latency test can be helpful in documenting hypersomnia or the presence of early-onset REM.

3. After the evaluation is complete, the clinician can initiate a strategy to address the sleep problem. This approach needs to take the addictive disorder into consideration because problems underlying the addiction must be addressed and treated.

REVIEW QUESTIONS

1. Which of the following is *not* an effect of stimulants on sleep?
   A. Reduced total sleep time
   B. Decreased sleep latency
   C. Reduced total REM time
   D. Rebound hypersomnia

2. True or False: Sleep need varies in individuals from 6 to 9 hours of sleep over a 24-hour period.

3. Bob is a 56-year-old male who is overweight, has diabetes, and drinks three to four alcoholic beverages per day. He experiences daytime sleepiness, decreased alertness, impaired concentration, and loud snoring at night. A sleep study ordered by his physician reveals multiple episodes of oxygen desaturation during the night. Which of the following is the most likely cause of his symptoms?
   A. Obstructive sleep apnea
   B. Poor sleep environment
   C. Insomnia
   D. Restless legs syndrome

ANSWERS

1. **B**
2. **False**
3. **A**

SUGGESTED READINGS

American Academy of Sleep Medicine. *The AASM Manual for the Scoring of Sleep and Associated Events. Version 2.0.* Darien IL: American Academy of Sleep Medicine, 2012.

American Academy of Sleep Medicine. *The International Classification of Sleep Disorders: Diagnostic & Coding Manual.*

2nd ed. Rochester, MN: American Academy of Sleep Medicine, 2005.

Aurora RN, Kristo DA, Bista SR, et al. The treatment of restless legs syndrome and periodic limb movement disorder in adults—an update for 2012: practice parameters with an evidence-based systematic review and meta-analyses: an American Academy of Sleep Medicine Clinical Practice Guideline. *Sleep.* 2012;35(8):1039-1062.

Baird CR, Fox P, Colvin LA. Gabapentinoid abuse in order to potentiate the effect of methadone: a survey among substance misusers. *Eur Addict Res.* 2014;20(3):115-118.

Bosker WM, Kuypers KP, Conen S, et al. MDMA (ecstasy) effects on actual driving performance before and after sleep deprivation, as function of dose and concentration in blood and oral fluid. *Psychopharmacology (Berl).* 2012;222(3):367-376.

Jaehne A, Unbehaun T, Feige B, et al. How smoking affects sleep: a polysomnographical analysis. *Sleep Med.* 2012;13(10):1286-1292.

Schierenbeck T, Riemann D, Berger M, Hornyak M. Effect of illicit recreational drugs upon sleep: cocaine, ecstasy and marijuana. *Sleep Med Rev.* 2008;12(5):381-389.

Thorpy MJ. The clinical use of the multiple sleep latency test. The Standards of Practice Committee of the American Sleep Disorders Association. *Sleep.* 1992;15(3):268-276.

88

Traumatic Injuries Related to Alcohol and Other Drug Use: Epidemiology, Screening, and Prevention

Summary by Walter Green, Deepa Camenga, Gail D'Onofrio, and Federico E. Vaca

Based on THE ASAM PRINCIPLES OF ADDICTION MEDICINE, 6th edition chapter by Federico E. Vaca, Deepa Camenga, and Gail D'Onofrio

Alcohol and other drug use contributes to a substantial proportion of injury events. These events lead to significant morbidity and mortality, with far-reaching implications for the individual, their family, their workplace, and society. As the prevalence of these events becomes better understood, so does the importance of implementing screening tools and interventions to identify and treat populations at risk. Emergency departments (EDs) have proven to be an important setting to both recognize and treat these patients.

EPIDEMIOLOGY OF ALCOHOL- AND OTHER DRUG-RELATED INJURIES

Alcohol is a factor in nearly 50% of major trauma cases and in 22% of minor trauma cases. Alcohol is a major risk factor for virtually all categories of unintentional and intentional injuries. Data show that persons who drink alcohol have an increased risk of fatal injury from a multitude of injury mechanisms, including drowning, firearm homicide, suicide, and unintentional poisoning. Of note, nearly one third of fatal motor vehicle crashes (MVCs) in the United States are related to alcohol use. In a study of injured versus noninjured patients in the ED, injured patients were more likely to test positive for alcohol use, to report heavy drinking, to report prior alcohol-related injuries, and to report prior treatment for consequences of alcohol consumption. These findings held true in both county and community hospital EDs.

Studies have shown that both patients with trauma in the ED and those admitted to the hospital have higher rates of substance use. In injured patients presenting to the ED, one study found this population to be five times more likely to report a higher quantity and frequency of alcohol consumption than control subjects. Similarly, patients with trauma admitted to the hospital were found to have significantly higher rates of substance dependence when compared to control samples.

Traumatic injury and its association with alcohol use has been explored more so than its relationship with other illicit substance use. However, studies do show that other drug use is linked to traumatic injury. Cocaine was shown to be a factor in as many as 25% of MVC fatalities. Additionally, marijuana, benzodiazepines, opiates, and amphetamines have all been shown to be associated with a higher risk for MVCs.

SCREENING FOR ALCOHOL PROBLEMS IN THE EMERGENCY DEPARTMENT

The proven association between alcohol use and traumatic injury calls for the importance of screening and intervention. These two processes may take place at any time during the ED visit. Ideally, there should be a protocol for screening and intervention that is based on the resources of the ED. If standardized, the screening process can often be carried out by various members of the ED treatment team. Interventions, on the other hand, often vary based on where the patient is on the clinical spectrum of alcohol use.

Alcohol use exists on a spectrum consisting of three categories of classification: at-risk use, harmful use, and dependent use. The National Institute on Alcohol Abuse and Alcoholism (NIAAA) differentiates between men and women when defining at-risk use. At-risk use is classified for females as having three or more drinks per day or seven or more drinks per week. For men, at-risk use is classified as having 4 or more drinks per day or 14 or more drinks per week. When compared to normal controls, people whose use is classified as at risk are more likely to experience consequences of their alcohol use in the future. The second category on the alcohol use spectrum is harmful use. People whose use is considered harmful currently experience negative consequences as a result of their alcohol consumption. These include medical, social, and/or legal problems. Most commonly, these problems are related to poor work or school performance, familial conflicts, car crashes, and even driving under the influence. Finally, patients whose use is on the severe end of the spectrum of alcohol use disorders is classified as dependent use. These individuals often experience significant and repeated negative physical and social effects from their alcohol use, including the cardinal signs of tolerance and withdrawal. These diagnostic classifications are useful to clinicians because they allow patients to be stratified according to disease severity and are useful in making treatment recommendations. In addition, these classifications affect the selection of a screening tool for application in identifying patients with unhealthy alcohol use in the clinical setting.

Historically, the most common alcohol screening tools utilized in the ED include the CAGE, TWEAK, and the Alcohol Use Disorders Identification Test systems. These screening tools do well to identify people with harmful and dependent alcohol use, but are not designed to screen for use that is at risk. More recently, the Screening Brief Intervention and Referral to Treatment (SBIRT) model has done well to identify patients with at-risk use. This system utilizes brief, formal screening questionnaires such as the NIAAA quantity and frequency questions, the Alcohol Use Disorders Identification Test-C, and the Alcohol, Smoking and Substance Involvement Screening Test.

The NIAAA single-item screening test requires the interviewer to ask the patient how many times in the past year they have had four or five drinks in a single day when questioning women or men, respectively. A response of one or more is considered positive. The Alcohol Use Disorders Identification Test-C consists of three multiple-choice questions that assess the quantity, frequency, and intensity of the patient's drinking behavior. The patient is given a score based on his or her answers to these questions.

These screening tools are quick and easy to administer, making them ideal for use in the ED. They successfully identify people who drink across the entire spectrum of alcohol use, thereby allowing for the proper intervention to be put into action.

INTERVENTIONS WITH INJURED PATIENTS

Alcohol- or other drug-related injuries provide a unique opportunity for intervention. The negative consequences of the injury can create what has been described as a "teachable moment," a unique opportunity to motivate patients to change their behavior or to encourage them to seek further treatment. The ED presents rich opportunities for such interventions because research shows that a higher proportion of patients in emergency settings than in other settings have unhealthy alcohol use. One study found that more than one third of ED patients who had been drinking alcohol and were subsequently injured in MVCs connected their alcohol use to the injury event. This association is crucial in creating a setting for successful intervention. One systematic review showed that brief interventions could not only be beneficial at reducing risky driving and alcohol-related crashes but was also effective at reducing alcohol-related injuries 6 to 12 months after the intervention was delivered. Brief interventions may not only reduce alcohol use but also may reduce the incidence of alcohol-related injuries. Another systematic review, which assessed 19 randomized controlled trials, found that addressing problem drinking was associated with a reduction in suicide attempts, domestic violence, falls, drinking-related injuries, hospitalizations, and deaths. The ED provides an ideal setting to incorporate these interventions into practice.

Brief interventions involve counseling sessions that require 5 to 45 minutes of time. Such interventions often involve the six elements summarized by the mnemonic FRAMES: Feedback, Responsibility, Advice, Menu of options, Empathy, and Self-efficacy. Additional components, including goal setting, follow-up, and timing, have also been shown to support the effectiveness of brief interventions. Behavior changes are agreed upon with the patient and vary based on where the individual falls on the alcohol use spectrum.

Numerous ED SBIRT studies have investigated the effectiveness of this model in patients presenting to the ED. One study showed that ED patients receiving a brief intervention consumed 3.25 fewer drinks per week when compared to controls at the 3-month follow-up. Another study demonstrated

TABLE 88-1	A Brief Intervention for Injured Patients
• **Raise the Subject:** "I would like to take a few minutes to talk to you about your alcohol use."	
• **Give Feedback:** "I am concerned about your drinking. Our screen indicates that you are above what we consider the safe limits of drinking. This level places you at risk for alcohol-related illness, injury, and death."	
• **Compare to Norms:** Compare with the NIAAA guidelines for low-risk alcohol consumption.	
• **Make a Connection:** "Do you see a connection between your visit and your alcohol use?"	
• **Assess Readiness:** "On a scale of 1 to 10 (1 being not ready to change and 10 being very ready), how ready are you to change your drinking pattern?"	
• **Develop Discrepancy:** "So, you enjoy drinking, but you also want to avoid getting hurt."	
• **Elicit a Response:** "How does all this sound to you?"	
• **Negotiate a Goal:** "What would you like to do?"	
• **Give Advice:** "If you stay within the recommended limits (NIAAA guidelines), you will be less likely to experience further illness or injury related to alcohol use. You should never drink and drive."	
• **Summarize and Provide an Agreement Form (ie, a plan for change) and Primary Care Follow-Up:** "This is what I heard you say. . . . Thank you for your time."	

NIAA, The National Institute on Alcohol Abuse and Alcoholism.

this significant reduction to persist at both 6 and 12 months following the intervention. At-risk drinkers seem to benefit the most from these brief interventions. Other studies have shown that adolescents exposed to brief interventions have a lower incidence of drinking and driving, alcohol-related injuries, and alcohol-related social problems when measured at the 6-month follow-up. An additional randomized control trial found that brief interventions performed by emergency practitioners significantly reduced hazardous and harmful drinking in ED patients. The intervention group in this study had a reduction from a baseline of 7.4 drinks compared to a 3.3 drink reduction in the control group when measured at 12 months. A reduction in the rates of driving after drinking more than three drinks was also demonstrated in the intervention group.

There is considerably less data available on the efficacy of SBIRT in relation to other drug use. One study did show brief interventions to reduce marijuana consumption and promote marijuana abstinence. Another study showed reduced illicit opioid use in patients receiving a brief intervention in conjunction with ED-initiated buprenorphine and referral to primary care follow-up.

INCORPORATING SCREENING AND BRIEF INTERVENTION INTO PRACTICE

In most settings where injured patients are treated such as EDs and trauma centers, competing priorities and lack of time make screening and brief interventions a challenge. Therefore, screening tools that are short, simple, and easily administered by a variety of providers have a greater chance of being utilized.

Screening for unhealthy alcohol use in injured patients should address the entire spectrum of alcohol use disorders. Interventions will vary depending on where the patient falls on this spectrum. For the person with at-risk alcohol use or the patient who has sustained an alcohol-related injury but does not have an alcohol use disorder, setting goals within safe limits coupled with a referral to the patient's primary care physician may be all that is needed. For the person with harmful alcohol or drug use, negotiating abstinence or harm reduction, such as not using while driving, with a referral to a primary care physician may be sufficient. For the patient who is dependent on alcohol or drugs or when the clinician is uncertain as to where a patient fits on the continuum of unhealthy substance use, the brief intervention becomes a negotiation process to seek further assessment, referral to a specialized treatment program, or repeat interventions in the primary care setting. The contents of such a brief intervention are outlined in Table 88-1.

EMERGING CONSIDERATIONS: ELECTRONIC CIGARETTE USE AND INJURIES

Electronic cigarettes (e-cigarettes), including vapes, vape pens, mods, tanks, and e-hookahs, are novel tobacco products that have rapidly risen in popularity over the past decade. In 2015, 3.5% of all US adults reported past-month e-cigarette use with cigarette reduction being the primary motivation for use. Additionally, 11.3% of US high school students reported e-cigarette use, exceeding the rate of cigarette use in this population.

As its use has become more prevalent, there has been an associated rise in e-cigarette–related injuries. Battery overheating in combination with the inherent flammability of the e-liquid creates an explosion capability that has led to unintentional injuries among users. Recent case series have reported burns and traumatic injuries of the oral/maxillofacial region (from explosions during e-cigarette use) and the extremities (from spontaneous explosions while users were storing the device in pockets). Overall, the burden of traumatic injuries secondary to e-cigarette systems is most likely underestimated due to the lack of a standardized surveillance system for such injuries. In August 2016, the US Food and Drug Administration gained the authority to regulate the manufacturing of e-cigarettes in an effort to protect public health. Therefore, it is possible that improved safety standards and manufacturing oversight could be enacted to reduce traumatic injuries.

KEY POINTS

1. Alcohol and other drug use is a major risk factor for virtually all categories of unintentional and intentional injuries.
2. The emergency department is an ideal setting to screen for alcohol and other drug use and to provide subsequent intervention because individuals are more likely to make behavior changes following an injury event.
3. Screening tools must be quick and easy to administer while still identifying drinkers across the entire spectrum of alcohol use; this allows for the proper intervention to be put into action.
4. As use of e-cigarettes has become more prevalent, there has been an increased rate of traumatic injury associated with their use.

REVIEW QUESTIONS

1. An individual whose alcohol use is more likely to lead to negative consequences in the future would be classified as:
   A. at-risk use.
   B. harmful use.
   C. dependent use.
   D. functional use.

2. Which of the following factors are useful characteristics of screening tools utilized in the emergency department?
   A. The screening tool is short.
   B. The screening tool is easy to use.
   C. The screening tool can be administered by multiple members of the treatment team.
   D. All of the above.

3. The primary motivation for e-cigarette use is:
   A. cost-effectiveness compared to cigarettes.
   B. recreational use.
   C. cigarette use reduction.
   D. the health benefits of e-cigarette use.

ANSWERS

1. **A**
2. **D**
3. **C**

SUGGESTED READINGS

Bernstein E, Bernstein J, Feldman J, et al. An evidence based alcohol screening, brief intervention and referral to treatment (SBIRT) curriculum for emergency department (ED) providers improves skills and utilization. *Subst Abus.* 2007;28(4):79-92.

Brady JE, Li G. Trends in alcohol and other drugs detected in fatally injured drivers in the United States, 1999-2010. *Am J Epidemiol.* 2014;179(6):692-699.

D'Onofrio G, O'Connor PG, Pantalon MV, et al. Emergency department-initiated buprenorphine/naloxone treatment for opioid dependence: a randomized clinical trial. *JAMA.* 2015;313(16):1636-1644.

Meernik C, Williams FN, Cairns BA, Grant EJ, Goldstein AO. Burns from e-cigarettes and other electronic nicotine delivery systems. *BMJ.* 2016;354:i5024.

Saitz R, Palfai T, Cheng DM, et al. Screening and brief intervention for drug use in primary care: the ASPIRE randomized clinical trial. *JAMA.* 2014;312(5):502-513.

Endocrine and Reproductive Disorders Related to Alcohol and Other Drug Use

Summary by Felipe Bolivar Rincon

> Based on THE ASAM PRINCIPLES OF ADDICTION MEDICINE, 6th edition chapter by Alan Ona Malabanan and Gwendolyne Anyanate Jack

Alcohol and other drugs have myriad effects on the endocrine system. Hormone synthesis, secretion, effect, and metabolism are affected in the hypothalamus, hypophysis, thyroid, adrenal glands, pancreas, gonads, as well as other target organs and cells. The pharmacologic properties of the substances and factors such as gender and pattern of substance use add to this complexity. Table 89-1 summarizes the most relevant endocrinologic clinical effects.

DISORDERS RELATED TO ALCOHOL

Hypoglycemia/Hyperglycemia

Alcohol causes hypoglycemia by decreasing gluconeogenesis, producing malnourishment and blunting the response to hypoglycemia through impaired release of cortisol, growth hormone, and glucagon. Hazardous use may cause pancreatitis, pancreatic insufficiency, and diabetes mellitus with resulting hyperglycemia complicating management due to the risk of hypoglycemia with alcohol intake.

Reproductive Consequences

In men, alcohol may disrupt the hypothalamic–pituitary–gonadal axis resulting in hypogonadism. Men with cirrhosis can have gynecomastia through the increase in prolactin and androstenedione. In women, through the increase in estradiol, it can cause amenorrhea, dysmenorrhea, metrorrhagia, and a possible delay in menopause as well as an increase in the risk of infertility and breast cancer. In pregnant women, there is a higher risk of miscarriage, placental abruption, preterm deliveries, stillbirths, and postpartum decreased milk production.

Bone Health Consequences

The effect of alcohol on bone is a continuum that ranges from increased bone mineral density with low intake to a decrease in vitamin D, decrease in bone mineral density, increased risk of fracture, and osteonecrosis of the bone at the end of the spectrum with hazardous use.

Other Endocrinologic Consequences

Alcohol use increases triglycerides, high-density lipoprotein (HDL), adrenocorticotropic hormone (ACTH), and cortisol, the latter of which can result in pseudo-Cushing syndrome, which reverses with alcohol abstention. Alcohol may also decrease vasopressin, norepinephrine and decrease melatonin as well, resulting in diluted diuresis, elevated blood pressure, and sleep cycle disturbances, respectively.

DISORDERS RELATED TO TOBACCO

Thyroid Consequences

Cigarette smoking increases the risk of Graves disease and Graves ophthalmopathy. It also appears to lower thyroid-stimulating hormone and thyroid autoantibodies and decreases the risk of thyroid cancer.

Insulin Resistance and Dyslipidemia

Current, former, and passive cigarette smokers have an increased risk to develop impaired glucose tolerance and diabetes mellitus. Increased levels of triglycerides and lower levels of HDL have also been evidenced in cigarette smokers.

Reproductive Function

In women, cigarette smoking may decrease estrogen levels. It has been associated with early menopause,

TABLE 89-1	Endocrine Associations and Clinical Effects of Alcohol and Other Drugs	
Substance	**Effect on Hormones**	**Clinical Effects**
Alcohol	↓ glucose, ↑ NADH, ↓ testosterone, ↑ prolactin, ↑ estradiol, ↓ oxytocin, ↓ leptin, ↓ ghrelin, ↑ triglycerides, ↓ HDL, ↑ ACTH, ↑ cortisol, ↓ vasopressin, ↑ norepinephrine, ↓ melatonin	Hypo/hyperglycemia, pancreatic insufficiency, diabetes mellitus, diabetes insipidus, hypogonadism/infertility, gynecomastia, hyperlipidemia, hyperadrenalism, osteoporosis
Amphetamines	↑ catecholamines, ↑ growth hormone, ↓ leptin	Hyperadrenalism, SIADH (ecstasy), appetite suppression
Anabolic Steroids	↓ LH, ↓ FSH, ↓ testosterone, ↑ estrone, ↓ HDL, ↑ LDL	Gynecomastia, hyperlipidemia, hypogonadism/infertility, virilization, hyperthyroidism[a]
Barbiturates	↓ thyroid hormone, ↓ hydrocortisone, ↓ vitamin D	Hypoadrenalism,[a] hypothyroidism,[a] osteoporosis
Benzodiazepines	↓ cortisol	Hypoadrenalism,[a] hypoglycemia,[a] SIADH[a]
Caffeine	↑ epinephrine, ↑ cortisol, ↑ growth hormone, ↑ urinary calcium, ↓ IGF-1	Hyperglycemia, ↓ diabetes mellitus, osteoporosis[a]
Cocaine	↑ catecholamines, ↑ glucose, ↑ prolactin (acutely), ↑ ACTH (acutely), ↑ FSH (acutely), ↑ LH (acutely)	Hyperglycemia, hyperprolactinemia, suppresses appetite
Inhalants	↑ phosphate, ↓ calcium (through renal damage)	Hypogonadism/infertility, hypothyroidism,[a] osteoporosis[a]
Marijuana	↑ leptin, ↑ ghrelin, ↓ LH,[a] ↓ testosterone[a]	Appetite stimulant, gynecomastia,[a] hypoadrenalism, hypogonadism/infertility[a]
Opioids	↓ FSH, ↓ LH, ↑ prolactin, ↓ ACTH, ↓ cortisol, ↓ estradiol, ↓ progesterone	Hyperprolactinemia, hypogonadism/infertility, osteoporosis, adrenal insufficiency[a]
Tobacco/Cigarette Smoking	↓ TSH, ↑ HDL, ↑ triglycerides, ↓ estrogen, ↑ FSH, ↑ vasopressin, ↑ prolactin, ↑ ACTH, ↑ cortisol	Hyperthyroidism, insulin resistance, hyperlipidemia, hypogonadism/infertility, osteoporosis, SIADH[a]

↓, decrease; ↑, increase; NADH, nicotinamide adenine dinucleotide; HDL, high-density lipoprotein; ACTH, adrenocorticotropic hormone; SIADH, syndrome of inappropriate antidiuretic hormone secretion; LH, luteinizing hormone; FSH, follicle-stimulating hormone; LDL, low-density lipoprotein; IGF-1, insulin-like growth factor 1; TSH, thyroid-stimulating hormone.
[a]Possible effect.

increased follicle-stimulating hormone (FSH) levels, increased ovarian age, and poorer outcomes with assisted reproduction. In men, it is associated with quantitative and qualitative decrements in sperm and increases in serum estrogen.

Bone Health

Cigarette smoking is associated with decreased levels of vitamin D_2 and D_3, parathyroid hormone, osteocalcin, as well as bone mineral density. It is also associated with osteoporotic fracture and osteonecrosis.

Other Endocrinologic Effects

Cigarette smoking is associated with increased antidiuretic hormone release and increased stimulation of the noradrenergic system, resulting in hyponatremia in susceptible groups and hypertension, respectively.

DISORDERS RELATED TO OPIOID USE
Gonadal Function

Opioids disrupt the hypothalamic–pituitary–gonadal axis through an increase in prolactin, a decrease in gonadotropin-releasing hormone and a consequent decrease in gonadotropins. In men, a dose-dependent decrease in total testosterone can be evidenced with resulting hypogonadism. In women, decreased levels of FSH, luteinizing hormone (LH), progesterone, and estradiol have been found to cause menstrual irregularities, including amenorrhea.

Bone Health

Opioids are associated with an increased risk of vitamin D deficiency, decreased bone mineral density, osteoporosis, and bone fracture.

Other Endocrinologic Effects

Opioids have been associated with hypoadrenalism; they may inhibit the effect of corticotropin-releasing hormone on ACTH, decrease cortisol levels, increase growth hormone and thyroid-stimulating hormone release, as well as increase the risk of developing glucose tolerance.

DISORDERS RELATED TO OTHER DRUGS

Marijuana

Marijuana increases appetite. It might affect male fertility and increase the risk of testicular germ cell tumors; nevertheless, the effects on hormonal levels and pregnancy outcomes in women are inconsistent. Evidence suggests that hazardous use might cause hypoadrenalism in those with preexisting adrenal disease.

Cocaine

Cocaine increases catecholamine concentrations, which antagonize insulin regulation resulting in an increased risk of hyperglycemia, diabetic ketoacidosis, and hyperosmolar nonketotic hyperglycemia. Chronic cocaine use is associated with hyperprolactinemia after dopamine has been depleted. Increases in ACTH, FSH, and LH associated with acute use have not been evidenced chronically.

Amphetamines

Amphetamines suppress appetite. They are associated with an increased release of corticosteroids and growth hormone acutely. Ecstasy has been associated with severe hyponatremia due to syndrome of inappropriate antidiuretic hormone secretion and an increased risk of death in patients with hyperthyroidism.

Caffeine

Caffeine effects are dose dependent. It is associated with epinephrine release with a resulting increase in blood pressure; increased response to tilt table testing; and increased epinephrine, norepinephrine, and cortisol response to hypoglycemia. Ingestion of 400 mg of caffeine has been associated with decreased insulin sensitivity in tolerant young adults, and 500 mg might increase average and postprandial glycemia in those with type 2 diabetes. Nevertheless, chronic coffee intake has been consistently associated with a decreased risk of type 2 diabetes mellitus. Lastly, coffee may impair L-thyroxine absorption, altering the management of hypothyroidism.

Benzodiazepines

Benzodiazepines might cause hypoadrenalism and persistent hypoglycemia in those with preexisting adrenal disease by suppressing basal cortisol levels and the body's cortisol and ACTH response to exercise, insulin-induced hypoglycemia, and corticotropin-releasing hormone. They also blunt the response to hypoglycemia through impaired growth hormone, glucagon, and catecholamine release.

Barbiturates

Through the induction of the P450 enzyme system, barbiturates can increase the metabolism of thyroid hormones, hydrocortisone, vitamin D, and methadone resulting in possible increased thyroid hormone and hydrocortisone requirements, osteomalacia, and risk of opioid withdrawal, respectively.

Inhalants

Through occupational exposure, inhalant use has been associated with skeletal fluorosis, infertility, increased risk of spontaneous abortion, and multiple birth defects (fetal solvent syndrome). Also, by provoking renal tubular dysfunction, solvents may lead to hyperphosphatemia and alter calcium and bone metabolism; nephrolithiasis has also been described with inhalant use.

Anabolic Steroids

Anabolic–androgenic steroids suppress the hypothalamic–pituitary–gonadal axis. In men, this can result in decreased testosterone, LH, and FSH, testicular atrophy, gynecomastia, and infertility. In women, menstrual abnormalities, deepening of the voice, acne, and hirsutism can be found. Other hormones may be affected by the decrease in hepatic binding globulin synthesis such as thyroid and sex hormones, but these changes are not clinically relevant without an underlying pathology. Lipid changes might include an increase in low-density lipoprotein and a decrease in HDL, although a consistent association with heart disease has not been established.

Other Drugs

Although lysergic acid diethylamide acutely increases blood pressure, cortisol, epinephrine, oxytocin, and prolactin, no clinically relevant significance has been found. Phencyclidine has not been associated with relevant endocrinologic effects. Further research is required.

KEY POINTS

1. Alcohol and other drugs have complex interactions with the endocrine system. Clinically relevant effects are summarized in Table 89-1.
2. Alcohol is associated with hypo- and hyperglycemia, infertility, adverse pregnancy outcomes, diabetes insipidus, pseudo-Cushing syndrome, and an increased risk of bone fracture.
3. Opioids are associated with hypogonadotropic hypogonadism, increased risk of bone fracture, and hypoadrenalism.

REVIEW QUESTIONS

1. Cocaine increases the risk of developing which of the following conditions?
   A. Diabetes insipidus
   B. Hypogonadism
   C. Vitamin D deficiency
   D. Diabetic ketoacidosis

2. Which of the following is *not* associated with male infertility?
   A. Opioids
   B. Amphetamines
   C. Marijuana
   D. Anabolic steroids

3. Which of the following is associated with severe hyponatremia?
   A. Benzodiazepines
   B. Ecstasy
   C. Alcohol
   D. Cocaine

ANSWERS

1. **D.** Cocaine has been associated with diabetic ketoacidosis in patients without any other identified precipitant factors.
2. **B.** Opioids and anabolic steroids cause hypogonadism, whereas marijuana is associated with decreased sperm count and motility.
3. **B.** Ecstasy causes syndrome of inappropriate antidiuretic hormone secretion, which in combination with profuse water intake, might lead to severe hyponatremia.

SUGGESTED READINGS

Ali K, Raphael J, Khan S, Labib M, Duarte R. The effects of opioids on the endocrine system: an overview. *Postgrad Med J.* 2016;92(1093):677-681.

Brown TT, Dobs AS. Endocrine effects of marijuana. *J Clin Pharmacol.* 2002;42(S1):90S-96S.

Dimitri P, Rosen C. The central nervous system and bone metabolism: an evolving story. *Calcif Tissue Int.* 2017;100(5):476-485.

Rachdaoui N, Sarkar DK. Pathophysiology of the effects of alcohol abuse on the endocrine system. *Alcohol Res.* 2017;38(2):255-276.

Tziomalos K, Charsoulis F. Endocrine effects of tobacco smoking. *Clin Endocrinol (Oxf).* 2004;61(6):664-674.

Alcohol and Other Drug Use during Pregnancy: Management of the Mother and Child

Summary by Michael F. Weaver, Hendrée E. Jones, and Martha J. Wunsch

Based on THE ASAM PRINCIPLES OF ADDICTION MEDICINE, 6th edition chapter by Michael F. Weaver, Hendrée E. Jones, and Martha J. Wunsch

APPROACH TO THE PREGNANT WOMAN

Women who use substances during pregnancy often do so in the context of intricately complex individual, social, and environmental factors, including poor nutrition, extreme stress, violence of multiple forms, poor housing conditions, exposure to environmental toxins and diseases, and depression, all of which can impact postnatal outcomes. Women using tobacco, alcohol, prescription medications, and illicit substances may have irregular menstrual cycles yet still have the ability to conceive. Perinatal substance use disorders (SUDs) affect women of all races, ethnicities, and socioeconomic levels. Pregnancy motivates some, but not all, women to quit using. Others may have difficulty stopping due to the severity of their SUD or fear of withdrawal. Pregnant women who use psychoactive substances experience more prejudice and are much more stigmatized than nonpregnant women, so clinicians should explicitly discuss the need for and limits around confidentiality.

Screening

Screening, followed when appropriate by a brief intervention and referral to treatment, especially for alcohol and tobacco, is recommended in obstetric settings and is effective. The combination of screening questions and urine toxicology is more effective for detection than either one alone. Screening is done at the first prenatal visit and repeated every trimester if necessary. Validated screening instruments for pregnant women include the T-ACE, the TWEAK, and the AUDIT-C (Alcohol Use Disorders Identification Test—Consumption) for alcohol, and the 4Ps (parents, partner, past, pregnancy). Those at low risk can simply receive brief advice, and those at high risk should be referred for definitive SUD treatment. Women at moderate risk (ie, those who have a history of SUDs with high quantities, recent SUD treatment, those who stopped using during pregnancy, and those who continue sporadic low-level use during pregnancy) benefit most from a brief intervention delivered by the clinician.

Laboratory Testing

Infant urine, meconium, and cord tissue, as well as maternal urine, are biological matrices that have been tested for use of legal and illegal drugs. A positive biological test does *not* diagnose a current SUD, provide a result of parenting ability, or indicate amount, frequency, or route of substance use.

Meconium, a dark-green odorless substance produced by the fetal gastrointestinal tract beginning at 13 to 14 weeks of gestation, may be tested for medications, alcohol, and other drugs. It is passed by the newborn in bowel movements shortly after birth. The advantage of testing meconium is information about a long window of prenatal exposure, beginning in the second trimester. Cord tissue sampling can be used to test for in utero exposure with no significant differences in detection rates of nonmedical substances (amphetamines, cannabis, and opiates) versus meconium and has a similar cost.

Alcohol biomarkers include ethyl glucuronide, ethyl sulfate, and fatty acid ethyl esters in urine. They may be present from 72 hours to 7 weeks after use.

Results indicate exposure to alcohol throughout pregnancy, which is an indicator of maternal risk, but not an assessment of parenting ability.

Teratogenicity

A teratogen is a substance that may produce an alteration in the offspring's physical structures and/or behavior when used during gestation. The time and amount of exposure affects whether congenital malformations or neurobehavioral problems will occur that persist throughout life. In many cases, a "subthreshold exposure" will not lead to malformations, whereas in others, a small dose during critical embryogenesis can lead to significant teratogenicity. It is difficult to attribute causation to exposure when there are confounding variables such as malnutrition, severe stress, and concurrent use of other substances. Alcohol and tobacco, alone and in combination with other substances, are known to have the most potential to cause teratogenicity in the human.

Exposure in the first trimester can result in significant problems, including pregnancy loss. The majority of development and organogenesis occurs in the first 12 weeks of pregnancy; however, exposure can cause problems during any trimester of pregnancy. Multiple factors affect the determination of fetal substance exposure, such as substances used in combination and recall bias.

NEONATAL ABSTINENCE SYNDROMES

In the newborn, signs of intoxication as well as withdrawal from illicit and legal psychoactive substances are all characterized by autonomic instability, central nervous system irritability, and feeding difficulties, and possibly poor weight gain, instability in heart rate, respiratory rate, and temperature as well as hyperactivity, irritability, hypertonia or hypotonia, difficulty sucking or excessive sucking, sleep disturbance, and high-pitched cries. The duration and severity of intoxication and the onset of withdrawal syndrome depend on the time of the last drug exposure, the combination of substances, and the metabolism of the drug.

When substance use is under consideration, newborns should have a regular assessment for withdrawal or intoxication beginning at birth. Initial treatment of the neonate experiencing neonatal abstinence syndrome (NAS) should be primarily supportive. Minimize ambient light exposure and noise, use swaddling and frequent small feedings, and consider intravenous fluids. Indications for pharmacotherapy include seizures; poor feeding, diarrhea, or vomiting resulting in dehydration or excessive weight loss; inability to sleep; or significant autonomic instability with bradycardia or tachycardia, apnea or tachypnea, or temperature instability not due to infection. Consider pharmacotherapy if the infant is too ill to assess possible withdrawal signs, if comorbid medical problems dictate that the infant will not tolerate NAS, or if the infant is not eating well and not thriving. The differential diagnosis for NAS includes sepsis, hypoglycemia, perinatal anoxia, intracranial bleeding, and hyperthyroidism.

Neonates with intrauterine drug exposure should be followed up with in the hospital for at least 72 to 96 hours after birth. If discharged prior to this time, the mother and her support network should be informed about signs of NAS.

TOBACCO

All pregnant women should be asked directly about tobacco (all forms) or use of electronic cigarettes. Strongly advise all who are pregnant and using tobacco and/or nicotinc to quit. Nicotine replacement has not been found to be successful with pregnant women. Varenicline has limited safety data for use in pregnancy. Bupropion showed no significant improvement in abstinence rates at the end of pregnancy. Focus on brief office-based interventions coupled with referral to tobacco and/or nicotine treatment programs specifically developed for pregnant women.

Cigarette use causes disruption of growth and developmental neurologic problems, and an inverse relationship exists between birth weight and number of cigarettes smoked per day. Generally, no differences in body weight or length are observed among these infants at 1 year of age. Infants exposed to tobacco are more excitable and hypertonic with indications of disturbance in the central nervous system, gastrointestinal system, and visual response. Nearly one third of deaths due to sudden infant death syndrome may be prevented with the cessation of smoking in pregnancy.

ALCOHOL AND SEDATIVES

Women who are pregnant or considering pregnancy should not drink alcohol. More than 60% of women who use alcohol quit during pregnancy. Women with sedative use disorder may take multiple drugs, including benzodiazepines, barbiturates, and other sleeping pills as well as drink alcohol.

Normal physiologic changes that accompany pregnancy can make it difficult to recognize early withdrawal. Uncontrolled withdrawal symptoms may be life threatening to both the mother and fetus. Treatment for acute withdrawal from sedatives (including alcohol) in pregnancy should be accomplished in an inpatient setting that allows for medical supervision in collaboration with an obstetrician.

Neurobehavioral Disorder Associated With Prenatal Alcohol Exposure

There is no known safe amount of alcohol to consume while pregnant. Alcohol is found in significant levels in amniotic fluid even after a single moderate dose and is not eliminated from the amniotic fluid as rapidly as from maternal circulation.

Fetal alcohol syndrome is a spectrum of structural anomalies and neurocognitive disabilities associated with teratogenic exposure to alcohol. A new diagnostic classification is proposed in the *Diagnostic and Statistical Manual of Mental Disorders*, 5th edition (*DSM-5*), neurobehavioral disorder with prenatal alcohol exposure, which includes impairments in neurocognitive, self-regulatory, and adaptive functioning.

The use of benzodiazepines during pregnancy appears to have a low teratogenic risk. Maternal misuse of sedatives near term has resulted in poor muscle tone and respiratory depression in the neonate. Neonatal sedative withdrawal syndrome usually resolves spontaneously and does not require specific treatment.

OPIOIDS
Maternal Pharmacotherapy

Naloxone should not be given to a pregnant woman maintained on an opioid-agonist medication or using opioid agonists illicitly, except as a last resort in life-threatening opioid overdose, because withdrawal precipitated by an opioid antagonist can result in spontaneous abortion, premature labor, or stillbirth.

Opioid withdrawal syndrome during pregnancy can lead to fetal distress and premature labor. Medically assisted withdrawal is not recommended because of high rates of relapse. Opioid-agonist maintenance with methadone has served as the long-time standard of treatment, and buprenorphine has emerged as a safe alternative to methadone as a first-line medication. Elimination of opioid use with adequate doses of an opioid-agonist medication prevents harm to the fetus, improves maternal health and nutrition, reduces obstetric complications, reduces criminal activity, decreases disruption of the maternal–child dyad, and enhances the woman's ability to participate in prenatal care and SUD treatment.

A pregnant woman may be able to enter treatment sooner than if she were not pregnant.

Maternal methadone dose does not correlate with neonatal abstinence symptoms, so the maternal benefits of methadone are not offset by harm to the newborn. The methadone dose requirement may increase during the third trimester of pregnancy due to larger plasma volume, decreased plasma protein binding, increased tissue binding, increased methadone metabolism, and increased clearance. The woman may experience mild withdrawal symptoms unless adjustments are made to her dose.

Buprenorphine has been well tolerated by pregnant women. Newborns have had a similar incidence of NAS compared to mothers on methadone yet appear to require less medication to treat and have a shorter duration of treatment. The onset of NAS may be longer compared to methadone but still within 4 days of hospital observation.

Neonatal Withdrawal

Neonatal opioid withdrawal syndrome occurs in 60% to 80% of infants with intrauterine exposure to heroin or prescription opioids, including methadone and buprenorphine. The most comprehensive assessment is provided by the Maternal Opioid Treatment: Human Experimental Research (MOTHER) NAS Measure. Newborns are evaluated at 2 hours after birth and then every 4 hours. Pharmacotherapy is usually initiated when the total score is ≥9 for 2 consecutive evaluations or ≥13 on a single evaluation, until the score remains ≤8 for 48 hours. Newborn treatment with an opioid agonist, such as oral morphine sulfate or methadone, reduces time to regain birth weight but may increase hospital length of stay.

There is no evidence that prescribed and illicit opioids are teratogenic. Other than a possible transmission of infection secondary to injection and intranasal insufflation, the most common ill effect of opioid use in pregnancy is intrauterine growth restriction. The most common complication in these infants is emergence of NAS.

CANNABIS

Delta-9-tetrahydrocannabinol easily crosses the placenta, and the fetus is exposed to this as well as carbon monoxide from the smoking of cannabis. Numerous studies have documented neurodevelopmental deficits in children prenatally exposed to cannabis. There is a small reduction in fetal growth and a higher risk of stillbirth and impaired regulatory control, including irritability, tremors, and sleep disturbances. Children exposed in utero have demonstrated behavioral problems and reduced attention spans, lower scores on tests of visual problem solving, visual–motor coordination, and visual analysis compared to unexposed children.

STIMULANTS

Preterm labor, premature rupture of membranes, placental abruption, or intrauterine growth restriction may indicate prior complications of stimulant use, especially cocaine or methamphetamines. Because an abrupt discontinuation of stimulants does not cause gross physiologic sequelae, they are not tapered off or replaced with a cross-tolerant drug during medically supervised withdrawal treatment. Pregnant women withdrawing from stimulants should not receive medication except in cases of extreme agitation. Low doses of a benzodiazepine may be used if necessary.

Effects of cocaine intoxication on neurobehavioral status include irritability with feeding and quieting difficulties. Cocaine is concentrated in the amniotic fluid, causing neurologic, developmental, and behavioral deficiencies in the child exposed prenatally to cocaine. Newborns exposed to methamphetamines in utero may be small for gestational age and at risk for neurodevelopmental abnormalities.

MATERNAL SUBSTANCE USE DISORDER TREATMENT

SUD treatment is more likely to be effective when begun during, rather than after, pregnancy. The possibility of being reunited with children that may have been placed with another family member or in temporary foster care is often an incentive for a mother to enter treatment. This also reduces the burden on the foster care system. Specialty residential treatment programs, specifically those that provide care for infants, are economically justified because comprehensive treatment programs for this population are successful.

Some forms of long-term SUD pharmacotherapy are not appropriate in pregnancy. Disulfiram is contraindicated during pregnancy because of the association with specific birth defects. Acamprosate and naltrexone have not been studied in pregnancy. Due to limited data on nicotine replacement or prescribed medication (varenicline, bupropion) for tobacco/nicotine use during pregnancy, clinicians should focus on office-based brief behavioral interventions. Buprenorphine or methadone treatment is a first-line therapy for pregnant women using opioids and requires dose monitoring throughout pregnancy; maintenance until after delivery is recommended as opposed to tapering off during pregnancy.

LABOR AND DELIVERY

Women may relapse as they near the end of pregnancy. They may confuse early signs of labor with signs of acute opioid withdrawal and may use illicit opioids during early labor. Staff on a labor and delivery units should be aware that women who use stimulants may display bizarre and potentially abusive behavior. The delivery method should be selected based solely on obstetric considerations.

Patients who use illicit drugs are subject to pain in the same manner as any other patient and can benefit from appropriate treatment for pain; however, if the drug used is an opioid, they may have tolerance and thus require higher doses of opioids for pain relief. Reassurance of access to adequate analgesia may allay some fears. Regional anesthesia may be the procedure of choice during delivery and for postpartum pain. Placement of an epidural catheter with infusion of a local anesthetic can reduce the need for opioid analgesics. Pain medication should not be withheld based on the presence of a current or past SUD. There is no reason to withhold or alter opioid agonist therapy given to women with an opioid use disorder in labor and delivery or postpartum. Administering the daily dose of buprenorphine every 6 hours may take advantage of the analgesic properties of the medication. Women who are using heroin or prescription opioids or who are prescribed chronic opioids (including methadone maintenance) should not receive opioid agonist/antagonist pain medications (such as pentazocine or butorphanol) for acute pain because these medications may cause acute opioid withdrawal.

BREASTFEEDING

Women actively engaged in recovery, including those in SUD treatment, should be encouraged to breastfeed as long as urine drug screens are negative and the mother is negative for HIV. Women infected with either hepatitis B or hepatitis C may also breastfeed as long as the nipple and surrounding areola are not cracked and/or bleeding to avoid exposing the child to direct contact with maternal blood. Breastfeeding builds a strong mother–infant bond while providing optimal nutrition and passive immunization for the child.

Women can breastfeed while on methadone or buprenorphine maintenance. There is insufficient information about the extent to which naloxone passes into breast milk to provide guidance for breastfeeding, so clinicians should discuss options regarding continuing buprenorphine without or with naloxone. Breastfeeding should be discouraged during maternal use of benzodiazepines, cocaine, and cannabis.

The substance-exposed nursing infant will display signs similar to those in adults using a substance. Exposure to nicotine causes irritability and poor feeding and disrupts sleep in the infant. Similarly, infants can become intoxicated and irritable with exposure to stimulants such as cocaine and amphetamine; the infant may feed and sleep poorly, may have gastrointestinal disturbance with vomiting or diarrhea, and may present with a seizure. Infants exposed to opioids may display intoxication with sedation and poor feeding or may exhibit withdrawal signs and become tremulous, restless, and feed and sleep poorly. Infants exposed to alcohol may feed and grow poorly, become diaphoretic, and have poor muscle tone.

LEGAL ISSUES

Laboratory screening for substances in a pregnant woman and/or newborn child should not be done without the patient's (ie, the woman's) knowledge and accompanied by informed consent. Some states have laws that equate positive drug testing with child abuse or criminal offenses, which can interfere with SUD treatment. However, in many cases across the nation, legislators and courts have ruled that SUDs in pregnancy is not a criminal matter, and there is no evidence that punitive approaches work.

A positive toxicology screen in a mother or infant warrants a Child Protective Services (CPS) evaluation. The federal Child Abuse Prevention and Treatment Act requires states to have policies and procedures to notify CPS of substance-exposed newborns. The mandate to report varies significantly; therefore, clinicians should be familiar with legislation in their state and community. CPS workers are responsible for investigating risks to the child, thus relieving the clinician from the task of optimizing the postpartum home environment.

Mandatory reporting of positive maternal drug screens or aggressive prosecution may cause women to avoid disclosure of SUDs during pregnancy or avoid prenatal care and hospital delivery because they fear the loss of their child, particularly if they have other children in the custody of CPS or living with relatives. However, mandatory reporting legislation may provide an incentive to enter treatment prior to delivery to avoid potential prosecution. Continued custody of the child may be contingent on adherence to a treatment plan determined by CPS. Use of the criminal justice system for coercion to initiate SUD treatment is supported by improved outcomes when women are allowed to retain custody of their infant. Every effort should be made to coordinate appropriate placement of the infant (eg, with the mother, another family member, or in foster care) when a mother needs SUD treatment. With such support, the mother can continue to bond with her infant, and it provides positive motivation for the mother to attend treatment and enter recovery.

POSTPARTUM CARE

Effectively treating a parent is the most important intervention for the child exposed to substances, both prenatally and during childhood. The stresses of meeting the developmental needs of a newborn, possibly rearing older children, lack of family and social support, depression and other psychiatric problems, inadequate housing or homelessness, exposure to violence, and financial difficulties may pose as much risk to successful child-rearing as SUDs. Comprehensive ongoing maternal SUD treatment, tailored to help the woman address other stressors besides the SUD, reduces the chance of an adverse outcome for both mother and child. If a mother is successful in treatment, she may be able to retain custody of her children. For the woman whose children have been removed from her home, a goal of treatment and recovery should be reunification of her family.

Following birth, maternal treatment plans should be expanded to address newborn medical problems such as infection and developmental problems due to substance exposure. Bonding with the infant may be more difficult, so the mother may need to be taught specific skills to calm and feed her infant. Older children may need to be evaluated for developmental problems if the mother is concerned or gives a history of substance use in earlier pregnancies. This can have a positive impact on the development of every child in the family and may prevent another substance-exposed pregnancy.

KEY POINTS

1. Screening with a brief intervention for substance use along with laboratory testing should be performed for all pregnant women at the initial prenatal visit and repeated if necessary; several validated screening tools are available.
2. Clinicians must be aware of mandated reporting requirements in their jurisdiction during pregnancy or after delivery, which may help motivate pregnant women to consider appropriate treatment for substance use.
3. Pregnant women should be offered appropriate pharmacotherapy for maternal withdrawal

syndromes, especially for alcohol, sedatives, and opioids.

4. Pregnant women should be offered appropriate options for pain management during labor and delivery.

5. Pregnant women should be offered education about breastfeeding as well as postpartum care and support.

REVIEW QUESTIONS

1. A 29-year-old pregnant woman is actively using legal and illicit substances daily. She has not seen a doctor for this pregnancy because she is ashamed and afraid that Child Protective Services will take the baby away from her after the delivery. She quit using substances 3 days ago because she does not want her baby "to be addicted" at birth. She comes to the emergency department in active labor and is determined by ultrasound and dates to be at about 30 weeks' gestation. Which of the following substances is most likely to cause fetal distress and premature labor?
   A. Alcohol
   B. Cocaine
   C. Opioids
   D. Phencyclidine

2. The obstetrics team is able to stabilize the pregnancy and halt the premature labor, and the patient enters a residential program for pregnant women with a substance use disorder. She follows the treatment plan successfully with all urine drug tests negative. At the last prenatal visit, she asks about being able to nurse her baby. Which of the following is a contraindication to breastfeeding?
   A. Maternal serum is positive for hepatitis B.
   B. Maternal serum is positive for HIV.

C. Maternal serum is positive for anti-DNA antibodies.
D. Maternal serum is positive for hepatitis C.

3. She delivers a healthy 3500-g female infant at 39 weeks, having abstained from all psychoactive legal and illegal substances. She was particularly worried about sudden infant death syndrome and the baby being "retarded" (ie, developmentally delayed). Which of the following substances are most likely to cause teratogenicity and are associated with an increased incidence of sudden infant death syndrome?
   A. Tobacco and alcohol
   B. Alcohol and cocaine
   C. Cocaine and tobacco
   D. Opioids and alcohol

ANSWERS

1. **C**
2. **B**
3. **A**

SUGGESTED READINGS

Chabarria KC, Racusin DA, Antony KM, et al. Marijuana use and its effects in pregnancy. *Am J Obstet Gynecol*. 2016;215(4): 506.e1-7.

Hudak ML, Tan RC. Neonatal drug withdrawal. *Pediatrics*. 2012;129(2):e540-e560.

Jones HE, Terplan M, Meyer M. Medically assisted withdrawal (detoxification): considering the mother-infant dyad. *J Addict Med*. 2017;11(2):90-92.

Kable JA, O'Connor MJ, Olson HC, et al. Neurobehavioral disorder associated with prenatal alcohol exposure (ND-PAE): proposed DSM-5 diagnosis. *Child Psychiatry Hum Dev*. 2016;47(2):335-346.

Wright TE, Terplan M, Ondersma SJ, et al. The role of screening, brief intervention, and referral to treatment in the perinatal period. *Am J Obstet Gynecol*. 2016;215(5):539-547.

91

Perioperative Management of Patients with Alcohol- or Other Drug Use

Summary by Daniel P. Alford

Based on THE ASAM PRINCIPLES OF ADDICTION MEDICINE, 6th edition chapter by Daniel P. Alford and Zoe M. Weinstein

Surgery may be required for complications of alcohol and other drug use. Substance use and its associated chronic medical conditions can increase the risk of postoperative complications. Hospitalization for surgery may be the first time that a patient with a substance use disorder does not have access to alcohol or other drugs, putting him or her at risk for withdrawal. Acute withdrawal syndromes may complicate surgery and the postoperative course. Treating physicians should not expect to cure the patient's substance use disorder during the perioperative hospitalization but should focus on getting the patient through the surgery safely and then offering the patient referral to long-term addiction treatment.

PERIOPERATIVE CARE OF PATIENTS WITH UNHEALTHY ALCOHOL USE

The prevalence of alcohol use disorders is as high as 40% in emergency room and various surgical inpatient settings and up to 50% in patients with trauma. The incidence of symptomatic alcohol withdrawal in hospitalized patients is as high as 8% and is two to five times higher in hospitalized trauma and surgical patients. Chronic alcohol use can increase the risk of postoperative mortality and morbidity through immune suppression, reduced cardiac function, and dysregulated homeostasis, including alterations in platelet production, aggregation, and changes in fibrinogen levels. Preoperative alcohol use is an independent predictor of pneumonia, sepsis, superficial surgical site infection, wound complications, and longer hospital stays.

Preoperative Evaluation

The preoperative evaluation should assess the patient for the risk of acute alcohol withdrawal and the presence of diseases associated with heavy alcohol use. Adults undergoing a preoperative evaluation should be screened using validated questionnaires such as the Single Item Screening Question (SISQ), CAGE, Alcohol Use Disorders Identification Test—Consumption (AUDIT-C). The AUDIT-C can identify patients at risk not only for postoperative complications but also for increased postoperative healthcare utilization (ie, hospital length of stay, more intensive care unit days, and increased probability to return to the operating room).

It is also important to note that sedatives (eg, benzodiazepines) and analgesics (eg, opioids) given during surgery and the postoperative period may delay, partially treat, or obscure some symptoms of alcohol withdrawal. Physical examinations should evaluate for evidence of liver, pancreatic, nervous system, and cardiac disease. The spectrum of alcoholic liver disease ranges from fatty liver with normal or mild elevations in liver function tests (ie, transaminases) to acute hepatitis and cirrhosis. Pancreatitis can present as acute and chronic abdominal pain as well as exocrine (ie, malabsorption) and endocrine dysfunction (ie, glucose intolerance to diabetes mellitus). Alcohol-associated dementia, Korsakoff syndrome, hepatic and Wernicke encephalopathy, myelopathies, and polyneuropathies can worsen during the perioperative period and may be confused with other postoperative neurologic complications. Preoperative evaluations for congestive heart failure should be considered because up to one third of patients with long-standing heavy alcohol use have a decreased cardiac ejection fraction. Because of the association between heavy alcohol use/alcohol use disorders and nicotine use disorder, smoking-related comorbidities such as coronary heart disease and chronic obstructive pulmonary disease (COPD) should also be evaluated for. Preoperative laboratory studies should include electrolytes, liver function tests, coagulation studies, and a complete blood count. Anemia is common in patients with alcohol use disorders as well as decreased platelet count from alcohol-associated bone marrow suppression and splenic sequestration. It is also important to identify patients who are in recovery from alcohol or other drug use preoperatively because they may have concerns and questions about perioperative exposure to sedative–hypnotics and opioid analgesics.

Management of Alcohol Withdrawal

Withdrawal symptoms may appear within hours of decreased intake; however, during the perioperative period, the administration of anesthetics, sedatives, and analgesics may delay the onset of withdrawal. Because alcohol withdrawal is especially dangerous during the postoperative period, asymptomatic but at-risk patients should receive prophylactic treatment (eg, benzodiazepines) to prevent withdrawal. Use of the Clinical Institute Withdrawal Assessment Scale for Alcohol, revised, may be difficult to use in the postoperative period in patients unable to verbally communicate and may be less reliable in patients with acute medical or surgical illnesses. Alternatively, for patients who are in severe withdrawal and unable to respond to questions, the Minnesota Detoxification Scale protocol, which has been studied in intensive care unit settings, could be used.

Alcohol Use and Surgical Risk

Heavy alcohol use even in the absence of clinical liver disease or alcohol use disorder per se is an independent risk factor for postoperative complications. There is a dose–response effect, with increased alcohol consumption in grams being associated with both increased postoperative complications and prolonged hospital stays. Five possible pathologic mechanisms have been identified to account for the increased rate of postoperative complications: immune incompetence, subclinical cardiac insufficiency, hemostatic imbalances, abnormal stress response, and wound healing dysfunction. Abstinence before surgery decreases postoperative morbidity.

Alcoholic Liver Disease

The spectrum of liver disease associated with the spectrum of unhealthy alcohol use (ie, risky use to alcohol use disorder) includes asymptomatic fatty liver, acute hepatitis, and finally, chronic cirrhosis. Each form of liver disease carries some degree of surgical risk and requires special preoperative considerations.

Alcoholic Fatty Liver

Patients with fatty liver seem to tolerate surgery well; however, there are no known studies evaluating perioperative risks in these patients. It is prudent to delay elective surgery until resolution of clinical signs and symptoms and, if possible, abstinence is achieved.

Alcoholic Hepatitis

Surgical risk is very high in this group, with 100% mortality rates reported in older series. Therefore, alcoholic hepatitis should be considered a contraindication to elective surgery. It is recommended that elective surgery be delayed until clinical and laboratory parameters normalize, sometimes taking up to 12 weeks.

Alcoholic Cirrhosis

The need for surgery is common in patients with cirrhosis, with up to 10% requiring a surgical procedure during the last 2 years of life. Depending on the severity of cirrhosis, surgery can be extremely risky. The most common causes of perioperative mortality in patients with cirrhosis are sepsis, hemorrhage, and hepatorenal syndrome. Although currently used anesthetic agents are not hepatotoxic, surgical stress in itself causes hemodynamic changes in the liver, resulting in an increased risk for hepatic decompensation during surgical stress. Anesthetic agents decrease hepatic blood flow by as much as 50% and therefore decrease hepatic oxygen uptake. Intraoperative traction on abdominal viscera may also decrease hepatic blood flow.

Effect of Cirrhosis on Surgical Risk

The preoperative factors associated with increased surgical morbidity and mortality include emergent surgery, upper abdominal surgery, poor hepatic synthetic function, anemia, ascites, malnutrition, and encephalopathy. These patients are at an increased risk for uncontrolled bleeding, infections, and delirium. Coagulopathies and thrombocytopenia result in difficulty achieving a perioperative hemostasis. Ascites increases the risk of intra-abdominal infections, abdominal wound dehiscence, and abdominal wall herniation. Nutritional deficiencies result in poor wound healing and an increased risk of skin breakdown, and encephalopathy decreases the patient's ability to effectively participate in postoperative rehabilitation. The action of anesthetic agents may be prolonged and increases the risk of delirium. In trying to risk stratify patients preoperatively, it is important to look for clinical signs of cirrhosis and portal hypertension. There are two scoring systems in use to predict whether patients with advanced liver disease will survive surgery. Using a multivariable clinical assessment, the Pugh (modified Child–Turcotte) classification stratifies patients with cirrhosis into three classes based on "hepatic reserve" and therefore surgical risk. Using pooled surgical data, the Pugh classification scheme has proven to be good for stratifying a patient's preoperative risk. A second scoring system is the Model for End-Stage Liver Disease, which is used to prioritize patients for liver transplantation and, more recently, as a predictor of survival after nontransplant surgery.

Preoperative Considerations in Patients With Cirrhosis

Preoperative abstinence should be the goal before all elective procedures. Coagulopathies should be corrected. Ascites should be optimally managed. Infectious risk should be mitigated as best as possible with prophylactic preoperative broad-spectrum antibiotics (eg, norfloxacin, ciprofloxacin) to protect against secondary and spontaneous bacterial peritonitis. Renal function should be monitored closely. Aggressive preoperative treatment of hepatic encephalopathy using lactulose and dietary protein restriction is recommended. Patients with known gastroesophageal varices should be monitored closely for gastrointestinal bleeding and should be considered for β-blocker prophylaxis preoperatively. Nutritional status should be optimized. From a pulmonary standpoint, patients should be kept on continuous oxygen saturation monitoring.

Management of Patients on Naltrexone (Opioid Antagonist) Pharmacotherapy

Because naltrexone is an opioid antagonist and will block the effects of coadministered opioid agonists, patients requiring opioid analgesics during the perioperative period will need to discontinue naltrexone. Oral naltrexone is typically discontinued at least 72 hours before surgery. Because a degree of opioid resistance will remain, patients should be observed closely for respiratory depression and sedation as well as analgesia efficacy. For patients on extended-release depot naltrexone, elective surgery should be postponed, if possible, for a month after the last naltrexone injection. Patients requiring opioids for pain management after emergent surgery should have their naltrexone discontinued and opioids analgesics administered under close observation. An anesthesiologist should be consulted to

assist with perioperative pain management, including the use of nonopioid alternatives and regional analgesia.

PERIOPERATIVE CARE OF PATIENTS WITH AN OPIOID USE DISORDER

Persons with an opioid use disorder are at high risk for medical complications that often require surgical intervention. Chronic diseases associated with opioid misuse, such as pulmonary hypertension secondary to talc granulomatosis, renal insufficiency secondary to heroin-associated nephropathy, and congestive heart failure from valvular heart disease secondary to endocarditis, HIV, and chronic hepatitis B and C, can all increase surgical risk. Acute opioid withdrawal can also complicate the perioperative period.

Preoperative Evaluation

Patients with current or past injection drug use should be evaluated for past endocarditis and the need for antibiotic prophylaxis. These patients should also be evaluated for HIV/AIDS and active hepatitis B and C. Hospitalized patients with an opioid use disorder are at risk for acute opioid withdrawal. Active opioid use can be verified using urine drug tests, whereas injection drug use can be identified by examining the skin for "track marks." Patients who have an opioid use disorder may also be using other drugs, such as cocaine, alcohol, or benzodiazepines.

Management of Patients on Opioid Agonist Pharmacotherapy

Patients on opioid agonist therapy (OAT) with methadone or buprenorphine should be maintained on their usual maintenance dose equivalent during the perioperative period.

Management of Acute Pain in Patients on Opioid Agonist Therapy

The daily methadone or buprenorphine dose a patient receives for opioid use disorder abstinence is not adequate analgesia for acute pain because of the patient's high tolerance to opioids and the pharmacodynamics of methadone and buprenorphine. The appropriate treatment of acute pain in these patients includes uninterrupted OAT to address the patient's baseline opioid requirement for their opioid use disorder treatment and aggressive acute pain management (Table 91-1). As with all patients suffering acute pain, nonopioid analgesics should be aggressively implemented first line. However, severe

TABLE 91-1	Recommendations for Treating Acute Pain in Patients on Opioid Agonist Therapy[a]

Addiction Treatment Issues

- Reassure the patient that his or her addiction history will not prevent adequate pain management.
- Continue the usual dose (or equivalent) of opioid agonist therapy.
- Methadone or buprenorphine maintenance doses should be verified.
- Notify the addiction treatment program or prescribing physician regarding the patient's admission and discharge and confirm the time and amount of last maintenance opioid dose.
- Inform the addiction treatment maintenance program or prescribing physician of any medications given to the patient during hospitalization because they (eg, opioids, benzodiazepines) may show up on routine urine drug screens.

Pain Management Issues

- Relieve patient anxiety by discussing, in a nonjudgmental manner, the plan for pain management.
- Use conventional analgesics, including opioids, to aggressively treat the painful condition.
- Opioid cross-tolerance and patients' increased pain sensitivity will necessitate higher opioid analgesic doses at shorter intervals.
- Write for continuous scheduled dosing rather than as needed orders.
- Avoid using mixed agonist/antagonist opioids as they will precipitate an acute withdrawal syndrome.

If on Methadone Maintenance

- Continue methadone maintenance dose and consider dividing the dose to every 6–8 h to take advantage of the analgesic properties.
- Use short-acting opioid analgesics.

If on Buprenorphine Maintenance

- Continue buprenorphine maintenance and consider dividing the dose to every 6–8 h to take advantage of the analgesic properties.
- Titrate short-acting opioid analgesics.

[a] These recommendations are applicable only when opioid analgesic treatment is determined to be necessary for the treatment of acute pain.

acute pain may require opioid analgesics. Because of cross-tolerance with OAT, adequate pain control will generally necessitate higher opioid doses at shorter intervals.

PERIOPERATIVE CARE OF PATIENTS WITH BENZODIAZEPINE USE DISORDER

Benzodiazepine use has been associated with higher rates of postoperative mechanical ventilation among trauma surgery patients. Patients with physical dependence to prescribed benzodiazepines should be maintained on their usual dose during the perioperative period to prevent acute withdrawal and subsequent postoperative complications. Patients physically dependent on illicit benzodiazepines should be maintained on an equivalent dose of long-acting benzodiazepine (eg, diazepam, chlordiazepoxide) during the perioperative period with psychiatric and addiction specialist consultation for guidance on a safe benzodiazepine taper during the postoperative period.

PERIOPERATIVE CARE OF PATIENTS WHO SMOKE TOBACCO OR CANNABIS

People who smoke have greater odds of postoperative cardiovascular events (ie, cardiac arrest, myocardial infarction, stroke), infections (ie, pneumonia, incision infections, sepsis, septic shock), and unplanned intubation. Preoperative evaluations should include an assessment of their physical dependence on nicotine and the risk of withdrawal. In addition, preoperative evaluations should include an assessment for evidence of cardiovascular disease and COPD. Patients with COPD have an increased risk of postoperative pulmonary complications, including pneumonia bronchospasm, respiratory failure with prolonged mechanical ventilation, and COPD exacerbations. Intensive preoperative interventions for nicotine/tobacco use have been shown to reduce the incidence of postoperative complications. Pharmacotherapy, including nicotine replacement, bupropion, and varenicline, consistently increases abstinence rates and should be considered preoperatively. An aggressive perioperative treatment of airflow obstruction should be achieved with inhaled steroids and β-agonists. Preoperative patient education regarding postoperative incentive spirometry use decreases the incidence of postoperative pulmonary complications. Nicotine replacement therapy also should be postoperatively offered to patients at risk for nicotine withdrawal. Compared with nicotine cigarettes, the airway effects of smoking cannabis are mild, but with acute use, upper airway edema can occur and a chronic cough and mild airflow obstruction can develop with long-term use.

PERIOPERATIVE CARE OF PATIENTS WITH STIMULANT USE DISORDER

People with stimulant use disorders may require surgical interventions due to the acute and chronic effects of these drugs. All patients who use cocaine should be screened for concurrent heavy alcohol use. Depression and hypersomnolence are common in stimulant withdrawal and may mimic or be confused with other postoperative neurologic complications.

ORGAN TRANSPLANTATION IN PATIENTS WITH SUBSTANCE USE DISORDERS

In the United States, hepatitis B and C infections from injection drug use and alcoholic liver disease are the most common causes of end-stage liver disease, requiring liver transplantation. In the past, patients with a history of substance use disorders have been kept off of transplantation lists not only because of fears of posttransplant nonadherence with subsequent loss of graft but also because of moralistic arguments that the patients had a "self-inflicted" disease. The transplant community continues to evolve in their treatment of patients with substance use disorders.

KEY POINTS

1. Heavy alcohol use, even in the absence of clinical liver disease and even in the absence of an

alcohol use disorder, is an independent risk factor for postoperative complications.
2. Patients with alcohol-associated cirrhosis can have their surgical risk assessed using the Pugh classification or Model for End-Stage Liver Disease score.
3. Perioperative morbidity associated with acute abstinence syndromes can be prevented with proper preoperative screening, assessment, and treatment.
4. Patients with an opioid use disorder treated with opioid agonist therapy (ie, methadone, buprenorphine) should be maintained on their usual maintenance dose equivalent during the perioperative period, whereas patients treated with opioid antagonist therapy (naltrexone) will need to discontinue the opioid antagonist preoperatively in order to achieve benefit from postoperative opioid analgesics.
5. Management of patients with substance use disorders going for surgery often requires consultation with addiction and pain specialists.

REVIEW QUESTIONS

1. Which of the following is a proposed mechanism for the increased rate of postoperative complications in patients with heavy daily alcohol use even in the absence of liver disease?
   A. Immune incompetence
   B. Subclinical kidney dysfunction
   C. Subclinical hypothyroidism
   D. Hypercoagulable state
   E. Elevated number of platelets

2. The preoperative factors associated with increased surgical morbidity and mortality in a patient with cirrhosis include all of the following *except*:
   A. emergent surgery.
   B. lower extremity surgery.
   C. poor hepatic synthetic function.
   D. encephalopathy.
   E. ascites.

3. For a patient on methadone maintenance treatment undergoing a total hip replacement, what is recommended regarding his or her methadone maintenance treatment and acute postoperative pain management?
   A. Discontinue methadone and treat acute pain with morphine intramuscularly every 6 hours as needed.
   B. Discontinue methadone and treat acute pain with morphine patient-controlled analgesia.

C. Double once-daily methadone dose to treat both opioid use disorder and pain.

D. Continue usual methadone dose and treat acute pain with morphine patient-controlled analgesia.

E. Discontinue methadone, start oral naltrexone, and treat acute pain with morphine intramuscularly every 6 hours as needed.

ANSWERS

1. **A**
2. **B**
3. **D**

SUGGESTED READINGS

Bradley KA, Rubinsky AD, Sun H, et al. Alcohol screening and risk of postoperative complications in male VA patients undergoing major non-cardiac surgery. *J Gen Intern Med.* 2011;26(2):162-169.

Donroe JH, Holt SR, Tetrault JM. Caring for patients with opioid use disorder in the hospital. *CMAJ.* 2016;188(17-18): 1232-1239.

Moran S, Isa J, Steinemann S. Perioperative management in the patient with substance abuse. *Surg Clin North Am.* 2015;95(2):417-428.

Oppedal K, Møller AM, Pedersen B, Tønnesen H. Preoperative alcohol cessation prior to elective surgery. *Cochrane Database Syst Rev.* 2012;(7):CD008343.

Thomsen T, Villebro N, Møller AM. Interventions for preoperative smoking cessation. *Cochrane Database Syst Rev.* 2014;(3):CD002294.

Co-Occurring Addiction and Psychiatric Disorders

Substance-Induced Mental Disorders

Summary by Christine Yuodelis-Flores, R. Jeffrey Goldsmith, and Richard K. Ries

Based on THE ASAM PRINCIPLES OF ADDICTION MEDICINE, 6th edition chapter by Christine Yuodelis-Flores, R. Jeffrey Goldsmith, and Richard K. Ries

Substance-induced psychiatric disorders mimic traditional psychiatric illnesses such as depressive, anxiety, bipolar, and psychotic disorders. The *Diagnostic and Statistical Manual of Mental Disorders,* 5th edition (*DSM-5*), published in 2013, did not change *DSM-IV* guidelines for diagnoses but does include changes to groupings of the disorders so that substance-induced disorders are discussed in general terms in the chapter "Substance-Related and Addictive Disorders," whereas the specific substance-induced psychiatric disorder is discussed in the chapter discussing that specific disorder (ie, substance-induced depressive disorder is found in the chapter on depressive disorders). In addition, there are two additional substance-induced psychiatric disorders in *DSM-5*: substance-induced bipolar and related disorder and substance-induced obsessive-compulsive and related disorder. Eleven substance-induced mental disorders (SIMD) are given in the *DSM-5* (Table 92-1).

DIAGNOSIS OF SUBSTANCE-INDUCED MENTAL DISORDERS

There are several classes of substances that may induce mental disorders as well as a variety of toxins and medications. The addictive substances that can induce mental disorders are alcohol, cannabis, phencyclidine and other hallucinogens, inhalants, opioids, sedative-hypnotic/anxiolytic drugs, stimulants, 3,4-methylenedioxymethamphetamine (MDMA, ecstasy), substituted cathinones ("bath salts"), synthetic cannabinoids ("Spice"), caffeine, and tobacco. According to the *DSM-5*, there are five criteria (A through E) for the diagnosis of all SIMDs:

A. The disorder represents a clinically significant symptomatic presentation of a relative mental disorder.

B. There is evidence from history, physical examination, or laboratory findings of both of the following:
1. The disorder developed during or within 1 month of a substance intoxication or withdrawal or taking a medication; and
2. The involved substance/medication is capable of producing the mental disorder.

C. The disorder is not better explained by an independent mental disorder. Such evidence of an independent mental disorder could include the following:
1. The disorder preceded the onset of severe intoxication or withdrawal or exposure to a medication.
2. The full mental disorder persisted for a substantial period of time (eg, at least 1 month) after the cessation of acute withdrawal or severe intoxication or taking the medication. This criterion does not apply to substance-induced neurocognitive disorders or hallucinogen-persisting perception disorder, which persist beyond the cessation of acute intoxication or withdrawal.

D. The disorder does not occur exclusively during the course of a delirium.

E. The disorder causes clinically significant distress or impairment in social, occupational, or other important areas of functioning.

PREVALENCE AND COURSE OF SUBSTANCE-INDUCED MENTAL DISORDERS

Substance-Induced Depressive Disorder

People with substance use disorders (SUDs) commonly present with depressive symptoms comparable to those seen in individuals hospitalized for

TABLE 92-1 *DSM-5* Substance/Medication-Induced Mental Disorders
Substance-induced depressive disorder
Substance-induced bipolar disorder and related conditions
Substance-induced anxiety disorder
Substance-induced obsessive–compulsive disorder and related conditions
Substance-induced psychotic disorder
Substance-induced major and minor neurocognitive disorder   Amnestic-confabulatory type
Hallucinogen-persisting perception disorder
Substance intoxication delirium
Substance withdrawal delirium
Substance-induced sexual dysfunction
Substance-induced sleep disorder

DSM-5, *The Diagnostic and Statistical Manual of Mental Disorders*, 5th edition.

affective disorder. Symptoms usually abate quickly over the first 2 to 4 weeks of abstinence. Using the Psychiatric Research Interview for Substance and Mental Disorders (PRISM-IV), it was found that among those with comorbid substance use and psychiatric disorders, 41% had psychiatric disorders considered to be independent of their substance use, 7% had substance-induced disorders only, and 38% had both independent and substance-induced disorders (Langås A-M et al., 2012).

It can be very difficult to differentiate between substance-induced depressive disorder (SIDD) and independent major depressive disorder (MDD), and the diagnosis may change if the patient is followed over time. In one study (Ramsey SE et al., 2004), over a course of a year, 26.4% of those diagnosed with SIDD were reclassified as having an independent MDD because of meeting the full criteria for the diagnosis of MDD after 1 month of sobriety. Those with a history of past independent MDD were five times more likely to be reclassified from SIDD to independent MDD. Patients who had lower severity of alcohol dependence were also more likely to be reclassified as having independent MDD. E.V. Nunes and colleagues (2006) studied depressive disorders in patients with alcohol use disorder who were admitted to an inpatient psychiatric unit using the PRISM-IV and found that 51% of patients with MDDs were classified as having SIDD and 49% were diagnosed as

having co-occurring major depression; however, after following them for a year, 32% of those with SIDD were reclassified as having independent depression.

In those with cocaine use disorder, findings suggests a lifetime prevalence of about 30% for cocaine-induced depressive disorder (Rounsaville, 1991). They also reported a 16% current rate and a 21% lifetime rate of anxiety disorders. People with methamphetamine use disorders are also reported to have high rates of depressive symptoms and suicidal behavior during active use as well as during withdrawal and early abstinence.

Substance-Induced Anxiety Disorder

Several studies have reported high rates of anxiety symptoms among patients with alcohol use disorder in withdrawal, with up to 80% of subjects with a dependence on alcohol experiencing repeated panic attacks during alcohol withdrawal, and over 50% of subjects with alcohol use disorder had symptoms of generalized anxiety and social phobia. Symptoms of substance-induced anxiety disorder abate rapidly after 2 to 4 weeks of abstinence.

Substance-Induced Psychotic Disorders

Psychosis during intoxication is common among those using psychotomimetic drugs of abuse, which include cannabis, cocaine, amphetamines and related stimulants, substituted cathinones, synthetic cannabinoids, hallucinogens, and dissociative drugs such as phencyclidine (PCP) and ketamine. A study evaluating individuals with psychosis and SUD presenting to a psychiatric emergency department reported a prevalence of 44% for substance-induced psychotic disorder (SIPD), whereas the other 56% had primary psychotic disorder (PPD) (Caton CL et al., 2005). In a later study, the PRISM-IV differentially diagnosed 56% of patients with first-episode psychosis with SIPD and 44% with PPD (Fraser S et al., 2012). Although SIPD is thought to have a better prognosis than PPD, a recent study concluded that SIPD transitions to a permanent schizophrenia spectrum disorder in about 11% to 24% of cases (Chen W-L et al., 2015). In another study of over 18,000 inpatients with SIPD, the 8-year cumulative risk of SIPD converting to a diagnosis of schizophrenia spectrum disorder was 46% for those diagnosed with cannabis-induced psychosis and 30% for those with amphetamine-induced psychosis (Niemi-Pynttäri JA et al., 2013).

Substance-Induced Bipolar and Related Disorder

According to *DSM-5*, substance-induced bipolar and related disorder is defined as a prominent and persistent disturbance in mood characterized by elevated, expansive, or irritable mood with or without depressed mood or markedly diminished interest or pleasure in almost all activities. The *International Classification of Diseases and Related Health Problems*, 10th edition, Clinical Modification (*ICD-10-CM*) codes for specific substance-induced bipolar and related disorders list substances such as alcohol, phencyclidine, hallucinogens, steroids, sedative–hypnotics/anxiolytics, and stimulants as inducing this disorder as well as medications such as dexamethasone. The prevalence of substance-induced bipolar and related disorder is unknown due to no epidemiologic studies. The *DSM-5* specifically mentions that antidepressant- or electroconvulsive-induced mania is not included in this diagnosis because they are indicative of true bipolar disorder.

Substance/Medication-Induced Obsessive Compulsive and Related Disorders

Obsessions, compulsions, skin picking, hair pulling, and other body-focused repetitive behaviors can occur during substance intoxication or withdrawal, use of a medication, or exposure to heavy metals or toxins. Stimulants such as methamphetamine, amphetamine, cocaine, and substituted cathinones are associated with this diagnosis (eg, methamphetamine-induced excoriation [skin-picking] disorder). The prevalence of substance/medication-induced obsessive-compulsive and related disorders is considered rare; however, one study of amphetamine-induced obsessive–compulsive disorder in Iran showed the prevalence to be 6.9%.

Substance-Associated Suicidal Behavior

SIDD can dissipate rapidly, but it is as dangerous as MDD in terms of the risk of suicide and self-injurious behavior. Both independent and substance-induced depressions are associated with suicidal ideation, planning, and attempts.

SPECIFIC SUBSTANCES: SUBSTANCE-INDUCED PSYCHIATRIC SYMPTOMS

See Table 92-2.

DIFFERENTIAL DIAGNOSIS AND TREATMENT

Substance-Induced Depressive and Anxiety Disorders

It is important to take a careful history and to seek confirmation of the history from collateral informants, especially family and friends, in addition to other healthcare professionals. Establishing a relationship between the use of psychoactive substances and the symptoms is important. Chronic use of alcohol, sedatives, and opiates can cause depressed mood, as can withdrawal from stimulants and sedatives. Exploring the mood and degree of anxiety during periods of sustained abstinence from all drugs and alcohol is critical. In making a diagnosis of SIMD, it is important to order a toxicology screen.

Substance-Induced Psychotic Disorders

A drug screen is especially important because the subject may not have accurate knowledge of what substances were ingested. Hallucinations or delusions must be prominent and are not counted if the individual has insight into the substance-induced nature of his or her psychiatric symptoms. Among young people, substance use is common in first-episode psychosis, and the differentiation of SIPD from PPD is challenging and requires a careful psychiatric and substance use history, drug screen, and collateral information from family and friends. The differential diagnosis of methamphetamine psychosis and PPD is difficult, and a recent multisite international study has concluded that the severity of psychotic symptoms observed in patients with methamphetamine-induced psychosis and patients with schizophrenia is almost the same. Using the PRISM-IV to diagnose individuals with first-episode psychosis admitted to a psychiatric ward, a study (Fraser S et al., 2012) found that 56% had SIPD. Those with SIPD had higher rates of substance use and SUDs, had higher levels of insight, were more likely to have a forensic and trauma history, and had more severe hostility and anxiety symptoms compared to those with non–drug-induced psychosis. In treatment, benzodiazepines can be used to manage acute agitation during intoxication. Atypical antipsychotics should be used if the psychosis is severe or not resolved within 1 to 2 weeks after the cessation of drug use. Most cases of SIPD are short lived and resolve within a few days to 2 weeks, with the exception of methamphetamine psychosis—persistent psychotic symptoms after heavy and/or long-term use has been well documented in several studies.

TABLE 92-2	Substance-Induced Symptoms			
Substance	**Source**	**Intoxication Symptoms**	**Withdrawal Symptoms**	**Miscellaneous**
Caffeine	Energy drinks, coffee, tea	Anxiety, restlessness, insomnia, gastrointestinal upset, tremors, tachycardia, cardiac arrhythmias	Headache, fatigue, drowsiness, impaired concentration, depressed mood	Withdrawal begins 12–24 h after cessation and reaches a peak after 20–48 h.
Nicotine	Tobacco, nicotine medication, e-cigarettes	Nausea; increased heart rate, blood pressure, and cardiac output; enhanced concentration; improved mood	Irritability, craving, depressed mood, insomnia, impaired concentration; acute withdrawal symptoms reach maximum intensity 24–48 h after cessation	There may be nonnicotine chemicals that exaggerate cravings and improve moods.
Alcohol	Alcoholic beverages, vitamins and medicinal liquids, mouthwash, cough syrup	Euphoria, sedation/relaxation, depressed mood, suicidal feelings, violent behaviors, psychomotor imbalance, lack of coordination	Hyperadrenergic state with agitation, anxiety, tremor, malaise, hyperreflexia, mild tachycardia, increased blood pressure, sweating, insomnia, nausea or vomiting, perceptual distortions, seizures	There can be protracted withdrawal symptoms persisting more than a week from the last drink. Some people have brain damage from chronic alcohol consumption.
Sedatives-Hypnotics	Anxiolytic medications, prescription sleep aids, barbiturates, benzodiazepines	Euphoria, sedation, reduction in anxiety, psychomotor imbalance, lack of coordination	Panic attacks, anxiety and depression, insomnia, autonomic hyperactivity, tremor, nausea or vomiting, tinnitus, transient hallucinations or illusions, seizures	There can be a protracted withdrawal syndrome lasting for weeks with symptoms including anxiety, depression, paresthesias, perceptual distortions, muscle pain and twitching, tinnitus, headache, derealization, depersonalization, and impaired concentration.
Stimulants	Cocaine, amphetamine, methamphetamine	Intense euphoria with hyperactive behavior and speech, hypersexuality, anorexia, insomnia, inattention, labile mood, psychotic symptoms	Depression, cognitive problems, hypersomnia, decreased energy, increased appetite	After binging, some may become hostile and agitated, paranoid, and delusional. Some have a chronic dysphoric state and concentration difficulties that can last for years, and some have a chronic psychotic state resembling paranoid schizophrenia.
Opiates	Pain pills, heroin	High or rush, euphoria, sedation, depression if used for long periods of time	Irritability, craving, muscle aches, flu-like syndrome, nausea, cramps and/or diarrhea; some have hypertension and tachycardia	Some report depression and anhedonia if used chronically.

TABLE 92-2	Substance-Induced Symptoms *(Continued)*			
Substance	**Source**	**Intoxication Symptoms**	**Withdrawal Symptoms**	**Miscellaneous**
THC: cannabis, marijuana, hashish, hash oil	Variety of products	Euphoria, augmented appetite, sedation, time distortion, depersonalization	Mild anxiety, irritability, physical tension, decreased appetite, restlessness, craving	Heavy users can have more severe depression. Early onset of psychosis can occur in vulnerable individuals.
Ecstasy (MDMA), synthetic cathinones (includes MDPV, mephedrone, methylone, etc.)	"Molly" "Bath salts"	Similar to stimulant intoxication; possible serotonin syndrome and psychotic symptoms	Similar to stimulant withdrawal	Residual dysphoric states and concentration difficulties can occur.
PCP, ketamine, designer drug analogues	PCP, anesthetics, methoxetamine	Hallucinations, dissociative states, violent behavior, amnesia	Not known	NMDA antagonists
Salvia divinorum	Mint family herb	Hallucinations, visual distortions, perceptual disturbances, anxiety, confusion, dysphoria	Not known	κ-Opioid receptor agonist
Synthetic cannabinoids	"Spice," "K2," "incense," etc.	Alterations in mood, perception, anxiety, agitation, nausea, vomiting, tachycardia, elevated blood pressure, tremor, seizures, hallucinations, paranoid behavior, nonresponsiveness	Not known; likely similar to cannabis withdrawal	A comprehensive national ban was enacted in 2012. Some are now Schedule I classified, including JWH-018, JWH-073, CP 47,497, and homologues.
Classical hallucinogens	LSD, mescaline, dimethyltryptamine, psilocybin	Visual distortions and hallucinations; sometimes, anxiety/panic, paranoia, and delusional states	None	There can be prolonged psychotic states, depression, flashbacks, or exacerbation of existing psychiatric illness.

MDMA, 3,4-methylenedioxymethamphetamine; MDPV, methylenedioxypyrovalerone; NMDA, *N*-methyl-D-aspartate; LSD, lysergic acid diethylamide; PCP, phencyclidine; THC, tetrahydrocannabinol.

CONCLUSIONS

Substance-induced mental disorders are common illnesses and frequently short lived. Most patients with SIMD can be diverted away from traditional psychiatric inpatient treatment, either to dual diagnosis units or to inpatient or outpatient addiction treatment programs in which adequate assessment and appropriate treatment are available. Dual diagnosis clinics play an important role when there is diagnostic confusion or when the patient does not respond to routine psychiatric treatment.

Achieving diagnostic clarification through a comprehensive evaluation is important as well as evaluating for suicidal behavior. Abstinence is a critical factor in recovery from SIMD. When a patient's behavior is unsafe or aggressive, a psychiatric unit may be necessary until the patient's behavior is less risky.

KEY POINTS

1. Most patients with substance-induced mental disorders can be diverted away from traditional

psychiatric inpatient treatment, either to dual diagnosis units or to inpatient or outpatient addiction treatment programs in which adequate assessment and appropriate treatments are available.

2. Dual diagnosis clinics and residential units that specialize in patients with a dependence on substances with a comorbid psychiatric illness play an important role when there is diagnostic confusion or when the patient does not respond to routine psychiatric treatment.

3. Achieving clarification through a comprehensive evaluation is essential after safety is addressed.

4. Abstinence is a critical factor in recovery from a substance-induced mental disorder.

REVIEW QUESTIONS

1. "Bath salts" commonly consist of synthetic analogues of:
   A. LSD.
   B. cathinone.
   C. methamphetamine.
   D. ecstasy (MDMA).
   E. PCP.

2. Substance-induced panic attacks are frequently seen with:
   A. alcohol withdrawal.
   B. cannabis withdrawal.
   C. LSD intoxication.
   D. cocaine withdrawal.
   E. A and C.

3. Substance-induced depression can be distinguished from independent major depression by:
   A. the absence of insight.
   B. the absence of a family history of depression.
   C. the presence of drugs or alcohol in the urine.
   D. the resolution of depressive symptoms within the first month of abstinence.
   E. None of the above.

ANSWERS

1. **B.** "Bath salts" are substituted cathinones.
2. **E.** Substance-induced panic attacks are common during alcohol withdrawal, sedative-hypnotic or benzodiazepine withdrawal, and LSD intoxication.
3. **D.** If depressive symptoms resolve within the first month of abstinence, they are considered to be substance induced.

SUGGESTED READINGS

American Psychiatric Association: Diagnostic and Statistical Manuel of Mental Disorders, Fifth Ed. Arlington, VA: APA, 2013.

Caton CL, Drake RE, Hasin DS, et al. Differences between early-phase primary psychotic disorders with concurrent substance use and substance-induced psychosis. *Arch Gen Psychiatry*. 2005;62:137-145.

Chen WL, Hsieh CH, Chang HT, Hung CC, Chan CH. The epidemiology and progression time from transient to permanent psychiatric disorders of substance-induced psychosis in Taiwan. *Addict Behav*. 2015;47:1-4.

Fraser S, Hides L, Philips L, Proctor D, Lubman DI. Differentiating first episode substance induced and primary psychotic disorders with concurrent substance use in young people. *Schizophr Res*. 2012;136(1-3):110-115.

Hides L, Dawe S, McKetin R, et al. Primary and substance-induced psychotic disorders in methamphetamine users. *Psychiatry Res*. 2015;226(1):91-96.

Langås A-M, Malt UF, Opjordsmoen S. Substance use disorders and comorbid mental disorders in first-time admitted patients from a catchment area. *Eur Addict Res*. 2012;18:16-25.

Niemi-Pynttäri JA, Sund R, Putkonen H, et al. Substance-induced psychoses converting into schizophrenia: a register-based study of 18,478 Finnish inpatient cases. *J Clin Psychiatry*. 2016;160:157-162.

Nunes EV, Liu X, Samet S, Matseoane K, Hasin D. Independent versus substance-induced major depressive disorder in substance-dependent patients: observational study of course during follow-up. *J Clin Psychiatry*. 2006;67(10):1561-1567.

Ramsey SE, Kahler CW, Read JP, Stuart GL, Brown RA. Discriminating between substance-induced and independent depressive episodes in alcohol dependent patients. *J Stud Alcohol*. 2004;65(5):672-676.

Rounsaville BJ, Anton SF, Carroll K, et al. Psychiatric diagnoses of treatment-seeking cocaine abusers. *Arch Gen Psychiatry*. 1991;48:43-51.

Co-occurring Mood and Substance Use Disorders

Summary by Laura Diamond

Based on THE ASAM PRINCIPLES OF ADDICTION MEDICINE, 6th edition chapter by Edward V. Nunes and Roger D. Weiss

OVERVIEW AND DIAGNOSTIC CRITERIA

Significance

Depressive disorders, major depression, and dysthymia are among the most common psychiatric disorders in the general population. Evidence shows that over 10% of the general population has experienced a depressive disorder at some point in their life span. Major depression is the most common co-occurring psychiatric disorder encountered among patients who present for treatment of substance use disorders (SUDs), with lifetime prevalence rates ranging from 15% to 50% across samples studied from numerous treatment settings. Among patients with SUDs, major depression has been correlated with worse outcome, including worse substance use outcome, worse psychiatric symptoms, and augmented suicide risk. Clinical trials suggest that treating depression with medication or behavioral therapy can improve outcomes among patients with co-occurring SUDs.

In contrast with depression, bipolar disorder is more scarce in the general population, with estimates of the lifetime prevalence of bipolar I disorder ranging from 1% to 3% and another 1% for bipolar II disorder. Bipolar disorder is also less common than major depression in samples of patients seeking treatment for SUDs in routine outpatient settings. However, the strength of the association between bipolar disorders and SUDs is greater than for depressive disorders, and the presence of a bipolar disorder increases the likelihood of an SUD by a factor of at least 4 or greater. The co-occurrence of bipolar disorder and SUD is associated with worse prognosis, and clinical trials indicate that the proper treatment of bipolar disorder improves the outcome of the SUD.

Substance-induced mood disorder (depressive or bipolar) is a persistent mood disturbance that impairs functioning and warrants clinical attention but which has occurred only in the context of active substance use. Research suggests that substance-induced depression has prognostic significance and may convert to independent depression following a period of abstinence from substances.

Disruptive mood dysregulation disorder is a new diagnosis, added in the *Diagnostic and Statistical Manual of Mental Disorders,* 5th edition (*DSM-5*), consisting of severe persistent temper outbursts and accompanied by persistent irritable or angry mood for the majority of time. It is important to note that a differential diagnosis of irritability among patients with SUDs must be considered because irritability and aggression can be features of a number of intoxication or withdrawal syndromes and is also common in antisocial personality, which has comorbidity with SUDs.

Distinguishing Substance-Related Mood Symptoms from Mood Disorders

One of the pivotal challenges for clinicians working with patients with SUDs is distinguishing mood symptoms caused by substance intoxication, withdrawal, or chronic exposure to substances from independent mood disorders themselves. Mood symptoms (eg, sadness, apathy, irritability, pessimism, hopelessness, fatigue, appetite changes, anxiety, insomnia or hypersomnia, euphoria, hyperactivity) are extremely common in patients with SUDs. Often, such symptoms are symptoms of substance intoxication or withdrawal and will resolve with abstinence, in which case the substance use problem should be aggressively treated. At other times, the mood symptoms are symptoms of an independent mood disorder that needs to be treated in addition to treating the SUDs. Initiating treatment for the SUD and efforts to achieve abstinence should always be a first step in the treatment of a patient with co-occurring mood disorders and SUDs. The clinician should examine the course of mood symptoms in relation to substance use over the patient's lifetime and look for onset of a mood disorder syndrome prior to the onset of substance use issues or the persistence or emergence of a mood disorder during abstinent periods over the lifetime.

PREVALENCE AND PROGNOSTIC EFFECTS OF CO-OCCURRING MOOD AND SUBSTANCE USE DISORDERS

General Population

Odds ratios reflecting the strength of association of SUDs and affective or other disorders are at least 2.0 for most combinations of disorders, thereby showing that the presence of unhealthy alcohol or drug use at least doubles the odds of a mood disorder or other disorder being present. For bipolar disorder, the odds ratios are substantially higher than for major depression or dysthymia.

Common anxiety disorders such as social phobia, panic disorder with or without agoraphobia, and posttraumatic stress disorder have substantial associations with SUDs of at least the same magnitude as major depression or dysthymia. Attention deficit hyperactivity disorder has strong associations with harmful alcohol and drug use. Antisocial personality disorder also has a strong association with SUDs. The presence of antisocial features or antisocial personality disorder does not rule out the presence of a mood or anxiety disorder, and these often co-occur.

Psychiatric and Primary Care Populations

The majority of individuals with SUDs, depression, and other common mental disorders do not seek care at specialty treatment settings such as SUD treatment programs. They often present at the offices of primary care physicians where SUDs and depression are more likely to go undetected.

Etiologic Relationships Between Mood and Substance Use Disorders

There are multiple different plausible etiologic relationships between mood symptoms or syndromes and SUDs. All mood symptoms are not caused by toxic and withdrawal effects of substances, nor are all SUDs a result of underlying psychopathology (as in "self-medication"). It is important to be vigilant in formulating casual mechanisms between co-occurring disorders.

MANAGEMENT OF CO-OCCURRING MOOD AND SUBSTANCE USE DISORDERS

Antidepressant medication is the most thoroughly studied treatment modality for co-occurring mood disorders and SUDs with numerous placebo-controlled trials reported in the literature. Two meta-analyses reached similar conclusions: Antidepressant medication is more effective than placebo at improving outcomes among patients with a dependence on alcohol with depressive disorders, although the evidence was less clear for patients with co-occurring cocaine or opioid use disorders.

Meta-analyses suggest that the treatment of depression with antidepressant medication is helpful at reducing SUDs when the depression improves, but it is not a stand-alone treatment and cannot be expected to resolve substance use issues when used alone. Concurrent treatment for the SUD (counseling or medication) is of equal importance.

Behavioral Treatments for Depression and Substance Use Disorders

Studies support the effectiveness of behavioral therapies for patients with depression with SUDs and suggest that an appropriate behavioral intervention, particularly cognitive–behavioral approaches that target depressive symptoms and promote behaviors that may improve depression, should be initiated from the outset with patients with depression who are dependent on substances.

Medication Treatments for Substance Use Disorders

Although medication treatments for SUDs have received less attention and study in terms of their effects among patients with co-occurring depression and SUDs, the evidence is favorable. Naltrexone and disulfiram have been shown to be safe and effective among patients with alcohol dependence with co-occurring psychiatric disorders, including major depression. Depressive symptoms have been shown to decrease substantially during the first 1 to 2 weeks of methadone maintenance treatment for individuals with opioid use disorders, and approximately half of major depressive syndromes in patients presenting for methadone maintenance can be expected to resolve during the initial weeks of treatment. The effect of these treatments is likely attributable to a reduction in substance use (which, in turn, reduces substance-induced depressive symptoms).

Adolescents and Treatment of Co-Occurring Depression and Substance Use Disorders

Onset of SUDs and mood disorders often occurs in adolescence, and the co-occurrence of these disorders is associated with risk factors such as a history of physical or sexual abuse. Effective intervention early in the course of these disorders can improve functioning during adolescence and prevent progression to chronic mood disorders and SUDs during adulthood.

Late Life and Treatment of Co-Occurring Depression and Substance Use Disorders

SUDs may be an underrecognized problem in the elderly, who particularly struggle with polypharmacy and potential iatrogenic addiction. Effective treatment of depression may improve sleep, pain tolerance, and general functioning, thereby possibly reducing the need for prescription medications.

Suicidal Behavior and Co-Occurring Depression/Substance Use

Depression and substance use are important risk factors for suicide, and the potential for suicide needs to be carefully assessed in any patient presenting with this combination of disorders. Recent evidence suggests that depression and substance-induced depression are both associated with increased suicidal thinking and behavior in patients with SUDs.

Depression and the Treatment of Tobacco Use Disorder

The prevalence of tobacco use disorder is elevated among patients with mood disorders and is very high among patients with SUDs. Evidence suggests that patients in treatment for SUDs are interested in attempting to quit smoking and that treatment with pharmacotherapy and counseling is effective. Patients with depression with or without concurrent SUDs should be assessed for tobacco use disorder, encouraged to quit smoking, and assisted in attempting to quit with pharmacotherapy and counseling.

Summary of Treatment Recommendations for Co-Occurring Depression and Substance Use Disorders

1. *Treat the SUD*: Clinicians should consider the full range of treatment options, including different levels of care, evidence-based behavioral interventions, and medications.

2. *Evaluate the mood symptoms*: All patients presenting for treatment of SUDs should receive a brief screening for depression. When screening indicates the presence of depression, patients should receive a thorough psychiatric evaluation that assesses severity of depression, suicide risk, and symptoms of bipolar disorder, anxiety disorders, and attention deficit hyperactivity disorder.

3. *Treat the depression and other co-occurring disorders*: Psychotherapy and pharmacotherapy should be offered.

Bipolar Disorder

Pharmacologic Treatments

Pharmacologic treatment is the mainstay of treatment of bipolar disorder and can be divided into management of acute mania or hypomania, management of bipolar depression, and maintenance medication to prevent relapse. Substance use often accompanies acute mania or hypomania, and brief hospitalization may be required to control symptoms, establish initial abstinence, and determine if manic symptoms are reflective of substance intoxication. Fewer studies have been conducted on pharmacotherapy for co-occurring bipolar disorder and SUDs than for co-occurring unipolar depression and SUDs.

Behavioral Treatments

The goals of behavioral and psychosocial treatment for bipolar disorder include maintaining a treatment alliance and continuity of care, securing adherence to medication treatment, and coping with symptoms and addressing stressors or other circumstances that may lead to symptomatic exacerbations. Because bipolar disorder usually runs a chronic waxing and waning course, maintaining continuity of care is an essential challenge. Several specific behavioral/psychosocial treatments for bipolar disorder have been developed and have shown evidence of efficacy, including psychoeducation, cognitive–behavioral therapy, interpersonal social rhythm therapy, and family-focused therapy.

KEY POINTS

1. Major depression is the most common co-occurring psychiatric disorder encountered in patients presenting for treatment for SUDs.

2. The co-occurrence of bipolar disorder and SUD is associated with worse prognosis, and clinical trials indicate that proper treatment of bipolar disorder improves outcomes of the SUD.

3. A carefully completed diagnostic assessment and lifetime clinical history will help clinicians

distinguish between independent mood disorders and substance-induced mood disorders and will also inform treatment decisions.

4. Independent depressive or bipolar disorders respond to the same medication or behavioral treatments that are effective for mood disorders in people without SUDs.

REVIEW QUESTIONS

1. Which psychiatric disorder is most common among those with SUDs?
   A. Schizophrenia
   B. Major depressive disorder
   C. Bipolar disorder
   D. Anxiety disorder

2. Which of the following disorders is associated with worse prognosis when it co-occurs with an SUD?
   A. Bipolar disorder
   B. Major depressive disorder
   C. Anxiety disorder
   D. Schizophrenia

3. What type of medication is the most thoroughly studied treatment modality for co-occurring mood disorders and SUDs and has been found to be more effective than placebos at improving outcomes among patients with

a dependence on alcohol and with depressive disorders?
   A. Antipsychotics
   B. Antidepressants
   C. Anxiolytics
   D. Mood stabilizers

ANSWERS

1. **B**
2. **A**
3. **B**

SUGGESTED READINGS

Hasin D, Nunes E, Meydan J. Comorbidity of alcohol, replace and psychiatric disorders: epidemiology. In: Kranzler HR, Tinsley JA, eds. *Dual Diagnosis and Treatment: Substance Abuse and Comorbid Disorders*. 2nd ed. New York: Marcel Dekker, 2004:1-34.

Hides L, Samet S, Lubman DI. Cognitive behaviour therapy (CBT) for the treatment of co-occurring depression and substance use: current evidence and directions for future research. *Drug Alcohol Rev*. 2010;29(5):508-517.

Nunes EV, Levin FR. Treatment of depression in patients with alcohol or other drug dependence: a meta-analysis. *JAMA*. 2004;291(15):1887-1896.

Nunes EV, Liu X, Samet S, Matseoane K, Hasin D. Independent versus substance-induced major depressive disorder in substance-dependent patients: observational study of course during follow-up. *J Clin Psychiatry*. 2006;67(10):1561-1567.

Vornick LA, Brown ES. Management of comorbid bipolar disorder and substance abuse. *J Clin Psychiatry*. 2006;67 (suppl 7):24-30.

Co-Occurring Substance Use and Anxiety Disorders

Summary by Andrea L. Maxwell, Alyssa M. Braxton, and Karen J. Hartwell

Based on THE ASAM PRINCIPLES OF ADDICTION MEDICINE, 6th edition chapter by Karen J. Hartwell, Dennis E. Orwat, and Kathleen T. Brady

Research indicates that substance use disorders (SUDs) and anxiety disorders commonly co-occur. Anxiety disorders may be a risk factor for the development of SUDs. Additionally, anxiety and substance use can modify the presentation and treatment outcomes for both disorders.

PREVALENCE

In the primary care population, 20% of patients have at least one anxiety disorder, with generalized anxiety disorder (GAD) at 8%, panic disorder (PD) at 7%, and social anxiety disorder (SAD) at 6%. There is a significant association (odds ratio, 1.3) between any lifetime SUD with GAD, PD, and SAD. Interestingly, the diagnosis of one or more anxiety disorders preceded the substance dependence 80% of the time. However, because anxiety disorders and SUDs are complicated by symptom overlap, the estimates of co-occurring disorders in treatment settings are variable and dependent on diagnostic techniques and the disorder being assessed.

SCREENING AND DIFFERENTIAL DIAGNOSIS

Substance use and withdrawal can mimic nearly every psychiatric disorder, as they have profound effects on the neurotransmitters involved in the pathophysiology of anxiety disorders and SUDs. The best way to differentiate transient substance-induced symptoms from a primary anxiety disorder is through careful history of time course of anxiety and substance use and observation during a period of abstinence. The duration of abstinence can vary on the diagnosis being assessed and substance used. Several screening tools such as the Mini-International Neuropsychiatric Interview, Four Dimensional Symptoms Question, and the Hospital

Anxiety and Depression Scale can help with the diagnosis. However, a detailed interview may still be needed to fully differentiate symptoms.

GENERAL TREATMENT CONSIDERATION

With co-occurring disorders, it is important to maximize the use of nonpharmacologic agents with cognitive–behavioral therapy (CBT) among the most effective for both disorders. If pharmacotherapy is warranted, it is important to be mindful of the potential toxic drug interactions between prescription medications and illicit drugs and alcohol in case of relapse as well as the addictive property of the medication. Selective serotonin reuptake inhibitors (SSRIs) are considered first-line agents with serotonin norepinephrine reuptake inhibitors being an alternative first-line agent due to effectiveness, tolerability, and safety (Table 94-1). Mirtazapine has also improved symptoms in open trials with PD and GAD. Tricyclic antidepressants and monoamine oxidase inhibitors are typically reserved for treatment-resistant cases due to lethality in overdose. Buspirone has been helpful in uncomplicated GAD, and pregabalin has had good support in randomized controlled trials for SAD and GAD. Medications that should be avoided or used on a limited basis included atypical antipsychotics due to side effect burden and benzodiazepines due to addiction potential and side effects.

ALCOHOL AND ANXIETY DISORDERS

Although the relationship between alcohol and anxiety disorders varies, drinking to self-medicate anxiety may make both the occurrence and persistence of alcohol use disorders (AUDs) more likely. The relationship between anxiety and alcohol use may predispose young people to develop an AUD, with

TABLE 94-1	Recommended Treatment for Anxiety Disorders		
First-Line Agents	**Second-Line Agents**	**Possible Adjunct Agents**	**Avoided/Limited Use**
SSRIs (all anxiety disorders), serotonin norepinephrine reuptake inhibitors (GAD, SAD), mirtazapine (PD, GAD)	Tricyclic antidepressants, monoamine oxidase inhibitors	Buspirone (GAD), pregabalin (GAD), hydroxyzine	Atypical antipsychotics, benzodiazepines

GAD, generalized anxiety disorder; PD, panic disorder; SAD, social anxiety disorder; SSRIs, selective serotonin reuptake inhibitors.

early-onset anxiety disorders associated with an earlier age of first alcohol use. The short-term relief of anxiety from alcohol use, in combination with longer term anxiety induction from chronic drinking and withdrawal, may also initiate a feed-forward cycle of increasing anxiety symptoms and alcohol consumption.

A recent Cochrane review concluded that the evidence base of pharmacotherapy for comorbid alcohol and anxiety disorders was of poor quality and inconclusive. Research indicates that alcohol use appears to attenuate the efficacy of anxiety disorder treatment. There is less evidence regarding integrated treatment that improves outcomes for both alcohol and anxiety disorders. Psychosocial interventions have an established role in anxiety disorders and SUDs.

Generalized Anxiety Disorder

In the recent National Epidemiologic Survey on Alcohol and Related Conditions (NESARC-III) survey, those with a lifetime history of AUDs were found to have weakly increased odds of also having a lifetime history of GAD. Alcohol withdrawal symptoms and GAD symptoms have considerable overlap. Ongoing assessments of anxiety in recovery will help clarify the diagnosis and need for continued treatment. There is minimal research to direct treatment decisions for individuals with GAD and comorbid AUDs. Although SSRIs have not been well studied in individuals with co-occurring GADs and SUDs, they are efficacious in the treatment of GAD and relatively safe to use in individuals with SUDs. Pregabalin has demonstrated efficacy for GAD and alcohol withdrawal syndrome but has not been evaluated in patients with comorbid AUD and GAD. Because GAD has a relapsing-remitting quality, long-term treatment of GAD is often indicated.

Social Anxiety Disorder

SAD may be a risk factor for AUDs in individuals who use alcohol to self-medicate, with SAD symptoms typically preceding onset of SUDs. The key symptom of SAD, fear of performance or social situations, is specific to SAD and not associated with substance use or withdrawal and can aid in clarifying the diagnosis. There are few studies examining treatment options in comorbid populations. Two small studies of paroxetine in co-occurring AUD and SAD demonstrated significant improvement in social anxiety with paroxetine treatment but no significant group differences in alcohol use. A more recent controlled trial integrating a brief alcohol intervention into treatment failed to demonstrate decreased alcohol use or drinking behavior in at-risk drinkers with SAD. In an investigation of group therapy in patients with AUD, with and without SAD, no difference was found between groups in treatment adherence and outcomes. Individual therapy may be better tolerated than group therapy, and a period of sobriety and skills training may be important before increasing exposure to social situations.

Obsessive–Compulsive Disorder

The association of obsessive–compulsive disorder (OCD) and AUDs is less robust than for other anxiety disorders. Previous research found that OCD was negatively correlated with AUDs. Craving in SUDs can be intrusive and recurrent; however, the thoughts and compulsions in individuals with AUDs are generally restricted to alcohol use and easily distinguished from OCD. One recent study of intensive OCD-oriented residential treatment found that lower past-year alcohol use predicted a better treatment response.

Panic Disorder

A lifetime history of an AUD has been associated with increased odds of PD. In one review, the presence of an AUD increased the risk of PD by as much as fourfold. Individuals with panic attacks may use alcohol to decrease panic symptoms and subsequently develop an AUD. Because alcohol withdrawal may increase anxiety to the point of panic-like severity, a diagnosis of PD should only be made following several weeks of abstinence if distinguishing the onset of PD and AUD cannot be readily done. Current guidelines for pharmacologic treatment of PD recommend against routine benzodiazepine, antihistamine, and antipsychotic prescribing in favor of SSRIs. The risk of relapse to drinking is increased without treatment. CBT has been found to be effective in the treatment of comorbid PD and AUD. In a study of Internet-based CBT for PD, harmful alcohol use attenuated, but did not eliminate, the benefits of the CBT intervention. One study comparing CBT targeting both alcohol and panic versus treatment as usual demonstrated CBT improved both drinking and PD outcomes.

TOBACCO PRODUCTS AND ANXIETY DISORDERS

Between 2004 and 2011, smoking rates significantly declined among individuals without mental illness (20% to 16%); however, similar declines ($P = .50$) were not seen in individuals with mental illness (29% to 27%), including anxiety disorders. An earlier onset of anxiety disorders has been found among smokers who start smoking at a younger age. Some studies have suggested that smoking and nicotine can alleviate anxiety; in contrast, other studies have found nicotine use and withdrawal can cause anxiety.

Differential Diagnosis

The anxiety associated with nicotine withdrawal can be distinguished from independent anxiety disorders by the time course. Nicotine withdrawal symptoms typically return to baseline within 10 days, and anxiety typically decreases within 4 weeks of quitting among smokers. Anxiety symptoms that persist beyond the withdrawal period warrant further investigation.

Panic Disorder

PD with and without agoraphobia has been associated with heavy smoking ($\geq$1 pack of cigarettes per day), nicotine dependence, and failed quit attempts. Early smoking and current smoking have been found to increase the risk for PD, and typically the initiation of smoking precedes the onset of PD by more than a decade. Current explanations of the associations include a shared vulnerability to both disorders, the release of norepinephrine by nicotine producing panic-like symptoms, self-medication, and the result of respiratory abnormalities from smoking.

Social Anxiety Disorder

Few studies have investigated the relationship between SAD and smoking. Some studies have failed to demonstrate a relationship; however, one prospective longitudinal study found both social fears and

SAD were significantly associated with higher rates of nicotine dependence, with about 50% reporting the onset of SAD before smoking. Among individuals with SAD, cigarette smoking may be used to attenuate social anxiety in anticipation of and during social situations.

Generalized Anxiety Disorder

Likewise, the prevalence of severe nicotine dependence has been associated with an increased risk of GAD. Heavy smoking ($\geq$20 cigarettes per day) in adolescence and young adulthood has been associated with an increased risk of GAD. GAD is about twice as common in women than in men, but men are more likely to have nicotine addiction, more likely to use alcohol and nonprescribed medications to relieve symptoms, and are less likely to seek treatment. A confounding issue is the high rate of co-occurrence of GAD between other anxiety and depressive disorders.

Obsessive–Compulsive Disorder

The prevalence of smoking is significantly lower among adults with OCD and parents of youth with OCD compared to those with other psychiatric disorders and the general population. These results suggest that the low prevalence of smoking may be familial, and the stimulating effect of nicotine may exacerbate OCD symptoms. OCD is a heterogeneous disorder, however, and smoking status differs based on the distinct subcategories of OCD.

Tobacco/Nicotine Treatment

Current guidelines for treating tobacco/nicotine use disorders recommend a combination of counseling and medication. Pharmacotherapy is recommended for all individuals attempting to quit unless there is a contraindication. Medications that reliably increase long-term smoking abstinence include sustained-release bupropion, all forms of nicotine replacement therapy (nicotine gum, nicotine inhaler, nicotine nasal spray, nicotine lozenge, and nicotine patch), and varenicline. The black box warning regarding neuropsychiatric adverse effects of varenicline was lifted in 2017. Further meta-analyses found that varenicline did not increase the rates of depression, suicidal events, agitation, or aggression. No differences in adverse events have been found between the standard nicotine patch, extended, flexible, combination (nicotine patch with gum or inhaler), or varenicline, including individuals with comorbid medical and psychiatric problems; this suggests smokers with anxiety disorders may safely be offered standard treatment. As bupropion can cause anxiety, it should be used with caution in anxious patients. Some but not all research has suggested that smokers with anxiety disorders may be less successful. Individuals with a history of anxiety disorders were about twice as likely to endorse stress and almost four times as likely to endorse negative affect as reasons for relapse. Interoceptive exposure therapy, cognitive therapy, mindfulness, and acceptance-based therapies hold some promise.

OPIOIDS AND ANXIETY DISORDERS

The 12-month and lifetime prevalence rates of non-medical use of prescription opioids increased from 0.9% to 4.1% and 2.1% to 11.3%, respectively, between NESARC-I and NESARC-III. Likewise, the 12-month and lifetime rates prevalence of non-medical prescription opioid use disorders increased from 0.4% to 0.8% and 1.4% to 2.9%, respectively. The lifetime prevalence of anxiety disorders has been found to be doubled in individuals with opioid use disorders. The presence of a comorbid SUD decreased the likelihood of recovery from GAD by nearly fivefold and increased the risk of recurrence threefold.

Diagnosis

The relationship between anxiety and opioid use disorders is complex. The release of endogenous opioids in response to stress has a modulating effect on anxiety, and blocking the opioid system with an antagonist produces anxiety symptoms in human volunteers and anxiety-linked behaviors in animal models. Additionally, anxiety is a key feature of opioid withdrawal.

Treatment

Stabilization in treatment including pharmacotherapy and psychosocial treatments can significantly reduce withdrawal-related symptoms in as little as a week. No clinical trials of treatments for co-occurring anxiety disorders have been conducted. Initial treatment should include medical detoxification and consideration of buprenorphine or methadone treatment. If anxiety persists after detoxification and stabilization, then specific treatments for anxiety should be considered.

CANNABIS AND ANXIETY DISORDERS

The NESARC-III survey of adults indicated the prevalence of past-year cannabis use was 9% and past-year cannabis use disorders was 3%. In 2010, there were 17.4 million current American cannabis users, and cannabis was the most commonly used drug (77%) by current illicit drug users and the only drug used by 60% of the illicit drug users surveyed. The relationship between cannabis and anxiety remains unclear. Most research has found an association between anxiety and cannabis use and use disorders, although causality and degree of mediation by confounders is not determined. Studies suggest the onset of anxiety occurs prior to cannabis use disorder onset for the majority of comorbid adults. Cannabis use can cause acute anxiety during intoxication, develop as part of withdrawal, and is associated with an increased lifetime risk of panic attacks and PD. The use of cannabis as a coping strategy may enhance anxiety through an avoidance-anxiety cycle; persons who report using cannabis to cope may use cannabis more often and have more cannabis-related problems and distress. Higher anxiety has been associated with increased cannabis-related problems at baseline and follow-up. Anxiety reduction is associated with improved cannabis outcomes; patients with cannabis use disorder may benefit from treatment focused on anxiety management skills. Successful quitters have been found to employ coping strategies such as alternative ways to relax and deal with unpleasant emotions than unsuccessful quitters.

STIMULANTS AND ANXIETY DISORDERS

Cocaine, methamphetamines, and amphetamines stimulate noradrenergic systems, and acute intoxication is commonly associated with anxiety. As a result, individuals who are vulnerable to anxiety may be less likely to misuse or become addicted to this class of drugs. Careful attention to the time course of anxiety symptoms relative to stimulant use is critical to determine an accurate diagnosis.

Prevalence

Previous research has suggested about 30% to 40% of individuals with amphetamine and cocaine use disorders report a lifetime history of an anxiety disorder. Conversely, among individuals with anxiety disorders, approximately 5% report a lifetime amphetamine or cocaine use disorder. Anxiety disorders are relatively less common in patients with cocaine use disorders compared with patients with AUDs and other SUDs seeking treatment. In the Methamphetamine Treatment Project, methamphetamine use was associated with greater general anxiety and phobic anxiety severity, with women reporting higher levels of anxiety than men. At a

3-year follow-up, 26% of participants met the criteria for current or past anxiety disorder, with GAD being most common. Treatment adherence and methamphetamine use was significantly worse in those with a comorbid anxiety disorder.

Diagnosis

The compulsive foraging for misplaced cocaine and skin-picking behavior has been noted in patients with cocaine dependence. These symptoms generally occur only during acute intoxication and withdrawal and do not meet diagnostic criteria for OCD. OCD and related disorders should be considered when such substance-related behavior is clinically relevant. Cocaine has been reported to precipitate panic attacks in patients without previous PD. Because stimulant withdrawal symptoms include low levels of anxiety, a period of abstinence is warranted before diagnosing an anxiety disorder.

Treatment

There is a paucity of research focused on the treatment of co-occurring stimulant use and anxiety disorders. Symptom improvement has been found with carbamazepine, valproate, and clonazepam in the treatment of PD. Benzodiazepines should be avoided as previously discussed. Psychosocial treatments have demonstrated efficacy in the treatment of stimulant dependence and include contingency management and CBT.

KEY POINTS

1. Anxiety disorders and SUDs commonly co-occur.
2. Symptoms of an anxiety disorder commonly occur both during intoxication and withdrawal. Careful history of the time course of SUDs and anxiety with observation during a period of sobriety can clarify the presence of an independent anxiety disorder.
3. Unless contradicted, SSRIs are effective first-line treatments of anxiety disorders.
4. Benzodiazepines should be avoided for the treatment of comorbid anxiety disorders and SUDs.
5. First-line pharmacotherapy for smoking cessation can be utilized in patients with anxiety disorder unless there is a contraindication.

REVIEW QUESTIONS

1. Which of the following disorders has the weakest association with an increased risk of SUDs?
   A. Panic disorder
   B. Social anxiety disorder
   C. Obsessive–compulsive disorder
   D. Generalized anxiety disorder

2. All of the following medications are first-line treatments for anxiety disorders with co-occurring SUDs *except*:
   A. alprazolam.
   B. fluoxetine.
   C. diazepam.
   D. citalopram.
   E. both A and C.

3. Which of following suggests an independent anxiety disorder co-occurring with an SUD?
   A. Onset of panic attacks occurred as a teenager prior to using opioids.
   B. Anxiety persists 1 month after sobriety.
   C. Heavy alcohol drinking began in college to ease long-standing discomfort in social settings with the opposite sex.
   D. Anxious mood occurs during outpatient medical detox for alcohol withdrawal.
   E. A, B, and C.

ANSWERS

1. **C.** Epidemiologic data indicates that GAD, SAD, and PD have a higher association with SUDs than OCD.
2. **E.** Benzodiazepines should be avoided in the treatment of co-occurring disorders.
3. **E.** An evaluation of anxiety symptoms during a period of sobriety and in the absence of intoxication and withdrawal is critical to clarify the diagnosis. The time course of symptoms in relation to substance use is also helpful.

SUGGESTED READINGS

Baldwin DS, Anderson IM, Nutt DJ, et al. Evidence-based pharmacological treatment of anxiety disorders, post-traumatic stress disorder and obsessive-compulsive disorder: a revision of the 2005 guidelines from the British Association for Psychopharmacology. *J Psychopharmacol.* 2014;28(5):403-439.

Fatséas M, Denis C, Lavie E, Auriacombe M. Relationship between anxiety disorders and opiate dependence—a systematic review of the literature: implications for diagnosis and treatment. *J Subst Abuse Treat.* 2010;38(3):220-230.

Glasner-Edwards S, Mooney LJ, Marinelli-Casey P, et al. Anxiety disorders among methamphetamine dependent adults: association with post-treatment functioning. *Am J Addict.* 2010;19(5):385-390.

Ipser JC, Wilson D, Akindipe TO, Sager C, Stein DJ. Pharmacotherapy for anxiety and comorbid alcohol use disorders. *Cochrane Database Syst Rev.* 2015;1:CD007505.

Tulloch HE, Pipe AL, Els C, Clyde MJ, Reid RD. Flexible, dual-form nicotine replacement therapy or varenicline in comparison with nicotine patch for smoking cessation: a randomized controlled trial. *BMC Med.* 2016;14:80.

Co-Occurring Addiction and Psychotic Disorders

Summary by Douglas Ziedonis, Celine Larkin, Xiaoduo Fan, Stephen A. Wyatt, and David Smelson

Based on THE ASAM PRINCIPLES OF ADDICTION MEDICINE, 6th edition chapter by Douglas Ziedonis, Xiaoduo Fan, Celine Larkin, Stephen A. Wyatt, and David Smelson

CO-OCCURRING ADDICTION AND PSYCHOTIC DISORDERS

Co-occurring substance use and psychotic symptoms pose special diagnostic and treatment challenges for clinicians in all treatment settings, including mental health, addiction, emergency room, and primary care settings. This chapter summarizes issues related to the assessment, diagnosis, and acute and long-term treatment considerations of co-occurring substance use and psychotic disorders.

CO-OCCURRENCE OF SUBSTANCE USE AND PSYCHOTIC SYMPTOMS

Substance use and psychotic symptoms often co-occur, both because individuals who use substances may experience psychotic symptoms as a result and because individuals with psychotic disorders are more likely to use substances. In addition, certain medical conditions can cause psychotic symptoms.

Psychotic symptoms can be induced by a variety of substances, such as alcohol, cocaine, cannabis, amphetamines, dissociatives, and hallucinogens, often in combination. Individuals who develop methamphetamine psychosis may experience persistent psychotic symptoms and even require hospitalization, despite months of abstinence. Conversely, psychosis persisting for more than several days after cocaine use is suggestive of an underlying psychotic disorder. In the addiction treatment setting, a differential diagnosis that includes a psychiatric disorder should be considered if psychotic symptoms persist for more than 1 month after cessation of substance use; less than 15% of individuals with a substance-induced psychosis will have psychotic symptoms after 1 month of abstinence. Delayed symptom clearance may be attributed to factors such as the type of substance, the duration of use, and preexisting psychiatric vulnerability.

Several studies have examined rates of co-occurring substance use disorders and schizophrenia and found that up to half of individuals with schizophrenia have a lifetime history of substance use disorders, excluding tobacco/nicotine use disorder. The National Epidemiologic Survey on Alcohol and Related Conditions suggested that schizophrenia is associated with increased transition from abstinence to substance use, particularly for cannabis. The odds of those with schizophrenia also carrying a substance use disorder diagnosis are many times higher than those of the general population. Some data suggest that the use of drugs or alcohol can lead to the earlier onset of schizophrenia in an already vulnerable individual. Substance use is also associated with an increased duration of untreated schizophrenia, noncompliance with treatment, and increased readmission. In first-episode patients, substance use is also associated with poorer functional responses, more frequent relapses, and a greater symptom burden. Nicotine/tobacco use disorder is very common (70% to 90%) and represents a major cause of increased morbidity and mortality in patients with psychotic disorders.

MANAGEMENT AND ASSESSMENT OF ACUTE SUBSTANCE-RELATED PSYCHOTIC SYMPTOMS

At the time of an individual's initial presentation for treatment of acute substance-related psychotic symptoms, the clinician should have four primary goals: patient safety, staff safety, elicitation of the patient's history, and formulation of initial impressions that will lead to a set of treatment recommendations about managing agitation and psychotic symptoms while also considering the need for potential detoxification. Providing a setting in which external stimuli are minimized can help increase the physical safety of patients and staff members and supports treating all with respect and dignity. If the patient is distressed, it may be helpful and supportive to allow family to accompany the patient. An initial assessment of vital signs should be obtained because variations in pulse, blood pressure, and respiratory function are not uncommon in the presentation of many toxic states.

The patient's mental status should be assessed in a longitudinal manner, with particular attention given to cognitive impairments and fluctuations of mental status. Protection of the airway is paramount. Physical restraints are used less frequently in mental health settings, and there is an increased use of a quiet room to reduce a patient's level of anxiety and agitation.

Medications for sedation may be warranted in an attempt to reduce distress and to prevent harm from self or others due to agitation. Options include a low-dose benzodiazepine (such as diazepam) or, if the patient is severely agitated with persistent psychotic symptoms, an atypical antipsychotic medication. These medications should be given only after the primary assessment has taken place because the sedative effect of these medications may disguise the presenting clinical symptoms and the effects of these medications may interact negatively with substances previously used by the patient. The assessment will also benefit from a collateral history obtained from family, friends, and emergency personnel.

For an individual who experiences psychotic symptoms and is actively using a substance at the same time, it is often challenging to determine whether the psychotic symptoms are due to a primary psychotic disorder or are substance induced, especially in the emergency room setting. Collateral information may help. One study showed that clinicians in psychiatric emergency rooms have a tendency to attribute psychotic symptoms to a primary psychotic disorder rather than to co-occurring substance use. In addition to a primary psychotic disorder, clinicians must consider the possibility that these symptoms are caused by a general medical condition or substance intoxication or withdrawal; cognitive disorders, such as delirium or dementia; or other categories of mental disorders, particularly affective disorders. In addition to ruling out mood disorders, substance-induced syndromes, and other medical causes, the type and duration of psychotic symptoms can help in making a differential diagnosis. Psychotic symptoms that have a sudden onset and that last more than 1 day but less than 1 month suggest a brief psychotic disorder. If the symptoms

have been present for less than 6 months, a diagnosis of schizophreniform disorder may be considered. If the symptoms last longer than 6 months and include prominent delusions or hallucinations, a diagnosis of schizophrenia or schizoaffective disorder (the latter if a major depressive or manic episode co-occurs) should be considered.

LONGER TERM MANAGEMENT OF CO-OCCURRING SUBSTANCE USE AND PSYCHOTIC SYMPTOMS

The major challenge in treating co-occurring psychosis and substance use is to provide integrated treatment that helps with both issues simultaneously. Often, treatment of the co-occurring disorder also requires a multidisciplinary treatment team and a systematic approach to issues that may be of lesser concern in other settings, such as housing, entitlements, rehabilitation, and use of community services. Clinicians who are nonjudgmental, empathic, and hopeful are most helpful to patients in the treatment and recovery processes. The long-term treatment of patients with a first episode of psychosis in the context of substance use is complicated by the fact that the diagnosis of up to one quarter of such patients changes from substance-induced psychotic disorder to a primary psychotic disorder, especially in individuals with a significant family history of psychotic disorder, poor premorbid adjustment, and/or less insight into the mental illness. Importantly, patients who misuse substances may be poorly compliant in taking their medications so that a presenting psychotic relapse may be the result of non-compliance of antipsychotic medication treatment.

The first step in medication management of a co-occurring substance use disorder and an established diagnosis of schizophrenia is to consider the best approach to treating the patient's schizophrenia. This should be followed by a consideration of the potential interactions between the substances used and the possible medication choices. In general, avoiding medications that cause sedation is recommended when treating patients who misuse sedating substances. In addition, clinicians generally should avoid prescribing medications with misuse liability. Antipsychotic medications are often an important component of the treatment of psychotic disorders in reducing long-term positive symptoms. Medications should be complemented by psychosocial therapy that engages patients, offers them practical training in interpersonal communication and crisis management, and develops their rehabilitation and recovery skills. Engaging the family or support network in the treatment process can also be helpful.

Over the past decades, atypical antipsychotic medications have been approved by the US Food and Drug Administration for the treatment of schizophrenia. Some of these drugs also have been studied for the treatment of substance use disorders, although none are approved for the treatment of substance use disorders. Clinical judgment based on the individual patient's situation should guide the choice of which antipsychotic medication to use. Substances, including tobacco and caffeine, can interact with antipsychotic medications and affect their efficacy and side effects in schizophrenia treatment.

Psychosocial approaches can ameliorate co-occurring substance use and psychotic disorders. Modifications of conventional substance use disorder treatments should take into account the common features among individuals with schizophrenia, including apathy and lethargy as well as low motivation and self-efficacy, isolation and loneliness, cognitive deficits, and maladaptive interpersonal skills. These psychosocial issues highlight the need for and difficulty in establishing a strong treatment alliance.

Bearing in mind the high prevalence of tobacco use disorder in individuals with psychotic disorders, effective strategies to address tobacco use in mental health and addiction treatment settings require changing clinician practices through broader system level changes, training, and alignment with wellness and recovery goals. Treatment of co-occurring nicotine/tobacco use disorder among individuals with schizophrenia can be effective and often requires a combination of medications and psychosocial treatment approaches, including continuity of care between primary care providers and community tobacco treatment resources.

SUMMARY

Individuals with substance use disorders may experience psychotic symptoms as a result of specific types and methods of substance use, and individuals diagnosed with psychotic disorders are disproportionately likely to misuse substances. In managing both groups, clinicians should be mindful of the complex and interacting pharmacology of medications and underlying disorders as well as the unique psychosocial challenges experienced by such patients.

KEY POINTS

1. Psychotic symptoms can occur in the context of acute intoxication or longer standing substance use as well as with a co-occurring psychiatric or medical conditions.

2. Short-term management of psychotic symptoms associated with intoxication should include creating a safe environment and administering medications (such as benzodiazepines and/or antipsychotics) as required.

3. Longer term management of co-occurring psychotic disorders and substance use disorders requires an integrated psychosocial approach to address both problems.

REVIEW QUESTIONS

1. Management of a patient who is intoxicated and who has delusions should start with:
   A. providing a safe supportive space for the patient.
   B. administering a high dose of benzodiazepines.
   C. placing the patient in physical restraints.
   D. an immediate computed tomography scan.

2. If a patient with schizophrenia is experiencing hallucinations after discontinuing heavy alcohol use, the patient:
   A. does not require special treatment because this is normal.
   B. should receive counseling to reduce alcohol consumption.
   C. should be treated with a tapering course of benzodiazepines.
   D. should be evaluated by a psychiatrist for a potential adjustment of antipsychotic medication.

3. Which of the following is specifically approved by the US Food and Drug Administration for the treatment of alcohol use disorder in patients with schizophrenia?
   A. Acamprosate
   B. Naltrexone
   C. Disulfiram
   D. None of the above

ANSWERS

1. **A**
2. **C**
3. **D**

SUGGESTED READINGS

Gregg L, Barrowclough C, Haddock G. Reasons for increased substance use in psychosis. *Clin Psychol Rev.* 2007;27(4): 494-510.

Lubman DI, King JA, Castle DJ. Treating comorbid substance use disorders in schizophrenia. *Int Rev Psychiatry.* 2010;22(2):191-201.

Wisdom JP, Manuel JI, Drake RE. Substance use disorder among people with first-episode psychosis: a systematic review of course and treatment. *Psychiatr Serv.* 2011;62(9):1007-1012.

Co-occurring Substance Use Disorder and Attention Deficit Hyperactivity Disorder

Summary by Leila M. Vaezazizi and Frances R. Levin

Based on THE ASAM PRINCIPLES OF ADDICTION MEDICINE, 6th edition chapter by Frances R. Levin and John J. Mariani

This chapter examines two common psychiatric problems: attention deficit hyperactivity disorder (ADHD), a disorder that manifests itself in childhood with symptoms that typically persist into adulthood, and substance use disorders (SUDs), which often occur in adolescence or early adulthood. ADHD is overrepresented among individuals with SUDs, and the coexistence of ADHD and SUD can reduce the effectiveness of treatment for either condition. In this chapter, we provide an overview of the etiology, epidemiology, diagnosis, and treatment of ADHD. We discuss the overlap of ADHD and SUDs and outline a treatment approach for patients who present with co-occurring ADHD and SUD.

ETIOLOGY OF ATTENTION DEFICIT HYPERACTIVITY DISORDER AND IMPLICATIONS FOR VULNERABILITY TO SUBSTANCE USE DISORDERS

ADHD is a highly heritable, polygenic disorder, and its etiology includes genetic, neuroanatomic, neurochemical, and environmental factors with complex interactions between genetic and environmental risks. Molecular genetic studies support the theory that ADHD is a heterogeneous disorder, dependent on interacting genes such as those involved in dopamine functioning, including the dopamine transporter and the dopamine receptor D4. Genetic aberrations of the dopamine transporter genotype are associated with ADHD as well as certain SUDs. Medications that inhibit the dopamine transporter, including methylphenidate and amphetamine, increase synaptic dopamine levels and ameliorate symptoms of ADHD.

The hypothesis that dysfunction in frontal-subcortical pathways occurs in ADHD is supported by brain imaging studies, implicating regions of the basal ganglia that provide feedback to the cortex for motor control regulation, behavior inhibition, and reward modulation. These abnormalities may contribute to SUD vulnerability among those with ADHD. Common findings in structural imaging studies of ADHD include smaller volumes in the dorsolateral prefrontal cortex, the cerebellum, and the subcortical structures. Neuroanatomic studies of patients with ADHD have demonstrated reduced volume of the prefrontal cortex, a region densely populated with both dopamine and norepinephrine receptors; balanced dopamine tone in the prefrontal cortex is essential for normal working memory function and attention regulation.

Certain environmental risks have also been associated with both ADHD and SUDs, including maternal smoking during pregnancy, premature birth, and low birth weight. Prenatal environmental tobacco smoke is a strong risk factor for ADHD, and overall, the adjusted risk for ADHD is 2.5-fold higher for children prenatally exposed to tobacco smoke. It is possible that there are shared underlying risk factors for individuals with ADHD with comorbid tobacco use disorder or other SUDs.

EPIDEMIOLOGY OF CO-OCCURRING ATTENTION DEFICIT HYPERACTIVITY DISORDER AND SUBSTANCE USE DISORDERS

ADHD is the most common behavioral disorder of children, affecting 8% to 18% of children and adolescents worldwide. A National Comorbidity Survey Replication study estimated the prevalence of adult ADHD at 4.4%, although there is variation in prevalence estimates across studies due, in part, to differences in how ADHD is assessed.

Among adults with and without ADHD, the rate of SUDs is 15.2% versus 5.6%, respectively, according to a National Comorbidity Survey Replication study. According to the National Epidemiologic Survey on Alcohol and Related Disorders, both substance use and SUDs are associated with having ADHD symptoms (ie, without the full diagnosis) and ADHD regardless of subtype (inattentive, hyperactive-impulsive, or combined), although the highest rates of SUDs are consistently among those with the ADHD combined subtype. Adolescents with ADHD demonstrate an earlier onset of substance use, particularly those with hyperactive-impulsive symptoms.

Perhaps more striking is the overrepresentation of ADHD in SUD treatment populations. According to one study conducted in 10 countries, the mean rate of adult ADHD among those seeking treatment for SUDs was 17%. In another meta-analysis of 23 studies that included adolescents and adults, ADHD prevalence was estimated at 23%.

POSSIBLE REASONS FOR LINKS BETWEEN ATTENTION DEFICIT HYPERACTIVITY DISORDER AND SUBSTANCE USE DISORDERS

There are several possible pathways to explain the overlap between ADHD and SUDs that have been studied, such as the possible mediation of childhood ADHD and later SUDs by other disruptive behavior disorders, the developmental vulnerabilities associated with childhood ADHD that may lead to later substance use (eg, neurocognitive deficits, impulsive anger), or shared biological factors such as diminished dopamine signaling or prefrontal hypodopaminergic functioning. Recent large registry and epidemiologic studies based on aggregate data support that stimulant medication decreases the risk of substance-related problems. The question remains whether ADHD alone confers a risk for later substance use and SUDs in adolescents. Regardless, once regular substance use is established, the presence of ADHD symptoms may increase the likelihood of heavy and impaired substance use even in the absence of a disruptive disorder.

Even when ADHD is diagnosed among those with SUDs, many clinicians are reluctant to treat ADHD in patients presenting with SUDs because stimulant medications are a primary treatment modality. However, an individual's response to SUD treatment is adversely affected by ADHD, and it has been shown that adults with ADHD are more likely to transition from an alcohol use disorder to a drug use disorder and to continue to use substances compared to similar patients without ADHD. Individuals with ADHD may have greater difficulty sitting through group meetings (a common format for SUD treatment) and may be more likely to drop out of SUD treatment because of increased impulsivity that is characteristic of ADHD. Beyond alleviating the attentional and behavioral problems associated with ADHD, treatment outcomes for SUDs may be improved by appropriately treating ADHD.

DIAGNOSIS OF ATTENTION DEFICIT HYPERACTIVITY DISORDER

ADHD is a clinical diagnosis characterized by inattention, impulsivity, and hyperactivity. To meet the *Diagnostic and Statistical Manual of Mental Disorders,* 5th edition (*DSM-5*) criteria for ADHD, individuals must have (1) six symptoms of inattention in childhood or five symptoms at age 17 years or older (inattentive presentation), (2) six symptoms of impulsivity and hyperactivity in childhood or five symptoms at age 17 years or older (impulsive/hyperactive presentation), or (3) both (combined presentation). Individuals who met the full criteria in childhood but currently have fewer than six symptoms of inattention or hyperactivity/impulsivity are described as having ADHD in partial remission. Some ADHD symptoms need to occur prior to the age of 12 years. In addition, some impairments from these symptoms need to be present in two or more settings, and the symptoms must produce clear evidence of significant impairment. The symptoms cannot be more readily accounted for by another mental disorder.

ADHD is common among those with SUDs but is frequently not assessed. A cost-effective and practical approach in clinical settings is to administer a reliable screening instrument followed by a standardized diagnostic interview for likely cases. Three commonly used instruments are the Wender Utah Rating Scale, which screens for childhood ADHD; the Conners Adult ADHD Rating Scale; and the Adult ADHD Self-Report Scale Version 1.1.

Difficulties in Diagnosing Adult Attention Deficit Hyperactivity Disorder in Populations that Use Substances

ADHD is a clinical diagnosis that is best made by carrying out a comprehensive assessment that includes a developmental history, a learning history, an evaluation of other psychiatric comorbidities, and a medical evaluation. However, diagnostic ambiguities can arise when attempting to assess for ADHD in an individual with a hazardous use of alcohol and/or drugs. Some general guidelines include the following:

- Assess individuals for ADHD when they have been abstinent from substances for 2 to 4 weeks so that substance intoxication or withdrawal symptoms are not confounding the diagnostic assessment. If a patient is unable to abstain, this should not preclude a diagnosis, especially in the outpatient setting.

- Making a diagnosis of ADHD requires establishing the symptom onset prior to 12 years of age. If a patient cannot recall and reliable collateral from a family member is not available, you can assess for symptoms in high school to make a late-onset ADHD, not otherwise specified diagnosis.

- Taking a good longitudinal history is important to establish both a continuity of ADHD symptoms from childhood to adulthood and symptomatology that does not occur episodically (which may suggest that symptoms are better explained by another psychiatric or medical condition) or that occurs only after a period of regular drug use.

- The last criterion in the *DSM-5* for ADHD indicates that ADHD should not be diagnosed if the observed symptoms are better accounted for by another mental disorder. In reality, ADHD can coexist with other psychiatric conditions such as bipolar disorder or depression, although the symptoms may overlap.

- Individuals with ADHD typically do not exhibit psychotic symptoms. If present, psychotic symptoms indicate the likelihood of another mood disturbance and/or a substance-induced psychotic disorder.

- *Some individuals may "feign" ADHD symptoms* in order to get special considerations in school or to obtain stimulants for performance enhancement. In our clinical experience, those who use substances are more likely to be surprised when a clinician suggests they may have ADHD and require psychoeducation to understand why they may have ADHD.

TREATMENT OF CO-OCCURRING ATTENTION DEFICIT HYPERACTIVITY DISORDER AND SUBSTANCE USE DISORDER

Pharmacotherapeutic Treatment Options for Attention Deficit Hyperactivity Disorder

Currently, the US Food and Drug Administration (FDA) has approved medications for ADHD; they include stimulant medications (amphetamine and methylphenidate) and three nonstimulant medications (clonidine, guanfacine, and atomoxetine). Other, off-label medications prescribed for ADHD include modafinil (a long-acting stimulant approved for narcolepsy and shift-work sleep) and some antidepressants including bupropion, venlafaxine, monoamine oxidase inhibitors, and tricyclics. Amphetamine analogues and methylphenidate are the stimulant medications most commonly used to treat ADHD in children and adults in the United States. See Table 96-1 for a summary of commonly used medications for ADHD.

Pharmacotherapy Selection for Attention Deficit Hyperactivity Disorder and Co-Occurring Substance Use Disorder

At present, there are no clear-cut guidelines regarding the appropriate use of traditional stimulant medications (ie, methylphenidate and amphetamine analogues) in the treatment of adult ADHD and SUDs. To date, outpatient, double-blind treatment studies show mixed reports of efficacy for stimulant and nonstimulant medication treatment in patients with co-occurring ADHD and SUDs. Most of these studies show some reduction in ADHD symptoms, and a minority of studies show some benefit of medications at reducing substance use, particularly if there is a large ADHD response. Some reasons for the modest response in these studies may include inadequate medication dosing, lower treatment responsiveness if actively using substances, the use of poorly absorbed sustained-released stimulant formulations, or poor medication adherence. Two recent studies showed that higher-than-standard FDA-approved stimulant doses were effective at reducing ADHD symptoms and promoting abstinence in ADHD adults with amphetamine use and cocaine use disorder. These findings suggest that more robust stimulant doses may be needed to effectively treat both ADHD and stimulant use disorders; however, further replication studies are needed. It remains a question whether higher dose stimulants would be efficacious for the treatment of other SUDs (eg, alcohol use disorder, cannabis use disorder). These studies also demonstrate that under closely monitored conditions and for carefully selected populations, stimulant medications can be given safely to those who actively use substances.

When choosing between stimulant and nonstimulant medications for co-occurring ADHD and

TABLE 96-1	Medications Used in the Treatment of Attention Deficit Hyperactivity Disorder		
Medication Type	**Substance**	**Primary Mechanism**	**Side Effects**
Stimulants	Methylphenidate[a]	Dopamine reuptake blockade in striatum	*Common:* Insomnia, emotional lability, nausea/vomiting, nervousness, palpitations, elevated blood pressure, tachycardia *Rare:* Seizures, psychosis, myocardial infarction
	Amphetamine analogues[a] (methamphetamine, dextro-amphetamine, mixed amphetamine salts, lisdexamfetamine)	Stimulates the cerebral cortex and reticular activating system by enhancing dopamine release and blocking dopamine reuptake	
Nonstimulants	Atomoxetine[a]	Centrally acting noradrenergic reuptake inhibitor	*Common:* Sedation, reduced appetite, nausea/vomiting, headache *Rare:* Suicidal ideation, hepatotoxicity
	Clonidine[a]	α_2 agonist	Sedation, dry mouth, depression, confusion, electrocardiographic changes, rebound hypertension
	Guanfacine[a]	α_2 agonist	Sedation, dry mouth, headache, dizziness, insomnia, electrocardiographic changes, rebound hypertension
	Bupropion	Norepinephrine and dopamine reuptake inhibitor	*Common:* Insomnia, tremor, agitation, tachycardia, elevated blood pressure, weight loss, loss of appetite *Rare:* Seizures, suicidal ideation, anaphylactoid reaction
	Venlafaxine	Norepinephrine and serotonin reuptake inhibitor	*Common:* Insomnia, dizziness, sedation, diaphoresis, nausea, elevated blood pressure *Rare:* Seizures, suicidal ideation, hyponatremia
	Tricyclic antidepressants	Blocks reuptake of norepinephrine and serotonin	Orthostatic hypotension, cardiac arrhythmia, seizures, blurred vision, constipation, dry mouth, weight gain, confusion, delirium
	Monoamine oxidase inhibitors (MAOIs)	Blocks metabolization of serotonin, norepinephrine, and dopamine	Diet- and medication-induced hypertensive crisis, serotonin syndrome, weight gain, hypotension, agitation, sleep disturbance

[a]Approved by the FDA for use in ADHD.

SUDs, the risk of untreated ADHD symptoms versus the risk of stimulant misuse and diversion should be balanced. Similar to other areas of clinical uncertainty, good clinical judgment becomes crucial when deciding on who will benefit from a pharmacologic treatment intervention and which medication(s) should be used. With careful ongoing monitoring and surveillance, emergent problems can be identified early and the treatment plan modified.

To organize treatment planning and decision making, we propose classifying patients with co-occurring ADHD and SUD into three risk groups: low, moderate, and high (Table 96-2). The most important clinical variable when considering the use of stimulant medication is whether the SUD is *active* or *in remission*. Patients with a remote history of SUDs and a long period of abstinence from substance use likely represent a low-risk group for prescribing stimulant medications, whereas patients with current substance use (without meeting the criteria for SUD) or SUDs represent moderate and high-risk groups, respectively.

General precautions when prescribing stimulant medications include using delayed-release preparations, monitoring prescription renewal times, and surveilling for evidence of substance use. Providers should always keep clear records of prescriptions written and the number of pills provided. Patients in a low-risk group for stimulant medication treatment of ADHD should be counseled that their history of SUD puts them at increased risk of hazardous stimulant use, and general prescribing precautions should be followed. Patients in the moderate-risk group (using substances but not meeting criteria for SUDs) may require more frequent office visits, urine toxicology testing, and monitoring of substance use patterns. Nonstimulant medication may be considered, although there may be a less robust treatment response. For patients in the high-risk group (patients with active SUDs), nonstimulant medications are likely to be the first-line, but in some cases, stimulant medications may be considered (eg, patient has a suboptimal response to nonstimulant medication, patient is in an intensive structured/monitored outpatient treatment program).

Patients in the moderate- or high-risk category should be seen on a more frequent basis to more closely monitor the patient and to reduce the pills per prescription. Any potential interactions between the stimulant medication and other non-medically used substances can be identified during more frequent visits. It should be made clear to patients that urine toxicology screens will be conducted routinely and that if the patient does not show a clinically significant reduction in alcohol or drug use, other treatment strategies will be implemented. Patients should take medication on a regular basis rather than on an as-needed schedule to avoid inadequate and intermittent palliation of symptoms. In addition, the risks of diversion and nonmedical use should be discussed with the patient before a stimulant is prescribed. Possible signs and symptoms of nonmedical use of prescription stimulant medications include frequent lost prescriptions or discordant pill counts, demands for immediate-release preparations, continuously escalating doses, psychosis, agitation, and physiologic toxicity (hypertension, tachycardia, or chest pain).

TABLE 96-2	Suggested Treatment Stratification for Co-Occurring Attention Deficit Hyperactivity Disorder and Substance Use Disorder
Low-Risk Group (eg, 20-year abstinence from alcohol, no current illicit drug use)	
• Brief office intervention	
• Advise of the risk of combining prescription stimulants with other substances	
• Warn about diversion	
• Ongoing monitoring	
• ADHD response	
• Use vs. nonmedical use pattern	
• Use delayed absorption formulation when prescribing stimulants	
Moderate-Risk Group (eg, some substance use but not current use disorder; nonmedical use of stimulants in past)	
• Include strategies for the low-risk group	
• More frequent office visits	
• Very close attention to patterns of alcohol/drug use	
High-Risk Group (eg, active substance use disorder)	
• Include strategies for the moderate-risk group	
• May try nonstimulants first	
• If poor response to nonstimulant, switch to long-acting stimulant	
• Requires counseling, involvement with the self-help group, or referral to appropriate SUD treatment center	
• If severe, may refer patient to intensive intervention prior to starting medication	
• May need to avoid stimulants if patient has history of or current use disorder due to prescription stimulants or high risk of diversion of medication (eg, sold medication in past)	

We recommend using long-acting stimulant preparations for patients with ADHD with comorbid SUDs to reduce the potential for nonmedical use.

Psychotherapeutic Interventions for Attention Deficit Hyperactivity Disorder and Substance Use Disorders

With respect to psychotherapeutic interventions for individuals with ADHD and SUDs, there are less clinical data to suggest which nonpharmacologic approaches work best for this population. For adult ADHD, interventions studied include cognitive–behavioral therapy (CBT), mindfulness training, psychoeducation, and metacognitive training. Overall, some studies have shown that for ADHD, combination therapy (medication and mostly cognitive therapy) is more effective than medication alone or medication plus psychoeducation. To our knowledge, there has not been a study directly comparing psychotherapy or medication alone as a treatment for ADHD and SUDs. CBT is a standard, empirically based psychotherapeutic approach for the treatment of SUDs, and interestingly, some studies have shown that when comparing medication plus CBT versus placebo plus CBT in individuals with ADHD and SUDs, both groups do equally well at reducing substance use and ADHD symptoms. Based on these results, CBT may be an effective monotherapy for some individuals, although more work is needed in this area.

KEY POINTS

1. ADHD is overrepresented in substance-using populations, and conversely, persons with SUDs have higher-than-expected rates of ADHD.
2. Several ADHD instruments may have utility for screening patients who use substances with ADHD, but a comprehensive diagnosis is required to accurately diagnose this population.
3. Under closely monitored conditions and for carefully selected populations, stimulant and nonstimulant medications for the treatment of ADHD can be given safely to patients who actively use substances.
4. Although stimulant medications have proven useful for treating adult ADHD, their benefits in patients who actively use substances are mixed. However, recent trials suggest that robust dosing may lead to a reduction in both ADHD symptoms and drug use.
5. Fewer data exist to support the use of nonstimulants or nonpharmacologic treatment alone for adults with ADHD and SUDs.

REVIEW QUESTIONS

1. Which of the following is *not* a reason why ADHD is thought to be overrepresented in populations with SUDs?
   A. ADHD and SUDs share some common genetic aberrations primarily in genes related to dopamine regulation.
   B. There are shared environmental risk factors, including maternal smoking during pregnancy, premature birth, and low birth weight.
   C. Patients with SUDs are more likely to present to clinicians requesting treatment for ADHD so that they can obtain stimulant medications, leading to higher rates of diagnosis compared to patients without SUDs.
   D. Childhood developmental vulnerabilities associated with ADHD, such as neurocognitive deficits and impulsive anger, increase the risk for later development of SUDs.

2. A 29-year-old man presents to you for evaluation of concentration problems. You find that he has a risky, binge-type alcohol drinking pattern on weekends and a family history of substance use disorder, but he does not meet the criteria for an alcohol use disorder. You diagnose him with ADHD, combined type, and want to start treatment. How would you categorize this patient in terms of his risk for receiving stimulant medication treatment?
   A. Low risk
   B. Moderate risk
   C. High risk
   D. Very high risk

3. Which of the following is *true* regarding the assessment of a patient with an active SUD and long-standing symptoms of ADHD?
   A. A diagnosis of ADHD cannot be ascertained unless he or she is able to completely stop using substances for a period of time.
   B. Neuropsychological testing is required for a diagnosis of ADHD in patients with SUDs.
   C. Collateral from family is important to obtain during the evaluation stage in order to ascertain the presence of childhood-onset and longitudinal ADHD symptoms.
   D. A diagnosis requires a baseline brain scan to rule out organic causes for the patient's symptoms of ADHD.

ANSWERS

1. **C**
2. **B**
3. **C**

SUGGESTED READINGS

Biederman J, Wilens TE, Mick E, Faraone SV, Spencer T. Does attention-deficit hyperactivity disorder impact the developmental course of drug and alcohol abuse and dependence? *Biol Psychiatry*. 1998;44(4):269-273.

Humphreys KL, Eng T, Lee SS. Stimulant medication and substance use outcomes: a meta-analysis. *JAMA Psychiatry*. 2013;70(7):740-749.

Levin FR, Mariani JJ, Specker S, et al. Extended-release mixed amphetamine salts vs placebo for comorbid adult attention-deficit/ hyperactivity disorder and cocaine use disorder: a randomized clinical trial. *JAMA Psychiatry*. 2015;72(6):593-602.

Mariani JJ, Levin FR. Treatment strategies for co-occurring ADHD and substance use disorders. *Am J Addict*. 2007;16 Suppl 1:45-54.

Molina BS, Pelham WE Jr. Attention-deficit/hyperactivity disorder and risk of substance use disorder: developmental considerations, potential pathways, and opportunities for research. *Annu Rev Clin Psychol*. 2014;10:607-639.

Co-occurring Personality Disorders and Addiction

Summary by Adam R. Demner and Stephen Ross

Based on THE ASAM PRINCIPLES OF ADDICTION MEDICINE,
6th edition chapter by Stephen Ross and Adam R. Demner

Personality disorders (PDs) are defined by the *Diagnostic and Statistical Manual of Mental Disorders*, 5th edition (*DSM-5*) as enduring patterns of inner experience and behavior that deviate markedly from the expectations of the individual's culture that are deepseated; pervasive; and produce psychopathologic symptoms affecting cognition, emotion, interpersonal functioning, and impulse regulation. Such patterns cause repeated conflicts with one's social and occupational environment and lead to emotional distress; the onset of PDs are in late adolescence or early adulthood when personality trait patterns become stable. Although PDs tend to have a chronic course of illness, longitudinal studies have generally supported the notion that PDs tend to improve over time, although the evidence is more mixed for Cluster A and C disorders.

PDs and substance use disorders (SUDs) are highly associated with each other, especially in mental health and SUD treatment settings where they represent the norm in terms of comorbidity. Standardized assessment instruments are vital components of diagnostic formulations to determine the presence of a PD that is distinguishable from or co-occurring with an SUD. Given the epidemiologic data where the majority of patients with a PD have a co-occurring addictive disorder and vice versa, an a priori diagnostic assumption should be that there are two separate problems until proven otherwise. The presence of a PD negatively affects the course of treatment of the SUD and is associated with worse outcomes. It is important to provide comprehensive care optimally within a structured environment with a dual focus (ie, PD and SUD), utilizing psychosocial treatments for PDs and SUDs in an integrated system of care and providing symptom-targeted pharmacotherapy when appropriate as an adjunct.

DEFINITIONS AND CLASSIFICATION

The *DSM-5* employs a categorical classification system placing the PDs into three *clusters* (A, B, and C) based on symptom similarities, which produce 10 distinct disorders. There have been no significant changes in this classification system relative to the *DSM-IV-TR*.

- Cluster A (paranoid, schizoid, schizotypal): These disorders are characterized by odd or eccentric cognition and behavior related to the schizophrenia spectrum.
- Cluster B (antisocial, borderline, histrionic, narcissistic): These disorders are marked by emotional, dramatic, or erratic behavior and are related to trait impulsivity and/or affect dysregulation and are on the spectrum with impulse disorders.
- Cluster C (avoidant, dependent, obsessive–compulsive): These disorders are marked by anxious symptoms, are related to trait anxiety or compulsivity, and are on the spectrum with anxiety disorders.

This *categorical or typological system* was based on a variety of theoretical perspectives. It includes a list of symptoms with diagnoses made if a recommended threshold or cutoff level of a given number of diagnostic criteria are present. The *DSM-5* also includes a *dimensional model* as an emerging model for the diagnosis of personality disorders; however, these criterion are not universally utilized in clinical practice.

EPIDEMIOLOGY

PDs and SUDs are both prevalent in the general population. In looking at five well-designed (ie, use of *DSM-IV* or *International Statistical Classification of Diseases and Related Health Problems*, 10th edition [*ICD-10*] diagnostic criteria and structured or semistructured interviews) community surveys of PDs published since 2000 with sample sizes ranging from 214 to 43,093, the estimated prevalence of any PD in the general population ranged from 4.4%

to 13.4% with a median of 9.6%. Cluster C disorders (obsessive–compulsive and avoidant PD) were the most commonly diagnosed. In comparison, SUDs—including alcohol or illicit drugs—affect approximately 9.2% of the population in individuals 12 years of age or older. This does not include nicotine/tobacco use disorders, which affect approximately 21% of the population.

In addition to being prevalent conditions by themselves in the general population, both PDs and SUDs are intimately related in community samples. For instance, in a nonpatient sample of approximately 800 individuals who were relatives of both controls and psychiatric patients, of those who had any PD, 43% and 53% met the criteria for a lifetime alcohol use disorder or drug use disorder, respectively, and having a PD increased the risk of both alcohol use disorder and drug use disorder by a factor of four compared to individuals without a PD. Compared to the rates of PDs in community samples, the rates of PDs in psychiatric or addiction treatment settings are significantly increased.

Even though Cluster C diagnoses (obsessive–compulsive and avoidant PD) are the most common PD diagnoses in the general population, Cluster B disorders (antisocial personality disorder [ASPD] and borderline personality disorder [BPD]) are the most commonly associated with SUDs either in community or treatment samples (eg, SUD or traditional psychiatric). In a review of comorbidity data between BPD and SUDs, researchers reported that among those seeking addiction treatments, rates of BPD ranged from 5% to 65%, and conversely, among those receiving treatment for BPD, the prevalence of current SUDs was between 25% and 67%.

DIAGNOSIS: THEORETICAL ISSUES

Given the markedly high co-occurrence of SUDs and PDs (especially ASPD and BPD), a correlation between the two has long been assumed, theorized, and studied with the evidence for an association derived from genetic, epidemiologic, retrospective, and longitudinal studies. Two main classification systems to model PDs comorbid with SUDs are discussed: *co-occurring* and *etiologic*.

Co-Occurring Models

In co-occurring models, there is the presence of two distinct disorders: one psychiatric and one substance related. One possibility relating the two disorders is that both have unique and independent etiologic determinants and both disorders *co-occur randomly*. Alternatively, in the *common factor* model, the co-occurrence of both a PD and an SUD

is caused by shared vulnerabilities or risk factors, ranging from genetic to sociocultural. This model would be most applicable to the interaction between addiction and certain PDs (ASPD and BPD) because of the considerable comorbidity as mentioned previously. This model is best evaluated by twin, family, and adoption studies. If shared genetic risk factors to both a PD and addiction were to account for the increased comorbidity, an elevated incidence of the one disorder (eg, SUD) would be expected in relatives of individuals with the other disorder (eg, PD). However, there is little evidence to support this model other than some data suggesting common genetic influences on symptom clusters that account for a significant genetic etiology for both alcohol dependence and conduct disorder/ASPD.

Etiologic Models

Etiologic diagnoses come in two varieties: *secondary SUD* and *secondary psychopathological* models. In the *secondary SUD models*, the presence of a PD or pathologic personality traits is a risk factor contributing to the development of a substance use disorder. Because the traits within a PD usually have some early manifestations in childhood and adolescence, it is possible to prospectively examine the relationship between maladaptive traits, seen prior to exposure to addictive substances, and the subsequent development of addiction. A number of traits have been identified that appear commonly in patients with both SUDs and PDs (such as sensation seeking, novelty seeking, impulsivity, negative emotionality), and prospective studies with such traits identified in children or adolescents can assess for correlations with a later onset of SUDs.

Several pathways have been proposed that might explain how certain personality traits or symptoms of a PD might lead to addiction. In all of these models, substance initiation and continued use secondary to personality psychopathology eventually translates into an independent SUD; over a long enough period of time, the neurobiology of the normative reward system can be sufficiently hijacked and corrupted, leading to chronic neuroadaptive changes associated with the transition from at-risk substance use to increasingly severe SUD. Once physical dependence or other SUD-related criteria reach a collective threshold, the SUD is now established and can continue independent of its original relationship to the mental disorder causing it, even if the original offending psychiatric condition (eg, PD) is treated with remission of illness. However, there will remain negative bidirectional effects now that there are two distinct problems.

In the *secondary psychopathology model*, substance use precedes and causes PDs. Although this model has a paucity of empirical support relative to the secondary SUD models, it remains pertinent from a conceptual perspective to the overall understanding of co-occurring PDs and SUDs; furthermore, this model may be a key element to avoid misdiagnosis of PDs. It is a frequent clinical observation that active addiction generates significant characterologic symptoms that can be indistinguishable from the symptoms of a PD. An example of this would be secondary sociopathy, symptoms consistent with antisocial PD occasioned by drug use. Certain drugs (eg, intravenous heroin, crack cocaine), especially those that are illegal and perceived as very harmful, are associated with antisocial behaviors. These apparent symptoms of personality psychopathology should remit with sobriety without a preexisting PD.

DIAGNOSIS: PRACTICAL ISSUES

Screening is a crucial step prior to diagnostic formulation. Because patients with PDs tend to have more severe pathology and more frequent treatment contact, they are more likely to present in the situations with the least time for an assessment, such as emergency rooms or incarcerated settings. However, most screening questionnaires focus on specific PDs or require too much time to be used in routine clinical practice. The use of standardized assessment instruments is important in diagnosing PDs because traditional unstructured clinical diagnostic interviews are poorly reliable and are associated with missed and incorrect diagnoses. There are a number of formal assessment tools used in evaluating a personality pathology, although they were not specifically designed for an SUD population.

Any assessment tool must be considered along with other information sources, such as unstructured patient interviews, collateral information, and longitudinal assessments. Collateral contacts can be essential for elucidating long-standing behavior patterns, providing information that the patient is not able or willing to provide, and increasing the convergent validity of diagnoses. Risk assessments for suicidality, nonsuicidal self-injury, and violence deserve special attention, particularly in patients with BPD and ASPD. Given the high-risk nature of these patients, a team-based approach and access to referral services is ideal for optimal management.

In addition to a careful substance history and risk assessment, important areas of focus include a history of trauma (physical, sexual, and emotional abuse, neglect, conflict in the household), familial history of personality dysfunction, and quality/quantity of current and past interpersonal relationships (ie, object relations). Inflexible or maladaptive coping skills are the hallmark of a PD. Close attention to interpersonal style and transference/countertransference can yield important diagnostic information. For example, patients with BPD tend to develop transference quickly and intensely and to have extreme and rapid oscillations (eg, the clinician is experienced as all-good and ideal and then suddenly all-bad and malicious after a seemingly small disappointment). Schizoid or avoidant patients may be especially deferential or reserved in a clinical encounter. It is also important to rule out other co-occurring psychiatric disorders whose symptom presentation may mimic symptoms of various PDs. For example, bipolar disorders should be excluded before diagnosing BPD, and social anxiety disorder should be ruled out before diagnosing avoidant personality disorder. A detailed temporal history and longitudinal assessment is key to differentiate acute *state* phenomenon usually associated with nonpersonality psychopathologic disorders (eg, acute mood instability associated with mania or substance use) versus longer term *traits* associated with PDs. In addition to harmful use of drugs, there are other general medical conditions that can sufficiently alter physiologic brain processes to produce changes in personality, either acutely or over a longer period of time.

The ultimate goal of an assessment is to determine the presence of a PD, which is distinguishable from or co-occurring with an SUD. Given the epidemiologic data where the majority of patients with a PD (especially BPD and ASPD) have a co-occurring addictive disorder and vice versa, a diagnostic a priori assumption should be that there are two separate problems until proven otherwise by a process of exclusion. As a general clinical rule, symptoms that persist beyond 1 month of abstinence are more likely to be primary.

TREATMENT
General Treatment Guidelines and Treatment Outcomes

The best predictor of therapeutic outcomes for patients with PD is severity of illness, not the type of personality psychopathology. One would expect that with co-occurring PDs and SUDs, the presence of two distinct disorders, irrespective of etiologic commonality, would raise the issue of bidirectional interaction considering the ways that each disorder might influence the persistence, expression, or progression of the other, thus altering its course and failure to treat one disorder (either mental illness or the SUD) would be predicted to negatively affect the severity of illness and longitudinal course of the other.

However, when examining co-occurring PDs and SUDs, the data are mixed as to whether co-occurring PDs in individuals with SUDs predict a worse response to treatment. A growing number of studies have consistently demonstrated that personality psychopathology—although associated with pre- and posttreatment problem severity—is not a strong predictor of clinical improvement in this population. Alternatively, a number of studies have shown that PDs can predict a shorter time to relapse, worse SUD outcomes in general, and increased treatment drop-out rates or lack of aftercare compliance after discharge in patients with SUDs. One systematic review looking at 122 studies with nearly 200,000 participants revealed an increased vulnerability for dropping out of treatment associated with younger patients, those with cognitive dysfunction, and individuals having a diagnosis of ASPD and histrionic PD. Studies focusing on "normal" personality traits in individuals with SUDs have delineated low persistence, high novelty seeking, high neuroticism, and low conscientiousness as strong predictors of a shorter time to relapse.

Other factors that have been identified as positively affecting treatment outcomes in individuals with co-occurring PDs and SUDs include a higher level of motivation for change, a longer length of time in treatment, and increased therapist alliance. Regarding the comorbidity of PDs and other psychiatric disorders, it has been demonstrated that PDs are associated with worse outcomes for patients with a broad range of psychiatric and addictive disorders. Prospective longitudinal outcome studies of patients with SUDs with both a PD and another psychiatric disorder suggest that having a combination of both disorders predicted worse outcomes such as an increased likelihood of relapse or worse psychosocial outcomes. Co-occurring non-SUD psychiatric pathology in individuals with PDs and SUDs (triply diagnosed) has also been associated with worse treatment outcomes in terms of aftercare compliance.

KEY POINTS

1. PDs commonly occur in both traditional psychiatric and SUD treatment settings, and there is considerable co-occurrence between these disorders and SUDs, especially with ASPD and BPD.
2. Screening, standardized diagnostic assessments, family history, age of symptom onset, premorbid symptom patterns, temporal history of PD symptoms relative to substance initiation and use, periods of abstinence, collateral history, serial and longitudinal assessments, and ruling out harmful substance use or medical conditions that can masquerade as PD symptoms are key to establishing the diagnosis of a PD independent from an SUD.
3. Patients with co-occurring PDs and SUDs can benefit from treatment as much as those without PDs, but the presence of a PD does negatively affect the treatment course of the SUD and is associated with treatment noncompliance and relapse.
4. It is important to provide comprehensive care optimally within a structured environment (eg, coexisting disorder day programs, opioid treatment programs, therapeutic communities) with a dual focus (eg, PD and SUD) in an integrated system utilizing symptom-targeted pharmacotherapy when indicated as an adjunct to psychosocial interventions.
5. A focus on therapeutic alliance and risk assessment as well as addressing motivational, interpersonal, and perceptual problems are key to engaging patients in longer term treatments, which are associated with improved outcomes.

REVIEW QUESTIONS

1. Which of the following personality disorders has the highest rate of co-occurrence of a substance use disorder?
   A. Borderline personality disorder
   B. Antisocial personality disorder
   C. Paranoid personality disorder
   D. Narcissistic personality disorder
   E. Avoidant personality disorder

2. A 41-year-old woman with no previous history of conduct disorder or criminality gets arrested multiple times over a 6-month period for possession and use of crack cocaine in addition to prostitution and repeated episodes of shoplifting. What is the most likely diagnosis?
   A. Antisocial personality disorder
   B. Borderline personality disorder
   C. Narcissistic personality disorder
   D. Histrionic personality disorder
   E. Secondary sociopathy

3. All of the following are proven effective treatments for personality disorders co-occurring with substance use disorders *except*:
   A. dialectical behavioral therapy.
   B. Alcoholics Anonymous.
   C. psychoanalysis.
   D. dual focus schema therapy.
   E. therapeutic communities.

ANSWERS

1. **B**
2. **E**
3. **C**

SUGGESTED READINGS

Dixon-Gordon KL, Turner BJ, Chapman AL. Psychotherapy for personality disorders. *Int Rev Psychiatry*. 2011;23(3):282-302.

Paris J. Pharmacological treatments for personality disorders. *Int Rev Psychiatry*. 2011;23(3):303-309.

Siever LJ, Davis KL. A psychobiological perspective on the personality disorders. *Am J Psychiatry*. 1991;148(12): 1647-1658.

Verheul R. Co-morbidity of personality disorders in individuals with substance use disorders. *Eur Psychiatry*. 2001;16(5): 274-282.

Verheul R, van den Bosch LM, Ball SA. Substance abuse. In: Oldham JM, Skodol AE, Bender DS, eds. *Textbook of Personality Disorders*. Arlington, VA: American Psychiatric Publishing, 2005.

98 Posttraumatic Stress Disorder and Substance Use Disorder Comorbidity

Summary by Colette L. Haward

Based on THE ASAM PRINCIPLES OF ADDICTION MEDICINE, 6th edition chapter by Michael Saladin, Jenni Teeters, Daniel F. Gros, Amanda K. Gilmore, Kevin M. Gray, Emma Louise Barrett, Cynthia L. Lancaster, Therese Killeen, and Sudie Back

The high comorbidity of posttraumatic stress disorder (PTSD) and substance use disorders (SUDs) indicates that persons presenting to treatment for either PTSD or SUDs should be screened for both. Both civilian and combat veteran populations have a more complicated clinical course and worse treatment outcomes with comorbid PTSD and SUDs than with SUDs alone.

PHENOMENOLOGY

The *Diagnostic and Statistical Manual of Mental Disorders,* 5th edition (*DSM-5*) outlines the following criteria necessary to diagnose PTSD:

- The occurrence of a traumatic event (criterion A).
- Greater than 1 month of symptoms (criterion F) within the four symptom criteria of intrusion (criterion B), avoidance (criterion C), negative alterations in cognitions and mood (criterion D), and arousal and reactivity (criterion E).
- Impaired functioning or significant distress (criterion G).
- If the onset of symptoms is 6 months or more after the traumatic event, the disorder is considered to have a delayed expression or onset.

It has been estimated that between 39% and 90% of the population have been exposed to a traumatic event. Of those who experience a traumatic event, only 10% to 20% will develop PTSD. The *DSM-5* yielded a lifetime prevalence rate of 8.3%.

EPIDEMIOLOGY

The National Comorbidity Survey, a large-scale survey that took place in the early 1990s and used the *DSM-III-R* criteria, found the lifetime prevalence rate

for PTSD at 7.8%, and those with PTSD were two to four times more likely than those without PTSD to meet the criteria for an SUD. The National Comorbidity Survey Replication, which took place a decade later, found a similar lifetime prevalence rate of 6.8% using *DSM-IV* criteria. The National Epidemiologic Survey on Alcohol and Related Conditions Wave 2 assessed for PTSD using *DSM-IV-TR* from 2004 to 2005. Results showed that 1.6% of the US population meets the criteria for co-occurring alcohol dependence and PTSD. The National Epidemiologic Survey on Alcohol and Related Conditions III, which took place between 2012 and 2013, used a modified *DSM-5* criteria (requiring three or more symptoms in criteria D and E). It demonstrated that a modified *DSM-5* PTSD diagnosis odds ratio for a co-occurring SUD was 1.3 among those with this modified *DSM-5* PTSD in the past 12 months and 1.5 among those with PTSD in their lifetime. The National Survey on Drug Use and Health Mental Health Surveillance Survey assessed PTSD from 2008 to 2012 using the *DSM-IV-TR* criteria. It showed that adults exposed to potentially traumatic events were more likely to use substances than those who were not exposed. In a nationally representative sample of 1,484 US veterans in 2013, based on the *DSM-5* criteria, the lifetime PTSD probability was 8.1% and PTSD was associated with increased odds of SUDs.

ETIOLOGIC RELATIONSHIP BETWEEN POSTTRAUMATIC STRESS DISORDER AND SUBSTANCE USE DISORDERS

Various theories have characterized the development of comorbid PTSD and SUDs. One of the most prominent, the self-medication theory, postulates that substance use serves to alleviate PTSD symptoms, as in the case of primary PTSD (ie, the person first develops PTSD and then develops an SUD).

When the onset of an SUD precedes the development of PTSD, as in secondary PTSD, then there are three potential causal pathways for developing PTSD:

1. Through the cognitive impairments caused by using substances, such as impaired decision making and attenuated fear responses; combined, this can put individuals at risk of a potentially traumatic event while intoxicated
2. The lifestyle of a person who uses substances; often considered high risk with dangerous environments and behaviors
3. Increased anxiety and arousal that accompanies chronic substance use, which may increase vulnerability to developing PTSD after trauma exposure

Other factors may play a role in the development of comorbid PTSD and SUDs, such as brain structure and connectivity abnormalities, the hypothalamic–pituitary–adrenal axis, genetics, and psychosocial factors.

NEUROBIOLOGICAL FACTORS IN COMORBID POSTTRAUMATIC STRESS DISORDER AND SUBSTANCE USE DISORDERS

PTSD and SUDs are associated with changes in the corticolimbic structures, specifically, the amygdala (AMY) and the prefrontal cortex. Individuals with PTSD exhibit hypoactive executive functioning (in the prefrontal cortex) and hyperactive fear circuitry (in the AMY) activity. Disconnection between both structures explains the inability to extinguish fear responses. Alcohol and/or drug cues stimulate AMY and prefrontal cortex activity, and individuals with *DSM-IV*–defined alcohol dependence have a lower AMY volume, which is associated with increased craving and alcohol intake. Dysregulation in corticolimbic structures common to both PTSD and SUDs reduces the ability to regulate intrusive trauma-related memories and craving-related thoughts.

The hypothalamic–pituitary–adrenal axis and the autonomic nervous system are also integral in the development and maintenance of PTSD and SUDs. Both of these neurobiological systems regulate the physiologic response to stress. In such a response, the hypothalamic–pituitary–adrenal axis is activated, involving the release of corticotropin-releasing factor from the hypothalamus, which stimulates adrenocorticotropic hormone release from the anterior

pituitary, which then stimulates the release of cortisol form the adrenal glands. While in the autonomic nervous system, the response is to release epinephrine and norepinephrine. Individuals with PTSD have higher levels of corticotropin-releasing factor and corticotropin-releasing hormone and abnormalities in the autonomic nervous system compared to controls. With regard to SUDs, corticotropin-releasing factor and the noradrenergic pathways are involved in the stress-induced reinstatement of drug-seeking behaviors.

ASSESSMENT OF POSTTRAUMATIC STRESS DISORDER IN SUBSTANCE USE DISORDERS

The assessment of PTSD should occur after a patient has emerged from acute alcohol or drug intoxication or withdrawal. In contrast to other anxiety disorders, less abstinence may be required to diagnose PTSD among patients with SUDs due to unique diagnostic criteria (ie, the requirement of exposure to a traumatic event). Intrusive PTSD symptoms are more characteristic of PTSD and are unlikely to be mimicked by substance use or withdrawal. Other PTSD symptoms (eg, irritability or anger outbursts, sleep impairment) could be worsened by the use of, or withdrawal from, alcohol or drugs.

Interviewer-Rated Assessment of PTSD

The Clinician-Administered PTSD Scale for DSM-5 is the most widely used interviewer-rated PTSD assessment. It is a 30-item structured interview with a checklist of potentially traumatic events at the beginning of the interview. Items assessed include the frequency, intensity, onset, and duration of PTSD symptoms; social and occupational functioning; symptom change; overall response validity; overall PTSD severity; and specifications for the dissociative subtype. The assessment can be used to diagnose PTSD (past month), to give a lifetime diagnosis of PTSD, and to assess PTSD severity.

Other commonly used clinician-applied scales include the PTSD Symptom Scale Interview for DSM-5, the Structured Clinical Interview for DSM-5 Disorders, the MINI International Neuropsychiatric Interview PTSD Module, and the Composite International Diagnostic Interview.

Self-Reported Assessment of PTSD

Measures to monitor PTSD symptoms are generally brief, self-report assessments. These include the PTSD Checklist for DSM-5 and the Posttraumatic Diagnostic Scale for DSM-5.

TREATMENT OF POSTTRAUMATIC STRESS DISORDER AND POSTTRAUMATIC STRESS DISORDER/ SUBSTANCE USE DISORDER COMORBIDITY

Treatment for PTSD alone or PTSD/SUD comorbidity are either psychotherapy, pharmacotherapy, or both.

Cognitive–Behavioral Therapy for Posttraumatic Stress Disorder

Exposure-based therapy represents the longest standing, empirically validated psychotherapy for PTSD. It is based on conditioning and information processing theories of fear attenuation. Fear abatement results from behavioral extinction, whereby simply repeating exposure to a fear-eliciting cue (eg, physical location where a motor vehicle accident happened) in the absence of the feared outcome (eg, motor vehicle accident) will eventually subside the fear response. Individuals are either exposed to in vivo or imaginal fear-eliciting cues.

Prolonged exposure therapy involves didactic training about common reactions to traumatic events, relaxation via breathing retraining, prolonged imaginal exposure to trauma, and in vivo exposure to trauma-related situations.

Cognitive-focused therapy is composed of cognitive therapy and cognitive processing therapy. Cognitive therapy is built conceptually around the notion that it is the *meaning* that individuals assign to traumatic events that determines the duration and intensity of emotion/mood states that ensue. The goal of cognitive therapy is to help individuals implement corrective cognitive procedures to identify and challenge inaccurate and irrational thoughts and beliefs.

Cognitive processing therapy is a PTSD-specific treatment protocol that combines a cognitive focus with elements of exposure therapy. It consists of a psychoeducation component in which an information-processing model of PTSD is presented and a writing–reading task where the individual develops a detailed narrative of the traumatic experience.

One of the most studied anxiety management therapies is stress inoculation training. Coping skills are taught that can be practiced both inside and outside treatment sessions. Patients then practice these coping skills in increasingly anxiety-provoking situations, such as graduated exposures, as a method of "inoculation" against relapse.

Exposure therapy (in vivo and imaginal combined) is considered the dominant therapeutic approach for resolving PTSD. The Substance Abuse and Mental Health Services Administration has selected prolonged exposure therapy as its model program.

Integrated Cognitive–Behavioral Therapy for Posttraumatic Stress Disorder/Substance Use Disorder Comorbidity

Findings from "integrated" treatment models, in which both SUDs and PTSD are simultaneously treated, show that alcohol and drug use typically decrease significantly with the addition of trauma-focused interventions. To date, most research has fallen into two broad categories: (1) exposure-based trauma therapies concurrently provided with evidence-based SUD interventions and (2) non–exposure-based therapies that focus on CBT or coping skills. Seeking safety is a well-known integrated CBT. It is a present-focused, manualized treatment that provides psychoeducation and teaches coping skills. Substance dependence posttraumatic stress disorder therapy is a manualized treatment that utilizes relapse prevention, coping skills, psychoeducation, and in vivo exposure for individuals with PTSD.

Imaginal and in vivo exposure techniques for PTSD can be used safely and effectively with patients with SUDs. Addressing trauma does not worsen patients' symptoms but rather improves PTSD, substance use, and psychiatric distress.

Pharmacotherapy of Posttraumatic Stress Disorder

The primary goals of treating PTSD with medication include decreasing PTSD symptoms, improving overall functioning, improving resilience to future stressors, decreasing symptoms of comorbid psychiatric conditions, and reducing the risk of PTSD relapse. Long-term pharmacologic treatment (eg, 1 year) is recommended.

Two selective serotonin reuptake inhibitors (SSRIs) have been approved by the US Food and Drug Administration for the treatment of PTSD: sertraline (Zoloft) and paroxetine (Paxil). They are considered first-line pharmacologic treatments of PTSD. SSRIs improve all three symptom clusters of PTSD, improve quality of life, effectively treat comorbid conditions, and are relatively safe in overdose.

Dual-action serotonergic and noradrenergic medications are able to decrease PTSD symptoms and help with sleep disturbances. Tricyclic antidepressants and monoamine oxidase inhibitors improve PTSD symptoms but come with adverse side effects and risks. Mood stabilizers and anticonvulsants fail to show any benefit in treating PTSD. Antipsychotics such as risperidone have been shown to be beneficial as an augmentation medication to partial responders of SSRIs. Benzodiazepines are contraindicated as a mono therapy or a preventative strategy based on an increased risk of PTSD. Medications that reduce central nervous system activity (eg, clonidine, prazosin) help decrease nightmares and hyperarousal symptoms.

Currently, there are no medications that effectively curtail the development of PTSD. However, the strategic use of β-blocking agents (eg, propranolol) may dampen PTSD symptoms when combined with exposure-based therapy and selectively interfere with emotional memory.

Pharmacotherapy of Posttraumatic Stress Disorder/Substance Use Disorder Comorbidity

Most studies show that patients with PTSD and comorbid SUDs respond as well to standard PTSD pharmacotherapies as compared to patients without comorbid SUDs. Studies that examine SSRIs have shown a decrease in alcohol use severity and significant reductions in all three PSTD symptoms clusters. A study comparing US Food and Drug Administration–approved alcohol use disorder medications—disulfiram, naltrexone, and their combination in individuals with comorbid PTSD and SUD—found that patients receiving medication, relative to placebo, yielded better alcohol outcomes and that disulfiram appeared to reduce PTSD symptoms.

KEY POINTS

1. Theory and research about the nature of the causal relationship between SUDs and PTSD suggest that PTSD most often precedes the onset of an SUD.
2. PTSD and SUDs have shared causal processes such as dysregulation of both the hypothalamic–pituitary–adrenal axis and noradrenergic systems as well as deficits in neural circuitry related to executive functioning and limbic system regulation.
3. The effective management of PTSD/SUD comorbidity begins with a comprehensive assessment that includes interviews and self-report measures. Ensuring a sufficient period of abstinence prior to conducting the assessment will enhance the assessment's findings.
4. PTSD/SUD comorbidity is best treated concurrently. Exposure-based interventions (eg, prolonged

exposure therapy) are considered the gold standard of cognitive–behavioral therapies; other cognitive-focused and anxiety-focused therapies have also shown success. Investigations are underway to identify medications that may help reduce the symptoms of both disorders in individuals with PTSD/SUD comorbidity.

REVIEW QUESTIONS

1. What is the approximate lifetime prevalence of PTSD per the *DSM-5*?
   A. 1%
   B. 3%
   C. 8%
   D. 15%

2. Which two medications are approved by the US Food and Drug Administration and considered first-line pharmacotherapeutic treatment options for PTSD?
   A. Venlafaxine (Effexor XR) and sertraline (Zoloft)
   B. Paroxetine (Paxil) and sertraline (Zoloft)
   C. Imipramine and buspirone
   D. Venlafaxine (Effexor XR) and buspirone

3. Which neurobiological pathway or nervous system is *not* integral to the development and maintenance of both PTSD and SUD?
   A. The corticolimbic pathway
   B. The hypothalamic–pituitary–adrenal axis
   C. The autonomic nervous system
   D. The corticobasal ganglia pathway

ANSWERS

1. **C**
2. **B**
3. **D**

SUGGESTED READINGS

American Psychiatric Association. *Diagnostic and Statistical Manual of Mental Disorders*. 5th ed. Arlington, VA: American Psychiatric Association, 2013.

Jacobsen LK, Southwick SM, Kosten TR. Substance use disorders in patients with posttraumatic stress disorder: a review of the literature. *Am J Psychiatry*. 2001;158(8):1184-1190.

Ouimette P, Read JP, eds. *Trauma and Substance Abuse: Causes, Consequences, and Treatment of Comorbid Disorders*. 2nd ed. Washington, DC: American Psychological Association, 2014.

Sadock BJ, Sadock VA, Ruiz P. *Kaplan & Sadock's Synopsis of Psychiatry: Behavioral Sciences/Clinical Psychiatry*. 11th ed. Philadelphia: Lippincott Williams & Wilkins, 2014.

Schoenfeld FB, Marmar CR, Neylan TC. Current concepts in pharmacotherapy for posttraumatic stress disorder. *Psychiatr Serv*. 2004;55(5):519-531.

99 Co-occurring Substance Use Disorders and Eating Disorders

Summary by Lisa J. Merlo, William M. Greene, and Mark S. Gold

Based on THE ASAM PRINCIPLES OF ADDICTION MEDICINE, 6th edition chapter by Lisa J. Merlo and Mark S. Gold

Disorders related to eating (including anorexia nervosa [AN], bulimia nervosa [BN], binge eating disorder [BED], and obesity) exhibit many commonalities with substance use disorders. Comorbidity of these conditions complicates the assessment, diagnosis, treatment, and long-term recovery for both.

DEFINITIONS
Addiction

Addiction has been summarized by four Cs: compulsive use, loss of control, use despite adverse consequences, and craving. Although the concept of "food addiction" is not included in the *Diagnostic and Statistical Manual of Mental Disorders,* 5th edition (*DSM-5*), research has demonstrated that pathologic attachment to food (particularly foods high in sugar and fat) is similar to a substance use disorder in virtually all spheres, including neurobiological.

Feeding and Eating Disorders

The feeding and eating disorders comprise a category of psychiatric illnesses characterized by disturbed eating patterns and dysfunctional attitudes related to food, eating, and body shape.

Anorexia Nervosa

Individuals with AN are characterized by significantly low body weight, intense fear of gaining weight, and disturbed body image. Associated physical symptoms and medical complications include constipation, cold intolerance, lethargy, lanugo, hypothalamic–pituitary–adrenal axis dysfunction, pubertal delay, growth retardation, osteopenia/osteoporosis, hypotension, cardiac arrhythmias, mitral valve prolapse, metabolic alkalosis or acidosis, hypokalemia, hypoglycemia, leukopenia, anemia, carotenemia, acrocyanosis, thrombocytopenia, peripheral neuropathy, hypothermia, dehydration, and hair loss. The mortality rate for individuals with AN

is high, ranging from 7% to 10%. Rates of completed suicide in this population range from 0.9% to 6.3%.

Bulimia Nervosa

Individuals with BN are characterized by recurrent episodes of binge eating, along with compensatory behaviors to prevent weight gain (eg, self-induced vomiting; misuse of laxatives, diuretics, or other medication; fasting; excessive exercise). Unlike AN, low body weight is not a diagnostic feature. Medical complications of BN include dental enamel erosion, hypokalemia, metabolic alkalosis/acidosis, cardiac arrhythmias, parotid enlargement, submandibular lymphadenopathy, menstrual irregularity, constipation, and reproductive problems.

Binge Eating Disorder

Individuals with BED are characterized by recurrent episodes of binge eating without any compensatory measures to lose weight. Studies demonstrate 40.5% to 56.8% of individuals with BED can be classified as food addicted, and 72.2% of individuals with obesity with food addiction can be diagnosed with BED. Approximately 70% of individuals with BED are obese and about 20% are overweight. Common medical complications associated with BED include morbid obesity, hypertension, type II diabetes, cardiovascular disease, stroke, osteoarthritis and arthralgias, increased risk for cancers, irritable bowel syndrome, and early menarche.

Obesity

An individual's body mass index (BMI) score determines a diagnosis of obesity. A BMI between 30 and 35 is considered stage 1 obesity, between 35 and 40 is stage 2 obesity, and over 40 is stage 3 obesity (also called morbid obesity).

PREVALENCE OF EATING DISORDERS
General Population

Both AN and BN are much more prevalent in females, and eating disorders are often described as diseases of pediatric origin. The prevalence of subclinical AN among females aged 16 to 25 years is estimated to be approximately 10%, with lifetime prevalence of AN in females estimated to be 0.9% to 1.9%; lifetime prevalence of AN in males is estimated to be 0.29% to 0.3%. The lifetime prevalence of BN is estimated to be 1.5% to 2.9% in females and 0.5% in males. The lifetime prevalence of BED is estimated to be 1.9% to 3.5% in females and 0.3% to 2.0% in males. As of 2014, 17% of American youth and 36.5% of American adults aged 20 years or older are obese (ie, BMI $\geq$30).

Patients With Substance Use Disorders

Among individuals receiving treatment for SUDs, approximately 0.02% to 3.4% also currently suffer from an eating disorder. Lifetime co-occurrence of alcohol use disorders and eating disorders ranges from 24% to 25%, whereas lifetime co-occurrence between drug use disorders and eating disorders is 18% to 26%. Between 2% to 41% of patients with a mild SUD have a lifetime history of eating disorder behaviors. It is estimated that 17% to 25% of women with eating disorders have a lifetime history of SUDs. Binge eating is frequently associated with SUDs, with up to 57% of men and 28% of women with BED meeting the criteria for SUDs. Individuals with a history of overeating commonly develop alcohol or drug use disorders after improving their eating habits (eg, post bariatric surgery), and treatment for SUDs is often associated with weight gain.

Patients With Psychiatric Disorders

The most common psychiatric comorbidities among individuals with AN are mood disorders, with approximately 94% of patients with AN meeting the criteria for a depressive disorder. Between 56% and 66% of patients with an eating disorder have one or more anxiety disorders. Obsessive–compulsive disorder is especially common, with a prevalence rate of 29.5% to 41% among individuals with AN or BN. Comorbid personality disorders (especially cluster B and C) are present in 21% to 97% of cases. Individuals with BED are three times more likely to suffer from major depressive disorder than are individuals from the general population. Obesity is also associated with increased psychiatric comorbidity, including major depressive disorder and generalized anxiety disorder.

Primary Care or Other Healthcare Populations

Within a family practice setting, the prevalence of AN is estimated to be between 4.2% and 6.3%, and the prevalence of BN is estimated to be between 6.3% and 12.2%.

DIFFERENTIAL DIAGNOSIS
Identifying Eating Disorders

The majority of individuals with an eating disorder go undiagnosed because they often do not seek treatment, are in significant denial with respect to their illness, actively hide their symptoms, and present with nonspecific symptoms, which could be attributable to other medical conditions.

Eating Disorders in Patients With Substance Use Disorders

Regardless of whether an eating disorder is initially suspected, addiction medicine clinicians should inquire about eating disturbances as well as weight-related drug use (eg, use of "diet pills," laxatives, stimulants) because individuals with eating disorders are unlikely to offer this information spontaneously. The presence of a comorbid eating disorder may affect decisions regarding treatment of SUDs. All patients with SUDs would also benefit from an analysis of their diet, exercise routine, eating behaviors, and BMI. In particular, patients undergoing treatment for alcohol use disorder should always be evaluated for binge eating symptoms, those in treatment for a stimulant use disorder should always be assessed for purging behaviors and excessive dieting, and patients with unhealthy use of caffeine or laxatives should always undergo a general eating disorder screening. As treatment for the SUD progresses, the patient's weight and BMI should be tracked.

SCREENING INSTRUMENTS

The **Yale Food Addiction Scale Version 2.0** is used to screen for "food addiction" by applying *DSM-5* SUD criteria to food via a 35-item self-report questionnaire.

The **Eating Disorders Inventory, 3rd edition** has established psychometric properties and is the most widely used self-report measure of disordered eating and related symptoms of AN and BN.

The **Eating Disorder Diagnostic Scale** is a 19-item self-report questionnaire that assesses eating disorder symptoms over the previous 3 months.

The **Eating Disorder Examination Questionnaire** assesses disordered eating behaviors and attitudes in order to assist with a diagnosis of AN and BN.

The **Bulimia Test—Revised** is a 36-item self-report measure of BN symptoms used to assist with a diagnosis of BN.

The **Binge Eating Scale** is a 16-item measure used to assess binge eating symptoms and to assist with a diagnosis of BED.

The **Night Eating Symptom Scale** is a self-report instrument that contains 12 items that specifically assess symptoms related to overeating during the nighttime hours.

TREATMENT

Like the treatment of SUDs, the treatment of eating disorders can be a long and arduous process marked by alternating periods of relapse and recovery.

Acute Treatment

For serious cases, and particularly for adolescent patients, treatment may commence on a coerced or even involuntary basis through enrollment in an inpatient or residential program. A focus on refeeding takes precedence in order to medically stabilize patients and restore cognitive functioning so that they are able to participate in the treatment process.

Subacute Treatment

Patients are more likely to be successful if they agree to treatment and are motivated to change their behavior. As a result, motivational interviewing interventions may be useful for helping patients to recognize the need for treatment and to increase their willingness to enter and participate in a treatment program.

Long-term Treatment

The management of an eating disorder typically involves a multidisciplinary team and includes psychosocial, behavioral, and pharmacologic interventions. Psychotherapy is a key component and may include both individual and family sessions. Treatment may be administered in outpatient, partial hospitalization, residential, or inpatient settings.

BIOLOGICAL MANAGEMENT

Acute Biological Management of Anorexia Nervosa

Medically or psychiatrically unstable patients require inpatient care. Individuals with comorbid SUDs may also be referred for more intensive treatment. The medical management of AN begins with a comprehensive medical and neurologic evaluation and treatment of medical comorbidities; safely rehydrating and refeeding are key to early medical intervention. Although weight gain is a goal, it is important that electrolyte abnormalities, cardiac arrhythmias, or other disease processes do not kill the patient or compromise the patient's ability to be treated or recover.

Subacute Biological Management of Anorexia Nervosa

In cases of comorbid AN and SUDs, an integrative treatment targeting both disorders is recommended. SUD treatment may take priority unless the patient is at immediate medical risk due to malnutrition. Weight gain should be implemented gradually (eg, 0.5 to 1 lb per week). Nutritional counseling by a registered dietitian is an integral part of treatment for AN, and clinicians should establish referral sources. Referral to a mental health professional who specializes in eating disorders may also be beneficial.

Long-term Biological Management of Anorexia Nervosa

The process of gaining weight is often very stressful for patients with AN, and clinicians should consider closer monitoring during the weight restoration period to assess for signs of relapse to substance use. Although no pharmacologic treatments have proven effective in the treatment of the primary symptoms of AN, selective serotonin reuptake inhibitors (SSRIs) may help to decrease associated symptoms such as depression, obsessive–compulsive symptoms, and lack of interoceptive awareness. Off-label medications to promote weight gain may be judiciously used in order to avoid overwhelming the patient. Use of a multivitamin and a calcium supplement are recommended. Oral contraceptives or hormone replacement therapy may be prescribed to help regulate the menstrual cycle, mitigate the effects of hypoestrogenemia, and minimize bone loss. Benzodiazepines are not indicated for the treatment of any eating disorder and should be avoided if possible, especially when an SUD is co-occurring.

Acute Biological Management of Bulimia Nervosa

Management of medical complications associated with BN may be necessary. For example, estrogen replacement may be indicated to treat hypothalamic hypogonadism. Physicians should monitor patients with BN to assess for fluid and electrolyte abnormalities, cardiac arrhythmias, gastrointestinal symptoms, and reproductive problems. Patients with BN with comorbid SUDs are more likely to have medical complications and should be evaluated accordingly.

Subacute Biological Management of Bulimia Nervosa

Integrative, concurrent treatment is recommended for patients with comorbid BN and SUDs. If concurrent treatment is not available, treatment of the SUD should take priority due to the relatively higher mortality risk in SUDs. Biologic management of BN generally involves medication with SSRIs; in particular, fluoxetine (US Food and Drug Administration [FDA] approved; target dose 60 mg per day) has established efficacy in reducing the core symptoms of BN. Other medications with demonstrated off-label efficacy include desipramine (up to 300 mg per day), imipramine (up to 300 mg per day), and topiramate (up to 400 mg per day).

Long-term Biological Management of Bulimia Nervosa

It is recommended that any pharmacotherapy be combined with cognitive–behavioral therapy (CBT). Pharmacotherapy for comorbid psychiatric conditions should also be considered. Dental examinations are recommended for patients with BN who engage in self-induced vomiting as well as those with the binge eating/purging subtype of AN.

Biological Management of Binge Eating Disorder

Lisdexamfetamine dimesylate became the first FDA-approved medication for the treatment of BED in adults, and there are several options for off-label medication management. Several SSRIs (eg, sertraline, 50 to 200 mg per day; fluvoxamine, 50 to 300 mg per day; fluoxetine, 20 to 80 mg per day; citalopram, 20 to 40 mg per day) and other medications, including topiramate (50 to 400 mg per day), have demonstrated efficacy. Medical management may be necessary to prevent or treat associated conditions (eg, hypertension, type II diabetes, hypercholesterolemia, hyperlipidemia).

Acute Biological Management of Obesity

Biological management of obesity begins with changes in diet and increased exercise, followed by medication management. If more conservative measures fail, Roux-en-Y gastric bypass surgery or lap band surgery may be performed. These surgeries result in sustained weight loss with decreased prevalence of obesity-related health problems (eg, type II diabetes) but do pose considerable risk, including risk of developing postoperative SUDs. Other FDA-approved options include the Maestro Rechargeable System, the ReShape integrated gastric balloon system, the ORBERA intragastric balloon system, and the AspireAssist device.

Subacute Biological Management of Obesity

Two FDA-approved obesity medications—phentermine and diethylpropion—are appetite suppressants for short-term use only. A third option is orlistat, a fat-absorption inhibitor, which causes gastrointestinal distress upon consumption of a high-fat meal. Four other medications were recently approved. The first, a naltrexone hydrochloride and bupropion hydrochloride extended-release tablet, combines the FDA-approved medications bupropion SR and naltrexone SR, which have each demonstrated effectiveness at promoting weight loss. Next, lorcaserin is a selective serotonin receptor agonist that is believed to suppress appetite signals in order to promote weight loss. Third, liraglutide, which is FDA approved for the treatment of both obesity and type II diabetes, is a glucagon-like peptide-1 receptor agonist that requires close medical monitoring. The final, newly approved medication combines the drugs phentermine (an appetite suppressant) and topiramate XR (an anticonvulsant with weight loss side effects) as a treatment for obesity, but the FDA recommends monitoring patients for cardiovascular risk.

Long-term Biological Management of Obesity

Lifestyle changes, including improved diet and increased exercise, are recommended for long-term management of obesity in all patients who are obese, including those who are prescribed antiobesity medication or who undergo bariatric surgery.

PSYCHOLOGICAL MANAGEMENT
Acute Psychological Management

For patients with AN, both family therapy and individual therapy have demonstrated efficacy, although family therapy may be particularly beneficial for younger patients. CBT has consistently been shown to reduce the risk for relapse and improve outcomes for patients with AN. CBT is currently recommended as a first-line treatment for BN and can be administered either individually or in a group setting. Among patients with BED without comorbid SUDs, psychotherapy appears to be most successful when administered individually or in group CBT, although interpersonal psychotherapy has also demonstrated efficacy.

Subacute Psychological Management

Social support can be beneficial to individuals as they undergo treatment and recovery. As in SUD treatment, group therapy is generally a useful component of treatment. However, for some individuals involuntarily admitted to treatment (particularly those with AN), group therapy may be contraindicated.

Long-term Psychological Management

Among motivated individuals, particularly those who have participated successfully in Alcoholics Anonymous or Narcotics Anonymous, referral to a 12-step program for eating disorders may be beneficial. Such programs include Eating Disorders Anonymous and Overeaters Anonymous.

RECOVERY ISSUES
Co-Occurring Substance Use Disorders

Co-occurrence of SUDs and eating disorders may negatively affect treatment prognosis, and disordered eating behaviors may serve as maladaptive coping mechanisms for patients with SUDs. When an SUD co-occurs with AN, it is generally preferred that treatment occur in a residential setting where both issues can be addressed. Recovery rates for AN with co-occurring SUDs, especially involving alcohol, are generally poor. Suffering from these conditions in combination is a strong predictor of fatal outcome. Although studies have shown that patients with BN plus a co-occurring SUD have treatment outcomes similar to those without an SUD, patients with an SUD with binge eating symptoms have worse outcomes than those without binge eating. Presence of a co-occurring SUD appears to have less impact on treatment outcomes for patients with BED.

General Recovery Rates

Research has demonstrated recovery rates for eating disorders to be approximately between 40% and 94%, with better recovery rates and outcomes for BN than AN. BN is rarely fatal, whereas the mortality rate for those with AN is about 10%. As is seen among individuals recovering from SUDs, the vacillation between dieting (ie, "abstinence") and overeating (ie, "active use") is common among individuals struggling with obesity or BED.

Disordered Eating After Substance Use Disorder Treatment

After treatment for an SUD, some individuals may compensate for the lack of chemical reinforcement by overeating. The presence of an eating disorder is associated with an increased risk of relapse to substance use. Clinicians should be vigilant to symptoms of overeating or disordered eating among patients with SUDs and should provide all patients with preventive counseling and referral to a registered dietitian if indicated.

KEY POINTS

1. Eating disorders are serious, potentially life-threatening conditions that require timely detection and intervention. All patient treated for SUDs should be screened for disorders of eating.
2. Eating disorders and substance use disorders share common features, frequently occur together, and complicate the treatment of the other.
3. Treatments for eating disorders and substance use disorders are complementary, and the skills learned in the management of one can often be applied to the other.

REVIEW QUESTIONS

1. Which of the following symptoms clusters characterizes bulimia nervosa?
   A. Extremely low body weight with food restriction
   B. Average or above-average body weight with binge eating
   C. Extremely low body weight with binge eating and purging
   D. Average or above-average body weight with binge eating and purging

2. Which of the eating disorders has the highest mortality rate?
   A. Anorexia nervosa
   B. Bulimia nervosa
   C. Binge eating disorder
   D. Obesity

3. What is the recommended psychotherapy for eating disorders?
   A. Interpersonal therapy
   B. Cognitive–behavioral therapy
   C. Psychoanalysis
   D. Humanistic counseling

ANSWERS

1. **D.** Answer A describes anorexia nervosa, restricting subtype; answer B describes binge eating disorder; and answer C describes anorexia nervosa, binge eating/purging subtype.

2. **A.** The mortality rate for anorexia nervosa is approximately 10%, with high rates of completed suicide and fatality from medical complications of malnutrition.

3. **B.** Cognitive–behavioral therapy has demonstrated efficacy in the treatment of anorexia nervosa, bulimia nervosa, and binge eating disorder. Evidence for interpersonal therapy is less robust. There is no good support for the use of psychoanalysis or humanistic counseling in the treatment of eating disorders.

SUGGESTED READINGS

American Psychiatric Association. Treatment of patients with eating disorders, third edition. American Psychiatric Association. *Am J Psychiatry*. 2006;163(7 suppl):4-54.

Cohen LR, Greenfield SF, Gordon S, et al. Survey of eating disorder symptoms among women in treatment for substance abuse. *Am J Addict*. 2010;19(3):245-251.

Franko DL, Dorer DJ, Keel PK, et al. How do eating disorders and alcohol use disorder influence each other? *Int J Eat Disord*. 2005;38(3):200-207.

Pritts SD, Susman J. Diagnosis of eating disorders in primary care. *Am Fam Physician*. 2003;67(2):297-304.

Wilson GT. Eating disorders, obesity and addiction. *Eur Eat Disord Rev*. 2010;18(5):341-351.

SECTION

12

Pain and Addiction

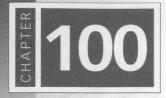
The Pathophysiology of Chronic Pain and Clinical Interfaces With Substance Use Disorder

Summary by David Son

> Based on THE ASAM PRINCIPLES OF ADDICTION MEDICINE, 6th edition chapter by Rollin M. Gallagher, Peggy Compton, and Adrian Popescu

This chapter focuses on the interface between chronic pain and substance use disorders (SUDs), discussing how the biopsychosocial factors are influenced by behavioral neuroscience and clinical practice.

Nociceptive pain involves the transduction of signal from one tissue to another, which is a normal response to actual tissue damage or injury. But neuropathic pain is a manifestation of a disease to the neural tissue, involving persistent activation and perception of pain. This is known as maldynia, which is contributed by the excitation of peripheral neurons and spinal microglial cells followed by structural reorganization of neural networks.

Pathophysiology of maldynia overlaps with the phenomenology of SUDs because neural/glial networks regulating pain perception and behavior interact with emotional regulation and reward systems. Pain, in conjunction with biopsychosocial factors, activates neural and inflammatory mechanisms in the central nervous system (CNS), interacting with neural networks via chemical messengers involved in cognitive–emotional processing and behavioral systems. This accounts for symptomatic and behavioral expression and psychosocial complexity in chronic pain and SUDs.

PAIN ANATOMY AND PHYSIOLOGY

Gate theory explains the phenomenology of pain perception and modulation. The perception of pain is shaped by neurotransmission that is gated by other neurophysiologic inputs rather than by tissue transduction processes. Environmental conditions and one's psychological state can affect the transmission of pain sensation and severity, thus altering the pain experience.

There are three main approaches to target different mechanisms in the pathophysiology of maldynia: (1) reduce the pain stimulus from musculoskeletal diseases by decreasing the transduction of nociceptor signaling via ergonomic modification, (2) block the transmission of the pain signal in the spinal cord via peripheral nerve blocks, or (3) target the CNS response to improve coping in the neuroplastic changes via cognitive–behavioral and psychomotor training. This multimodality treatment improves functional outcomes, not just pain control.

The phenomenology of pain can be characterized as three major stages: brief nociception, persistent/repeated nociception, and neurologic damage. These stages interact in various brain regions and in the body to produce chronic pain.

Stage 1: Nociception

Strong noxious stimulus activates nociceptors. This leads to depolarization of pain afferent fibers, transmitting the signal to the thalamus. Projections from the thalamus to the limbic system activate suffering and the emotional aspect of pain. Repetitive nociceptor stimulation in the periphery can trigger a hyperresponse, increasing pain perception despite no increase in nociceptor input.

Stage 2: Peripheral Sensitization

A noxious stimulus that is very intense and prolonged leads to tissue damage and inflammation, followed by a continuous release of inflammatory mediators, which causes nociceptors to spontaneously discharge and become more sensitive to peripheral stimulation. Eventually, this results in a low threshold for sensitized fibers to fire without noxious stimulus, increasing the pain signal from an innocuous light touch. Also, an adrenergic outflow due to psychological stress can damage the peripheral nerves, resulting in the spontaneous firing of pain fibers. Over time, this results in neuroplastic changes, where dendritic sprouting at the afferent fibers contributes to allodynia.

Stage 3: Central Sensitization

Persistent noxious input enhances dorsal horn neuron responsiveness, which is responsible for secondary hyperalgesia (pain away from the site of initial injury). Stage 3 pain also may involve genetic, cognitive, and emotional factors. Stimulating goal-directed activities and exercise suppress pain, enable functional ability improvement, and reduce central sensitization. This explains the effectiveness of comprehensive rehabilitation programs in treating chronic pain.

PAIN AND EMOTIONS

Emotional states that activate sympathetic arousal (anxiety or anger) can exacerbate both acute and chronic pain. Treating only pain without treating mood disorders increases the chance of treatment failure. SUDs lead to poor pain treatment outcomes because it interferes with the goal-oriented behavior needed for functional restoration.

Common environmental factors exist between depressive and anxiety disorders and chronic pain. The body demonstrates an impaired capacity to regulate depression and pain during stress. The stress of living with chronic pain increases the risk for depression. Major depression is more common in the setting of myofascial pain. Women with fibromyalgia had greater pain elevations during negative mood experiences and traumatic life events. Genetic studies show that fibromyalgia and depression share the same vulnerability of serotonin and norepinephrine transporter gene expression in response to stressful or traumatic life events.

PAIN AND ANXIETY

There is neuroanatomic evidence for an overlap in the processing and perception of pain and anxiety. People with chronic pain and anxiety have heightened brain chemistry interactions in the cortex, cingulate gyrus, and thalamus regions via the common shared neurochemical pathway. The cortex plays an essential role in reacting to fearful and painful stimuli. A greater cortical connection to conscious recognition provides more control over the primitive fight–flight response.

An association between anxiety and pain is also mediated by the amygdala, which regulates the emotional response to pain. The amygdala is influenced by environmental and internal stimuli from the hippocampus. The amygdala then places emotional value in the stimuli and feeds it back to the hippocampus. For this reason, events with high emotional content, such as painful injuries, tend to be remembered in greater detail. Posttraumatic stress disorder, which is comorbid with chronic pain, is associated with consistent reductions in hippocampal volume or blood flow.

Adult hippocampal neurogenesis, which is implicated in learning emotional functions, is disrupted both in negative mood disorders and during persistent pain. Blocking adult hippocampal neurogenesis has been observed to decrease postinjury neuropathic/inflammatory pain behaviors. Furthermore, behavioral and rehabilitative approaches in goal-oriented, motivating, engrossing activities and biofeedback have been observed to reverse hippocampal sensitization and to reduce pain.

PAIN AND SUBSTANCE USE DISORDERS

Because pain and drug rewards share a common neuroanatomic pathways, neurochemical substrates, and gene expression patterns, the physiologic response to addiction has clear effects on pain management. Although opioids bring analgesic properties, SUDs worsen the pain experience by bringing forth malaise, mood states, behavior, and social losses because opioids are imbued with both analgesic and hyperalgesic properties.

SUDs are defined as a chronic, relapsing disorder characterized by a compulsion to seek and take drugs, loss of control over drug intake, and emergence of a negative emotional state when the drug access is prevented.

SUDs represent a break from homeostatic brain regulatory mechanisms that control daily emotional and motivational states, which is known as allostasis (ability to achieve stability through change). SUDs worsen over time and cause dramatic changes in the brain reward and stress systems that potentiate emotional dysregulation and worsening pain experience. Pain is relevant to SUDs in two different allostatic states: tolerance and physical dependence.

Tolerance

Tolerance is defined as a reduction in response to a given dose of drug after repeated use. To maintain the homeostasis in a rewards system, an antireward system is recruited to counteract acute drug effects, which become stronger with each exposure and extinguish more slowly. Over the course of repeated exposure, a counteracting emotional or physiologic response develops, which eventually becomes the predominant feeling state in the absence of the drug.

Physiologic tolerance occurs by the uncoupling of opioid receptor transduction in the nucleus accumbens reward pathways. Neuroreceptors are being rendered as nonfunctional, thus making the drug less effective. Tolerance can take the form of an adaptation where another neurotransmitter circuit becomes activated in an attempt to restore homeostasis.

Physical Dependence

Physical dependence is a consequence of chronic drug use, and an allostatic state occurs where the opposite effect of the drug manifests when the drug is removed. Unopposed by the drug effects, this adaptive change becomes evident as drug withdrawal syndrome, which results in more generalized negative emotional states such as malaise, anxiety, emotional pain, and depression.

GENERAL EFFECTS OF SUBSTANCE USE DISORDERS ON PAIN

SUDs facilitate the experience of pain in multiple ways, including sympathetic arousal and negative mood states. Strong and persistent negative emotional states accompany a withdrawal from many drugs, which is attributed to dopamine depletion in the reward pathway and activation of brain stress systems. Interpersonal conflicts, role adjustments, and social support losses can worsen the experience of pain. Psychiatric illness and sleep disorders, which are characteristics of addiction, can contribute to the experience of chronic pain and decreased efficacy of analgesia. Depression, which commonly co-occurs with SUDs, increases pain perception and impairs function in patients with chronic pain.

ALLOSTATIC STATES OF SUBSTANCE USE DISORDERS AND PAIN

Allostatic states secondary to ongoing drug use can drive aberrant drug-seeking behaviors, which is mediated by increased glutamatergic activity in the mesocorticolimbic dopaminergic pathway projecting to the medial prefrontal cortex. However, chronic exposure to rewarding drugs can inhibit the prefrontal cortical activities and functional decision-making processes. Imprinting of memories associated with the drug reward can exclude other functional activities and allow for long-term vulnerability to relapse.

The development of negative emotional states in SUDs has been linked to a loss of function in the reward systems and the recruitment of an antireward system. Reward deficiency is identified by decreased sensitivity to natural reinforcers and decreased activity of dopaminergic pathways in the amygdala, where the reward function is diminished and persistent negative emotional states predominate.

OPIOID USE DISORDER AND PAIN

Opioid agonist activity at the μ-opioid receptor is central to both opioid addiction and pain systems. Patients chronically exposed to opioids have perturbation in the pain systems. Opioids activate the μ-opioid receptor shared by both drug reward and anesthesia systems to induce interrelated CNS changes in the medulla, cortex, thalamus, spinal cord, and peripheral sensory neurons.

Genetic factors account for tolerance and physiologic dependence. Polymorphisms in the μ-opioid receptor gene result in varying phenotypes for pain sensitivity, opioid analgesic response, and addiction that require different levels of morphine to achieve an analgesic response. Heritable differences in hepatic P450 isoenzyme activity affect both the reward and analgesia systems from opioids. High P450 activity results in less analgesia and reward, putting them at decreased risk for addiction but increased risk for unrelieved pain.

OPIOID-INDUCED HYPERALGESIA

Opioid-induced hyperalgesia (OIH) is defined by increased sensitivity to pain resulting from opioids, heightened external stimuli over time, and spreading of pain to locations beyond the initial pain site. OIH generalizes across nociceptive stimuli (thermal, chemical, electrical), causing a decreased nociceptive threshold. OIH is considered as an opioid withdrawal syndrome, which arises following single or chronic opioid exposure and is variable in duration and intensity depending on opioid, opioid dose, route of administration, and duration of use. Heightened pain perception is observed during abstinence. A hyperalgesic state can persist for up to 5 months in abstinent patients with SUDs, and those with more pain sensitivity also display greater craving.

Mechanisms of Opioid-Induced Hyperalgesia

A common pathway for the development of opioid tolerance that induces hyperalgesia is via activation of ionotropic N-methyl-D-aspartate receptors on dorsal horn spinal cord neurons.

OIH may be the result of activation in descending pain facilitation systems arising from μ-opioid receptors in the medulla, where the opioid increases the pronociceptive peptide cholecystokinin. This results in a spinal hyperalgesic response to nociceptive input. Hyperalgesia has been reversed by an antagonist agent to nociceptive neuropeptide substance P. This suggests that OIH has a neuroinflammatory component because substance P is active in pain of inflammatory origin. Opioids also bind to μ-opioid receptors on the astrocytes of the blood–brain barrier, which activates peripheral immune cells to induce specific central proinflammatory cytokines, resulting in heightened pain sensitivity.

CONCLUSIONS

The pain stimulus involves a dynamic interaction in both the peripheral and central nervous systems. The unique susceptibility of pain to neuromodulation and allostasis portends a significant role for SUDs in altering the pain experience. SUDs affect addiction physiology that processes motivational system encoding reward and antireward/stress. Overlap between chronic pain and addiction exists. This complexity is evident in psychosocial, cognitive, and cultural domains. Chronic use of reinforcing drugs alters the processing of noxious stimuli (stress response, withdrawal phenomena, opioid tolerance). Genetic and epigenetic influences on phenotype expression of pain and reward systems also play a role in the pain experience.

Specifically with opioid addictions, the presence of OIH complicates pain management strategies. Individuals vary in propensity to both addiction and pain responses due to differences in the endogenous opioid system or opioid-induced epigenetic changes that influence homeostatic and allostatic processes.

KEY POINTS

1. The pathophysiology of chronic pain overlaps with the phenomenology of SUDs because neural/glial networks regulating pain perception and behaviors interact with emotional regulation and behavioral systems.
2. Pain and drug rewards share the common neuroanatomic pathway, neurochemical substrates, and gene expression pattern. Therefore, a physiologic response to addiction has clear effects on pain management.
3. SUDs cause dramatic changes in the brain reward and stress systems that potentiate treatment resistance, which results in emotional dysregulation and a worsening pain experience.
4. There is a correlation between hypersensitive negative emotional states and OIH.
5. Opioid-agonist activity at the μ-opioid receptor is central to both opioid addiction and pain systems, and genetic factors involved in polymorphisms of the μ-opioid receptor account for opioid tolerance and physiologic dependence.

REVIEW QUESTIONS

1. Which theory provides the physiologic basis for pain perception and modulation phenomena, where small nerve fibers enter the dorsal horn of the spinal cord and transmit impulses to inhibit or allow stimulation from the spinal cord up to the brain?
   A. Sensory interaction theory (Noordenbos)
   B. Gate theory (Melzack and Wall)
   C. Central summation theory (Livingstone)
   D. Specificity theory (von Frey)
   E. Intensive theory (Erb)

2. Which physiologic mechanism in the brain is disrupted both in negative mood disorders and in persistent pain?
   A. Axon arborization
   B. Amygdala neurogenesis
   C. Neuronal synaptogenesis
   D. Hippocampal neurogenesis
   E. Hypothalamic–pituitary–adrenal axis

3. Which of the following is *true* regarding OIH?
   A. It usually resolves 1 week after opioid abstinence.
   B. It usually resolves 1 month after opioid abstinence.
   C. It usually resolves 1 year after opioid abstinence.
   D. It can persist up to 5 months after opioid abstinence.
   E. None of the above.

ANSWERS

1. **B**
2. **D**
3. **D**

SUGGESTED READINGS

Bourne S, Machado AG, Nagel SJ. Basic anatomy and physiology of pain pathways. *Neurosurg Clin N Am.* 2014;25(4):629-638.

Chou R, Fanciullo GJ, Fine PG, et al. Clinical guidelines for the use of chronic opioid therapy in chronic noncancer pain. *J Pain.* 2009;10(2):113-130.e22.

Edwards R. Clinical assessment tools. In: Mao J, ed. *Opioid-Induced Hyperalgesia.* Boca Raton, FL: CRC Press, 2009:38-60.

Smith HS. Role of opioid rotation and tapering in managing opioid-induced hyperalgesia. In: Mao J, ed. *Opioid-Induced Hyperalgesia.* Boca Raton, FL: CRC Press, 2009: 134-163.

Volkow ND, McLellan AT. Opioid abuse in chronic pain – misconceptions and mitigation strategies. *N Engl J Med.* 2016;374(13):1253-1263.

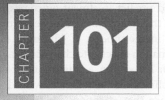

101

Psychological Issues in the Management of Pain

Summary by Martin D. Cheatle

Based on THE ASAM PRINCIPLES OF ADDICTION MEDICINE, 6th edition chapter by Martin D. Cheatle

Chronic pain remains a significant healthcare problem affecting approximately 30% of the American population, and this number continues to burgeon. The increasing prevalence of chronic pain not only causes individual suffering and disability but also affects the patient's family and society as well. The 2011 report by the National Academy of Medicine (formerly the Institute of Medicine), titled "Relieving Pain in America: A Blueprint for Transforming Prevention, Care, Education, and Research," emphasized that the chronic pain experience is complicated and multifaceted, stating "we believe pain arises in the nervous system but represents a complex and evolving interplay of biological, behavioral, environmental, and societal factors." Patients with chronic pain tend to be complex, and commonly, these patients have multiple medical and psychiatric comorbidities including mood and anxiety disorders, posttraumatic stress disorder, and substance use disorders (SUDs). When discussing psychological issues in pain management, there is a misconception that the typical patient is psychologically prone to develop chronic pain and to have poor coping skills that lead to disability. To the contrary, the majority of individuals that live with chronic pain develop coping mechanisms that support them in remaining functional and productive and maintaining a good quality of life. Pain and emotional states can be bidirectional, however, with pain exacerbating mood and anxiety and vice versa.

MIND–BODY CONNECTION

Cartesian dualism, mostly associated with the philosophy of René Descartes, suggested that the mind (mental function) and the body are distinct, separate entities, and therefore, it is feasible that one can exist without the other. Although there is robust literature on the effect of the mind–body connection in maintaining health or contributing to the development of illnesses, in many ways, the current medical methodology, including pain management, still practices this dualistic approach. There are many examples of the strong influence of an individual's emotional state, social milieu, and attitudes on physical symptoms and disability. The tendency to separate the mind from the body, the organic from the psychological, does not allow the clinician to fully understand the person's pain experience and biases the diagnosis and treatment of the whole person, leading to poorer outcomes. In spite of the incredible advances in diagnostic imaging, pharmacotherapy, pharmacogenetics, and refinement in surgical interventions, the number of individuals suffering and becoming disabled from chronic pain grows each year. This is the result, in part, of our failure to adequately address the psychological aspects of chronic nonmalignant pain (CNMP) and the focus of our healthcare system on the organic pathology rather than the person. This is in the face of compelling evidence that psychosocial variables predict onset, chronicity, and outcomes in back pain (one of the most prevalent pain conditions) more than somatic variables. These influences frequently supersede the extent of tissue damage in determining the experience of the person who has pain.

This chapter briefly reviews key psychological factors that can significantly affect an individual's pain experience and pain-related functional impairment and outline treatments that have been demonstrated to be efficacious in improving functionality and mood in this patient population.

PSYCHOLOGICAL MODULATION OF PAIN

Historically, clinicians have been trained in the biomedical approach to healthcare, which can erroneously lead clinicians either to doubt the reality of the symptoms or to assume that they were caused psychologically if there is no identified organic pathology. Although it has been well documented that beliefs, fears, expectations, and affects can both exacerbate and reduce the pain experience, this should not be taken as evidence that psychological processes are the root cause of the pain. Pain is primarily a function of the nervous system and, especially in the case of protracted and/or neuropathic pain, may bear little relation to the intensity of peripheral stimulation. The classical single pathway theory of pain as a signal transmitted from the receptor to the cortex is an oversimplification; it does not incorporate processes such as sensitization, descending inhibition and facilitation of pain, and neuroplastic changes.

A primary example of this misinterpretation is the condition of fibromyalgia. Patients with fibromyalgia present with a complaint of widespread musculoskeletal pain with diffuse hyperalgesia and/or allodynia with no apparent evidence of initiating trauma or tissue damage and patients with fibromyalgia tend to also experience other central nervous system (CNS)-mediated symptoms such as sleep disturbance, fatigue, memory problems, and mood disturbance. Fibromyalgia was initially considered a psychiatric or somatic disorder due to the paucity of an identifiable organic pathology and the diffuse nature of the pain complaints and related symptoms. Findings from functional neuroimaging studies have supported the theory that fibromyalgia is related to a problem with augmented pain or sensory processing in the CNS and imbalances in levels of neurotransmitters that affect pain and sensory transmission.

Animal studies have also demonstrated genetic vulnerability to developing neuropathic pain, and human studies have identified genetic variations that modify pain perception or opioid responsivity.

This emerging literature on the variability of pain perception and the predisposition to developing painful conditions having a strong genetic component should obviate the tendency of clinicians to attribute unexplained pain solely to psychological processes. However, there are a number of psychological factors that can alter an individual's pain experience. These factors include emotional distress, the ability to attend to or distract from a stimulus, expectations, kinesiophobia/fear avoidance, and cognitions and coping skills.

■ *Emotional Distress:* It is very common for patients with CNMP to experience concomitant mood and anxiety symptoms that often do not meet the criteria for a psychiatric diagnosis but can nonetheless exacerbate pain and contribute to the individual's suffering. Research has demonstrated that emotional states such as depression and anxiety can influence pain perception acutely, predict

its persistence, and predict treatment outcomes. There are also data that depression and anxiety are important factors in the process of "chronification," the transformation of acute to chronic pain.

■ *Attention and Pain Perception:* A number of experimental and clinical studies have revealed compelling evidence that attention can significantly alter pain perception. When an individual with either acute experimental pain or chronic pain is distracted from their pain by engaging in a competing cognitive task, pain is perceived as less intense. Neuroimaging studies have begun to elucidate the underlying neurobiologic mechanisms of these effects related to the influence of descending inhibitory and facilitatory pathways regulated by a number of brain regions.

■ *Expectations:* Although not often assessed, patient expectations can be important in influencing treatment outcomes and pain perception. Several studies have suggested that patients' expectations of recovery predicted their return to work and pain-related disability and that patients' expectations can influence their response to specific interventions. It is always critical to assess and reassess patient expectations regarding the treatment itself and potential outcomes.

■ *Kinesiophobia and Fear Avoidance:* A subgroup of patients will heal from an initial trauma but go on to develop chronic pain and related disabilities in part due to certain psychological processes. One that is common in patients with CNMP is kinesiophobia, defined as an irrational fear that movement or activity will lead to reinjury or heightened pain. If a patient interprets their pain as nonthreatening (ie, temporary), they tend to resume usual and therapeutic physical activities after the initial recovery from an injury. On the other hand, if a patient misinterprets their pain as a sign of a serious injury or pathologic state that they have little control over, this leads to catastrophic fear of pain or further injury, which can be generalized to fear of any physical activity. This fear-avoidance belief creates a vicious cycle of inactivity, which causes physical deconditioning, leading to more pain and disability.

■ *Cognitions and Coping:* The role of cognition in supporting healthy moods and attitudes and contributing to psychiatric conditions has been recognized for over three decades and has been extended to the area of chronic pain. The underlying premise of cognitive theories is that individuals react to their interpretation and understanding of events, rather than to the events themselves. In the patient with depression, the view of the world is clouded by irrational, maladaptive thoughts that perpetuate and deepen the depression. Maladaptive cognitions have the quality of being automatic and habitual so that they are rarely examined for validity. The patient accepts these distorted thoughts as real, even when clearly illogical to others. These theories on cognition form the basis for the well-validated treatment approach of cognitive–behavioral therapy (CBT), which is discussed later in the chapter.

PSYCHOLOGICAL PROCESSES AND PAIN

A number of psychological processes have been identified as potential mediators between pain and adaptive/maladaptive behavior. These include catastrophizing and helplessness versus self-efficacy.

- *Catastrophizing:* Catastrophizing is a well-studied cognitive factor that is associated with poor pain tolerance and coping, sleep disturbance, increased risk of opioid abuse, and suicidal ideation in patients with CNMP. Catastrophizing can be conceptualized as a negative cognitive–affective response to pain. Negative thoughts that reduce pain tolerance include those emphasizing the aversiveness of the situation, the inadequacy of the person to bear it, or the physical harm that could occur.
- *Helplessness Versus Self-Efficacy:* Cognitive influences include not only beliefs regarding pain but also those regarding the person experiencing it and their beliefs about their ability to control the pain. The model of learned helplessness in depression suggests that those who feel unable to control events in their lives will respond passively to them, become depressed, and experience increased disability and pain. Conversely, belief in self-efficacy is a major determinant of successful coping and predicts better functioning in fibromyalgia and arthritis. These beliefs are favorably associated not only with pain and functioning but also with treatment outcomes.

Understanding the psychological modulation and processes of pain provide valuable information to develop a comprehensive approach to assessing and treating patients with CNMP.

ASSESSING PSYCHOLOGICAL AND SUBSTANCE USE DISORDERS

Given the high prevalence of mood disturbance and anxiety in patients with CNMP and the effect of these psychological processes on the pain experience, it is important that every patient seen for chronic pain undergo at least a brief screening for the presence of anxiety and depression. There are a number of validated and reliable mental health screening tools that vary in length. In the pain population, two often recommended assessment tools are the Beck Depression Inventory and the Profile of Mood States. The Beck Depression Inventory is a 21-question self-report measure of depression severity over the past week. The Profile of Mood States has a full-length version (65 items) and a short-length version (35 questions), both of which are composed of seven scales. Three of these scales are very pertinent to the pain population (anger/hostility, depression/dejection, and tension/anxiety). In busy practices, the brief Patient Health Questionnaire-4, which is a four-item screening tool for depression and anxiety, can be used.

Assessing for SUDs in patients with CNMP can be challenging, especially if patients are legitimately prescribed medications that can have euphoric effects. Every patient with CNMP should be initially screened for opioid misuse or the presence of an SUD and, if prescribed opioids, periodically monitored long term for the development of aberrant drug-related behaviors. Examples of opioid screening tools and general substance abuse screening assessments are outlined in Table 101-1.

BIOPSYCHOSOCIAL APPROACH TO THE MANAGEMENT OF PAIN

A biopsychosocial program typically includes a graded exercise program, CBT, and rational pharmacotherapy.

Exercise

Exercise and physical therapy have been shown to *improve pain and functioning in those with CNMP.* An effective physical therapy program for patients with CNMP pain should involve (1) acquiring first aid techniques for pain relief at home for patients to self-manage pain flares (eg, use of transcutaneous electrical nerve stimulation, heat/cold packs, positioning), which can engender a sense of empowerment over their pain and independence, and (2) establishing a well-balanced, independent exercise program in a very graded fashion because these patients typically have had poor experiences with traditional physical therapy and tend to catastrophize. Weekly achievable goals should be established that will not lead to an increase in pain.

Cognitive–Behavioral Therapy for Chronic Nonmalignant Pain

Patients with CNMP often present with concomitant mood and anxiety disorders and maladaptive

TABLE 101-1 Examples of Opioid Misuse Risk and Substance Use Disorder Screening Tools

Screening Tool	Items	Administered by
Patients Considered for Long-Term Opioid Therapy		
Opioid Risk Tool (ORT)	5	Patient
Screener and Opioid Assessment for Patients With Pain (SOAPP)	24, 14, and 5	Patient
Diagnosis, Intractability, Risk, and Efficacy (DIRE) score	7	Clinician
Characterize Misuse Once Opioid Treatments Begins		
Pain Medication Questionnaire (PMQ)	26	Patient
Current Opioid Misuse Measure (COMM)	17	Patient
Prescription Drug Use Questionnaire (PDUQ)	40	Clinician
Not Specific to Pain Populations		
Cut Down, Annoyed, Guilty, Eye-Opener Tool, Adapted to Include Drugs (CAGE-AID)	4	Clinician
Relax, Alone, Friends, Family, Trouble (RAFFT) test	5	Patient
Drug Abuse Screening Test (DAST)	28	Patient
Screening, Brief Intervention, and Referral to Treatment (SBIRT)	Varies	Clinician
Alcohol Use Disorders Identification Test–Concise (AUDIT-C)	3	Patient

behaviors and thought processes that contribute to suffering. Patients with CNMP tend to engage in maladaptive thinking (catastrophizing) and maladaptive behavior (kinesiophobia), both of which contribute to depression, low self-efficacy, and disability. The process of CBT typically includes specific skill acquisition, such as mindfulness-based stress reduction, assertiveness training, and cognitive restructuring, followed by skill consolidation, rehearsal, and relapse training. The process of cognitive restructuring consists of identifying and modifying negative and/or irrational thought patterns and substituting more rational and functional cognitions to aid the patient in reframing and reconceptualizing his or her own personal view of pain, thus promoting being more proactive rather than passive and encouraging a sense of competence and self-efficacy. CBT has been found to be cost-effective and clinically effective at improving mood and functioning in a variety of chronic pain disorders.

SUMMARY

Compelling evidence demonstrates that dividing the mind from the body and treating them separately is not only ineffective at managing complex pain conditions but also does not allow for advancing our understanding of this complex interaction and developing novel interventions.

Psychological traumas can produce lasting alterations in the function and even the structure of the CNS. At the same time, studies have shown that numerous painful symptoms thought to be "psychogenic" or "somatic" have their explanation in central sensitization and neuroplasticity. A biopsychosocial-based, interdisciplinary pain care approach that includes rational pharmacotherapy; restorative, activating physical therapy; and psychological interventions has been demonstrated to significantly improve functional status and psychological well-being, reduce pain severity and opioid use, and decrease healthcare utilization. Access to these types of programs are limited, and we need further healthcare economics research to support improved access to interdisciplinary pain care, behavioral health, and SUD treatment. Other future directions include developing and testing novel delivery systems for psychological interventions for pain and additional research on the biological substrates of the mind–body interaction in pain.

KEY POINTS

1. Pain, like substance use disorders, should be considered a disease of the brain that can significantly affect not only the individual but also his or her family and society.
2. Patients with refractory pain often present with multiple psychiatric and medical comorbidities

and should be screened for depression, anxiety, and risk of substance misuse.

3. A biopsychosocial, interdisciplinary pain care model is the most efficacious treatment approach for managing complex pain disorders.

REVIEW QUESTIONS

1. A patient presents to the clinic and says, "This pain will eventually kill me" and "I may become paralyzed." Which of the following are these statements an example of?
   A. Helplessness
   B. Kinesiophobia
   C. Catastrophizing
   D. Emotional stress

2. Which of the following are typically included in cognitive–behavioral therapy?
   A. Cognitive restructuring
   B. Exercise
   C. Assertiveness training
   D. Relaxation training
   E. All of the above.
   F. A, C, and D.
   G. A, B, and D.

ANSWERS

1. **C.** Catastrophizing is a negative cognitive–affective response to pain. Negative thoughts that reduce pain tolerance include those emphasizing the aversiveness of the situation, the inadequacy of the person to bear it, or the physical harm that could occur.

2. **F.** Although exercise is a key component of a comprehensive pain management program, it is not part of a standard CBT approach.

SUGGESTED READINGS

Cheatle MD. Biopsychosocial approach to assessing and managing patients with chronic pain. *Med Clin North Am.* 2016;100(1):43-53.

Covington EC. Psychogenic pain: what it means, why it doesn't exist, and how to diagnose it. *Pain Med.* 2000;1(4):287-294.

Institute of Medicine. *Relieving Pain in America: A Blueprint for Transforming Prevention, Care, Education, and Research: A Call for Public Action.* Washington, DC: National Academies Press, 2011.

Rome HP Jr, Rome JD. Limbically augmented pain syndrome (LAPS): kindling, corticolimbic sensitization, and the convergence of affective and sensory symptoms in chronic pain disorders. *Pain Med.* 2000;1(1):7-23.

Woolf CJ. Central sensitization: implications for the diagnosis and treatment of pain. *Pain.* 2011;152(3 suppl):S2-S15.

102

Rehabilitation Approaches to Pain Management

Summary by Abigail J. Herron

Based on THE ASAM PRINCIPLES OF ADDICTION MEDICINE, 6th edition chapter by Steven P. Stanos and Randy L. Calisoff

Rehabilitation may be described as a "return to ability . . . the return to the fullest physical, mental, social, vocational, and economic usefulness that is possible for the individual." The focus is placed more on one's abilities rather than one's disabilities.

A rehabilitation-based approach focuses on a staged approach to addressing the range of acute to chronic pain conditions. Chronic pain and substance use disorders (SUDs) are highly prevalent conditions with potentially negative synergy between them. Although causative and developmental factors of SUDs and chronic pain may negatively impact each other, successful rehabilitation efforts for both conditions should focus on active interventions (eg, physical therapy [PT], exercise, occupational therapy [OT]), passive interventions (eg, heat and cold modalities, stretching, massage), and behavioral health interventions.

A number of chronic and acute pain conditions can benefit from a wide range of nonpharmacologic interventions. A rehabilitation-based approach focuses on a staged approach to addressing the range of acute to chronic pain conditions. A focused history and physical exam can help to identify areas of impairment and guide subsequent treatment interventions and the development of a comprehensive rehabilitation plan. More chronic presentations may need psychological and vocational interventions as well. In carefully selected patients, some interventional procedures (eg, epidural injections for acute radicular pain or trigger point injections for myofascial pain complaints) may provide additional tools for the pain clinician but is not the focus of this chapter.

A conceptual model based on disease management approaches similar to those for diabetes, heart disease, and asthma can be applied to the treatment of many chronic pain conditions. In this model, moving from parallel practice to integrative treatment includes moving from a biomedical, disease-focused approach to a collaborative integrative team-based treatment model. Moving across the continuum, the philosophy emphasizes the whole person and flexible roles among clinicians with little reliance on hierarchy. Parallel practice, for example, could involve an emergency team working efficiently on a patient presenting with cardiac pain. Individual roles are specifically defined, and extensive communication is not necessary. Collaborative models may involve a physician referring a patient to a different specialist for consultation. Coordinated models may include the additional use of a case manager to help coordinate delivery and communication of care. A "multidisciplinary" approach includes the use of one or a number of allied health disciplines, such as PT or OT directed by a senior provider. In a multidisciplinary care, clinicians need not be in the same facility, and communication may vary, as may the transfer of records and reports. As the presenting complaint becomes more chronic, a more collaborative approach involving the coordination of multiple caregivers defines an "interdisciplinary approach."

In an interdisciplinary model, care is usually provided at one facility, where patients participate in a number of therapies and work with multiple disciplines and healthcare providers. Treatments may include PT and OT, psychotherapy (eg, cognitive–behavioral therapy) and relaxation training, aerobic conditioning, education, vocational rehabilitation, medical management, and pain education. Outcomes from interdisciplinary treatment programs have demonstrated not only improvement in pain and psychophysical functioning but also significant weaning or elimination of opioids. Treatments focus on helping the patient acquire pain management skills, decrease pain, improve psychosocial functioning, and return to leisure and vocational function.

ACTIVE PHYSICAL THERAPY

PT includes the application of modalities, physical agents, therapeutic exercise, functional training in home and work activities, and manual therapy.

PT treatment primarily includes 1-hour sessions that can include patient education, instruction in exercises and stretches, core strengthening, gait training, manual therapy, and pool or aquatic therapy, with progression of activities over several therapy visits. Patients are given short- and long-term therapy goals and instruction in exercises and stretches.

The goal of any referral to a physical therapist is to establish a patient in an independent therapeutic exercise program. The basic principles of a therapeutic exercise prescription include:

- a functional evaluation and assessment of dysfunction and impairments,
- an evaluation and management of motor control (ie, strength and balance),
- the identification and management of bony and joint kinematic limitations (ie, joint contracture, soft tissue restrictions), and
- assessments of movement patterns followed by strategies for improvement or facilitation of synergistic movement patterns.

Physical Therapy Approaches to Stretching

The physical therapist can assess joint ranges of motion, soft tissue changes, and strength deficits as they relate to a functional unit of the body. Various stretching techniques can be used and guided by the therapist and, over time, performed individually by the patient.

Basic types of stretching include ballistic, passive, static, and neuromuscular facilitation. Ballistic stretching uses repetitive, rapid application of force in a jerking or bouncing manner in which momentum helps to carry the body part through a range of motion until muscles are stretched to their physiologic maximums. Static stretching techniques involve stretching an antagonist muscle passively by putting the segment in a maximal position of stretch and holding for 10 to 60 seconds, often incorporating the patient's own body weight, the assistance of a therapist, or stretching equipment.

More commonly used stretching for chronic pain includes static stretching and proprioceptive neuromuscular facilitation. Proprioceptive neuromuscular facilitation techniques can be also useful for improving flexibility. Myofascial release is a PT or OT technique that requires specific training and

can accomplish the stretching of deeper fascia and connective tissue.

A growing area of therapy, called "neurodynamic therapy," includes stretching the perineural tissues commonly used in cervical and lumbar radicular pain or peripheral nerve compression disorders.

Aquatic Therapy

Numerous studies have found aquatic therapy to be beneficial in a variety of acute and chronic pain conditions and can help to decrease peripheral edema, improve range of motion and strength, increase balance, and improve cardiovascular conditioning.

Lumbar and Cervical Stabilization

Stabilization exercises focus on strengthening weak and inhibited muscles and strengthening or "stabilizing" muscles that surround the spine, thereby improving muscular support. Assessing and improving the "core" is the cornerstone of any stabilization program for the lumbar spine, and similar principles can be applied to cervical and joint-related pain conditions. The *core* is defined as the lumbo–pelvic–hip complex, which is thought to include over 29 muscles attaching in this region of the body. A core strengthening therapy program could include strengthening exercises on an exercise ball or without specific equipment. The goals of core training include improving and increasing dynamic postural control, establishing optimal muscular balance and joint movement around the affected region, and maximizing functional strength and endurance.

Mechanical Diagnosis and Therapy (McKenzie Therapy)

Mechanical diagnosis and therapy, commonly referred to as McKenzie therapy, is a specialized approach in which specially trained therapists instruct patients through a number of active positions of motion in the lumbar spine and determine whether patients are able to decrease or change the pain referral pattern from the extremities to more "centralized" low back or neck pain. This is based on the theory that an intact nucleus pulposus (cervical or lumbar), responsible for generating referred pain to a limb, will produce different symptoms in certain positions with repeated standardized end-range test movements.

OCCUPATIONAL THERAPY

OT consists of assessments and training of patients in areas related to functional activities, which may include specific activities of daily living, posture, ergonomics, and body mechanics.

Posture and Body Mechanics

Many chronic musculoskeletal pain conditions of the cervical and lumbar spine may be aggravated by poor posture. A basic assessment of the patient's sitting and standing posture and retraining may be a focus of individual OT sessions and can be applied at home and work. Proper standing and sitting posture will help reduce stress and strain over bony and soft tissue structures. Ergonomics is the science of designing equipment with the aim of increasing productivity and reducing fatigue and discomfort. This is an additional area in which OT can be of value to a patient with chronic pain.

PSYCHOLOGICAL INTERVENTIONS AS PART OF A PAIN REHABILITATION PLAN

In addition to PT and OT, pain rehabilitation relies heavily on psychological interventions. The reader is referred to Chapter 101 on psychological therapies for pain.

MODALITIES USED IN ACUTE AND CHRONIC PAIN CONDITIONS

Passive modalities commonly used for acute musculoskeletal and soft tissue injuries include heat and cold therapies, ultrasound, electrical stimulation such as transcutaneous electrical stimulation and iontophoresis, and soft tissue massage.

Heat therapy applied to soft tissues produces an elevated temperature and an increase in blood flow to the affected region. With increased blood flow, hydrostatic pressure and increased capillary permeability lead to an increase in inflammatory mediators in the region, serving an important role in early healing. Ultrasound provides the deepest heat of all of the heat therapy modalities used. General indications for cold therapy include acute musculoskeletal trauma, pain, muscular spasm, and spasticity. Precautions and contraindications for cold therapy include ischemia, cold intolerance, Raynaud phenomenon, and skin sensitivity. Transcutaneous electrical stimulation is a form of electrotherapy that works by applying a low-voltage electrical pulse to the nervous system via surface electrodes placed onto the skin in the affected area. Iontophoresis uses transcutaneous electrical stimulation therapy and is commonly used for the treatment of bursitis or plantar fasciitis to drive topical medications into the affected tissues. Massage therapy involves pressure and

stretching provided in a rhythmic fashion to affected regions for approximately 5 to 15 minutes. The physiologic effects include reflex vasodilation with improvement in circulation, assistance in venous blood return from the periphery to the central nervous system, increased lymphatic drainage, decreased muscular tightness, and softening of adhesions and/or scars.

CONCLUSION

The patient with a prior or current SUD and co-occurring chronic pain can benefit from a wide array of active therapeutic interventions including PT and OT, passive treatments for acute and some chronic pain conditions, and participation in more comprehensive multi- and interdisciplinary treatment programs. The focus of care, as in SUD-related treatment, should encompass a biopsychosocial multimodal approach. Psychological interventions, including behavioral, cognitive–behavioral therapy, mindfulness training, and acceptance- and commitment-based therapies, may be integrated into rehabilitation-based programs.

KEY POINTS

1. Patients with a substance use disorder and co-morbid chronic pain can benefit from a wide array of active therapeutic interventions, including physical and occupational therapies.
2. The focus of care, as in substance abuse treatment, should encompass a biopsychosocial multimodal approach.
3. In some patients, the use of passive modalities may be used as an additional tool for treating acute musculoskeletal and soft tissue disorders or for ongoing maintenance management of chronic pain.

REVIEW QUESTIONS

1. Physical therapy sessions typically last for how long?
   A. 1 hour
   B. 30 minutes
   C. As long as is necessary to relieve pain
   D. 45 minutes

2. McKenzie therapy consists of which of the following?
   A. Transcutaneous electrical stimulation
   B. Hypnosis and psychotherapy
   C. Aquatic therapy
   D. Active positions of motion in the lumbar spine led by a specially trained therapist

ANSWERS

1. **A**
2. **D**

SUGGESTED READINGS

Fischer B, Lusted A, Roerecke M, Taylor B, Rehm J. The prevalence of mental health and pain symptoms in a population samples reporting nonmedical use of prescription opioids: a systematic review and meta-analysis. *J Pain*. 2012;13(11):1029-1044.

Hopkins HL, Smith HD, Tiffany EG. Rehabilitation. In Hopkins HL, Smith HD, eds. *Willard and Spackman's Occupational Therapy*. 6th ed. Philadelphia: JB Lippincott, 1983.

Turk DC. Efficacy of multidisciplinary pain centers in the treatment of chronic pain. *Prog Pain Res Manag*. 1996;7: 57-74.

World Health Organization. *International Classification of Functioning, Disability and Health (IFC)*. Geneva, Switzerland: World Health Organization, 2001.

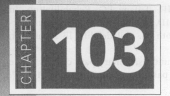

103 Nonopioid Pharmacotherapy of Pain

Summary by Simy K. Parikh, Michael Perloff, and James A.D. Otis

> Based on THE ASAM PRINCIPLES OF ADDICTION MEDICINE, 6th edition chapter by Simy K. Parikh, Michael Perloff, and James A.D. Otis

Pharmacotherapy can provide effective pain management in most patients. Traditionally, opioid therapy has been a principal treatment of somatic pain; now, there is a growing role for nonopioid analgesics and adjuvant analgesics in the treatment of somatic and neuropathic pain. Nonopioid primary analgesics include nonsteroidal anti-inflammatory drugs (NSAIDs), and nonopioid adjuvant analgesics include antidepressants, anticonvulsants, anesthetics, medical marijuana, α-adrenergic agonists, topical agents, and muscle relaxants. This summary provides an overview of the mechanisms and indications of nonopioid pharmacotherapy for the treatment of pain.

NONOPIOID ANALGESICS
Nonsteroidal Anti-Inflammatory Drugs

NSAIDs are indicated for somatic pain of mild-to-moderate intensity. Pain from bone or joint injury and fever-induced myalgias are responsive to NSAIDs, but neuropathic pain, with the exception of acute pain from migraine headache, and pain from other diffuse myalgias are usually not. The mechanism of NSAID analgesia is thought to be related to the inhibition of cyclooxygenase activity, which inhibits prostaglandin production; prostaglandins sensitize peripheral nerve endings to noxious stimuli and trigger an inflammatory cascade. Another mechanism of NSAID analgesia is modulation of pain in the central nervous system. Patients have variable responses to the different classes of NSAIDs, and individual titration is required to determine the maximally tolerated and effective dose for each patient. NSAIDs should be avoided or used with caution in the elderly and pregnant patient populations and in patients with

(1) hepatic and renal impairment or failure, (2) hematologic conditions, (3) a risk for gastrointestinal ulceration, and (4) cardiovascular risk factors. Finally, NSAIDs may have drug interactions with other medications, including lithium and prophylactic aspirin, and concomitant use should be done with caution. Cyclooxygenase-2 selective NSAIDs were developed to lessen the potential gastrointestinal side effects but were ultimately found to contribute to increased myocardial and cerebrovascular risk. Celecoxib is still available, but with a black box warning for cardiovascular risk.

Adjuvant Analgesics

Adjuvant analgesics are medications that have a primary indication other than analgesia but which have analgesic properties under certain conditions.

Antidepressants

Tricyclic antidepressants (TCAs) and selective serotonin-norepinephrine reuptake inhibitors (SNRIs) have an analgesic effect independent of their antidepressant actions. They are indicated for the treatment of neuropathic pain, including pain arising from fibromyalgia, migraine headache, diabetic peripheral neuropathy, radiculopathy, and postmastectomy pain syndrome. They are most effective for continuous, burning, or dysesthetic pain. The mechanism of antidepressant analgesia is secondary to enhancement of the body's own pain-modulating pathways. The greatest analgesic effect is seen with the older, tertiary amine antidepressants, such as amitriptyline, imipramine, and doxepin. Side effects seen with TCAs are related to their anticholinergic properties. Secondary amine tricyclics, such as desipramine and nortriptyline, are also effective and have less sedating and anticholinergic side effects. TCAs should be avoided or used with caution in patients with glaucoma, cardiac arrhythmias, prolonged QT syndrome, history of urinary outlet obstruction, and older adults.

Commonly used SNRIs include venlafaxine, duloxetine, and milnacipran. Compared to TCAs, SNRIs do not cause QT prolongation and have fewer anticholinergic side effects and less α blockade, leading to less risk of falls from orthostasis. SNRIs are also preferred for pain syndromes associated with depression.

Anticonvulsants

Carbamazepine, oxcarbazepine, valproic acid, gabapentin, and several other anticonvulsant and antiepileptic drugs are indicated for the treatment of allodynia or neuropathic pain syndromes that are characterized as paroxysmal, lancinating, or burning pain. The mechanism of action is variable, but generally, antiepileptic drugs reduce neuronal excitability and local neuronal discharges. Carbamazepine and oxcarbazepine are indicated for trigeminal neuralgia. Side effects of carbamazepine include hyponatremia, dizziness, somnolence, and significant leukopenia as well as Stevens-Johnson syndrome. In addition, carbamazepine dosage may need to be escalated over time due to significant autoinduction. Oxcarbazepine has fewer side effects and drug interactions than carbamazepine, and drug interactions, other than additive sedation and dizziness, are not a major concern. Valproic acid has been used for the management of lancinating pain, migraines, and diabetic neuropathy pain, but significant drug interactions and hepatic dysfunction can occur. Gabapentin is useful for both lancinating and continuous dysesthetic pain. Sedation during the dose titration period is a primary side effect. Gabapentin has a non-linear absorption at higher doses and a 5- to 7-hour half-life necessitating a three-times-a-day dosage. Pregabalin is indicated for neuropathic pain and fibromyalgia and is similar to gabapentin except that it has a linear pharmacokinetic profile. Lamotrigine has been shown to have modest efficacy in the treatment of diabetic and HIV neuropathy; however, it does require slow-dose titration to avoid Stevens-Johnson syndrome. Topiramate has well-established efficacy in migraine prophylaxis; it has little efficacy comparable to established agents for the treatment of lower back pain, radicular pain, or diabetic neuropathy. Clonazepam is a benzodiazepine with anticonvulsant properties that has been used for lancinating pain and muscle spasms. Side effects include sedation and dysphoria. The use of clonazepam should be used with caution in patients with a history of substance use disorder.

Anesthetics

Neuropathic pain has been found to respond transiently to high doses of intravenous anesthetics, such as lidocaine. The mechanism of action of intravenous lidocaine and the oral anesthetic mexiletine is thought to involve the suppression of sensory dorsal horn neuron activity. Side effects are dose related and commonly include nausea, dizziness, blurred vision, and tremors. Hematologic reactions are idiosyncratic and rare. Typically, oral and intravenous anesthetics are indicated for acute pain syndromes and their use is confined to inpatient settings. Ketamine, an N-methyl-D-aspartate receptor antagonist, also has a role in neuropathic pain. Limited evidence shows a benefit from the use of intranasal ketamine for breakthrough pain relief. Side effects include transient fatigue, dizziness, nausea, feelings of unreality, increases in blood pressure, change in taste, rhinorrhea, and nasal passage irritation. Topical ketamine has shown some promise for the use of refractory neuropathic pain, including chemotherapy-induced peripheral neuropathy and complex regional pain syndrome. Common systemic side effects have not occurred with topical ketamine use. The use of ketamine should be used with caution in patients with a past or current history of substance use disorder.

Medical Marijuana

Studies have shown a role for medical marijuana in the treatment of refractory chronic pain. The mechanism of action is thought to involve the activation of cannabinoid receptors, thereby causing dopaminergic increase and modulation of endogenous μ- and δ-opioid receptors. Side effects include somnolence, amnesia, cough, nausea, dizziness, euphoric mood, hyperhidrosis, and paranoia. The American Society of Addiction Medicine recommends its members and other physician organizations and their members reject responsibility for providing access to cannabis and cannabis-based products until such time that these materials receive marketing approval from the US Food and Drug Administration.

α-Adrenergic Agonists

The α_2-adrenergic agonists clonidine and tizanidine have been studied in a variety of pain syndromes including chronic neuropathic pain, myofascial pain, and complex regional pain syndrome. The mechanisms of action are thought to be secondary to the enhancement of endogenous pain-modulating systems and to a reduction of sympathetically maintained pain. Clonidine can be administered epidurally, intrathecally, orally, or transdermally. Major limiting side effects are hypotension and sedation. Tizanidine is useful for muscle and soft tissue pain and produces less muscle weakness than baclofen. Side effects include sedation. Concomitant use with other adrenergic agonists should be avoided.

Topical Agents

Topical agents have a localized action and are therefore most effective in peripheral pain syndromes, such as neuropathies, herpetic and postherpetic neuralgia, painful arthropathies, and for patients who experience adverse side effects from systemic medications. Capsaicin, a naturally occurring pepper extract, has been found to be useful for reducing diabetic neuropathic pain in combination with systemic therapy. Capsaicin's mechanism of action is thought to be related to the depletion of substance P. Side effects include burning pain. Topical lidocaine is indicated for postherpetic neuralgia. Side effects can include local irritation and hypersensitivity. Topical clonidine is useful for the treatment of painful diabetic neuropathy. Diclofenac is also formulated as a transdermal patch or gel and is used for arthritis pain localized to a specific joint. Side effects are the same as oral diclofenac, although they occur to a markedly lesser extent. Ketoprofen is also marketed in the United States as a topical gel, and topical ibuprofen is available in Europe.

EMLA (eutectic mixture of local anesthetics) is a 1:1 mixture of prilocaine and lidocaine, which can penetrate the skin and produce local anesthesia and is used in patients with peripheral nerve lesions and postherpetic neuralgia and for reducing pain associated with venipuncture. EMLA has been particularly helpful in postherpetic neuralgia. The combination of EMLA applied first, followed by capsaicin, may be better tolerated than capsaicin alone and may be more effective.

Muscle Relaxants

Several different classes of medications have muscle relaxant properties. Spasmolytic agents such as baclofen, tizanidine, and benzodiazepines are useful for conditions that produce flexor and extensor spasms because of neural injury as well as chronic muscle spasm. Cyclobenzaprine, carisoprodol, methocarbamol, and chlorzoxazone are agents that have no clear spasmolytic action, but may act through central nervous system depression. Baclofen is a γ-aminobutyric acid–affecting drug that suppresses excitatory transmitter release and action

at the spinal cord level and may block transmitter release at cutaneous nociceptive nerve endings. It is indicated for spasticity related to multiple sclerosis or for upper motor neuron lesions related to trauma, cerebrovascular disease, or degenerative disease. The major side effect of baclofen is sedation. Abrupt discontinuation can result in seizures. Cyclobenzaprine is a tricyclic agent for which the exact mechanism of action is unclear. It is indicated for short-term use only. Side effects include sedation, and it should be used with caution with other serotonin uptake inhibitors. Methocarbamol, carisoprodol, and chlorzoxazone are all older agents, the exact mechanism of action of which remains unclear. They do carry a potential for addiction and should be avoided.

KEY POINTS

1. There are multiple classes of nonopioid medications that produce varying degrees of pain reduction. They are associated with several different mechanisms of action. Nonopioid medication prescriptions require careful attention to side effects and drug–drug interactions.

2. The overarching goal of nonopioid therapy should be to improve function as opposed to only reducing pain.

3. Nonopioid medications have special utility in the patient with a past or current substance use disorder history.

REVIEW QUESTIONS

1. Amitriptyline should be avoided in patients with which of the following conditions?
   A. Prolonged QT syndrome
   B. History of urinary outlet obstruction
   C. Cardiac arrhythmias
   D. Both A and C.
   E. All of the above.

2. A patient with localized diabetic neuropathy may benefit from which of the following treatments?
   A. Clonidine patch
   B. Capsaicin
   C. Cyclobenzaprine
   D. Both A and B.
   E. All of the above.

3. Which agent acts as an N-methyl-D-aspartate receptor antagonist?
   A. Topiramate
   B. Mexiletine
   C. Ketamine
   D. Amitriptyline
   E. None of the above.

ANSWERS

1. **E**
2. **D**
3. **C**

SUGGESTED READINGS

Fishbain DA, Cutler R, Rosomoff HL, Rosomoff RS. Evidence-based data from animal and human experimental studies on pain relief with antidepressants: a structured review. *Pain Med*. 2000;1(4):310-316.

Snedecor SJ, Sudharshan L, Cappelleri JC, et al. Systematic review and meta-analysis of pharmacological therapies for painful diabetic peripheral neuropathy. *Pain Pract*. 2014;14(2):167-184.

Tremont-Lukats IW, Challapalli V, McNicol ED, Lau J, Carr DB. Systemic administration of local anesthetics to relieve neuropathic pain: a systematic review and meta-analysis. *Anesth Analg*. 2005;101(6):1738-1749.

Whiting PF, Wolff RF, Deshpande S, et al. Cannabinoids for medical use: a systematic review and meta-analysis. *JAMA*. 2015;313(24):2456-2473.

Wiffen PJ, Derry S, Moore R, et al. Antiepileptic drugs to treat neuropathic pain or fibromyalgia—an overview of Cochrane reviews. *Cochrane Database Syst Rev*. 2013;(11): CD010567.

Opioid Therapy of Pain

Summary by Tim K. Brennan

Based on THE ASAM PRINCIPLES OF ADDICTION MEDICINE,
6th edition chapter by Peggy Compton and
Friedhelm Sandbrink

Opioids are the most potent analgesic agents clinically available at this time. They have wide efficacy and utility in the treatment of acute and cancer-related pain. Although opioids may be helpful as one component within a multimodal pain management plan for chronic non–cancer-related pain in some patients, the risks of opioid therapy are considerable and, for most patients, likely outweigh the potential benefit, especially when used long term. Opioid pain medication use presents serious risks, including overdose and opioid use disorder (OUD), and patients with mental health disorders and a history of substance use disorder (SUD) are particularly vulnerable.

HISTORICAL PERSPECTIVE ON OPIOIDS

Opioids have been used for medicinal purposes for millennia. One of the first documented uses of opioids comes in the Sumerian ideogram of *hul gil*, the "plant of joy," inscribed more than 5000 years ago. Theophrastus, the Greek philosopher and popularizer of science, provides the first written account of the use of opium to relieve pain in 300 BC. In 1805, morphine was purified from opium, but its use did not become widespread until the development of the hypodermic syringe in 1853, which allowed morphine to be introduced directly into the circulatory system. This led to the widespread use of morphine for soldiers in the Civil War. Heroin was introduced as an over-the-counter drug by the Bayer Company in 1895 and was widely marketed as a panacea for numerous medical conditions.

By the early 1900s, both the appropriate therapeutic use and misuse of opioids were widespread in the United States. The Institute of Medicine estimates that about 300,000 Americans were opioid addicted at that time: With a total population of a little over 75 million in 1900, this would be about 1 in every 250 people. The medical community came to recognize the problem of opium addiction, and in a 1900 article in the *Journal of the American Medical*

Association, Dr. John Witherspoon, referring to opioids, exhorted physicians to "save our people from the clutches of this hydra-headed monster which stalks the civilized world, wrecking lives and happy homes, filling our jails and lunatic asylums."

Opioids were subsequently subjected to regulation and taxation through the Harrison Narcotics Tax Act in 1914, with legal use restricted to "legitimate medical purposes." In 1919, a federal ruling held that addiction treatment was "outside the realm of legitimate medical interest," creating a conundrum that allowed physicians to treat pain but not addiction that sometimes occurred in the context of medical use. The prescribing of opioids decreased and remained relatively low into the 1960s.

The hospice and palliative care movement blossomed in England in the mid-1960s under the leadership of Dame Cicely Saunders at St. Christopher's Hospice. With demonstration that opioid use could be safe and effective and could provide comfort at the end of life, the movement spread rapidly to the United States. With observation of favorable outcomes in hospice patients, aggressive management of acute pain emerged. The 1970 Controlled Substances Act classified controlled substances into risk categories and required the registration of providers; this provided a structure that both supported and allowed for the controlled use of opioids and other controlled substances. Cancer pain specialists noted favorable long-term results from opioid therapy of pain in cancer survivors without the inevitable evolution of tolerance or addiction. A one-paragraph letter by Porter and Jick to the editor of the *New England Journal of Pain* in 1980 reported on the low incidence of addiction in patients who did not have a history of addiction and who received opioid pain medication during hospitalization. Portenoy and Foley published a case series in 1986 with favorable outcomes in 24 of 38 patients with non–cancer-related pain, opening a debate about the use of opiate painkillers for a wider variety of pain.

In 1984, extended-release morphine was introduced and marketed for cancer pain. As of 1995, clinical practice guidelines recommended avoiding the long-term use of opioids for noncancer patients with chronic pain syndrome. The introduction of extended-release oxycodone in 1996 was associated with aggressive marketing for use in noncancer pain, with the argument that extended-release formulations would improve pain management by providing more stable blood levels and thus more consistent relief. Professional organizations and national initiatives began to promote more aggressive pain management including the use of opioid medications. In 1996, the president of the American Pain Society promoted the concept of pain as a vital sign in order to elevate awareness of pain treatment among healthcare professionals. The same year, the American Academy of Pain Medicine and the American Pain Society issued a consensus statement supporting long-term opioid therapy as an option for chronic noncancer pain, stating that the risk for de novo addiction was low, respiratory depression induced by opioids was short lived and was antagonized by pain, and tolerance was not a prevalent limitation to long-term opioid use. In 2000, the US Veterans Health Administration declared pain the fifth vital sign, and in 2001, the Joint Commission on Accreditation of Hospital Organizations implemented the evaluation and management of pain as a quality measure. Subsequently, state rules pertaining to opioid prescribing were relaxed. An era of aggressive pain management was born with increased utilization of opioid medications for patients with chronic non–cancer-related pain in combination with pressure on providers to document the lowering of pain scores, whereas at the same time, health insurance reimbursements for interdisciplinary pain management teams dwindled. The prescribing of opioid medication increased steadily from the 1980s until recently, and in the early 2000s, the first reports of increases in opioid overdoses emerged. In 2005, data was published from the Washington State workers' compensation system on opioid overdose deaths of injured workers and noted the association with escalating dosages of high-potency opioids including long-acting formulations. By 2007, deaths from overdoses of opioids exceeded the deaths from heroin and cocaine combined, and by 2008, drug overdoses, mostly from opioids, surpassed auto fatalities as the leading cause of accidental death in the United States. After approval of a risk evaluation and mitigation strategies program by the US Food and Drug Administration for transmucosal immediate-release fentanyl products in 2011, the US Food and Drug Administration implemented the extended-release/long-acting opioids risk evaluation and mitigation strategies program with voluntary training for prescribers in 2012, and even consumer groups published warnings about the dangers of opioid use for pain. Despite these efforts, opioid-related deaths continued to escalate, including a dramatic increase in overdoses from heroin since 2010 and fentanyl and its derivatives since 2013. On October 26, 2017, the US Department of Health and Human Services Acting Secretary Eric D. Hargan declared a nationwide public health emergency regarding the opioid crisis, as requested by President Donald Trump.

PREVALENCE OF PAIN

Pain is one of the most common ailments for which patients seek medical care. Chronic pain impacts the daily lives of fully one third of Americans older than 45 years, with 25 million (11.2%) US adults reporting daily chronic pain, and another 23 million (10.3%) reporting severe daily pain. It is estimated that between 5 and 8 million Americans use opioids on a daily basis for chronic pain management. According to a 2011 report by the Institute of Medicine, the costs of chronic pain is about US $600 billion per year when lost productivity and medical costs are combined, dwarfing the costs of other chronic illnesses. These numbers are expected to grow as baby boomers age, obesity rates rise, and persons increasingly survive traumatic injuries and cancer. A large systematic review of pain following a traumatic musculoskeletal injury found that a large proportion (28% to 93%) of patients experiencing traumatic musculoskeletal injury will develop persistent pain for a period of up to 84 months, although the severity of pain generally decreases over time.

The prevalence of pain among persons with SUDs may be significantly higher than that of the general population, with studies suggesting chronic pain occurring in up to 50% to 60% of patients on medication-assisted therapy (methadone, buprenorphine).

PREVALENCE OF USE AND MISUSE OF PRESCRIPTION OPIOIDS

Opioid prescribing, misuse, and opioid-associated harm have significantly increased in parallel over the past two decades. At the writing of this chapter, the United States is in the midst of what the US Department of Health and Human Services calls an epidemic of prescription drug abuse. In 2015, it is estimated that 12.5 million Americans misused a prescription opioid, with 2.1 million misusing the medication for the first time, and 2 million meeting the diagnostic criteria for a prescription opioid use disorder. This public health crisis has been fueled by the large supply of opioids being prescribed in our communities. The quantity of prescription opioids sold to pharmacies, hospitals, and doctors' offices was four times greater in 2010 than in 1999, and in 2012, clinicians wrote an estimated 259 million prescriptions for opioid analgesics. Evidence suggests 70% of persons who report misuse of opioids divert them from friends or relatives; however, 27% of the most frequent misusers obtain them with a physician prescription. Most concerning is that opioid-involved deaths continue to increase in the United States. Since 1999, the number of overdose deaths involving opioids (including prescription opioids and heroin) quadrupled, with an estimated 91 Americans dying every day from an overdose related to opioids.

POSITION OF OPIOIDS IN THE TREATMENT OF PAIN

Opioids are the most potent analgesic agents available. For severe acute postsurgical or trauma-induced pain, opioid therapy is usually included in the pain treatment plan, which also includes nonopioid analgesics and nonpharmacologic interventions as appropriate. Opioids are **not recommended** as first-line therapy in patients with mild-to-moderate acute pain, and the recommendation is always to keep the dosage as low and the duration as short as possible and as needed for the severity of the pain condition. Opioids remain standard in the treatment of advanced or progressive cancer-related pain, occupying steps 2 and 3 of the widely accepted "therapeutic ladder" developed by the World Health Organization, although recent meta-analyses suggest that their efficacy may be overstated and multimodal pain treatment is being implemented more widely.

Based on the assessments that there is a lack of evidence to suggest any long-term benefit in pain and function for patients with chronic pain treated with opioid therapy when compared to no opioids and that extensive evidence shows the possible harms of opioids (including OUD, overdose, and motor vehicle injury), the 2016 Centers for Disease Control and Prevention *Guideline for Prescribing Opioids for Chronic Pain* expresses great caution against long-term opioid therapy and recommends against dosage increases. Short-term use of opioid therapy as part of a multimodal comprehensive treatment approach, such as for acute exacerbation of a chronic pain condition, needs to be separated from long-term opioid prescribing (eg, >90 days) but

should also be kept at the lowest dosage and shortest duration possible and as appropriate for the pain condition, in awareness that even brief and low-dose opioid therapy increases the likelihood of developing an OUD, particularly in those with risk factors. The Centers for Disease Control and Prevention guideline draws attention to the lack of an evidence base to determine what patient characteristics, medications, dosing regimens, and other variables favor safe and effective opioid use and highlights the harms associated with their ongoing use in this population. The Department of Veterans Affairs' and Department of Defense's *Clinical Practice Guideline for Opioid Therapy of Chronic Pain,* published in 2017, recommends against the initiation of long-term opioid therapy in patients with non–cancer-related pain altogether and notes the particularly high risks of poor outcomes in patients younger than 30 years of age, with concurrent SUDs, and in the presence of benzodiazepine coprescribing.

SPECIAL ISSUES IN THE USE OF OPIOIDS

Like most medications, opioids have the potential for both benefit and harm. In addition to a range of physical side effects, however, opioids, like other controlled substances, deserve special consideration for their capacity to provide rewards (eg, euphoria) and to result in SUDs in certain at-risk individuals. These characteristics can lead to their misuse, diversion, and associated harm, including SUDs and overdose. In addition, opioids have specific pharmacologic effects, including physical dependence, tolerance, and hyperalgesia, which may complicate their use for pain treatment and require special care in management.

These issues may be of less significance in the treatment of acute and cancer pain, given the often time-limited duration of use in these contexts, than in the management of chronic non–cancer-related pain, but a thorough understanding of these issues may enhance decision making in all three contexts.

Physical Dependence

Physical dependence may be defined as a physiologic adaptation to the continuous presence of a drug that produces symptoms of withdrawal when the drug effect significantly diminishes or stops. Physical dependence occurs not only to drugs with reward potential, such as opioids and benzodiazepines, but also to those with little or no reward potential, such as α_2 adrenergic agonists (eg, clonidine) and tricyclic antidepressants. It is a drug class–specific withdrawal syndrome that can be produced by abrupt cessation, rapid dose reduction, decreasing blood level of the drug, and/or administration of an antagonist. Such dependence is an expected occurrence in all patients (with and without a co-occurring addiction) after 2 to 10 days of continuous administration of an opioid.

Tolerance

Tolerance is indicated by the need for increasing doses of a medication to achieve the initial effects of the drug. Tolerance may occur differentially to both to a drug's analgesic effects and to such side effects as respiratory depression, sedation, or nausea. Tolerance can be innate due to inherent biogenetic characteristics of the individual (in response the particular opioid), or it can be acquired in response to ongoing exposure to the opioid. Acquired tolerance may be due to both pharmacokinetic factors, such as changes in drug absorption and metabolism that reduce blood concentration, and to pharmacodynamic factors, such as receptor desensitization or other density changes at the level of opioid receptors.

Hyperalgesia

Opioid use may worsen pain in some contexts. Hyperalgesia is a physiologic state in which there is sensitization to nociceptive stimuli resulting in a lowered pain threshold and/or decreased tolerance to pain. There are many factors that may result in hyperalgesia and sensitization, including the long-term presence of pain itself, and physiologic and psychological stressors such as sleep deprivation, possibly mediated by aberrant glial activation.

Rewards

Commonly used analgesic opioids act primarily on μ-opioid receptors. μ Opioids produce rewards (eg, euphoria) in many, although not all, individuals. Some persons, in fact, experience dysphoria or no mood changes in association with opioid use. Pain relief of any kind is generally very rewarding. The potential for opioids to further activate and potentiate the reward system when used for pain is a critical factor to consider in all patients.

CLINICAL VARIABLES IN THE USE OF OPIOIDS

Opioids are often the mainstay of treatment of moderate-to-severe acute pain and pain associated with progressive or terminal illnesses. When used in the treatment of chronic, nonterminal pain, they should only be used as one component of multimodal and multidisciplinary pain, and only for the lowest dosage and shortest duration to achieve the pain treatment goals.

Drug Selection

Opioids produce their analgesia and side effects primarily through action on opioid receptors. Stimulation of the μ, κ, and δ receptors is associated with analgesia and side effects. Most of the commonly used opioid analgesics have predominantly μ-receptor activity; however, some analgesic opioids have agonist–antagonist or partial μ-agonist activity.

μ-Opioid agonists are the most commonly prescribed class of opioid analgesics and include morphine, oxycodone, hydromorphone, oxymorphone, methadone, hydrocodone, and fentanyl. Pure μ agonists usually have no ceiling analgesic effect and may be titrated as needed to achieve analgesia, limited by side effects and risks as discussed elsewhere. Tolerance to some side effects generally occurs more rapidly than tolerance to analgesia but is usually incomplete, and, in particular, monitoring for respiratory depression and sedation is always important, especially in opioid-naïve individuals, as doses are increased or as specific opioids are changed.

Although most μ agonists are interchangeable if attention is paid to relative potencies and the onset and duration of action, individuals may respond differently to different opioids in terms of both analgesia and side effects.

Methadone differs from other μ agonists in several ways. Although it may have potentially advantageous properties compared to other opioids used for pain management, methadone has been associated with a disproportionate high number of overdoses and deaths, in part due to its cardiac side effects and the complex pharmacokinetic and pharmacodynamic properties, including its variable half-life and multiple drug interactions, which make it more difficult to use safely than other opioids. Thus, methadone should only be initially prescribed or increased in dosage by providers thoroughly familiar and experienced with the use of this medication.

Agonist–antagonist opioids, or κ-agonist opioids, including pentazocine, nalbuphine, and butorphanol, have predominantly κ-agonist effects while antagonizing the μ receptor. These drugs have been widely regarded as having less potential for unhealthy use and addiction than the pure μ agonists, although elective use for rewards and the development of addiction to these medications have been observed.

Partial μ agonists, including buprenorphine and tramadol, provide analgesia via μ-opioid receptors but have relatively low intrinsic efficacy; that is, they bind to μ-opioid receptors but produce less receptor activation than full μ agonists. Clinically, they are very different medications. Tramadol and tapentadol are dual-mechanism opioids that combine action on the μ-opioid receptor with a second analgesic mechanism mediated by their inhibitory action on serotonin and norepinephrine reuptake. Buprenorphine is a partial agonist opioid with complex pharmacology that is available in parenteral, sublingual, and transdermal preparations. It has a long half-life and high receptor affinity and is of course useful in the treatment of OUD.

Routes of Administration

Opioids may be administered orally, rectally, transmucosally, nasally, intravenously, subcutaneously, transdermally, and intraspinally. The oral, enteral, or transdermal routes generally are preferred when feasible because they are not invasive and usually provide satisfactory analgesia, even when high doses are required.

Dose Titration and Scheduling

Measuring Efficacy

The serial use of a pain severity rating scale, such as a numerical 0 to 10 rating scale or the visual Faces Pain Scale, is helpful in assessing a response to pain treatment. In treating chronic pain, it is often helpful to inquire about worst pain, least pain, and average (or typical) pain experienced in a particular period of time, such as the past week.

Dose Requirements

Several factors must be considered when determining the dose and interval of administration that will provide effective analgesia in a given patient for a given problem; however, starting with short-acting formulations and using lower doses is always recommended. The pharmacokinetics and potencies of the drugs must be taken into consideration, along with idiosyncratic or individual patient responses to different opioids. Finally, the tolerance of individuals who have been exposed to opioids on a prolonged basis (whether therapeutically or due to addiction) must be accommodated.

Long-Acting Versus Short-Acting Medications

Long-acting medications include those that are intrinsically long acting, such as methadone, levorphanol,

and buprenorphine, and medications that are long acting by virtue of being formulated for slow release, such as controlled-release and transdermal preparations. Most other opioids are shorter acting and immediate release.

When patients have persistent pain on an around-the-clock basis, longer-acting medications at least theoretically offer the advantage of providing relatively stable drug blood levels and, therefore, more consistent analgesia than frequent doses of short-acting medications.

Scheduled Versus As-Needed (Rescue) Opioids

Shorter-acting medications may be considered for intermittent pain, for acute pain conditions and acute exacerbation of chronic pain, or for evoked increases of chronic pain when not sufficiently controlled by nonopioid pharmacologic and non-pharmacologic modalities. If pain is continuous, patient-controlled analgesia, a continuous parenteral infusion, or long-acting oral or transdermal medications, depending on the context, are appropriate. In acute or cancer pain, rescue doses of as-needed medications are usually provided for breakthrough pain or exacerbations of baseline pain.

Opioid Side Effects

Opioid side effects include respiratory depression, constipation, nausea and vomiting, urinary retention, and pruritus. Respiratory depression deserves special consideration because it can be life threatening. It is a potentially fatal side effect of opioid administration and demands awareness throughout treatment, particularly when opioids are first introduced, when doses are increased, or when specific opioids are changed. Side effects of long-term opioid use may include hyperalgesia, respiratory depression, and constipation as well as effects on the endocrine and immune systems. Effects of opioids on the immune system have been demonstrated, with numerous early studies both in animals and humans suggesting immunosuppressive effects, particularly on cell-mediated immunity. No clear clinically significant effects of opioids on immune function have been demonstrated to date, and the clinical relevance of these findings is therefore uncertain.

Changing Opioids

Because side effects often vary from one opioid to another in different patients, rotation from one opioid to another is sometimes helpful in resolving side effects that do not resolve over time or that do not respond to pharmacologic treatment. The transition from one opioid or form of opioid to another may be indicated in a number of circumstances: when tolerance occurs to a specific opioid with a loss of analgesic efficacy, when a patient on chronic oral opioids must be withheld food and fluids, or when significant side effects occur and persist.

PAIN MANAGEMENT IN PERSONS WITH AN ADDICTION

It is well accepted that inadequate treatment of pain increases morbidity after trauma and surgery, whereas optimal pain treatment appears to shorten hospitalizations in similar contexts. Pain increases distress and anxiety and may be a risk factor for relapse in those in recovery and for aberrant use in those with an active SUD. Individuals with an SUD often experience particularly high levels of anxiety in association with trauma, illness, or surgery because they fear that their pain will not be adequately managed. This, in turn, can affect how they experience and respond to pain. Attention to their concerns facilitates pain management. An open and nonjudgmental approach to the discussion of substance use concerns facilitates information exchange with patients, and it is especially important to include the patient in the clinical decision-making process.

Patients on methadone maintenance provided for OUD treatment should usually be continued rather than being entirely switched to an alternative opioid if opioid analgesia is required due to severity of the acute pain condition. If acute pain occurs due to trauma or illness in a patient on buprenorphine, μ opioids can usually be titrated to higher doses to overcome the buprenorphine blockade. Alternatively, a patient on a low dose of buprenorphine (2 to 8 mg per day) may receive acceptable analgesia from a temporarily increased daily dose that is often administered twice a day to achieve around-the-clock analgesia.

Universal Precautions in Opioid Therapy for Chronic Pain

Because the risk of opioid misuse for a given patient cannot be reliably determined, it is prudent to view all patients as having some level of risk and to employ a set of universal precautions in managing all patients. Commonly discussed universal precautions for opioid therapy include the following:

- A comprehensive pain assessment
- An assessment of risk for opioid misuse

- The formulation of a differential diagnosis of contributing factors to pain
- An informed consent for treatment following risk–benefit discussion
- Documentation of a clear plan of treatment
- The initiation of opioid therapy as a trial with clear goals
- A reassessment of pain, level of function, quality of life, and adherence to plan of care
- Urine drug testing prior to opioid prescribing and routinely during opioid therapy at random intervals
- Querying state prescription drug monitoring programs prior to opioid prescribing and routinely during opioid therapy in accordance with state and federal guidelines
- Documentation of decision making and care
- Opioid overdose education and prescribing of naloxone rescue medication

Opioid Treatment Agreements

A written opioid treatment agreement is a valuable tool that can help ensure that the patient understands the potential risks and benefits of treatment. It may also help to mitigate the risks of treatment, although there is limited evidence of improvement in treatment outcomes. Most often, the treatment agreement is between patient and clinical treatment providers, although engagement of the pharmacist and family in the treatment plan is likely to improve care. Usually, there are two components of an opioid treatment agreement: informed consent and a written plan of care that ensures mutual understanding of the treatment plan.

CONCLUSIONS

Opioids have an important role in relieving human suffering. At the same time, it is important to respect their potential to cause harm in vulnerable individuals. In order to use opioids effectively and safely when they are indicated, clinicians must understand pharmacologic and clinical issues related to opioids and carefully structure treatment with respect to the particular benefits and risks for individual patients. It is to be hoped that, over time, science and clinical experience will provide a fuller understanding of ways to harness the full potential of opioids to relieve suffering while eliminating the harmful consequences of their use. In the meantime, the art of pain care should be combined with the science of pain care to give patients the best quality of life possible, given the reality of their clinical diagnoses.

KEY POINTS

1. Opioids have not been proven to be efficacious in the treatment of nonmalignant chronic pain disorders.
2. Tolerance and dependence are inevitable in any patient receiving chronic opioid therapy.
3. A written opioid treatment agreement is a valuable tool that can help ensure that the patient understands the potential risks and benefits of treatment.

REVIEW QUESTIONS

1. Which of the following medications is approved by the US Food and Drug Administration for the treatment of opioid use disorder?
   A. Buprenorphine intravenous preparation
   B. Buprenorphine sublingual tablets
   C. Buprenorphine transdermal device
   D. Tramadol

2. Which of the following is *true* regarding prescribing methadone from a physician's office?
   A. It is only allowed if there is an opioid treatment contract.
   B. It is only allowed for patients using methadone for pain, not for addiction.
   C. It is allowed only for patients using methadone for addiction, not for pain.
   D. It is never allowed under any circumstance. All methadone must come from an opioid treatment program.

3. Which federal act regulated the use of opioids for "legitimate medical purposes"?
   A. The Harrison Act
   B. The Affordable Care Act
   C. The Opioid Reform Act
   D. The Patriot Act

ANSWERS

1. **A**
2. **B**
3. **A**

SUGGESTED READINGS

Booth M. *Opium: A History.* New York: St. Martin's Press, 1996.

Courtwright DT. A century of American narcotic policy. In: Gerstein DR, Harwood HJ, eds. *Treating Drug Problems.* Vol. 2. Washington, DC: National Academy Press, 1992:1-62.

Webb v United States, 249 US 96 (1919).

Wier MS. *Injuries of Nerves and Their Consequences.* Philadelphia: J. B. Lippincott, 1872.

Witherspoon JA. A protest against some of the evils in the profession of medicine. *JAMA.* 1900;34(25):1589-1592.

Co-Occurring Pain and Addiction

Summary by Anil Abraham Thomas

Based on THE ASAM PRINCIPLES OF ADDICTION MEDICINE,
6th edition chapter by William C. Becker and Declan T. Barry

In the past decades, clinicians have struggled with the dichotomy of assessing and treating of patients with pain and patients suffering from substance use disorders (SUDs). These two conditions are not mutually exclusive—each can increase the vulnerability to the other, obscure the diagnosis, and impede the treatment. Studies have shown that a significant percentage of patients seeking SUD treatment suffer from comorbid chronic pain.

PROBLEMS OF COMORBIDITY

Reciprocal Vulnerability

Epidemiology data imply that persons with SUDs are at higher risk of developing chronic pain conditions given that individuals with SUDs are more susceptible to incurring trauma and painful illnesses such as strokes, infections, peripheral artery diseases, pancreatitis, and cirrhosis. The converse also hold true: Having pain increases the vulnerability to SUDs by increased exposure to controlled substances. Several studies have concluded that substance misuse problems preceded therapeutic opioid exposure. Disabling chronic pain and SUDs share several risk factors including childhood trauma/neglect, adult trauma, and posttraumatic stress disorder.

Diagnostic Confounds

SUDs may complicate the diagnosis of pain, which may or may not be consciously appreciated by the patient. Most chronic pain is due less to peripheral nociception than to central sensitization. Therefore, the clinician is in a precarious situation in which the primary diagnostic finding guiding decision making is the patient report, which may be unreliable.

Pain complicates the diagnosis of SUDs because pain probably makes it harder for the patient to recognize that an SUD has developed. Unlike the person who initiated using substances recreationally, for euphoria, and gradually transitioned into using in order to prevent distress, persons

with pain initiated the substance use to stop feeling "bad," and so the transition to addictive behavior may be less apparent.

Treatment Impediments

Patients with an opioid use disorder (OUD) may not respond readily to nonopioid modalities of pain treatment, eg, other medications, injections, physical therapy, or cognitive–behavioral therapy. A patient-centered approach, one that is transparent and focused on patient education, can be effective. Patients may be dissatisfied with nonopioid treatment recommendations, but they will be more dissatisfied if they receive those recommendations having the perception that they were not listened to or their pain was not taken seriously.

The therapeutic relationship can be complicated with SUDs. Patients may believe that they are entitled to pain relief, whereas the prescriber may suspect that the pain complaints reflect drug-seeking behavior. Similarly, treating SUDs can be complicated by chronic pain. Patients with only pain may fail to identify with persons with only SUDs and no pain conditions as they lack "legitimate" reasons for use of opioids.

EVOLVING GUIDANCE ON THE USE OF OPIOIDS IN THE TREATMENT OF CHRONIC PAIN

In 2016, the Centers of Disease Control and Prevention (CDC) released the *Guideline for Prescribing Opioids for Chronic Pain*. This was in contrast to the 2009 guidelines by the American Pain Society and the American Academy of Pain Medicine's *Clinical Guidelines for the Use of Chronic Opioid Therapy in Chronic Noncancer Pain*, as decidedly "opioid avoidant" because the CDC guideline instead promotes nonopioid and nonpharmacologic treatment options for the treatment of chronic pain and recommends limits in dosage prescribed and vigilance in surveilling for indications to taper down or discontinue opioids among patients on long-term opioid therapy (LTOT) when benefits no longer outweighs harm.

The CDC guideline also places a greater emphasis on the lack of evidence demonstrating long-term efficacy of LTOT, unlike other treatments for chronic pain, and the evidence of potential harm, especially at higher doses.

As the impact of the CDC guideline evolves, it has already changed the conversation. There is an appreciation that quality pain care means a blend of nonpharmacologic and pharmacologic options, treatments where patients take an active role (eg, yoga), and promoting self-management and skill building for nonreliance on the healthcare system. In addition, it may be in the patient's best interest in the intermediate and long term to reduce or avoid opioids. For people on LTOT for whom the benefits outweigh the harm, LTOT should be continued with ongoing close monitoring. Involuntary tapering of patients not experiencing harm is not evidence based, not guideline concordant, and presents its own set of serious risks.

Monitoring for Misuse and Opioid Use Disorder

The CDC guideline does not proscribe the initiation of LTOT and advocated discontinuation of extant LTOT when benefits do not outweigh harm. Thus, the CDC guideline recommends ongoing monitoring of patients prescribed opioid analgesics for aberrant medication-taking behaviors and incident OUDs. The CDC guideline recommends risk-reduction strategies, seeing patients on LTOT every 3 months or sooner if the patient is at a high risk, querying the state prescription drug monitoring program, and performing random urine drug testing. For a detailed, non–consensus-based guidance on monitoring, published by Gourlay, Heit, and Almahrezi, see Table 105-1.

It is essential to communicate clearly to patients the specific plan for monitoring, to keep the patient as safe as possible, and the consequences if monitoring reveals unsafe use. This can be in the form of a written treatment agreement, a conversation with expectations clearly conveyed; however, a document should not supplant a conversation. Clinical pain care should follow best practices in safe opioid prescribing; there is a need to discontinue therapy when the benefit is not outweighing harm, which may be before a diagnosable SUD or if a benefit is absent or there is another appreciable harm.

TABLE 105-1	The Ten Steps of Universal Precautions in Pain Medicine
Diagnose the cause of pain
Psychological assessment, including addiction risk
Informed consent
Treatment agreement
Assess pain and function pre- and postintervention
Opioid trial ± adjunctive medication
Continued reassessment of pain and function
Regularly assess the "Four As": analgesia, activity, adverse effects, aberrant behavior ± affect
Periodically review diagnoses, including addiction
Careful documentation

Data from Gourlay DL, Heit HA, Almahrezi A. Universal precautions in pain medicine: a rational approach to the treatment of chronic pain. *Pain Med*. 2005;6(2):107-112.

Diagnosis of Opioid Use Disorder in Chronic Pain

The criteria for a diagnosis of OUD in patients with chronic pain are similar to those in patients without pain; however, they may be more difficult to discern because many of the OUD criteria may be in the context of undertreated pain. To resolve this, clear communication of what constitutes unsafe use must be provided.

The *Diagnostic and Statistical Manual of Mental Disorders,* 5th edition (*DSM-5*) diagnosis of opioid use disorder requires a maladaptive pattern of use leading to significant impairment or distress, as indicated by at least 2 of the 11 indicators within a 12-month period.

Iatrogenic OUDs (ie, occurring in the course of medically supervised opioid analgesic therapy) are more subtle than in recreational SUDs. Loss of control is manifested by the inability to ration and the patient runs out of medication early. The patient with an OUD may continue to use despite adverse consequences, such as losing the thread of a conversation or falling asleep at the dinner table. Having multiple prescribers may indicate the development of prescription OUD.

TREATING PAIN IN THE PRESENCE OF A SUBSTANCE USE DISORDER

SUDs are a challenge for the safe and successful treatment of both acute and chronic pain; most challenging is the management of acute-on-chronic pain. Optimal treatment is patient centered, whether the patient is actively using substances, is in abstinence-based recovery, or is in active treatment and whether the focus is acute or chronic pain management.

Acute Pain

Substance use increases the likelihood of developing acute pain by a number of mechanisms and increases the likelihood that the pain will not be optimally managed. Patients actively using licit or illicit opioids are frequently undermedicated by the prescriber due to the presence of tolerance or fear of being duped into "fueling the addiction." Patients with OUDs would benefit from multimodal analgesia.

Acute-on-Chronic Pain

Acute-on-chronic pain describes the presence of acute pain in a patient who has preexisting chronic pain. Patients who are on long-term high-dose opioids for pain, whether with a comorbid OUD or not, and who undergo surgery, are vulnerable to poor perioperative pain control. These patients require their typical maintenance dose and also additional doses for optimal control.

It is more difficult to achieve satisfactory analgesia in tolerant patients, and aggressive treatment is more hazardous. Tolerant patients have both more postoperative pain and more opioid-induced sedation. Tolerance develops to opioid effects at different rates: Tolerance to sedation and respiratory depression occurs more rapidly than to miosis and constipation. Tolerance to opioid toxicity and opioid analgesia develops at different rates: The therapeutic window in naïve users becomes narrower, and the effective dose approaches the lethal dose. Regional analgesia, nonopioid systemic analgesia, and non-pharmacologic interventions are often required. The phenomena of opioid-induced hyperalgesia should also be considered.

Acute or Acute-on-Chronic Pain Among Patients Receiving Opioid Agonist Therapy for Opioid Use Disorder

Patients receiving methadone (full μ agonist) maintenance treatment for OUDs should be assumed to receive no analgesic effects from it and, in the case of trauma, may require continuation of the methadone in addition to a greater that usual dose of opioid analgesia.

A similar phenomena is seen with buprenorphine (partial μ agonist) therapy with one difference: Buprenorphine has a higher binding affinity and will displace the full agonist for the receptor site. Buprenorphine can precipitate withdrawal when given to patients who are taking opioids and, thus, must be avoided in these situation. Conversely, a full agonist can be given to treat pain in a patient receiving buprenorphine; however, aggressive dose titration is required due to buprenorphine's avid receptor binding and the need for the new opioid to displace it at the receptor. Clinicians can wean buprenorphine off and replace it with a full μ agonist in preparation for a procedure, or if the patient is on a relatively low dose of buprenorphine, it can be titrated for analgesia.

Patients treated with oral or depot naltrexone (competitive opioid antagonist) experience an attenuated effect from the administered opioid; the blockade can be overcome with high-dose therapy. The risk of overdose is present because the dose of opioid needed to overcome the naltrexone block may become toxic as naltrexone is metabolized.

Frequent Emergency Department Visits

Emergency departments frequently encounter patients with SUDs who present with complaints of severe pain, often without evidence of acute illness. Ignoring suffering versus rewarding aberrant medication use are both unacceptable. Guidelines have been developed by hospitals and states that emphasize avoiding opioids for chronic pain in the emergency setting, avoiding prescriptions for long-acting opioids, not refilling lost or stolen prescriptions for opioids given for pain or OUDs, avoiding parenteral opioids, using nonopioids when possible, and creating a care plan for patients who visit frequently. When opioid are provided, emergency departments should give only small quantities.

Chronic Pain

Nonpharmacologic treatments for chronic pain include physical therapy, exercise, fitness, yoga, and other similar activities that reduce pain. Psychological treatments can not only reduce pain but can also increase the patients ability to cope with residual pain and improve overall quality of life. Transcutaneous electrical neurostimulation, massage, and osteopathic manipulative therapies also provide pain reduction.

Interdisciplinary pain rehabilitation programs have shown the best outcomes for disabling chronic pain. They improve pain, physical function, psychological distress, and healthcare utilization. Pain rehabilitation programs also demonstrate lasting benefits. These programs rely on behavioral treatment, cognitive therapies, physical reconditioning, and adjuvant analgesics.

Many adjuvant analgesics have important roles in providing pain relief. Regional anesthesia provides relief of sufficient duration to positively impact a patient's quality of life. Botulinum toxin, approved for chronic migraines, has a role in muscle spasms; celiac plexus blockade provides relief of pain from the upper abdominal viscera; spinal cord stimulation reduces chronic radicular pain, complex regional pain syndrome, and axial spine pain; peripheral nerve stimulation reduces pain from peripheral mononeuropathies; deep brain stimulation provides relief for intractable poststroke pain; and motor cortex stimulation provides relief for complex regional pain syndrome.

Numerous nonopioid pharmacologic treatments for chronic pain have shown to effective. Gabapentinoids are useful for neuropathic pain, fibromyalgia, and migraine prophylaxis. Other antiepileptic have shown benefits for neuropathic pains including tic douloureux and multiple sclerosis. Serotonin and norepinephrine reuptake inhibitors and tricyclic antidepressants (which also inhibit the uptake of serotonin and norepinephrine) are useful for neuropathic, migraine, and fibromyalgia pain. They have benefits for chronic low back pain, irritable bowel syndrome, temporomandibular joint syndromes, vulvodynia, and other hyperalgesic states. Topical analgesics, such as capsaicin, diclofenac gel and patches, and transdermal lidocaine are effective in select pains. Acetaminophen relieves minor pains and can reduce a patient's need for others. Anti-inflammatory medications are effective for nociceptive pain of inflammatory or bony origin and have opioid sparing effects when used after surgery or trauma.

There are little data for the use of LTOT in patients with a history of SUDs; LTOT provided less than 50% pain reduction to less than half of those entering treatment. In addition, there is a paucity of evidence of improved quality of life in most pain conditions. The safest treatment for patients with comorbid SUDs and chronic pain is to avoid controlled substances.

Sublingual buprenorphine, approved for the treatment of OUD, is an excellent analgesic and thus offers the side benefit of pain relief for patients receiving it for OUDs. Buprenorphine is less likely to produce respiratory depression, immune suppression, and analgesic tolerance than a full μ agonist. Suboxone is a combination buprenorphine and naloxone and is less subject to diversion and to altered routes of administration. Of note, the relative safety of buprenorphine is overcome if combined with benzodiazepine.

Chronic Pain Among Patients on Opioid Agonist Therapy for Opioid Use Disorder

Chronic pain is highly prevalent in patients receiving opioid agonist therapy for OUD. Opioid treatment programs target the OUD and often ignore chronic pain. Strategies for managing chronic pain in patients on opioid agonist therapy focus of pharmacotherapy. Consistent with the CDC guidance, non–opioid-based therapies should be favored when a patient receiving opioid agonist therapy needs pain management on a chronic basis.

Additional Reward Medications

Patients with chronic noncancer pain and SUDs often have comorbid psychiatric issues, commonly anxiety and/or depression. Anxiolytics and sedative–hypnotics create an added risk for overdose and are commonly used in unhealthy patterns. Most antidepressants have anxiolytic properties, are first-line therapies for anxiety disorders, and are not addictive. Antiepileptic drugs used in pain management also are not subject to addiction. Chronic pain is strongly associated with sleep disorders, which amplify pain; prolonged use of pharmacotherapies with addictive potential should be avoided.

TREATING ADDICTION IN THE PRESENCE OF PAIN

Chronic pain complicates addiction treatment. Most patients attribute the failure of treatment to pain, not to drug or other substance use. Patients and family members may be unsure whether rewarding drugs are an asset, liability, or both. In treating addiction in those with chronic pain, other means must be employed to manage patients' pain.

Agonist or Abstinence

Abstinence-based treatment of OUD has a high failure rate; pharmacotherapy is recommended for most. An interdisciplinary pain rehabilitation program should also be strongly considered. Addiction in those taking opioids for pain may have a more favorable prognosis than in those who began use for other reasons. This may reflect cultural factors such as less toxic social groups, friends who promote sobriety, and less situations where drug use is prevalent.

CONCLUSION

The concurrence of chronic noncancer pain and SUDs is challenging for patients and healthcare providers alike with regard to both assessments and treatments. Clinicians should appreciate that chronic pain often co-occurs with OUD. The CDC's new guideline aims to bring clarity to various interventions, and multimodal treatment approaches should be made available and accessible to all.

KEY POINTS

1. The diagnosis and treatment of comorbid pain and SUDs are difficult because pain increases patients' vulnerability to SUDs and patients with an SUD are vulnerable to chronic pain.
2. The CDC Guideline recommends risk reduction strategies for patients with comorbid pain and SUDs.
3. Treatment of comorbid pain and SUDs should be multimodal with pharmacologic, nonpharmacologic, and psychosocial interventions.

REVIEW QUESTIONS

1. Iatrogenic opioid use disorder indicators include:
   A. an inability to ration medications and running out of medications early.
   B. falling asleep at dinner table and losing the thread of a conversation.
   C. seeking or having multiple prescribers.
   D. All of the above.

2. Which statement is correct?
   A. Buprenorphine is a partial opioid agonist with a high binding affinity.
   B. Methadone is a reverse opioid agonist.

C. Naltrexone is a competitive opioid antagonist.
D. Both A and C.

3. Comorbid pain and SUDs are optimally managed by:
   A. long-term opioid therapy.
   B. a multimodal approach (pharmacologic and nonpharmacologic therapies).
   C. nonpharmacologic therapies for pain only.
   D. SUD treatment because the pain is a "drug-seeking behavior."

ANSWERS

1. **D**
2. **D**
3. **B**

SUGGESTED READINGS

American Psychiatric Association. *Diagnostic and Statistical Manual of Mental Disorders.* 5th ed. Arlington, VA: American Psychiatric Association, 2013.

Cheatle M, Comer D, Wunsch M, Skoufalos A, Reddy Y. Treating pain in addicted patients: recommendations from an expert panel. *Popul Health Manag.* 2014;17(2): 79-89.

Galanter M, Kleber HD, Brady KT, eds. *The American Psychiatric Publishing Textbook of Substance Abuse Treatment.* 5th ed. Arlington, VA: American Psychiatric Association, 2014.

Tompkins DA, Hobelmann JG, Compton P. Providing chronic pain management in the "Fifth Vital Sign" era: historical and treatment perspective on a modern-day medical dilemma. *Drug Alcohol Depend.* 2017;173(suppl 1): S11-S21.

Volkow ND, McLellan AT. Opioid abuse in chronic pain—misconceptions and mitigation strategies. *N Engl J Med.* 2016;374(13):1253-1263.

Legal and Regulatory Considerations in Opioid Prescribing

Summary by Julia Megan Webb, David J. Copenhaver, and Scott M. Fishman

Based on THE ASAM PRINCIPLES OF ADDICTION MEDICINE, 6th edition chapter by Julia Megan Webb, David J. Copenhaver, Wesley Prickett, and Scott M. Fishman

Chronic pain affects nearly 100 million American adults. Opioids are often used to treat chronic pain despite weak evidence of long-term efficacy and increasing evidence of significant risks associated with continued use. Prescription drug overdose, predominantly involving opioids, is a leading cause of accidental death in adults aged 25 to 64 years. This dilemma has prompted increased national attention on responsible opioid prescribing and the need to balance effective pain management with harm reduction. The wide range of risks associated with chronic opioid therapy requires prescribers to have a foundational understanding of evolving federal and state regulations governing the use of all controlled substances, not just opioids.

FEDERAL OPIOID REGULATIONS

Federal regulations governing controlled substances are intended to balance consumer protection from controlled substances with appropriate access to these substances for therapeutic use. Regulations are based on two major concepts: (1) truth in labeling and (2) the appropriate distribution/use of controlled substances. Truth in labeling protects consumers from an educational standpoint, and the appropriate distribution of controlled substances reduces inappropriate access to these substances, thereby protecting the public from drugs of abuse. The Controlled Substances Act governs the medical use of controlled substances in the United States. It divides controlled substances into five schedules based on eight characteristics: (1) potential for abuse, (2) pharmacologic effects, (3) scientific properties, (4) pattern of abuse, (5) public health risk, (6) psychologic or physiologic dependence, (7) liability, and (8) whether the

substance is an immediate precursor of a substance already classified under a Controlled Substances Act schedule.

Methadone and buprenorphine can be prescribed to treat pain without a special Drug Enforcement Administration (DEA) registration. However, when these medications are prescribed as therapy in the setting of detoxification and maintenance therapy for opioid use disorder (OUD), additional regulations may apply to ensure that the provider is appropriately trained in managing patients with an OUD. The Drug Addiction Treatment Act of 2000 amended the Controlled Substances Act to allow physicians to provide buprenorphine or methadone for maintenance or detoxification in patients with opioid dependency or OUD who are admitted for a primary problem other than opioid dependence and for whom opioid withdrawal would complicate treatment of the presenting medical or surgical condition, such as myocardial infarction, without obtaining an official waiver. The "3-day rule" allows clinicians who are not registered to treat OUD to administer, but not prescribe, opioids for a maximum of 72 hours to relieve acute withdrawal symptoms in a patient who is dependent on opioids while a referral is arranged for treatment.

STATE-CONTROLLED SUBSTANCE REGULATIONS

Physicians are expected to comply with both state and federal prescribing regulations. However, sometimes, state and federal laws are in conflict. The Supremacy Clause of the US Constitution Article VI and the doctrine of preemption suggests federal law prevails over state law. In general, where state and federal regulations conflict, clinicians are advised to adhere to the most conservative or restrictive standards. State and federal law may also conflict in cases where a physician must balance obligations to report a crime related to opioid prescriptions or misuse with mandated confidentiality of protected health information as set forth by the Health Insurance Portability and Accountability Act.

THE DRUG ENFORCEMENT AGENCY

Healthcare providers who wish to prescribe controlled substances must be registered and obtain a provider number through the DEA. The DEA is part of the US Department of Justice and does not directly regulate medical practice but does investigate practitioners who do not comply with the laws regarding distribution of controlled substances. These investigations can lead to revocation of the provider's DEA number or criminal prosecution. Behaviors that may result in investigation include issuing prescriptions for controlled substances without a physician–patient relationship, issuing prescriptions in exchange for sex, issuing several prescriptions at once for a highly potent combination of controlled substances, charging fees commensurate with drug dealing rather than providing medical services, and issuing prescriptions using fraudulent names and self-abuse by practitioners. Federal DEA numbers are valid for 3 years and must be kept at the registered location and be readily retrievable for inspection purposes. Currently, there are no continuing medical education requirements to obtain a DEA number.

The DEA limits the amount of Schedule II controlled substances that can be prescribed within a *single prescription to no more than a 90-day supply.* Refills on Schedule II drugs are never allowed, but multiple prescriptions can be issued and filled sequentially for the same Schedule II controlled substance without interval office visits. Issuing multiple prescriptions in this way is not permitted in every state. In 2010, the DEA determined that practitioners who are registered with the DEA can prescribe scheduled substances electronically through special procedures, although state laws vary with respect to electronic prescribing.

THE US FOOD AND DRUG ADMINISTRATION AND RISK EVALUATION AND MITIGATION STRATEGIES

The US Food and Drug Administration (FDA) has the authority to require manufacturers to develop risk evaluation and mitigation strategies to ensure that the benefits of a substance outweigh potential risks and also to provide drug class–specific education to prescribers. In response to increasing opioid overdose and misuse, the FDA requested certain manufacturers of long-acting opioids develop risk evaluation and mitigation strategies for their products and provide financial support for voluntary continuing medical education credits related to their products. The FDA has issued several consumer warnings on the disposal of controlled substances. These warnings highlight the need for prescribers to educate their patients and, if applicable, their patients' families or caregivers about the safe use, storage, and disposal of controlled substances, especially for those formulations that leave residual drugs to be discarded such as transdermal formulations of fentanyl. Responsible opioid prescribing necessitates that patient education about these topics be a part of every provider–patient opioid agreement.

THE CENTERS FOR DISEASE CONTROL AND PREVENTION AND THE 2016 OPIOID PRESCRIBING GUIDELINE

The 2016 Centers for Disease Control and Prevention's *Guideline for Prescribing Opioids for Chronic Pain* provides "recommendations to primary care physicians who are prescribing opioids for chronic pain outside of active cancer treatment, palliative care, and end-of-life care." It is not a federal statute. However, it is intended to shape opioid prescribing practices and influence the standard of care.

STATE REGULATIONS

State medical boards are responsible for licensing healthcare providers; however, the regulations and requirements regarding licensing can vary significantly from state to state. State medical boards are also responsible for determining the standards of medical practice and subsequent investigation of practitioners who may be practicing outside these standards.

PRESCRIPTION DRUG MONITORING PROGRAMS

Prescription drug monitoring programs (PDMP) help prescribers or law enforcement professionals prevent misuse and abuse of controlled substances by tracking the prescribing and dispensing of controlled substance prescriptions. PDMPs are state specific, and the information recorded, such as which drug schedules are tracked, varies by each PDMP.

Communication between states with PDMPs is uncommon, which creates difficulty for clinicians who service populations across state lines or when a patient initiates care from out of state.

KEY POINTS

1. The Controlled Substance Act is the primary federal regulation governing the medical use of controlled substances.
2. State and federal regulations regarding controlled substances may conflict. Physicians are advised to adhere to the most stringent standards or to seek legal advice in these cases.
3. The DEA limits the amount of Schedule II medications that can be prescribed within a single prescription to no more than a 90-day supply. Refills on Schedule II medications are not allowed.
4. Although not a federal statute, the 2016 Centers for Disease Control and Prevention's *Guideline for Prescribing Opioids for Chronic Pain* provides guidance to prescribers for prescribing opioids for chronic, noncancer pain.
5. The FDA has mandated that manufacturers of long-acting opioid preparations and transdermal immediate-release fentanyl develop risk evaluation and mitigation strategies.

REVIEW QUESTIONS

1. Which of the following is the primary federal regulation governing the medical use of controlled substances?
   A. The Pure Food and Drug Act
   B. The Harrison Narcotic Act
   C. The Marijuana Tax Act
   D. The Controlled Substances Act
2. Prescription drug monitoring programs are intended to monitor:
   A. the prescription of controlled substances between select states that have demonstrated a history of aberrant practitioner prescribing practices.
   B. the prescription of controlled substances between the Veteran Affairs hospital system and civilian medical facilities.
   C. the prescriptions of controlled substances nationally across the United States.
   D. and track the prescription of controlled substances on a state-by-state basis because the programs are individually state funded.
3. Marijuana is listed under which controlled substances schedule in the Controlled Substances Act?
   A. Schedule I
   B. Schedule II
   C. Schedule III
   D. Schedule IV
   E. Marijuana is legal and therefore not scheduled by the Controlled Substances Act.

ANSWERS

1. **D**
2. **D**
3. **A**

SUGGESTED READINGS

Bloodworth D. Opioids in the treatment of chronic pain: legal framework and therapeutic indications and limitations. *Phys Med Rehabil Clin N Am*. 2006;17(2):355-379.

Centers for Disease Control and Prevention, National Center for Injury Prevention and Control. Ten leading causes of death and injury. http://www.cdc.gov/injury/wisqars/leadingcauses.html. Reviewed April 13, 2018. Accessed December 11, 2018.

Dowell D, Haegerich TM, Chou R. CDC guideline for prescribing opioids for chronic pain—United States, 2016. *MMWR Recomm Rep*. 2016;65(1):1-49.

Federation of State Medical Boards. https://www.fsmb.org/. Accessed December 11, 2018.

US Department of Justice, Drug Enforcement Administration. Title 21 Code of Federal Regulations, §1306.7. Administering or dispensing of narcotic drugs. https://www.deadiversion.usdoj.gov/21cfr/cfr/1306/1306_07.htm. Accessed December 11, 2018.

Children and Adolescents

Preventing Substance Use Among Children and Adolescents

Summary by Kenneth W. Griffin and Gilbert J. Botvin

> Based on THE ASAM PRINCIPLES OF ADDICTION MEDICINE, 6th edition chapter by Kenneth W. Griffin and Gilbert J. Botvin

Substance use and substance use disorders are important public health problems that contribute significantly to morbidity and mortality in this country and throughout the world. Epidemiologic research shows that from a population perspective, the onset of substance use typically begins during the adolescent years. Many adolescents who use substances initiate use by experimenting with alcohol and cigarettes, and research demonstrates that this typically begins in a social context with one's peer group. National and international datasets show that the prevalence of alcohol, tobacco, and other drug use increases rapidly from early to late adolescence, peaking during the years of young adulthood. Furthermore, a large body of research has shown that early initiation of substance use is associated with higher levels of use later in life as well as negative outcomes such as violent and delinquent behavior, poor physical health, and mental health problems.

Given the well-established pattern of onset and developmental progression of substance use, a variety of prevention initiatives for children and adolescents have been developed. Initiatives to prevent youth substance use include programs in school, family, and community settings. A goal of many prevention initiatives is to prevent early-stage substance use or delay the onset of use. Most aim to prevent alcohol, tobacco, and marijuana use because these are widely used in our society and pose a great risk to public health. Most prevention programs target middle or junior high school–age youth to prevent substance use experimentation before it begins to occur. The most effective prevention approaches target salient risk and protective factors at the individual, family, and/or community levels and are guided by relevant psychosocial theories regarding the etiology of substance use.

PREVALENCE RATES AND PROGRESSION OF USE

In the United States, national survey data demonstrate that the prevalence rates of use for most substances have gradually declined among adolescents but remain problematic. The 2017 Monitoring the Future study found that among high school seniors, 62% of students reported lifetime alcohol use and 45% reported ever being drunk. The use of electronic vaporizers (including e-cigarettes) was reported by 36% of high school seniors, higher than the lifetime prevalence of cigarette smoking (27%). Findings showed that almost half of 12th graders (49%) reported ever using any illicit drug, and most of this was accounted for by marijuana use (45%). Lifetime prevalence rates were about 5% for each of the following substances: lysergic acid diethylamide, other hallucinogens, ecstasy (3,4-methylenedioxymethamphetamine), cocaine or crack, and inhalants. Lifetime prevalence rates were 1% to 2% for methamphetamine and crystal methamphetamine and 0.7% for heroin. The misuse of any prescription drug (ie, taking a medication "without a doctor telling you to use them") was reported by 17% of high school seniors, and this included the misuse of amphetamines (9%), narcotics other than heroin (7%), tranquilizers (8%), or sedatives/barbiturates (5%).

During early adolescence, substance use occurs largely in a social context. Experimentation often begins with substances that are readily available such as alcohol, tobacco, and inhalants. Eventually, some users of these substances may become regular users and/or progress to marijuana, hallucinogens, and other illicit drugs in a predictable pattern. A subset eventually develops patterns of use characterized by both psychological and physiologic dependence. The initial social motivations for substance use typically yield to those driven increasingly by pharmacologic, genetic, and psychological factors. Prevention programs that effectively target risk factors for alcohol and tobacco use may not only prevent the use of these substances but also may reduce or eliminate the risk of using other substances further along the progression.

ETIOLOGY AND IMPLICATIONS FOR PREVENTION

Substance use is frequently linked to important developmental goals and transitions that occur during adolescence. The degree of substance use involvement of any teenager is often a function of the negative prodrug social influences in his or her environment combined with his or her individual psychosocial vulnerabilities to these influences.

Developmental Aspects

A developmental perspective on the etiology of substance use is informative in understanding how best to prevent early experimentation with alcohol, tobacco, and other drugs. Adolescence is a key period for experimentation not only with substances but also with a wide range of behaviors and activities. Indeed, a great number of changes occur during the years of adolescence, and experimenting with new behavior occurs as part of a natural process of separating from parents, gaining acceptance and popularity with peers, developing a sense of autonomy and independence, establishing a personal identity and self-image, seeking fun and adventure, and/or rebelling against authority. However, from the point of view of an adolescent, engaging in alcohol, tobacco, and other drug use may be a functional way of achieving independence, maturity, or popularity.

The Importance of Social Influences

Research has shown that social influences are among the most powerful factors promoting experimentation or initiation of alcohol, tobacco, and other drug use among young people. Important types of negative social influence include the modeling of substance use behavior by important others (eg, parents, older siblings, and especially peers) and exposure to positive attitudes and expectations regarding substance use. The positive portrayal of substance use by celebrities in movies, television, and music videos is also a powerful negative social influence. Advertisements that communicate positive messages about alcohol and tobacco use are likely to promote pro–substance use attitudes, expectancies, and perceived positive consequences of use that can translate into increases in substance use among young people.

Risk and Protective Factors

Risk and protective factors for adolescent alcohol, tobacco, and illicit drug use occur at the level of the individual, family, school, and community.

Individual Level

These include cognitive, attitudinal, social, personality, pharmacologic, biologic, and developmental factors, including a lack of knowledge about the risks of substance use, believing that substance use is normative, and psychological characteristics such as poor self-esteem, low assertiveness, and poor behavioral self-control. Although most drugs of abuse have different molecular mechanisms of action, they affect the brain in a similar way by increasing strength at excitatory synapses on midbrain dopamine neurons. There are important individual differences in neurochemical reactivity to these drugs that place some individuals at a higher risk.

Family Level

These factors include the direct modeling of substance use behaviors and positive attitudes regarding use by family members, harsh disciplinary practices, poor parental monitoring, low levels of family bonding, and high levels of family conflict. Parenting practices characterized by firm and consistent limit setting, careful monitoring, and nurturing, open communication patterns with children are protective against substance use and other negative outcomes.

School and Community Level

Characteristics of schools have been found to be associated with levels of substance use among students. When large numbers of students feel disengaged from school, feel unsafe at school, or do not have good relationships with teachers, this has been found to be associated with greater substance use prevalence. Similarly, when young people feel disengaged from their communities or feel unsafe in their neighborhoods, this is associated with greater substance use.

TYPES OF PREVENTIVE INTERVENTIONS

Contemporary terminology classifies interventions along a continuum of care that includes prevention, treatment, and maintenance. In this framework, prevention refers only to interventions that occur prior to the onset of a disorder and is divided into three types. *Universal prevention* programs focus on the general population and aim to deter or delay the onset of a condition. *Selective prevention* programs target selected high-risk groups or subsets of the general population believed to be at high risk due to membership in a particular group (eg, pregnant women or children of drug users). *Indicated prevention* programs are designed for those already engaging in the behavior or those showing early danger signs or engaging in related high-risk behaviors.

There have been significant advances in the effectiveness of both drug treatment and prevention programs. However, treatment remains expensive, labor intensive, and suffers from high rates of recidivism. Prevention is therefore a key component in addressing the problem of drug abuse, especially given the increasing availability of effective programs. In recent decades, mounting empirical evidence from a growing number of methodologically sophisticated studies indicates that prevention can be highly effective.

School-Based Prevention Approaches

In the scientific literature on universal prevention programs targeting children and adolescents, schools are the most common implementation site for such programs. School settings are desirable because schools provide access to large numbers of young people, and substance use is inconsistent with the goals of educating our youth. Three types of contemporary approaches to school-based prevention of substance use are (1) social resistance skills training, (2) normative education, and (3) competence enhancement skills training. One or more of these approaches or components may be combined within a single preventive intervention.

Social Resistance Skills

These interventions are designed to increase the adolescent's awareness of the various social influences to engage in substance use and teach young people specific skills for effectively resisting both peer and media pressures to smoke, drink, or use drugs. Resistance skills training programs teach adolescents how to recognize situations in which they are likely to experience peer pressure to smoke, drink, or use drugs along with ways to avoid or otherwise effectively deal with these high-risk situations. Participants are taught ways of handling pressure to engage in substance use, including what to say (ie, the specific content of a refusal message) and how to deliver it in the most effective way possible. Resistance skills programs also typically include content to increase students' awareness of the techniques used by advertisers to promote the sale of tobacco products or alcoholic beverages and teach techniques for formulating counterarguments to the messages used by advertisers.

Normative Education

Because adolescents tend to overestimate the prevalence of smoking and drinking and the use of certain drugs, normative education approaches include content and activities to correct inaccurate perceptions regarding the high prevalence of substance use. This can be done by providing feedback from survey data showing actual prevalence rates collected locally in the classroom, school, or community or by showing the relatively low prevalence rates in national survey data for young teens. Normative education also attempts to undermine popular but inaccurate beliefs that substance drug use is considered acceptable and not particularly dangerous. This can be done by highlighting evidence from national studies showing strong antidrug social norms and generally high-perceived risks of drug use in the population. Materials on normative education is often included in social resistance programs.

Competence Enhancement

These programs recognize that social learning processes are important in the development of adolescent drug use. However, they also recognize that youth with poor personal and social skills are more susceptible to influences that promote drug use, and these youth may be more motivated to use drugs as an alternative to more adaptive coping strategies. Competence enhancement approaches typically teach some combination of the following life skills: general problem-solving and decision-making skills, general cognitive skills for resisting interpersonal or media influences, skills for increasing self-control and self-esteem, adaptive coping strategies for relieving stress and anxiety through the use of cognitive coping skills or behavioral relaxation techniques, general social skills, and general assertive skills. In contrast to the more focused drug resistance skills training approaches, competence enhancement programs are designed to teach the kind of generic skills that will have a relatively broad application. The most effective personal and social skills training programs emphasize the application of general skills to situations directly related to substance use and demonstrate that these same skills can be used for dealing with many of the challenges confronting adolescents in their everyday lives.

With regard to effectiveness, there have been several published meta-analyses of the prevention literature for school-based programs focused on preventing smoking, alcohol use, and illicit drug use among children and adolescents. A meta-analysis of school-based smoking prevention studies found that interventions that combined social resistance and social competence approaches were the only type that showed significant effects on smoking onset in both the short and long term. Programs that provided information only or social resistance skills only were not effective. Other reviews of school-based smoking prevention programs show that the strongest behavioral effects are typically observed for programs that include social resistance combined with cognitive and/or affective skills training activities and/or programs that included both schools and community components in their implementation.

A meta-analysis of universal school-based alcohol prevention programs found that fewer than half of the included studies produced significant reductions in alcohol use relative to a control group. Among the effective studies, the most commonly observed beneficial effects were for heavier levels of alcohol use (eg, drunkenness, binge drinking). A meta-analysis of school-based programs for preventing illicit drug use found that, compared to usual curricula, skills-based interventions significantly reduced marijuana and hard drug use and improved decision-making skills, self-esteem, peer pressure resistance, and drug knowledge. Knowledge and affective programs were not effective at changing behaviors.

In summary, the most effective school-based prevention programs are interactive in nature, focus on building skills in drug resistance and general competence skills, and are implemented over multiple years. School-based programs that have a substantive community component that includes mass media or parental involvement also tend to be more effective than school-only programs. However, only about one in four schools in the United States use one of the ten most effective prevention curricula available and less than one in five providers effectively deliver prevention program content.

Family-Based Prevention Approaches

Family-based prevention programs include training in parenting skills that may focus on ways to nurture, bond, and communicate with children; how to help children develop prosocial skills and social resistance skills; training on rule setting and techniques for monitoring activities; and ways to help children reduce aggressive or antisocial behaviors. Many prevention programs bring parents

and children together in order to improve family functioning, communication, and practice in developing, discussing, and enforcing family policies on substance abuse.

A meta-analysis of family-based programs for preventing smoking found that better trained program staff who delivered programs with high fidelity improved their effectiveness on smoking behavior. In summary, drug prevention programs that focus on both parenting skills and family bonding appear to be the most effective at reducing or preventing substance use. An important limitation of family-based prevention is the difficulty in getting parents to participate; families most at risk for drug use are least likely to participate in prevention programs.

Community-Based Prevention Approaches

Community-based drug prevention programs typically have multiple components, including some combination of school-based programs, family or parenting components, mass media campaigns, public policy components such as restricting youth access to alcohol and tobacco, and other types of community organization and activities. The multiple components of a community-based intervention may be managed by a coalition of stakeholders including parents, educators, and key leaders in the community.

Multicomponent community-based prevention programs can be effective at preventing adolescent substance use, particularly when the different components focus on a coordinated, comprehensive message. Limitations of community-based programs include the expense and the high degree of coordination needed to implement and evaluate the type of comprehensive program most likely to be effective.

SUMMARY AND CONCLUSIONS

Contemporary school-based prevention programs focus on skills building in the areas of drug resistance, life skills, and/or correcting inaccurate beliefs about the high prevalence of substance use. The most effective school-based prevention programs are theory driven, are interactive, focus on building skills in drug resistance and general competence skills, and are implemented over multiple years. School-based programs that include a substantive community component tend to be more effective than school-only programs. Family-based prevention programs include training in parenting skills and/or group interventions for the entire family that focus on improving family functioning, communication, and family policies on substance abuse. Family interventions that combine parenting skills and family bonding appear to be the most effective. Community-based drug abuse prevention programs typically include some combination of school, family, mass media, public policy, and community organization components. The most effective community programs present a coordinated, comprehensive message across multiple delivery components. Online resources helpful in identifying exemplary evidence-based prevention programs include Blueprints for Healthy Youth Development (www.blueprintsprograms.org) and the Social Programs That Work (http://evidencebasedprograms.org).

Despite the progress that has been made in the field of drug prevention for children and adolescents, there are several factors that reduce the public health impact of effective school, family, and community prevention programs. Most schools still use non–evidence-based prevention programs. Effective family programs often do not reach the families in greatest need. Community programs require substantial financial and human resources. In addition to refining our understanding of the risk and protective factors for substance use and translating this knowledge into improved interventions, future research is needed to find ways to effectively disseminate the most promising prevention programs to our schools, families, and communities.

KEY POINTS

1. Most young people who use substances first experiment with alcohol use and cigarette smoking or vaping during early or middle adolescence in a social context with one's peer group.
2. Prevention programs for youth aim to prevent early-stage substance use or delay the onset of use and typically focus on alcohol, tobacco, and marijuana use.
3. From the point of view of an adolescent, engaging in alcohol, tobacco, and other drug use may be seen as a functional way of achieving independence, maturity, or popularity.
4. Effective school-based prevention programs focus on skills building in the areas of drug resistance, life skills, and/or correcting inaccurate beliefs about the high prevalence of substance use.
5. The most effective community-based drug prevention programs present a coordinated,

comprehensive message across multiple settings that may include schools, families, mass media, and public policy components.

REVIEW QUESTIONS

1. Who do drug prevention programs most commonly target?
   A. Parents
   B. Middle school–aged youth
   C. Teachers
   D. Active drug users

2. What are some of the key characteristics of effective school-based prevention programs for adolescent alcohol, tobacco, and other drug use?
   A. Classroom sessions should be interactive rather than lecture based.
   B. Classroom lectures should be provided by peers rather than teachers.
   C. Classroom sessions should build students' social resistance skills.
   D. All of the above.
   E. A and C.

3. What is a particular challenge for schools engaging in drug prevention?
   A. Schools still use non–evidence-based prevention programs.
   B. Teachers are not comfortable delivering anti-drug messages.
   C. Kids are too distracted by other academic duties to listen to drug prevention programs.
   D. Parents resist prevention efforts

ANSWERS

1. **B**
2. **E**
3. **A**

SUGGESTED READINGS

Faggiano F, Minozzi S, Versino E, Buscemi D. Universal school-based prevention for illicit drug use. *Cochrane Database Syst Rev.* 2014;(12):CD003020.

Foxcroft DR, Tsertsvadze A. Universal school-based prevention programs for alcohol misuse in young people. *Cochrane Database Syst Rev.* 2011;(5):CD009113.

Johnston LD, Miech RA, O'Malley PM, et al. *Monitoring the Future national survey results on drug use: 1975-2017. 2017 overview. Key findings on adolescent drug use.* Ann Arbor, MI: Institute for Social Research, The University of Michigan, 2018.

Thomas RE, Baker PR, Thomas BC, Lorenzetti DL. Family-based programmes for preventing smoking by children and adolescents. *Cochrane Database Syst Rev.* 2015;(2):CD004493.

Thomas RE, McLellan J, Perera R. Effectiveness of school-based smoking prevention curricula: systematic review and meta-analysis. *BMJ Open.* 2015;5(3):e006976.

Governmental Policy on Cannabis Legalization and Cannabis as Medicine: Impact on Youth

Summary by Sion Kim Harris, Julie K. Johnson, and John R. Knight Jr.

Based on THE ASAM PRINCIPLES OF ADDICTION MEDICINE, 6th edition sidebar by Sion Kim Harris, Julie K. Johnson, and John R. Knight Jr.

The past two decades have seen a growing trend among US states toward a more liberal cannabis policy, first legalizing its use for medical conditions that purportedly benefit from its analgesic and antiemetic properties and, more recently, legalizing its recreational use by adults aged 21 years and older. As of February 1, 2018, 30 states, the District of Columbia (DC), Puerto Rico, and Guam have passed "medical marijuana" (also known as "cannabis as medicine") policies, and 8 states and DC have enacted "recreational marijuana" policies. (See http://www.ncsl.org /research/health/state-medical-marijuana-laws.aspx for up-to-date information on state laws.) At the federal level, cannabis remains classified as a Schedule 1 substance (ie, no currently accepted medical use, high abuse potential, lack of accepted safety data), making its possession, growth, medicinal prescribing, and distribution for any purpose illegal.

There remains considerable controversy in the scientific and medical communities regarding efficacy, safety, and the potential collateral effects of legalization. Some acute benefits of cannabinoids as medicine have been shown in placebo-controlled trials for nausea and vomiting, appetite loss, neuropathic pain, and muscle spasticity. However, the effects tend to be modest, and the risks of long-term use, addiction, and the adverse effects of smoke inhalation as a delivery system remain of substantial concern.

Recently, the National Academy of Sciences released a draft report, *The Health Effects of Cannabis and Cannabinoids: The Current State of Evidence and Recommendations for Research*, based on an expert panel's systematic review of published evidence. The panel organized its findings into five weighted "strength of evidence" categories: Conclusive, Substantial, Moderate, Limited, and No or Insufficient Evidence. Among its findings of health-risk correlations, they found evidence was *Substantial* for early age of initiation of use and increased risk of developing "problem cannabis use," increased risk of motor vehicle crashes, and the development of schizophrenia or other psychoses. Evidence was *Moderate* for the development of substance use disorders

involving alcohol, tobacco, and illicit drugs; for impairment in cognitive domains of learning, memory, and attention; increased incidence of suicidal ideation, suicide attempts, and suicide completions; and among pediatric populations where cannabis is legal, increased risk of overdose injuries, including respiratory distress.

Consequently, a number of leading medical professional organizations, including the American Medical Association, the American Psychiatric Association, the American Society of Addiction Medicine, and the American Academy of Pediatrics, continue to recommend against cannabis legalization policies. Instead, they all advocate for increased research into the development of standardized, rapid-onset cannabinoid-based pharmaceuticals using safe delivery systems.

Of particular concern is the effect that liberalization of cannabis laws would have on youth, for whom cannabis is the most commonly used illicit drug and the leading cause of their entering substance abuse treatment. It is feared that enactment of any cannabis liberalization policy legalizing cannabis for medicinal or recreational purposes, even if only legal for adults aged 21 years and older, may increase cannabis availability, lower the cost, and send the erroneous message to youth that cannabis is not harmful, thus increasing youth use.

CANNABIS AND THE ADOLESCENT BRAIN

A growing body of neuroscience research suggests that adolescent brains may be particularly vulnerable to the addictive potential of cannabis as well as its neurotoxic effects. In particular, adolescence appears to be the critical period for maturation of the prefrontal cortex and neural networks involving the prefrontal cortex. The prefrontal cortex is central to the performance of "executive" cognitive functions such as attentional control, impulse inhibition, working memory, risk–benefit appraisal, etc. Exposure to substances with addiction potential such as cannabis during this period could interfere with the development of these abilities, potentially with lifelong effects.

Continued

One study examined within-person intelligence quotient changes between the ages of 13 and 38 years and found significant decline in measures of memory, attention, processing speed, reasoning, and comprehension in a linear fashion according to the number of assessment time points in which at least weekly cannabis use was identified. Individuals with heavy cannabis use at three or more time points had the greatest average decline (a loss of approximately six points), whereas those who had never smoked cannabis showed little or no change. Interestingly, among cannabis users, those that had started using at least weekly before the age of 18 years had a much greater decline in their intelligence quotient, and had much less recovery of their neuropsychological functioning with cessation by 38 years of age, than those who had started regular use after 18 years of age.

Exogenous cannabinoids are also known to act in the same manner as other addictive substances like opioids and nicotine. They stimulate the dopaminergic reward pathway, in which neurons in the midbrain and ventral striatum release dopamine in response to rewarding behaviors, which in turn activates the prefrontal cortex, setting up cue-based expectations of and sensitization to those behaviors. Neuroimaging studies have revealed that, relative to the cortical control system, this incentive processing system undergoes more rapid change in adolescence, and may be more sensitive during adolescence to highly rewarding experiences, such as those associated with drug use. Thus, the asynchronous nature of brain system maturation is hypothesized to confer on adolescents a greater vulnerability to the addictive properties of drugs. Epidemiologic data attest to this heightened vulnerability; the National Survey on Drug Use and Health (NSDUH) showed that those starting cannabis use during adolescence had a greater likelihood of reporting cannabis dependence as defined by the *Diagnostic and Statistical Manual of Mental Disorders,* 4th edition, Text Revision (*DSM-IV-TR*), compared to those starting at age 21 years or older. Initiation before 16 years of age was associated with a fourfold increase in risk (17% vs. 4%) compared to initiation at 21 years of age.

In addition to a greater risk for addiction, there is a growing body of scientific evidence showing a clear association between early onset of cannabis use and the development of psychiatric disorders. There is now sufficient evidence for healthcare providers to warn their adolescent patients that using cannabis could result in major mental illness, particularly among those with familial risk.

One systematic review estimated a 40% increase in the risk of psychosis among youth who had ever tried cannabis, and larger effects (50% to 200% increase) were found with more frequent, heavy use.

In light of the growing evidence of the potential harms of early cannabis use, it is particularly concerning that the potency of cannabis products has increased dramatically in recent years, with the percent of tetrahydrocannabinol (THC; the psychoactive ingredient in cannabis) going from an average of 4% in 1995 to about 12% in 2014. The highest potency found in 2015 was in a leaf-based product from Southern California with 31.1% THC. Moreover, there is now widespread availability of THC edibles (cannabis-infused food and beverage products such as candies, cookies, brownies, and tea) and butane-extracted hash oil products (called "dabs," "budder," "shatter," "wax," etc.), which are designed to concentrate THC levels even more so. Cannabidiol (CBD), another component of the cannabis plant which does not have psychoactive properties, has been found to attenuate some of the adverse effects of THC, such as psychosis. However, with rising THC levels, the ratio of THC to CBD in the average cannabis plant and product has also dramatically changed, from a ratio of 14:1 in 1995 to nearly 80:1 in 2014. Thus, increased THC content combined with less CBD in today's cannabis poses a greater risk for users, particularly adolescents. Indeed, nationally, the rate of emergency department visits per 100,000 population for cannabis-related adverse reactions has seen a dramatic rise during this period of growing cannabis liberalization, from 96.2 in 2004 to 146.2 in 2011. Importantly, it is more often CBD and not THC that is associated with any purported medical benefits, raising real questions as to the value of these newer cannabis products being developed.

EFFECTS OF LIBERALIZED CANNABIS POLICY ON YOUTH: WHAT DO WE KNOW?

Eleven studies used nationally representative samples to investigate the potential effects of cannabis-as-medicine policies on youth. Findings have been mixed, with some studies reporting that cannabis-as-medicine states had higher youth cannabis use rates than other states, whereas others found little evidence that these policies significantly changed youth cannabis use. A study by Cerda and colleagues assessed cannabis use, abuse, and dependence rates among individuals aged 12 years or older participating in the NSDUH or National Epidemiologic Survey on Alcohol and Related Conditions. Analyzing all 50 states, this study reported that the average state-level prevalence of past-year use differed significantly in states with (7.1%) and without (3.6%) a cannabis-as-medicine law ($p < .01$), with the odds of past-year use 1.92 times higher and cannabis abuse or dependence 1.81 times higher among individuals living in states with legalized cannabis as medicine. A second study analyzed 2002 to 2008 NSDUH data and found a significantly higher mean adolescent cannabis use rate and lower perceived risk of harm in cannabis-as-medicine states compared to other states. In a replication study, however, this same NSDUH data was reanalyzed using a difference-in-differences approach, comparing trends in adolescent cannabis use before and after state cannabis-as-medicine law passage. In this study, adolescent past-month use rates showed little change after legalization, when additionally controlling for state fixed effects (ie, allowing for control of other unmeasured differences across states). The authors concluded that the associations found in the previous study are unlikely to be causal. Similarly, a more recent study using NSDUH data from 2004 to 2013 that included all 50 states found no significant increase in youth or young adult cannabis use with cannabis-as-medicine legalization but did report increased past-month prevalence among adults aged 26 years and older. Finally, a study that used data from the Monitoring the Future study found that cannabis use was more prevalent in states that passed cannabis-as-medicine laws but that passage of these laws was not associated with a significant change in cannabis use rates in those states.

A limitation of most prior studies is that they did not account for the considerable heterogeneity in cannabis-as-medicine law provisions (eg, dispensary systems, allowing home cultivation, possession limits, mandatory registration, enforcement fidelity, eligible conditions) across states in examining their effects. More recent studies, however, have begun to attempt to parse out the effects of specific provisions or account for law heterogeneity across states using index variables in predictive models. For example, only a few of the cannabis-as-medicine states have allowed commercialization of the dispensary system, allowing for-profit dispensaries to advertise their products and compete for customers. One recent study examined the effect of specific cannabis-as-medicine provisions on youth cannabis use and heavy use rates using state Youth Risk Behavior Survey data from 1991 to 2011 across 45 states. Findings indicated that allowing the possession of no more than 2.5 usable ounces of cannabis predicted significantly increased odds of past 30-day adolescent use compared to states that allowed less or none at all.

Recreational Cannabis Legalization

In 2012, Colorado and Washington were the first states to enact a recreational cannabis policy, followed by Oregon and Alaska in 2014, and California, Massachusetts, Maine, and Nevada in 2016. These laws allow for recreational use of a limited amount of cannabis (ranging from 1 to 2.5 oz) by adults aged 21 years or older. Given the relative newness of these recreational use laws, few studies to date have examined their impact. There have been a few preliminary studies gauging effects in Colorado and Washington. One exploratory study of 238 adolescents in Washington assessed the prevalence of lifetime and past-month cannabis use in two consecutive cohorts recruited in the eighth grade and followed up with in the ninth grade, with the second cohort experiencing the change to recreational use legalization during their follow-up period. They found that cannabis use was higher in the second cohort compared to the first cohort, but this difference was not statistically significant, perhaps due to the small sample size. A second study examined how the recreational law impacted the frequency and consequences of adolescent cannabis use in a sample of 262 Washington students participating in a school-based substance use intervention from 2010 to 2015. This study found similar rates of use among pre– versus post–recreational law participants, but reports of cannabis-related consequences were significantly higher after passage of the recreational law. In Colorado, a qualitative study of adolescent substance use treatment providers in the Denver metro area that explored their views and experiences related to the impact of the recreational law on youth found the following core consequences: Legalization has contributed to cannabis normalization among youth, its consumption has been validated, misperceptions have been reinforced in both adolescents and adults about its potential risks (including that cannabis is a less harmful alternative to tobacco and alcohol), and there is greater access to a large variety of highly potent THC products. Pre– and post–recreational law youth usage trends in Colorado are being closely monitored and disseminated by the Office of National Drug Control Policy's Rocky Mountain High Intensity Drug Trafficking Area Investigative Support Center. According to the

Continued

latest report published in September 2016, Colorado youth aged 12 to 17 years had a 20% increase in the 2-year average past-month cannabis use rate between 2011 and 2012 and between 2013 and 2014, with the 2013 to 2014 rate being the highest of any state in the country, and 74% higher than the national average.

KEY POINTS

1. Because adolescent brain development can be adversely affected by the early initiation of marijuana use, how changing laws surrounding cannabis affect youth usage is of special concern.

2. The changes in laws have resulted in a sharp increase in the potency of leaf marijuana and the wide availability of concentrated oils and edible forms containing THC. At the same time, the CBD content, which is largely responsible for marijuana's therapeutic effects, has been falling.

3. Usage rates among adolescents in states with medical or recreational use laws are higher than states that do not allow use, but research cannot definitively say whether this is a cause and effect relationship.

SUGGESTED READINGS

Committee on Substance Abuse, Committee on Adolescence. The impact of marijuana policies on youth: clinical, research, and legal update. *Pediatrics*. 2015;135(3):584-587.

D'Amico EJ, Tucker JS, Pedersen ER, Shih RA. Understanding rates of marijuana use and consequences among adolescents in a changing legal landscape. *Curr Addict Rep*. 2017;4(4):343-349.

Kilmer B. Recreational cannabis—minimizing the health risks from legalization. *N Engl J Med*. 2017;376(8):705-707.

Levine A, Clemenza K, Rynn M, Lieberman J. Evidence for the risks and consequences of adolescent cannabis exposure. *J Am Acad Child Adolesc Psychiatry*. 2017;56(3):214-225.

Squeglia LM, Gray KM. Alcohol and drug use and the developing brain. *Curr Psychiatry Rep*. 2016;18(5):46.

108

Translational Neurobiology of Addiction from a Developmental Perspective

Summary by Deborah R. Simkin and Ammar El Sara

Based on THE ASAM PRINCIPLES OF ADDICTION MEDICINE, 6th edition chapter by Deborah R. Simkin

BIOPSYCHOSOCIAL ANALYSIS

Prenatal Exposures

Prenatal exposure to nicotine increases a toddler's risk for attention deficit hyperactivity disorder (ADHD) and conduct disorders and has been associated with a lower performance on cognitive testing. Teenagers who had been exposed to marijuana in utero have higher rates of executive function and visual–spatial working memory deficits, attention deficit problems, externalizing behaviors, and psychiatric disorders, including substance use. Fetal alcohol syndrome is the most common nonhereditary cause of intellectual disability, with a prevalence of 0.5 to 3 per 1000 live births, and an incidence that has increased sixfold between 1979 and 1993. The diagnosis of alcohol-related neurodevelopmental disorder refers to children with fetal alcohol syndrome who lack the characteristic facial features and are thus underidentified despite the significant impairment in learning, memory, visual–spatial processes, executive function, and attention. Developmental delays due to prenatal exposure to cocaine are hard to separate from those caused by alcohol, tobacco, marijuana, and the quality of the child's environment. On the other hand, a nurturing environment was found to ameliorate a lower intelligence quotient found at age 4 years in babies exposed to cocaine.

Stress, Drugs, Reward, and the Hypothalamic–Pituitary–Adrenal Axis: Antireward System

Prenatal, postnatal, and early life stressors increase the risk for substance use disorders (SUDs) later in life via the epigenetic modulation of gene expression. Such stressors include fetal distress, hypoxia, prenatal exposure to addictive substances, poor nutrition, sexual abuse, parent's separation, undetected learning

disabilities, and early substance use itself. The role of these stressors is of considerable importance in adolescence, when the interaction between one's genetic background and the environment leads to dysregulation of the hypothalamic–pituitary–adrenal (HPA) axis and permanent neural circuitry changes.

Acute drug use is associated with the activation of the reward neural circuitry, increasing dopamine in the shell of the nucleus accumbens (NAc), as well as other areas, then reverting to a homeostatic state. In contrast, chronic drug use is driven by negative reinforcement, in which the drug is administered to restore the decreased function of the reward system. Chronic drug use is also driven by persistent recruitment of the brain stress system (also called the antireward system). The HPA axis, as well as several neurotransmitters (such as corticotropin-releasing hormone, norepinephrine, and dynorphin, especially in the extended amygdala), are activated during states of stress and during drug withdrawal, thus maintaining a vicious cycle that is furthermore exacerbated by dysregulation of the antistress system (neuropeptide Y). Each time drugs are used, the continued decrease in reward function in the brain reward system and the increased recruitment of the brain antireward system move the brain from a reversible state where homeostasis could have been reinstated to a more dysregulated state. This dysregulation occurs through a process known as allostasis. Rather than the allostatic state reaching stability, it instead causes chronic pathologic states and damage.

Changes in the Brain Reward Circuitry in the Transition to an Addicted State

Adolescence is a transition period that is characterized by an enhanced sensitivity to stress and considerable neurobiological changes, including maturation of the prefrontal cortex (PFC), which may explain a teenager's increased propensity for substance use. When an individual engages in a pleasurable event, like eating ice cream, there is a rapid increase in dopamine in the shell of the NAc. Later, just the anticipation of eating the ice cream would cause an associated release of dopamine, and more incentive salience is given to ice cream by the PFC. This same process occurs when anyone uses a drug of abuse for the first time. In contrast, chronic drug use is associated with the recruitment of glutamatergic efferents from the PFC to the core of NAc, with reduced salience to nondrug stimuli.

Role of Genes

Stressors can turn on genes that can lead to dysregulation of the HPA axis. The number of dopamine receptors genetically inherited may play another role in genetic vulnerability. Other inherited receptors may increase the risk of SUDs, including CB1, the μ-opioid receptor, the nicotinic receptor, as well as corticotropin-releasing factor receptors 1 and 2. Increasingly, molecular pathways that help maintain the SUD state are being identified. Although much more research is needed to further understand the molecular genetics of addiction, additional pharmacotherapies will be discovered.

STUDIES OF INHERITABILITY

Adoption studies have shown that genetic susceptibility seemed to be a stronger predictor of risk for an SUD than exposure to adoptive parents using substances. However, both genetic and environmental influences may be correlated to substance initiation, whereas progression to substance use and an SUD may be more related to genetic factors alone. In addition, studies have demonstrated greater tolerance in children of persons/patients with an alcohol use disorder.

Substance Use History

Young age is an important risk factor. A rapid progression of SUD generally occurs with earlier age of onset and frequency instead of duration of use. The age of onset of heavy drinking also predicts alcohol-related problems. Furthermore, an early age of onset also influences higher risks for the use of other substances.

Personality

Studies have found risk-taking behaviors (eg, smoking, drinking, drugs, sex, driving, gambling) to be associated with specific personality traits (eg, impulsivity, sensation seeking, aggression, sociability) but not to others (eg, neuroticism, anxiety). Other studies have described specific personality types that are associated with a more negative prognosis, including Cloninger Type II and Babor Type B personality.

Comorbidity

Many neuropsychiatric disorders can affect executive function, which is further affected once substance use begins, subsequently interfering with and undermining treatment.

Mood and Conduct Disorders

The antireward system is hyperfunctioning in both untreated depression and chronic drug use, and this may explain why depressed people self-medicate. Although patients with bipolar disorder may use substances to self-medicate their manic symptoms, it is clear that the use of multiple substances, such as marijuana and alcohol, may in reality exacerbate manic symptoms. A unique feature of girls with conduct disorders, SUDs, and depression has been identified. These girls have more anxiety disorders and elevated cortisol levels near sleep onset (when the hypothalamic–pituitary system is expected to be more active) than depressed girls without SUDs. The role that this may play in treatment, if any, is unclear at this time.

Anxiety Disorders

The role of dopamine in the development of social anxiety may help to explain the increased risk of developing an SUD if a social phobia goes untreated. Striatal dopamine reuptake sites were markedly lower in patients with social phobias as compared to controls. The combination of shyness and aggressiveness in boys has been found to be a more valid predictor of future cocaine use than a history of aggressiveness alone. For African American as well as Caucasian women patients, childhood traumatic events were related to the development of adolescent SUDs.

Attention Deficit Hyperactivity Disorder

It is well recognized that patients with co-occurring ADHD and conduct disorders have a much greater risk for developing an SUD than just with ADHD alone. Furthermore, children with untreated ADHD were found to have a two times higher risk of substance use compared to those who were treated with stimulants. Untreated ADHD seems to involve an underactive anterior cingulate and PFC, which could increase the risk of using substances and lead to an SUD.

Exposure to Stimulants for Attention Deficit Hyperactivity Disorder and Attention Deficit Disorder Treatment

There is so much controversy over the use of stimulants in the treatment of ADHD and attention deficit disorder. First and foremost, one must consider the speed with which a drug (recreational or medication) moves through the blood–brain barrier because the addiction liability of a drug is directly related to its speed of entry into the brain and resultant reinforcing effects. Unlike intranasal cocaine, oral methylphenidate does not produce this rapid high because it enters the brain barrier more slowly. Many have postulated that even oral use of stimulant medications may result in dopamine system alterations, which in turn may increase sensitivity to the reinforcing effects of the drug and, hence, increase the risk of later substance use. However, initiation of methylphenidate at an earlier age for the treatment of ADHD was not associated with the development of an SUD and may be protective. It is hypothesized that perhaps the trophic effect on myelination, dendritic branching, and length of spines in the treated youth with ADHD was somehow protective, perhaps by providing a greater brain functional reserve that may be associated with a decreased risk of SUDs.

Learning Disorders

Beyond early onset of use, poor academic achievement, poor social skills, and competence, learning disorders and poor self-esteem were found to be associated with SUDs. Too often, ADHD is assumed to be the reason for school problems, and a comorbid learning disorder goes undetected. In addition, ADHD can be confused with processing problems. Although early detection of learning disorders is essential for reducing the risk for developing an SUD, the timing of the intervention may also be crucial.

DEVELOPMENT OF THE ADOLESCENT BRAIN

It has been suggested that perhaps researchers should consider adolescence as a period wherein two separate entities are independently working: lack of cognitive control and risk taking. These systems have different developmental trajectories, with limbic systems developing earlier than prefrontal control regions.

DEVELOPMENT OF GOAL-DIRECTED BEHAVIOR

Impulsivity generally diminishes with age across childhood and adolescence and is associated with

protracted development of the PFC. In contrast to PFC impulse inhibition/cognitive control, risk taking appears to increase during adolescence relative to childhood and adulthood and is associated with subcortical systems known to be involved in the evaluation of rewards.

EVIDENCE FROM NEUROIMAGING STUDIES OF HUMAN DEVELOPMENT

Magnetic Resonance Imaging Studies of Human Development

Data from longitudinal magnetic resonance imaging studies indicate that gray matter volume has an inverted U-shape pattern, with greater regional variation than white matter. In contrast to gray matter, white matter volume increases in a roughly linear pattern and does so throughout development well into adulthood. These changes presumably reflect ongoing myelination. Some of the largest changes in the brain across development are seen in subcortical regions, particularly in the basal ganglia, especially in males. Magnetic resonance imaging–based prefrontal cortical and basal ganglia regional volumes have been associated with measures of cognitive control.

Diffusion Tensor Imaging Studies of Human Brain Development

In multiple studies, diffusion tensor imaging has shown associations between measures of prefrontal white matter development and cognitive control in children. These findings underscore the importance of examining not only regional but also circuitry-related changes when making claims about age-dependent changes in neural substrates of cognitive development.

Functional Magnetic Resonance Imaging Studies of Behavioral and Brain Development

The ability to measure functional changes in the developing brain with magnetic resonance imaging has significant potential for the field of developmental science. Collectively, these studies show that children recruit distinct but often larger, more diffuse prefrontal regions when performing tasks than do adults. In addition, during adolescence, relative to adulthood, an immature ventral PFC may not provide sufficient top-down control of robustly activated reward processing regions (eg, accumbens), resulting in less influence of prefrontal systems (orbitofrontal cortex) relative to the accumbens in reward valuation.

Why Would the Brain Be Programmed to Develop This Way?

Evolutionarily speaking, adolescence is the period in which independence skills are acquired to increase success upon separation from the protection of the family. Specifically, risk taking and novelty seeking may provide a mechanism for increasing exposure to the environment. However, high-risk behaviors increase the chances for harmful circumstances (eg, injury, depression, anxiety, drug use, SUDs).

BIOLOGIC PREDISPOSITIONS, DEVELOPMENT, AND RISK

Although adolescents may be more prone to risky choices as a group, some are more prone than others due to individual and developmental differences. Such differences are postulated to include variations in dopaminergic mesolimbic circuitry as well as allelic variants in dopamine-related genes.

THE ROLE OF FAMILY AND PEERS DURING KEY DEVELOPMENTAL STAGES

Modeling the use of substances by parents when children are young increases the notion that alcohol and other drugs are not harmful substances, which may increase the risk of using as a teen. Peers have a stronger influence on adolescents than their parents and influence not only initiation of use but also rates of relapse.

OTHER FACTORS INFLUENCING THE HYPOTHALAMIC–PITUITARY–ADRENAL AXIS

New research is beginning to reveal associations between alcohol use and early developmental factors that increase intestinal permeability, including prematurity, lack of breastfeeding, cesarean sections, early exposure to antibiotics, and signs of food sensitivities including being colicky and eczema. Increased gut permeability can influence the afferent vagus nerve found in the gut. This stimulates the stress system in the HPA axis and can result in depression and anxiety, subsequently influencing alcohol consumption. The use of probiotics and other interventions in those with an alcohol use disorder may allow for another avenue for treatment interventions.

EFFECTS OF EARLY ONSET AND PERSISTENT MARIJUANA USE

In one birth cohort study, persistent cannabis users showed global neuropsychological decline. Furthermore, this decline was still apparent after controlling for years of education and after ruling out multiple other alternative explanations. Interestingly, memory dysfunction induced by cannabis was generally robust, particularly for those using cannabis with a lower proportion of cannabidiol and a higher proportion of Δ9-tetrahydrocannabinol. Because the hippocampus appears to have the highest density of CB1 receptors, higher tetrahydrocannabinol in today's cannabis may cause more neurotoxic effects on the developing brain.

KEY POINTS

1. Adolescence is a transition period that is characterized by enhanced sensitivity to stress and considerable neurobiological changes, which inherently increases the risk for substance use.
2. Understanding risk factors for addiction can guide efforts aimed toward early interventions.

REVIEW QUESTIONS

1. Which area of the brain develops the latest in adolescents and may be responsible for the inability to inhibit the drive to seek out pleasurable experiences?
   A. Basolateral amygdala
   B. Prefrontal cortex
   C. Nucleus accumbens
   D. HPA axis

2. Which of the following changes to the antireward system would increase the risk of developing an addiction?
   A. An increase in neuropeptide Y
   B. Decreased norepinephrine
   C. A decrease in corticotropin-releasing hormone
   D. A decrease in neuropeptide Y

3. Which statement is *true* about adoption studies examining the risk of developing an SUD?
   A. Both genetic susceptibility and exposure to adoptive parents using substances equally predicted the risk for an SUD.
   B. Exposure to adoptive parents who use substances is a stronger predictor of risk for an SUD than genetic susceptibility.
   C. Genetic susceptibility is a stronger predictor of risk for an SUD than exposure to adoptive parents who use substances.
   D. Genetic susceptibility but not exposure to adoptive parents who use substances predicted the risk for an SUD.

ANSWERS

1. **B**
2. **D**
3. **D**

SUGGESTED READINGS

Biederman J, Wilens T, Mick E, Spencer T, Faraone SV. Pharmacotherapy of attention-deficit/hyperactivity disorder reduces risk for substance use disorder. *Pediatrics*. 1999;104(2):e20.

Blum K, Braverman ER, Holder JM, et al. Reward deficiency syndrome: a biogenetic model for the diagnosis and treatment of impulsive, addictive, and compulsive behaviors. *J Psychoactive Drugs*. 2000;32(suppl i-iv):1-112.

Casey BJ, Tottenham N, Liston C, Durston S. Imaging the developing brain: what have we learned about cognitive development? *Trends Cogn Sci*. 2005;9(3):104-110.

Koob G. The neurobiology of addiction: a neuroadaptational view relevant for diagnosis. *Addiction*. 2006;101(suppl 1): 23-30.

Zuckerman M, Kuhlman DM. Personality and risk-taking: common biological factors. *J Pers*. 2000;68(6):999-1029.

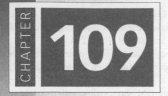

Screening and Brief Intervention for Adolescents

Summary by Traci L. Brooks, John R. Knight Jr., and Sion Kim Harris

Based on THE ASAM PRINCIPLES OF ADDICTION MEDICINE, 6th edition chapter by Traci L. Brooks, John R. Knight Jr., and Sion Kim Harris

Substance use usually begins during childhood and adolescence, making addiction a pediatric-onset disorder. Primary care offices offer an excellent venue for reaching adolescents; greater than three in four adolescents see a physician yearly and many have trusting, long-term relationships with their providers. The annual wellness visit also affords an important opportunity for preventive guidance or to identify substance use early and intervene before a serious problem occurs.

There are several goals for screening: (1) to determine whether a teen has used alcohol or drugs during the past 12 months, (2) to determine whether teens who have used alcohol or drugs are at low risk or high risk for developing substance use disorders, (3) to give pertinent health advice to teens who are at risk of acute consequences of alcohol or other drug use as well as give positive feedback to teens who have never used, and (4) to refer teens who are at high risk of long-term consequences of substance use to the appropriate level of intervention. These goals can be summarized as screening, brief intervention, and referral to treatment.

SCREENING FOR USE

The National Institute on Alcohol Abuse and Alcoholism recommends screening children as young as 9 years of age. However, for children younger than 12 years of age, we recommend first asking, "Do you know what alcohol is?" and "Do you know what marijuana is?" Those who reply with "no" may not be appropriate candidates for additional questions.

For those 12 years of age and older, first meet with the parent and patient together to review the ground rules of confidentiality. Emphasize that the details discussed will remain confidential unless they have immediate concerns about the safety of the patient or others. Injection drug use, reports of overdose, or substance-related injuries are likely to trigger safety concerns, whereas sporadic use of alcohol or marijuana by themselves may not. Reassure the adolescent that if it becomes necessary to inform a parent about an acute risk to safety, you will first discuss it with them, so the patient does not feel blindsided or betrayed. After everyone agrees, then ask the parent(s) to leave the room.

Screening for drug and alcohol use is best accomplished with a structured interview or validated questionnaire, rather than an informal history and one's own clinical impressions. The most sensitive approach is to ask "presumptive" questions such as "During the past 12 months, on how many days have you had a drink containing alcohol?" Similar questions follow on the use of marijuana and other drugs (Fig. 109-1). Many adolescents prefer to answer questions about substance use on paper or on a computer immediately before seeing their providers. This must be done in a private location where parents cannot see their child's responses.

SCREENING FOR RISKS AND PROBLEMS

Several tools have been developed to screen patients for high-risk use of alcohol and other drugs. In general, these tools are either self-completion questionnaires (such as the Alcohol Use Disorders Identification Test, or AUDIT, and the Problem Oriented Screening Instrument for Teenagers, or POSIT), or

The CRAFFT Interview (version 2.1)

To be orally administered by the clinician

Begin: *"I'm going to ask you a few questions that I ask all my patients. Please be honest. I will keep your answers confidential."*

Part A

During the PAST 12 MONTHS, on how many days did you:

1. Drink more than a few sips of beer, wine, or any drink containing **alcohol**? Say "0" if none.

   # of days

2. Use any **marijuana** (weed, oil, or hash, by smoking, vaping, or in food) or "**synthetic marijuana**" (like "K2," "Spice") or "vaping" **THC oil**? Put "0" if none.

   # of days

3. Use **anything else to get high** (like other illegal drugs, prescription or over-the-counter medications, and things that you sniff, huff, or vape)? Say "0" if none.

   # of days

Did the patient answer "0" for all questions in Part A?

Yes ☐   No ☐

↓   ↓

Ask CAR question only, then stop   **Ask all six CRAFFT* questions below**

Part B

		No	Yes
C	Have you ever ridden in a **CAR** driven by someone (including yourself) who was "high" or had been using alcohol or drugs?	☐	☐
R	Do you ever use alcohol or drugs to **RELAX**, feel better about yourself, or fit in?	☐	☐
A	Do you ever use alcohol or drugs while you are by yourself, or **ALONE**?	☐	☐
F	Do you ever **FORGET** things you did while using alcohol or drugs?	☐	☐
F	Do your **FAMILY** or **FRIENDS** ever tell you that you should cut down on your drinking or drug use?	☐	☐
T	Have you ever gotten into **TROUBLE** while you were using alcohol or drugs?	☐	☐

*Two or more YES answers suggest a serious problem and need for further assessment. See back for further instructions ➡

NOTICE TO CLINIC STAFF AND MEDICAL RECORDS:
The information on this page is protected by special federal confidentiality rules (42 CFR Part 2), which prohibit disclosure of this information unless authorized by specific written consent. A general authorization for release of medical information is NOT sufficient.

Figure 109-1. The CRAFFT Interview (version 2.1).

oral interviews (such as the CAGE). One screening tool, the CRAFFT can be administered either way. It begins with presumptive questions on use, and then goes on to screen for substance-related risks and problems.

CRAFFT is a mnemonic acronym composed of the first letters of key words in its six questions: Car, Relax, Alone, Forget, Family/Friends, and Trouble (see Fig. 109-1). Each "yes" response is scored 1 point. A score of 2 or greater is a positive screen and indicates that the adolescent is at a high risk for having an alcohol- or drug-related disorder. All adolescents, including those who report abstinence from alcohol and drugs, should be asked whether they have ever ridden in a car with a driver who was high or had used alcohol or drugs. To increase time efficiency, clinicians can ask the remaining questions only to those who report use.

SCREEN-SPECIFIC STRATEGIES
Physician Brief Advice

Brief advice is 2 to 3 minutes of clinician counseling that occurs at the time of the screening. It is aimed at reinforcing the choices of those at low risk, encouraging risk reduction in those at medium risk, and encouraging those at high risk to try to stop their use at least until a return visit. A suggested guiding framework for brief advice includes five Rs: review of the screening results, recommend not to use, riding/driving risk counseling, response (elicit self-motivational statements), and reinforce self-efficacy (Fig. 109-2).

Low Risk: No Use/Car Question Negative

Adolescents that have been abstinent from alcohol and drugs should receive praise and encouragement from their clinicians. Statements such as, "It sounds as if you have made healthy choices by not using drugs or alcohol. If that ever changes, I hope you will feel comfortable enough to talk to me about it" aim both to praise the young person's abstinence and avail the opportunity for open communication in the future.

Medium Risk: No Use/Car Question Positive

All adolescents who have ridden with a driver who is intoxicated should receive a copy of the "Contract for Life," a document that asks adolescents never to ride with a driver who has been drinking or using drugs and also asks parents to promise to provide safe, sober transportation home without any discussion until the next day.

Medium Risk: Use Question Positive/ CRAFFT <2

Adolescents who report alcohol or other drug use but screen negative (0 or 1 on the CRAFFT) should receive brief advice to stop using, such as: "My recommendation is not to use alcohol or drugs at all, because they can harm your brain development, interfere with learning, place you in dangerous situations, and pose a serious risk to your health." The clinician could challenge the patient to a time-limited trial of abstinence (eg, 1 week to 3 months) and ask him or her to come for a return visit to discuss how it went.

High Risk: CRAFFT ≥2

Adolescents who screen positive (CRAFFT score of 2 or more) need further assessment. When there is insufficient time to perform a more detailed assessment, the best strategy is a return visit. First show the bar graph at the top of Figure 109-2 to the patient and ask, "Your score was X; where does that place your level of risk?" Then make a statement such as, "I am concerned about you and would like us to have an appointment next week to talk again. Is that ok?" Ask the patient to agree to no alcohol or drug use until the return visit but clarify this statement with "Even if you do use, I'd still like for you to come back. We can discuss why it was so difficult for you to abstain."

ASSESSMENT
Interviewing Adolescents

For any patient, a nonjudgmental, empathetic interviewing style encourages more information sharing than an interrogative style. The interviewer should use open-ended questions to begin the conversation, with an emphasis on the pattern of drug use over time. At times, cues from the clinician may help the adolescent make connections between drug use and consequences. For example, statements such as, "It seems that your grades started to fall at the same time that you started using more marijuana" may help the adolescent associate the two occurrences.

Physical Exam

Adolescents who have a positive screen for high-risk substance use should have a physical exam to look for signs of intoxication or withdrawal (eg, changes in pupil size, blood pressure or heart rate, diaphoresis, slurred speech, difficulty with balance or walking). Signs of chronic drug use, such as injection

1. Show your patient his/her score on this graph and discuss level of risk for a substance use disorder.

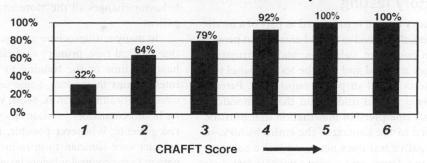

Percent with a DSM-5 Substance Use Disorder by CRAFFT score*

CRAFFT Score ➡

*Data source: Mitchell SG, Kelly SM, Gryczynski J, Myers CP, O'Grady KE, Kirk AS, & Schwartz RP. (2014). The CRAFFT cut-points and DSM-5 criteria for alcohol and other drugs: a reevaluation and reexamination. Substance Abuse, 35(4), 376–80.

2. Use these talking points for brief counseling.

1. **REVIEW** screening results
   For each "yes" response: *"Can you tell me more about that?"*

2. **RECOMMEND** not to use
   "As your doctor (nurse/health care provider), my recommendation is not to use any alcohol, marijuana or other drug because they can: 1) Harm your developing brain; 2) Interfere with learning and memory, and 3) Put you in embarrassing or dangerous situations."

3. **RIDING/DRIVING** risk counseling
   "Motor vehicle crashes are the leading cause of death for young people. I give all my patients the Contract for Life. Please take it home and discuss it with your parents/guardians to create a plan for safe rides home."

4. **RESPONSE** elicit self-motivational statements
   Non-users: *"If someone asked you why you don't drink or use drugs, what would you say?"* Users: *"What would be some of the benefits of not using?"*

5. **REINFORCE** self-efficacy
   "I believe you have what it takes to keep alcohol and drugs from getting in the way of achieving your goals."

3. Give patient Contract for Life. Available at www.crafft.org/contract

Figure 109-2.

"track marks" or nasal septum erosions, are rare in teens but should be discussed with the adolescent and recorded in the chart if present.

Laboratory Testing

If laboratory testing is to be used as part of a medical workup, the clinician should ensure that proper specimen collection, validation, and confirmation techniques are used and that the testing panel will include tests for all suspected substances. Parents and patients should understand that a laboratory test is only one piece of information that must be interpreted in the context of the entire history—a single negative test does not prove that a teenager is not using drugs, and a single positive test does not confirm a substance use disorder. Ethical and confidentiality issues as they relate to drug testing in adolescents are reviewed in the sidebars of Chapter 111.

REFERRAL TO TREATMENT

Brief Interventions

Brief interventions consist of several counseling sessions delivered over a few weeks or months, aimed at reducing substance use and its related health risks. They have been shown to have modest but significant effects in the range of 25% to 30%. Brief interventions have been shown to be effective for adolescents in reducing both alcohol use and marijuana use in multiple settings such as schools, emergency departments, and primary care settings.

Most brief interventions are based on motivational interviewing (MI), a nonconfrontational counseling style that seeks to create conditions necessary for positive behavioral change. MI is based on a core assumption that motivation is a product of interpersonal interaction and not an innate character trait. Confrontation leads to resistance, whereas empathy and understanding leads to change. Core strategies of MI include developing a discrepancy between goals or values and current behavior, avoiding arguments, rolling with resistance, empathy as a counseling style, and supporting self-efficacy.

One application of MI to a medical encounter is the Brief Negotiated Interview, originally created for the emergency department. According to Boston University School of Public Health, "The [brief negotiated interview] helps health care providers explore health behavior change with patients in a respectful, non-judgmental way within a finite time period. Instead of telling the patient what changes

he/she should make, the [brief negotiated interview] is intentionally designed to elicit reasons for change and action steps from the patient. It gives the patient voice and choice, making any potential behavior changes all the more empowering to the patient."

In many settings where adolescents receive routine medical care, primary care clinicians may not have the time or the training to implement brief interventions themselves. Some settings may have colocated health educators, social workers, or mental health counselors to whom they can refer high-risk patients. Whenever possible, it is best for the primary care clinician to introduce the adolescent patient to the counselor before leaving the office. Referrals for subsequent appointments have high rates of noncompletion. In one study, none of 75 patients of an adolescent clinic kept follow-up appointments with a clinic social worker.

KEY POINTS

1. Easily implemented substance use screens can quickly and reliably identify teens at high risk of having a substance use disorder.
2. Teens at low risk can be effectively counseled in a primary care setting with just a few minutes of clinician advice.
3. For teens with more serious substance use disorders, experienced clinicians can follow up with a brief assessment to determine the appropriate level of care and make referrals.

REVIEW QUESTIONS

1. Screening adolescents for drug and alcohol use is best accomplished by:
   A. asking parents if they're aware of any substance use.
   B. collecting an observed urine specimen for immunoassay testing.
   C. asking a presumptive question such as, "During the past 12-months, how many times have you used alcohol?"
   D. asking a nonspecific question such as, "What kinds of experiences have you had with drug and alcohol use?"

2. Adolescents who report no use of drugs or alcohol during the past 12 months should be asked:
   A. nothing more.
   B. all six CRAFFT questions.
   C. the Alone question only.
   D. the Car question only.

3. Core strategies of motivational interviewing include:
   A. developing a discrepancy between goals or values and current behavior.
   B. developing an improved understanding of what triggers substance use.
   C. learning the warning signs of a developing addictive disorder.
   D. listing alternatives to attending a party where there will be drug and alcohol use.

ANSWERS

1. **C**
2. **D**
3. **A**

SUGGESTED READINGS

Boston University School of Public Health. *The Brief Negotiated Interview (BNI)*. Boston, MA: BNI ART Institute. https://www.bu.edu/bniart/sbirt-in-health-care/sbirt-brief-negotiated-interview-bni/. Accessed November 30, 2018.

D'Amico EJ, Parast L, Meredith LS, et al. Screening in primary care: what is the best way to identify at-risk youth for substance use? *Pediatrics.* 2016;138(6):e20161717.

Harris SK, Louis-Jacques J, Knight JR. Screening and brief intervention for alcohol and other abuse. *Adolesc Med State Art Rev.* 2014;25(1):126-156.

Miller WR, Rollnick S. *Motivational Interviewing: Helping People Change.* 3rd ed. New York: Guilford Press, 2012.

Naar-King S, Suarez M. *Motivational Interviewing with Adolescents and Young Adults.* New York: Guilford Press, 2010.

National Institute on Alcohol Abuse and Alcoholism. *Alcohol Screening and Brief Intervention for Youth: A Practitioner's Guide.* Washington, DC: National Institutes of Health, 2015. NIH Publication No. 11-7805.

CHAPTER 110

Assessing Adolescent Substance Use

Summary by Ken C. Winters, Andria M. Botzet, and Randy Stinchfield

Based on THE ASAM PRINCIPLES OF ADDICTION MEDICINE, 6th edition chapter by Ken C. Winters, Andria M. Botzet, Randy Stinchfield, and Walker H. Krepps

Adolescent onset of drug use greatly increases the estimated risk for developing a substance use disorder (SUD) and can lead to a variety of other negative consequences, including failing in school, risky sexual behavior, delinquency, incarceration, suicidality, motor vehicle injuries/fatalities, possible damage to the brain's memory region, and significant medical healthcare costs. A precise assessment of adolescent drug use is essential to gain an accurate understanding of the nature and extent of adolescent drug use and to inform possible intervention or treatment needs.

PRINCIPLES OF ASSESSMENT

Screening is the first step in identifying whether a youth may be involved with drugs. Screening results should be used to determine the need for a comprehensive assessment. The comprehensive assessment is used to explore the extent and nature of the drug involvement, consequential problems, and treatment needs.

Screening

For adolescents, the assessment process should begin with screening questions pertaining to recent drug use quantity and frequency (eg, How often did you use the following drugs in the past 6 months?), the presence of adverse consequences of use (eg, Has your drug use led to problems with your parents?), and situations in which drug use is common.

Comprehensive Assessment

If the screening suggests a possible drug use problem, a more comprehensive assessment can determine details of drug use history, consequences, whether criteria is met for an SUD, and what other behavioral and mental co-occurring problems may exist. This assessment, which may involve interviews, questionnaires, or both, should include a detailed inquiry into the age of onset and progression of use for specific substances; circumstances; and the type, frequency, and variability of drugs used recently and historically. Additional areas to assess are context of use; mode of administration; use patterns of peers; environmental factors that promote or prevent use; triggers associated with drug use; the negative consequences of use in the domains of school, social, family, psychological functioning, and physical/medical problems; and the adolescent's problem recognition and readiness for treatment.

DEVELOPMENTAL CONSIDERATIONS

Identifying Clinical Significance

Most often, adolescent substance use involves alcohol, tobacco, or both. However, the use of marijuana among youth is increasing in recent years; it is the most commonly used illicit drugs among adolescents. Although the majority of youth will not progress beyond the recreational use of drugs, it is estimated that between 5% and 15% will meet the formal criteria for an SUD during adolescence. Two major factors that increase the risk of an SUD are (1) early onset of drug use and (2) a preexisting behavioral or mental disorder, such as attention deficit hyperactivity disorder (ADHD), conduct disorder, or trauma.

Substance Use Disorder Criteria

The *Diagnostics and Statistical Manual of Mental Disorders*, 5th edition (*DSM-5*) criteria for an SUD include changes from the *DSM-IV* that are relevant to adolescents and supported by research and clinical observation: the elimination of the abuse and dependence categories, the elimination of the "legal problems" symptom, and the addition of the symptom pertaining to craving and a strong desire to use. But some of the criteria are problematic when applied to adolescents. For example, the two physiologic symptoms, tolerance and withdrawal, are not highly relevant to young people who are going through neurodevelopmental changes and are not yet chronic users.

Neurobiology

The brain, particularly the prefrontal cortex region that is responsible for judgment, goes through significant neurodevelopment during adolescence. The young brain does not fully develop until early adulthood, and research supports the view that the developing adolescent brain is more vulnerable to the effects of drug use compared to a fully mature brain.

METHODS OF ASSESSMENT

Self-Reporting

Self-reporting is a hallmark of a clinical assessment given its convenience, comprehensiveness, low cost, and the perception that the individual is the most knowledgeable reporter. Self-reporting formats include self-administered questionnaires, interviews, timeline follow-backs, and computer-assisted interviews. Self-administered questionnaires and interviews are the primary approaches used by clinicians. Research on the concordance of self-administered questionnaires, interviews, timeline follow-backs, and computer-assisted interviews suggests that, for the most part, the various formats yield similar levels of disclosure.

Underreporting of the quantity and type of drug use on self-report measures by adolescents can occur. In response, improved drug testing techniques (discussed in the following sections) are available to corroborate adolescent self-reporting of drug use. Youth may also see the self-report assessment as an opportunity to "cry for help" or exaggerate their responses. Despite possible limitations, the validity of self-reporting for adolescent drug use has been supported by several lines of evidence: Only a small percentage of youth are detected by scales intended to detect faking tendencies; adolescent self-reports agree with corroborating sources of information such as archival records and, for the most part, urinalyses; and the base rate of elevations on "faking good" and "faking bad" scales is relatively low.

Also, an important condition for detailed and valid self-disclosures is good rapport between the client and clinician.

Drug Testing

Urinalyses, hair analyses, saliva testing, and sweat testing are all used to detect exposure to drugs. Newer biomarkers for alcohol, such as ethyl glucuronide (urine or hair) and phosphatidylethanol (blood), hold promise of detecting alcohol for longer periods (days) compared to standard procedures and with greater accuracy. The primary aspect that distinguishes these specimens is the period or window of time for which the drug can be detected. Additional considerations are cost, access, tampering vulnerability, invasiveness, and reliability.

Other Sources

Observable signs of use may indicate the acute effects of or withdrawal from drug use (eg, sweating, pupil size). Information from peers also may be a valuable resource, especially if the peers are not currently using drugs or are in recovery. Whereas parents are usually willing to provide a report about their adolescent, it is not likely that they can provide detailed reports about drug use by their child.

CLINICAL CONTENT

Psychosocial Factors

Psychosocial dimensions provide valuable information and should be included in the assessment protocol. Variables include interpersonal relationships, school and employment, history of criminal justice involvement and delinquency, recreational activities, and sexual behavior. Details of core psychosocial variables are presented as follows.

Peer Factors

Peer variables are one of the most prominent factors contributing to the onset and maintenance of drug use. Youth who associate with peers who use drugs are far more likely to use drugs than those who do not associate with peers who use drugs.

Family Factors

Family influences encompass several variables, including familial genetic risk and parenting practices. Children whose parents suffer from an SUD have been shown to be at increased risk for the development of an SUD. The importance of parenting factors cannot be understated; increased drug use among adolescents is associated with families that lack closeness or affection, lack effective discipline, lack supervision, have excessive or weak parental control, and have inconsistent parenting. Also, parental antisocial behavior history is relevant in offspring SUD liability.

Psychological Benefits

Many adolescents use drugs because these serve psychological need states including mood enhancement, stress reduction, and relief from boredom.

Co-Occurring Mental or Behavioral Disorders

Most adolescents who are involved with drugs have co-occurring behavioral or mental disorders, and when present, they often are associated with poorer recovery from a drug problem compared to adolescents without a co-occurring disorder. Childhood aggression, rebelliousness, theft, and destructiveness, along with related externalizing disorders such as conduct disorder and oppositional defiant disorder, are common among youth with an SUD as well as among children who have a parent with a history of an SUD. Antisocial behaviors and ADHD during childhood are moderately predictive of adolescent-onset drug use. However, the complex relationship between these externalizing disorders most certainly involves the impact by other variables (eg, youth with ADHD who are receiving pharmacotherapy tend to have lower SUD liability compared to youth with ADHD who do not receive treatment). Internalizing disorders such as anxiety disorders, posttraumatic stress disorder, and mood disorders (eg, major depression) may be another pathway associated with SUDs. These disorders may contribute to the adolescent seeking psychological relief. Also, in some instances, drug use may further aggravate these very negative states that the teenager is striving to address.

Impact on Treatment Outcome

Many of the variables discussed have been found to predict the course of drug involvement among adolescents who are receiving drug treatment. Pretreatment characteristics that are associated with more favorable substance use outcomes include a lower substance use severity level at admission, greater readiness to change, and fewer conduct problems or other co-occurring psychopathology. Factors influencing better outcomes during treatment include a longer length of treatment and family involvement in treatment. Posttreatment predictors of better outcome include participation in aftercare, low levels of peer substance use, ability to use coping skills, and continued commitment to abstain.

INSTRUMENTATION

Several psychometrically sound screening and comprehensive tools exist to evaluate adolescents suspected of substance use and also can be administered at the conclusion of treatment to evaluate treatment outcome. A select group of tools are summarized in Table 110-1. Two instrument categories are discussed in the following sections.

Screening Tools

A screener is a brief and efficient method that indicates if a client is in need of a more comprehensive assessment. The CRAFFT interview is a specialized six-item screen designed to be administered verbally during a primary care interview to address both alcohol and drug use. The Global Appraisal of Individual Needs—Short Screener consists of 20 items that screen for drug use and related problems. The 40-item Personal Experience Screening Questionnaire consists of a problem severity scale, drug use history, select psychosocial problems, and response distortion tendencies ("faking good" and "faking bad"). The Screening to Brief Intervention tool utilizes frequency of use items to categorize the adolescent's substance use into different risk categories.

Comprehensive Assessment Instruments

If an initial screening indicates the need for a further assessment, clinicians and researchers can employ various diagnostic interviews, problem-focused interviews, and multiscale questionnaires. Diagnostic interviews, which focus on *DSM*-based criteria, address numerous psychiatric disorders, including SUDs. One example is the Global Appraisal of Individual Needs. As opposed to the Short Screener version, this more robust semistructured interview covers recent and lifetime functioning in several areas, including substance use, legal and school functioning, and psychiatric symptoms. Other comprehensive tools are self-administered and measure several problem areas associated with adolescent drug involvement; an example is the Personal Experience Inventory.

ACKNOWLEDGMENTS

The authors wish to extend gratitude to Tamara Fahnhorst and Ali Nicholson for their contributions to an earlier version of this chapter.

TABLE 110-1 Select Screening and Comprehensive Tools

Screening Tools

Instrument	Study Settings	Format	Administration Time	Manual Available	Scoring Time	Computer Scoring	Fee for Use	Source
CRAFFT	Clinic, drug treatment	6 items	5 min	Yes	2 min	No	No	https://www.integration.samhsa.gov/clinical-practice/sbirt/CRAFFT_Screening_interview.pdf
Global Appraisal of Individual Needs—Short Screener (GAIN-SS)	Clinic, drug treatment	20 items	10 min	Yes	2 min	Yes	No	http://gaincc.org/instruments/
Personal Experience Screening Questionnaire (PESQ)	Clinic, drug treatment, school	40 items	10 min	Yes	5 min	No	Yes	http://lib.adai.washington.edu/instruments
Screening to Brief Intervention (S2BI)	Pediatric clinic	3-7 items	5 min	No	2 min	Yes	No	http://www.ncbi.nlm.nih.gov/pmc/articles/PMC4270364

Comprehensive Tools

Instrument	Study Settings	Format	Administration Time	Manual Available	Scoring Time	Computer Scoring	Fee for Use	DSM-5	Source
Global Appraisal of Individual Needs (GAIN)	Clinic, drug treatment, juvenile detention	Semistructured interview	75-100 min	Yes	15 min	Yes	Yes	Yes	http://gaincc.org/instruments/
Teen Addiction Severity Index (T-ASI)	Clinic, drug treatment, juvenile detention	Semistructured interview	25-45 min	Yes	10 min	No	No	Yes	http://www.emcdda.europa.eu/attachements.cfm/att_4008_EN_tt-asi.pdf
Personal Experience Inventory (PEI)	Clinic, drug treatment, juvenile detention	Self-report	45-60 min	Yes	10 min	Yes	Yes	No	http://lib.adai.washington.edu/instruments

KEY POINTS

1. An assessment of adolescent drug involvement and SUDs is a critical first step when addressing the possible preventive intervention or treatment needs for the teenager. Drug use during adolescence significantly elevates the risk to develop an SUD compared to those who wait until adulthood to use.
2. Brain development during adolescence is incomplete, especially in the prefrontal cortex, which governs judgment. This and many other factors unique to adolescents demand assessments that are tailored to youth.
3. Many factors can influence the onset of adolescent drug use and the course of use and resulting consequences, including peer influences, parenting practices, and the presence of co-occurring mental health conditions, including externalizing and internalizing disorders.

REVIEW QUESTIONS

1. True or False: Parents are a very reliable source of their child's possible drug use.

2. Which of the following is not one of adjustments in the *DSM-5* with regard to adolescent substance use disorders?
   A. The distinction between abuse and dependence was eliminated.
   B. An adolescent definition of SUD is provided.
   C. Legal problems resulting from drug use criteria are eliminated.

3. What is another option to the self-report method?
   A. Drug testing
   B. Parent report
   C. Peer report
   D. All of the above.

ANSWERS

1. **False**
2. **B**
3. **D**

SUGGESTED READINGS

Alcohol and Drug Abuse Institute Library. Substance use screening & assessment instruments database. http://lib.adai.washington.edu/. Updated August 2018. Accessed October 25, 2018.

Brown SA, McGue M, Maggs J, et al. A developmental perspective on alcohol and youth 16 to 20 years of age. *Pediatrics*. 2008;121(suppl 4):S290-S310.

National Institute on Drug Abuse. *Principles of Adolescent Substance Use Disorder Treatment: A Research-Based Guide*. Bethesda, MD: National Institute on Drug Abuse, 2014.

Tanner-Smith EE, Wilson SJ, Lipsey MW. The comparative effectiveness of outpatient treatment for adolescent substance abuse: a meta-analysis. *J Subst Abuse Treat*. 2013;44(2):145-158.

Winters KC, Kaminer Y. Screening and assessing adolescent substance use disorders in clinical populations. *J Acad Child Adolesc Psychiatry*. 2008;47:740-744.

Placement Criteria and Strategies for Adolescent Treatment Matching

Summary by Marc Fishman

Based on THE ASAM PRINCIPLES OF ADDICTION MEDICINE, 6th edition chapter by Marc Fishman

Although the fields of adolescent treatment in general and adolescent treatment outcomes research in particular are still in their early stages, recent progress has been considerable. Much has been learned about the effectiveness and limitations of current adolescent treatment methods and programs. Reviews of the published literature have shown favorable outcomes up to 1 year after treatment and beyond across various modalities and levels of care. But little is known about the differential effectiveness of various treatment strategies, intensities, and treatment program components.

DEVELOPMENTAL CONSIDERATIONS IN ADOLESCENT PLACEMENT

One of the most important advances in the field of adolescent treatment is the articulation of approaches that are developmentally specific to the adolescent population. These respond to the principle that adolescents must be approached differently from adults because of differences in their levels of emotional, cognitive, physical, social, and moral development. Substance use can prevent a young person from completing the maturational tasks of adolescence, which involve formation of personal relationships, acquisition of social skills, psychologic development, identity formation, individuation, education, employment, and family role responsibilities. Adolescent treatment thus often requires habilitative rather than rehabilitative approaches, emphasizing the acquisition of new capacities rather than the restoration of lost ones.

Among adolescents, there may be special populations to take into consideration. Younger adolescents have a very narrow view of the world, with little capacity to think of future implications of present actions. Some adolescents may adopt a pseudomature ("streetwise") posture, despite their overall immaturity. Adolescents who live in a chaotic family system may have difficulties with normative expectations of behavioral contingency. Adolescents who have various cognitive difficulties may be delayed or impaired in acquiring abstract thinking. Most adolescents struggle with emotional regulation, but this is especially problematic in those with co-occurring psychiatric disorders.

In general, for a given degree of severity or functional impairment, adolescents require greater intensity of treatment than do adults. This is reflected in clinical practice by a greater tendency to place adolescents in more intensive levels of care.

The mixed features of both adolescence and adulthood for young adults or transition age youth require a special approach. Some providers have begun to develop specialized programming for this group and its unique clinical needs. Eventually, the separation of a third category (adolescent, adult, and transition age youth) of developmental programming may become standard. The tensions inherent in their transition often require a balancing act, especially between emerging independence and persistent dependence. For example, issues of confidentiality versus open sharing of information with parents/caregivers are common. Other common issues include financial support, shared living environments with parents, and extension of standard insurance coverage under parental policies until age 26 years with the Affordable Care Act. These tensions and the dynamic interplay between youth and parents are dramatized in the caricatured quotes: "I'm old enough to take care of myself" versus "You may think you're all grown up, but as long as you're living under my roof."

THE AMERICAN SOCIETY OF ADDICTION MEDICINE CRITERIA

The American Society of Addiction Medicine's (ASAM's) *The ASAM Criteria: Treatment Criteria for*

Addictive, Substance-Related, and Co-Occurring Conditions, 3rd edition, is a clinical guide that has been widely adopted to assist in matching patients to appropriate treatment settings. In contrast to previous editions that had separate sections for adolescents and adults, this edition has an integrated approach that emphasizes common features and then calls special attention to those features that differ for adolescents. The criteria rest on the concept of enhancing the use of multidimensional assessments in placement decisions by organizing the assessment of the adolescent who uses substances into six dimensions and specifying appropriate placements according to gradations of problem severity within each dimension.

Assessment-Based Treatment Matching and Clinical Appropriateness

The ASAM Criteria use decision rules to guide placement in specified levels of care, which exist along a continuum. These also attempt to standardize some of the program specifications for each level of care. The principal goal of *The ASAM Criteria* is to facilitate the process of matching patients in need of treatment for substance use disorders (SUDs) with appropriate treatment services and settings to maximize the accessibility, effectiveness, and efficiency of the treatment experience. The reality of limited availability of services is, of course, a major problem, particularly in the treatment of adolescents.

The ASAM Criteria outline a full range of treatment services appropriate to the needs of all adolescents involved with drugs, whether they are privately insured, publicly insured, underinsured, or uninsured. Although they may not have access to it, many adolescents who are marginalized or homeless and those in the juvenile justice system may need an even broader continuum of services than do those with greater resources. In general, adolescents with fewer supports, less resiliency, and lower levels of baseline functioning may need a higher intensity of services and longer lengths of service at all levels of care than do those with the benefits conferred by economic advantage.

Placement and Treatment Considerations by Assessment Dimension

Dimension 1: Intoxication and Withdrawal Potential

Severe physiologic withdrawal and the need for its management are seen less frequently in adolescents than in adults, given typical patterns of use and duration of exposure. The exception to this has been increasing rates of presentation for opioid treatment with withdrawal in the context of the current opioid epidemic. The provision of detoxification as a stand-alone service is less common and less needed with adolescents versus adults. Services to manage the withdrawal in a setting separate from other treatment services for adolescents with SUDs are also clinically undesirable because of the developmental issues involved in the care of adolescents. This phase of treatment frequently requires an initial intensity to establish treatment engagement that will lead to the next steps of recovery.

Dimension 2: Biomedical Conditions and Complications

Although the medical sequelae of addiction generally are not as common or as severe in adolescents as in adults, these sequelae certainly need to be considered in treatment placement decisions. Some of the acute and subacute medical complications of substance use include traumatic injuries associated with any substance intoxication, respiratory depression and death caused by opioid overdose, acute alcohol poisoning, hypoxia and cardiac arrhythmia from inhalants ("sudden inhalant death syndrome"), complications of injection drug use such as hepatitis C, cellulitis and endocarditis, sexually transmitted diseases, gastritis caused by alcohol use, and exacerbation of reactive airway disease caused by smoking marijuana. Another notable area of medical complication in adolescents is the exacerbation of chronic illness (such as diabetes, asthma, or sickle cell disease) that results from impaired self-care and poor compliance with indicated medical treatments.

The special needs and medical vulnerabilities of pregnant teenagers who use substances require particular care in selecting treatment services. Overall, the need for contraception and other medical prevention and treatment services related to sexual behaviors in adolescents involved with drugs cannot be overemphasized.

Dimension 3: Emotional, Behavioral, and Cognitive Conditions and Complications

Drug-involved adolescents typically demonstrate a very high degree of co-occurring psychopathology, which frequently does not remit with abstinence. Many experts estimate that rates of psychiatric comorbidity, or dual diagnosis, are higher in adolescents than in adults. The treatment of co-occurring psychiatric disorders and sequelae is vital in youth with SUDs. Many issues should be taken into consideration, including:

- Previously diagnosed psychiatric illnesses;
- High rates of depressive disorders, typically characterized by irritability, moodiness, overreactivity, and anxiety, rather than sadness;
- Subsyndromal symptoms such as mood lability or anger issues;
- The nonspecific features of immature or impaired executive functioning including impulsiveness, explosiveness, poor affective self-regulation, or poor strategic planning;
- Cognitive functioning and problems such as borderline intellectual functioning, fetal alcohol effects, assorted attentional deficits, or learning disorders;
- Complications of substance use (such as marijuana-induced amnestic disorder);
- Behavioral issues;
- Adolescent learning in normal adolescent development as well as in those with the delayed development and immaturity that often accompanies drug use and co-occurring psychiatric disorders; and
- Cannabis-induced or cannabis-exacerbated psychosis.

Dimension 4: Readiness to Change

Placement decisions based on Dimension 4 include consideration of whether the adolescent (and related systems, such as the family) is in the "precontemplation," "contemplation," "preparation," or "action" stage of change. Motivational interviewing and other motivational enhancement techniques have formed the basis of a variety of intervention models at various levels of care, including early intervention and outpatient treatment.

Dimension 5: Relapse, Continued Use, or Continued Problem Potential

Dimension 5 entails an estimation of the likelihood of resumption or continuation of substance use. Four subdomains have been proposed as issues to take into consideration: (1) historical pattern of use (including amount, frequency, chronicity, and treatment response), (2) pharmacologic response to the effects from particular substances (including positive reinforcement such as pleasure with use and cravings and negative reinforcement such as relief from withdrawal or other negative experiences), (3) response to external stimuli (including reactivity to environmental triggers and acute or chronic stress), and (4) cognitive and behavioral

vulnerability and resiliency factors (including traits of impulsivity, passivity, locus of control, and overall coping capacities). Responses to past treatment also may be a way of using individualized treatment effectiveness as a guide to placement.

Dimension 6: Recovery/Living Environment

Dimension 6 aims to assess the ability of the adolescent's home environment to support or impede treatment and recovery. For adolescents, the most important features of the recovery environment generally involve family and peers.

There is an acute shortage of availability of services that provide recovery environment support for youth. These structured, protective living environments are frequently vital to support ongoing treatment that might be integrated into the living environment itself or more commonly coordinated with programming off site. Frequently, these environments serve the function of a supervised context where adolescents can sustain and rehearse therapeutic gains initiated at a more intensive level of care. This need for step down, lower intensity residential support is perhaps even more vital in the continuum of care for youth than for adults because of their lack of independence and reliance on the full or partial support of caregiving adults. For younger adolescents, these programs would typically be Level 3.1 (see the following section for a description of that level of care), often in group homes or similar programs. For young adults, these programs could also be Level 3.1. But there is also a need for less intensive recovery housing programs with more supervision than typical adult-style self-organized sober housing (eg, Oxford Houses), or adult-style recovery house boarding houses that have minimal supervision but perhaps with less intensity than the typical Level 3.1 or halfway house.

Placement and Treatment Considerations by Levels of Care

The adolescent levels of care in ASAM's *Patient Placement Criteria for the Treatment of Substance-Related Disorders,* second edition, revised (*PPC-2R*), are similar to the levels of care described and endorsed in other expert consensus documents.

Level 0.5: Early Intervention

Early intervention services are designed to explore and address the adolescent's problems or risk factors that appear to be related to early stages of substance use. Their goal is to help the adolescent recognize the potentially harmful consequences of substance use before such use escalates into substance abuse or dependence. Level 0.5 services may be delivered in a variety of settings, including primary care medical clinics, schools, social service and juvenile justice agencies, and driving under the influence intervention programs. Early intervention services are intended to combine prevention and treatment services for youth. Populations that warrant special attention at Level 0.5 are children with parents or siblings who harmfully use substances, and adolescents with other emotional or behavioral problems. Early intervention is not appropriate for adolescents who qualify for a diagnosis of an SUD.

Level 1: Outpatient Treatment

Outpatient treatment is by far the most frequently used level of care. It is often the initial level of care for an adolescent with a low severity of illness. Level 1 also may be employed as a "step-down" program for the adolescent who has made progress at a more intensive level of care, eg, aftercare from a residential program. One of the advantages of outpatient treatment is the possibility of achieving therapeutic goals in the context of the patient's own home environment, where new behaviors can be practiced and solidified in real-life circumstances. Ongoing treatment at less intensive levels of care to consolidate gains initiated at more intensive levels of care is a critical feature of successful treatment across a continuum of care. The need for "booster" doses of treatment should be anticipated. Some adolescents will need a longer term (sometimes indefinite) maintenance phase of treatment. Treatment successes, such as a period of abstinence or improvement in functioning, sometimes are misinterpreted as completion of treatment, but actually, long-term maintenance and monitoring of short-term successes are essential goals of active outpatient treatment.

Level 2: Intensive Outpatient Treatment/ Partial Hospitalization

Intensive outpatient programs (Level 2.1) generally offer at least 6 hours of structured programming per week (eg, "day programs"). Adolescent intensive outpatient programs generally meet after school hours.

Partial hospitalization (Level 2.5) programs often have direct access to or close referral relationships with psychiatric and medical services. Partial hospitalization may occur during school hours, and many programs, especially if longer term, have access to educational services for their adolescent patients.

Level 3: Residential Treatment

Although earlier editions of *The ASAM Criteria* treated all adolescent residential treatment as one broad undifferentiated level of care, the *PPC-2R* divides Level 3 into three sublevels.

- Level 3.1: Clinically managed low-intensity residential treatment: Programs typically provided in halfway houses and group homes, offering several hours a week of low-intensity treatment sessions for adolescents who require a longer term, structured, and safe environment to learn recovery skills, relapse prevention, and improved social functioning.
- Level 3.5: Clinically managed medium-intensity residential treatment: These programs are designed to provide relatively extended subacute treatments with the goal of achieving fundamental personal change for the adolescent who has significant social and psychologic problems or highly unstable home environments. Such programs are characterized by their reliance on the treatment community as a therapeutic agent of change.
- Level 3.7: Medically monitored high-intensity residential/inpatient treatment. This level is appropriate for adolescents whose problems are so severe that they require medically monitored residential treatment but do not need the full resources of an acute care hospital or medically managed inpatient treatment program (Level 4). Medically monitored services are provided under the supervision of physicians who are specialists in addiction medicine. Services typically provided include crisis stabilization, medical detoxification, diagnostic clarification of a co-occurring disorder with initiation of abstinence, attempts to remediate psychosocial chaos including toxic home environments, titration of a psychopharmacologic regimen, and high-intensity behavior modification.

Level 4: Medically Managed Intensive Inpatient (Hospital) Treatment

Delivered in an acute care inpatient setting in which the full resources of a general or psychiatric hospital are available, Level 4 treatment tends to be brief and generally consists of emergency or crisis interventions aimed at stabilization in preparation for transfer to a less intensive level of care for ongoing treatment.

Linkages Between Levels of Care

Issues regarding continuity of care, continuing care, and longitudinal follow-up are critical, especially for adolescents because they are so dynamic in their developmental changes and needs. *The ASAM Criteria* emphasize the concept of treatment as a dynamic, longitudinal process rather than a discrete episode of care or particular program enrollment. However, current treatment delivery systems do not generally support the necessary continuum of care. Long-term relationships with youth and families, with the expectation of accommodating dropping in and dropping out, with changing needs over time, should be standard. Although the fantasy notion that patients should be expected to be "fixed" after a discrete episode of care (eg, residential rehab) is both common and absurd in all ages, it is even more common for youth, who are too often assumed to have "learned their lesson" or "grown out of it." The need for facilitating a continuity between linked episodes of care at different levels of care based on need is vital and includes role induction, coordination, communication, warm handoffs, assertive outreach, and overlapping levels of care.

KEY POINTS

1. Developmentally specific and youth-friendly approaches to adolescent treatment are critical to success in the treatment of adolescent SUDs.
2. The adolescent section of *The ASAM Criteria* provides a guide to assessment, treatment, placement, and treatment matching strategies for youth.
3. Assessing and treating co-occurring psychiatric disorders are critical to success in the treatment of adolescent SUDs.
4. Continuity of care, linkages between levels of care, longitudinal treatment, and monitoring are all essential in the treatment of adolescent SUDs.
5. Promotion of family engagement, monitoring, and supervision has high yield in the treatment of adolescent and young adult SUDs and needs to be balanced skillfully with considerations of patient confidentiality.

REVIEW QUESTIONS

1. Which of the following statements about adolescent treatment is true?
   A. Adolescent treatment usually requires rehabilitative rather than habilitative approaches, emphasizing the restoration of lost capacities rather than the acquisition of new capacities.
   B. Adolescent substance use in the form of normative experimentation is frequent and often misdiagnosed as a substance use disorder. There is a shortage of treatment capacity for adolescents because the demand created by referrals from the healthcare system outstrips supply.

C. Historically, adolescent treatment has often consisted of adult-style components without sufficient developmental adaptation, attention to adolescent learning styles, or focus on youth-friendly features.

2. Which of the following are important factors in assessing co-occurring mental health problems (Dimension 3) in youth?
   A. High rates of depressive disorders, typically characterized by irritability, moodiness, overreactivity, and anxiety, rather than sadness
   B. Subsyndromal symptoms such as mood lability or anger issues
   C. The nonspecific features of immature or impaired executive functioning including impulsiveness, explosiveness, poor affective self-regulation, or poor strategic planning
   D. Cognitive functioning and problems such as borderline intellectual functioning, fetal alcohol effects, assorted attentional deficits, or learning disorders
   E. Complications of substance use (such as marijuana-induced amnestic disorder)
   F. Behavioral issues such as disruptive behavior and peer aggression
   G. All of the above.

3. Which of the following characterizes features of adolescent levels of care?
   A. Although there is evidence for safe and effective ambulatory detoxification for adults, most withdrawal management techniques for adolescents that require medical intervention are best accomplished at the residential/inpatient level of care (Level 3.7D).
   B. Transitional, lower intensity residential settings (Level 3.1) are frequently needed following higher intensity, residential/inpatient treatment for youth to provide continued recovery environment support for ongoing outpatient treatment. These settings often require more supervision an structure and higher levels of staffing than do the corresponding levels of care for adults.
   C. Longitudinal treatment and linkages between levels of care are less important for adolescents than for adults. Discrete episodes of care are usually sufficient for most adolescents because they have high levels of insight and are developmentally resilient, often "growing out of" their problems.
   D. A, B, and C.
   E. A and B.
   F. B and C.

4. All of the following statements about family involvement in treatment are true *except*:
   A. Adolescents and young adults may sometimes object inappropriately to the disclosure of information to their families that might be clinically helpful to them.
   B. Families may sometimes inappropriately demand information about their adolescent's or young adult's treatment in a way that is overly intrusive.
   C. Out of respect for confidentiality and emerging autonomy, it is important that an adolescent's or young adult's family never be involved in treatment.

ANSWERS

1. **C**
2. **G**
3. **E**
4. **C.** Although adolescents may push unilaterally for no disclosure, and parents may push for indiscriminate disclosure, prudent and thoughtful family involvement with "brokered" disclosure improves treatment outcomes.

SUGGESTED READINGS

Fishman M. Placement criteria and strategies for adolescent treatment matching. In: Ries RK, Fiellin DA, Miller SC, Saitz R, eds. *Principles of Addiction Medicine*. 5th ed. Philadelphia: Lippincott Williams & Wilkins, 2014:1627-1646.

Fishman M. Placement criteria and treatment planning for adolescents with substance use disorders. In: Kaminer Y, Winters KC, eds. *Clinical Manual of Adolescent Substance Abuse Treatment*. Washington, DC: American Psychiatric Publishing, 2010:113-142.

Fishman, M. Relationship between substance use disorders and psychiatric comorbidity: implications for integrated health services. In Kaminer Y, ed. *Youth Substance Abuse and Co-Occurring Disorders*. Arlington, VA: American Psychiatric Association, 2016:21-48.

Fishman MJ, Winstanley EL, Curran E, Garrett S, Subramaniam G. Treatment of opioid dependence in adolescents and young adults with extended release naltrexone: preliminary case series and feasibility. *Addiction*. 2010;105:1669-1676.

NIDA for Teens. Teens: drug use and the brain. http://teens.drugabuse.gov. Updated September 5, 2018. Accessed September 5, 2018.

Partnership for Drug-Free Kids. http://www.drugfree.org. Accessed September 5, 2018.

Sampl S, Kadden R. *Motivational Enhancement Therapy and Cognitive Behavioral Therapy for Adolescent Cannabis Users: 5 Sessions. Cannabis Youth Treatment Series. Volume 1.* Rockville, MD: Substance Abuse Mental Health Services Administration, 2001.

Confidentiality in Dealing with Adolescents

Summary by Margaret R. Moon

Based on THE ASAM PRINCIPLES OF ADDICTION MEDICINE, 6th edition sidebar by Margaret R. Moon

Confidentiality is an essential component of healthcare for adolescents. Key principles underlying the approach to confidentiality include an *intrinsic* duty to respect autonomy—in particular, to respect, protect, and promote the developing autonomy of adolescents—and the *instrumental* value of establishing an environment for care that encourages access and disclosure.

Although autonomy, in terms of decision-making capacity, cannot be presumed for adolescents, there is evidence that by age 14 to 15 years, most children make decisions about healthcare issues in a manner similar to adults. However, more recent work on the neurodevelopment and neurophysiology of adolescence emphasizes that adolescents have specific vulnerabilities, including less capacity to incorporate long-term outcomes into decisions, weaker impulse control, and heightened reactivity to stress.

For both adolescents and adults, the threshold level of capacity needed for autonomous decision making increases with the risk and complexity of the decision. An important challenge for those providing care for adolescents is to assess decisional capacity *specific* to the medical choice to be made.

The instrumental value of confidential care continues to be supported by evidence that adolescents, especially those at highest risk, will avoid seeking care for sensitive issues if they cannot anticipate privacy. Although all US states permit confidential care for minors seeking treatment of sexually transmitted illnesses, state regulations regarding confidential care for reproductive health, mental health, and substance use disorders vary. Federal confidentiality regulations have generally supported confidentiality around substance use treatment. However, clinicians must be knowledgeable about specific state regulations.

Balancing the intrinsic and instrumental value of confidential care for adolescents with the duty to promote well-being and avoid harm can present a complex challenge. Parental involvement in an adolescent's healthcare is most often a benefit. Working to help the adolescent safely engage with parents around health concerns can create the necessary balance. There will be circumstances in which a clinician feels compelled to disclose information for the adolescent's safety. Accordingly, most experts agree that promises of confidentiality should be *conditional* instead of absolute. Clinicians should make it clear that there are limits beyond which confidentiality will not be ensured, and those limits should be specified. When confidentiality must be breached, the adolescent must be informed and engaged in the process to the extent possible.

Drug Testing Adolescents in School

Summary by J. Wesley Boyd

Based on THE ASAM PRINCIPLES OF ADDICTION MEDICINE, 6th edition sidebar by J. Wesley Boyd and John R. Knight Jr.

Substance use among adolescents is associated with the leading causes of death and other adverse health and behavioral outcomes. Because schools are generally tasked with keeping children safe, it is not surprising that schools have been a target of efforts to reduce youth drug and alcohol use by implementing involuntary testing for these substances.

Reasonable steps should be taken to ensure that adolescents have as little exposure to these substances as possible. However, the question remains: What constitutes "reasonable"? In particular, is it acceptable to drug test children in school settings?

The US Supreme Court weighed in on this issue with its ruling in the 2002 *Board of Education v Earls* case, which gave public schools the legal right to randomly test middle and high school students who participate in extracurricular activities for illicit substances. This ruling overrode students' rights to privacy given "the School District's important interest in detecting and preventing drug use among its students."

Not long after this ruling, the White House Office of National Drug Control Policy published a booklet entitled *What You Need to Know About Drug Testing in Schools* in support of school drug testing. This document stated, "Testing can also be an effective way to prevent drug use. The expectation that they may be randomly tested is enough to make some students stop using drugs—or never start in the first place."

In response to the US Supreme Court ruling and the Office of National Drug Control Policy booklet, the American Academy of Pediatrics (AAP) issued two policy statements in 2007. The first noted a number of potentially harmful effects of mandatory drug testing in schools. "Drug testing poses substantial risks—in particular, the risk of harming the parent-child and school-child relationships by creating an environment of resentment, distrust, and suspicion." Additionally, "there is little evidence of the effectiveness of school-based drug testing in the scientific literature." The AAP statement concludes that further study of the efficacy of school- and home-based testing is necessary, that such testing should not be implemented at present, and that if parents are concerned about the possibility that their children are using harmful substances, they should consult their primary care physician or another healthcare provider rather than rely on drug screening at home or in the school.

In the second policy statement, the AAP acknowledged that despite some advantages, problematic aspects of mandatory drug testing include the fact that students using illicit drugs might decrease their involvement in extracurricular activities in order to avoid drug testing, that positive tests might worsen family conflict, that the money spent on testing might be better used for drug counseling and/or prevention programs, and that forcing every child to test might be perceived as unfair and thus increase levels of distrust by youth toward their school. Not surprisingly, given their positions in these policy statements, the AAP concludes that pediatricians should not support drug testing in schools.

Continued

Instead, the AAP believes that physicians should serve as a resource for their patients and their families about substance use and offer primary and secondary prevention as well as identify youth who are at risk for misuse of substances. The AAP also states that physicians should also promote awareness about the changing patterns of substance use in their communities and serve as a conduit into substance use treatment when needed.

Although compelling arguments can be made to both support and reject such compulsory drug testing, overall, the judgment and recommendations of the pediatric community ought to be given more weight than those of the judicial or executive branches of the government. Therefore, mandatory drug testing in the school setting ought not occur.

SUGGESTED READINGS

Committee on Substance Abuse, Council on School Health. Testing for drugs of abuse in children and adolescents: addendum—testing in schools and at home. *Pediatrics.* 2007;119(3):627-630.

Council on School Health, Committee on Substance Abuse. The role of schools in combating illicit substance abuse. *Pediatrics.* 2007;120(6):1379-1384.

Office of National Drug Control Policy. *What You Need to Know About Drug Testing in Schools.* Washington, DC: US Government Printing Office, 2002.

112 Adolescent Treatment and Relapse Prevention

Summary by Steven L. Jaffe and Ashraf Attalla

Based on THE ASAM PRINCIPLES OF ADDICTION MEDICINE,
6th edition chapter by Steven L. Jaffe and Ashraf Attalla

TREATMENT MODALITIES

A longer duration of treatment, increased readiness to change substance use behavior, and family involvement are associated with a better outcome during treatment. In a recent review, three treatment approaches—multidimensional family therapy (MDFT), functional family therapy (FFT), and group cognitive–behavioral therapy (CBT)—emerged as well-established models for treatment of this population. The researchers pointed out that none of the treatment approaches appeared clearly superior and that other therapeutic modalities were efficacious as well. Because studies of various treatment modalities report similar outcomes, positive treatment effects may be due to common nonspecific factors. These appear to include the change elements of motivational interviewing (ie, feedback, personal responsibility, clear advice, a menu of change options, therapist empathy, and enhancing self-efficacy).

FAMILY THERAPY

A recent meta-analysis of the family treatment of delinquent adolescents with substance use examined the efficacy of four family therapies, that is, brief strategic family therapy (BSFT), FFT, MDFT, and multisystemic therapy (MST). All four had statistically significant but modest effects compared to treatment as usual or alternate therapies.

Multidimensional Family Therapy

Liddle's MDFT has established the most empirical support for efficacy. MDFT is an outpatient family-based treatment that combines substance use treatment with multiple system assessments and interventions within the family and the surrounding psychosocial environment. MDFT usually involves therapy sessions one to three times per week over 3 to 6 months both in the home and at the clinic. Treatment domains of

the adolescent, parents, family, and other social groups are addressed.

Brief Strategic Family Therapy

BSFT is a manualized family therapy with a structural and strategic approach developed for Hispanic families with youth with behavior problems. A recent randomized trial comparing BSFT to group therapy showed that BSFT treatment resulted in a significant reduction of self-reported marijuana use and parent-reported conduct problems.

Multisystemic Therapy

Henggeler's MST integrates family therapy with direct interventions in the multiple interacting systems involving the individual, school, peer group, and community. This treatment approach promotes responsible behavior among all family members and attempts to develop each individual's capacity to manage his or her own problems. Therapists work intensively with each adolescent and family in the home, school, and even neighborhood peer group. MST has demonstrated excellent retention rates and favorable outcomes. A randomized clinical trial of 118 juvenile offenders with a diagnosis of substance use disorder (SUD) examined MST compared to community service provided through the local office of the state substance abuse commission. MST significantly reduced substance use at posttreatment, but the effect was not found at the 6- or 12-month follow-up. It appears that MST has significant effects for the treatment of conduct disorder but very modest effects for the treatment of adolescent SUD.

Functional Family Therapy

FFT integrates behavioral and cognitive interventions with ecological–family relationship strategies. A recent study showed FFT and FFT with CBT to be efficacious at 4 months compared to individual CBT or group psychoeducational therapy.

Behavioral Family Therapy

Azrin combined family therapy with behavior therapy such that parents reinforced drug-incompatible activities, supervised home urge control assignments, and employed written specifications of desired behaviors with contingent reinforcers. Abstinence rates at 6 months were 73%, whereas the control group of supportive counseling was only 9%. A more recent study showed equal efficacy to cognitive problem-solving therapy.

COGNITIVE–BEHAVIORAL THERAPY

This therapeutic modality combines the learning principles of classical and operant conditioning with approaches to correct cognitive distortions and underlying negative belief systems. Treatment involves teaching the adolescent specific techniques to deal with drugs and alcohol. Specific skills to refuse alcohol and drugs are taught and practiced in role-playing exercises. Cognitive–behavioral coping skills to deal with urges, to manage thoughts of alcohol or drug use, and to handle emergencies and lapses are taught and practiced. Because deficits in coping skills for negative feelings and life stresses contribute to continued substance use, more general coping strategies (such as communication skills, problem-solving strategies, anger and mood management, and relaxation training) also are taught and practiced.

A number of randomized clinical trials provide empirical support for the efficacy of CBT in the treatment of adolescents with SUDs. It should be noted that with CBT, interventions improved self-efficacy (ie, confidence in the ability to refrain from drug use as a proximal outcome was directly associated with better outcomes).

TWELVE-STEP APPROACHES

Twelve-step approaches are now considered an effective adjunct to SUD treatment among adults. Although the 12-step–based treatment is one of the most common treatment models for adolescents, there has been little research into its efficacy. This approach is suitable for teens who have developed severe drug problems.

The 12 steps guide changes in actions, thoughts, feelings, and beliefs that an individual slowly undergoes in order to establish a state of recovery and abstinence from alcohol and drugs. Twelve-step groups and supervision of working the steps are often a treatment component of residential or intensive outpatient programs. Actively working a program (ie, writing and presenting the steps, meeting with a sponsor, meditating and praying, attending and participating in Alcoholics Anonymous [AA] or Narcotics Anonymous [NA] meetings while in intensive treatment) results in a higher rate of teens continuing in the program after discharge and in aftercare. The adolescent needs to be actively linked to the 12 steps and not just told to go to a meeting. The following descriptions present the first five steps, modified to make them developmentally meaningful for adolescents.

Step 1

"We admitted we were powerless over alcohol—that our lives had become unmanageable." The adolescents write and examine in detail the negative consequences of their alcohol or drug use. Putting their own and others' lives in danger and effects on their family, school, work, mood, and self-esteem in relationship to alcohol and drug use are explored. The major issue is whether drugs and alcohol are destroying their lives such that they need to stop using to make their lives better. Although many adult programs emphasize the concept of "surrendering" and admitting one is an addict, these are not useful for adolescents. Rather, enhancing power by doing what one needs to do (ie, stop using alcohol and drugs) instead of doing what one wants to do (ie, use alcohol and drugs) is emphasized.

Step 2

"We come to believe that a power greater than ourselves could restore us to sanity." In the development of an addictive state, alcohol and drugs have become a negative higher power that has taken over the adolescent's life. Stopping the alcohol and drugs leaves a void that needs to be filled by a positive higher power. The higher power concept is not a religious belief but a spiritual feeling that one can trust something positive (eg, the group, another person, God, nature) to take care of those aspects of one's life that one cannot control. For many adolescents, the concrete positive feelings of their relationships to other members (love) become the first higher power.

Step 3

"We make a decision to turn our will and our lives over to the care of God as we understand Him." The adolescent workbook interprets this step to involve having adolescents make a decision to commit themselves to working the steps and having a positive spiritual power. Teenagers are helped to recognize that they turned over their lives to alcohol and drugs. Now they are being asked to turn their lives over to a positive program. Learning to meditate and pray is an important part of this step.

Step 4

"We made a searching and fearless moral inventory of ourselves." Here, adolescents answer numerous detailed questions covering all aspects of their childhood and present life.

Step 5

"We admitted to God, to ourselves, and to another human being the exact nature of our wrongs." In this step, adolescents verbalize an inventory to a counselor or sponsor.

Twelve-step programs also provide the opportunity to attend free AA or NA meetings, which are conducted several times a day in almost every city and town in the United States and most other countries. Twelve-step programs provide the opportunity of being part of a recovering peer group and mentoring relationships in the form of sponsors. An older member with at least a year of sobriety, the sponsor provides support and guidance on how to work the program to achieve sobriety. Twelve-step programs accept the concept of addiction as a chronic progressive disorder that renders the addict unable to control and moderate his or her drinking or drug use. The only viable alternative is complete abstinence.

There is a significant research base that supports the efficacy of 12-step programs. The major mechanism identified was that 12-step attendance maintained and enhanced motivation for abstinence. Limitations of these studies include lack of random assignment and that only inpatient and residential treatment programs were studied. Benefits of AA or NA participation were shown in a follow-up of 8 years for a sample of inpatient youth. Attending one meeting per week was associated with significant benefit and attending two to three meetings was associated with abstinence. In one study, greater contact with a sponsor outside of meetings and more verbal participation during meetings were especially important components. It also appears that teens that reported feeling connected to others, engaged in a higher frequency of meditation and prayer, and who endorsed a more spiritual orientation to life were those who expressed a greater preference for spirituality and the 12-step approaches.

MOTIVATIONAL TREATMENT

Prochaska and DiClemente have described a series of stages that mark the progress of an individual toward ceasing alcohol or drug use. These stages are designated as (1) precontemplation, in which the person is not even thinking about stopping and does not recognize any problem with alcohol or drug use; (2) contemplation, which is marked by ambivalence in which the person goes back and forth between reasons to change and reasons not to change; (3) preparation, in which the person increases the commitment to change; (4) action, in which the person stops using alcohol and drugs; and (5) maintenance, in which the person develops a lifestyle to avoid relapse. Individuals exhibit different levels of motivation depending on their stage of change. Therapeutic intervention involves helping the patient in an empathetic, nonconfrontational manner to move along the stages.

Miller and Rollnick developed motivational enhancement therapy (MET), which used the strategies of expressing empathy, developing discrepancy, avoiding argumentation, rolling with resistance, and supporting self-efficacy to enhance changes along the stages. Studies show that higher motivation to change relates to lower substance use. Brief motivational interventions consist of one to four sessions following an assessment, in which direct feedback and advice are given in a nonconfrontational manner that respects the person's personal responsibility for making a decision. Although brief motivational therapy may not be sufficient for those with severe alcohol or drug use, MET is often used prior to other psychosocial treatments.

Adolescent Community Reinforcement Approach

The community reinforcement approach is a treatment approach originally developed for adults in which the individual's life is rearranged so that abstinence is more rewarding than drinking. This modality has been adapted for adolescents and has been manualized and evaluated as part of the Cannabis Youth Treatment Study, where efficacy was demonstrated. This therapeutic approach is warm, enthusiastic, and nonjudgmental as therapists identify adolescents' and parents' reinforcers. They then work toward learning and practicing new skills to obtain these positive rewards. Adolescents and their parents are seen separately and together in flexible sessions. A functional analysis of substance use and prosocial behavior identifies triggers. Short-term positive consequences and long-term negative consequences are also noted. Other sessions my involve problem solving, communication skills, and how to achieve healthy social and recreational activities, making their environment increasingly supportive of recovery. Clinical effectiveness has been shown in independent replications.

Enthusiastic Sobriety Approach

The enthusiastic sobriety approach uses a modified 12-step structure with young, energetic, enthusiastic, recovering, and well-trained counselors who are role models who demonstrate that one can live a fun life without drugs or alcohol. The adolescent is asked to try 30 days without drugs or alcohol. In the intensive outpatient program, the adolescent participates in daily groups, meetings, individual counseling, weekend social activities, and frequent contact with their sponsor and positive peers who are active in the aftercare support group. They work their steps and learn it is "cool" to meditate and pray. Parents are seen in a weekly parents group.

Mindfulness-Based Approaches

Mindfulness-based approaches have been successfully applied to the treatment of severe SUDs. They include mindfulness-based cognitive therapy, acceptance and commitment therapy, dialectical–behavioral therapy (DBT), mindfulness-based relapse prevention (MBRP), and mindfulness-based therapeutic community treatment.

The basis for mindfulness-based approaches is the cultivation of a nonjudgmental awareness, curiosity, openness, and acceptance of internal and external experiences, with the intended goal of eliciting greater reflection and acceptance, especially with regard to negative affect. Mindfulness seeks to diminish the escalation of negative emotional reactivity (ie, a secondary negative affect in reaction to transient negative emotion) during stressful periods. During mindfulness training, individuals learn to become more aware of habit-linked affective states and cravings, thus "deautomating" this largely habitual process.

Improving distress tolerance is an important target of mindfulness-based substance use treatment. In behavioral terms, mindfulness-based approaches for SUDs are described as a process of desensitization to negative affect through exposure, which helps to extinguish automatic avoidance of negative emotions and consequential substance use.

DBT is an empirically validated therapy developed by Linehan that is effective at decreasing self-harming and self-defeating behaviors. This psychotherapy is now being applied to patients with SUDs, including adolescents. DBT combines the CBT techniques for emotional regulation with the skills of mindfulness, distress tolerance, and interpersonal effectiveness.

Contingency Management

Contingency management (CM) is based on the premise that drug seeking and drug use are directly modifiable by manipulating the relevant environmental contingencies. CM uses concrete positive rewards to enhance attendance, participation, and abstinence. Numerous studies have demonstrated CM's efficacy in adult populations. It is just beginning to be studied with adolescents who use substances.

Neurofeedback

Along with major advances in technology, there has been significant progress in the development of neurofeedback as a treatment for SUDs. Using real-time functional magnetic resonance imaging, adults dependent on nicotine were able to reduce the activity of the anterior cingulate cortex, which correlated with decreased cravings. Using electroencephalogram neurofeedback, adults with alcohol use disorder were able to increase their alpha and theta brain rhythms, resulting in decreased depression scores and relapse percentage compared to a control group. Electroencephalogram neurofeedback can also be combined with other treatments. This is a promising area to be explored with adolescents.

Pharmacotherapy

Nicotine replacement therapy for nicotine dependency, disulfiram aversion therapy for alcohol use disorders, naltrexone as a blocker of opiates or to decrease cravings for alcohol, and methadone/buprenorphine as substitution therapy for opiate dependency are some of the strategies being tried. Pharmacotherapy of the comorbid disorders—that is, attention deficit hyperactivity disorder, posttraumatic stress, anxiety, and affective disorder—have been more extensively studied. With adolescents, pharmacologic interventions should always be used with psychosocial treatments.

USING MULTIPLE THERAPIES

No single treatment modality has been demonstrated to be clearly superior. All therapies have a significant percentage of failures. Multiple approaches are being integrated in an attempt to improve outcomes.

Relapse and Continued Care

The most pressing problems in adolescent substance abuse treatment are the large number of treatment noncompleters, which range from 30% to 50% in clinical settings, and the extremely high relapse rate (40% to 60% regardless of the treatment used.) Continued care for noncompleters should involve either a different treatment modality or a stepped-up, more intensive intervention of the failed treatment. Relapse is common and should be expected. With this frame of reference, it is extremely important not to allow a lapse (ie, return to alcohol or drug use for a few days) to develop into a full relapse (ie, return to use for weeks or months). Relapse perception themes include emotional reasons that involved coping with negative feelings, life stresses that included parental criticism and failing school, socialization processes that included peer pressure, cognitive factors that included poor motivation and cravings, and environmental issues that included availability and triggers.

A commonly used treatment modality especially in adult studies is cognitive–behavioral relapse prevention (RP). High-risk situations that may precipitate a relapse are identified, and cognitive and behavioral skills are taught. In MBRP, the patient is taught awareness of environmental cues as well as cognitive and emotional states that triggered the relapse. This includes learning to tolerate negative affects, which are often a precursor to relapse. Sitting meditation is an essential part of MBRP. A recent clinical trial compared adults who completed an initial treatment and were then randomized to receive 8 weeks of RP, MBRP, or group 12-step–based treatment as usual. Although the 3-month follow-up showed no difference between groups, both the RP and the MBRP groups significantly reduced relapse compared to treatment as usual at 6 months, and at the 12-month follow-up, the MBRP group did better than the RP group. The success of MBRP in this adult population indicates it should be studied in adolescents in aftercare.

Recovering adolescents working a 12-step program who relapse need to examine the strength of their program and recognize the need for a solid sponsor, a nonusing peer group, and frequent (two or more each week) attendance at AA/NA meetings. All relapsing adolescents should be evaluated for comorbid disorders, such as depression or posttraumatic stress disorder, which may require specific treatment.

A recent development is assertive continuing care, where continued contact is the responsibility of the therapist. Education, support, and reintervention are done via monitoring by telephone and/or home visits. A study of postresidential adolescents yielded a 52% abstinent rate for marijuana at 3 months for the assertive continuing care group compared to 32% for the usual continuing care group. Another study compared 50-minute individual MET/CBT sessions, 15-minute MET/CBT therapeutic phone contacts, and a no intervention control group. There were positive results for both active interventions, and sessions were maintained over 12 months. Importantly, the phone intervention was feasible and acceptable.

KEY POINTS

1. Family therapy, especially MDFT, has been the most studied treatment modality and has demonstrated significant efficacy.
2. CBT, adolescent community reinforcement approach, MET, DBT, and CM also show positive but limited results.
3. Twelve-step approaches modified for adolescents, including enthusiastic sobriety, have some positive studies but lack random assignment.
4. All studies show similar outcomes, and no treatment modality has been demonstrated superior to the others.
5. The most difficult challenge to adolescent treatment is the high percentage of treatment noncompleters (30% to 50 %) and the high relapse rate (40% to 60%).

REVIEW QUESTIONS

1. Which of the following statements are true? (Select all that apply.)
   A. Confrontation is helpful to prove the adolescent has a problem.
   B. Approaching the adolescent according to their stage of change gets the best results.
   C. No treatment approach is clearly superior to the others.
   D. Effective pharmacotherapy is sometimes sufficient to treat adolescent substance use disorders.

2. If relapse occurs, which of the following should be done?
   A. Discharge the patient from the program because he or she is unmotivated.
   B. Send the patient to a residential program.
   C. Promote shame and guilt in the patient to enhance motivation.
   D. Approach the patient as to what he or she can learn from the relapse.

ANSWERS

1. **B** and **C**
2. **D**

SUGGESTED READINGS

Dennis M, Godley SH, Diamond G, et al. The Cannabis Youth Treatment (CYT) study: main findings from two randomized trials. *J Subst Abuse Treat.* 2004:27(3):197-213.

Jaffe SL. *Step Workbook for Adolescent Chemical Dependency Recovery: A Guide to the First Five Steps.* Washington, DC; American Psychiatric Press, 1990.

Kaminer Y, ed. *Youth Substance Abuse and Co-Occurring Disorders.* Arlington, VA: American Psychiatric Association, 2016.

Kaminer Y, Winters KC, eds. *Clinical Manual of Adolescent Substance Treatment.* Arlington, VA: American Psychiatric Publishing, 2011.

113

Pharmacotherapies for Adolescents with Substance Use Disorders

Summary by Ashwin Jacob Mathai and Samar Ali Mirzaei

Based on THE ASAM PRINCIPLES OF ADDICTION MEDICINE, 6th edition chapter by Geetha A. Subramaniam and Kevin M. Gray

Exposure to alcohol, tobacco, and illicit substances during adolescence increases the risk of developing substance use disorders (SUDs). According to the annual, school-based Monitoring the Future survey (2017), past month (ie, current) use among 12th graders was reported at 33%, 10%, and 25% for alcohol, tobacco, and any illicit substance, respectively. Among the illicit substances, cannabis is most prevalent, with 23% of 12th graders, 16% of 10th graders, and 6% of 8th graders reporting past month (ie, current) use. Prescription medication misuse, including stimulants and opioid analgesics, was second most common with 6% and 2% reporting past-year nonmedical use of prescription stimulant Adderall and opioid analgesic Vicodin, respectively. Despite this, there are limited studies evaluating the efficacy of pharmacologic treatment of SUDs in youth. Moreover, psychosocial approaches to treatment are limited by modest effect sizes. In the following sections, we outline available evidence for pharmacologic treatments of SUDs in youth, alone or in combination with psychosocial interventions.

EMPIRICAL SUPPORT FOR PHARMACOTHERAPIES IN THE TREATMENT OF ADOLESCENT SUBSTANCE USE DISORDERS

As in adults, medications for SUDs in youth work as agonists and partial agonists or antagonists. In other cases, they produce aversive symptoms or work to relieve cravings or withdrawal.

Nicotine/Nicotine

Smoking during adolescence is associated with poorer physical fitness, SUDs, and psychiatric illnesses like conduct disorder. Although adolescents who smoke tend to smoke fewer cigarettes and at a lesser frequency than adults who smoke, teens who smoke intermittently resemble daily smokers in a number of ways including their motivation to quit, attitudes toward smoking, and quit history. It is also concerning that nicotine addiction can develop rapidly in youth, with one in four adolescents who smoke developing dependence within a month of smoking. Quit rates are extremely low among adolescents who smoke who try to quit on their own. None of the pharmacologic interventions approved for nicotine use disorder in adults (nicotine replacement therapies, bupropion, or varenicline) are approved for individuals younger than 18 years. Overall, the evidence suggests that they are safe and well-tolerated in this population, but long-term quit rates have not been demonstrated. However, several studies have demonstrated a reduction in the number of cigarettes used with these interventions.

Nicotine Replacement Therapies

Nicotine replacement therapies act as agonists at nicotine receptors and thus decrease cravings and withdrawal symptoms. Of the five placebo-controlled trials evaluating the efficacy of nicotine replacement therapies in youth, none were able to establish any long-term efficacy with regard to abstinence rates. Three studies evaluating the efficacy of nicotine patches relative to placebo did not find any discernible difference between the two groups with regard to long-term rates of abstinence. One of these studies demonstrated that subjective craving and withdrawal symptoms were lower in the group that received nicotine patches. Another study demonstrated that abstinence rates were lower at 2 weeks into treatment in the group that received the patch but not at end of treatment.

Moreover, end-of-treatment abstinence rates were dependent on adherence. A study that compared nicotine gum, patches, and placebo showed that adherence was better with patches.

Bupropion

Bupropion acts as a nicotine receptor antagonist and norepinephrine/dopamine reuptake inhibitor. Bupropion was previously associated with a black box warning regarding risk of depression and suicidal thoughts but has since been removed. Preliminary evidence suggests that bupropion has some efficacy in treating nicotine use disorder in adolescents. Higher rates of self-reported abstinence was shown with bupropion in a double-blind, placebo-controlled trial. Upon comparing 150 mg and 300 mg doses of bupropion with placebo, there was a more significant reduction in smoking in the group receiving the higher dose, although rates were lower than outcomes observed with comparable doses in adults. In a study that compared the efficacy of nicotine patches plus bupropion and nicotine patches alone, both interventions produced a reduction in smoking, but combination therapy did not result in any improved outcome relative to patches alone. Another study compared outcomes in four groups: bupropion plus contingency management (CM), bupropion alone, CM alone, and placebo with no CM. The combination of bupropion with CM resulted in better abstinence rates than either treatment alone or placebo. Adverse effects were slightly more common in the group receiving bupropion.

Varenicline

Varenicline acts as a partial agonist at the nicotine receptor to reduce cravings and withdrawal symptoms. Like bupropion, the black box warning regarding the risk of neuropsychiatric adverse events including suicidal thoughts with the use of varenicline has been revised in light of recent findings, suggesting that this risk was lower than previously thought. The only randomized double-blind trial comparing the effectiveness of varenicline and bupropion did not reveal any differences in outcomes between the two groups, although both interventions decreased smoking. No serious adverse effects were reported in both groups. Therefore, the evidence for use of this medication in this population is very preliminary.

Alcohol

Alcohol use during adolescence is associated with negative outcomes like academic underachievement and relationship difficulties within families.

A majority of teens use alcohol before completing high school. Three medications have been approved for the treatment of alcohol use disorder (AUD) in adults: disulfiram, naltrexone, and acamprosate.

Disulfiram

Disulfiram interferes with the metabolism of alcohol and leads to the accumulation of an intermediary product that produces unpleasant and aversive symptoms upon consumption of alcohol. Disulfiram has been evaluated in two small trials in adolescents, one in comparison with placebo and another with μ-opioid antagonist naltrexone. Both trials demonstrated efficacy for this medication, although using this medication is limited by an individual's commitment to abstinence and the need for close medical supervision due to the likelihood for hepatotoxicity and lethal symptoms with combination of alcohol and disulfiram.

Naltrexone

Naltrexone is a μ-opioid antagonist that decreases craving and severity of drinking. In both an open-label study and crossover trial, both with small sample sizes, naltrexone was found to be effective. In the first open-label trial with a sample size of five, naltrexone was effective at reducing the number of drinks and subjective cravings. In the second randomized trial with crossover design (n = 22), naltrexone decreased cravings, the likelihood of heavy drinking, and altered subjective responses to alcohol, thus demonstrating some preliminary evidence for efficacy of this medication in youth.

Acamprosate

No published studies are available for acamprosate in youth with alcohol use disorders.

Ondansetron

A small open-label study conducted over 8 weeks evaluating the efficacy of this 5-hydroxytryptamine type 3 (5-HT$_3$) antagonist showed that this medication decreased the number of drinks consumed and increased the number of abstinent days, primarily by decreasing cravings.

Other medications like topiramate, acamprosate, and baclofen, which have shown promise in adults with alcohol use disorder, have not been systematically evaluated in adolescents.

Marijuana/Cannabis

Cannabis is the most widely used illicit substance in youth. Cannabis use before the age of 17 years is associated with a significantly increased risk of SUDs in adulthood. Cannabis use in youth is also associated with poorer cognitive functioning, poorer academic and occupational achievement, and comorbid psychopathology. To date, no medications have been approved for the treatment of cannabis use disorder in adults.

N-Acetylcysteine, a glutamate-modulating agent sold as an over-the-counter dietary supplement in the United States, has some preliminary evidence for reducing cannabis use in a recent randomized controlled trial. Topiramate also showed some benefit in reducing cannabis use in youth in combination with motivation enhancement therapy in a recent pilot study, although dropout rates were high, likely due to poor tolerability.

Opioids

The high prevalence of prescription opioid analgesics misuse has paralleled the increasing availability and prescription of these medications in adults in the United States. In 2015, 276,000 adolescents were current nonmedical users of opioid analgesics, and 5000 were current heroin users.

Buprenorphine

The partial μ-receptor agonist, buprenorphine, has been studied in a number of rigorous trials in youth meeting opioid dependence as defined by the *Diagnostic and Statistical Manual of Mental Disorders*, 4th edition (*DSM-IV*). It has shown considerable promise in this population. A double-blind randomized controlled trial comparing Subutex (sublingual buprenorphine) and clonidine showed markedly better abstinence rates and treatment retention with buprenorphine, although both medications appeared safe and well tolerated. In another randomized controlled trial, 12 weeks of sublingual buprenorphine (in a 4:1 combination of buprenorphine to naloxone) up to a max of 24 mg per day (most frequently 16 mg per day) was superior to 2 weeks of sublingual buprenorphine/naloxone with regard to rates of opioid-negative urines. In youth with more advanced illness, those who received ancillary treatments to buprenorphine and those who were successful in the first 2 weeks and completed 12 weeks of treatment have been shown to particularly benefit from buprenorphine. As per the US Food and Drug Administration (FDA), there are no safety data for this medication in patients younger than 16 years.

Naltrexone

No controlled studies are available evaluating the efficacy of the μ-receptor antagonist, naltrexone, although it has shown promise in preventing relapse in youth who are dependent on opioids but are abstinent. A case series of 16 adolescents who were treated with monthly deep intramuscular injections of extended-release naltrexone (380 mg every 4 weeks) provided preliminary evidence for the tolerability, feasibility, and clinical utility of this medication. This approach also has the advantage of better adherence to treatment.

Methadone

There are no controlled trials evaluating the efficacy of methadone in adolescents. Moreover, methadone is administered in specialty treatment programs that usually do not offer this intervention to youth younger than 18 years. Youth between the age of 16 and 18 years need to meet specific criteria for admission, which includes two documented detoxification treatments or drug-free treatment and a specific FDA consent form signed by a parent or legal guardian.

Cocaine

Cocaine use among teens has been declining over the last decade. There are no FDA-approved medications for the treatment of cocaine use disorder in adults. There are no placebo-controlled trials evaluating the efficacy of medications for the treatment of cocaine use disorder in teens. Two case reports examining the efficacy of the tricyclic antidepressant, desipramine, in teens with cocaine dependence produced inconclusive evidence.

Over-the-Counter Medications and Other Drugs

Synthetic drugs ("bath salts," cathinone derivatives) and over-the-counter substances (dextromethorphan) are being abused by adolescents. Literature regarding toxicity and patterns of use are only just emerging, and currently, there is no evidence supporting the use of medications for the use or abuse of these substances, especially in youth.

Psychosocial Treatments

Many of the studies previously described for the treatment of SUDs in youth combined medications with psychosocial interventions like motivational enhancement therapy, family-based therapies, community reinforcement approaches, CM, and behavioral interventions. Medication-assisted treatment is not meant to function as a stand-alone option. Pharmacologic interventions are routinely combined with the aforementioned psychosocial interventions for improved outcomes.

CLINICAL CONSIDERATIONS

■ Early identification and treatment of adolescent SUDs is warranted because adolescent-onset use of substances is invariably linked to negative outcomes.

■ As outlined, evidence for the treatment of teen SUDs with medications is preliminary (except buprenorphine in opioid use disorder). Therefore, psychosocial interventions should be the first line of treatment.

■ If the teen may benefit from medication-assisted treatment, the physician should conduct a physical exam, order relevant blood work, and review all prescribed and over-the-counter medications before initiation.

■ Providers should review relevant state rules and regulations regarding parental consent for the treatment of minors with SUDs.

■ Physicians should engage the parent or caregiver frequently to enhance adherence, monitor for adverse effects, and to have an additional source of feedback regarding efficacy.

■ Most published studies of medication-assisted treatments have been conducted for 4 to 16 weeks. The duration of treatment should be tailored based on factors like adherence, adverse events, ability to achieve and maintain abstinence, and improvement of functioning.

Withdrawal Management/ Detoxification

There is very limited available literature regarding withdrawal syndromes and the management of withdrawal symptoms in youth, with the exception of some studies characterizing withdrawal symptoms in frequent and heavy users of marijuana, alcohol, and opioids. Common withdrawal symptoms across most categories of substances include irritability/negative affect, sleep disturbances, and cravings, which are most pronounced during the first 2 weeks after cessation of use. Behavioral interventions and, if indicated, medications for symptomatic relief of these symptoms should be used in order to prevent early relapse. Youth presenting with symptomatic alcohol or sedative-hypnotic withdrawal may require treatment in specialized detoxification settings with cardiovascular monitoring and benzodiazepine administration. Some youth with heavy use of nicotine may benefit from nicotine replacement therapy, varenicline, or bupropion (with parental consent if younger than 18 years) in addition to counseling. Patients 16 years and older who present with opioid withdrawal symptoms can

be safely and successfully inducted to buprenorphine in an office-based setting. Depending on the degree of withdrawal symptoms (assessed using a validated tool like the Subjective Opiate Withdrawal Scale), patients may be started on 2/0.5 mg of sublingual buprenorphine/naloxone combination, and an additional dose (2/0.5 to 4/1 mg) after 2 hours. Subsequent titration may be performed, based on response, to a dose of 8/2 mg to 16/4 mg daily but not to exceed 24/6 mg daily (which is only required in rare instances).

Overdose Management

Overdose management of alcohol, opioids, stimulants, and/or hallucinogens is generally handled no differently than with adults. The high incidence of anxiety, psychosis, seizures, and cardiovascular toxicity with exposure to synthetic cannabinoids is of particular concern, considering that a majority of reported cases involved patients younger than 25 years. Similarly, the toxicity from synthetic cathinones stimulants ("bath salts") can also result in psychosis, agitation, and cardiovascular toxicity. These patients may require emergency management with cardiovascular support, sedation (with benzodiazepines and/or antipsychotics), intravenous fluids, and, in some rare instances, intubation. Establishing a diagnosis in these cases is complicated by the fact that these compounds (ie, "K2," "Spice," "bath salts") are not detected on routine urine drug screens.

FUTURE DIRECTIONS

Pilot and adequately powered replication studies are required to examine the efficacy and tolerability of FDA-approved medications for SUDs in adults for youth populations. Moreover, elucidating neurobiologic and genetic underpinnings of deficits that predispose youth to developing SUDs will be crucial for preventative efforts.

KEY POINTS

1. Adolescent substance use is associated with a multitude of negative outcomes, including an increased risk of developing SUDs in the future. Alcohol, nicotine, marijuana, and tobacco are some of the most frequently abused substances in this population.

2. Although there are FDA-approved medications for the treatment of SUDs in adults, none of them have been approved for individuals younger than 18 years (with the exception of buprenorphine, which has been found to be safe in individuals older than 16 years).

3. There is evidence establishing the safety, tolerability, and efficacy of medications (which are approved for use in adults) in youth, especially with regard to nicotine replacement therapies, bupropion, varenicline, and buprenorphine.
4. Medications are best offered in conjunction with evidence-based psychosocial and behavioral interventions.

ACKNOWLEDGMENTS

The authors do not report any conflict of interest and are not beneficiaries of funding from any organization. Dr. Mathai would like to thank Kings County Hospital, Brooklyn, New York, for their continued support in completing this chapter. Dr. Mirzaei would like to acknowledge the support of Rutgers University School of Medicine, Newark, New Jersey.

REVIEW QUESTIONS

1. Which of the following medications are approved by the FDA for use in individuals younger than 18 years?
   A. Naltrexone
   B. Acamprosate
   C. Varenicline
   D. Buprenorphine

2. There are controlled trials evaluating the safety, tolerability, and efficacy of the following medications for the treatment of SUDs in youth *except*:
   A. varenicline.
   B. buprenorphine.
   C. naltrexone.
   D. methadone.

3. To date, research evaluating the safety, tolerability, and efficacy of pharmacotherapies for the management of adolescent SUDs has produced some promising findings for the treatment of all of the following *except*:
   A. opioid use disorder.
   B. cocaine use disorder.
   C. nicotine use disorder.
   D. alcohol use disorder.

ANSWERS

1. **D**
2. **D**
3. **B**

SUGGESTED READINGS

Bailey SR, Crew EE, Riske EC, et al. Efficacy and tolerability of pharmacotherapies to aid smoking cessation in adolescents. *Paediatr Drugs.* 2012;14(2):91-108.

Clark DB. Pharmacotherapy for adolescent alcohol use disorder. *CNS Drugs.* 2012;26(7):559-569.

Subramaniam GA, Gray KM. Pharmacotherapies for adolescents with substance use disorders. In: Ries RK, Fiellin DA, Miller SC, Saitz R, eds. *The ASAM Principles of Addiction Medicine,* 6th ed. Philadelphia: Lippincott Williams & Wilkins, 2018:1683-1692.

Subramaniam GA, Warden D, Minhajuddin A, et al. Predictors of abstinence: National Institute of Drug Abuse multisite buprenorphine/naloxone treatment trial in opioid-dependent youth. *J Am Acad Child Adolesc Psychiatry.* 2011;50(11):1120-1128.

Tanner-Smith EE, Wilson SJ, Lipsey ML. The comparative effectiveness of outpatient treatment for adolescent substance abuse: a meta-analysis. *J Subst Abuse Treat.* 2013;44(2):145-158.

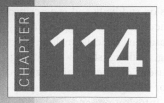
Co-occurring Psychiatric Disorders in Adolescents

Summary by Kelly S. Mulé

Based on THE ASAM PRINCIPLES OF ADDICTION MEDICINE, 6th edition chapter by Ramon Solhkhah and Muhammad A. Abbas

Adolescents with substance use disorders (SUDs) are more likely also to have psychiatric disorders than their peers, with research studies indicating that 50% to 90% of teens with SUDs also have psychiatric distress.

The use of terms such as *comorbidity* and *co-occurring disorders* are used in this chapter to describe individuals who meet the symptom criteria for SUDs and psychiatric disorders based on the *Diagnostic and Statistical Manual of Mental Disorders*, 5th edition (*DSM-5*). Adolescents who present for treatment for SUDs may symptomatically and behaviorally present differently from their peers who are treated only for psychiatric disorders. This chapter focuses on an increasing awareness of trends in teen comorbidities as well as recommendations for the treatment of this high-risk population.

INCIDENCE AND PREVALENCE

The Substance Abuse and Mental Health Services Administration published the National Survey on Drug Use and Health in 2016. Per the report, in 2015, approximately 3.4% of adolescents between the ages of 12 and 17 years had an SUD with the substance being from the following 10 categories: marijuana, cocaine/crack, heroin, hallucinogens, inhalants, methamphetamines, prescription pain relievers, tranquilizers, stimulants, and sedatives.

Longitudinal study data supported that alcohol and marijuana are the most common substances that adolescents use. Marijuana was the most commonly used illicit substance, with prescription amphetamines and other stimulants being the second most widely used illicit substance by teens. The general prevalence of teen substance use is decreasing.

Another study examined electronic medical records of patients aged 2 to 17 years at a large university hospital in inpatient and outpatient settings and found that 25% of teens aged 13 to 17 years met the criteria for SUDs, with marijuana being the

identified substance for 80% of those with substance disorders. Patients who met the *DSM-IV* criteria for substance abuse or dependence had comorbid anxiety and mood disorders, externalizing disorders of attention deficit hyperactivity disorder (ADHD) and conduct disorders, personality disorder symptoms, impulse-control disorders, psychotic disorders, and learning disorders as well as intellectual disability.

DIAGNOSIS AND MANAGEMENT

Given the likelihood of comorbidity and the overlap of patients who present with SUD symptoms and other psychiatric illnesses, the following guidelines are suggested for best practice. First, engage in a comprehensive clinical interview with the adolescent regarding all substances used (including nicotine/tobacco) and obtain collateral information. Second, assume comorbidity may exist for those patients whose psychiatric symptoms do not remit with appropriate treatment and engagement. Third, customize treatment to tailor interventions that address both psychiatric conditions and SUD symptoms. Finally, consult with an appropriate specialist clinician when comorbid diagnoses are met or suspected.

Depressive Disorders

Research indicates that for adolescents, like adults, there are two distinct presentations of depression: a primary depressive disorder or a substance-induced mood disorder. Individuals with a substance-induced mood disorder can present similarly to those with major depressive disorder. Studies indicate that it is important to parse out depressive disorder from substance-induced mood disorder. Signs of a substance-induced mood disorder are seeming reserved, intermittent or poor eye contact, poor grooming, denial of sad mood, and tearfulness during the session or interview. Research indicates that for adults who are abstinent, substance-induced mood disorder symptoms will decrease or remit.

Research indicates a strong overlap between depressive symptoms and SUDs in adolescents, with study data indicating that girls with a history of SUDs are three times more likely to develop a depressive disorder than girls without a history of SUDs. Regarding suicidality, research suggests that having a comorbid psychiatric illness and an SUD contributes to suicide attempt risk, which should be closely monitored.

Bipolar Disorder

Bipolar disorder has a typical onset of older adolescence. It is difficult to diagnose bipolar disorder in children and teens, especially when a comorbid SUD is present. Side effects of frequent substance use resemble bipolar disorder (eg, mood dysregulation, erratic sleeping patterns). Bipolar disorder may be present if binging is part of a teen's substance use profile. Adolescents who present with bipolar disorder are at a higher risk of developing an SUD, especially if they develop bipolar disorder as an adolescent rather than as a child. Best practice is to engage in substance abuse prevention work with youth at risk or who meet the criteria for bipolar disorder.

Adolescents sometimes use substances, specifically alcohol, to regulate mania. For these patients, medication treatment for bipolar symptoms should be considered.

Anxiety Disorders

Co-occurring anxiety and SUDs are quite common for teens and adults. There are many anxiety disorders that may be comorbid, including generalized anxiety, panic disorder, social anxiety, obsessive-compulsive disorder, and posttraumatic distress disorder. When a patient presents with an SUD, it can be difficult to diagnose and, therefore, treat comorbid anxiety symptoms.

It is a well-supported view that anxiety disorders are successfully treated via behavioral therapy. Psychopharmacologic treatment for anxiety disorder is a more disputed treatment approach with comorbid SUD presentation. Benzodiazepines are not advised for someone with active SUD symptoms or a history of SUD given their addictive nature. Physicians can adopt the following clinical stance when comorbidity of anxiety and an SUD exists and the patient requests benzodiazepines: Work to achieve abstinence and engage in cognitive–behavioral therapy, then offer alternative medication options.

Panic Attacks

An individual must endure persistent panic attacks in order to meet the criteria for a panic disorder. A panic attack comes on suddenly and is described as feeling intensely uncomfortable for approximately 10 minutes. Body sensations typically include heart palpitations, sweating, shaking, shallow breathing, chest tightness, nausea, disorientation/dizziness, and a fear of dying or losing control. These symptoms also describe intoxication and withdrawal from various substances; therefore, abstinence must be achieved in order to consider if an individual meets the criteria for a panic disorder.

Posttraumatic Stress Disorder

Incidents of trauma occur at higher rates in clinical adolescent populations than in nonclinical populations. Teens may use substances to avoid recollections and symptoms of posttraumatic stress disorder. Clinical tools to treat SUDs and trauma include implementing self-care strategies and using a harm reduction model in a group setting to reduce life-threatening aspects of behavior. Integration of posttraumatic stress disorder and SUD treatment that involves family work shows success as well as including the manualized treatment of Seeking Safety.

Substance-Induced Mental Disorders

Several substances have been identified as contributing to acute and long-term cognitive issues including alcohol, methamphetamines, marijuana, cocaine, ecstasy, hallucinogens, and inhalants. Symptoms in the acute phase include poor concentration ability, language deficits, and an irritable mood. Residual symptoms include memory and executive functioning impairments. Patients who develop these symptoms may gain back cognitive functioning when they establish abstinence, although this can take a year or more, and sometimes, functioning never returns to baseline. If cognitive deficits remain, the patient should be referred for cognitive rehabilitation and educational and vocational planning as well as neuropsychological assessment.

It is important to educate adolescents and their guardians of the possible effects of substance use on cognitive functioning without eliciting hopelessness from the patient regarding their substance use.

Schizophrenia

Teens who experience psychotic symptoms at a younger age frequently use substances to cope with their symptoms. It is highly recommended to simultaneously treat psychosis and SUDs in a co-occurring treatment model. The most frequently used substances for teens with psychosis are marijuana and alcohol, and marijuana may further enhance psychotic symptoms and increase the likelihood of onset of schizophrenia. Individuals with severe SUDs and schizophrenia have a poorer prognosis, and therefore, it is recommended that treatment includes a harm reduction approach and long-term access to care.

Attention Deficit Hyperactivity Disorder

There is high comorbidity for adolescents who have ADHD and SUDs. A study found that an ADHD diagnosis strongly predicted substance use.

Medication treatments for ADHD in teens who have SUDs have had a mixed reception, with only some endorsing stimulant medication. If a stimulant medication is being considered, a physician should consider the current length of sobriety; educate the family about the risks of prescribing stimulants; assess compliance and reliability of the patient and family regarding dispensing of medication; assess what motivates the patient for abstinence; and, if there is a history of stimulant use without a prescription, assess the motive for seeking the prescription.

Conduct Disorder

Conduct disorder is very common in individuals with SUDs, with comorbidity in adolescents that is supported by research. The best practice for treating comorbid conduct and SUD behaviors in adolescents includes family involvement and establishing clear rules and limits.

Eating Disorders

The prevalence of adolescents who are substance users and have disordered eating behaviors has increased. Research indicates that 25% of patients who have an eating disorder also have a history of SUDs or current substance use. Bulimia is more common and more associated with SUDs than anorexia.

KEY POINTS

1. Similar to adults, psychiatric disorders and substance use disorders are highly comorbid in adolescents.
2. Although adolescent substance use is declining in the United States, many adolescents who meet the criteria for comorbid substance use disorders and psychiatric illness are not in treatment or are only in treatment for one issue. A tailored intervention to treat comorbid issues is essential.
3. Gold standard treatments and psychiatric medications are often warranted for the treatment of

comorbid presentations including antidepressants, mood stabilizers, antipsychotics, and psychostimulants. Pharmacologic therapies need to be closely monitored with populations who use substances due to the interaction between use of the prescribed medication and use of substances.

REVIEW QUESTIONS

1. Which of the following guidelines will help detect and provide earlier interventions for comorbid substance use and psychiatric disorders?
   A. Perform a clinical interview of the parent and adolescent. Do not begin a treatment regimen until it is clear if a comorbidity exists because this can be dangerous to the patient. Consult others as needed.
   B. Perform a clinical interview with the adolescent, obtain collateral information, assume comorbidity is present for patients whose symptoms do not remit with the gold standard treatment, customize the treatment to address comorbid symptoms, collect information regarding current and history of all substances used, consult with addiction medicine specialist as needed.
   C. Clinically assess for substance use disorder and history of use, provide supportive and pharmacologic treatments, always prescribe psychotropic medication.
   D. Perform a clinical interview only with the adolescent because parents do not have a sense of whether their teen is actively using substances.

2. What is the best description of the difference between major depressive disorder and substance-induced mood disorder?
   A. Major depression is prevalent for teens and adults, whereas a substance-induced mood disorder only occurs in adults.
   B. Clinicians can tell the difference based on length of time and frequency of symptoms.
   C. Patients with major depressive disorder have suicidal tendencies, whereas patients with a substance-induced mood disorder do not.
   D. Patients with a substance-induced mood disorder may present slightly differently than teens with major depressive disorder, including tearfulness, poor grooming, or denial of sad mood.
   E. They are two derivations of the same disorder.

3. A 17-year-old male enters the emergency room after he wandered into a restaurant requesting alcohol at 11 am. He appears to have mood fluctuations and dysregulation (sometimes answering

your questions, sometimes looking away and grunting or shouting). He reports a lack of sleep for the "past few days" and feeling "great." His shirt smells of alcohol, although he does not appear intoxicated. What is the best course of action?

A. Contact his guardian to let them know that he is in the emergency room and release him to them.

B. Request a urine toxicology report and lab workup to assess if he taking psychiatric medication. Keep him in the comprehensive psychiatric emergency program for observation and monitor symptoms because alcohol use is commonly used to cope with manic symptoms. When he is sober, do a clinical interview for substance use history and to rule out bipolar disorder.

C. He is too young to present with bipolar disorder; therefore, refer him to inpatient rehabilitation to treat alcohol use disorder.

D. Have a consult with a pediatrician regarding a hormonal imbalance.

ANSWERS

1. **B**
2. **D**
3. **B**

SUGGESTED READINGS

Hovens JG, Cantwell DP, Kiriakos R. Psychiatric comorbidity in hospitalized adolescent substance abusers. *J Am Acad Child Adolesc Psychiatry.* 1994;33(4):476-483.

Riggs P, Levin F, Green AI, Vocci F. Comorbid psychiatric and substance abuse disorders: recent treatment research. *Subst Abus.* 2008;29(3):51-63.

Riggs PD, Mikulich-Gilbertson SK, Davies RD, et al. A randomized controlled trial of fluoxetine and cognitive behavioral therapy in adolescents with major depression, behavior problems, and substance use disorders. *Arch Pediatr Adolesc Med.* 2007;161(11):1026-1034.

Wu LT, Gersing K, Burchett B, Woody GE, Blazer DG. Substance use disorders and comorbid axis I and II psychiatric disorders among young psychiatric patients: findings from a large electronic health records database. *J Psychiatr Res.* 2011;45(11):1453-1462.

Ethical, Legal, and Liability Issues in Addiction Practice

Based on THE ASAM PRINCIPLES OF ADDICTION MEDICINE, 6th edition chapter by Tim K. Brennan and H. Westley Clark

Ethics amount to a set of moral principles that govern an individual's behavior, regardless of whether that person is a clinician or a patient. In fact, the ethical principles that apply to addiction research and practice are similar to the ethical principles that apply to general medical care. Simply stated, ethics provide us with light to navigate the sometimes dark roads of clinical care. The long tradition of Western medicine that evolved from Hippocrates in the fifth century BC has matured through the activities of various professional organizations such as the American Medical Association, the American Hospital Association, the American Nurses Association, the American Psychiatric Association, the American Psychological Association, and the National Association of Social Workers, to name a few. These organizations have promulgated codes of conduct and behavior predicated on the imperative that clinicians must behave in an ethical manner in their interactions with patients and in the conduct of health-related matters.

In this regard, it is important to recognize that what is deemed to be *ethical* may sometimes conflict with what is deemed to be *legal*. What is *legal* is governed by laws or regulations that are codified and published, whereas what is *ethical* is governed by a unique situation that is specific to a particular clinician and patient. However, ethical principles are commonly encoded as standards by organized medicine and other professional organizations related to law, divinity, education, finance, etc. Many people enter the practice of medicine guided by a spirit of altruism—that is, acting with regard to others. This is a near-universal trait among physicians and one that is easy to embody because people who are sick generate empathy in others quite easily. However, within addiction medicine, where many practitioners have preconceived notions of certain moral implications of the disease of addiction, an ethical framework becomes much more essential and worthy of continued inquiry.

CORE ETHICAL PRINCIPLES

There are five general principles that provide a basis from which to explore the ethical questions and concerns that arise in the treatment of substance use disorders (SUDs): autonomy, beneficence, nonmaleficence, justice, and fidelity.

Autonomy

A primary principle in modern medicine is that clinicians should respect the right of individuals to determine what course of action is appropriate for themselves. In other words, a person acts in his or her own self-interest as a rational actor. Thus, the clinician is obligated to treat the patient as autonomous and avoid actions that would diminish the patient's ability to exercise personal liberty. Customarily, the patient's capacity to decide is presumed. However, the underlying assumption of competent self-determination may be questioned when a patient is suffering from an SUD because psychoactive substances interfere with cognitive processes and decision-making ability. Compromised competence is an important consideration for clinicians because it can influence how the clinician should respond to the exercise of autonomy by a patient.

Thus, a clinician should have some means to assess the ongoing competence of a patient being treated for an SUD. Conditions that cause competence to wax and wane may be especially vexing for both patient and clinician. Conditions that have a progressively deteriorating effect on competence also can create dilemmas because it becomes critical to assess the course and rate of the deterioration in order to determine the degree to which the clinician should respect the patient's autonomy and right to self-determination.

A growing number of patients in addiction treatment have been forced or compelled into such treatment by their families, employers, or the criminal justice system. For example, a spouse may give his or her partner an ultimatum: "Get help or else." An employer may require treatment as a condition of retaining a job. A criminal justice agency may require a defendant to enter treatment as a condition of probation, parole, or suspension of charges. Critics of coerced treatment contend that it is unethical because it violates the principle of autonomy. Some critics are particularly concerned when the criminal justice system mandates treatment or offers inducements such as the possibility that a criminal defendant will avoid incarceration because they view the power imbalance in such circumstances as especially annihilative to the principle of autonomy.

Proponents of coerced treatment counter that although such coercion unquestionably impinges on a patient's autonomy, it does not violate it altogether, even in the context of the criminal justice system. The patient may not wish to enter treatment but always has a choice about whether to do so and retains the right to refuse. The patient may not like the consequences of refusal (losing a spouse, losing a job, or being incarcerated on criminal charges) but still retains the autonomy to make the decision in question.

Much of the discussion presented here dovetails with the concept of *informed consent*. As a critical component of autonomy, informed consent is the process of communication between a patient and a clinician that allows the clinician to provide specific medical treatments to the patient. As the American Medical Association has pointed out, the communication process associated with informed consent is both a legal requirement and an ethical obligation.

Beneficence

The principle of beneficence assumes that an individual wishes to help others and implies a moral obligation to act for the benefit of the patient. Inherent in the physician–patient relationship is an obligation on the part of the physician to aid the patient and avoid harming him or her. However, there are limits to this obligation, and the practitioner should guard against becoming overinvolved with the patient.

Defining the boundaries of what is "good for the patient" also is tied to the notion that a licensed practitioner is, in part, an agent of the state and, as such, an agent of social good. If the "good" in addiction medicine is recovery, then the boundaries of that "good" could become limitless, with the life of the clinician intertwined with the life of the patient. Such an outcome would invoke paternalism and a diminution of patient autonomy. Consequently, beneficence must have natural, ethical limits. Although there may not be a natural boundary to the legitimate practice of addiction medicine, involving the patient in shared decision making about his or her care can lead to consensus between the clinician and patient as to the way forward.

Nonmaleficence

This ethical principle means "to do no harm." In treating patients with SUDs, the clinician must not knowingly provide ineffective treatments or act with malice toward a patient. This principle is *not* about avoiding exposing a patient to the known or unknown risks of a particular therapeutic intervention; in fact, there are risks associated with many effective treatments. Rather, the principle suggests that a clinician's bias for or against a particular type of treatment should be informed by best practices, scientific research, and/or objective clinical experience.

An example of nonmaleficence is seen in the actions of a primary care physician who prescribes opioid analgesics for the treatment of pain. Because there is an inherent risk of dependence and/or addiction associated with the long-term use of opioids, the failure to explain that risk to a patient would be "doing harm." Further, the physician could be seen as causing harm because he or she lacks the knowledge needed to monitor the patient's progress and adjust the analgesic as indicated. It is clear, then, that the intersection of doing good (the principle of beneficence) and causing no harm (nonmaleficence) can produce a conundrum of sorts for the addiction medicine specialist. A clinician whose moral values argue against the use of methadone or buprenorphine for the treatment of opioid dependence will be faced with a decision whether to limit the options available to patients. Although clinicians who hold this view have access to naltrexone, care must be exercised in discussing clinical options with patients in order to avoid violating the principle of nonmaleficence. Stated differently, patients should be aware of *all treatment options available to them*, regardless of the personal beliefs of the clinician who is treating them.

Justice

This ethical principle requires that, at a macrolevel, society distributes goods and services—including medical goods and services—fairly. At the microlevel, it means that clinicians will treat patients with equal conditions equally. In a normative sense, the principle of justice would require that medical needs are determined according to (1) the benefit that would accrue to a patient from the services offered, (2) the acuity of the patient's need, (3) the potential enhancement of the patient's quality of life, and (4) the duration of the benefit. In an ideal world, nonmedical criteria would not limit the services that a patient would receive. The American Medical Association's *Code of Medical Ethics* affirms that "non-medical criteria, such as ability to pay, age, social worth, perceived obstacles to treatment, patient contribution to illness, or past use of resources should not be considered." Despite these views, there are wide disparities in the ability of patients to pay for services, just as there is a wide difference in the cost of services offered by addiction treatment providers. Fortunately, a wide spectrum of treatment facilities and services are available, from volunteer non–profit-run organizations to government-financed programs to privately operated facilities.

A larger issue may be the absence of demand for services. Data collected by the Substance Abuse and Mental Health Services Administration show that more than 90% of those who meet the clinical criteria for SUDs do not seek or receive such treatment. Moreover, although there is a hope that enactment of federal parity laws will allow millions more people to access mental health and addiction services, there is a difference between having financial access to services and perceiving a need for such services. It has been argued that healthcare practitioners have a responsibility to advocate for their patients and to be involved in establishing humane policies of resource allocation at both the institutional and societal levels. Thus, in order to give meaning to the principle of justice in the context of addiction, practitioners should make efforts to educate their colleagues and patients and to promote societal awareness of the need for addiction treatment.

Fidelity

The principle of fidelity focuses on the quality of being faithful or loyal to the duties and obligations of a caregiver to a patient. It encompasses telling the truth and keeping actual and implicit promises to the patient—that is, veracity. It also involves not representing fiction as truth. In establishing a relationship with a patient, the clinician creates a set of expectations. These include honoring the treatment agreement, adhering to professional codes of ethics, maintaining an acceptable level of competence through training and continuing education, and following the policies and procedures of the treatment organization and all applicable laws. It also means that the information provided to the clinician will remain confidential to the extent permitted by law. Among other things, fidelity invokes the Hippocratic oath: "What I may see or hear in the course of the treatment or even outside of treatment of the patient in regard to the life of men, which on no account one must spread abroad, I will keep to myself, holding such things to be shameful to be spoken about."

Although US Code 42 CFR Part 2, Confidentiality of Substance Use Disorder Patient Records, provides a legal framework for confidentiality that governs federally funded treatment programs, it is not the law alone on which a patient relies in his or her relationship with a clinician. Confidentiality is both an implicit and explicit promise by the clinician not to divulge a patient's personal information without that patient's permission. If a physician is going to maintain fidelity by keeping promises, it is essential to be clear in advance about which promises may have to be broken and the circumstances under which that might occur. Federal regulations offer a limited list of exceptions to confidentiality in the context of addiction treatment. For example, if a patient appears to be suicidal or homicidal, confidentiality may need to be breached. Also, if a patient violates certain aspects of the treatment agreement, the relationship between the clinician and patient may be terminated. It is important that the clinician be very clear about the limits to fidelity, so there are no surprises at a later date.

DEALING WITH DENIAL

Historically, practitioners in primary care settings did not inquire about a patient's substance use unless it was directly related to the presenting complaint, and annual physical examinations rarely included questions about alcohol or drug use. In fact, guidelines from the US Preventive Services Task Force recommend only that primary care physicians screen for depression and alcohol misuse. The US Preventive Services Task Force guidelines state that "screening in primary care settings can accurately identify patients whose alcohol consumption does not meet criteria for alcohol dependence, but places them at risk for increased morbidity and mortality. Brief behavioral counseling interventions with follow-up produce small to moderate reductions in alcohol consumption that are sustained over 6 to 12 months or longer." In contrast, the US Preventive Services Task Force concluded that current evidence is insufficient to support recommended screening of adolescents, pregnant women, and other adults for drug misuse. If the opioid use disorder pandemic continues, these guidelines may change.

Nevertheless, when a clinician suspects that a patient may be misusing alcohol or drugs, he or she must take the initiative to raise the issue, even if the patient has not previously disclosed it. Similarly, if a clinician suspects that a patient may have an abdominal mass, he or she is obligated to share that finding with the patient and make a referral for an appropriate clinical workup. SUDs are no different. The clinician has an ethical duty to act if there is reason to believe that the patient's use of alcohol or drugs is negatively affecting that patient's health.

In such situations, a difficulty commonly encountered by clinicians is that raising the issue may not be enough. Denial is an integral part of SUDs. Individuals in denial fail to recognize or are reluctant to acknowledge their problem or find ways to deny or minimize the extent of their substance use because they are ambivalent about changing that use. In such situations, what is the proper balance between respect for the principle of autonomy and the physician's responsibility for the patient's health? Should the physician raise the issue and then drop it if the patient is resistant?

Talking to the Patient

To fulfill the ethical responsibility to the patient, the clinician must do more than simply raise an issue. He or she should provide relevant information, engage the patient in discussion, and, if the patient shows resistance, follow-up during future visits in a compassionate and nonconfrontational manner. Unless a firm foundation of trust and understanding has been established, persistent questions or a forceful confrontation can backfire and ultimately reinforce the patient's resistance.

Ordering Laboratory Tests

Must, or should, a patient's consent be obtained before a drug screen is ordered? It is likely that the law does not require the patient's consent. Ordinarily, a clinician does not ask a patient to sign a consent form before sending blood or urine for other types of testing. However, ordering laboratory tests to screen patients for SUDs has different implications, and failing to consult the patient can damage the physician–patient relationship and undermine efforts to induce the patient to acknowledge the presence of a problem. A second reason that physicians should obtain a patient's permission before ordering laboratory drug screens has to do with the patient's right to privacy. If the physician orders a test, the patient's insurance company or other third-party payer will know about the test and perhaps even its result, so even the decision to order a drug screen discloses a good deal, regardless of whether the test result is positive or negative. Therefore, it is the patient, not the physician, who should decide whether it is necessary and appropriate for the health insurer to have that information.

Older Patients

The clinician who suspects that an older adult is misusing alcohol or other drugs should proceed with caution. As we age, we become more sensitive to perceived threats to our autonomy. Because of the stigma surrounding SUDs, a patient whose clinician suggests that he or she may be drinking too much or misusing drugs (whether legal or illegal) may conclude that the physician is suggesting that whatever brought the patient to the physician's office for a medical visit has an emotional basis or that the patient's functioning or capacity is diminished. If an older adult thinks that his or her autonomy is being threatened, the patient may point to the "normal" infirmities of old age as the source of the difficulty, rather than acknowledging a problem with alcohol or other drugs.

ESTABLISHING AN ETHICAL STANCE

Clinicians can avoid or minimize potential ethical dilemmas if they remain aware of the sources of potential conflicts of interest, keep the purposes of the ethical principles in mind, discuss potential conflicts with patients at the beginning of treatment, and take steps to reduce the potential for conflicts. Resources for obtaining professional guidance on ethical issues can be found through consultation with colleagues, accessing professional standards or codes of ethics, and obtaining legal consultation. Each has strengths and drawbacks, and each is more relevant to some types of ethical dilemmas than are others.

Consultation

Consultation can involve peers, senior staff, or other providers within the community. Confidentiality needs to be ensured when seeking consultation. If there is a chance that information cannot be shared without accidentally divulging confidential information, the provider should find a consultant in another geographic locale. Identifying information must not be shared without the patient's consent.

Professional Standards or Codes of Ethics

Professional standards are another resource. Many medical organizations have adopted professional standards and codes of ethics, as have organizations in social work, nursing, and psychology. Although such standards do not provide answers to every ethical dilemma, they do provide useful parameters for acceptable and unacceptable professional behavior. They also may help the professional frame questions that clarify the underlying issues and thus move the situation toward a decision.

LEGAL CONSULTATION

For many providers, obtaining legal advice may seem unrealistic given limited resources, but there are low-cost strategies for obtaining advice in certain situations. Most bar associations have a pro bono legal component that may provide consultation at no charge or at a reduced rate. Legal service agencies that operate as a social service to the community may have expertise regarding certain ethical dilemmas. In addition, every state has a department of substance abuse and/or mental health services that are charged with funding and regulating addiction treatment. Such an entity may have an attorney available who can assist with legal issues related to treatment.

FUTURE DEVELOPMENTS

The coming decades promise exciting breakthroughs in the treatment of SUDs. Yet, if the past is any guide to the future, each new discovery will bring with it new challenges to the core ethical obligations of honoring informed consent, protecting confidentiality, and respecting justice while also protecting the public from harm and ensuring good care of individual patients. With the growth of managed care, the physician and patient no longer have an exclusive relationship. Third-party payers have intruded into the relationship in multiple ways, such as by shifting some financial risk to the physician or awarding bonuses to physicians whose patients do not use expensive (or extensive) services. Under other plans, contracts limit the services for which a physician will be reimbursed. (Note that such contracts do not limit the services the physician can provide, only those for which they will be paid.) In this way, many managed care plans create incentives that can impinge on sound medical judgment.

If a clinician allows financial incentives or disincentives to influence his or her treatment recommendations, or lead the clinician to discharge a patient who has exhausted benefits under a health insurance contract, that clinician has placed financial interests before his or her obligation to the patient, which is a clear ethical violation. Because health insurers and other third-party payers place (often hidden) limits on certain forms of treatment, ethicists have begun to suggest that clinicians should inform their patients about any economic issues that could influence either the clinician's recommendation or the patient's decision. Providing an opportunity for the patient to give "economic informed consent" ensures that the patient knows about such limitations before making a decision about the proposed course of care. If clinicians can adapt to the "new normal," these unprecedented paradigm shifts can influence healthcare decision making in a reasoned and balanced fashion, and there is real hope that the cultural stigma and disenfranchisement underlying health disparities in addiction treatment may move in the direction of compassionate and competent care for all those who suffer from addiction.

KEY POINTS

1. There are five general principles that provide a basis from which to explore the ethical questions and concerns that arise in the treatment of SUDs: autonomy, beneficence, nonmaleficence, justice, and fidelity.
2. When a clinician suspects that a patient may be misusing alcohol or drugs, he or she must take the initiative to raise the issue, even if the patient has not previously disclosed it.
3. Clinicians can avoid or minimize potential ethical dilemmas if they remain aware of the sources of potential conflicts of interest, keep the purposes of the ethical principles in mind, discuss potential conflicts with patients at the beginning of treatment, and take steps to reduce the potential for conflicts.

REVIEW QUESTIONS

1. Which of the following is the definition of beneficence?
   A. Acts of mercy, kindness, and charity
   B. One ought not to inflict evil or harm
   C. Being free from controlling authority
   D. To each person an equal share

2. Which of the following is the best description of nonmaleficence?
   A. One should always report colleagues if they appear to be doing harm.
   B. To each according to their greatest need
   C. Do no harm.
   D. Being free from controlling authority

3. When you suspect a cocaine use disorder in a patient you are treating for primary care, which is the best course of action?
   A. Obtain a urine toxicology first. If negative, do nothing; if positive, speak to the patient.
   B. Ask the patient about his or her cocaine use.

C. Ask for a urine specimen and state, "I get this for all of my patients as a routine test."

D. Speak to his or her spouse to see if they have noticed anything suspicious.

ANSWERS

1. **A**
2. **C**
3. **B**

SUGGESTED READINGS

American Medical Association. *Code of Medical Ethics*. Chicago: American Medical Association, 2008.

Center for Substance Abuse Treatment. *Substance Abuse Treatment for Persons With HIV/AIDS. Treatment Improvement Protocol (TIP) 37*. Rockville, MD: Substance Abuse and Mental Health Services Administration, 2000. HH Publication No. (SMA) 12-4137.

Fisher CB. Addiction research ethics and the Belmont principles: do drug users have a different moral voice? *Subst Use Misuse*. 2011;46(6):728-741.

Page K. The four principles: can they be measured and do they predict ethical decision making? *BMC Med Ethics*. 2012;13:10.

Schaler JA. *Addiction Is a Choice*. Chicago: Open Court Publishers, 2000.

116 Consent and Confidentiality Issues in Addiction Practice

Summary by R. Corey Waller

> Based on THE ASAM PRINCIPLES OF ADDICTION MEDICINE, 6th edition chapter by Louis E. Baxter Sr., Mark F. Seltzer Esq, and Bonnie B. Wilford

As the personal lives of the average American become more and more intertwined with the delivery of healthcare services, the personal information contained within health-related documents has the ability to improve patient care, allow for more efficient healthcare systems, and increase the convenience for patients significantly. However, the other side of this coin is the use of this information for more nefarious reasons that can lead to a patient losing custody of their child, losing their job, or having an increased risk of incarceration from an unrelated crime. With a combination of logic, federal laws, state laws, and regulations, we have attempted to create a balanced approach to the utilization of sensitive patient information pertaining to substance use disorders (SUDs). However, there are still many areas that are very gray and many laws and regulations that need to be updated to meet modern medical standards in the age of the electronic health record (EHR). This chapter attempts to give a succinct overview of the concepts of confidentiality, informed consent, the laws pertaining to these issues, the approach to special populations, as well as the answers to the more commonly asked questions. The author of this chapter must state clearly and concisely that "I am not a lawyer, and this is not a legal opinion." For questions about implementation into a specific program or healthcare apparatus, an in-house counsel or an appropriately trained and licensed individual should be utilized to help make decisions about patient confidentiality.

BASIS OF CONFIDENTIALITY

Medical records tend to lay bare the more human moments of a patient's life. This includes a cadre of bad luck, bad decisions, or both. The most basic aspect of building a therapeutic alliance is trust. One of the key components of trust is knowing that the information patients divulge to medical practitioners in confidence (the root word of confidentiality) will

not come back to cause them harm. This becomes even more important when speaking of highly stigmatized conditions such as mental health disorders, SUDs, and infectious diseases. As a society, there has been a constant struggle with balancing the need for the individual's privacy and how it relates to the safety of the population at large. It is also important to recognize that confidentiality does not only pertain to that which a patient has disclosed but also other information such as toxicologic evaluations, laboratory studies, medication lists, and information about other medical specialties being utilized. With all of these being relevant, and a bit confusing, the federal government and many state governments have enacted laws and regulations, to varying degrees of specificity, that attempt to guide the medical field through what pieces of information may be shared and to whom they may be shared with. In the remainder of this chapter, these pathways are delineated and guidance is provided as clearly as humanly possible.

INFORMED CONSENT

Although informed consent may be considered as only pertaining to a test or procedure that may result in a serious adverse physical or psychological consequence, it actually begins the minute a patient walks into a healthcare office or hospital. The first consent a patient gives is the ever-present consent to treat. This allows for the initial engagement of the patient and typically is the first time in which the basics of confidentiality come into play. Although the consent to treat form is the most superficial version of an informed consent, in many ways, the patient feels obligated to sign (and is generally obligated) to be evaluated by a healthcare professional, unless in the direst of situations. In a more practical sense, informed consent must have three basic components: knowledge, competency, and voluntary acceptance.

The first component, knowledge, is usually the one least attended to prior to initiating treatment. However, it is of the utmost importance that the provider delivers the risks and benefits of the treatment being offered as well as any alternative treatments and the most likely (nonhyperbolic) consequences if they decline treatment. In practical terms, all patients will receive differing levels of this based on the knowledge of the provider delivering the information, the communicative skill of that provider, and the expediency of the situation in which it needs to be delivered.

The competency portion of informed consent is directed at the patient and or caregiver's capacity to make a rational decision based on the information given to them. For a minor, this test may also require them to be the age of consent. Generally, if the patient is able to understand the explanation given, comprehend the treatment options, and associated risks and benefits, they are deemed to be competent to enter into an informed consent agreement. See later in the chapter for a discussion of this issue as it pertains to patients with mental illness and patients with cognitive impairment.

The third component revolving around voluntary acceptance is where ethics can become a bit murky. Given the inherent perceived power of a physician, many patients do not feel that they have the ability to question their authority and many times are told as much by the practicing provider. Given this, it is important to allow for the patient or guardian to express their concerns and desires of a second opinion when it comes to highly risky treatments or interventions.

FEDERAL LAWS GOVERNING CONFIDENTIALITY

Health Insurance Portability and Accountability Act of 1996

In 1996, the US Congress enacted a set of standards for confidentiality surrounding individually identifiable health information: Public Law 104 to 191, or the Health Insurance Portability and Accountability Act (HIPAA). In 2000, the US Department of Health and Human Services issued its initial set of regulations in 45 CFR Parts 160 and 164. The entities covered by HIPAA are

- health plans,
- healthcare providers,
- businesses associated with healthcare providers (eg, hospitals, surgical centers), and
- healthcare clearing houses (supporting business to healthcare infrastructure).

Life insurers, employers, workers compensation carriers, schools, state agencies like child protective services, law enforcement, and municipal offices are not required to follow HIPAA guidelines.

In a nutshell, HIPAA allows for the release of information, after patient consent is given, to those entities involved in healthcare-related treatment, payment, and operations. Again, the consent for agreement to HIPAA is usually part of the initial consent to treat and, thus, is generally not called out explicitly.

The Rehabilitation Act of 1973 and The Americans With Disabilities Act of 1990

Both the Rehabilitation Act and the Americans with Disabilities Act afford specific protections for individuals with disabilities. The former is focused on federal employees and contractors, whereas the Americans with Disabilities Act is for the general public and applies to all entities in the nongovernmental United States. The reason that these are mentioned in a chapter about confidentiality is twofold. (1) Release or utilization of healthcare records relating to addiction to make a determination of employment would be a breach of these acts. (2) A memo written by the US Attorney for the Southern District of New York on October 3, 2017, stated very clearly that the Americans with Disabilities Act protects patients who are on medication-assisted treatment (https://lac .org/wp-content/uploads/2018/02/DOJ-SDNY -ltr-to-OCA-10.3.17.pdf). Making sure that the utilization of information pertaining to addiction-related conditions is not utilized to discriminate is of the utmost importance to maintaining both trust and engagement in treatment. The next section explains how this information is protected under the current statute.

42 CFR PART 2

History

In 1972, Congress enacted the Drug Abuse Prevention, Treatment, and Rehabilitation Act (DAPTRA). Although DAPTRA was statutorily vague, it did make confidential "records pertaining to identity, diagnosis, prognosis, or treatment of any patient which are maintained in connection with the performance of any program or activity relating to substance abuse education, prevention, training, treatment, rehabilitation, or research, which is conducted, regulated, or directly or indirectly assessed by any department or agency of the United States."

DAPTRA also required consent for disclosure, except for:

- medical personnel in the case of a "bona fide medical emergency,"
- qualified personnel conducting "scientific research, management audits, financial audits, or program evaluation," or
- as authorized by a court order, including in cases to avert a substantial risk of death or serious bodily harm.

It was made clear in the statute that DAPTRA does not apply to the military, veteran affairs, or in cases of reporting suspected child abuse to local authorities.

Because DAPTRA was both short and without detail, 42 CFR Part 2 was written in 1975 to further define the process by which information may be released. This code was further updated in 1987 and then most recently in 2016, 2017, and then again in the spring of 2018. The remainder of this discussion is around the most recent "final rule" and should be considered an accurate description as of October 25, 2018. As of the writing of this chapter, there was a bill passed by the House of Representatives and one being considered by the US Senate that would align 42 CFR Part 2 with HIPAA.

Covered Entities

There are three basic requirements to be considered an "covered entity" under 42 CFR Part 2. The first requires very little interpretation and states that the record must "identify a patient as having or having had an SUD either directly, by reference to publicly available information, or through verification of such identification by another person." The other two are less straightforward and include that the record must of been obtained by a "program" and that this "program" must be "federally assisted."

To qualify as a "program," one must provide SUD services. This can be an individual, an entity, or an entity that has an identified unit that "holds itself out" as providing SUD services. To be clear, the unit does not have to have a physical distinction and should be considered to exist if there are staff whose "primary function is the provision of SUD diagnosis, treatment or referral for treatment and is identified as such specialized medical personnel or other staff by the general medical facility." In practical terms, an entity is not considered covered if it merely treats patients in a general practice who happen to have addiction as a secondary diagnosis or are admitted to the hospital for a non-SUD diagnosis but are being treated concurrently for an SUD. The Substance

Abuse and Mental Health Services Administration has specifically stated that having a Drug Treatment Act of 2000 waiver or "X-waiver," does not automatically qualify a person or entity as a "covered entity."

In a situation where an individual or an entity meets both the first and second requirement, they may still not be considered subject to Part 2 requirements. This would occur if the individual or entity is not federally assisted in any capacity. However, it is rare that an entity would not have some version of federal assistance such as having a tax-exempt status, receiving any other support from the federal government, or having a providing prescriber that maintains a Drug Enforcement Administration registration.

Exceptions to 42 CFR Part 2

As is the case with the original statute, DAPTRA, there are limited exceptions to Part 2 regulation. With the exception made to the military and the veterans affairs, all Part 2 programs must obtain consent for the release of SUD information except under the following conditions:

- responding to a bona fide emergency,
- for the purposes of child abuse reporting,
- when conducting research,
- performing audit evaluations, or
- pursuant to a court order.

A second area that the Part 2 disclosures do not apply are "within a Part 2 program or between a Part 2 program and an entity that has direct administrative control over the program."

A third qualifier that does not require a new consent to disclose Part 2 information is to a qualified service organization. Most importantly, this includes a health information exchange (see the following for a full explanation), and also includes basic structures of healthcare delivery "such as data processing, bill collecting, dosage preparation, laboratory analysis, or legal, accounting, population health management, medical staffing, or other professional services."

With regard to a health information organization (HIO) or health information exchange (HIE), the program that falls under 42 CFR Part 2 may upload patient records to these entities if the patient directly consents to this or if there is a qualified service organization agreement in place. In order for the HIO/HIE to redisclose the information and have members obtain an electronic copy of the records, the patient would need to *agree* and sign a consent form that states that the "patient agrees for the records to be released through the HIO/HIE to other entities and individuals for the purposes of treatment and care coordination."

If the patient *does not agree* to have their records redisclosed, then the information would be uploaded to the HIO/HIE with the statement "this information has been disclosed to you from records protected by Federal confidentiality rules (42 CFR Part 2). The federal rules prohibit you from making any further disclosure of this information unless further disclosure is expressly permitted by the written consent of the person to whom it pertains or as otherwise permitted by 42 CFR Part 2. A general authorization for the release of medical or other information is not sufficient for this purpose. The Federal rules restrict any use of the information to criminally investigate or prosecute any alcohol or drug abuse patient."

Using an Electronic Medical Record

When DAPTRA and 42 CFR Part 2 were first written, only the military, colleges, and fortune 100 companies owned computers. Unfortunately, the regulations have not kept up with the rapid expansion of electronic health records and are vague at best. So, in this section, a conservative approach is required. As stated at the beginning of the chapter, I recommend engaging with qualified legal professionals when making an EHR policy.

For medical professionals with their own office and "closed" EHRs, then this is quite easy. A standard EHR can be used to input all biopsychosocial information, and only when the patient consents can this information be shared with other providers. It starts to get muddy when work is done in a health system or larger office.

For medical professionals working in an office or hospital system with multiple providers who are not "Part 2 providers," there are some general approaches to complying with 42 CFR Part 2 with your EHR. The most important is the segregation of addiction-related information from the main EHR. Once completed, access can be blocked to records that are labeled as "Part 2" unless the employee is associated with the program. Another path is adding a "break the glass" feature that allows only those with a defined exception (eg, medical emergency) or an explicit consent to view the data and have the ability to enter this portion of the patient's chart. The third approach is to develop specific policies and procedures for controlling access to Part 2 records without consent. This would need to have Quality Improvement attached and reports kept. The other approach is to simply have a separate EMR for the Part 2 program. All of these approaches will work but are generally unnecessary if consent development is robust.

Consent Utilization

If a consent document is written well, it can allow for movement of information to the necessary treatment teams, increase accessibility through an EHR or HIO/HIE, as well as maintain the trust garnered by the all-important therapeutic alliance. The requirements of a 42 CFR Part 2 compliant consent to release protected health information is as follows. First, a consent to a disclosure under Part 2 regulations *must be in writing* and include the following items:

1. the specific name or general designation of the program or person permitted to make the disclosure;
2. the name or title of the individual or the name of the organization to which disclosure is to be made;
3. the name of the patient;
4. the purpose of the disclosure;
5. how much and what kind of information is to be disclosed (eg, treatment history, toxicology studies, admission summaries, discharge summaries, prescriptions);
6. the signature of the patient, and when required for a patient who is a minor, the signature of a person authorized to give consent under § 2.14, or when required for a patient who is incompetent or deceased, the signature of a person authorized to sign under § 2.15 in lieu of the patient;
7. the date on which the consent is signed;
8. a statement that the consent is subject to revocation at any time except to the extent that the program or person who is to make the disclosure has already acted in reliance on it—acting in reliance includes the provision of treatment services in reliance on a valid consent to disclose information to a third-party payer; and
9. the date, event, or condition upon which the consent will expire if not revoked before, which must ensure that the consent will last no longer than reasonably necessary to serve the purpose for which it is given.

These are the nine major components required in a Part 2 compliant consent. Of note, the most recent changes to Part 2 allow for the utilization of a general designation when SUD information is exchanged through a qualified service organization such as HIO/HIE and can read simply, "All of the providers that provide me with treatment." With this designation an HIO/HIE can both disclose and redisclose SUD information to someone with a "treating provider" relationship.

In the newest regulation, there is also no specification with regard to whether the consent needs to be opt in or opt out. Thus, simply listing all of the entities or individuals that the patient's records may need to be disclosed to for coordination of care and having them initial next to the ones that they do not want to give their records to is commensurate with the current regulatory interpretation. The opt-out pathways make it more likely, by a large margin, that a patient will agree to allow for collaborative treatment between the Part 2 program and the ever more complex healthcare system.

Special Populations

As if HIPAA, DAPTRA, the Americans with Disabilities Act, and 42 CFR Part 2 were not confusing enough, a few special populations result in additional caveats. The most common special populations that require discussion are adolescents, patients with a cognitive impairment, patients with a severe and persistent mental illness, and patients in safety sensitive professions. Although some of these issues revolve around competency, others revolve around specific "rights" garnered by statute.

Legal consent to treat questions may seem dicey to adolescents. However, making the decision to do the right thing for the patient's well-being is always the best first step. Not every state's approach to this population can be discussed here; however, most fall into two categories: (1) those that give an adolescent the right to consent to screening, assessment, and/or treatment for SUDs and (2) those that do not. If the state gives the right to consent, then the state-specific age of consent should be known before applying all the above information. In those that do not give adolescents the right to consent, any of the following three approaches may be used:

■ Treat the adolescent without consulting the parent.
■ Try to obtain consent to treatment from the adolescent's parent.
■ Refuse to treat the adolescent.

Although the physician who treats an adolescent without parental consent or notification is acting in accordance with the ethical principles of putting the patient's health first and respecting the patient's autonomy (and privacy), they may be violating the law. The physician who is considering whether to offer treatment without parental consent or notification in a state that requires it should consider the following factors:

■ the adolescent's age,
■ the adolescent's maturity,

■ the adolescent's family situation,
■ the severity of the adolescent's addictive disorder,
■ the kind of treatment to be provided,
■ the physician's possible liability for refusing to treat the patient, and
■ the financial consequences.

Although violation of the parental consent/notification law most likely is not a criminal offense, it could put the physician's professional license at risk or expose them to a lawsuit by the adolescent's parents. This, however, is unlikely given the benefit of treatment for the patient presenting to the physician.

If attempting to obtain consent from the parent, the physician will be complying with the letter of the law; however, this clearly violates the adolescent's right to privacy. An added complication is the federal and/or state privacy rules regarding release of information about SUDs without the patient's consent. This again leads us back to the previous definitions of informed consent and competency.

Patients with cognitive impairments include those with a history of traumatic brain injury, those with intellectual disabilities, patients who have moderate-to-severe spectrum disorders, and those with chronic brain injury from SUDs. It is important to asses the support systems and the availability of a guardian when appropriate for this group. It is appropriately difficult to have a guardianship granted, given that this takes away basic human rights but is sometimes necessary. If that is unavailable or inappropriate, then there are basic approaches that may be helpful. (1) Make sure and present the information in such a way that they can understand it. This can be determined by their ability to do a "teach back" of the information given. (2) Attempt to find a friend or family member who can help "translate" more complex information. (3) Attempt to obtain case management for the patient so they may have surrogate support during their decision-making process and beyond.

Patients with a severe and persistent mental illness have components of those listed previously but usually have specific state laws associated with obtaining guardianship. In addition, most mental illness is waxing and waning by nature, so they may drift in and out of "competence" depending on the cycle of their illness or their compliance with medications. Either way, it is important to do consistent checks on their mental capacity and have a plan for an official evaluation if it begins to wane. Also, having a designated family member or designate can be helpful in predicting the need for help.

Safety sensitive professionals, including health professionals, are a generally protected set and care should be taken to evaluate all the specific rules and regulations surrounding their health information. For instance, any pilot who has a syncopal episode has a specific set of career safety rules that have to be followed. An eligible healthcare professional can choose an anonymous pathway of treatment where they are assigned a code and is followed only by this code without names. Other state licensing boards "require" disclosure by the treating physician. However, once involved in treatment at a "covered entity," 42 CFR Part 2 applies.

No matter who is being treated or where, it is important to balance the patient's right to privacy and the "duty to warn." There are no perfect rules to follow; therefore, use of this information and in-house council should be followed to make the best decision for individual patients in their situation, at that time.

KEY POINTS

1. Confidentiality is key to helping form a therapeutic alliance.
2. Informed consent requires knowledge, competency, and voluntary acceptance by the patient.
3. 42 CFR only pertains to covered entities that hold themselves out as addiction treatment providers, are federally assisted, and have SUD information in the record.
4. Exceptions to 42 CFR Part 2 are medical emergencies, in cases of suspected child abuse, in duty-to-warn situations, when performing audits, for research, or to fulfill a court order.
5. Many states have laws that are more protective than 42 CFR Part 2, so it is necessary to know your state's rules and regulations.
6. Special populations need to have an extra layer of care when signing an informed consent.

REVIEW QUESTIONS

1. Which of the following constitutes the components of informed consent?
   A. Knowledge
   B. Competency
   C. Involuntary consent
   D. Both A and B

2. When consenting an adolescent for addiction treatment, which of the following offers the least legal risk?
   A. Treat the adolescent without consulting a parent.
   B. Attempt to obtain consent to treatment from the adolescent's parent.

C. Refuse to treat the adolescent.
D. Wait until the adolescent is 18 years old.

3. Which of the following laws covers confidentiality pertaining to all healthcare records?
   A. The Americans with Disabilities Act
   B. The Health Insurance Portability and Accountability Act
   C. 42 CFR Part 2
   D. The Rehabilitation Act of 1973

4. Which of the following is a *true* statement concerning the treatment of health professionals for a substance use disorder?
   A. Health professionals are not covered by 42 CFR Part 2.
   B. Health professionals may be eligible for an "anonymous" treatment pathway.
   C. Health professionals are required to disclose all information concerning their addictive disorder.
   D. Health professionals are required to disclose their diagnosis to all of their patients.

5. Which of the following is a circumstance under which information may be disclosed?
   A. When a disclosure identifies the patient as an individual with a substance use disorder
   B. When there is a medical emergency
   C. When a patient presents for treatment at a covered program
   D. All of the above.

ANSWERS

1. **D**
2. **B**
3. **A**
4. **B**
5. **B**

SUGGESTED READINGS

Center for Substance Abuse Treatment. *Substance Abuse: Administrative Issues in Outpatient Treatment. Treatment Improvement Protocol (TIP) Series, No. 46.* Rockville, MD: Substance Abuse and Mental Health Services Administration, 2006. DHHS Pub. No. (SMA) 06-4151.

Center for Substance Abuse Work Group, Federation of State Medical Boards. Model policy for opioid addiction treatment in the medical office. *Pain Physician.* 2003;6(2): 217-221.

US Department of Health and Human Services. *Confidentiality of Patient Records for Alcohol and Other Drug Treatment. Technical Assistance Publication (TAP) Series 13.* Rockville, MD: Substance Abuse and Mental Health Services Administration, 1994. DHHS Pub. No. (SMA) 95-3018.

Clinical, Ethical, and Legal Considerations in Prescribing Drugs With Potential for Nonmedical Use and Addiction

Summary by Theodore V. Parran Jr., James W. Finch, and Bonnie B. Wilford

Based on THE ASAM PRINCIPLES OF ADDICTION MEDICINE, 6th edition chapter by Theodore V. Parran Jr., James W. Finch, and Bonnie B. Wilford

Many medications in common use have a clearly documented potential for nonmedical use and addiction. These include opioid analgesics, stimulants, sedative–hypnotics, and cannabinoid-like medications. Although widely varying in terms of their primary effects on the brain, all at least indirectly trigger an acute surge of dopamine from the ventral tegmental and nucleus accumbens regions of the brain to the prefrontal cortex, resulting in brain reward and euphoria. This is what gives them their potential for nonmedical use and addiction.

It is equally important to understand that controlled medications, despite their potential for nonmedical use, are valuable therapeutic tools in the treatment of pain, anxiety, insomnia, attention deficit disorder, and other medical and psychiatric conditions. This challenging interplay of potential risk and benefit requires that *any* and *every* decision to prescribe such medications must be made judiciously and with attention to appropriate patient assessment, informed consent, and meticulous risk/benefit analysis, followed by careful patient monitoring.

The decision as to whether to prescribe a controlled substance is further complicated by prescribers' understandable concerns about legal and regulatory scrutiny. For this reason, it is important to recognize the fact that although the concern is understandable, the actual risk of investigation is extremely small. The overwhelming majority of physicians who prescribe controlled substances do so in a legitimate manner that does not warrant,

or receive, scrutiny by federal or state law enforcement or regulatory agencies. In fact, fewer than 1 in 10,000 physicians has lost a Drug Enforcement Administration (DEA) registration to prescribe controlled substances on the basis of a DEA investigation of his or her prescribing.

Patients who have an active substance use disorder (SUD) or a history of such disorders pose a special challenge when considering the use of controlled medications. Such patients are at a substantially elevated risk for nonmedical use of controlled substances such as opioid analgesics, benzodiazepines, and stimulants. They also are at risk of experiencing increased cravings and even relapse, which may occur even with short-term medication use. Nonmedical use can range from diversion (with legal ramifications including arrest and incarceration) to binge-type behaviors and accidental overdose. Risks also include increased disinhibition and associated dangerous interpersonal behaviors.

On the other hand, individuals with SUDs also are at an elevated risk of physical and emotional trauma, chronic pain, debilitating mood disorders, attention deficit hyperactivity disorders, and stressful life conditions. Untreated pain and psychiatric conditions not only cause suffering in and of themselves but also are strong triggers for relapse to substance use.

Fortunately, at least in the realm of chronic conditions, there are reasonable alternatives to virtually all controlled drugs. The risk/benefit calculation becomes critical in these circumstances.

FACTORS THAT CONTRIBUTE TO INAPPROPRIATE MEDICATION PRESCRIBING AND USE

Factors that frequently contribute to over- or under-prescribing of controlled medications and their nonmedical use include:

- physician uncertainty as to prevailing standards of care,
- inadequate medical evaluation and workup of the patient's disorder,
- unclear or conflicting clinical guidelines,
- physician concerns that prescribing adequate amounts of medication will result in unnecessary scrutiny by regulatory authorities,
- physician misunderstanding of the causes and manifestations of SUDs,
- physician fear of causing addiction or being deceived by a patient,
- physician behaviors that have been described as "confrontation phobia" and "hypertrophied enabling," and
- inadequate physician education about regulatory policies and processes.

The goals of treatment with controlled medications, or any medication, ought to involve, in descending order of importance: (1) patient safety; (2) reasonably attainable improvement in symptoms and quality of life; (3) improvement in associated symptoms such as sleep disturbance, depression, and anxiety; (4) maintenance or improvement of function; and (5) avoidance of unnecessary or excessive use of medications.

Patients share with physicians a responsibility for the appropriate use of prescribed medications, which encompasses providing the physician with complete and accurate information, including permission to access other sources of clinical information. Some patients, either intentionally or unintentionally, are less than forthcoming about their health history or have unrealistic expectations regarding the need for therapy or the amount of medication required. Other patients may begin to use medications as prescribed and then slowly deviate from the therapeutic regimen. Still others may not comply with the treatment plan because they misunderstood the physician's instructions. Some patients share their medications with others without intending harm. There also are patients who deliberately use medications excessively or, because of an SUD involving prescription medications, either mislead, deceive, or fail to disclose information to their physicians in order to obtain such medications in an effort to sustain their out-of-control, dangerous behavior and avoid the symptoms of withdrawal.

Also of concern, patients' carelessness in leaving controlled medications where they can be stolen by visitors, workers, and family members is another important source of diversion. The prescribing physician's duty includes not only appropriate prescribing but also appropriate education of patients regarding the secure storage of medications and their safe disposal.

A more problematic individual is the patient with criminal intent, whose primary purpose is to obtain drugs for resale. Whereas most patients with an addiction seek a long-term relationship with one or more prescribers, patients with criminal intent sometimes move rapidly from one prescriber (or dispenser) to another. Such individuals often visit multiple practitioners in a day—a practice known as "doctor shopping"—and travel from one geographic area to another in search of unsuspecting targets. Physician attention to patient assessment, obtaining and reviewing records from past prescribers, and the routine use of state prescription drug monitoring programs (PDMPs) have been cited as effective ways to identify individuals who engage in such criminal activities.

LEGAL AND REGULATORY REQUIREMENTS WHEN PRESCRIBING CONTROLLED MEDICATIONS

To legally prescribe, dispense, or administer a controlled medication, a physician must be (1) registered with the DEA, (2) licensed by the state in which he or she practices, and (3) acting in compliance with all applicable federal and state laws and regulations. The legal requirements for prescribing controlled medications generally rest on the principles of the "usual course of medical practice," which involves an appropriate patient evaluation and a legitimate medical purpose.

The DEA addresses this issue by placing certain medications into "schedules" that relate to their presumed relative risk of nonmedical use and addiction. It is important for clinicians to recognize that the DEA's schedules provide only a rough estimate of a specific medication's potential for nonmedical use, addiction, and diversion and that regardless of schedule, all controlled medications have some potential for evoking nonmedical use and addiction in certain patients. Notably, an array of nonscheduled medications (approved by the FDA for prescription and over-the-counter use) also have some potential for nonmedical use.

The DEA's *Practitioner's Manual* and any relevant documents issued by the physician's state medical board should be consulted for specific rules and regulations governing the prescribing of controlled substances. Additional resources are available on the DEA's website (at www.deadiversion.usdoj.gov) as well as from the medical licensing board in each state.

The Prescription Order

The federal Controlled Substances Act defines a "lawful prescription" as one that is issued for a legitimate medical purpose by a practitioner acting in the usual course of professional practice. By law, every prescription order must include at least the following information:

- Name and address of the patient
- Name, address, and DEA registration number of the physician
- Signature of the physician
- Name and quantity of the drug prescribed
- Directions for use
- Refill information

Many states impose additional requirements, which the physician can determine by consulting the medical licensing board in his or her state. In addition, there are special requirements for drugs in different schedules of the federal Controlled Substances Act, particularly those in Schedule II.

Patients who are seeking controlled substances for nonmedical use are constantly on the lookout for blank prescription forms and often use the names of physicians who recently retired, left the state, or died. Therefore, storing blank prescription order forms in a safe place (such as behind a locked door or in a locked cabinet) as opposed to leaving the pads in examining rooms is a sound practice. All states now have the capacity for electronic prescribing, which eliminates most of the risk of theft or forgery of prescriptions for controlled substances.

Medical Records

In the event of a legal, regulatory, or civil (malpractice-related) challenge, detailed medical records documenting what was done and why are the foundations of the physician's defense. Every physician needs to know and understand the federal requirements for record-keeping as well as the laws and regulatory requirements of the state in which

he or she practices. At a minimum, patient records should contain the following information:

1. *Patient history and physical examination:* The patient record must include a history of all controlled medications used to treat the patient, any history of illicit substances, and any patient allergies. Medical records obtained from providers who have treated the patient in the past should be included. The medical record also must include information about the patient's personal and family history of alcohol, tobacco, and other drug use as well any personal history of major depression or other psychiatric disorder.
2. *Treatment plan:* The treatment plan and goals should be documented in the record so that there is evidence of clear-cut, individualized objectives to guide the choice of therapy.
3. *Consultation reports:* Generally, the results of the consultation should be discussed with the consulting physician and a written consultation report added to the patient's medical record.
4. *Prescription orders:* The patient record must include all prescription orders, whether written or telephoned. The prescription order itself should specify both the milligram dose and the volume of medication to be taken. Confusion related to ambiguous orders can lead to tragic outcomes, especially early in treatment. The physician should clearly specify the dose and formulation and how often the medication should be used.
5. *Informed consent or treatment agreement:* As noted earlier, a written informed consent and a treatment agreement signed by both the patient and physician can be helpful in establishing a set of "ground rules" and appropriate expectations.
6. *Monitoring visits:* Medication monitoring visits are billable and can be performed by a nurse. They should be carefully documented in the medical record, in the same manner as a visit with the physician. A long-term controlled drug prescription flow sheet provides an efficient format for this documentation.
7. *Treatment progress/outcomes:* The patient's record should clearly reflect the decision-making process that led to any given medical outcome.

UNIVERSAL PRECAUTIONS WHEN PRESCRIBING CONTROLLED MEDICATIONS

Judicious prescribing of medications that have a potential for nonmedical use requires thoughtful application of several broadly accepted elements of good medical care to this particular area of practice. Wherever possible, the strategies for safe and appropriate prescribing presented here are supported by the weight of clinical evidence.

1. Conduct an Initial Patient Assessment and Risk Stratification, and Make a Diagnosis With an Appropriate Differential

This involves identifying a clear *indication* for potential prescribing and ruling out *contraindications* to such prescribing. An assessment also involves determining whether a medication is appropriate in terms of its potential *efficacy* relative to available alternatives.

An assessment of the patient's history of alcohol, tobacco, or other nonmedical drug use and relative risk for nonmedical medication use or SUD is an absolutely essential component of the initial evaluation. This can be done through a careful clinical interview, which also should include questions about any history of physical, emotional, or sexual abuse, because those are risk factors for SUDs. The patient history also should involve the use of validated screening tools (such as the full or concise Alcohol Use Disorders Identification Test), PDMP review, and toxicology testing, and contacting family members to corroborate the functional assessment as well as to screen for SUDs (Family CAGE).

Another step in an assessment is *risk stratification*, which includes screening for relative or absolute contraindications to the use of controlled medications and evaluating the risks posed by other available therapies or no use of pharmacologic therapies. Use of a screening tool such as the Screener and Opioid Assessment for Patients With Pain, the Opioid Risk Tool, or the three-question PEG (pain, enjoyment, and general activity) scale can save time in collecting and evaluating information and determining the patient's level of risk, although these tools have not been well validated in primary care populations.

For every patient, the initial workup should include a system review and relevant physical examination as well as appropriate laboratory tests.

The physician's decision as to whether to prescribe a controlled medication should reflect the totality of the information collected as well as the physician's own knowledge and comfort level in prescribing such medications (area of expertise) and the available resources for patient support. In reaching such a decision, it is important to recognize that not every substance use history indicates the same level of risk. The presence of an active SUD carries different risks than does a history of SUD, and a history of SUD with appropriate treatment and attention to ongoing recovery poses different risks than does a past SUD with no active attention. The issue of "cross-addiction"—the concept that an SUD with one class of drugs substantially raises the risk (as much as sevenfold) of an SUD involving a different class of drugs—must not be minimized, especially given the high level of morbidity associated with an SUD relapse.

2. Discuss the Proposed Treatment Plan With the Patient, and Obtain His or Her Informed Consent

Once established, the treatment plan and goals should provide clear-cut, individualized objectives to guide the choice of therapies. It also should specify the objectives that will be used to evaluate treatment progress, such as patient safety, relief of symptoms, and improved physical and psychosocial function.

The plan should document the need for any further diagnostic evaluations, consultations, or referrals and list other therapies that have been considered. Use of a written informed consent whenever longitudinally prescribing any controlled drugs is strongly recommended.

Once established, the treatment plan and goals should provide clear-cut, individualized objectives to guide the choice of therapies. The treatment plan should contain information supporting the selection of all therapies, both pharmacologic and nonpharmacologic. It also should specify the objectives that will be used to evaluate the treatment progress, such as patient safety, relief of symptoms, and improved physical and psychosocial function. The plan should document the need for any further diagnostic evaluations, consultations, or referrals and list other therapies that have been considered. Use of a written informed consent whenever longitudinally prescribing any controlled drugs is strongly recommended.

3. Execute a Written Informed Consent Form or Treatment Agreement that Sets Forth the Expectations and Obligations of Both the Patient and the Treating Physician

Treatment agreements or written informed consent forms are used to outline the joint responsibilities of the patient and physician. Typically, they address the following:

- The goals of treatment in terms of symptom management, restoration of function, and safety
- The patient's responsibility for safe medication use (as by not using more medication than prescribed

or using the medication in combination with other substances, by storing the medication in a secure location, and by safe disposal of any unused medication)

- The patient's responsibility to obtain his or her prescribed medication from only one physician or practice
- The patient's permission for the physician to contact corroborators to support the initial history as well as to corroborate reports of ongoing functional improvement
- The patient's agreement to periodic drug testing (as of blood, urine, hair, or saliva)
- The physician's responsibility to be available or to have a covering physician available to care for unforeseen problems and to prescribe scheduled refills

The medical record should document the presence of one or more recognized medical indications for prescribing and reflect an appropriately detailed patient evaluation, including risk stratification and screening for contraindications. Even when sound medical indications have been established, for safety reasons, physicians *must* consider four additional factors before deciding to prescribe:

- The *level of risk associated with the use of the controlled medication* within the context of *the patient's history of SUDs* (presence of contraindications): The physician must assess a patient's vulnerability to SUDs before prescribing any medication that poses the risk of addiction and weigh the benefits against the risks.
- The *severity of symptoms*, in terms of the patient's ability to accommodate them: Relief of symptoms is a legitimate goal of medical practice, but using medications with addiction liability in an effort to achieve *complete* relief of symptoms, or relief of more *minor or mild* symptoms, usually is unrealistic and may be dangerous.
- The patient's *reliability in taking medications and adhering to treatment plans*, noted through observation and careful history-taking: Patients who have had major problems in adhering to treatment plans, because of mental health or other factors, are at increased risk when prescribed controlled medications.
- The *addiction liability of the medication*: The physician should consider whether a drug with less potential for producing an SUD, or even a nondrug therapy, would provide comparable benefits.

4. If a Decision Is Made to Prescribe Medications, Initiate an Appropriate Trial of Medication Therapy

Rational pharmacotherapy demands that the efficacy and safety of *all* potentially useful medication classes be reviewed for their relevance to the patient's disease or disorder as well as the patient's risk for nonmedical medication use and SUDs.

When the optimal medication has been selected, the *dose, schedule*, and *formulation* should be determined. Decisions involve (1) the *dose*, based not only on the patient's age, weight, and size but also on the severity of symptoms, possible loading dose requirements, the presence and extent of drug tolerance, and the presence of potentially interacting medications; (2) the *timing of administration*, as by using a bedtime dose to minimize problems associated with sedative effects; (3) the *route of administration*, chosen to improve compliance/adherence as well as to attain peak drug concentrations at the desired time and speed; and (4) the *drug formulation* (eg, selecting a patch in preference to a tablet or an extended-release rather than an immediate-release formulation).

At the time a drug is prescribed, patients should be informed that it is illegal to sell, give away, or otherwise share their medication with others, including family members. The patient also should be informed that his or her obligation extends to keeping the medication in a locked cabinet or otherwise restricting access to it, as well as safely disposing of any unused supply.

5. Monitor the Patient's Response to Therapy

Frequent monitoring visits should be scheduled while the treatment plan is being initiated and the medication dose adjusted. The use of a standardized monitoring strategy, much like that used for patients with diabetes, facilitated by a monitoring flowchart, is strongly recommended.

The frequency of follow-up visits should reflect the stability of the patient, with more frequent visits scheduled during initiation and initial titration of controlled medication, less frequent visits during maintenance periods, and then more frequent visits during periods of dose adjustments/tapering or concerning patient behavior. The patient can play an active role in this monitoring by keeping a log of signs, symptoms, side effects, and other treatment issues.

Important areas to track on a longitudinal controlled substance/medication flow sheet include scores on validated patient questionnaires such as the Current Opioid Misuse Measure, or COMM; prescription refills; toxicology results; contact with significant others to corroborate function and safety; as well as the patient's adherence to referrals, medications prescribed and dose, pill counts, ongoing use of a single pharmacy, patient and family education regarding safety issues, and more. Periodic checks with corroborators regarding the patient's level of function, adherence to the treatment plan, and risk behaviors are essential in ensuring the ongoing safety of prescribing.

Another significant source of information is the state PDMP. At this writing, 49 states have enacted laws that establish PDMPs to facilitate the collection, analysis, and reporting of information on the dispensing of controlled substances. Most such programs employ electronic data transfer systems, under which prescription information is transmitted from the dispensing pharmacy to a state agency, which collates and analyzes the information. Where data are available in real time, routine use of PDMPs can help to prevent nonmedical prescription drug use and diversion by allowing the physician to learn whether a patient is receiving prescriptions for controlled substances from other physicians, as well as whether the patient has filled or refilled prescriptions for any controlled substances the physician has ordered. PDMP information can be very helpful in assessing the patient's level of physical tolerance and thus is an important contributor to patient safety.

Therapeutic drug testing also is a necessary part of long-term prescribing of controlled medications. Drug testing is an important monitoring tool because patients' self-reports of medication use can be unreliable, and behavioral observations may detect some problems but not others. However, physicians need to be aware of the limitations of available tests (such as their limited sensitivity to many opioids) and know how to order tests appropriately. Because of the complexities involved in interpreting drug test results, it is advisable to verify significant or unexpected results through confirmatory studies and consultation with the testing laboratory's toxicologist or a clinical pathologist.

Test results that suggest possible nonmedical use of the prescribed medication or other drugs should be discussed with the patient. It is helpful to approach such a discussion in a positive, supportive manner, so as to strengthen the physician–patient relationship and encourage healthy behaviors (as well as behavioral changes where needed). Both the test results and subsequent discussion with the patient should be thoroughly documented in the medical record.

Whenever the physician is concerned about a patient's behavior or clinical progress (or the lack thereof), it is advisable to seek a consultation with an expert in the disorder for which the patient is being treated. If there is concern about possible nonmedical use or diversion of a prescribed medication, consultation with an expert in addiction medicine also is advised. Physicians place themselves and their patients at risk if they continue to prescribe controlled medications in the presence of concerning patient behaviors, and consultation with an addiction specialist can be very helpful in protecting both the patient and the physician.

6. Decide Whether to Continue, Modify, or End Medication Therapy

No treatment regimen should be left open-ended. Throughout the course of therapy, the physician and patient should regularly weigh the potential benefits and risks of continued treatment and determine whether such treatment remains appropriate. Continuation, modification, or termination of medication therapy should be contingent on *both* (1) evidence of the patient's progress toward the established treatment objectives *and* (2) the absence of substantial risks or adverse events.

A satisfactory response to treatment would be indicated by reduced severity of symptoms, increased level of function, and/or improved quality of life in the absence of dangerous or concerning behaviors. Information from family members and the use of measurement tools to reassess the patient's level of pain, function, and quality of life is important in documenting therapeutic outcomes and should be recorded on the monitoring flow sheet.

If a decision is made to continue medication therapy, the treatment plan may need to be adjusted to reflect the patient's changing physical status and needs as well as to support safe and appropriate medication use. Steps such as simplifying the drug regimen and offering additional patient education can improve adherence, as can phone calls to patients, home visits by nursing personnel, convenient packaging of medication, and monitoring of serum drug levels. On the other hand, it is *not* advisable to have family or friends supervise the patient's medication use (except for pediatric or geriatric patients), because placing such an individual between a patient who demonstrates aberrant medication use behaviors and the patient's supply of medications can be dangerous for both parties.

If the results of ongoing monitoring indicate that the treatment plan needs to be modified (eg, because the patient's symptoms are not responding to the medication or because there is evidence of problematic medication use behaviors), the treatment agreement may need to be adjusted to include more frequent visits, smaller prescriptions with fewer or no refills, callbacks for pill counts or random drug screens, or referral for adjunctive addiction-related or psychotherapeutic treatment.

Reasons for discontinuing medication therapy include resolution of the condition being treated, emergence of intolerable side effects, inadequate medication effect, failure to improve the patient's quality of life despite adequate dosing, evidence of deteriorating function, or significant aberrant medication use.

Evidence of nonmedical use of prescribed medications requires prompt intervention. Patient behaviors that require such intervention typically involve multiple early requests for refills, multiple reports of lost or stolen prescriptions, obtaining controlled medications from multiple sources without the physician's knowledge, patient intoxication or impairment (either observed or reported), and pressuring or threatening behaviors. The presence of illicit or nonprescribed drugs in drug tests also requires action on the part of the prescriber.

Documented drug diversion or prescription forgery, obvious impairment, and abusive or assaultive behaviors require a firm, immediate response, which typically involves immediate cessation of all controlled medication prescribing. Indeed, failure to respond can place the patient, his or her family, the community, and the prescriber at significant risk of adverse consequences, including violence, accidental overdose, suicide attempts, arrests and incarceration, or even death.

When such events arise, it is important to separate the *person* of the patient from the *behaviors* triggered by the SUD by demonstrating a positive regard for the person but no tolerance for the behaviors. The essential steps are to (1) stop prescribing, (2) inform the patient that continued prescribing is not clinically supportable and thus not possible, (3) urge the patient to accept a referral for assessment by an addiction specialist, (4) educate the patient about signs and symptoms of spontaneous withdrawal and urge the patient to accept referral for medically managed withdrawal management or to go to the emergency department if withdrawal symptoms occur, and (5) assure the patient that he or she will continue to receive care for the presenting symptoms or condition but without continued prescribing of controlled medications.

7. Know How to Discontinue Medication Therapy

Any patient who has become physically dependent on a prescribed medication should be provided with a safely structured tapering regimen and referred for medical management of withdrawal or, at a minimum, educated about the signs and symptoms of withdrawal in combination with an offer to help treat such symptoms. The physician must determine whether such discontinuation constitutes a clinical emergency (requiring referral for inpatient withdrawal management or education about withdrawal and an offer of outpatient withdrawal management), an urgent situation (requiring a rapid structured taper over several weeks as an outpatient), or a nonurgent situation (involving a gradual taper over several months).

When tapering, it is important to be realistic regarding the patient's ability to comply and tailor the program accordingly. Much smaller prescription allotments, more frequent check-ins and drug screens, and greater involvement of family or other caregivers may be required. If the patient is not able to comply with the tapering plan, alternatives such as discontinuation of prescribing and referral for inpatient or outpatient withdrawal management or referral for opioid agonist therapy with methadone or buprenorphine typically are necessary.

Patients should be given the benefit of the physician's concern and attention. It is important to remember that even patients with drug-seeking behaviors can have very real medical problems that demand and deserve the same high-quality medical care offered to any patient. Also, the termination of therapy with a controlled medication should not mark the end of treatment, which should continue with other modalities, through either direct care or referral to a specialist, as appropriate. Physicians who abruptly terminate their relationship with the patient at the time they stop prescribing controlled medications run the risk of breaching accepted medical ethics and can be reported for patient abandonment.

Special Precautions With New Patients

Many experts recommend that additional precautions be taken when prescribing a controlled medication to a new patient.

■ *Assessment:* The physician should determine which physician(s) have been caring for the patient, what medication(s) have been prescribed for which indications, how recently such medications were prescribed, and what substances (including alcohol, illicit drugs, and over-the-counter products) the patient has used and how recently. Medical and pharmacy records should be obtained (with the patient's consent) to verify this information.

■ *Quantities:* In nonemergency situations, the physician should prescribe only enough of a controlled medication to meet the new patient's needs until the next appointment.

■ *Emergencies:* In emergency situations, the physician should prescribe no more than a 1-day supply of a medication and arrange for a return visit.

As presented here, the concept of universal precautions recognizes that all patients are at some level of risk for nonmedical use of prescribed medications, however small, and that the risk level initially can only be estimated, with the estimate modified over time as additional information is obtained. The concept of universal precautions encourages a consistent and respectful approach to all patients, thus minimizing stigma, improving patient care, and reducing overall risk.

KEY POINTS

1. Like all clinical tools, medications with the potential for nonmedical use must be considered in terms of potential risks and benefits. Judicious use of these medications—with attention to proper assessment, collaborative informed consent and treatment planning, adequate monitoring, and intervention as needed—can minimize the likelihood of nonmedical use of medications and the attendant risks.

2. The decision as to whether to prescribe a controlled substance is further complicated by prescribers' understandable concerns about legal and regulatory scrutiny. Although the concern is understandable, the actual risk of investigation is extremely small. The overwhelming majority of physicians who prescribe controlled substances do so in a legitimate manner that does not warrant, or receive, scrutiny by federal or state law enforcement or regulatory agencies.

3. Adoption of the "universal precautions" approach in deciding whether to prescribe controlled medications, coupled with careful patient monitoring, is an excellent way to systematically ensure that medications are prescribed for a legitimate medical purpose, within the usual course of medical practice, and with patient safety as the most

important clinical consideration. Attention to these elements, along with careful record-keeping, serves to improve patient outcomes and reduce physicians' concerns about regulatory or legal scrutiny.

REVIEW QUESTIONS

1. Universal precautions when prescribing controlled drugs includes all of the following principles *except*:
   A. establishing an indication (diagnosis).
   B. screening for contraindications.
   C. reporting patient drug diversion to authorities.
   D. monitoring adherence.
   E. stopping if evidence of patient danger emerges.

2. Legal and licensure agencies are required to monitor for all of the following *except*:
   A. that controlled drug prescriptions are only prescribed by those with an active DEA number.
   B. that controlled drug prescriptions are done within the usual course of medical practice.
   C. that only physicians prescribe controlled drug prescriptions.
   D. that controlled drug prescriptions are done for a legitimate medical purpose.
   E. that oversight does not create an undue burden on the practice of medicine.

3. Which of the following is the pharmacologic characteristic of a medication that results it in being classified as a controlled drug?
   A. Potency
   B. Half-life
   C. Street value
   D. Physical dependence/withdrawal
   E. Dopamine surge from midbrain to forebrain

4. Which of the following is the strongest contraindication to long-term prescribing of controlled drugs?
   A. Schizophrenia
   B. Chronic obstructive pulmonary disease
   C. Old age
   D. Current or prior substance use disorder
   E. Obstructive sleep apnea

ANSWERS

1. **C**
2. **C**
3. **E**
4. **D**

SUGGESTED READINGS

Ballantyne JC. Opioids for the treatment of chronic pain: mistakes made, lessons learned, and future directions. *Anesth Analg.* 2017;125(5):1769-1778.

Berrettini W. A brief review of the genetics and pharmacogenetics of opioid use disorders. *Dialogues Clin Neurosci.* 2017;19(3):229-236.

Federation of State Medical Boards. Guidelines for the chronic use of opioid analgesics. https://www.fsmb.org/globalassets/advocacy/policies/opioid_guidelines_as_adopted_april-2017_final.pdf. Published April 2017. Accessed December 11, 2018.

Heit HA, Gourlay DL. Using urine drug testing to support healthy boundaries in clinical care. *J Opioid Manag.* 2015;11(1):7-12.

Kaye AD, Jones MR, Kaye AM, et al. Prescription opioid abuse in chronic pain: an updated review of opioid abuse predictors and strategies to curb opioid abuse: Part 1. *Pain Physician.* 2017;20(2S):S93-S109.

Drug Control Policy: History and Future Directions

Summary by John J. Coleman and Robert L. DuPont

Based on THE ASAM PRINCIPLES OF ADDICTION MEDICINE, 6th edition sidebar by
John J. Coleman and Robert L. DuPont

Modern drug control in the United States traces its origins to the early 20th century when, not long after the Spanish–American War, the United States annexed the Philippines. The colonial administration of Governor William Howard Taft, alarmed by the number of people addicted to opium he found in his newly acquired territory, dispatched emissaries to Shanghai to learn how China was dealing with a similar problem.

In 1908, Taft became the 27th president of the United States, and in the following year, the United States summoned a meeting of colonial powers in Shanghai to address the opium problem in Asia. At the initial meeting of the Shanghai Opium Commission, the parties agreed that opium should be produced, traded, and used solely for medicinal and scientific purposes.

The second meeting of the commission took place at The Hague where, under the elected leadership of the United States, the parties agreed to a treaty calling for international and domestic controls on opium and cocaine. However, the World War I interrupted the commission's work. The Treaty of Versailles that ended the war in 1919 established the League of Nations as a forum for resolving international conflicts. The Opium Commission and the treaty negotiated before the war were transferred to the League of Nations. Although the United States did not join the league, it was influential as an observer nation in its work, including the work of the Opium Commission.

In 1914, in response to the first US heroin epidemic, the United States enacted the Harrison Narcotic Tax Act, in part to comply with the treaty it signed at The Hague, which was ratified by the Senate in 1913. The act imposed "a special tax on all persons who produce, import, manufacture, compound, deal in, dispense, sell, distribute, or give away opium or coca leaves, their salts, derivatives, or preparations. . . ." The most controversial among its provisions was that the dispensing of a covered drug was lawful only if done by a registered person "in the course of his [*sic*] professional practice only." This effectively ended a common practice at the time of providing individuals with drugs for the sole purpose of maintaining their addiction.

In 1931, the League of Nations proposed a treaty to regulate the production and trade in manufactured drugs. Noteworthy was the classification of opiates into two tiers or *schedules* based on their potential addictive properties. The United States joined this treaty in 1932, and it became domestic law in July 1933.

World War II effectively ended the League of Nations. Many of its responsibilities, including those of the Opium Commission, were transferred to the newly created United Nations (UN). In 1961, the UN proposed the Single Convention on Narcotic Drugs, a comprehensive treaty intended to prohibit the production and sale of controlled substances except for medical and scientific purposes. The convention increased the number of drug schedules to four, and in 1964, the Single Convention was entered into force after being ratified by 40 nations, including the United States.

In 1970, the United States enacted the Controlled Substances Act (CSA), in part to comply with its obligations under the Single Convention. The CSA adopted the convention's scheduling schema and added an additional schedule to designate drugs and other substances that are *not* approved for medicinal use in the United States. Forty-six states adopted the Uniform Controlled Substances Act, a version of the federal CSA. The CSA permits the Attorney General and the Secretary of Health, Education, and Welfare (subsequently renamed the US Department of Health and Human Services) to schedule or classify existing and new drugs according to their abuse potential and medical use. The act also regulates importers, exporters, manufacturers, distributors, prescribers, dispensers, and others who handle controlled substances.

In 1971, responding to the second US heroin epidemic, President Richard M. Nixon established the first White House Special Action Office for Drug Abuse Prevention, adding a major demand reduction component to national drug policy and emphasizing a need to focus on drug abuse prevention, treatment, and research, in addition to focusing on law enforcement. A year later, methadone was approved for use by the US Food and Drug Administration as a substantial component of opioid addiction treatment. Since the 1970s, US drug control policy has represented a balance of supply and demand reduction strategies designed to reduce illicit drug use, with leadership for this important work shared among the US Department of Justice, the US Department of Health and Human Services, and the Office of National Drug Control Policy.

The current drug epidemic is headlined by a devastating rise in opiate-related overdose deaths.

Prescribed medications, especially opioids and benzodiazepines, play a central role in this along with imported drugs that are illegally produced and sold such as fentanyl analogues, heroin, and cocaine. State governments, too, are playing a larger role today in regulating access to abusable prescription drugs. Some measures adopted by states hit most hard by this epidemic have inadvertently hindered the delivery of care and services for legitimate pain patients. As evidenced over the years since the Shanghai meeting more than a century ago, the success of national efforts to reduce this epidemic will primarily depend upon cooperation among domestic stakeholders in the public and private sectors as well as improved support from our international partners.

SUGGESTED READINGS

Hanes WT III, Sanello F. *The Opium Wars: The Addiction of One Empire and the Corruption of Another*. Naperville, IL: Sourcebooks, 2002.

McAllister WB. *Drug Diplomacy in the Twentieth Century: An International History*. New York: Routledge, 2000.

Musto DF. *The American Disease: Origins of Narcotic Control*. 3rd ed. New York: Oxford University Press, 1999.

Musto DF. The history of legislative control over opium, cocaine, and their derivatives. In: Hamowy R, ed. *Dealing With Drugs: Consequences of Government Control*. Lexington, MA: D.C. Heath and Company, 1987:37-50.

Spillane JF. Debating the Controlled Substances Act. *Drug Alcohol Depend*. 2004;76(1):17-29.

United Nations Office on Drugs and Crime. *A Century of International Drug Control*. Vienna: United Nations, 2008. http://www.unodc.org/documents/data-and-analysis/Studies/100_Years_of_Drug_Control.pdf. Accessed January 5, 2018.

Guidance on the Use of Opioids to Treat Chronic Pain

Summary by James W. Finch and Bonnie B. Wilford

Based on THE ASAM PRINCIPLES OF ADDICTION MEDICINE, 6th edition sidebar by James W. Finch and Bonnie B. Wilford

In response to the current public health crisis involving opioid overdoses and deaths, a number of national organizations and federal agencies have developed and disseminated clinical guidelines as a means of mitigating the risks related to the use of prescribed opioids. Similarly, at the state level, growing public concern has prompted medical boards and state agencies to recommend or mandate risk mitigation strategies.

These efforts reverse a trend toward encouraging opioid prescribing, which emerged in the late 20th and early 21st centuries in response to significant concerns that clinicians were not providing their patients with adequate pain management. At the time, clinicians sometimes were characterized as "opioid phobic" and accused of allowing patients to suffer needlessly. It was in this spirit that pain began to be described as the "fifth vital sign." In response,

Continued

guideline writers viewed preventing the underuse of prescription opioids as a very high priority.

Although well-intended, the resulting guidelines may have inadvertently opened the door to excessive use of opioids. This has led to the current flurry of activity to revise and update guidelines, laws, and regulations. However, even with the current concern over opioid misuse and abuse, inadequate treatment of chronic pain continues to be a serious public health concern, as documented in a 2012 report by the Institute of Medicine.

On the positive side, some comprehensive approaches have been shown to achieve dramatic reductions in overdose deaths through community-wide collaborative approaches that engage prescribers, pharmacists, educators, law enforcement personnel, and community leaders. Data also support a wider use of state prescription drug monitoring programs (PDMPs), which are associated with reductions in "doctor shopping" for opioids. These results remind us that laws, regulations, and guidelines are only part—albeit an essential part—of the comprehensive approach needed to solve the current crisis involving prescription and illicit opioids and other drugs.

CHALLENGES CONFRONTING THE DRAFTERS OF GUIDELINES, LAWS, AND REGULATIONS

There is not yet sufficient evidence to demonstrate widespread improvement in clinical outcomes as a result of the updated guidelines, laws, and regulations. Given the need to respond to the current opioid crisis without waiting for empirical validation, the revised policies are being recommended on the basis of their "face validity."

This situation requires careful monitoring of patients for unanticipated adverse consequences. For example, injudicious or exploitative promotion of expensive drug screening and confirmation testing have been shown to generate excessive laboratory costs. Further, there is concern that if the requirements imposed on clinicians become too time-consuming or costly, some practitioners will respond by avoiding or turning away patients who present with chronic pain. Developers of guidelines and drafters of legislation and regulations thus face the challenge of providing guidance that protects access to opioids when medically justified while minimizing the risk of untoward outcomes, all in the setting of a woefully inadequate research base.

COMMON FEATURES OF RECENT GUIDANCE

The updated guidelines, laws, and regulations are largely consistent in their core recommendations. For example, most endorse the following constructs:

- Clinicians need to conduct an initial *risk assessment* and also determine the source and severity of the patient's pain before deciding whether to prescribe opioid analgesics.
- Clinicians are advised to obtain the patient's written *informed consent*, which should include explicit information about risks associated with the use of opioids and recognized limits to the effectiveness of opioids in reducing pain.
- Clinicians should be aware that opioids *should not be used as first-line therapy* and, ideally, always should be part of a *multimodal treatment plan*.
- High doses of opioids should be avoided.
- Whenever an opioid is initiated, the patient should be informed that the medication is being prescribed as a *therapeutic trial*, in which continued prescribing will be contingent on the successful management of pain, as well as functional improvement and evidence of safe use.
- Clinicians should conduct *ongoing monitoring* of patients to whom they have prescribed opioids in order to assess relative risks and benefits as well as to identify and respond to aberrant drug use behaviors.

Specific risk mitigation strategies that are found in a majority of the guidance documents include the following:

- Before and during prescribing, clinicians should consult their state's *PDMP* to determine whether the patient has been or is obtaining prescriptions for opioids from other practitioners.
- *Urine drug screening* should be employed on a regular basis to determine whether the patient is following the clinician's instructions for opioid use.
- Clinicians who prescribe opioids must be willing and able to seek *consultation from, or make referrals to,* specialists in the treatment of pain and/or addiction whenever there are indications that the patient would benefit from such a step.

VARIATIONS IN EMPHASIS ACROSS RECENT GUIDELINES

Although there is a great deal of congruence among the current guidelines, variations also are found. Most of these involve the degree of emphasis and/or specificity on certain points, such as dosage limits. Variations most often relate to the following points:

- Guidance as to *when and for how long* opioids are indicated for the treatment of chronic pain
- Specific advice on *patient monitoring* (eg, what to monitor, how often)
- Use of morphine milligram equivalents to define *acceptable or excessive doses*
- Differences in the use of *short-acting* and *long-acting* opioid analgesics
- Advice on the use of opioids to treat *acute pain*
- Guidance as to the advisability of prescribing *naloxone* to pain patients along with prescriptions for opioid analgesics so that the naloxone will be available to treat an opioid overdose if one should occur
- Advice regarding the treatment of patients diagnosed with *opioid use disorder*, including specific advice about the use of medication-assisted treatment
- Recommendations regarding the use of *methadone* for pain management

NATIONAL GUIDELINES, LAWS, AND REGULATIONS

Among many documents on this topic, two are worthy of special mention because of their national prominence. The first is a guideline published in 2017 by the federal Centers for Disease Control and Prevention (CDC). The other is a model policy, also published in 2017, by the Federation of State Medical Boards (FSMB), which has been disseminated to every state medical licensing board.

CENTERS FOR DISEASE CONTROL AND PREVENTION GUIDELINE

Given the level of public concern about opioid misuse and overdose, the CDC created a guideline for the safe and appropriate prescribing of opioids for chronic pain. The resulting *CDC Guideline for Prescribing Opioids for Chronic Pain* was released in May 2017. Important features of the document are as follows.

Dosing: Recommended doses of opioid analgesics are lower than in previous CDC guidelines.

Assessing risks and harms: Whereas earlier guidelines recommended safety precautions only for so-called "high-risk patients," the new guidelines point out that the use of opioid analgesics poses some degree of risk to *all* patients. The 2017 guideline

therefore contains recommendations for delivering safe care to all patients. It also encourages the use of recent technological advances, such as electronic PDMPs.

Monitoring and discontinuing opioids: The 2017 CDC guideline contains more specific recommendations on monitoring and discontinuing opioids than those seen in earlier versions.

FEDERATION OF STATE MEDICAL BOARDS GUIDELINES

The FSMB represents all US medical licensing boards. One of the FSMB's most significant activities involves convening expert panels to develop consensus statements or model policies. These are forwarded to individual state medical boards for review and adoption. As part of this process, state boards can, and often do, modify their version of the policy to be more or less restrictive than the national model.

FSMB released its *Guidelines for the Chronic Use of Opioid Analgesics* in April 2017. The new guidelines feature updated criteria for:

- patient assessments, evaluations, and ongoing monitoring;
- use of written treatment agreements;
- accessing state PDMPs;
- initiating, continuing, or discontinuing opioid therapy;
- risks inherent in concurrent use of opioids and benzodiazepines; and
- special considerations in prescribing naloxone or methadone.

STATE-SPECIFIC GUIDELINES, LAWS, AND REGULATIONS

In response to similar concerns, a number of state-level professional organizations and public health agencies have produced guidance documents for clinicians practicing in their state. For example, Arizona published updated opioid prescribing guidelines in 2017. The Arizona initiative is noteworthy because its guidelines are intended not only for physicians but also for nurse practitioners, physician assistants, and pharmacists.

At present, most state medical licensing boards have opioid prescribing regulations that are based on FSMB's 2013 *Model Policy on the Use of Opioid Analgesics in the Treatment of Chronic Pain*. However, states are likely to update their existing policies to reflect the changes in FSMB's 2017 guidelines.

Continued

Physicians are advised to check regularly with their state medical licensing board to access the most current guidance.

SUGGESTED READINGS

Dowell D, Haegerich TM, Chou R. CDC guidelines for prescribing opioids for chronic pain—United States, 2016. *MMWR Recomm Rep.* 2016; 65(RR-1):1-49.

Federation of State Medical Boards. *Guidelines for the Chronic Use of Opioid Analgesics.* Washington, DC: Federation of State Medical Boards, 2017. https://www.fsmb.org/globalassets /advocacy/policies/opioid_guidelines_as_adopted_april -2017_final.pdf. Accessed December 11, 2018.

Franklin GM, Mai J, Turner J, et al. Bending the prescription opioid dosing and mortality curves: impact of the Washington State opioid dosing guideline. *Am J Ind Med.* 2012;55(4):325-331.

Joranson DE, Gilson AM, Dahl JL, Haddox JD. Pain management, controlled substances, and state medical board policy: a decade of change. *J Pain Symptom Manage.* 2002; 23(2):138-147.

Trescot AM, Boswell MV, Atluri SL, et al. Opioid guidelines in the management of chronic non-cancer pain. *Pain Physician.* 2006;9:1-39.

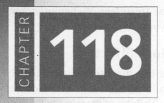

118

Medicinal Uses of Cannabis and Cannabinoids

Summary by Jag H. Khalsa

Based on THE ASAM PRINCIPLES OF ADDICTION MEDICINE, 6th edition chapter by Jag H. Khalsa, Gregory C. Bunt, Marc Galanter, and Norman W. Wetterau

Plants and plant-derived chemical constituents have been used as medicine by humans for thousands of years. Of the many varieties of cannabis cultivated in various parts of the world, three are most commonly used: *Cannabis sativa Linn*, *Cannabis indica Linn*, and *Cannabis ruderalis Janisch*, corresponding to useful, Indian, and wild cannabis plants. Cannabis is defined as the flowering tops of the cannabis plant from which resin has not been extracted. Generally, European authors tend to use the terms *cannabis* and *medicinal* or *medical* cannabis, whereas American authors tend to simply use *marijuana* or *medical marijuana*. The term *marijuana* refers to the desiccated leaves, flowers, stems, and seeds of the hemp plant, *C. sativa Linn*.

FACTS ABOUT CANNABIS

The Epidemiology of Cannabis Use and Misuse

Cannabis is the most frequently used illegal drug in the world today. In 2013, an estimated 181 million *persons (3.9% of the global population 15 to 64 years of age)* used cannabis for nonmedical purposes. In 2015, an estimated 22.2 million Americans, or 8.9% of the population aged 12 years or older, used cannabis in the preceding month. Approximately 2 to 3 million new users of marijuana are added each year, with an estimated 9.1% of users developing pre–substance dependence as defined by the *Diagnostic and Statistical Manual of Mental Disorders,* 5th edition. The risk of developing pre–substance dependence may be as high as 17% among those who begin in adolescence and 25% to 50% of those who smoke marijuana daily. In 2016, an estimated 5.4%, 14.0%, and 22.5% of 8th-, 10th-, and 12th-grade students, respectively, smoked cannabis in the preceding month. Rates of cannabis use by young people have risen and declined at various points over the past decade, possibly due to the increasing potency of cannabis, which has been on the rise, from about 4% concentration

of Δ9-tetrahydrocannabinol (THC, marijuana's active chemical constituent) in 1995 to about 12% in 2014. The increase also could be driven by changes in young peoples' perception of marijuana's dangers. Cannabis use usually peaks in the late teens to early 20s and then declines with increasing age.

The Chemistry of Cannabis

The cannabis plant has hundreds of chemical constituents, of which only a few are pharmacologically active. Of the 525 identified and characterized chemicals in cannabis, 104 are classified as cannabinoids; the rest are terpenes and flavonoids. Only two cannabinoids—THC and cannabidiol (CBD)—have been extensively studied for their potential therapeutic applications and thus have been discussed in relation to medical care. THC is the most active psychoactive component, and CBD has been postulated to have many pharmacologic mechanisms of action, including immunosuppressive, anti-inflammatory, analgesic, neuroprotective, antiepileptic, and antipsychotic effects. However, the data from case reports or randomized clinical trials have been limited to just a few of these indications. The other cannabinoids such as tetrahydrocannabivarin, cannabichromene, cannabicyclol, and Δ8-THC have yet to be thoroughly studied for pharmacologic activity and medicinal value. In addition to phytocannabinoids, some endocannabinoids are neurotransmitters within the brain or its periphery and act on cannabinoid receptors in the brain (cannabinoid type 1 [CB1] receptor) or periphery (cannabinoid type 2 [CB2] receptor). The synthetic cannabinoids are structurally similar to endocannabinoids and act by similar mechanisms.

CANNABIS OR CANNABINOIDS AS MEDICINE

Since the first description of the medicinal value of cannabis by the Chinese Emperor Shen-Nung in

2737 BC, many preparations of cannabis have been used for recreational and medicinal purposes. The biological plausibility of cannabis as medicine is based on the fact that the endocannabinoid system is believed to be involved in functions like analgesia, vomiting, immune system regulation, appetite, cognitive processes, and motor control. THC and CBD exert their effect by interacting with CB1 and CB2 receptors. The CB1 receptor is widely distributed in the hippocampus, cerebellum, basal ganglia, and neocortex, in addition to peripheral nerve terminals. Although CB1 receptors reportedly possess analgesic, antispasmodic, antitremor, anti-inflammatory, appetite stimulant, and antiemetic properties, the CB2 receptors, found largely within the periphery including cells of the immune system, reportedly possess anti-inflammatory, analgesic, anticonvulsant, antipsychotic, antioxidant, and neuroprotective properties. As a result, both THC and CBD have been tested for their therapeutic potential.

Currently, the two synthetic cannabinoids similar to THC, dronabinol and nabilone, have been approved by the US Food and Drug Administration (FDA). Dronabinol is approved for the treatment of anorexia associated with weight loss in patients with AIDS and chemotherapy-induced nausea and vomiting, and nabilone has been approved for the treatment of chemotherapy-induced nausea and vomiting. An oral spray containing THC and CBD in a 1:1 ratio, has been approved in 28 countries (but not in the United States) for moderate-to-severe spasticity due to multiple sclerosis in patients who have not responded adequately to other treatments. In addition, data from a double-blind randomized phase III clinical trial on cannabis-derived CBD for the treatment of Lennox-Gastaut syndrome—a rare form of epilepsy in children—are being evaluated by the FDA.

Many investigators have presented data from clinical studies with a few to hundreds of patients treated with a single cannabinoid like THC, CBD, or a combination of the two for clinical conditions including chemotherapy-induced nausea and vomiting, loss of appetite, pain, multiple sclerosis, spinal cord injuries, Tourette syndrome, epilepsy, glaucoma, Parkinson disease, dystonia, and posttraumatic stress disorder (PTSD). These clinical data are summarized in the following sections.

Antiemetic Effects

Data from numerous clinical trials involving hundreds of patients have clearly shown that nabilone and dronabinol are effective as antiemetics and have been approved for the treatment of chemotherapy-induced nausea and vomiting.

Appetite Stimulant Effect

Oral THC stimulates the appetite and significantly improves weight gain in patients who are on cancer therapy or infected with human immunodeficiency virus, who often develop cachexia.

Analgesic Effect

Oral cannabis plant extract, sublingual spray, intravenous THC, and single cannabinoids such as THC or CBD or a combination thereof have been tested for analgesic activity in several small clinical studies or trials.

Multiple Sclerosis

Several formulations of marijuana have been successfully tested in clinical studies/trials involving hundreds of patients with symptoms of multiple sclerosis.

Epilepsy

Several anecdotal observations and data from three clinical trials suggest that cannabidiol has positive effects on epilepsy. Additional trials are under way.

For conditions like spinal cord injuries, Tourette syndrome, glaucoma, dystonia, and Parkinson disease, limited data from a small number of patients are available to show that cannabis products have a potential, but are not yet approved, as medicine. Although a few state governments have approved cannabis for the treatment of multiple psychiatric conditions, including PTSD and agitation in Alzheimer disease or Tourette syndrome, there is no credible evidence from several studies to support the use of cannabis for any of these conditions. Although there may be a biological basis for use of cannabis to treat psychiatric conditions including PTSD, caution is advised. Additional research is urgently needed to assess the efficacy and safety of cannabis or cannabinoids for psychiatric disorders.

THE PHYSICIAN'S ROLE IN PRESCRIBING CANNABIS OR CANNABINOIDS FOR MEDICINAL PURPOSES

Despite the widespread publicity and many testimonials as to the effectiveness of cannabis as medicine, an objective review of all available data suggests that it is premature to draw any definitive conclusions regarding the efficacy of cannabis or cannabinoids as medicine for many of the proposed clinical indications. Nevertheless, 23 states have adopted some form of legalization of marijuana for medical use. In some states, the practice is reasonably well regulated, but other states have very permissive laws—all based on the same evidence.

The Institute of Medicine, the American Society of Addiction Medicine (ASAM), and other scientific and medical organizations have adopted policies stating that more research is needed before physicians prescribe marijuana, marijuana extract, CBD, or any of the 100+ cannabinoids of marijuana. ASAM has endorsed the use of cannabinoids and cannabis for medicinal purposes only when such use is governed by appropriate safety and monitoring regulations, such as those established by the FDA. According to ASAM, cannabis, cannabis-based products, and cannabis delivery devices should be subject to the same safety and efficacy standards that are applied to other prescription medications and medical devices, and that such products should not be distributed or otherwise provided to patients until they have been approved by the FDA. However, ASAM rejects smoking as a means of drug delivery.

ASAM recommends that physicians assess patients to whom they have prescribed or recommended marijuana for the following signs of problems: (1) Is the patient already addicted to marijuana before asking for a prescription for marijuana for medical reasons? (2) Is the patient addicted to other substances, such as opioids for pain? If yes, has he or she reduced or discontinued the opioid? (3) Is the patient showing signs of a substance use disorder involving marijuana? And (4) is marijuana causing negative effects in the patient's life?

Physicians who recommend cannabis to patients should do so within the context of a physician–patient relationship that includes the creation of a medical record and follow-up visits to assess the results of the recommended clinical intervention, and the treatment plan should be amended as indicated. In 2016, the Federation of State Medical Boards outlined several expectations of licensed physicians who recommend or prescribe marijuana. Those expectations involve the presence of a physician–patient relationship; a patient evaluation; decision making; a treatment agreement to document other measures used to relieve the patient's symptoms; the qualifying conditions; ongoing monitoring; consultation with and referral to a specialist in psychiatry, addiction, or mental health; maintenance of detailed medical records; the absence of physician conflict of interest; and abstention of the physician from personal use of marijuana. Additionally, state prescription drug monitoring program databases should be checked before recommending cannabis and periodically thereafter. The physicians who do not approve of the use of marijuana for any medical purpose should maintain a cordial relationship with physicians who do prescribe medicinal marijuana so that they can help prevent harm to patients and accept referrals for treatment.

CONCLUSIONS

In summary, there is little doubt that cannabis constituents such as THC, CBD, or a combination of the two have the *potential* to treat a wide range of clinical conditions. *Smoked marijuana is not approved for any clinical indication.* However, there has been a strong movement in the United States and elsewhere to use or promote marijuana as medicine and to legalize its use outside of regular channels and laws. This effort has been very successful. Nevertheless, the Institute of Medicine, ASAM, and other medical organizations have recommended that additional research be conducted before cannabis is prescribed for an unapproved clinical indication. Physicians are generally allowed to prescribe an FDA-approved medication for the approved indication or an off-label indication. However, those who prescribe or recommend cannabis or cannabinoids for medical use—or who are contemplating doing so—should realize that although some courts have upheld physicians' right to do so, federal law prohibits the use of marijuana for either recreational or medical purposes. The American Bar Association has provided additional guidance in cautioning physicians who are considering involvement with cannabis as medicine. Under federal law, marijuana and its components are classified as Schedule I substances under the Controlled Substances Act of 1970, which was reaffirmed in 2016. Accordingly, marijuana cannot be knowingly or intentionally distributed, dispensed, or possessed, and an individual who aids and abets another person in violating federal law—or who engages in a conspiracy to purchase, cultivate, or possess marijuana—may be punished to the same extent as the individual who commits the crime.

ACKNOWLEDGMENTS

We appreciate very much the thoughtful suggestions from Dr. Robert DuPont, the first director of the National Institute on Drug Abuse.

KEY POINTS

1. The cannabis plant has many chemical constituents that have therapeutic potential and should be tested in well-designed clinical studies or randomized, double-blind, placebo-controlled clinical trials.

2. Synthetic THC alone or in combination with another cannabinoid, such as CBD, has been approved by the FDA and other international regulatory agencies for certain indications.

3. The clinical evidence is limited for the use of cannabis, cannabis extract, or isolated cannabinoids such as THC, CBD, or combination of the two, in the treatment of conditions including multiple sclerosis, dystonia, glaucoma, Parkinson disease, and PTSD. Therefore, none of these products is approved by the FDA or any regulatory body for physicians to prescribe. Many more well-designed clinical studies and trials are needed to achieve such a goal.

REVIEW QUESTIONS

1. Which of the following is a cannabis compound?
   A. Megestrol
   B. Dronabinol
   C. Candesartan
   D. Ondansetron
   E. Dronedarone

2. Which of the following drugs are approved for multiple sclerosis by the FDA?
   A. Dronabinol
   B. Marinol
   C. Nabilone
   D. All of the above.
   E. None of the above.

3. Which of the following is *true* regarding the safety of smoked cannabis?
   A. It has not been approved by the FDA, although it is legal in some states.
   B. It has been approved by the FDA, but it is legal in only some states.
   C. It has not been approved by the FDA, and it is illegal in all states except Oregon.
   D. It has been approved by the FDA and it is legal in all 50 states.
   E. It has not been approved by the FDA, and it is illegal in all states except Oregon and Colorado.

ANSWERS

1. **B**
2. **E**
3. **A**

SUGGESTED READINGS

American Society of Addiction Medicine. Public policy statement on marijuana, cannabinoids and legalization. https://www.asam.org/docs/default-source/public-policy-statements/marijuana-cannabinoids-and-legalization-9-21-2015.pdf?sfvrsn=0. Published September 21, 2015. Accessed October 5, 2017.

American Society of Addiction Medicine. Public policy statement on medical marijuana. https://www.asam.org/docs/default-source/public-policy-statements/1medical-marijuana-4-10.pdf?sfvrsn=3110df6b_0. Published April 2010. Accessed October 5, 2017.

Ben Amar M. Cannabinoids in medicine: a review of their therapeutic potential. *J Ethnopharmacol.* 2006;105(1-2):1-25.

Kumar RN, Chambers WA, Pertwee RG. Pharmacological actions and therapeutic uses of cannabis and cannabinoids. *Anaesthesia.* 2001;56(11):1059-1068.

Whiting PF, Wolff RF, Deshpande S, et al. Cannabinoids for medical use: a systematic review and meta-analysis. *JAMA.* 2015;313(24):2456-2473.

119

Practical Considerations in Drug Testing

Summary by Gary M. Reisfield, Roger L. Bertholf, Bruce A. Goldberger, and Robert L. DuPont

Based on THE ASAM PRINCIPLES OF ADDICTION MEDICINE, 6th edition chapter by Gary M. Reisfield, Roger L. Bertholf, Bruce A. Goldberger, and Robert L. DuPont

Drug testing brings a measure of objectivity to patients' reports regarding their drug and alcohol use. Patients are not always truthful with their physicians, and physicians cannot reliably tell when patients are telling the truth. Drug testing serves to verify adherence with prescribed medications and to detect the unauthorized use of other drugs. It may also serve to deter drug use, but the literature on its effectiveness for this purpose is conflicting.

Clinical drug testing thus informs medical diagnosis and treatment. However, it is not a standalone technique for monitoring recovery from a substance use disorder (SUD) or the safety of pharmacotherapies involving controlled substances. It should be integrated, as necessary, with patient conversations and physical examinations, information from collaterals, queries of prescription drug monitoring program databases, and medication reconciliation.

This chapter provides an overview of the uses of drug testing in clinical settings, with a focus on optimizing the application of these technologies to enhance efforts to prevent SUDs, as well as the identification, treatment, and long-term management of individuals who have such disorders.

THE SCIENCE OF DRUG TESTING

Laboratory Test Results Assessments

Laboratory tests are intended to inform the clinician of pathologic conditions. Toward that objective, the performance of a test can be characterized by its clinical sensitivity and specificity. *Clinical* sensitivity and specificity are distinct from *analytical* sensitivity and specificity, which refer to the smallest concentration of substance detectable and the degree to which the method is free from interferences, respectively.

For the purpose of this discussion, the following definitions apply:

- True positive (TP): An abnormal result in a patient who has the suspected disease
- True negative (TN): A normal result in a patient who does *not* have the suspected disease
- False positive (FP): An abnormal result in a patient who does *not* have the suspected disease
- False negative (FN): A normal result in a patient who does have the suspected disease

Given these parameters, the *sensitivity* of a laboratory test is defined as:

$$\text{Sensitivity} = \frac{TP}{TP + FN}$$

The denominator in this equation, $TP + FN$, corresponds to all patients who have the suspected disease; thus, the sensitivity is the fraction of patients with the suspected disease who produce a positive test result. Sensitivity is sometimes called "positivity in the presence of disease."

The *specificity* of a laboratory test is defined as:

$$\text{Specificity} = \frac{TN}{TN + FP}$$

In this case, the denominator of the equation, $TN + FP$, corresponds to all patients who do *not* have the suspected disease. In this case, the specificity is the fraction of patients without the suspected disease who produce a negative test. Specificity is sometimes called "negativity in the absence of disease."

To determine sensitivity, the test is applied to specimens confirmed to contain the drug at a concentration above the positive threshold. Although the assessment provides a measure of the ability of the assay to reliably detect the drug when present, it does not give a reliable estimate of the likelihood that a patient taking the drug will test positive because the latter may be affected by multiple factors, including absorption, metabolism, and clearance of the drug; drug dose and pattern of administration; and hydration status.

The specificity of a drug screening test is also difficult to evaluate because potential cross-reactivity is difficult to predict for immunoassay-based assays, and there is a practical limit to the number of compounds that can be tested for interference. Therefore, estimates of specificity are necessarily inflated because there always are compounds that might interfere but were not tested. Experience in drug testing teaches that screening methods sometimes produce positive test results that are not confirmed by more specific analytical methods.

A more useful measure of the clinical performance of a laboratory test is its *predictive value*. The predictive value of a positive test (PV_+) is defined as:

$$\text{Predictive Value } (+) = \frac{TP}{TP + FP}$$

The denominator in this equation is the total number of positive results, so the PV_+ represents the likelihood that a positive test result is a true positive (ie, correctly identifies a patient with the suspected disease). Unlike sensitivity and specificity, which characterize the performance of a test when the patient already has been classified as positive or negative, the predictive value is an estimate of the probability that a patient who tests positive has the suspected disease. For a laboratory test with established specificity, the number of false-positive results it produces depends on the frequency of negative specimens. If all specimens are negative, then all positive results will be false positives.

However, if all specimens are positive, then all positive results will be true positives. Therefore, the FP in the equation, and consequently the predictive value of the test, depends on the frequency of patients who test positive among the population being tested. As a result, the predictive value of drug screening tests will vary from one practice to another, depending on the frequency with which patients meet the expectations that prompted use of the drug test. Studies that have assessed the predictive value of positive urine drug test results have produced estimates ranging from 10% to 100% depending on the drug being screened.

In drug screening immunoassays, the extent of cross-reactivity with other compounds varies among methods. Amphetamine screening immunoassays, for example, are susceptible to cross-reacting analytes because there are many drugs with the same or similar phenethylamine structure. Other screening immunoassays, as for the cocaine metabolite (benzoylecgonine) and cannabinoids, are relatively specific, so false-positive test results are rare.

Although it sometimes leads to false-positive test results, the cross-reactivity of antibodies with similar chemical structures also has a beneficial aspect. Certain immunoassay methods react with multiple drugs within a class, obviating the need to test for each individual drug. For example, opiate immunoassays typically detect morphine, codeine, hydromorphone, and hydrocodone. Barbiturate and benzodiazepine immunoassays detect several drugs within their respective classes. An immunoassay may be more reactive with one drug than another within the same class. For example, opiate screens typically have high reactivity to morphine and codeine, but are less reactive to hydrocodone and hydromorphone, and may react negligibly with oxycodone and oxymorphone. Therefore, when using an immunoassay to monitor adherence, the reactivity of the immunoassay toward that drug and/or its metabolite(s) must be considered. The performance specifications of immunoassays, including cross-reactivity data, are included in the manufacturer's product insert. Laboratories performing drug screens also can provide this information on request.

Mass Spectrometry

Mass spectrometers identify compounds by fragmenting them into ions that can be separated through use of a mass filter. Separation of the molecular fragments can be achieved by several methods, including one or more magnetic sectors, one or more quadrupole filters, or a time-of-flight mass filter.

Liquid chromatography (LC) combined with mass spectrometry (MS) is considered a confirmatory (or definitive) method to assess for drugs because no other analytical method has greater specificity. When properly configured, drug analyses by MS-based methods have a vanishingly small chance of producing a false-positive test result.

Drug testing by LC-MS/MS methods is becoming increasingly common, and because little specimen preparation is required, some laboratories now eliminate immunoassay screening tests altogether.

Screening tests alone can be useful, but positive screening test results should not be considered proof that a drug or drug metabolite is present in the specimen. Likewise, negative screening results do not rule out the presence of a drug because the drug may be present at a concentration below the detection threshold of the screening test.

CHOICE OF TESTING MATRIX

There is no universal "best" matrix for drug testing. The choice of testing matrix should be based on situational considerations, including the particular drugs of interest, the desired window of detection, and the available clinical resources.

Urine

Urine is the most commonly used matrix for clinical drug testing. Its advantages include its rapid production, noninvasive collection, high concentration of analytes relative to blood (thus providing a wider window of detection of up to several days for many drugs or weeks in the case of long-term use of lipid-soluble drugs), relatively simple preparation of samples for analysis, and decades of accumulated knowledge about the disposition of a large number of drugs and their metabolites.

The most important limitation to urine as a testing matrix is that its collection is generally unobserved, thus providing the opportunity for test subversion. This can be minimized through observed collections, but this is widely considered intrusive and is not commonly used in clinical testing. Subversion often can be detected by assessing specimen integrity—including its color, pH, temperature, specific gravity, creatinine, and presence of oxidants—at the point of collection. Specimen integrity measures are commonplace features of inexpensive collection cups.

Compared to blood, one limitation of urine is the inability to correlate the concentration of drug and drug metabolite with drug dose and schedule of administration. Determinants of drug and metabolite concentrations include the specific drug of interest, dose and route of administration, chronicity of use, time between last drug administration and collection of urine sample, the donor's pharmacokinetic profile, urinary pH, and hydration status.

Oral Fluid

Using oral fluid as a testing matrix addresses the most important limitation of urine: privacy concerns. With oral fluid, the donor can be observed throughout the collection process, thus minimizing opportunities for test subversion.

Oral fluid shares some of urine's other advantages, including its ability to be easily collected and

prepared for analysis. Compared to urine, oral fluid has a narrower temporal window of detection. Some drugs may be detected earlier in oral fluid (eg, within minutes of administration) but at the expense of diminished sensitivity for later detection.

Oral fluid has a propensity to accumulate 6-acetylmorphine following heroin administration, making it advantageous in detecting heroin use. On the other hand, relative to urine, it appears to be inferior for the detection of several opiates (including buprenorphine), benzodiazepines, and cannabis. The ability of MS techniques to detect these and other analytes in oral fluid is highly dependent on the cutoff concentrations of the analytical method. Technology improvements and lower cutoff concentrations have the potential to greatly narrow the sensitivity gap between oral fluid and urine for the detection of drugs.

Hair

Because drugs and their metabolites are incorporated, in varying degrees, into the developing hair follicle, hair offers the widest window of detection of the commonly used matrices. Hair is unaffected by short-term abstinence. Additional advantages include simple, noninvasive collection and stability at room temperature.

Hair typically is collected from the vertex posterior section of the scalp, where growth is rapid and uniform. Because it takes approximately 7 to 10 days for hair from the follicle to emerge from the scalp, it is unsuitable for assessing recent drug use; although, in actuality, hair also incorporates drug from sweat and sebum as well as from environmental exposure.

Laboratories typically test the proximal 3 cm—corresponding roughly to the most recent 3 months of growth—because with longer samples, the natural washout of drug over time could dilute analytes of interest to below the cutoff concentration of the assay. Some laboratories offer to "fractionate" hair into segments in order to provide greater temporal resolution of drug use. Other laboratories demur because axial diffusion of the drug/metabolite along the hair shaft and incorporation of drug/metabolite into hair from sweat and other secretions may potentially confound an interpretation of results.

There are limitations to the use of hair as a testing matrix. Most studies have reported the lack of a linear relationship between drug dose and drug concentration in hair. A drug's concentration in hair depends on several factors, including dose and frequency of administration, metabolic factors, basicity of the drug, hair color, percentage of collected hairs in the anagen and telogen phases, prolonged exposure to sunlight or other sources of ultraviolet radiation, and cosmetic treatments.

The ability to detect drugs and metabolites in hair is critically dependent on the cutoff concentrations of the assays. Suggested cutoff concentrations for drug and alcohol testing in hair have recently been published.

LIMITATIONS OF DRUG TESTING

A "general" drug test does not exist. It is impossible for any laboratory to develop a validated method for the detection of every drug with a potential for abuse, the list of which is vast and continually growing. However, individuals with SUDs often are indiscriminate in their drug use and may use several drugs concurrently, including those detected by common screening assays. The inability to detect use of every drug is not usually necessary for the purposes of assessing recovery status and/or the need to modify a patient's treatment plan.

As noted earlier, drug testing typically begins with a screening immunoassay, the results of which sometimes require confirmation with a definitive technique. Screening immunoassays have inherent limitations based on the imperfect specificity of antigen–antibody reactions. Thus, all nonnegative immunoassay screening test results are labeled "presumptive positive" and require MS-based testing if a definitive identification of an analyte is necessary.

In addition, screening immunoassays often have clinically important sensitivity limitations, particularly with regard to the class-specific assays (such as those for amphetamines, barbiturates, benzodiazepines, and opiates) in which an antibody directed against a specific member of the drug class will have varying, but usually lesser, degrees of cross-reactivity with other class members. Thus, negative immunoassay results, particularly when the results are unexpected, are more properly regarded as "presumptive negative" results.

MS-based definitive techniques are highly specific. Their sensitivity, however, is defined by the administrative cutoff concentration, which might be defined by the lower limit of quantification. These limits vary by analyte, matrix, and laboratory.

For drugs that are represented on a laboratory's menu of assays, the temporal limits of detection are determined by several factors, including quantity, frequency, and recency of drug use; the testing matrix; and the analytical capabilities of the assay.

With regard to the testing matrix, oral fluid and urine typically have windows of detection of up to several days. Head hair provides a window of detection of approximately 3 months.

Drug test results do not permit the clinician to determine the drug dose, quantity or frequency of administration, the specific time of last use, or the route of administration. Despite claims to the contrary by some commercial laboratories, there is no peer-reviewed scientific basis for the use of propriety algorithms to determine adherence with prescription medication instructions. Moreover, drug test results involving the analysis of urine and hair do not permit inferences about drug-related impairment, nor do tests involving the analysis of blood for any substance except alcohol.

A confirmed positive drug test result verifies the presence of a drug or drug metabolite at or above a cutoff concentration, but a diagnosis of SUD is made on the basis of a constellation of signs and symptoms. Hence, an unexpected drug test result should prompt a conversation with the patient about the meaning of the test result.

Similarly, a negative drug test result does not prove that a drug or metabolite of interest was absent from the testing matrix. Rather, it means that, *if* the drug or metabolite is present, it is present below the cutoff concentration for the test. An *unexpected*, confirmed negative drug test requires a behavioral explanation for the test result. For example, the differential diagnosis includes running out of the medication several days or more prior to the test because of an SUD, as-needed medication use with little or no use in the days preceding the drug test, sample adulteration, and medication diversion.

MS-based drug testing techniques are capable of providing results of exquisite sensitivity and specificity, but they have the aforementioned limitations. Thus, although drug testing is an essential component of the care of individuals with SUDs and individuals who are prescribed long-term controlled substance therapies, it is not a sufficient stand-alone monitoring technique and does not obviate the need for spending time talking with patients about how they are doing in life, speaking with the patients' loved ones (with the patient's permission), checking state prescription drug monitoring databases, and performing medication reconciliations.

BIOMARKERS OF ALCOHOL CONSUMPTION

Until recently, alcohol testing was limited almost entirely to the measurement of blood and breath in cases of acute intoxication and suspected impairment. This was true, in part, because of its rapid metabolism by first-order kinetics, so that even in the setting of chronic, heavy use, it generally cannot be detected in the blood, breath, and urine more than several hours after use.

Knowledge of an individual's alcohol consumption beyond acute use or intoxication is important in several clinical contexts, including alcohol and drug use disorder treatment programs and post-treatment monitoring programs. It should be regarded as important in patients receiving long-term treatment with opioids or benzodiazepines because the co-consumption of alcohol plays an important role in the morbidity and mortality associated with those medications. None of the traditional, indirect biomarkers of heavy alcohol use—carbohydrate-deficient transferrin, γ-glutamyltransferase, or mean corpuscular volume—have the necessary sensitivity and specificity for these purposes.

In recent years, ethyl glucuronide (EtG), ethyl sulfate (EtS), and more recently phosphatidylethanol (PEth) have been identified as widely available, longer lasting, direct biomarkers of alcohol consumption.

Ethyl Glucuronide and Ethyl Sulfate

EtG and EtS are minor ethanol metabolites, which are formed by the conjugation of ethanol with glucuronic acid and sulfate, respectively. They can be detected in a variety of biological matrices. EtG and EtS are commonly measured in the urine; EtG is also commonly measured in hair. They appear in the urine within 1 hour of alcohol consumption and, depending on the drinking pattern and the cutoff concentration of the assay, may be detected for 72 hours or more after the last drink.

It has been demonstrated that EtG can be synthesized in vitro in the presence of alcohol; as a result, in patients with glycosuria and *Escherichia coli* urinary tract infections, clinical false-positive EtG test results can be produced. Conversely, *E. coli* also can hydrolyze EtG in vitro. Genetic polymorphisms of the *UGT1A1* gene, which encodes several uridine 5′-diphospho-glucuronosyltransferases, have the potential to interfere with EtG production. EtS is neither produced nor degraded by bacteria or is it vulnerable to known genetic polymorphisms, making it a useful complementary biomarker of alcohol consumption.

It has been suggested that verifying alcohol abstinence requires urinary EtG and EtS cutoffs of 100 ng/mL and 25 ng/mL, respectively. These low cutoffs

reduce the specificity of the source of alcohol because EtG and EtS are detectable following the consumption of nonalcoholic beer and wine, fruit juices, and ripe bananas as well as ethanol-containing mouthwashes and hand sanitizers. Therefore, patients for whom there is a zero tolerance for alcohol consumption should be counseled to avoid such exposures.

In head hair, it has been proposed that EtG concentrations of <7 pg/mg indicates either abstinence or low intake of alcohol, 7 to 30 pg/mg suggests repeated alcohol consumption, and >30 pg/mg suggests chronic heavy use (ie, >60 g per day).

Phosphatidylethanol

PEth comprises a group of phospholipids, each consisting of a glycerol backbone, a phosphoethanol head group, and two fatty acid chains, which are produced in red blood cell membranes by the action of enzyme phospholipase D on phosphatidylcholine in the presence of ethanol. Dozens of PEth homologues have been identified in humans; commonly, only the predominant 16:0/18:1 species is analyzed. PEth becomes detectable in the blood within hours of a drinking episode and has an elimination half-life of 4.5 to 12 days. It can be measured in whole blood, including capillary blood collected on filter paper ("dried blood spot"), which simplifies collection, transport, and storage.

Originally described as a biomarker for detecting heavy alcohol consumption (eg, ≥50 g per day of alcohol for several weeks), with the development of LC-MS/MS methods, PEth has been shown to distinguish binge drinkers from moderate drinkers and abstainers and to identify a single heavy drinking occasion for up to 12 days.

KEY POINTS

1. Immunoassay-based drug screens are rapid and inexpensive, but are sometimes limited by their sensitivity, specificity, or both. Thus, results are considered *presumptive*. Mass-spectrometry-based drug tests are highly specific and usually highly sensitive. The results are considered *definitive*.

2. There is no universal "best" drug testing matrix. The choice of matrix should be based on the situational considerations.

3. The temporal windows of detection of drugs and their metabolites are determined by several factors, including quantity, frequency, and recency of drug use; the testing matrix; and the analytical capabilities of the assay.

4. The confirmed presence of a drug or its metabolite does not diagnose a substance use disorder,

the diagnosis of which is based on a constellation of signs and symptoms.

5. Although drug testing is a vital component of the evaluation and management of individuals with substance use disorders, it is not a sufficient standalone monitoring technique.

REVIEW QUESTIONS

1. An immunoassay-based urine drug screen yields a presumptive positive result for amphetamine. Subsequent testing by liquid chromatography-tandem mass spectrometry fails to confirm the result. The screening result is an example of:
   A. True positive
   B. True negative
   C. False positive
   D. False negative

2. Which of the following is true of urine drug tests:
   A. The window of detection is longer than that of blood
   B. Preparation of samples for analysis is complex and time-consuming
   C. They permit correlation of drug concentration with drug dose and time of administration
   D. Sample subversion is difficult

3. The most useful test for detection of past-three-week alcohol consumption is:
   A. Urine ethyl glucuronide (EtG)
   B. Urine ethyl sulfate (EtS)
   C. Blood phosphatidylethanol (PEth)
   D. Blood γ-glutamyl transferase (GGT)

ANSWERS

1. **C.** A false positive screening result is one in which the *presumptive* positive result fails to confirm by analysis with a *definitive* mass spectrometry-based technique.

2. **A.** Urine is a highly concentrated ultrafiltrate of blood and it generally offers a longer window of detection than blood.

3. **C.** Blood PEth can remain positive for several weeks, depending on quantity and pattern of alcohol consumption. The urinary conjugates may be positive for up to several days, depending on the quantity of recent drinking. At low concentrations, it can be difficult to distinguish alcohol consumption from incidental exposures. Blood GGT lacks the necessary sensitivity and specificity of the direct biomarkers.

SUGGESTED READINGS

Bertholf RL, Sharma R, Reisfield GM. Predictive value of positive drug screening results in an urban outpatient population. *J Anal Toxicol.* 2016;40(9):726-731.

Cabarcos P, Alvarez I, Tabernero MJ, Bermejo AM. Determination of direct alcohol markers: a review. *Anal Bioanal Chem.* 2015;407(17):4907-4925.

Cooper GA, Kronstrand R, Kintz P. Society of Hair Testing guidelines for drug testing in hair. *Forensic Sci Int.* 2012;218(1-3):20-24.

Reisfield GM, Bertholf R, Barkin RL, Webb F, Wilson G. Urine drug test interpretation: what do physicians know? *J Opioid Manag.* 2007;3(2):80-86.

Reisfield GM, Maschke KJ. Urine drug testing in long-term opioid therapy: ethical considerations. *Clin J Pain.* 2014;30(8):679-684.

Workplace Drug Testing and the Role of the Medical Review Officer

Summary by James L. Ferguson and Robert L. DuPont

Based on THE ASAM PRINCIPLES OF ADDICTION MEDICINE, 6th edition sidebar by James L. Ferguson and Robert L. DuPont

The role of the medical review officer (MRO) for workplace drug testing programs is an area of practice frequently overlooked by addiction medicine physicians. MROs are physicians who are impartial gatekeepers and advocates for the accuracy and integrity of many different drug testing programs. We focus here on workplace testing, but the need for MRO knowledge, impartiality, and objectivity has been recognized by many other programs, including addiction treatment programs and recovery monitoring programs and in courts and pain clinics.

Workplace drug testing is built on the military testing during the post–Vietnam era as a means not only to deter illegal drug use but also to identify individuals with drug dependency in order to provide treatment for them. Following the lead, in 1989, the US Department of Transportation issued drug testing regulations requiring employers in transportation industries to implement drug testing of applicants and employees in safety-sensitive positions.

The Omnibus Transportation Employee Testing Act came in 1991, which was the first federal law that mandated drug testing of private and public sector employees in safety-sensitive positions. This focused drug testing programs on safety-sensitive employees and carefully avoided Fourth Amendment concerns by identifying "illegal" drugs. In 2018, these regulations were expanded to include Schedule II opioids as well.

Federal workplace testing is a legally defensible program to be administered in safety-sensitive positions in the general workplace population where the vast majority of those being tested do not have a substance use disorder. It is designed to act as a deterrent to the use of impairing drugs in the workplace as well as to promote evaluation and treatment.

The federal workplace drug testing program protects donors, their workplaces, the integrity of the program, and the public. Testing is done under strict chain of custody protocols, and all samples that screen positive are confirmed by a definitive analysis. When confirmed, the result is then verified by an MRO before it is considered positive and reported to the employer who ordered the test. In the federal workplace drug testing program, donors found to be positive for drug use are referred for evaluation by a qualified substance abuse professional. These employees must not only be compliant with the substance abuse professional's recommendations but must also pass a return-to-duty test and enter into a more rigorous follow-up testing program.

Addiction medicine physicians are the ideal professionals to enter MRO practice. The federal regulations require MROs to be "knowledgeable about and have clinical experience in controlled substances abuse disorders." In addition to the specific qualifications of those certified to practice addiction medicine, there are additional training and certification requirements for those who want to be MROs in the federal programs. There are two MRO certification organizations accredited by the Substance Abuse and Mental Health Services Administration (SAMHSA): the American Association of Medical Review Officers and the Medical Review Officer Certification Council. Both require an initial

comprehensive training course that varies between 12 and 20 continuing medical education credits in length and then continuing CME and recertification every 5 years. The training includes the metabolism of drugs being tested for and how that varies in the different body specimens being tested. The training covers procedures used in forensic specimen collection, including the different strategies that donors may use to manipulate the drug test, laboratory technology, and applicable regulatory requirements. MRO training and certification contains the basic information that physicians, especially addiction medicine physicians, need to understand to use drug testing in clinical practice. Unlike in the practice of addiction medicine, MROs do not have physician–patient relationships with sample donors. Addiction medicine physicians understand that they must consider the whole patient, not just a laboratory result. MROs must know what laboratory reports mean and what they do not mean. They must be able to identify which results are valid and which aren't by understanding specimen validity testing. MROs must understand the stages of laboratory testing that all specimens undergo and what it means when a result is confirmed and also what it means when a result cannot be confirmed. MROs use appropriate interview techniques to discuss those laboratory results with the donors of the specimens before deciding whether the confirmed laboratory positive was consistent with licit or illicit drug use. MROs must understand the different testing techniques for urine, hair, nails, blood, and oral fluids and what different specimens are best used for particular circumstances.

Workplace drug testing, unlike drug testing in clinical practice, is primarily a prevention or deterrent program. It understands that most workplace drug tests, unlike most clinical tests, are negative. The program is not intended to detect every use of drugs in the workplace. It is intended to help prevent nonmedical use of impairing drugs. Many protections are built into workplace programs to prevent the false accusation of someone who does not use drugs illicitly. These protections have existed since the 1980s. Because the window of detection for workplace drug tests is short and the testing is infrequent, most of those testing positive are frequent drug users. For this reason, if someone cannot pass a workplace drug test, there is a significant likelihood that a substance use disorder exists.

Continued

SUGGESTED READINGS

DuPont RL, Griffin DW, Siskin BR, Shiraki S, Katze E. Random drug tests at work: the probability of identifying frequent and infrequent users of illicit drugs. *J Add Dis.* 1995;14(3):1-17.

Substance Abuse and Mental Health Services Administration. Mandatory guidelines for federal workplace drug testing programs. *Fed Reg.* 2017;82(13);7920-7970.

Substance Abuse and Mental Health Services Administration. *Medical Review Officer Guidance for Federal Workplace Drug Testing Programs.* Rockville, MD: US Department of Health and Human Services, 2017.

Swotinsky RB. *The Medical Review Officer's Manual: MROCC's Guide to Drug Testing.* 5th ed. Beverly Farms, MA: OEM Press, 2015.

US Department of Transportation. Procedures for transportation workplace drug and alcohol testing programs. 49 CFR Part 40, 2018. https://www.transportation.gov/odapc/part40. Updated September 4, 2018. Accessed October 9, 2018.

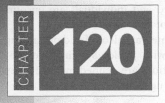

CHAPTER

120

Reducing Substance Use in Criminal Justice Populations

Summary by Peggy Fulton Hora

Based on THE ASAM Principles of Addiction Medicine, 6th edition chapter by Beau Kilmer, Jonathan P. Caulkins, Robert L. DuPont, and Keith Humphreys

In the criminal justice system, the tide is slowly turning away from a "lock 'em up and throw away the key" mentality toward an emphasis on treatment. A recent poll reported by the MacArthur Foundation found that 60% of Americans believe that "rehabilitating or treating the person" is the most appropriate response to nonviolent offenses as opposed to "punishing the person for committing the crime" or "keeping the person off the street so they can't commit more crimes." Support for rehabilitation rises to 71% for nonviolent offenses by those who suffer from mental illness.

This phenomenon is so dramatic that over 24 states have reduced their prison population and at least 13 states have closed prisons. In 2011, the Bureau of Justice Statistics reported the first decline in the overall state prison population since 1977. Over the past two decades, it has become abundantly clear that incarceration alone is totally ineffective at addressing substance use disorders (SUDs) and mental illness. It also does not reduce recidivism rates. Society is coming to realize that prison is a scarce resource best employed to isolate violent offenders from the community. Such a change in philosophy, coupled with an increased knowledge of the neurobiology of SUDs and their treatment, has led to an understanding by the community and the criminal justice system that collaborative approaches such as drug treatment courts (DTCs) are the most intelligent way to address this issue.

The link between criminal activity and alcohol and other drug use is clear. In a 2011 study of arrestees, 60% tested positive for one or more drugs (other than alcohol) within 48 hours of apprehension. At all but one test site, almost 80% of arrestees had been arrested previously and many had been arrested more than once in the preceding 12 months.

A DTC is a collaborative program of judicially supervised treatment and recovery within the criminal justice system. This specialized system of courts was created to address spiraling numbers of drug-related offenses and offenders, which have swelled court dockets over the past two decades. DTCs represent a major retooling of the criminal justice system as well as a new role for the courts as an interdisciplinary, problem-solving community institution with therapeutic implications—in short, a partner in public health.

From fewer than a dozen in 1991, the number of DTCs has increased to over 3000 today. DTCs are found in all states, in all federal districts, and in American Indian reservations in tribal courts (called Healing to Wellness Courts). Justice Speakers International reports that there are 22 countries outside of the United States that also run such programs. More are in the planning stage. There are about 127,000 DTC participants at any given time in the United States.

DEFINITIONS

A DTC is a judicially supervised, treatment-driven program for high-risk, high-need criminal offenders who have SUDs. It is a collaborative effort that involves judges, prosecutors, defense attorneys, probation officers, law enforcement, treatment providers, and other persons or agencies that interact with individuals whose behavior has brought them into the criminal justice system. DTCs have been in operation for almost 30 years. Participation by the offender is voluntary and is set forth as a condition of diversion, probation, or parole.

DTCs are as varied in form and format as the diverse legal and treatment cultures from which the DTCs spring. Some courts divert offenders from the criminal justice system entirely; 82% operate in a postplea modality, whereas others accept only

667

misdemeanants and yet others only felons. There are DTCs solely for people with alcohol use disorders or, of late, solely opioid users. Other DTCs accept anyone whose criminal involvement is related to substance use. There are courts that focus on those who drive while impaired or serial inebriants with arrest records dating back decades. There are gender-specific courts and courts that enroll only juveniles. Reentry DTCs serve adjudicated offenders with SUDs who are returning to society on parole or probation. There are about 350 veterans' courts that have emerged for returning warriors, many of whom have SUDs and co-occurring mental health issues such as posttraumatic stress disorder and physical problems such as traumatic brain injury.

As varied as these courts may be, there are a set of underlying principles that must be adhered to for a court to be called a DTC, which are the 10 Key Components of a Drug Court (see the following section) and the Adult Drug Court Best Practice Standards. Some states have certification programs that ensure compliance.

DTCs rely on the principle that the coercive powers of the court system can contribute to recovery from alcohol and other drug disorders. Contrary to the popular notion that offenders who have SUDs are best dealt with by adjudication and sanctions, DTCs embrace the scientific premise that SUDs are chronic, often relapsing medical conditions. The authoritative and supervisory power of a judge is critical to this approach to treatment. However, the participation of a judge in the rehabilitation process represents a dramatic shift in legal thought and judicial behavior.

A NEW APPROACH TO AN OLD PROBLEM

Through the collaborative efforts of defense attorneys and prosecutors, treatment providers, court coordinators or case managers, community policing agencies, and community corrections officials, a criminal defendant in a DTC is given an opportunity to engage in an alternative to the criminal "business as usual", and, in its place, to pursue a program of treatment and recovery.

DTCs employ a series of incentives and sanctions to induce treatment compliance and lifestyle changes in criminal defendants. The ultimate reward for the participants is dismissal of charges, having a sentence set aside, or imposition of a lesser penalty. By choosing to participate in a DTC, criminal defendants avoid serving a substantial period of incarceration and gain sobriety and crime-free lifestyles. As the federal Bureau of Justice Assistance has defined it: "A [DTC] establishes an environment that the participant can understand: a system in which clear choices are presented and individuals are encouraged to take control of their own recovery."

Further, DTCs integrate alcohol and other drug treatment services with justice system case processing. Their operations are defined by the 10 Key Components of a Drug Court:

1. Drug courts integrate alcohol and other drug treatment services with justice system case processing.
2. Using a nonadversarial approach, prosecutors and defense counsel work together to promote public safety while protecting participants' due process rights.
3. Eligible participants are identified early and promptly placed in the drug court program.
4. DTCs provide access to a continuum of alcohol, drug, and related treatment and rehabilitation services.
5. Abstinence is monitored through frequent alcohol and other drug testing.
6. A coordinated strategy governs DTC responses to participants' compliance.
7. Ongoing judicial interaction with each DTC participant is essential.
8. Monitoring and evaluations measure the achievement of program goals and gauge its effectiveness.
9. Continuing interdisciplinary education promotes effective DTC planning, implementation, and operations.
10. Forging partnerships among DTCs, public agencies, and community-based organizations generates local support and enhances the DTC's effectiveness.

When these components are employed, the courtroom is transformed into an arena in which a judge is the central figure of a team that is focused on the participants' recovery. The prosecutor screens each candidate for eligibility and verifies that he or she is appropriate for participation in a DTC. The defense counsel verifies that the client understands that DTC participation is voluntary and that he or she is aware of all legal options and makes a knowing and intelligent waiver of rights, including his or her confidentiality rights. The opposing counsel thus focuses on the participants' progress, rather than on the merits of the pending case. A close, interpersonal, and therapeutic relationship develops between the judge and the participants, who are encouraged to develop the tools they need to maintain sobriety and recovery.

Participants often enter into written contracts, agreeing to certain behaviors. A typical contract covers on-time appearances at treatment sessions, court dates, peer support meetings, and other appointments; compliance with all rules; waivers of confidentiality; payment of fees and fines; participation in urine tests without water-loading, adulteration, or counterfeiting; an agreement to refrain from alcohol or other drug use or contact with individuals who engage in such use; an agreement to abstain from taking over-the-counter or prescription medications without prior approval or other conduct that could yield a positive result on a urine test; and agreement to a 12- to 18-month commitment to treatment.

Although judges remain the final arbiter of all issues, they receive input from the entire team; they also receive input from the participants. If a problem arises, such as a use episode, it is not unusual for a participant to arrive in court having already discussed the problem with the treatment provider and a probation officer or court coordinator, who presents a recommendation to the judge. When participants themselves propose the sanctions, they are more likely to comply with them, less likely to feel coerced by the "system" or the judge, and more likely to consider them fair.

Confidentiality waivers are mandatory, as are waivers of judicial ethical issues such as the prohibition on ex parte communications, simply because the treatment providers, mental health professionals, and physicians must be able to communicate with the court coordinator/case manager and the team. Written waivers that comply with federal statutes such as 42 CFR confidentiality and the Health Insurance Portability and Accountability Act are mandatory. Judges must be able to talk to team members individually throughout the week without inhibition. Participants must understand their rights to confidentiality and the judges' prohibition on ex parte communication and be willing to provide a written waiver as a condition of entering the DTC.

Most DTCs have three phases: (1) an initiation of abstinence phase, in which participants come to court weekly or fortnightly; (2) a treatment phase, in which participants meet with the judge twice a month; and (3) a relapse prevention or sobriety maintenance phase, with monthly court dates.

Frequent contact with and monitoring by the judge is essential to the success of DTC participants. As the ultimate authority figure in this system, the judge also is important in motivating and encouraging participants. Treatment may be delivered in a variety of settings, including community-based programs; in day treatment; in a variety of outpatient, inpatient, and residential settings; and in custody.

Using graduated sanctions, the court usually begins with the least restrictive model using the American Society of Addiction Medicine (ASAM) Criteria, as indicated by an assessment tool such as the Addiction Severity Index. Participants are moved to more or less restrictive placements as needed. Placing participants in a more restrictive environment is not phrased in terms of punishment or a sanction; rather, participants are encouraged to see the change as necessary to their recovery. Likewise, a move to outpatient treatment is presented as a reward for desired behaviors. At intake, a social needs assessment is completed, along with an alcohol assessment and other drug use assessments. Mental health, housing, physical health, employment, education, and other legal entanglements are addressed. Periods of abstinence are required for phase advancement—typically 30, 90, and 180 days before moving to an advanced phase.

DTCs provide aftercare planning, and participants petition the court to "graduate," typically at about 180 days of sobriety. To receive approval to graduate, participants must demonstrate insight into their addiction and have a plan for relapse prevention/sobriety maintenance. To graduate, participants must have a clean and sober living environment as well as full-time employment or full-time student status or, if disabled, a source of income such as Social Security, and all fees and fines must be paid or substantial amounts of volunteer work completed. Graduating participants also must have a driver's license, insurance, and proof of registration of all vehicles and be able to show that they have no outstanding tickets or warrants. They must have a high school diploma or GED (unless they are unable to obtain one because of cognitive deficits or lack of numeracy or literacy skills) and either take literacy classes, if they are English speaking, or enroll in a class for students learning English as a second language. Abstinence alone is not enough.

When a participant submits a positive urine test, misses meetings or appointments, fails to participate, or otherwise breaks program rules, sanctions are imposed immediately. There is a distinction made between proximal goals such as arriving on time for all appointments and distal goals such as sobriety or becoming employed. Sanctions are applied accordingly so that there is a high sanction for breach of a proximal goal and a low sanction for breach of a distal goal. This may result in participants engaging in the same behavior (eg, a use episode), but having different sanctions imposed. The delivery of a sanction must be fully explained so that the participant is left with a sense of procedural fairness and trust in the process. Such sanctions may include paying the cost of the urine test, increased meeting attendance, a temporary demotion to an earlier phase of the program, a requirement to perform volunteer work, or short stints of jail time. The ultimate sanction is removal from the program and reentry into the criminal system or sentencing, including incarceration. Consistent noncompliance may trigger a mental health assessment because many DTC participants have undiagnosed comorbid mental health problems. Program dismissal is reserved for the most serious offenses, such as attempts to falsify or adulterate a urine sample, leaving without permission, threatening staff, or arrest for a violent offense.

The focus of the DTC team is on treatment compliance and program retention rather than punishment. It is the goal of the DTC team to keep participants in treatment, to support their recovery, and to encourage participants by emphasizing their abilities and strengths. Rewards may include a reduction of program fees, a reduction in the number of court appearances, and awarding of certificates (with much cheering and applause from the audience) to mark the completion of each phase. Simple praise from a judge is a potent incentive, as is a drawing for a small gift. One study showed that the opportunity to draw from a fish bowl increased stimulant users' success in treatment fourfold.

At any point in the process, participants may opt out of the DTC and into the traditional criminal justice case processing system, with all the attendant rights and remedies.

WHY DRUG TREATMENT COURTS WORK

There is support for DTCs on many fronts and from all points on the political spectrum. First, it is clear that coerced treatment works. Research indicates that a person coerced to enter treatment by the criminal justice system is likely to do as well as one who enters voluntarily. In fact, there is debate about the "voluntariness" of any addiction treatment because most people come to treatment as the result of legal or marital problems, other concerns in their personal lives, problems with job performance, or for health reasons. Second, addiction treatment is as successful as treatment for other chronic diseases and saves $7 in criminal justice costs for every $1 spent on treatment. Moreover, because of the requirement for interdisciplinary training, DTC judges and other team members are aware of the likelihood of relapse and know how to respond appropriately. DTCs are in a unique position to recognize these temporary setbacks as learning experiences for the participant and the treatment team.

A study that assessed the effectiveness of DTCs examined nine adult drug courts in California. Using a transactional and institutional costs analysis approach, the investigators calculated costs based on every subject's transactions within the drug court or the traditional criminal justice system. This method allowed the calculation of costs and benefits by agency. Results in the nine sites showed that the majority of agencies saved money when offenders were processed through a drug court. Overall, participation in drug courts saved the state more than $9 million in criminal justice and treatment costs (largely from reduced recidivism among drug court participants). Similar results have been found in studies of family DTCs. Long-term follow-up studies are needed to reach definitive conclusions about the effectiveness of family drug courts.

The largest studies of the efficacy of DTCs have been undertaken by NPC Research in Portland, Oregon. Data they have collected on hundreds of DTCs show that when there is fidelity to the 10 Key Components (described previously) and compliance with the Adult Drug Court Best Practice Standards, DTCs reduce both cost and recidivism rates. The US Government Accountability Office found that participants in DTCs have rearrest rates that are 12% to 58% lower than those in a comparison group of arrestees who did not participate in DTCs.

Courts have come to accept that their role is changing from that of a neutral, uninvolved arbiter to a problem solver that deals with cases holistically. There also is support for the proposition that judicial job satisfaction is increased if judges work therapeutically. In 2001, the US Conference of Chief Justices and the Conference of State Court Administrators adopted a joint resolution endorsing DTCs and problem-solving courts based on the drug court model, the first resolution of its kind. The resolution commits all 50 chief justices and state court administrators "to take steps nationally and locally to expand the principles and methods of well-functioning drug courts into ongoing court operations." It also pledges to "encourage the broad integration, over the next decade, of the principles and methods employed in problem-solving courts into the administration of justice."

Law enforcement support for DTCs is strong because officers see that recovery presents a long-term solution to a community's and an individual's problems with alcohol or other drugs. Formal liaisons between community police and DTCs are encouraged.

THE COURTS AND PHYSICIANS WORKING TOGETHER

DTCs and the criminal justice system can be powerful allies for addiction medicine specialists. Through DTCs, physicians and judges have initiated a new dialogue about alcohol and other drug problems. The partnership has extended to other venues as well: Judges have participated in congressional and US mayoral briefings. Judges have presented programs at ASAM meetings. Addiction medicine specialists teach courses on alcohol and other drug problems at the National Judicial College and in many state training programs. The time is ripe for local coalitions of judges and other leaders in the criminal justice system to collaborate with addiction medicine specialists to educate one another on how to be more effective at working with their mutual clients/patients. Judges in the criminal justice system may have more to say about a patient's treatment than the physician does, whereas physicians may wish to add questions relating to involvement with the justice system to patient assessments as a case-finding tool for alcohol and other drug problems.

Physicians should acquaint themselves with their local DTCs and, if none are available locally, join a community coalition to ask that one be established. Most courts have long-range strategic, operational, and action plans developed with community input; DTCs should be part of those plans. Local grand juries, with the help of addiction medicine specialists, should study DTCs and make recommendations for appropriate use of such courts in their own communities. State chapters of ASAM should make experts available to judges who have questions about alcohol and other drug issues. Judges have the power to appoint such physicians as expert advisors to the court. Although the number of DTCs has increased exponentially, there are 1.2 million people who would be eligible for a DTC who remain unserved.

KEY POINTS

1. DTCs are a proven solution to the revolving door of alcohol and other drug-fueled crime.
2. When using evidence-based practices, DTCs have shown to reduce recidivism and save money.
3. Physicians and DTCs should be partners in helping court-involved patients.

REVIEW QUESTIONS

1. Crime rates are:
   A. falling.
   B. rising.
   C. static.

2. Drug treatment courts (DTCs) are:
   A. soft on crime.
   B. collaborative in nature and focused on the treatment and recovery of offenders.
   C. supported by Democrats but not Republicans.

3. Addiction professionals are:
   A. a welcome addition to the drug treatment court team.
   B. given little voice in their patients' care.
   C. seen as making excuses for criminal offenders.

ANSWERS

1. **A.** Crime rates are going down as the demand for "tough on crime" responses are reduced and the "war on drugs" is unwinding.
2. **B.** DTCs combine accountability and effective practices. The collaborative nature strengthens the information given to the judge in order to make a good decision. Support for DTCs comes from "both sides of the aisle."
3. **A.** Treatment and criminal justice work hand in hand to support the changes necessary for offenders to remain crime free.

SUGGESTED READINGS

Marlowe DB, Hardin CD, Cunningham V, et al., eds. Best practices in drug courts. *Drug Court Rev.* 2012;8(1):1-151.
Marlowe DB, Meyer WG, eds. *The Drug Court Judicial Benchbook.* Alexandria, VA: National Drug Court Institute, 2011.
National Association of Drug Court Professionals. *Principles of Evidence-Based Sentencing and Other Court Dispositions for Substance Abusing Individuals.* http://www.nadcp.org. Accessed October 23, 2018.

Treatment of Substance Use Disorders During Incarceration

Summary by Lori D. Karan

Based on THE ASAM PRINCIPLES OF ADDICTION MEDICINE, 6th edition sidebar by Lori D. Karan

INCARCERATION AS A PUBLIC HEALTH OPPORTUNITY

Incarceration holds promise for advancing individual and public health because those who are not seen in the healthcare system can receive screening, diagnosis, and treatment in jail and prison. The ability to ensure retention in care and to perform directly observed therapy holds promise for improving disease management such as diabetic control and for limiting the spread of infections like HIV and hepatitis C virus.

Continued

Theoretically, correctional facilities have the potential to provide addictions treatment of greater intensity than intensive outpatient programs for patients for whom probation, drug courts, and other less intensive treatments have not been successful.

ESTELLE V GAMBLE

The foundation of inmates' constitutional right to healthcare is the Supreme Court's 1976 decision in *Estelle v Gamble,* in which the Court ruled that "deliberate indifference" to a prisoner's health was "cruel and unusual punishment" and thus prohibited by the Eighth Amendment to the US Constitution. The overall requirement is that inmates are given access to medically necessary services, and that these services are in accordance with a community standard of care.

CHALLENGES FOR ADDICTIONS TREATMENT

Optimally, prison settings could be utilized when probation, drug courts, and other less intensive treatments do not halt harmful drug use. The reality is that it is difficult to promote a culture of support and rehabilitation in a setting where drugs can be rampant, gang leaders have significant influence, and criminal behavior is revered.

Correctional settings are highly structured and prescriptive. Imprisonment takes away inmates' initiative, responsibility, and choice. This is in contrast to motivational interviewing, which recognizes that individuals may be in a precontemplation or contemplation phase rather than in the action phase of behavioral change. Motivational interviewing works to resolve ambivalence by collaboration rather than confrontation, autonomy rather than authority, and exploration rather than explanation. In authoritarian environments, correctional staff can confuse a healthcare provider's need to understand the inmate's world and create a therapeutic partnership with that of being "overfamiliar."

Withdrawal Management

Although accreditation standards by the National Commission on Correctional Health Care, Clinical Practice Guidelines from the Federal Bureau of Prisons and policies and standards from the American Society of Addiction Medicine and the California Society of Addiction Medicine may be referenced during litigation, it is case law that determines constitutional care. There is no constitutional right to rehabilitation from alcoholism and/or drug addiction, although some consent decrees by the US

Department of Justice have had more sweeping requirements than the constitutional minima.

Deaths from alcohol and drug withdrawal continue to occur despite over 20 years of knowledge and advocacy. There can be up to a 72-hour delay between an individual's arrest and their eventual incarceration. Although some people experience few symptoms, others are admitted to jail or readmitted to prison with severe substance withdrawal. Unfortunately, many healthcare workers, police, and custody officers are inadequately trained to take a substance use history and to assess and treat withdrawal.

Persons with opioid use disorder, including those who are on opioid agonist treatment, often experience overly rapid detoxification as well as the undertreatment of withdrawal. This is such a significant problem internationally that Juan E. Mendez, Special Rapporteur on the United Nations Human Rights Council, presented a statement to the United Nations General Assembly on February 1, 2013, which stated that the denial of opioid substitution in jails and prisons is "a violation of the right to be free from torture and ill treatment."

CHRONIC PAIN MANAGEMENT

Offenders frequently request treatment for their chronic pain. They often have long histories of trauma and injury. The concrete and steel environment they live in is unforgiving.

A functional assessment of the inmate-patient with chronic pain includes determining if she or he can get in and out of their bunk, shower, dress, groom and toilet, walk to meals, participate in yard activities, get down for alarms, and stand up for counts.

In addition to assessing the nociceptive, mechanical, and neuropathic components of the patient's pain, the patient needs to be evaluated and treated for substance use disorders, depression, anxiety, other mental health issues, stress, and insomnia, which can complicate his or her pain.

A "whole person" approach to treating pain in inmate-patients is optimal, although correctional facilities have less restorative resources to offer patients. Psychological and physical therapy are preferred, but there is often limited availability of these services. Psychologic therapies include coping skills, relaxation training, guided imagery, diaphragmatic breathing, and cognitive–behavioral therapy (to reduce negative thought content and promote heightened self-concept). Physical therapies work on stretching, core strengthening, endurance, balance, and flexibility. Although ice packs may be allowed, TENS units and other forms of electrical stimulation are often not permitted.

Acupuncture and chiropractic treatment are rarely obtainable. Nonsteroidal anti-inflammatory agents and acetaminophen are first-line medications when they are not contraindicated by the inmate's underlying medical concerns. Antidepressants and anticonvulsants for neuropathic and radicular pain are often crushed and floated in water, and given as directly observed therapy.

Drugs with sedative or stimulant effects such as gabapentin (Neurontin), quetiapine (Seroquel), bupropion (Wellbutrin), loperamide (Imodium), and diphenoxlate/atropine (Lomotil) have increased nonmedical use liability and street value within the corrections environment. Topical medicine such as lidocaine may be expensive and capsaicin can be dangerous. Opioids are challenging because of problems of tolerance and hyperalgesia, as well as security concerns and the tendency for addiction and relapse in this high-risk population. Even psyllium (Metamucil) can be fermented and used as an ingredient for inmate-brewed alcohol.

Inmates may need special dispensation so that they do not have to climb to an upper bunk, and they may need extra time to get to the dining hall or eat their food. Correctional physicians must be careful that they are not played off against one another for differences in how they prescribe accommodations and other pain therapies.

The Importance of Relapse Prevention

More than 600,000 individuals are released each year from jails and prisons. Newly released offenders face substantial challenges when they reenter society. Release from prison is associated with increased mortality from accidental drug-induced deaths, suicide, accidental injury, and violence. The Washington State Department of Corrections conducted a landmark study of 30,237 persons who were newly released from prison between July 1999 and December 2003. Investigators found that the risk of death in the first 2 weeks after release was more than 12 times that of the general population. Drug overdoses can be due to an intentional response to the problems of reentry and/or due to an accidental result of decreased tolerance.

Pharmacotherapy for Opioid Use Disorders During Incarceration and Release

Jails and prisons have been slow to adopt treatment with opioid agonists for opioid use disorder. Methadone and buprenorphine maintenance are well researched and have been shown to engage persons in treatment, decrease opioid relapse, decrease the transmission of infectious diseases, and diminish crime. The results of a large, landmark study in South Wales replicated in England and also in Rhode Island, US, demonstrated that opioid agonist pharmacotherapy in prison and immediately postrelease was highly protective against mortality during both these time periods. Lower crime rates were observed during periods in pharmacotherapy, with the greatest reductions observed among people who were retained longer in treatment.

In other studies, releasing inmates on methadone or buprenorphine helped facilitate continuity of care, with a maintenance clinic more than merely referring individuals without starting them on this medication. Nonetheless, jails and prisons in the United States are reticent to employ opioid agonist pharmacotherapy due to fears of surreptitious use, diversion, and the potential for violence if there is opioid diversion. In the criminal justice system, pharmacotherapy is most available for pregnant women because concerns about the health of the fetus take precedence in decision making. Through 2018, opioid agonist pharmacotherapy has been rarely available to inmates in the United States. American judicial and law enforcement communities accept naltrexone to a greater degree than other pharmacotherapies.

Nicotine and Marijuana

Many inmates quit nicotine/tobacco use during incarceration because of the absence of conditioned cues. Unfortunately, a majority of inmates relapse to cigarette use in work-release programs, where the environment is more permissive and also upon discharge from incarceration.

Cannabis poses another challenge for newly released inmates. When individuals with substance use disorders and/or mental illness are given medical permission to use marijuana, it is difficult for judges, parole officers, and prison healthcare workers to counter this authorization. Therefore, legal use of cannabis for purported medical purposes is a growing concern for this at-risk population.

Newly released offenders have high rates of chronic illness, and they have difficulty navigating and engaging in health care. In one study, 80% of released individuals had chronic medical, psychiatric, or substance use problems at the time of their release, yet only 15 to 25% reported visiting a physician outside of the emergency department in the first year after their release.

Continued

Newly released offenders face substantial challenges when they reenter society. They often experience poor social support, financial stress, debts, and continued exposure to drugs in the neighborhoods to which they return.

THE VALUE OF A SYSTEMS APPROACH

The goals of corrections include deterring members of society from committing wrongful acts, punishing those that do, and separating criminals from society to ensure public safety. However, the goals of rehabilitation and punishment can run counter to each other. Corrections healthcare providers work within an environment that is monitored and maintained by custody, and healthcare providers rely on custody officers for their personal safety. Nonetheless, healthcare providers have a duty to honor the doctor–patient relationship and to optimize the health of their patients.

If continuity of care prevailed, individuals would receive a set of essential core assessments just after their arrest in the police holding cells, in jails, and in prison reception centers. Their withdrawal from alcohol or other substances would be appropriately managed, and treatment designed to meet their individual needs would be initiated. Supplementary material based on additional observations and evaluations would be added to an inmate patient's record over time to complement and fine-tune his or her core assessment(s). Case management would proceed on a continuous basis through institutions at the county, state, and federal levels. Family and support systems would be kept intact. After undergoing rehabilitation, parolees would reenter society with a recovery plan, a relapse prevention plan, appropriate resources, community engagement, and therapeutic monitoring. Unfortunately, the judicial, correctional and public health systems of care are fragmented. Both redundancies and omissions occur in the assessments of justice-involved individuals, as they undergo independent evaluations by parole and probation officers, intake staff of the facilities, jail and prison counselors, medical and psychiatric correctional care providers, and community health care and service providers.

Targeting recidivism holds the promise of reducing crime, increasing public safety, and curbing correctional costs. It is not enough for wardens to meet constitutionally minimal standards of confinement, prevent riots, thwart escapes, and keep the staff safe. Rather, reducing recidivism ought to be the criterion by which the success of incarceration is measured.

CONCLUSIONS

Incarceration can be an opportunity to improve both the individual's health and public health because persons who are not seen in the healthcare system can receive screening, diagnosis, and treatment. Healthcare and rehabilitation can be optimized in an environment that is highly controlled. Alcohol, drug, and mental health rehabilitation could be magnified by the intensity of services.

However, the reality is that the US system of incarceration is very large and difficult to change. Jails and prisons are poorly funded. It is difficult for taxpayers to want to invest in the rehabilitation of those they fear. Addiction continues to be poorly treated.

KEY POINTS

1. When addressing the needs of incarcerated persons who have substance use disorders, the mixed missions of retaliation, punishment, and public safety are at odds with rehabilitation.
2. Improvements in screening, assessments, withdrawal management, treatment, and relapse prevention are critically needed in US jails and prisons.
3. A systems approach that furthers continuity of care for justice-involved individuals can benefit offenders, their families, taxpayers, the community, and overall public health.
4. Measures of treatment success should include the absence of illicit drug use; reductions in recidivism; vocational placement; and improvements in mental, physical, family, and public health.

SUGGESTED READINGS

Binswanger IA, Nowels C, Corsi KF, et al. "From the prison door right to the sidewalk, everything went downhill," a qualitative study of the health experiences of recently released inmates. *Int J Law Psychiatry*. 2011;34(4):249-255.

Binswanger IA, Stern MF, Deyo RA, et al. Release from prison: a high risk of death for former inmates. *N Engl J Med*. 2007;356(2):157-165.

Detoxification of Chemically Dependent Inmates, Clinical Guidance. Washington, DC: Federal Bureau of Prisons, 2014.

Green TC, Clarke J, Brinkley-Rubinstein L, et al. Post incarceration fatal overdoses after implementing medications for addiction treatment in a statewide correctional system. *JAMA Psychiatry*. 2018;75(4):405-407.

Kendig NE. The potential to advance health care in the US criminal justice system. *JAMA*. 2016;316(4):387-388.

121

Preventing and Treating Substance Use Disorders in Military Personnel

Summary by Kenneth Hoffman, Robert M. Bray, and Janet H. Lenard

Based on THE ASAM PRINCIPLES OF ADDICTION MEDICINE, 6th edition chapter by Kenneth Hoffman, Robert M. Bray, and Janet H. Lenard

HISTORICAL PERSPECTIVE ON SUBSTANCE USE DISORDERS IN THE MILITARY

The military's policy on the prevention and treatment of substance use disorders (SUDs) began in 1967 when the US Department of Defense (DoD) convened a task force to investigate the problem of drug use in the military. With congressional direction, the task force also studied the problem of hazardous alcohol use. During this time, in the Vietnam theater, the 4th Infantry Division piloted a Drug Amnesty and Rehabilitation Program for soldiers who, although not otherwise identified as using or involved with illicit drugs, had voluntarily presented themselves as drug users to their chaplain, unit surgeon, or commander. Without punishment or adverse personnel actions, these soldiers were provided with (1) rapid medical assessment, (2) individual counseling and group therapy, and (3) a "buddy" who was assigned to them who could deliver positive reinforcement for abstinence. Throughout treatment, soldiers were expected to continue full duty. The results were very positive, and the success of this approach became the model for a US Army–wide program implemented 2 years later.

A study of 451 Army enlisted men who had returned from duty in Vietnam found that before their deployment, half had used alcohol regularly and one in four had engaged in risky drinking. Once in Vietnam, the prevalence of risky drinking in this group declined, but their nonmedical use of opioids rose sharply. Half of the personnel surveyed reported that they had tried opioids, and 20% said they had become physically dependent or addicted. When these personnel returned to the United States, their use of opioids declined sharply (with only 2% reporting

physical dependence or addiction), whereas their rate of hazardous alcohol use increased.

Since 1970, the DoD's policies and service-specific regulations have supported the prevention and treatment of SUDs through education and enforcement procedures that focused on detection, early intervention, and treatment of risky use of alcohol and nonmedical use of drugs, with an emphasis on helping those engaged in such use return to service. Policy has also been specific to ensure no adverse personnel or legal action is taken against an individual in treatment using any information collected within the treatment program.

The comprehensive approach to the prevention and treatment for SUDs illustrates a "healthcare continuum," as shown in Figure 121-1. Since the beginning, personnel and command have had responsibility for educating the general population on risks related to the hazardous use of alcohol and use of illicit drugs. With medical support, personnel and command have had responsibility for health promotion and employee assistance programs for early identification of individuals at risk for alcohol misuse and early intervention. With a "zero tolerance" policy for illicit drug use, personnel and command developed a deterrence drug testing program that set current standards for current civilian drug-free workplace programs. With command support, medical services have been expected to provide treatment for all active duty personnel who have been identified as dependent on alcohol or other drugs. The underlying assumption is that those in treatment can achieve full sustained remission.

With support for "responsible" use of alcohol and "zero tolerance" for illicit drug use, the military developed a bifurcated approach toward individuals

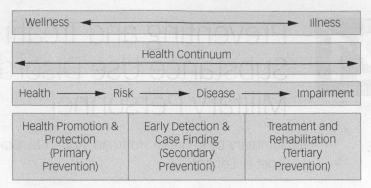

Figure 121-1. Healthcare continuum. (From US Department of Defense. *Population Health Improvement Plan and Guide. DoD TRICARE Management Activity.* Washington DC: TRICARE Management Activity, Government Printing Office, 2001:10.)

who had developed alcohol problems and individuals who were using illicit drugs. Military personnel with an alcohol use disorder were evaluated by trained alcohol and drug counselors at the individual's assigned post or base for possible referral for treatment. Personnel who were using illicit drugs but not yet detected by command could also volunteer for treatment, under a "safe harbor" policy and would be assessed for referral.

From 1970 through 2000, treatment programs for active duty personnel were initiated by referral from a patient's assigned post or base to a covered residential treatment facility (RTF). The RTF program was initially designed for 6 weeks and then shortened to 4 weeks to achieve early remission. Within that time, craving and withdrawal symptoms were managed, while the individual worked with other patients to learn skills that would sustain longer-term recovery. Emerging comorbid medical or psychiatric conditions were identified with appropriate interventions initiated. At the end of the RTF program, patients successfully completing the program would "graduate" in a ceremony that connected them back to the referring post or base. Treatment personnel at the post or base continued to work with "graduates" over the following year to sustain remission. In a study of patients treated at one RTF, the 1- to 2-year period of patient follow-up showed that 77% maintained abstinence with 90% still on active duty.

With an emerging opioid problem among service members and a presidential directive in 1971, the military developed a drug testing program to detect active duty personnel in Vietnam who were using heroin and expanded it to random testing for all service members to identify those using specific illicit Schedule I or highly addictive Schedule II drugs. Individuals testing positive on these drug

screens were offered treatment either within the military's or the US Department of Veterans Affair's healthcare system but also could be discharged from active duty under honorable conditions. The testing program was discontinued in the late 1970s due to limitations in the testing procedures.

In the 1980s, the DoD adopted a "zero tolerance" illicit drug use policy after discovering continuing significant prevalence of illicit drug use among active duty personnel. This was followed by reinitiating random and "for cause" forensic drug urine test methodology (that resolved prior limitations) to deter use. Forensic urine drug testing was designed to have a 100% test specificity for 100% positive predictive value. Personnel identified with a urine positive for tested drugs could be subject to adverse command action to include discharge without the need for additional evidence. For specific drugs that had medical indications for prescribed use, a medical officer reviewed the individual's medical record and/or interviewed the individual to determine if there had been prescribed use (eg, valid prescription for amphetamine, surgical use of cocaine). With valid medical use, the urine test result was recorded as "negative" in a report to command.

For individuals using illicit drugs who wanted treatment, a "safe harbor" policy allowed for self-disclosure to medical personnel. An initial urine test could be ordered by medical personnel to screen for drugs but, if positive, was not reported to command and not used for any adverse action. Subsequent follow-up forensic drug tests could be ordered through command and, if positive, were allowed to be used in adverse command action.

This drug testing methodology continues in use today within the military and within the federal Drug-Free Workplace Program.

PREVALENCE OF SUBSTANCE USE DISORDERS AMONG MILITARY PERSONNEL

To better understand and monitor substance use in the active duty military, the DoD initiated a series of comprehensive surveys of personnel in the Army, Navy, Marine Corps, Air Force, and (more recently) the Coast Guard. The surveys are cross-sectional studies conducted every 3 to 4 years, with a random sample of personnel selected for each survey. The studies are particularly valuable because they are population-based surveys with large sample sizes (ranging from 12,000 to nearly 25,000 participants) that are representative of the DoD active duty population. Respondents are asked to answer all questions anonymously to encourage honest answers to sensitive questions. Ten surveys were conducted between 1980 and 2008. An 11th survey was completed in 2011, but the findings are not readily comparable with the earlier surveys because the data collection methods and many of the questions had changed substantially.

Figure 121-2 presents trend data from 1980 through 2008 that show the percentage of active duty military personnel who engaged in heavy alcohol use and illicit drug use during the 30 days prior to the survey. As seen in Figure 121-2, heavy alcohol use (defined as five or more drinks on one occasion at least once a week in the preceding 30 days) declined between 1980 and 1988, showed some fluctuation between 1988 and 1998, increased significantly from 1998 to 2002, and continued to increase gradually between 2005 and 2008. The heavy drinking rate for 2008 was not significantly different from that in 1980, when the survey series began, although heavy alcohol use showed a gradual and significant increase during the decade from 1998 to 2008 (from 15% to 20%). Similar changes occurred in the rate of binge drinking (five or more drinks on a single occasion for men, four or more for women, at least once in the preceding month), which increased from 35% to 47% during the 10-year period from 1998 to 2008.

Higher levels of drinking were associated with higher rates of alcohol-related problems, but problem rates were notably higher for those who drank heavily. Those with heavy alcohol use showed nearly three times the rate of self-reported serious consequences and more than twice the rate of self-reported productivity loss than did moderate-to-heavy drinkers.

The prevalence of illicit drug use including prescription drug misuse (see Fig. 121-2) declined from 28% in 1980 to 3% 2002 and then rose again to 5% in 2005 and 12% in 2008. The higher rates in the latter two surveys are largely a function of increases in reported nonmedical use of prescription opioids but also may be due, in part, to improved wording of the questions.

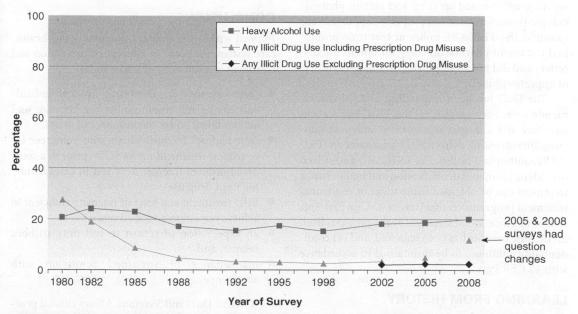

Figure 121-2. Trends in Use of Illicit Drug and Alcohol Use Over the Past 30 Days Among Active Duty Personnel, 1980-2008. (From Bray RM, Pemberton MR, Hourani LL, et al. *Department of Defense Survey of Health Related Behaviors Among Active Duty Military Personnel: A Component of the Defense Lifestyle Assessment Program [DLAP].* Research Triangle Park, NC: RTI International, 2009.)

TREATMENT OF SUBSTANCE USE DISORDERS IN THE MILITARY MEDICAL SYSTEM

Since the late 1980s, SUD treatment programs for military personnel have been required to meet The Joint Commission Behavioral Health Standards. Under TRICARE, which was established in 1997, more intensive levels of care were contracted out to civilian programs. As a result, many of the intensive military RTFs closed. Intensive outpatient programs also were contracted out under TRICARE, whereas military SUD facilities primarily offered care at American Society of Addiction Medicine Levels 0.5 and 1.0. Only a few military programs offered care at Levels 2.0 or 2.5.

In 2013, the Institute of Medicine (IOM) released a comprehensive review entitled *Substance Use Disorders in the U.S. Armed Forces*. The report described significant deficiencies in the diagnosis and treatment of SUDs under TRICARE as a defined health benefit within the direct care and contract support systems. Although the military services include SUD prevention programs, most such programs either have not been evaluated or shown to be effective. The IOM report also described the military's policies on access to care as outdated and charged that they actually created barriers to care. The expert panel that prepared the report also found that some evidence-based treatments, such as intensive outpatient services, office-based services, and certain pharmacologic therapies, were not properly supported. For example, the TRICARE policy at that time prohibited the use of pharmacotherapy for opioid use disorders and did not allow provider training in the use of buprenorphine.

The DoD has been responding to IOM recommendations. For example, (1) the TRICARE benefit structure has changed significantly and now contains incentives to deliver SUD treatment in TRICARE-authorized facilities by TRICARE-authorized providers; (2) opioid detoxification and maintenance treatment can be obtained in inpatient or residential treatment programs certified under 42 CFR Part 8, as well as in office-based settings; (3) the previous limit on lifetime benefits has been removed, and (4) confidentiality continues to be maintained in accordance with 42 CFR Part 2.

LEARNING FROM HISTORY

From the initial observations in 1969 through the 1990s, the military's alcohol and drug treatment programs operated separately from behavioral health services. Senior leadership positions, senior

consultants, and specific treatment services existed at the DoD Health Affairs and offices of the Surgeon General. Policies and directives covering command and medical responsibilities were considered general rather than specific to medical or behavioral health needs.

Beginning in 1991, and consistent with the multidimensional Addiction Severity Index and the American Society of Addiction Medicine Criteria, health status began to be viewed multidimensionally, with strengths and problems assessed within biological, psychological, social, and environmental domains. Problems then could be matched to appropriate interventions at a convenient location and delivered by appropriate providers. At any level of care and location, treatment modalities could be grouped into one of four areas: (1) physiologic (eg, medication), (2) psychological (eg, individual/group therapy), (3) health promotion (eg, physical fitness, nutrition, stress/time management), and (3) case management (eg, other specialty care needed).

Figure 121-3 highlights an optimized approach to patient care within the Army's alcohol and drug treatment program in the 1990s. This assessment was done for all individuals to identify specific problems that would become a focus for treatment intervention no matter where the beneficiary was located. Each problem or barrier to recovery was addressed in treatment planning and follow-up.

CONCLUSIONS

Implicit within the military command and healthcare system has been the concept of prevention and treatment of addiction, which includes:

- "zero tolerance" for illicit drug use with individuals having full responsibility for behavior and actions taken under the influence of drugs,
- "safe harbor" for individuals who volunteer for or request treatment for an SUD (prior to a command-ordered forensic drug test in cases involving illicit drug use),
- SUD treatment at a level of intensity sufficient to achieve remission and abstinence,
- an expectation of return to full duty without relapse, and
- maintenance of sustained remission with abstinence.

Current DoD and Veterans Affairs clinical practice guidelines no longer require abstinence as a successful outcome and are more tolerant of relapse. IOM recommendations are being integrated into the TRICARE policy manual, and there is growing

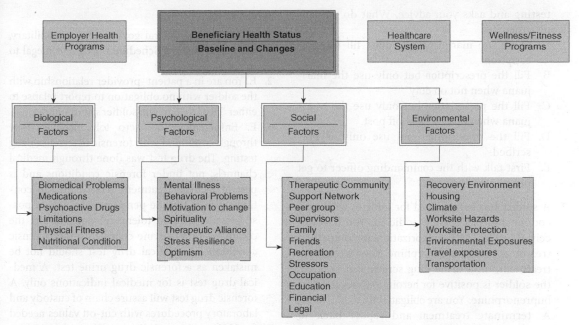

Figure 121-3. A multidimensional approach to individual and population health improvement: measuring baseline multidimensional health status and changes through population-based and individual interventions. (From Hoffman KJ. Demystifying mental health information needs through Integrated Definition [IDEF] activity and data modeling. *Proc AMIA Annu Fall Symp.* 1997:111-116; Hoffman KJ, Neven T. *The Alcohol and Drug Prevention and Control Program [ADAPCP] Clinical Information System [ACIS]. Guide Prototype Instruction Manual: User Manual for the ADAPCP Prototype Electronic Patient Record.* Bethesda, MD: Center for Training and Education in Addiction Medicine, Uniformed Services University of the Health Sciences/Henry M Jackson Foundation, 1995.)

recognition of the need for more TRICARE network physicians who are educated, trained, and skilled in the practice of addiction medicine.

KEY POINTS

1. Beginning with the opioid epidemic in the 1960s, the military response covered a healthcare continuum that integrally involved both command and medical personnel to deter the use of illicit drugs and prevent the misuse of alcohol, and a medical program to identify and treat all active duty personnel who were dependent on alcohol or other drugs.

2. Military commands have had responsibility for preventing the use of illicit drugs and hazardous use of alcohol through education, deterrence forensic drug testing, and the potential use of adverse personnel action.

   a. For all active duty, education has stressed "responsible" use of alcohol.

   b. Adverse personnel actions assume that individuals remain fully responsible for their behavior and actions taken under the influence of alcohol or other drugs.

   c. Random and "for cause" deterrence forensic drug testing are designed to have a 100%

positive predictive value; a positive urine test reported to command is sufficient evidence that the individual has used an illicit Schedule I drug or a nonprescribed Schedule II drug.

   d. Support treatment is provided for personnel identified with an alcohol or other use disorder, and "safe harbor" is provided for personnel asking for treatment of an illicit drug prior to being selected for random forensic drug testing.

3. Medical treatment providers have a responsibility for evaluating and treating TRICARE beneficiaries (that include all active duty personnel) who have a substance use disorder, following best standards of care needed to achieve full sustained remission and with the same privacy and confidentiality provided to any other patient in treatment for an SUD.

REVIEW QUESTIONS

1. An active duty sailor has a prescription for medical marijuana from a medical provider licensed and allowed to prescribe medical marijuana. The sailor is subject to randomized deterrence drug

testing and asks your advice. What do you advise them?

A. Don't use marijuana and don't fill the prescription.
B. Fill the prescription but only use the marijuana when not on duty.
C. Fill the prescription but only use the marijuana when on leave and off post.
D. Fill the prescription and use only as prescribed.
E. First talk with the commanding officer to get permission to use.

2. A soldier has been treated for injuries with oxycodone and has become addicted. You have received a TRICARE authorization for outpatient treatment using buprenorphine. Four weeks into treatment, on a urine drug screen you ordered, the soldier is positive for heroin and negative for buprenorphine. You are obligated to:

A. terminate treatment and report back to TRICARE that the patient has relapsed.
B. terminate treatment and report to the soldier's commander that the soldier has failed treatment.
C. continue treatment but report back to TRICARE that the patient has relapsed.
D. continue treatment but report to the soldier's commander that the soldier has had a positive urine test for heroin.
E. discuss the drug test results with the soldier and reassess the current treatment plan but don't report back to TRICARE or the soldier's commander.

3. An active duty airman, fearing an upcoming random drug test, asks to be treated for a methamphetamine addiction. You receive TRICARE authorization to assess and treat the soldier. In your medical assessment, you collect a urine sample and send the sample to a laboratory for drug testing. It is positive for methamphetamines. Knowing there is a "zero tolerance" policy, you are required to:

A. report the positive drug test to the airman's commander.
B. order a forensic drug test to be reported to the airman's commander.
C. report the positive drug test to TRICARE.
D. terminate treatment.
E. none of the above.

ANSWERS

1. **A.** Within the federal government and military, marijuana is still a Schedule I drug and illegal to use or possess.

2. **E.** You are in a patient–provider relationship with the soldier with no obligation to report relapse to either TRICARE or the soldier's commander.

3. **E.** Enforcement of "zero tolerance" is done through command with forensic deterrence drug testing. The drug test was done through medical channels, not under forensic conditions and is part of medical treatment. Treatment can continue even if adverse personnel actions are possible under a "zero tolerance" policy when the command orders urine collected under forensic conditions. A medical drug test should not be mistaken as a forensic drug urine test. A medical drug test is for medical indications only. A forensic drug test will assure chain of custody and laboratory procedures with cut-off values needed for 100% positive predictive value with a positive result being sufficient for adverse personnel/legal actions.

SUGGESTED READINGS

Bray RM, Pemberton MR, Hourani LL, et al. *Department of Defense Survey of Health: Related Behaviors Among Active Duty Military Personnel: A Component of the Defense Lifestyle Assessment Program (DLAP)*. Research Triangle Park, NC: RTI International, 2009. http://prhome.defense.gov/Portals/52/Documents/RFM/Readiness/DDRP/docs/2009.09%202008%20DoD%20Survey%20of%20Health%20Related%20Behaviors%20Among%20Active%20Duty%20Military%20Personnel.pdf. Accessed November 2, 2018.

Military Health System. Chapter 7, section 3.20: medication assisted treatment (MAT). In: *TRICARE Policy Manual 6010.57-M, February 1, 2008*. Falls Church, VA: Military Health System, 2017. http://manuals.tricare.osd.mil/DisplayManualPdfFile/TR08/145/ChangeOnly/tp08/c7s3_20.pdf. Accessed November 2, 2018.

Military Health System. Survey of health-related behaviors. https://www.health.mil/Military-Health-Topics/Access-Cost-Quality-and-Safety/Health-Care-Program-Evaluation/Survey-of-Health-Related-Behaviors. Accessed November 2, 2018.

National Institute on Drug Abuse. DrugFacts: substance abuse in the military. https://www.drugabuse.gov/publications/drugfacts/substance-abuse-in-military. Revised March 2013. Accessed November 2, 2018.

Office of the Under Secretary for Personnel and Readiness. Drug Demand Reduction Program. http://prhome.defense.gov/Readiness/ForceResiliency/DDRP/. Accessed November 2, 2018.

Risk Factors for Military Families

Summary by Joan E. Zweben and Susan A. Storti

Based on THE ASAM PRINCIPLES OF ADDICTION MEDICINE, 6th edition sidebar by
Joan E. Zweben and Susan A. Storti

Military families have their own constellation of stressors and issues that put them at great risk for both substance use and mental health problems and often turn to local providers for help. It is important for community practitioners to be attuned to the unique features of military culture that affect willingness to seek help and engage in treatment. They need preparation to provide care for service-related conditions. It is especially important that primary care providers are alert to the presence of these patients because they are in an excellent position to identify behavioral issues in a population reluctant to seek care. Familiarity with the key issues of military members and their families will strengthen the process of assessment and treatment planning and promote more effective assistance.

Over 2.3 million US forces have been deployed to Iraq and Afghanistan since 2001, the majority (76%) of which are between 18 and 30 years of age. Over half (51%) are married, and 45% have children. The military uses a narrow definition of family: "heterosexual marriages and parents with dependent children who live with them at least part of the time," and thus, studies do not reflect the diversity of the families affected. This is particularly true of those families serving with the National Guard or reserve component. In some cases, both parents are deployed simultaneously, leaving parents, grandparents, or guardians responsible for the care of children.

Up to 75% of our all-volunteer military has been deployed more than once, and many have longer deployments and shorter times in between than in previous wars. There has been increased deployment of women, parents of young children, and Reserve and National Guard troops. Although many readjust without great difficulty, significant numbers have trouble adapting to family life, resuming education, and finding employment. Many military personnel and their families feel that other Americans are oblivious to their situation.

Specific circumstances determine the nature of the stressors. The military member in theater faces difficult living conditions, periods of intense violence followed by inactivity, multiple demands, sleep deprivation, great human suffering, and death. Family members must adapt to living with ambiguity, great anxiety, and little communication with the person on active duty. Initially, there can be intense fear and worry, followed by an adjustment period that includes loneliness, sadness, and fear of the unknown. Ambiguity and uncertainty are dominant. Children's reactions vary with their age, developmental stage, and preexisting problems. Homecoming presents additional challenges. Family roles have usually shifted, and new roles have become established. Couples have learned to live apart and independently, and a new relationship needs to be explored upon return. Family members may feel emotionally disconnected and alone, especially when trying to assist their loved one who has sustained a serious wound or other medical condition. Providing adequate pain control while maximizing functioning can be difficult. Family members struggle with not knowing what will trigger their loved one, and if triggered, how they will react and when is it time to ask for help. All these elements are risk factors for substance abuse. These risk factors are heightened for National Guard and Reservists, who typically have fewer benefits and support from the military.

Family members are an essential support to military service members, playing an important role in readiness and effective functioning while deployed, and support and care upon returning home. Assisting them with meeting their challenges is essential for the service member on active duty as well as those who return. In the absence of sensitive care, spouses, partners, and children are likely to become collateral damage over the long term. Although resources are offered through the military, these are often inadequate in particular locations, and community providers will make a major contribution when they are prepared to meet the needs of this group.

SUGGESTED READINGS

Ahmadi H, Green SL. Screening, brief intervention, and referral to treatment for military spouses experiencing alcohol and substance use disorders: a literature review. *J Clin Psychol Med Settings*. 2011;18(2):129-136.

Continued

Armstrong K, Best S, Domenici P. *Courage After Fire: Coping Strategies for Troops Returning from Iraq and Afghanistan and Their Families.* Berkeley, CA: Ulysses Press, 2006.

Institute of Medicine. *Returning Home from Iraq and Afghanistan: Assessment of Readjustment Needs of Veterans, Service Members, and Their Families.* Washington, DC: National Academies Press, 2013.

Laudet A, Timko C, Hill T. Comparing life experiences in active addiction and recovery between veterans and non-veterans: a national study. *J Addict Dis.* 2014;33(2):148-162.

Nazarian D, Kimerling R, Frayne SM. Posttraumatic stress disorder, substance use disorders, and medical comorbidity among returning U.S. veterans. *J Trauma Stress.* 2012;25(2):220-225.

Shen YC, Arkes J, Williams TV. Effects of Iraq/Afghanistan deployments on major depression and substance use disorder: analysis of active duty personnel in the US military. *Am J Public Health.* 2012;102(suppl 1):S80-S87.

Wooten NR. A bioecological model of deployment risk and resilience. *J Hum Behav Social Environ.* 2013;23(6):6.

Index

NOTE: Page numbers followed by the letter *f* refer to figures; those followed by the letter *t* refer to tables.

A

AA. *See* Alcoholics Anonymous
AAAP. *See* American Academy of
    Addiction Psychiatry
AASs. *See* Anabolic–androgenic steroids
ABAM. *See* American Board of
    Addiction Medicine
Abraham, Karl, 149
Absorption, 40
    anabolic–androgenic steroids,
        105–106
    stimulants, 61
Abstinence
    alcohol, 156, 391, 391*t*
    opioid use disorders and, 576
    smoking, 345
Abstinence syndrome
    cannabis, 79–80
    neonatal, 329, 495
    opioid, 327–328
ACA. *See* Affordable Care Act
Acamprosate, 317, 621
Accreditation, treatment programs, 198
Acetylcholine nicotinic receptors, 46,
    74, 342
N-Acetylcysteine, 622
Action stage of change, 355
Active physical therapy, 559
Acupuncture, 187, 339
Acute-on-chronic pain, 575
Acute pain, 575
Adderall, 132
Addiction, 8–9, 541
    anatomy of, 16–20, 18*f*
    blockade of, 24*f*, 25–26
    brain reward circuitry changes and,
        591–592
    challenges for society, 5
    comorbid disorders in (*See* Comorbid
        psychiatric disorders)
    cycle of, 2, 3*f*
    as developmental disorder, 2
    mechanisms (*See* Mechanisms of
        addiction)
    medical and surgical complications of
        alcohol, 435–438
        hospitalization care, 435
        medical history for, 433–434
        opiates, cocaine, and other drugs,
            438–441
        tobacco, 438

neurobiology of (*See* Neurobiology)
pain management with, 571
prevention of, 4–5
vulnerability to, 4
Addiction counselors, 381
Addiction liability
    alcohol, 47–48
    anabolic–androgenic steroids, 105
    dissociatives, 94
    e-cigarettes, 109
    hallucinogens, 89
    inhalants, 99
    nicotine and tobacco, 74
    opioids, 57–58
    sedative–hypnotics, 52
Addiction medicine
    consent and confidentiality in,
        636–641
    ethical principles for, 630–632
    history of, 147–151
    as medical subspecialty, 33, 151–152
    terminology use in, 7–9, 9*t*, 10
    WHO and UNODC initiatives in,
        207–208
Addiction medicine physician
    in creating transformational change,
        35–36
    drug treatment courts and, 671
    in effecting change in health care,
        36–38
    in facilitating twelve-step
        participation, 422
    family interactions with, 396
    group therapy input and support
        by, 362
    as medical review officer, 665
    in protecting and promoting public
        health, 33–34
    responsibility and role of, 33–35
Addiction nurse, 204
Addiction recovery. *See* Recovery
Addiction specialist, 136–137
Addiction treatment, 5. *See also specific
        treatments*
    accreditation of programs for, 198
    alternative therapies, 186–188
    ASAM Criteria and matching
        patients to, 172–177, 174*t*, 175*t*,
        176*f*
    blockade of addiction process, 24*f*,
        25–26

blockade of drug targets, 22–24,
    23*t*, 24*f*
brain neuromodulation, 351–352
chronic care management model for,
    167–170, 168*t*
consent and confidentiality in,
    636–641
in criminal justice populations,
    667–671
cultural issues in, 240–243, 242*t*
in drug treatment courts, 667–671
ethical principles for, 630–632
failure of, 173
for gambling disorder, 257–258
goals of, 161, 172
harm reduction integration with,
    189
history of, 147–151
during incarceration, 672–674
integrated care (*See* Integrated care)
integrating behavioral with
        pharmacologic interventions
        in, 412–416
international perspectives on,
    206–208
lapse, relapse, and recovery in, 402
linking other medical and
        psychiatric services with,
        179–184, 180*t*, 182*t*
maternal, 497
for microprocessor-based disorders,
    269–270
in military personnel, 675–682, 676*f*,
    677*f*, 679*f*
mimicry of drug action, 24–25, 24*f*
nursing roles in, 202–205
for older adults, 237–238
outcome prediction for, 604
overview of
    SUDs, 161–165
    unhealthy alcohol use, 154–159,
        159*f*
for patients with TBI, 227
for physicians, 280–283
physician's office, 163
for prescription medication use
        disorders, 217
in presence of pain, 576
quality improvement for, 196–200,
    197*f*
services of, 163–164

Addiction treatment (*Continued*)
  settings of, 161–163
  unprecedented historical moment
    for, 166–167
  for women, 219–223
Adenosine, 47
Adenosine receptors, 66–67
Adenosine triphosphate–gated ion
  channels, 46
ADHD. *See* Attention deficit
  hyperactivity disorder
Adherence
  collaborative care to achieve,
    415–416
  to group therapies, 362
  medication, 413
  in relapse prevention, 406
Adjuvant analgesics, 562–564, 576
Adolescents
  in AA, 425
  antireward system, 591
  biological predispositions, 594
  brain development of, 593, 603
  brain reward circuitry changes and
    addiction in, 591–592
  cannabis and brain of, 587–588
  cocaine use disorder in, 340–341
  community reinforcement approach
    for, 372
  confidentiality in dealing with,
    612–613
  co-occurring mood and SUDs in,
    515
  family and peer roles during
    developmental stages, 594
  family therapy for, 396
  inheritability studies, 592–593
  neuroimaging studies of
    development of, 593–594
  placement criteria and strategies for,
    607–611
  school drug testing of, 613–614
  screening and brief intervention in,
    122, 596–600, 605*t*
Adolescent substance use
  cannabis legalization and, 587–590
  DXM, 94–95
Adolescent substance use disorders
  assessment of, 602–604, 605*t*
  comorbid psychiatric disorders in,
    604, 625–627
  prevalence rates and progression of,
    582–583
  prevention of, 582
    etiology and implications for, 583
    types of, 583–585
  treatment of
    cognitive–behavioral therapy, 616
    family therapy, 615–616
    modalities for, 615
    motivational, 617–618

    multiple therapies for, 618–619
    overdose management in, 623
    pharmacotherapy, 618, 620–623
    psychosocial, 622
    twelve-step approach to, 616–617
    withdrawal management in, 623
Adult ADHD Self-Report Scale
  Version 1.1, 526
Adverse effects
  anabolic–androgenic steroids,
    104–105
  caffeine, 69–70
  cannabinoids, 80–81
  dissociatives, 94–95
  inhalants, 99–100
Affordable Care Act (ACA), 179, 181,
  196, 198
Aftercare programs, for substance use
  disorders, 162
Age, substance use disorder risk and,
  13
Al-Anon, 421
Alateen, 421
Alcohol
  for alcohol withdrawal, 294
  biomarkers for consumption of,
    662–663
  caffeine interactions, 70
  drug target blockade, 23, 23*t*, 24*f*
  endocrine and reproductive
    disorders with, 437, 490, 491*t*
  intoxication with, 290
  laboratory testing for, 131–132, 285
  pharmacology, 44–48
  prenatal exposure to, 591
  prescription medication interactions
    with, 233
  psychiatric symptoms induced by,
    510*t*
  toxic, 455
Alcoholic cardiomyopathy, 442–443
Alcoholic fatty liver, 449, 501
Alcoholic heart disease, 442
Alcoholic hepatitis, 501
Alcoholics Anonymous (AA), 150,
  364, 419
  effectiveness of, 422–423, 426
  mechanisms of change in, 426–427
  in network therapy, 380
  outcome studies of, 422
  physician facilitation of participation
    in, 422
  population subgroups and, 425–426
  predecessors to, 420–421
  in professional context, 431
  spirituality in, 429–431
  successful affiliation with, 424–425
  twelve steps of, 399
  utilization of, 424
Alcohol-related liver disease (ALD),
  448–450

Alcohol-sensitizing agents, 318–319
Alcohol use
  in adolescents, 582
  cardiovascular system and, 435,
    442–444
  college student, 245–249
  environmental prevention
    approaches to, 142–144
  epidemiology, 44–45, 128
  gastrointestinal system and, 435,
    460–461
  gender differences with, 219
  harm reduction interventions for,
    192
  herbal remedies reducing, 187
  historical features, 44
  international policy frameworks
    for, 207
  liver and, 435, 448–452, 501
  medical consequences of, 435–438
  metabolic disorders and, 436,
    454–455
  by military personnel, 675–679,
    676*f*, 677*f*, 679*f*
  neurologic disorders and, 436,
    470–473
  perioperative patient and, 438,
    500–502
  in pregnancy, 219–220, 495–496
  renal effects of, 436, 454–455
  respiratory system and, 436,
    467–468
  scope of problem, 141–142
  screening and brief intervention
    for, 119
    adults, 120
    current evidence, 121
    individual studies, 122
    in older adults, 128–129, 129*t*
    for pregnant women, 123–124
    systematic reviews and
      meta-analyses, 122
    in trauma centers, hospitals,
      and emergency departments,
      125–126
    youth, 121
  sleep and, 438, 480–482
  surgical risk and, 501–502
  TBI and, 224–227
  trauma and, 437, 486–487
  by women, 219–220
  worldwide prevalence of, 206
Alcohol use disorder (AUD)
  anxiety disorders and, 517–519
  aversion therapy for, 390–391, 391*t*
  biomarkers of, 132
  cocaine use disorder with, 340
  in college students, 245
  in criminal justice populations,
    667–671
  epidemiology of, 11–14, 44–45, 128

nicotine association with, 76
in older adults, 233–238, 234t, 237t
  screening and brief intervention
    for, 128–129, 129t
  opioid use disorder with, 349
  pharmacologic interventions for
    alcohol-sensitizing agents,
      318–319
    medications for comorbid
      psychiatric disorders, 319–320
    medications for reducing or
      stopping alcohol consumption,
      316–318
  physicians with, 278–279
  screening and assessment of,
    120–121
  spectrum of severity in, 154, 159f
    tailoring treatment to, 156–158
  tobacco use disorder with, 348, 377
  treatment of
    acupuncture, 187
    in adolescents, 621
    behavior change and, 158
    community reinforcement
      approach, 372
    defining and measuring outcomes
      in, 155–156
    digital health interventions for,
      408–409
    herbal remedies, 187
    integrating evidence and
      personalizing practice in,
      158–159, 159f
    modern approaches to, 154–155
    systems of care in, 158
    tailoring of, 156–158
    twelve-step programs for (See
      Alcoholics Anonymous)
Alcohol Use Disorders Identification
  Test—Concise (AUDIT-C),
  124, 500
Alcohol withdrawal syndrome (AWS),
  291, 292t
  assessment tools for, 138–139
  clinical assessment for risk of, 125
  common treatment issues in, 296
  initial management of, 125, 501
  management of, 292–296
ALD. See Alcohol-related liver disease
Alkyl nitrites, 97–100, 98t
Allostatic states of substance use
  disorders and pain, 550
α2-Adrenergic agents
  for opioid use disorder, 326–327
  for opioid withdrawal, 306, 327
α-Adrenergic agonists, 563–564
Alternative therapies, 186–188
American Academy of Addiction
  Psychiatry (AAAP), 151
American Association of Medical
  Review Officers, 665

American Board of Addiction
  Medicine (ABAM), 151
American Indians, addiction medicine
  of, 147
American Society of Addiction
  Medicine (ASAM), 151
  cannabinoid policy of, 657
  criteria for matching patients
    to treatment (See ASAM
    Criteria)
  detoxification goals of, 286
  standards workgroup, 197–198
Americans with Disabilities Act of
  1990, confidentiality, 637
Amphetamines
  for ADHD treatment, 527, 528t
  cardiovascular system and, 445–446
  drug action mimicry, 24f, 25
  drug target blockade, 23, 23t, 24f
  endocrine and reproductive
    disorders with, 491t, 492
  epidemiology, 61
  gastrointestinal system and, 462
  laboratory testing for, 132–133
  neuroanatomy of reinforcement,
    17–19
  neurologic disorders and, 470–473
  pharmacology, 60–65
  physician addiction to, 279
  respiratory system and, 467
Amphetamine use disorder, 339, 392
Amyl nitrite, 97–98, 98t
AN. See Anorexia nervosa
Anabolic–androgenic steroids (AASs)
  endocrine and reproductive
    disorders with, 491t, 492
  pharmacological interventions for,
    347
  pharmacology, 102–106
  respiratory system and, 469
Analgesia, cannabinoid effects, 82, 656
Analytical sensitivity, 659
Anatomy of addiction. See
  Neuroanatomy
Androstenedione, 102
Anesthetics
  inhalants, 97–100, 98t
  for pain, 563
Anorexia nervosa (AN), 541, 543
Antabuse. See Disulfiram
Antagonists, 41
Anticholinergics, 462
Anticipation stage, of addiction cycle,
  3f, 4
Anticonvulsants
  for alcohol use disorder, 318
  cannabinoids, 81
  for cocaine use disorder, 339
  for pain, 563
  for sedative–hypnotic withdrawal,
    323

Antidepressants
  in alcohol use disorder, 319
  for cocaine use disorder, 338, 340
  for co-occurring mood and SUDs,
    514
  ketamine, 94–95
  for pain, 562–563
Antiemetics, cannabinoids, 81, 656
Antiparkinson agents, 338
Antipsychotics, 338–340
  Antireward system and, 591–592
Antisocial personality disorder
    (ASPD), 514, 533
Anxiety, pain and, 549
Anxiety disorders
  in adolescents, 626
  co-occurring SUDs and
    alcohol and, 517–519
    cannabis, 520
    opioids, 520
    prevalence of, 517
    screening and differential
      diagnosis for, 517
    stimulants, 520–521
    tobacco products, 519–520
    treatment considerations for, 517,
      518t
  substance-induced, 508–509
  SUD development and, 592
  in women with addictive disorders,
    220–221
Appetite, 81, 656
Aquatic therapy, 559
Arrhythmias, 443–444
Arylcyclohexylamines, 91–95
ASAM. See American Society of
  Addiction Medicine
ASAM Criteria
  assessment dimensions, 173, 174t
    for adolescents, 608–609
  features and guiding principles of
    choice of treatment levels, 173
    clinical versus reimbursement
      considerations, 173
    concept of treatment failure, 173
    continuum of care, 173
    goals of treatment, 172
    individualized treatment plan, 172
    length of stay, 173
    progress through treatment levels,
      173
  levels of care, 173–174, 175t
    for adolescents, 609–610
    linkages between, 610–611
  placement criteria and strategies for
    adolescent treatment
    assessment-based treatment
      matching and clinical
      appropriateness, 608
    by assessment dimension,
      608–609

ASAM Criteria (*Continued*)
  developmental considerations, 607
  by levels of care, 609–610
  levels of care linkages, 610–611
  in 3rd edition, 607–608
  placement dilemmas
    assessment of imminent danger, 174
    co-occurring disorders, 174
    ensuring individualized treatment, 177
    logistical impediments, 177
    mandated care, 176
  selecting appropriate services, 174, 176*f*
  software, 177
  in withdrawal management, 288
ASPD. *See* Antisocial personality disorder
Aspiration syndromes, 465
Assessment
  by addiction specialist, 136–137
  of adolescent substance use, 602–606, 605*t*
  of alcohol and nonmedical prescription medication use in older adults, 236–237
  cultural aspects of, 241
  of gambling disorder, 256
  information sources for, 137–138
  of microprocessor-based disorders, 268–269
  of physician addiction, 280
  by primary care provider, 136
  of problematic sexual behavior, 263
  of SUD in patients with TBI, 226–227
  by SUD researcher, 137
  by SUD treatment provider, 137
  tasks of, 137, 137*t*
  tools
    for comorbid conditions and functioning, 139
    diagnostic, 138
    for intoxication and withdrawal, 138–139
    screening, 138
Assessment dimensions, ASAM Criteria, 173, 174*t*
  for adolescents, 608–609
Atelectasis, 440, 465
Athletes
  anabolic–androgenic steroid use in, 103
  college drinking by, 246
  TBI in, 225
Atomoxetine, 527, 528*t*
Atrial fibrillation, 443–444
At-risk drinking, 120, 121, 156
At-risk use, 120

Attention and pain perception, 554
Attention deficit hyperactivity disorder (ADHD)
  in cocaine use disorder, 340
  co-occurring SUD and, 525–530, 528*t*, 529*t*
  diagnosis of, 526–527
  pharmacotherapeutic treatment for, 527, 528*t*, 593
  SUD development and, 592–593, 604, 627
AUD. *See* Alcohol use disorder
AUDIT-C. *See* Alcohol Use Disorders Identification Test—Concise
Autonomy
  in addiction practice, 630–631
  older patients and, 633
Aversion therapy
  for alcohol use disorder, 390–391, 391*t*
  further research needed in, 393–394
  for marijuana use disorder, 391
  for nicotine and tobacco use disorder, 391
  for opioid use disorder, 392
  as part of established care for SUDs, 393
  as part of multimodality treatment program, 389
  reinforcement (booster) treatment use in, 392
  safety of, 393
  for stimulant use disorder, 392
  support programs and 12-step meetings after, 392–393
AWS. *See* Alcohol withdrawal syndrome
Ayahuasca, 87

B
BAC. *See* Blood alcohol concentration
Baclofen, 317–318, 564
Barbiturates
  for alcohol withdrawal, 293
  endocrine and reproductive disorders with, 491*t*, 492
  intoxication, 298, 322–323
  laboratory testing for, 133
  misuse and abuse, 322
  pharmacology, 321
  physical dependence and tolerance, 322
  withdrawal, 323–324
Basal ganglia, 16
Bath salts, 113–114, 313
  laboratory testing for, 134–135
  renal effects of, 457
Beck Depression Inventory, 555
BED. *See* Binge eating disorder
Behavior, cannabinoid effects, 80

Behavioral addiction
  binge eating disorder, 251–252
  chemical addiction features shared with, 274–275
  compulsive buying disorder, 253–254, 272–273
  compulsive sexual behavior, 252–253
  definition of, 250
  diagnostic challenges in, 275
  excessive tanning, 273
  impulse control disorders, 250
  kleptomania, 273–274
  pathologic gambling, 250–251
  problematic Internet use, 253
  problematic video game playing, 253
  substance use co-occurrence with, 275
  treatment models for, 275–276
Behavioral conditions, for adolescent placement criteria, 608–609
Behavioral couples therapy, 396
Behavioral family therapy, 616
Behavioral interventions. *See also* Psychotherapy
  integrating pharmacologic interventions with, 412–416
  for nicotine and tobacco use disorder, 374–377
Behavioral pharmacology, stimulants, 62
Behavior change
  AUD treatment and, 158
  enhancing motivation for, 354–358, 357*t*
Beneficence, 631
Benezet, Anthony, 147
Benzodiazepines
  in alcohol use disorder, 319
  for alcohol withdrawal, 292–296
  for insomnia in older adults, 235
  intoxication, 298, 322–323
  laboratory testing for, 133
  misuse and abuse, 322
  nonmedical prescription use, 213–215
  for pain, 564
  perioperative patient and, 503
  pharmacology, 50–53, 321
  physical dependence and tolerance, 322
  physician addiction to, 279
  sleep and, 483
  withdrawal, 299–302, 302*t*, 323–324
  in women with addictive disorders, 221
β-Adrenergic–blocking agents, for alcohol withdrawal, 294
Binge drinking, 245–249
Binge eating disorder (BED), 251–252, 541, 544
Binge stage, of addiction cycle, 2–3, 3*f*

Bioavailability, 40
Biochemical markers
    alcohol use disorder, 132
    nicotine, 72–73
Biomedical conditions and
        complications, for adolescent
        placement criteria, 608
Biopsychosocial analysis, 591–592
Bipolar disorder
    in adolescents, 626
    in cocaine use disorder, 340
    co-occurring SUDs, 513–515
    substance-induced, 509
Bisexual persons, 263
Blinding, clinical trials, 29
Blockade
    of addiction process, 24f, 25–26
    of drug targets, 22–24, 23t, 24f
Blood
    alcohol use and, 437
    drug testing, 130
    substance use and, 440
Blood alcohol concentration (BAC),
        131–132, 290, 292t
BN. See Bulimia nervosa
Body mechanics, 560
"Body packing," 463
Bone health, 490–491
Borderline personality disorder (BPD),
        221–222, 533
Brain
    adolescent development of, 593, 603
    anatomy (See Neuroanatomy)
Brain neuromodulation, 351–352
Breastfeeding, 497–498
Breath alcohol testing, 131–132
Brief advice, 366
Brief alcohol interventions, for older
        adults, 237
Brief interventions. See Screening and
        brief intervention
Brief motivational interventions, for
        college student drinking, 247
Brief strategic family therapy (BSFT),
        615
Bulimia nervosa (BN), 541, 543–544
Buprenorphine (Subutex), 41
    in adolescents, 622
    for cocaine use disorder, 338
    drug action mimicry, 24f, 25
    federal regulations on, 578
    HIV pharmacotherapy interactions
        with, 329
    in HIV primary care settings, 182
    for mixed cocaine and opioid use
        disorder, 339–340
    in multiple use disorders, 349
    for opioid use disorder, 326,
        328–330, 334–335
    for opioid withdrawal, 307, 327
    pain treatment and, 575

pharmacology, 55, 57
    for pregnant women, 220
    for prescription medication use
        disorders, 217
    prescription training for, 199
    for preventing injection and
        overdose risks, 192
Bupropion
    for ADHD, 527, 528t
    in adolescents, 620–621
    for cocaine use disorder, 340
    for microprocessor-based disorders,
        270
Bupropion sustained release, for
        tobacco use disorder, 343–346,
        345t
Buspirone, 319–320, 517, 518t
Butane, 97–98, 98t
Buying, compulsive, 253–254, 272–273

C
Caffeine
    endocrine and reproductive
        disorders with, 491t, 492
    epidemiology, 66
    historical features, 66
    neurologic disorders and, 470
    pharmacology, 66–70
    psychiatric symptoms induced by,
        510t
    respiratory system and, 467
    sleep and, 483
Caffeine use disorder, 69
Calcium channel blockers, 339
Calcium channels, alcohol effects,
        46–47
California Diversion Program, 283
Cancer
    alcohol use and, 437, 461
    screening for, 433–434
    substance use and, 440
    tobacco use and, 462
Cannabidiol (CBD), 472, 655
Cannabinoid receptors, 78–79,
        655–656
Cannabinoids. See also Δ9-
        Tetrahydrocannabinol
    chemistry of, 655
    drug target blockade, 23t, 24
    endo-, 47, 78–80, 655
    historical features, 78
    intoxication, 81, 311, 311t
    as medicine, 655–656
    neuroanatomy of reinforcement, 20
    pharmacology, 79–82
    physician prescription of, 656–657
    phyto-, 655
    renal effects of, 458
    synthetic (See Synthetic
        cannabinoids)
    withdrawal, 79–80, 311

Cannabis, 78
    abstinence syndrome, 79–80
    adolescent brain and, 587–588
    anxiety disorders and, 520
    cardiovascular system and, 446
    chemistry of, 655
    electronic delivery of, 111
    epidemiology of, 655
    gastrointestinal system and, 462–463
    during incarceration, 673
    laboratory testing for, 133
    legalization of, adolescent impact of,
        587–590
    as medicine, 655–656
    neurologic disorders and, 471–473
    older adults using, 233–234
    perioperative patient and, 503–504
    pharmacotherapy for, 621–622
    physician prescription of, 656–657
    physician use of, 279
    potency of, 588–589
    during pregnancy, 496–497
    psychiatric symptoms induced by,
        511t
    screening and brief intervention, 126
    sleep and, 483
Cannabis sativa, 78
Cannabis use disorder (CUD)
    aversion therapy for, 391
    digital health interventions for, 409
    pharmacological interventions for,
        347
Capsaicin, 564
Carbamazepine, 563
    for alcohol use disorder, 318
    for alcohol withdrawal, 294
    for cocaine use disorder, 340
    for sedative–hypnotic withdrawal,
        323
Carcinogens, tobacco, 74–75
Cardiomyopathy, alcoholic, 442–443
Cardiovascular system
    alcohol use and, 435, 442–444
    anabolic–androgenic steroid effects,
        104
    cannabinoid effects, 80
    preventive medication for, 434
    stimulant effects, 62
    substance use and, 440, 445–446
    tobacco use and, 444
Care integration. See Integrated care
Carfentanil, 305
CARN. See Certified Addictions
        Registered Nurse
Case management, for substance use
        disorders, 162
CAT. See Computer-assisted therapy
Catastrophizing, 555
Cathinones, synthetic, 113–114, 313
CB$_1$ receptor, 78–79
CB$_2$ receptor, 78–79

CBD. *See* Cannabidiol; Compulsive buying disorder
CBT. *See* Cognitive–behavioral therapy
CCM. *See* Chronic care management
Centers for Disease Control and Prevention (CDC), opioid guidelines of, 579, 653
Centralized models, of linked services, 181–183, 182t
Central nervous system (CNS)
  alcohol effects, 45
  stimulant effects, 62
Central sensitization, 549
Central sleep apnea, 480
Certified Addictions Registered Nurse (CARN), 204
Cervical stabilization, 559
Change
  mechanisms of, 426–427
  motivation to, 354–358, 357t
  principles and processes of, 356–358, 357t
  stages of, 354–358, 357t
  theory of, 269, 400
Chemical addiction, behavioral addiction features shared with, 274–275
Child Protective Services, 498
Chinese medicine, traditional, 186–188
Chlordiazepoxide (Librium), 50, 293
Chloroethane, 98t
Chronic care management (CCM)
  linked services model, 183
  stage model of, 167–170, 168t
Chronic nonmalignant pain (CNMP). *See* Chronic pain
Chronic pain
  allostatic states of SUDs and, 550
  anatomy and physiology of, 548–549
  anxiety and, 549
  biopsychological approach to management of, 555–556
  emotions and, 549
  mind–body connection in, 553
  modalities in, 560
  opioid-induced hyperalgesia, 550–551, 569
  opioid use disorder and, 550
    diagnosis of, 574
    monitoring for, 574, 574t
    treatment with, 574–576
  opioid use for, 571, 651–654
    evolving guidance for, 573–574
    monitoring for misuse, 574, 574t
  prevalence of, 567
  psychological issues in, 553
  psychological modulation of, 553–555
  psychological processes of, 555
  rehabilitation approaches to, 558–560

SUDs and, 549–550, 555, 556t
  nonopioid pharmacologic treatments, 576
  nonpharmacologic treatments for, 575
  opioid agonist therapy and, 576
  problems of comorbidity, 573
  rehabilitation programs for, 575–576
  treatment with, 574–576
Cigarettes, electronic. *See* Electronic cigarettes
Cigarette smoking. *See also* Tobacco use
  achieving abstinence of, 345
  caffeine interactions, 70
  e-cigarettes as gateway to, 110
  reduction of, 345
Cirrhosis, 433, 449–450, 501–502
CIWA. *See* Clinical Institute Withdrawal Assessment—Alcohol
Clearance, 40–41
Clinical Institute Withdrawal Assessment—Alcohol (CIWA), 291, 292t
Clinical management, in therapeutic communities, 385
Clinical monitoring, 163
Clinical monitoring/management stage, of chronic care management, 168t, 169
Clinical sensitivity, 659
Clinical skills, for addiction treatment, 412
Clinical trials
  efficacy versus effectiveness, 29
  elements of, 28
  features
    blinding, 29
    design, 30
    monitoring and quality control, 31
    outcomes, 30–31
    randomization, 29
    sample size, power, effect size, and feasibility, 29–30
  phases, 28–29
  types, 28–29
Clomiphene (Clomid), 102
Clonazepam, 563
Clonidine, 484, 527, 528t
  for opioid use disorder, 326–327
  for opioid withdrawal, 306, 327
Club drugs, 84–85
  intoxication and withdrawal, 312–314
  laboratory testing for, 134–135
  pharmacokinetics, pharmacodynamics, and subjective effects, 88–89
CM. *See* Contingency management
CNMP. *See* Chronic pain

CNS. *See* Central nervous system
Cocaine
  cardiovascular system and, 444–445
  drug action mimicry, 24f, 25
  drug target blockade, 23, 23t, 24f
  endocrine and reproductive disorders with, 491t, 492
  epidemiology, 61
  gastrointestinal system and, 462
  laboratory testing for, 133
  liver and, 452
  medical consequences of, 438–441
  neuroanatomy of reinforcement, 17–20
  neurologic disorders and, 470–473
  pharmacology, 60–65
  pharmacotherapy for, 622
  prenatal exposure to, 591
  renal effects of, 456–457
  respiratory system and, 467
Cocaine Anonymous, 421
Cocaine use disorder
  alcohol use disorder with, 340
  aversion therapy for, 392–393
  digital health interventions for, 409
  goals of treatment, 337
  opioid use disorder with, 339–340, 349
  pharmacotherapy for, 337–341
  tobacco use disorder with, 348–349
Cocaine vaccine, 23
Codeine, 55, 133–134, 134t
Codependence, 395
Codes of ethics, 633–634
Cognitive–behavioral relapse prevention therapy, 366
Cognitive–behavioral therapy (CBT), 163, 616
  for chronic nonmalignant pain, 555–556
  for comorbid PTSD and SUDs, 539
  for co-occurring mood and SUDs, 514–515
  for co-occurring SUDs and ADHD, 530
  for eating disorders, 544–545
  for gambling disorder, 258
  in network therapy, 379
  for problematic sexual behavior, 263–264
  for PTSD, 539–540
  for relapse prevention, 366
Cognitive conditions
  for adolescent placement criteria, 608–609
  chronic pain and, 554–555
Cognitive disorders, 471
Cognitive distortions, in relapse prevention, 405
Cognitive function, cannabinoid effects, 80

Collaborative care, 414–416
College student drinking
  future directions in, 248–249
  individually focused interventions
    for, 247–248
  prevalence and consequences of,
    245–246
  prevention strategies for, 247
  risk factors for, 246–247
  structural interventions for, 248
College students, screening and brief
    intervention in, 122
Colon, 461
COMM. *See* Current Opioid Misuse
    Measure
Communication skills, in relapse
    prevention, 405
Community as method, in therapeutic
    community approach, 385
Community-based prevention programs
  approaches to, 585
  ecologic research emergence and, 144
  efficacy trials of, 143–144
  individual approaches versus,
    142–143
  medical professionals role in, 144
  risk and protective factors in, 583
  scope of problem and, 141–142
Community clinics, extending
    contingency management into,
    371
Community reinforcement approach
    (CRA), 163, 366–372
  to adolescent substance use
    treatment, 617
Comorbid psychiatric disorders
  addiction with, 4–5
  ADHD, 525–530, 528t, 529t
  in adolescents, 604
    diagnosis and management of,
      625–627
    incidence and prevalence of, 625
  in alcohol use disorder, 319–320
  anxiety disorders, 517–521
  assessment tools for, 139
  behavioral addiction and substance
    use, 275
  in cocaine use disorder, 340
  eating disorders, 541–545
  in gambling disorder, 257
  in high-volume sexual behavior, 261
  in microprocessor-based disorders,
    269
  mood disorders, 513–515
  nonmedical prescription medication
    use and, 214
  in older adults, 235, 515
  personality disorders, 532–535
  in physician addiction, 279
  psychotic disorders, 522–524
  SUD development and, 592

TBI, 225–227
therapeutic communities for,
    384–388, 387t
  in tobacco use disorder, 377
  treatment placement and, 174
  in women with addictive disorders,
    219–222
Competence enhancement, 584–585
Comprehensive assessment, of
    adolescents, 602, 604, 605t
Compulsive buying disorder (CBD),
    253–254, 272–273
Compulsive sexual behavior (CSB),
    260–261
  as behavioral addiction, 252–253
  in combination with substance use,
    262–263
Computer-assisted therapy (CAT), 164,
    367–368
Conditioned tolerance, 42
Conduct disorders, 592, 627
Confidentiality
  Americans with Disabilities Act, 637
  as barrier to linked services, 181
  basis of, 636
  consent utilization, 639–640
  in dealing with adolescents, 612–613
  electronic medical records, 639
  42 CFR Part 2 and, 637–639
  HIPAA, 637
  Rehabilitation Act, 637
  young patients, 121
Conners Adult ADHD Rating Scale, 526
Consent. *See* Informed consent
Consultation, for ethical issues, 633
Contaminants
  consumer drug testing for, 192–193
  in e-cigarettes, 108
  respiratory complications of, 466
Contemplation stage of change, 354
Contingency management (CM),
    366–372
  for adolescent substance use
    treatment, 618
Continued use or problem potential,
    adolescent placement criteria
    and, 609
Continuum of care, 173, 618–619
CONTINUUM software, 177
Controlled medications
  considerations for, 642
  continuation, modification, or
    termination of, 647–648
  discontinuation of, 648
  inappropriate prescription and use
    of, 643
  informed consent for, 645–646
  initial patient assessment and risk
    stratification for, 645
  legal and regulatory requirements
    for, 578–580, 643–644

new patient precautions with, 648–649
response monitoring, 646–647
trial therapy for, 646
universal precautions for, 644
Controlled Substances Act (CSA)
  history of, 650–651
  lawful prescription under, 644
  marijuana under, 657
Coping
  in relapse prevention, 404
  substance use for, 241–242
Coping skill groups, 360
Coping skills, 365
Coronary artery disease, 443
Correctional settings. *See* Incarceration
Corydalis yanhusuo, 187
Cotinine, biochemical assessment, 72–73
Counseling groups, 360
Counselors, collaborative care with,
    414–415
Counterconditioning. *See* Aversion
    therapy
Couples therapy, 396
Court-ordered referral. *See* Drug
    treatment courts; Mandated
    treatment
Covert sensitization, 390–391
CRA. *See* Community reinforcement
    approach
CRAFFT interview, 597f, 598, 599f,
    604, 605t
Cravings
  alternative therapies for, 187
  aversion therapy effects on, 391, 391t
  in relapse prevention, 405
Craving stage, of addiction cycle, 3f, 4
Criminal justice system
  drug treatment courts, 667–671
  incarceration and SUD treatment in,
    672–674
  mandated SUD treatment in, 163
  women patients in, 223
Cross-tolerance, 42
CSA. *See* Controlled Substances Act
CSB. *See* Compulsive sexual behavior
CUD. *See* Cannabis use disorder
Cues, in relapse prevention, 405
Cultural coping, 241–242
Cultural history, 241
Culture
  addiction treatment and
    assessment, 241
  definitions related to substance
    use, 240–241
  patterns of substance use, 241
  substance use for cultural coping,
    241–242
  treatment and recovery, 242–243,
    242t
  military, 230
  treatment, 222

Current Opioid Misuse Measure
(COMM), 647
Cyclohexamine, 91
Cyclohexyl nitrite, 98t
CYP450. See Cytochrome P450
Cyproterone acetate, 264
Cytochrome P450 (CYP450), 51, 72

D
DA. See Dopamine
DAPTRA. See Drug Abuse Prevention,
Treatment, and Rehabilitation
Act
DEA. See Drug Enforcement
Administration
Death. See Mortality
Dehydroepiandrosterone, 102
Delirium tremens (DTs), 291, 295–296
Denial, 632–633
Dependence, 8–9. See also Pre–substance
dependence
alcohol, 47–48
opioids, 568–569
physical, 42, 322, 550
stimulants, 60–61
Depression
in cocaine use disorder, 340
in older adults, 235
in women with addictive disorders,
221
Depressive disorders
in adolescents, 625–626
co-occurring SUDs, 513–515
substance-induced, 507–509
tobacco use disorder and, 515
Design, clinical trials, 30
Designer drugs, 113–116, 116t
Desipramine, 622
for cocaine use disorder, 338, 340
Desomorphine, 115–116
Detoxification
in adolescents, 623
behavioral therapies in context of,
413
goals of, 286
opioid, 306–307, 327–328
relapse after, 288
settings of, 287–288
Development
adolescent brain development, 593
adolescent placement and, 607
adolescent substance use and
assessment of, 602–603
prevention of, 583
biological predispositions and, 594
family and peer roles during, 594
neurobiology of addiction from
perspective of, 591–594
neuroimaging studies of, 593–594
Developmental disorder, addiction
as, 2

Dextromethorphan (DXM), 91–95,
311, 622
*Diagnostic and Statistical Manual of
Mental Disorders* (*DSM*)
addiction and SUD terminology
in, 8–9
substance-induced mental disorders,
507, 508t
Diagnostic assessment tools, 138
Diazepam, 51, 293, 295–296
Diclofenac, 564
Dietary guidelines, caffeine, 69
Differential therapeutics, 367
Diffusion tensor imaging studies, 593
Difluoroethane, 98t
Digital health interventions
for alcohol use disorder, 408–409
for cannabis use disorder, 409
for cocaine use disorder, 409
in diverse samples with SUDs,
409–410
future opportunities for, 410–411
Dilaudid. See Hydromorphone
Dimethyltryptamine (DMT), 84–86,
87, 349
Disruptive mood dysregulation
disorder, 513
Dissociatives
epidemiology, 92
historical features, 91–92
intoxication, 95, 311
pharmacology, 91–95
withdrawal, 311–312
Distribution, 40
stimulants, 61
Distributive models, of linked services,
182t, 183–184
Disulfiram (Antabuse), 155, 389, 514,
621
for alcohol use disorder, 318–319
for cocaine use disorder, 338
in multiple use disorders, 349
Divalproex, 318–319, 340
DMT. See Dimethyltryptamine
"Doctor shopping," 643
Dole, Vincent, 150
Domestic violence, 220, 222
Dopamine (DA)
alcohol effects, 45–46, 47
drug reinforcement and, 16–20, 18f
gambling effects, 251
stimulant effects, 64
TBI effects on, 226
Dopamine (DA) agonists, 338
Dopamine (DA) receptors, 187
Dose response, 41–42
Drinking. See also Alcohol use; Alcohol
use disorder
college student, 245–249
continuum of severity of, 154,
156–158, 159f

herbal remedies reducing, 187
screening and assessment of,
120–121
treatment outcomes and measures
of, 155–156
Dronabinol (Marinol), 133, 656
Dropout, from group therapies, 362
Drug Abuse Prevention, Treatment,
and Rehabilitation Act
(DAPTRA), 637–639
Drug action
mimicry of, 24–25, 24f
nicotine and tobacco, 73–74
Drug Addiction Treatment Act of
2000, 578
Drug consumption venues, 191
Drug Control Policy, 650–651
Drug–drug interactions
alcohol, 45
caffeine, 70
cannabinoids, 82
dissociatives, 93
nicotine and tobacco, 73
opioids, 51–52, 58
sedative–hypnotics, 51–52
stimulants, 61–62
Drug Enforcement Administration
(DEA)
controlled medications and, 578,
642–643
opioid prescriptions and, 579
Drug reinforcement. See
Reinforcement
Drug targets, blockade of, 22–24, 23t,
24f
Drug testing
in adolescent assessment, 603
alcohol biomarkers for, 662–663
consumer, 192–193
controlled medication and, 647
laboratory, 130–135, 131t, 134t
limitations of, 662
mass spectrometry for, 660–661
matrix selection for, 661–662
results assessments for, 659–660
in school, 613–614
in workplace, 131, 664–665
Drug treatment courts (DTCs),
667–671
Drug use. See also specific drugs
in older adults, 233–234
screening and brief intervention for,
119–125
by women, 220
Drug use disorders. See also specific
disorders
in criminal justice populations,
667–671
epidemiology of, 12–14
*DSM. See Diagnostic and Statistical
Manual of Mental Disorders*

DTCs. *See* Drug treatment courts
DTs. *See* Delirium tremens
DUI enforcement programs, 143
DXM. *See* Dextromethorphan
Dyslipidemia, 490

E
Early identification/intervention stage,
    of chronic care management,
    167–168, 168*t*
Early intervention, for adolescent
    substance abuse, 609–610
Eating disorders
    in adolescents, 627
    binge eating, 251–252
    biological management of, 543–544
    definitions for, 541
    differential diagnosis of, 542
    prevalence of, 542
    psychological management of,
        544–545
    recovery issues with, 545
    screening instruments for, 542–543
    SUDs with, 542, 545
    treatment of, 543
    in women with addictive disorders,
        221
e-cigarettes. *See* Electronic cigarettes
Ecologic research, 144
Ecstasy. *See* 3,4-Methylenedioxy-
    methamphetamine
ED. *See* Emergency department
Education
    overdose risk, 189–190, 190*t*
    prescriber, 215, 216*t*
    SUD risk and, 14
    in therapeutic communities, 385
Effectiveness, efficacy versus, 29
Effect size, clinical trials, 29–30
Efficacy
    of controlled medications, 645
    drug, 41–42
    effectiveness versus, 29
Elderly. *See* Older adults
Electronic cigarettes (e-cigarettes),
    72, 345
    adolescent use of, 582
    cardiovascular system and, 444
    constituents, 108–109
    as gateway to combustible cigarettes,
        110
    health effects, 110
    injury and, 488–489
    nicotine delivery and addiction
        potential, 109
    other substance use with, 111
    patient recommendations, 111
    prevalence, 109–110
    regulation of, 111
    secondhand and thirdhand
        exposure, 109

in smoking cessation, 110
types, 108, 109*f*
Electronic medical record (EMR),
    confidentiality with, 639
Electronic nicotine delivery systems
    (ENDS), 345
Elimination, 40
    stimulants, 61
Emergency department (ED)
    alcohol screening in, 486–487
    opioid use disorders and, 575
    screening and brief intervention in,
        125–126
    SUD treatment in, 161
Emetic therapy. *See* Aversion therapy
EMLA. *See* Eutectic mixture of local
    anesthetics
Emotional conditions
    for adolescent placement criteria,
        608–609
    chronic pain and, 549
Emotional distress, 554
Employment status, substance use
    disorder risk and, 14
EMR. *See* Electronic medical record
Enabler, 395
Endocannabinoids, 78–79
    alcohol effects, 47
    cannabinoid receptors and, 655
    toxicity and adverse effects, 80
Endocarditis, 439, 475–476
Endocrine system
    alcohol use and, 437, 490, 491*t*
    cannabinoid effects, 81
    stimulant effects, 63
    substance use and, 440, 491–492, 491*t*
    tobacco use and, 490–491, 491*t*
Endogenous opiates, stimulant effects,
    64
ENDS. *See* Electronic nicotine delivery
    systems
Energy drinks, alcohol and, 70
Entactogens, 84, 88–89
Enthusiastic sobriety approach, to
    adolescent substance use
    treatment, 617–618
Environment, college drinking risk
    and, 246–247
Environmental prevention
    ecologic research emergence and,
        144
    efficacy trials of, 143–144
    individual approaches versus,
        142–143
    medical professionals role in, 144
    scope of problem and, 141–142
Ephedra, 60–61
Ephedrine, 60, 63
Epidemiologic principles, 11
Epilepsy, cannabinoids and, 656
Esophagus, 460

Estelle v Gamble, 672
Eszopiclone, 50–51, 299, 321
EtG. *See* Ethyl glucuronide
Ethanol. *See* Alcohol
Ether, 97, 98*t*
Ethics
    autonomy, 630–631
    beneficence, 631
    codes of, 633–634
    consultation for, 633
    denial, dealing with, 632–633
    establishing stance on, 633–634
    fidelity, 632
    future developments and, 634
    justice, 631–632
    in laboratory testing, 135, 633
    legal consultation for, 634
    nonmaleficence, 631
    professional standards for, 633–634
Ethnicity
    addiction treatment and, 240
    college drinking risk and, 246
    SUD risk and, 13–14
Ethyl glucuronide (EtG), 663
Ethyl sulfate (EtS), 663
Eutectic mixture of local anesthetics
    (EMLA), 564
Excessive tanning, 273
Excretion, 40
Exercise, for chronic nonmalignant
    pain, 555
Expectancy challenge interventions, for
    college student drinking, 247
Expectations
    drinking, 246
    pain and, 554
Exposure therapy, 539

F
Fagerström Test for Nicotine
    Dependence, 74
Failure, treatment, 173
False negative, 659–660
False positive, 659–660
Family
    involvement in addiction, 395–396
    military, 681–682
Family history
    of gambling disorder, 257
    SUD risk and, 14, 603–604
Family prevention, 583, 585
Family psychoeducational workshops,
    361–362
Family therapy, 164, 396–397, 615–616
Faradic aversion, 390
FCTC. *See* Framework Convention for
    Tobacco Control
FDA. *See* US Food and Drug
    Administration
Fear avoidance, 554
Feasibility, clinical trials, 29–30

Federal laws
  concerning confidentiality, 637–641
  for opioid use, 578, 653
Federation of State Medical Boards
    (FSMB), 579, 653, 657
Feedback-only interventions, for college
    student drinking, 247–248
Fentanyl, 214
  intoxication and overdose, 304–305
  laboratory testing for, 133–134, 134t
Fentanyl analogues,
    nonpharmaceutical, 113–115
Fentanyl derivatives, 57
Fetal alcohol syndrome, 123, 219–220,
    496, 591
Fetal health
  alcohol use and, 123, 219–220, 437,
    496, 591
  inhalant effects, 100
  stimulant effects, 63
  substance use and, 441
Fetal solvent syndrome, 100
FFT. See Functional family therapy
Fidelity, in addiction practice, 632
Flavorants, in e-cigarettes, 108
Flumazenil, 298, 321, 324
Flunitrazepam (Rohypnol), 134–135,
    313
Fluoxetine, 340
Folate, 434
Fomepizole, 455
Formulations
  alcohol, 44
  cannabinoids, 78
  dissociatives, 91
  nicotine and tobacco, 72
  stimulants, 60–61
42 CFR Part 2, confidentiality, 637–639
Fox, Ruth, 147, 151
Framework Convention for Tobacco
    Control (FCTC), 207
Fraternity organizations, college
    drinking in, 246
Freud, Sigmund, 364
FSMB. See Federation of State Medical
    Boards
Fuels, inhalants, 97–100, 98t
Functional family therapy (FFT), 615
Functional impairment, in gambling
    disorder, 256–257
Functional magnetic resonance
    imaging studies, 593

G
γ-Aminobutyric acid (GABA),
    291–292, 298–299
GABA_A receptors, 46, 50, 321
Gabapentin, 483–484, 563
GAIN-SS. See Global Appraisal of
    Individual Needs—Short
    Screener

Gamblers Anonymous, 421
Gambling disorder
  assessment of, 256
  as behavioral addiction, 250–251
  clinical characteristics of, 256
  epidemiology of, 255–256
  family history of, 257
  functional impairment, quality of
    life, and legal difficulties in,
    256–257
  pharmacotherapy for, 258
  psychiatric comorbidity with, 257
  psychologically based treatments for,
    257–258
  treatment recommendations for, 258
Gaming disorder, Internet, 267–268
γ-Hydroxybutyric acid (GHB),
    134–135, 312–313
Gastrointestinal malignancy, 462
Gastrointestinal system
  alcohol use and, 435, 460–461
  infections of, 476–477
  stimulant effects, 62–63
  substance use and, 439, 461–463
  tobacco use and, 462
Gateway effect, e-cigarettes, 110
Gay persons, problematic sexual
    behavior among, 263
Gender
  cocaine use disorder and, 340
  college drinking risk and, 246
  differences in alcohol and substance
    use based on, 219
  SUD risk and, 3, 13
Gene doping, 106
Generalist nurse, in addiction care,
    203–204
Generalized anxiety disorder, 517–519
Genes, stressors and, 592
GHB. See γ-Hydroxybutyric acid
Ghrelin, 252
Gingivitis, 475
Glaucoma, cannabinoid treatment, 81
Global Appraisal of Individual Needs—
    Short Screener (GAIN-SS),
    604, 605t
Glutamate, 25, 64
Glutamate-activated ion channels,
    alcohol effects, 46
Glycine receptors, alcohol effects, 46
Goal-directed behavior development,
    593
G protein–coupled receptors, 26, 79
Graves disease, 490
Group therapies, 361–362
Guanfacine, 527, 528t
Guidance for opioid use, 651
  CDC, 579, 653
  challenges for, 652
  common features of, 652
  DEA, 579

FDA, 579
  FSMB, 653
  national, 578, 653
  PDMPs, 579–580, 643, 647, 652
  state-specific, 578–579, 653–654
  variations in emphasis across,
    652–653
Gum, nicotine, 342

H
HAART. See Highly active
    antiretroviral therapy
Hair, drug testing, 661–662
Halazepam, 51
Half-life, 40–41
Hallucinations, alcohol withdrawal,
    291
Hallucinogens
  drug target blockade, 23t
  epidemiology, 85
  intoxication, 310
  neurologic disorders and, 471–472
  pharmacology, 84–89
  psychiatric symptoms induced by,
    511t
  withdrawal, 310–312
Hallucinogen use disorder, 85, 349–350
HAN. See Heroin-associated
    nephropathy
Hangover, 290
Harm reduction
  addiction treatment integration
    with, 189
  definition and principles of, 189
  interventions
    access to clean injection
      equipment, 190–191, 191t, 216
    consumer drug testing to reduce
      risk of contaminant ingestion,
      192–193
    managed alcohol programs, 192
    medications to prevent injection
      and overdose risks, 192
    naloxone to prevent overdose,
      189–190, 215–216
    opioid antagonists for alcohol
      use, 192
    overdose risk education, 189–190,
      190t
    pre- and post–HIV exposure
      prophylaxis medication,
      191–192
    strategies and mechanisms of, 190t
    supervised drug consumption
      venues, 191
  for nonmedical prescription
      medication use, 215–217, 216t
Harrison Narcotic Tax Act, 650
Hashish, 78
Hash oil, 78
HBV. See Hepatitis B virus

hCG. *See* Human chorionic
    gonadotropin
HCV. *See* Hepatitis C virus
HDV. *See* Hepatitis D virus
Head, stimulant effects, 63
Headache, 470–471
Health care
    effecting change in
        action, 37
        multispecialty interdisciplinary
            team, 36–37
        shared purpose and plan of
            action, 37
        strategy for evaluation and
            improvement, 37
        systems approach, 36
    incarceration and, 672
Health information exchange (HIE), 42
    CFR Part 2 and, 638–639
Health information organization
    (HIO), 42 CFR Part 2 and,
    638–639
Health Insurance Portability and
    Accountability Act (HIPAA) of
    1996, confidentiality, 637
Healthy living, therapeutic community
    view of, 385
Heart failure, 443
Heat-not-burn (HNB) devices, 111
Heat therapy, 560
Heavy drinking, 154–156
    college student, 245–249
Helplessness versus self-efficacy, 555
Hepatitis, 433, 435, 448–452
Hepatitis B virus (HBV), 450–451
Hepatitis C virus (HCV), 451–452
    harm reduction interventions for,
        190–191, 191*t*
    nonmedical prescription medication
        use and, 213–214
Hepatitis D virus (HDV), 452
Hepatorenal syndrome (HRS), 455
Hepatotoxicity
    anabolic–androgenic steroids, 104
    inhalants, 100
Hepatotoxins, 448
Herbal remedies, 186–188, 339
Herbs of abuse, 313
Heroin, 214
    aversion therapy for, 392
    laboratory testing for, 133–134
    neuroanatomy of reinforcement,
        19–20
    neurologic disorders and, 470–473
    pharmacology, 55–56
    withdrawal, 306
Heroin-associated nephropathy
    (HAN), 456
HIE. *See* Health information exchange
Highly active antiretroviral therapy
    (HAART), 329

High-risk situations, relapse prevention
    and, 404
High-volume sexual behaviors
    (HVSBs), 260–261
HIO. *See* Health information
    organization
HIPAA. *See* Health Insurance Portability
    and Accountability Act
Histone deacetylases, 26
HIV. *See* Human immunodeficiency
    virus
HIV-associated nephropathy (HIVAN),
    455–456
HNB devices. *See* Heat-not-burn
    devices
Holiday heart, 443–444
Homeless, community reinforcement
    approach for, 372
Hormonal therapies, for paraphilic
    disorders, 264
Hormonal treatments, for anabolic–
    androgenic steroid use, 347
Hospitals
    adolescent substance abuse in, 610
    care at, 435
    screening and brief intervention in,
        125–126
    SUD treatment in, 161–162
Host defenses, 475
HPA axis. *See* Hypothalamic–
    pituitary–adrenal axis
HRS. *See* Hepatorenal syndrome
5-HT. *See* Serotonin
5-HT₃ receptors. *See*
    5-Hydroxytryptamine type 3
    receptors
5-HT receptors. *See*
    5-Hydroxytryptamine
Human chorionic gonadotropin
    (hCG), 102
Human development. *See* Development
Human growth hormone, 102
Human immunodeficiency virus
    (HIV), 5, 477
    harm reduction interventions for,
        190–192, 191*t*, 216–217
    linked services for, 182, 184
    nonmedical prescription medication
        use and, 213
    pharmacotherapy for, opioid agonist
        interactions with, 329
    women with, 220
Huss, Magnus, 148
HVSBs. *See* High-volume sexual
    behaviors
Hydrocodone (Vicodin)
    laboratory testing for, 133–134, 134*t*
    pharmacology, 55–56
Hydromorphone (Dilaudid)
    laboratory testing for, 133–134, 134*t*
    pharmacology, 55–56

5-Hydroxytryptamine (5-HT)
    receptors, 84
5-Hydroxytryptamine type 3 (5-HT₃)
    receptors, 46
Hyperalgesia, opioid-induced,
    550–551, 569
Hyperglycemia, 490, 491*t*
Hypersexual disorder, 260–261
Hypertension, 443
    pulmonary, 466
Hyperuricemia, 437
Hypnotics. *See* Sedative–hypnotics
Hypoglycemia, 490, 491*t*
Hypomagnesemia, 455
Hypothalamic–pituitary–adrenal
    (HPA) axis
    alcohol use and, 594
    antireward system and, 591
    stressors, genes and, 592

I
ICCE. *See* International Centre for
    Credentialing and Education of
    Addiction Professionals
ICDs. *See* Impulse control disorders
IDC. *See* Individual drug counseling
IGD. *See* Internet gaming disorder
Imipramine, 340
Imminent danger, residential treatment
    for, 174
Immune system
    cannabinoid effects, 80
    stimulant effects, 63
Immunoassay
    predictive value of, 660
    urine, 130–135, 131*t*, 134*t*
Impulse control disorders (ICDs), 250.
    See also Behavioral addiction
Incarceration, SUD treatment during,
    672–674
Incidence, 11
Individual drug counseling (IDC), 367
Individualized treatment plans, 172,
    177
Individual prevention
    environmental approaches versus,
        142–143
    risk and protective factors in, 583
Individual treatment
    for college student drinking,
        247–248
    network therapy and, 381
    psychotherapies (*See* Psychotherapy)
Infectious diseases
    alcohol use and, 436–437
    endocarditis, 475–476
    gingivitis, 475
    harm reduction interventions for,
        190–192, 191*t*, 216
    hepatic and gastrointestinal,
        476–477

Infectious diseases (*Continued*)
  HIV (*See* Human immunodeficiency
    virus)
  nervous system, 477
  neurologic complications of,
    473–474
  noncardiac vascular, 476
  nonmedical prescription medication
    use and, 213–214
  respiratory, 465–466, 476
  sexually transmitted diseases, 433,
    477
  skin and soft tissue, 475
Inflammatory bowel disease, 462
Informed consent
  in addiction medicine, 636–637
  controlled substances and, 645–646
  for special populations, 640–641
Inhalants
  drug target blockade of, 23*t*
  endocrine and reproductive
    disorders with, 491*t*, 492
  epidemiology of, 98–99
  historical features of, 97–98
  intoxication with, 312
  pharmacological interventions for,
    348
  pharmacology, 97–100, 98*t*
  renal effects of, 457
  respiratory system and, 466
  withdrawal from, 312
Inhalation of drugs, 439
Inhaler, nicotine, 343
Inheritability studies, 592–593
Injection drug use, 438–439
  access to clean equipment for,
    190–191, 191*t*, 216
  infectious diseases with, 475–477
  respiratory complications of, 466
  SUD treatment medications for
    preventing, 192
  supervised drug consumption
    venues for, 191
Injury. *See* Trauma
Inpatient detoxification, 287–288
Insomnia, 235, 480
Institute of Medicine (IOM), 196, 657
Insulin resistance, 490
Integrated care
  chronic care management model for,
    167–170, 168*t*
  implementation and sustainability
    of, 170
  integrating behavioral with
    pharmacologic interventions
    in, 412–416
  linked services, 181–183, 182*t*
  unprecedented historical moment
    for, 166–167
Intensive outpatient treatment, for
  adolescent substance abuse, 610

Interdisciplinary team, for effecting
  change in health care, 36–37
International addiction management
  medical association roles in, 208
  policy frameworks for, 206–207
  WHO and UNODC roles in,
    207–208
  worldwide prevalence of substance
    use and, 206
International Centre for Credentialing
  and Education of Addiction
  Professionals (ICCE), 200
International medical associations, 208
International Society of Addiction
  Medicine (ISAM), 208
Internet addiction, 253, 267–270
Internet gaming disorder (IGD),
  267–268
Interpersonal functioning, 365
  in relapse prevention, 404–405
Intimate social network (ISN), 242,
  242*t*
Intoxication
  for adolescent placement criteria,
    608
  alcohol, 290
  assessment tools for, 138–139
  caffeine, 68
  cannabinoids, 81, 311, 311*t*
  club drugs, 312–314
  dissociatives, 95, 311
  hallucinogens, 310
  identification of, 285
  inhalants, 312
  management of, 285–286, 309
  opioids, 304–305
  sedative–hypnotics, 298, 322–323
  stimulants, 62, 309–310
Intoxication stage, of addiction cycle,
  2–3, 3*f*
IOM. *See* Institute of Medicine
ISAM. *See* International Society of
  Addiction Medicine
ISN. *See* Intimate social network

J
Justice, in addiction practice, 631–632

K
Kennedy, Foster, 149
Ketamine (Ketalar)
  epidemiology of, 92
  historical features of, 91–92
  intoxication and withdrawal, 311
  laboratory testing for, 134–135
  for pain, 563
  pharmacological interventions for,
    348
  pharmacology, 91–95
  psychiatric symptoms induced by,
    511*t*

Ketones, 97–100, 98*t*
Khat, 60, 313
Kidneys, 81. *See also* Renal effects
Kinesiophobia, 554
Kleptomania, 273–274
Kolb, Lawrence, 149
Korsakoff syndrome, 295
Kratom, 115
Krokodil, 115–116
Kudzu plant, 187

L
LAAM. *See* Levo-alpha-acetylmethadol
Labor and delivery, 497
Laboratory testing
  in adolescents, 600
  approach to, 130–131, 131*t*
  ethical considerations in, 135, 633
  identification of intoxication, 285
  for older adults, 237
  for pregnant women, 494–495, 498
  results assessments for, 659–660
  substance-specific tests, 131–135,
    134*t*, 285
Lactation, 52, 75
Lamotrigine, 340, 563
Lapse, 402
Laughing gas, 91–92, 97
Laws
  cannabis legalization, youth and,
    587–590
  federal (*See* Federal laws)
  for opioid use (*See* Guidance for
    opioid use)
Laxatives, 462
Learned tolerance, 42
Learning disorders, SUD development
  and, 593
Legal consultation, for ethical issues,
  634
Legal difficulties, in gambling disorder,
  256–257
Legalization, of recreational cannabis,
  589–590
Length of stay (LOS), 173, 176
Lennox-Gastaut syndrome, 656
Leptin, 251–252
Lesbian persons, problematic sexual
  behavior among, 263
Levels of care
  ASAM Criteria, 173–174, 175*t*
  for adolescents, 609–610
  linkages between, 610–611
  mandated treatment and, 176
  transition between, in relapse
    prevention, 406
Levo-alpha-acetylmethadol
  (levomethadyl acetate, LAAM),
  56–57, 326
Liability, addiction. *See* Addiction
  liability

Librium. *See* Chlordiazepoxide
Licensed providers, collaborative care with, 414–415
Lidocaine, 563–564
Lifestyle, in relapse prevention, 405–406
Limbic system, 16–21, 17*f*
Linked services, 179–184, 180*t*, 182*t*
Lithium, 340
Liver
    alcohol use and, 435, 448–452, 449*t*, 501
    cannabinoid effects, 80
    infections of, 476–477
    stimulant effects, 63
    substance use and, 452
Living environment, adolescent placement criteria and, 609
Lofexidine, 306, 326–327
LOS. *See* Length of stay
Lozenges, nicotine, 342
LSD. *See* Lysergic acid diethylamide
Lumbar stabilization, 559
Lysergic acid diethylamide (LSD), 84–86, 133, 349

M

Magnesium, for alcohol withdrawal, 295
Magnetic resonance imaging studies, 593
Maintenance stage of change, 355
Maldynia, 548
Managed alcohol programs, 192
Mandated treatment, 163, 176
MAOIs. *See* Monoamine oxidase inhibitors
Marijuana, 78. *See also* Cannabinoids; Cannabis
    adolescent use of, 582
    early onset and persistent, 594
    endocrine and reproductive disorders with, 491*t*, 492
    epidemiology, recent trends, 13
    intoxication, 311, 311*t*
    laboratory testing for, 133
    older adults using, 233–234
    for pain, 563
    pharmacotherapy for, 621–622
    physician use of, 279
    potency of, 588–589
    prenatal exposure to, 591
    respiratory system and, 467
    sleep and, 483
    withdrawal, 311
Marijuana Anonymous, 421
Marijuana use disorder, 347, 391, 409
Marinol. *See* Dronabinol
Marital status, substance use disorder risk and, 14
Martha Washington Society, 420

Massage therapy, 560
Mass spectrometry (MS), for drug testing, 660–661
Maximal efficacy, 41
McKenzie therapy, 559
MDFT. *See* Multidimensional family therapy
MDMA. *See* 3,4-Methylenedioxy-methamphetamine
Mechanical diagnosis and therapy, 559
Mechanisms of addiction
    alcohol, 45–47
    binge/intoxication stage, 2–3, 3*f*
    caffeine, 67
    nicotine and tobacco, 74, 342
    opioids, 57–58
    preoccupation/anticipation (craving) stage, 3*f*, 4
    stimulants, 63–64
    withdrawal/negative affect stage, 3–4, 3*f*
Mechanisms of change, 426–427
Medically integrated therapeutic communities, 388
Medically managed intensive inpatient treatment, for adolescent substance abuse, 610
Medically supervised withdrawal, opioid, 327–328
Medical management, 367, 413
Medical records
    confidentiality of, 636
    controlled medications and, 644
Medical review officer (MRO), 664–665
Medical Review Officer Certification Council, 665
Medical training, as barrier to linked services, 179
Medical treatment services, linking addiction treatment with, 179–184, 180*t*, 182*t*
Medication adherence, 413
Mendez, Juan E., 672
Mental disorders. *See* Psychiatric disorders; Substance-induced mental disorders
Mental healthcare, linking addiction treatment with, 179–184, 180*t*, 182*t*
Mental Health Parity and Addiction Equity Act (MHPAEA), 181, 196, 198
Men who have sex with men (MSM), 262–263
Meperidine, 56
Mescaline, 84–85
    pharmacokinetics, pharmacodynamics, and subjective effects, 87–88

Metabolic disorders
    alcohol use and, 436, 454–455
    substance use and, 440
Metabolism, 40–41
    anabolic–androgenic steroids, 105–106
    benzodiazepines, 51
    nicotine, 72
    stimulants, 61
Methadone, 214
    in adolescents, 622
    approval of, 651
    drug action mimicry, 24*f*, 25
    federal regulations on, 578
    HIV pharmacotherapy interactions with, 329
    intoxication and overdose, 304–305
    laboratory testing for, 134, 134*t*
    for mixed cocaine and opioid use disorder, 339
    in multiple use disorders, 348–349
    for opioid use disorder, 326
        maintenance treatment, 328–330, 332–333
    for opioid withdrawal, 306–307, 327
    pain treatment and, 575
    pharmacology, 56
    for pregnant women, 220
    for prescription medication use disorders, 217
    for preventing injection and overdose risks, 192
Methadone-to-buprenorphine transfer, 307, 329–330
Methamphetamine, 61, 63–64, 132–133
Methylene chloride, 98*t*
3,4-Methylenedioxymethamphetamine (MDMA), 84–85
    intoxication, 312
    neurologic disorders and, 470–473
    pharmacokinetics, pharmacodynamics, and subjective effects, 88–89
    psychiatric symptoms induced by, 511*t*
    renal effects of, 452, 457
    sleep and, 482
Methylphenidate
    for ADHD treatment, 527, 528*t*
    pharmacology, 62, 64
    SUD development and, 593
MHPAEA. *See* Mental Health Parity and Addiction Equity Act
MI. *See* Motivational interviewing
Microprocessor-based disorders
    assessment of, 268–269
    as behavioral addiction, 253
    definition of, 267
    diagnostic dilemmas in, 267–268

Microprocessor-based disorders (*Continued*)
epidemiology and comorbidity of, 269
historical perspective on, 267
neuroimaging and neuropsychological correlates in, 268
pretreatment issues in, 269–270
treatment model for, 269
treatment planning for, 269
treatment research in, 270
Milieu groups, 360
Military families, 681–682
Military personnel
college drinking in, 246
family therapy for, 397
SUDs in
historical perspective on, 675–676, 676f
learning from history and, 678
military medical system treatment of, 678, 679f
prevalence of, 677, 677f
risk factors for military families, 681–682
TBI in, 225
Military sexual trauma (MST)
barriers to reporting of, 229–230
clinical issues of, 230–231
getting VA help for, 231, 231t
military culture and, 230
Mimicry, of drug action, 24–25, 24f
Mindfulness-based approaches, to adolescent substance use treatment, 618
Minerals, 434
Minnesota Model, 154, 431
Minors, sex with, 262
Mirtazapine, 517, 518t
Misuse, 322
Mitragynine, 115
Modafinil, 527
Modified therapeutic communities (MTCs), 386–388, 387t
Monitoring, clinical trials, 31
Monoamine oxidase inhibitors (MAOIs), 338, 527, 528t
Mood disorders. *See also* Bipolar disorder; Depressive disorders
co-occurring SUD, 513–515
in physicians, 279
substance-related, 513–514
SUD development and, 592
in women with addictive disorders, 221
MOPr. *See* μ receptor
Morbidity
of microprocessor-based disorders, 269
nicotine and tobacco, 76
Morphine, 55, 133–134, 134t

Mortality
alcohol-related causes, 141–142
of microprocessor-based disorders, 269
nicotine and tobacco, 76
Motivation
to change, 354–358, 357t
in microprocessor-based disorder treatment, 269–270
neurobiology of, 2–5, 3f
to quit smoking, 375
to reduce or stop substance use and adhere to treatment, 365
in relapse prevention, 403–404
in twelve-step facilitation, 400–401
Motivational enhancement therapy, 163, 365–366
Motivational interventions, for college student drinking, 247
Motivational interview groups, 362
Motivational interviewing (MI), 365–366, 412
Motivational treatment, adolescent substance use treatment, 617–618
Motives, drinking, 246
Motor vehicle crashes, 142
Movement disorders, 81, 473
MRO. *See* Medical review officer
MS. *See* Mass spectrometry
MSM. *See* Men who have sex with men
MST. *See* Military sexual trauma; Multisystemic therapy
MTCs. *See* Modified therapeutic communities
Multicomponent skills-based interventions, for college student drinking, 247
Multidimensional family therapy (MDFT), 164, 615
Multiple sclerosis, 656
Multiple use disorders, pharmacotherapy for, 339–340, 348–349
Multisystemic therapy (MST), 615
μ receptor (MOPr), 19, 55, 58, 186–188, 304
Muscle relaxants, 50, 564
Musculoskeletal system
alcohol use and, 437–438
stimulant effects, 63

N
NA. *See* Narcotics Anonymous
Nabilone, 81, 656
NAcc. *See* Nucleus accumbens
Nalmefene (Revex), 55
Naloxone (Narcan), 434
for opioid overdose, 58, 304–305
for opioid use disorder, 326, 334
overdose prevention with, 189–190, 215–216

pharmacology, 55
for pregnant women, 220
synthetic opioid treatment, 114–115
Naltrexone (Trexan, ReVia, or Vivitrol)
in adolescents, 621–622
for alcohol use disorder, 155, 316–317, 621
alcohol use reduction with, 192
for amphetamine use disorder, 339
for co-occurring mood and SUDs, 514
drug target blockade, 23, 24f
in multiple use disorders, 349
for opioid use disorder, 326, 328
for opioid withdrawal, 306–307
pharmacology, 55
for prescription medication use disorders, 217
for problematic sexual behavior, 264
surgery and, 502
for tobacco and alcohol use disorders, 348
Narcan. *See* Naloxone
Narcotics Anonymous (NA), 421
NAS. *See* Neonatal abstinence syndrome
Nasal spray, nicotine, 342
National Academy of Medicine, 196
National Epidemiologic Survey on Alcohol and Related Conditions (NESARC), 11–15
National Institute on Drug Abuse (NIDA), 150
National Quality Forum (NQF), 197, 197f
National Survey on Drug Use and Health (NSDUH), 12–14
cannabis legalization and, 588–589
Nausea aversion, 390
Neck, stimulant effects, 63
Needles, access to clean, 190–191, 191t, 216
Negative affect, relapse prevention and, 404–405
Negative affect stage, of addiction cycle, 3–4, 3f
Neonatal abstinence syndrome (NAS), 329, 495
Neonatal health
alcohol use and, 437
stimulant effects, 63
substance use and, 441
Neonatal opioid withdrawal syndrome, 496
Nephritic–nephrotic syndromes, 456
Nephritic syndromes, 456
Nephrology, 454
Nephrotic syndromes, 455–456
Nervous system infections, 477
NESARC. *See* National Epidemiologic Survey on Alcohol and Related Conditions

Network therapy (NT), 379–382
Neuroanatomy
    of drug addiction, 20
    of drug reinforcement, 16
        cannabinoids, 20
        opioids, 19–20
        psychostimulants, 17–19, 18*f*
        primer on, 16, 17*f*
Neurobehavioral disorders, 471, 496
Neurobiology
    of addiction
        binge/intoxication stage, 2–3, 3*f*
        preoccupation/anticipation
            (craving) stage, 3*f*, 4
        withdrawal/negative affect stage,
            3–4, 3*f*
    of addiction from developmental
            perspective
        adolescent brain development,
            593, 603
        biologic predispositions,
            development, and risk, 594
        biopsychosocial analysis, 591–592
        early onset and persistent
            marijuana use, 594
        family and peers role during, 594
        goal-directed behavior
            development, 593
        inheritability studies, 592–593
        neuroimaging studies, 593–594
    alcohol, 45–47
    caffeine, 67
    cannabinoids, 79
    cannabis and adolescent brain,
        587–588
    in comorbid PTSD and SUDs, 538
    dissociatives, 93–94
    gambling, 250–251
    hallucinogens, 84
    microprocessor-based disorders,
        268
    nicotine and tobacco, 74, 342
    opioids, 57–58
    stimulants, 63–65
Neurofeedback, for adolescent
        substance use treatment, 618
Neuroimaging studies
    of human development, 593–594
    in microprocessor-based disorders,
        268
Neuroimmune modulators, 47
Neuroleptic agents, 294
Neurologic disorders
    alcohol use and, 436, 470
    cannabinoid effects, 81
    substance use and, 439
Neuromodulation, 351–352
Neuromuscular disorders, 472–473
Neurotoxicity
    inhalants, 100
    stimulants, 65

Neurotransmitters. *See also specific*
        neurotransmitters
    alcohol effects, 47
    gambling effects, 251
NIATx Model, 198–199
Nicotine
    in adolescents, 620–621
    alcohol use disorder association
        with, 76
    caffeine interactions, 70
    drug action mimicry of, 24*f*, 25
    drug target blockade of, 23, 23*t*, 24*f*
    in e-cigarettes, 108–109
    during incarceration, 673
    neurobiology of, 74, 342
    pharmacology, 72–76
    pregnancy effects of, 75, 495
    prenatal exposure to, 591
    psychiatric symptoms induced by,
        510*t*
    sleep and, 482–483
    stroke and, 472
    withdrawal from, 74, 438
Nicotine replacement therapy (NRT),
        342–343, 343*t*
    in adolescents, 620–621
    clinical decisions about, 346
    combination pharmacotherapy with,
        344–345, 345*t*
    in multiple use disorders, 348
Nicotine use
    aversion therapy for, 391
    behavioral interventions for,
        374–377
    older adult use of, 234
    by physicians, 278–279
Nicotinic receptors
    alcohol effects, 46
    tobacco effects, 74, 342
NIDA. *See* National Institute on Drug
        Abuse
Nitrous oxide
    dissociative effects, 91–94
    inhalant abuse, 97–100, 98*t*
    respiratory system and, 468–469
N-methyl-D-aspartate (NMDA)
        receptors, 46, 91, 93–94
Nociception, 548
Nonalcoholic fatty liver disease, 448
Nonbenzodiazepine hypnotics, 50–53
Noncardiac vascular infections, 476
Nonmaleficence, 631
Nonmedical prescription medication
        use. *See* Prescription
        medications
Nonmedical use. *See* Controlled
        medications
Nonopioid analgesics, 562–564
Non–rapid eye movement (NREM), 479
Nonsteroidal anti-inflammatory drugs
        (NSAIDs), 562

Norepinephrine
    in alcohol withdrawal syndromes,
        292
    drug reinforcement and, 16–19, 18*f*
    gambling effects, 251
    stimulant effects, 64
Normative education, 584
Norms
    cultural, 240–241
    social, 246
Novel psychoactive substances (NPS),
        113
    examples, 114–116
    harm reduction interventions for,
        192–193
    identifying and accessing
        information on, 116, 116*t*
    intoxication management and, 286,
        309
    laboratory testing for, 134–135
    screening and brief intervention, 126
    treatment, 114
NPI-025, 186–187
NPI-028, 187
NPs. *See* Nurse practitioners
NPS. *See* Novel psychoactive
        substances
NQF. *See* National Quality Forum
NREM. *See* Non–rapid eye movement
NRT. *See* Nicotine replacement therapy
NSAIDs. *See* Nonsteroidal anti-
        inflammatory drugs
NSDUH. *See* National Survey on Drug
        Use and Health
NT. *See* Network therapy
Nucleus accumbens (NAcc), 16, 19–20,
        250–252
Nurse practitioners (NPs), 202–203
Nursing, addiction care roles of
    addiction nurse, 204
    current substance use trends and,
        202–203
    generalist's roles, 203–204
    history of development of, 202
    levels of nursing education and
        practice in, 203
    workforce available for, 204–205
Nutritional supplements, 339
Nyswander, Marie, 150

O
OAT. *See* Opioid agonist therapy
Obesity, 448, 541, 544
Obsessive-compulsive disorder (OCD),
        509, 518–519
Obstructive sleep apnea, 480–482
Occupation, substance use disorder
        risk and, 14
Occupational therapy, 559–560
OCD. *See* Obsessive-compulsive
        disorder

Odds ratio, 11
OFC. *See* Orbitofrontal cortex
Office-based opioid treatment, 332–335
OIH. *See* Opioid-induced hyperalgesia
Older adults
alcohol use in, 128–129, 129*t*, 233–238, 234*t*, 237*t*
autonomy and, 633
co-occurring mood and SUDs in, 515
family therapy for, 397
screening and brief intervention for, 122, 128–129, 129*t*
sleep in, 235
SUDs in
co-occurring disorders with, 235, 515
formal addiction treatment for, 237–238
intervention strategies for, 237
issues unique to, 234–235, 234*t*
relapse reduction for, 238
scope of problem, 233–234
screening and detection of, 235–237, 237*t*
treatment outcome research for, 238
Omnibus Transportation Employee Testing Act, 665
Ondansetron, 621
On-site models, of linked services, 181–183, 182*t*
On-site testing, 130
Opiates
endogenous, 64
laboratory testing for, 133–134, 134*t*
medical consequences of, 438–441
psychiatric symptoms induced by, 510*t*
Opioid agonists, HIV pharmacotherapy interactions with, 329
Opioid agonist therapy (OAT)
for opioid use disorder, 326, 328–330
for opioid withdrawal, 306–307, 327
pain treatment with, 575–576
perioperative period, 502–503, 503*t*
Opioid antagonists
alcohol use reduction with, 192
for opioid use disorder, 326, 328, 330
for opioid withdrawal, 307
for problematic sexual behavior, 264
Opioid-induced hyperalgesia (OIH), 550–551, 569
Opioid peptides, 47
Opioid receptors
addiction liability and, 58
drug reinforcement and, 19–20
in intoxication and overdose, 304
opioid effects, 55, 58
traditional medicines blocking, 186–188

Opioids
abstinence syndrome, 327–328
drug action mimicry, 24*f*, 25
drug–drug interactions of, 51–52, 58
drug target blockade, 23, 23*t*, 24*f*
epidemiology, 13, 57–58
intoxication, 304–305
laboratory testing for, 133–134, 134*t*
neuroanatomy of reinforcement, 19–20
nonmedical prescription use of, 122, 211–217, 212*f*, 213*f*, 216*t*
overdose, 304–305
naloxone for, 189–190, 215–216
risk education for preventing, 189–190, 190*t*
SUD treatment medications for preventing, 192
pharmacology, 55–59
prevalence of use and misuse of, 567–568
side effects of, 570–571
synthetic (*See* Synthetic opioids)
Opioid therapy
clinical variables in, 569–571
dose titration and scheduling, 570
drug selection for, 569–570
evolving guidance on, 573–574
historical perspectives on, 566–567
legal and regulatory considerations for, 578–580
physical dependence, 568–569
position of, 568
rewards, 569
routes of administration, 570
side effects, 570–571
special issues in use of, 568–569
tolerance, 569
universal precautions in, 571
use and misuse of, 567–568
written agreement for, 570
Opioid use
cardiovascular system and, 445
for chronic pain, 651–654 (*See also* Opioid therapy)
endocrine and reproductive disorders with, 491–492, 491*t*
gastrointestinal system and, 461–462
guidelines, laws, and regulations for (*See* Guidance for opioid use)
harm reduction interventions for (*See* Harm reduction)
by military personnel, 675–679, 676*f*, 677*f*, 679*f*
monitoring for misuse, 574, 574*t*
neurologic disorders and, 470–473
nonmedical prescription, 122, 211–217, 212*f*, 213*f*, 216*t*
nursing care roles in, 202
by physicians, 279
in pregnancy, 496

prevalence of, 567–568
renal effects of, 455–456
respiratory system and, 467–468
sleep and, 482
worldwide prevalence of, 206
Opioid use disorder (OUD)
alcohol use disorder with, 349
anxiety disorders and, 520
aversion therapy for, 392
chronic pain and, 550, 573–576
cocaine use disorder with, 339–340, 349
epidemiology, 57–58
herbal remedies for, 186–187
monitoring for, 574, 574*t*
perioperative patient and, 502–503, 503*t*
pharmacologic interventions for, 326
abstinence syndromes and medically supervised withdrawal, 327–328
in adolescents, 622
during incarceration and release, 673
long-term maintenance therapies, 328–330
in multiple drug use disorders, 349
office-based treatment, 332–335
tobacco use disorder with, 348
treatment for, 520
Opioid withdrawal, 305
alternative therapies for, 187
assessment tools for, 138–139
during incarceration, 672
initial management of, 125
pharmacologic therapies for, 306–307, 327–328
Opium Commission, 650
Oral cavity, 460
Oral contraceptives, 73
Oral fluids, drug testing, 130, 661
Orbitofrontal cortex (OFC), 226
Orexin, 252
Organ systems, cannabinoid effects, 80–81
Organ transplantation, 504
O'Shaughnessy, William, 78
Osteoporosis, 434
OUD. *See* Opioid use disorder
Outcome expectancies, in relapse prevention, 403
Outcomes
clinical trials, 30–31
contingency management, 371–372
of modified therapeutic communities, 388
quality improvement, 197–198, 197*f*
of twelve-step programs, 422
for unhealthy alcohol use, 155–156

Outpatient detoxification, 288
Outpatient programs, 162, 610
Overdose
  in adolescents, 623
  cannabinoids, 81
  dissociatives, 95
  opioid, 304–305
    naloxone for, 189–190, 215–216
    risk education for preventing,
      189–190, 190*t*
    SUD treatment medications for
      preventing, 192
  prevention of
    naloxone, 189–190, 215–216
    risk education, 189–190, 190*t*
    SUD treatment medications for,
      192
    supervised drug consumption
      venues for, 191
  sedative–hypnotics, 298
Oxcarbazepine, 563
Oxford Group, 420
Oxycodone (OxyContin), 55–56,
  133–134, 134*t*
Oxymorphone, 133–134, 134*t*

P
PA. *See* Protracted abstinence
Pain. *See also* Chronic pain
  addiction and management of, 571
  addiction treatment in presence
    of, 576
  during hospitalization, 435
  nonopioid analgesics for, 562–564
  opioid prescription guidelines for,
    215, 216*t*
  opioid therapy for, 568–572
  physicians with, 279
  prevalence of, 567
Pancreas, 460–461
Pancreatitis, 460–461
Panic attacks, 626
Panic disorder, 517–519
Paraphilias, 261–262
Paraphilic disorders, 261–262, 264
Parental involvement, confidentiality
  and, 121
Parotid glands, 460
Paroxetine (Paxil), 539
Partial hospital programs, 162
Particles, in e-cigarettes, 109
Patch, nicotine, 343, 343*t*
Pathologic gambling (PG), 255–258
  as behavioral addiction, 250–251
  Internet, 267–268
Patient, avoiding stigmatizing
  terminology, 7–8, 9*t*, 10
Patient self-management stage, of
  chronic care management, 168*t*,
  169–170
Paxil. *See* Paroxetine

Payment systems, as barrier to linked
  services, 180–181
PCP. *See* Phencyclidine
PDMPs. *See* Prescription drug
  monitoring programs
PDs. *See* Personality disorders
Pedophilia, 262
Peer factors, 603
Pentazocine, 56
Performance, caffeine effects, 68
Performance-enhancing drugs.
  See Anabolic–androgenic
    steroids
Perioperative patient
  alcohol use and, 438, 500–502
  opioid use disorder and, 502–503,
    503*t*
  substance use and, 440–441,
    503–504
  tobacco use and, 438, 503–504
Peripheral sensitization, 548–549
Person, therapeutic community view
  of, 384–385
Personal Experience Screening
  Questionnaire (PESQ), 604,
    605*t*
Personality, 592
Personality disorders (PDs), 532–535
Personal management stage, of chronic
  care management, 168*t*,
  169–170
PESQ. *See* Personal Experience
  Screening Questionnaire
PEth. *See* Phosphatidylethanol
Peyote cactus plant, 85, 87–88
PFC. *See* Prefrontal cortex
PG. *See* Pathologic gambling;
  Propylene glycol
Pharmacodynamics, 41–42, 85–89
  alcohol, 45
  cannabinoids, 79–80
  inhalants, 99
  stimulants, 62–63
Pharmacodynamic tolerance, 42
Pharmacogenomics, 41, 51
Pharmacokinetics, 40–41, 85–89
  alcohol, 45
  caffeine, 67
  cannabinoids, 79
  inhalants, 99
  nicotine and tobacco, 72
  sedative–hypnotics, 51
  stimulants, 61
Pharmacokinetic tolerance, 42
Pharmacology
  alcohol, 44–48
  anabolic–androgenic steroids,
    102–106
  caffeine, 66–70
  cannabinoids, 79–82
  dissociatives, 91–95

hallucinogens, 84–89
  inhalants, 97–100, 98*t*
  nicotine and tobacco, 72–76
  opioids, 55–59
  sedative–hypnotics, 50–53, 321
  stimulants, 60–66
Phencyclidine (PCP), 84
  drug target blockade, 23*t*
  epidemiology, 92
  historical features, 91–92
  intoxication and withdrawal, 311
  laboratory testing, 134
  pharmacological interventions for,
    348
  pharmacology, 91–95
  psychiatric symptoms induced by,
    511*t*
Phenobarbital
  for alcohol withdrawal, 293
  for sedative–hypnotic withdrawal,
    301–302, 302*t*, 323–324
Phentermine, 64
Phosphatidylethanol (PEth), 663
PHPs. *See* Physician health programs
Physical abuse, 222
Physical assault, college drinking and,
    245
Physical dependence, 42, 322, 550
Physical examination, 433
Physical therapy, active, 559
Physician. *See* Addiction medicine
  physician
Physician addiction
  characteristics of, 278
  comorbid disorders in, 279
  controversies over, 281–282
  drugs misused in, 278–279
  identification, intervention, and
    assessment of, 280
  prevalence of, 278
  risk factors for, 279
  theories of, 280
  treatment of, 280–283
Physician health programs (PHPs),
    278, 280–283
Physician's office, substance use
  disorder treatment in, 163
Phytocannabinoids, 655
PIU. *See* Problematic Internet use
Plan–Do–Study–Act cycles, 198–199
Plant-derived cannabinoids, 78
Plant-derived stimulants, 60
Point-of-care testing, 130
Policy, addiction treatment impact
  of, 198
Postacute withdrawal syndrome,
  benzodiazepines, 299
Postcessation weight gain, 345
Post–HIV exposure prophylaxis
  medication, 191–192
Postpartum care, 498

Posttraumatic stress disorder (PTSD)
  in adolescents, 626
  epidemiology of, 537
  phenomenology of, 537
  physicians with, 279
  SUD and, 537–540
  treatment of, 539–540
Posture mechanics, 560
Postwithdrawal treatment, sedative–
    hypnotic use disorder, 324
Potassium channels, 46–47
Potency, 41–42
  of cannabis, 588–589
Power, clinical trials, 29–30
PPD. *See* Primary psychotic disorders
Practitioner's Manual (DEA), 644
Precontemplation stage of change, 354
Predictive value, 660
Prefrontal cortex (PFC), 16, 20
  cannabis and adolescent, 587–588
  maturation of, 591–592
Pregabalin, 517, 518*t*, 563
Pregnancy
  alcohol use during, 219–220, 495–496
  benzodiazepine effects, 52
  cannabinoid effects, 81
  family therapy for substance use
      in, 397
  inhalant effects, 100
  laboratory testing for, 494–495
  legal issues in, 498
  nicotine and tobacco effects, 75, 495
  opioid agonist treatment during, 329
  opioid use in, 496
  screening and brief intervention in,
      123–125, 494
  substance use during, 496–498
Pre–HIV exposure prophylaxis
    medication, 191–192
Prenatal alcohol exposure, 219–220
Prenatal exposures, 591
Preoccupation stage, of addiction cycle,
    3*f*, 4
Preparation stage of change, 354–355
Prescriber education, 215, 216*t*
Prescription drug monitoring
    programs (PDMPs), 215,
    579–580, 643, 647, 652
Prescription medications
  alcohol interactions with, 233
  nonmedical use of
    epidemiology of, 211–214, 212*f*,
        213*f*
    evidence-based treatment for, 217
    major drug classes in, 211, 212*f*,
        214–215
    in older adults, 233, 235–237, 237*t*
    prevention and harm reduction
        strategies for, 215–217, 216*t*
    screening and brief interventions
        for, 122

Prescription medication use disorders,
    211, 217
Prescription order, 644
Prescription take-back programs, 217
Pre–substance dependence, 655
Prevalence, 11
Preventive counseling, 434
Primary care
  linking addiction treatment with,
      179–184, 180*t*, 182*t*
  screening and brief intervention in,
      119–120, 122
Primary care provider
  identification, treatment, or referral
      and monitoring of SUDs by,
      199–200
  substance use assessment by, 136
Primary care settings, co-occurring
    mood and SUDs in, 514
Primary psychotic disorder (PPD),
    508
Principles of change, 356–358, 357*t*
Problematic Internet use (PIU), 253
Problematic sexual behavior (PSB)
  assessment of, 263
  as behavioral addiction, 252–253
  compulsive sex in combination with
      substance use, 262–263
  high-volume, 260–261
  historical and cultural context of,
      260
  among lesbian, gay, bisexual, and
      transgender persons, 263
  paraphilias and paraphilic disorders,
      261–262, 264
  pedophilia and sex with minors, 262
  pharmacotherapy, 264
  treatment of
    CBT, 263–264
    twelve-step and self-help groups,
        264
Problematic video game playing
    (PVG), 253
Problem-solving therapy groups, 361
Processes of change, 356–358, 357*t*
Professionalism, 35
Professional standards, for ethical
    issues, 633–634
Profile of Mood States, 555
Project MATCH, 413–414
Prolapse, 402
Prolonged withdrawal,
    benzodiazepines, 299, 302, 324
Propofol, 279
Propylene glycol (PG), in e-cigarettes,
    108
Protective effects, caffeine, 70
Protective factors, for adolescent
    substance use, 583
Protracted abstinence (PA), opioid,
    327–328

PSB. *See* Problematic sexual behavior
Pseudoephedrine, 60, 63
Psilocybin, 84–85, 349
  pharmacokinetics,
      pharmacodynamics, and
      subjective effects, 86
Psychiatric disorders. *See also specific
    disorders*
  comorbid (*See* Comorbid psychiatric
      disorders)
  eating disorders and, 542
  substance-induced, 509, 510*t*
Psychiatric treatment services, linking
    addiction treatment with,
    179–184, 180*t*, 182*t*
Psychiatry residents, network therapy
    provided by, 381
Psychoeducational recovery groups, 360
Psychological benefits, of substance
    use, 604
Psychomotor functions, cannabinoid
    effects, 80
Psychopathology, cannabinoid effects,
    80
Psychostimulants, 17–19, 18*f*, 462
Psychotherapists, collaborative care
    with, 414–415
Psychotherapy
  common elements of, 365
  development of, 364
  evidence-based, 365–367
  history of, 364
  matching patients with, 367
  training clinicians to deliver, 368
  virtual and computer-delivered,
      367–368
Psychotic disorders
  co-occurring addiction and,
      522–524
  substance-induced, 508–509,
      522–523
PTSD. *See* Posttraumatic stress
    disorder
Public health
  addiction medicine physician as
      agent of
    effecting change in health care,
        36–38
    physician responsibility, 33
    physician role, 34–35
    protecting and promoting public
        health, 33–34
    transformational change, 35–36
  incarceration and, 672
Pueraria lobata, 187
Pulmonary effects, stimulants, 62
Pulmonary hypertension, 466
PVG. *See* Problematic video game
    playing
Pyramiding, anabolic–androgenic
    steroids, 104

Q

Quality control, clinical trials, 31
Quality improvement
  accreditation for treatment
    programs, 198
  building system capacity to deliver
    effective treatments, 198–199
  defining and measuring quality
    treatment and outcomes,
    197–198, 197f
  ensuring primary care providers
    can identify, treat, or refer and
    monitor SUDs, 199–200
  evaluating policy impact on
    treatment, 198
  framework for change, 196–197
  international efforts in, 200
Quality of life, gambling disorder
  effects on, 256–257
Quitting smoking. *See* Smoking cessation

R

Race, substance use disorder risk and,
  13–14
Randomization, clinical trials, 29
Rapid eye movement (REM), 479
Rapid opioid detoxification, 327–328
RBS programs. *See* Responsible
  beverage service programs
Readiness to change, adolescent
  placement criteria and, 609
Receptors, drug, 42
Recombinant human growth hormone,
  102
Recovery, 402
  cultural aspects of, 242–243, 242t
  spirituality role in, 429–431
  therapeutic community view of, 385
  twelve-step programs in, 419–423
Recovery coaches, for substance use
  disorders, 162
Recovery environment, adolescent
  placement criteria and, 609
Recovery group sessions, 361
Recovery social network, 405
Recruitment, into addiction treatment,
  356
Referral to treatment, by primary care
  providers, 199–200
Registered nurses (RNs), in addiction
  care, 203
Regulations for opioid use. *See*
  Guidance for opioid use
Rehabilitation Act of 1973,
  confidentiality, 637
Rehabilitation approaches, to chronic
  pain, 558–560
  with opioid use disorders, 575–576
Reimbursement considerations
  as barrier to linked services, 180–181
  clinical considerations versus, 173

Reinforcement, 365
  caffeine effects, 68
  neuroanatomy of, 16
    cannabinoids, 20
    opioids, 19–20
    psychostimulants, 17–19, 18f
Relapse
  after detoxification, 288
  potential of, adolescent placement
    criteria and, 609
  prevention of
    in adolescent substance abuse
      treatment, 618–619
    clinical interventions, 404–406
    cognitive–behavioral therapy
      for, 366
    definitions in, 402–403
    determinants of relapse and,
      403–404
    effectiveness and efficacy of, 403
    incarceration and, 673
  as process and event, 404
  reduction of
    alternative therapies for, 187
    for older adults, 238
Relative risk, 11
Religious experience, 430
REM. *See* Rapid eye movement
Remission, 13
Renal clinical syndromes, 454
Renal effects
  of alcohol use, 436, 454–455
  of MDMA, 452, 457
  stimulants, 62
  of substance use, 440, 455–458
  of tobacco use, 458
Repetitive TMS (rTMS), 351–352
Reproductive system
  alcohol use and, 490, 491t
  cannabinoid effects, 81
  stimulant effects, 63
  substance use and, 491–492, 491t
  tobacco use and, 490–491, 491t
Research. *See* Clinical trials
Researchers, assessment by, 137
Residential interventions, modified
    therapeutic communities,
    387t
Residential programs
  for adolescent substance abuse, 610
  for stabilization of imminent danger,
    174
  for SUDs, 162
Respiratory depression, 465
Respiratory infections, 465–466, 476
Respiratory system
  alcohol use and, 436, 467–468
  cannabinoid effects, 80
  common complications of, 465–466
  substance use and, 466–469
  tobacco use and, 466–467

Responsible beverage service (RBS)
    programs, 143
Restless legs syndrome (RLS), 479
Retention, women patients and, 222
Revex. *See* Nalmefene
ReVia. *See* Naltrexone
Reward circuits, 22, 251–252
  changes in, 591–592
  drug use and, 591
Rhabdomyolysis, 457
Rimonabant, 24, 78, 80
Risk education, overdose, 189–190,
    190t
Risk stratification, 645
RLS. *See* Restless legs syndrome
RNs. *See* Registered nurses
Rohypnol. *See* Flunitrazepam
Roid rage, 105
rTMS. *See* Repetitive TMS
Rush, Benjamin, 147

S

S2BI. *See* Screening to Brief
    Intervention
Safer injection practices, 190–191,
    191t, 216
Salvia divinorum, 85, 88, 116, 511t
Salvinorin A, 84–85, 88, 116
Sample size, 29–30
SBI. *See* Screening and brief
    intervention
SBIRT. *See* Screening, brief
    intervention, and referral to
    treatment
Schizophrenia, 340, 626–627
School prevention, 583–585
Screening
  for cancer, 433–434
  in older adults, 122, 128–129, 129t,
    235–237, 237t
Screening, brief intervention, and
    referral to treatment (SBIRT),
    199
  nursing role in, 204
  for SUD in patients with TBI,
    226–227
Screening and brief intervention (SBI),
    163
  in adolescents
    assessment, 598, 600
    for risks and problems, 596, 598
    screen-specific strategies, 598,
      599f
    treatment referral, 600
    for use, 596, 597f
  clinical guidelines for, 119–121
  in clinical settings using quality
    improvement principles,
    126–128, 127f
  current evidence on, 121–122
  individual studies on, 122–123

Screening and brief intervention (SBI)
(*Continued*)
national recommendations for, 119
in older adults, 122, 128–129, 129*t*
for pregnant women, 123–125, 494
systematic reviews and meta-
analyses on, 122
for trauma, 488, 488*t*
in trauma centers, hospitals, and
emergency departments,
125–126
Screening assessment tools, 138
adolescents, 602, 604, 605*t*
Screening to Brief Intervention (S2BI),
604, 605*t*
Screening urine immunoassays,
130–135, 131*t*, 134*t*
Secondhand smoke (SHS), 75–76
e-cigarette, 109
Sedative–hypnotics
for alcohol withdrawal, 292–296
intoxication with, 298, 322–323
misuse and abuse of, 322
neurologic disorders and, 470–471
nonmedical prescription, 211, 212*f*,
215
pharmacology of, 50–53, 321
physical dependence on, 322
physician addiction to, 279
psychiatric symptoms induced by, 510*t*
respiratory system and, 468
tolerance to, 51–52, 322
withdrawal from, 51–53
common treatment issues in, 302
evaluation and management of,
300–302, 302*t*
host factors affecting, 300
pharmacologic characteristics
affecting, 300
pharmacologic interventions for,
323–324
signs and symptoms of, 298–299,
299*t*
Sedative–hypnotic use disorder,
321–324
Seiberling, Henrietta, 420
Seizures, 471–472
alcohol withdrawal, 291–295
Selective serotonin reuptake inhibitors
(SSRIs), 517, 518*t*, 539–540,
543, 562–563
for cocaine use disorder, 338
for problematic sexual behavior, 264
Selegiline, 338
Self-efficacy, 403
Self-efficacy versus helplessness, 555
Self-help groups, 264
Self-management procedures, in
smoking cessation, 375–377
Self-management stage, of chronic care
management, 168*t*, 169–170

Self-medication theory, 537–538
Self-monitoring, of smoking behavior,
375
Self-reporting, 538, 603
Sensitivity, of laboratory test, 659–660
Sensitization, 42
alcohol, 47
in chronic pain, 548–549
covert, 390–391
stimulants, 64–65
Septic thromboemboli, 466
Serotonin (5-HT)
alcohol effects, 47
in binge eating disorder, 252
drug reinforcement and, 16–19, 18*f*
gambling effects, 251
stimulant effects, 6
Serotonin syndrome, 93, 314
Sertraline (Zoloft), 539
Sexual abuse, 222, 261
Sexual addiction, 260–261
Sexual assault
college drinking and, 245
in military (*See* Military sexual
trauma)
Sexual behavior. *See* Problematic
sexual behavior
Sexual function, stimulant effects, 63
Sexually transmitted diseases, 433, 477
Sexual minorities, 222
Sex with minors, 262
Shanghai Opium Commission, 650
Shoemaker, Sam, 420
Short Michigan Alcoholism Screening
Test–Geriatric version, 236, 237*t*
SHS. *See* Secondhand smoke
SIDD. *See* Substance-induced
depressive disorders
SIFs. *See* Supervised injection facilities
Significant others, community
reinforcement approach for, 372
Silkworth, William D., 420
Single Convention on Narcotic Drugs,
650–651
SIPDs. *See* Substance-induced
psychotic disorders
Skin and soft tissue infections, 475
Sleep
alcohol use and, 438, 480–482
disorders of, 479–480
in older adults, 235
substance use and, 441, 482–484
Small intestine, 461
SMART Recovery, 421–422
Smith, Robert, 147, 150, 420–421
Smokeless tobacco, 345
Smoking. *See* Tobacco use
Smoking cessation
aversion therapy for, 391
behavioral interventions for,
374–377

benefits, 76
choosing quit date, 375–376
e-cigarette use in, 110
motivation for, 375
pharmacologic interventions for,
342–346, 343*t*, 345*t*, 348–349
planning of, 374
preparing for, 374–375
self-monitoring in, 375
weight gain after, 345
SNAPs. *See* Syringe needle access
programs
Sober coaches, for substance use
disorders, 162
Social anxiety disorder, 517–519
Social influences, adolescent substance
use prevention and, 583
Social medicine, 35
Social network, 242, 242*t*, 379–382,
405
Social norms, drinking, 246
Social resistance skills, 584
Social support, 365, 379
Society, addiction challenges for, 5
Sociocultural interventions, 243
Sodium valproate, 294, 340
Software, ASAM Criteria, 177
Solvents, 97–100, 98*t*
Somatotropin, 102
Sorority organizations, college
drinking in, 246
Specificity, laboratory test, 659–660
Specimen collection, 130
Spectrum of use, 7–8
Spirituality, 423, 429–431
Sports, TBI in, 225
SSRIs. *See* Selective serotonin reuptake
inhibitors
Stabilization stage, of chronic care
management, 168*t*, 169
Stacking, anabolic–androgenic
steroids, 103
Stages of change, 354–358, 357*t*
Steatosis, 449
Steroids, AASs. *See* Anabolic–
androgenic steroids
Stigma
as barrier to linked services, 181
terminology for avoiding, 7–8, 9*t*, 10
Stimulants
for ADHD treatment, 527, 528*t*, 593
anxiety disorders and, 520–521
for cocaine use disorder, 338
drug action mimicry, 24*f*, 25
drug target blockade, 23, 23*t*, 24*f*
eating disorders and use of, 221
epidemiology, 61
historical features, 61
intoxication, 62, 309–310
neuroanatomy of reinforcement,
17–19, 18*f*

nonmedical prescription, 211, 212*f*, 214–215
perioperative patient and, 504
pharmacology, 60–66
during pregnancy, 497
psychiatric symptoms induced by, 510*t*
respiratory system and, 467
sleep and, 482
treatment for, 521
withdrawal, 62, 310
Stimulant use disorder, 337–341, 392
Stomach, 460
Stress inoculation training, 539
Stressors, 591
Stretching, 559
Stroke, 443, 472
Structural interventions, for college student drinking, 248
Student drinking. *See* College student drinking
Subcultures, addiction treatment and, 240
Subjective effects, hallucinogens, 86–89
Substance abuse, 7, 9
Substance-associated suicidal behavior, 509
Substance-induced anxiety disorder, 508–509
Substance-induced bipolar disorder, 509, 513
Substance-induced depressive disorders (SIDD), 507–509, 513
Substance-induced mental disorders, 626
   in *DSM-5*, 507, 508*t*
   prevalence and course of, 507–509, 510*t*–511*t*
Substance-induced psychiatric symptoms, 509, 510*t*–511*t*
Substance-induced psychotic disorders (SIPDs), 508–509, 522–523
Substance/medication-induced obsessive compulsive, 509
Substance-related mood disorders, 513–514
Substance-specific history, 241
Substance use. *See also specific substances*
   in adolescents (*See* Adolescent substance use)
   assessment of, 136–140, 137*t*
   compulsive sex in combination with, 262–263
   cultural coping with, 241–242
   cultural definitions related to, 240–241
   cultural patterns of, 241
   gender differences with, 219
   harm reduction and (*See* Harm reduction)

international policy frameworks for, 206–207
liver and, 452
medical consequences of, 438–441
metabolic disorders and, 440
neurologic disorders and, 470
perioperative patient and, 440–441, 503–504
during pregnancy, 496–498
screening and brief intervention for (*See* Screening and brief intervention)
sleep and, 441, 482–484
TBI and, 224–227
terminology for discussing spectrum of, 7–8
trauma and, 440, 486–487
trends in, 286
by women, 219–223
worldwide prevalence of, 206
in youth, 121
Substance use disorders (SUDs). *See also specific substance use disorders*
   ADHD co-occurring in, 525–530, 528*t*, 529*t*
   in adolescents (*See* Adolescent substance use disorders)
   anxiety disorders co-occurring in, 517–521
   ASAM Criteria for, 172–177, 174*t*, 175*t*, 176*f*
   behavioral addiction co-occurrence with, 275
   behavioral addiction features shared with, 274–275
   chronic pain and, 549–550, 555, 556*t*, 573–577, 574*t*
   comorbidity of PTSD, 537–540
   consent and confidentiality with, 636
   controlled medications and challenges with, 642–643
      risk stratification for, 645
      termination of, 647–648
   criteria for, 602–603
   denial in, 632–633
   drug testing and, 659–662
   eating disorders co-occurring in, 541–545
   epidemiology of, 11–14
   42 CFR Part 2 and, 638
   harm reduction and (*See* Harm reduction)
   inheritability and, 592–593, 604
   integrated care for (*See* Integrated care)
   mental disorders co-occurring with, therapeutic communities for, 384–388, 387*t*
   in military personnel, 675–679, 675–682, 676*f*, 677*f*, 679*f*

mood disorders co-occurring in, 513–515
   in older adults, 233–238, 234*t*, 237*t*, 515
   personality disorders co-occurring in, 532–535
   physician responsibility in, 33
   physicians with, 278–283
   prevention, 34
   primary care provider identification, treatment, or referral and monitoring of, 199–200
   psychotic disorders co-occurring in, 522–524
   public health promotion and, 33–34
   screening and assessment of, 120
   stressors and, 591
   substance use history and, 592
   TBI co-occurrence with, 225–227
   terminology for discussing, 8–9
   therapeutic community view of, 384
   transformational change and, 35–36
   treatment overview, 161–165 (*See also* Addiction treatment)
   unprecedented historical moment for, 166–167
   in women, 219–223
   worldwide prevalence of, 206
Substance use disorder treatment provider, assessment by, 137
Substance withdrawal. *See* Withdrawal
Substitution and tapering, sedative–hypnotics, 301, 302*t*
Subutex. *See* Buprenorphine
SUDs. *See* Substance use disorders
Suicidal behavior
   co-occurring mood and SUDs in, 515
   substance-associated, 509
Suicidality, in older adults, 235
Supervised injection facilities (SIFs), 191
Support groups, after aversion therapy, 392–393
Supportive–expressive therapy, 366
Support services, for substance use disorders, 162
Surgical risk, alcohol use and, 501–502
Sweetser, William, 147–148
Synthetic cannabinoids, 78, 80, 113–114
   adverse effects and toxicity, 81
   cardiovascular system and, 446
   chemistry of, 655
   clinical uses, 81
   laboratory testing for, 134–135
   as medicine, 656
   neurologic disorders and, 471
   ongoing preclinical studies, 81–82
   psychiatric symptoms induced by, 511*t*
   screening and brief intervention, 126
Synthetic cathinones, 113–114, 313, 622

Synthetic opioids, 113–115
    laboratory testing for, 133–134, 134*t*
    screening and brief intervention, 126
Synthetic stimulants, 60
Syringe needle access programs
        (SNAPs), 190–191, 191*t*, 216
Systems approach
    effecting change in health care, 36
    incarceration and, 673
Systems-based practice, 34–35

T

T-ACE questionnaire, 124
Take-back programs, 217
Talk therapy, 163–164
TAMF. *See* The Addiction Medicine
        Foundation
Tamoxifen, 102
Tanning, excessive, 273
Tapering, sedative–hypnotics, 301–302,
        302*t*, 323
Tapering regimen, 648
TBI. *See* Traumatic brain injury
TCAs. *See* Tricyclic antidepressants
TCs. *See* Therapeutic communities
Technology-based interventions, 122,
        367–368, 408–411
Technology model, for developing
        psychotherapies, 364
Telemedicine, 164
Teratogenicity, 495
Termination stage of change, 355
Terminology
    for avoiding stigma, 7–8, 9*t*, 10
    for discussing spectrum of use, 7–8
    for discussing SUDs, 8–9
    for discussing treatment, 9
Testosterone, 102–106
Tetrachloroethylene, 98*t*
Tetrafluoroethane, 98*t*
Δ9-Tetrahydrocannabinol (THC), 78–79
    changes in concentration of, 655
    chemistry of, 655
    laboratory testing for, 133
    during pregnancy, 496–497
    psychiatric symptoms induced by,
        511*t*
L-Tetrahydropalmatine (L-THP),
        186–187
THC. *See* Δ9-Tetrahydrocannabinol
The Addiction Medicine Foundation
        (TAMF), 152
*The ASAM Criteria: Treatment Criteria
        for Addictive, Substance-Related,
        and Co-Occurring Conditions,*
        172
Thebaine, 55
Theory of change, 269, 400
Therapeutic communities (TCs), 162
    modified, 386–388, 387*t*
    traditional, 384–386

Therapeutic ladder, 568
Therapy groups, 360
Thiamine deficiency, 294–295
Thirdhand smoke, 109
Thought disorders, in physicians, 279
L-THP. *See* L-Tetrahydropalmatine
Thyroid, 490
Tizanidine, 564
TMS. *See* Transcranial magnetic
        stimulation
Tobacco
    neurobiology of, 74, 342
    pharmacology of, 72–76
    pregnancy effects of, 75, 495
    withdrawal from, 74, 438
Tobacco use
    cancer and, 462
    cardiovascular system and, 444
    endocrine and reproductive
        disorders with, 490–491, 491*t*
    epidemiology of, 12–13
    gastrointestinal system and, 462
    international policy frameworks
        for, 207
    medical consequences of, 438
    in older adults, 234
    perioperative patient and, 438,
        503–504
    renal effects of, 458
    respiratory system and, 466–467
    screening and brief intervention for,
        119–120
    stroke and, 472
    worldwide prevalence of, 206
Tobacco use disorder
    alcohol use disorder with, 348, 377
    anxiety and, 519–520
    aversion therapy for, 391
    behavioral interventions for, 374–377
    depressive disorders and, 515
    neurobiology of, 342
    pharmacologic interventions for
        clinical decisions about, 346
        combination pharmacotherapy,
            344–345, 345*t*
        electronic nicotine delivery
            systems, 345
        genetics and, 345
        in multiple drug use disorders,
            348–349
        nicotine replacement therapy,
            342–343, 343*t*
        nonnicotine medications, 343–344
        postcessation weight gain and, 345
    treatment for, 519–520
Tolerance, 42
    alcohol, 47–48
    caffeine, 68
    cannabinoids, 79
    opioids, 58, 569
    pain and SUDs and, 550

sedative–hypnotics, 51–52, 322
stimulants, 64–65
Toluene, 97, 98*t*
Topiramate, 318, 339, 563, 622
Toxic alcohols, 455
Toxicity
    alcohol, 48
    cannabinoids, 80–81
    dissociatives, 94–95
    e-cigarettes, 110
    inhalants, 99–100
    nicotine and tobacco, 74–75
    novel psychoactive substances,
        114–115
    opioids, 58
    sedative–hypnotics, 52–53
    stimulants, 65
Toxicology screens, 285
Traditional Chinese medicines, 186–188
Transcranial magnetic stimulation
        (TMS), 351–352
Transcutaneous electrical acupuncture,
        187
Transformational change, 35–36
Transgender persons, 263
Trauma
    alcohol use and, 437, 486–487
    e-cigarettes and, 488–489
    interventions for, 487–488
    screening and brief intervention for,
        488, 488*t*
    substance use and, 440, 486–487
Trauma centers, screening and brief
        intervention in, 125–126
Traumatic brain injury (TBI), 224–227,
        225*t*, 470
Treatment. *See* Addiction treatment
Treatment agreements, 645–646
Treatment alliance, 365
Treatment culture, 222
Treatment failure, 173
Trexan. *See* Naltrexone
TRICARE, 678
Trichloroethane, 98*t*
Tricyclic antidepressants (TCAs), 338,
        527, 528*t*, 562–563
Triptorelin pamoate, 264
True negative, 659–660
True positive, 659–660
TSF. *See* Twelve-step facilitation
Tuberculosis, 433
TWEAK questionnaire, 124
Twelve-step approaches, 616–617
Twelve-step facilitation (TSF), 367,
        399–401
Twelve-step programs
    in addiction recovery, 419–423
    after aversion therapy, 392–393
    for problematic sexual behavior, 264
    recent research into, 424–427
    spirituality in, 429–431

U

U-47700, 305
Ultrarapid opioid detoxification,
327–328
Uncaria rhynchophylla, 187
Unhealthy alcohol use. *See* Alcohol
use
Unhealthy substance use. *See* Substance
use
United Nations Office on Drugs and
Crime (UNODC), 206, 207
Urine
identification of intoxication, 285
screening immunoassays, 130–135,
131*t*, 134*t*, 661
US Food and Drug Administration
(FDA)
approved dissociative formulations,
91
e-cigarette regulation, 111
on opioids, 579

V

VA. *See* Veterans Administration
VA. *See* Veterans Affairs
Vaccination, cocaine, 23
Valium, 50
Valproic acid, 563
Vaping. *See* Electronic cigarettes
Vapors. *See* Inhalants
Varenicline
in adolescents, 620–621
drug action mimicry, 25
for tobacco use disorder, 343–346,
345*t*, 348
Vasculitis, 456
Vegetable glycerin (VG), 108
Venlafaxine, 527, 528*t*
Ventral striatum, 16, 19–20
Ventral tegmental area (VTA), 17–20,
18*f*
Veterans. *See* Military personnel
Veterans Administration (VA),
screening and brief
intervention implementation
by, 126–128, 127*f*
Veterans Affairs (VA)
getting help for MST at, 231, 231*t*
MST screening in, 230
VG. *See* Vegetable glycerin

Vicodin. *See* Hydrocodone
Video game addiction, 253
Viral hepatitis, 450–452
Virtual therapy, 367–368
Vitamins, 434, 438
Vivitrol. *See* Naltrexone
VOCs. *See* Volatile organic compounds
Volatile chemicals, 97–100, 98*t*, 468
Volatile organic compounds (VOCs),
108–109
Voucher-based reinforcement therapy,
163–164
Vouchers intervention, 370–371
VTA. *See* Ventral tegmental area
Vulnerability, to addiction, 4
Vulnerable populations, linked services
for, 184

W

WADA. *See* World Anti-Doping
Agency
Warning signs, of relapse, 404
Washington Circle Group, 197
Washingtonian Total Abstinence
Society, 420
Weight gain, after smoking cessation,
345
Wender Utah Rating Scale, 526
Wernicke disease, 294–295
WHO. *See* World Health
Organization
Wilson, Bill, 420–421
Wilson, Lois, 421
Withdrawal
for adolescent placement criteria,
608
for adolescent SUDs, 623
alcohol (*See* Alcohol withdrawal
syndrome)
assessment tools for, 138–139
caffeine, 68–69
cannabinoids, 79–80, 311
clinical assessment for risk of, 125
club drugs, 312–314
dissociatives, 311–312
hallucinogens, 310–312
during hospitalization, 435
during incarceration, 672
inhalants, 312
initial management of, 125

management of, 309
ASAM Criteria use in, 288
goals and general principles of,
286–287
pharmacologic, 287
relapse after, 288
settings of, 287–288
in special populations, 288–289
medical consequences of, 439
nicotine and tobacco, 74, 438
opioid (*See* Opioid withdrawal)
sedative–hypnotics, 51–53, 298–302,
299*t*, 302*t*, 323–324
sleep in, 481
stimulant, 62, 310
Withdrawal stage, of addiction cycle,
3–4, 3*f*
Women. *See also* Pregnancy
in AA, 425
addiction treatment for, 219–223
Women for Sobriety, 422
Woodward, Samuel, 148
Workforce, nursing, 204–205
Workplace drug testing, 131, 664–665
World Anti-Doping Agency (WADA),
106
World Health Organization (WHO),
206, 207–208
World Medical Association, 208
Worldwide prevalence, of substance
use, 206
Written informed consent, 645–646

X

Xylene, 98*t*

Y

Yan hu so, 186
YGT (NPI-025), 186–187
Youth. *See also* Adolescents
cannabis legalization and, 587–590
screening and brief intervention in,
121–122

Z

Zaleplon, 50–52, 321
Zero-order elimination, 41
Zoloft. *See* Sertraline
Zolpidem, 50–52, 299, 321
Zopiclone, 299

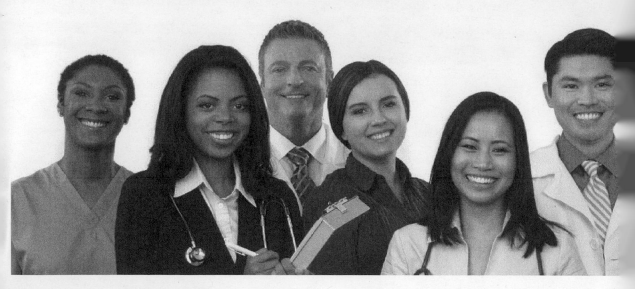

Join ASAM Today!

The American Society of Addiction Medicine (ASAM), founded in 1954, is a professional society representing physicians, clinicians, and associated professionals in the field of addiction medicine. ASAM is dedicated to increasing access and improving the quality of addiction treatment, educating physicians and the public, supporting research and prevention, and promoting the appropriate role of physicians in the care of patients with addiction.

Benefits Include:

The Journal of Addiction Medicine:
The Journal of Addiction Medicine, the official peer-reviewed Journal of ASAM, promotes excellence in the practice of addiction medicine and in clinical research as well as supports addiction medicine as a mainstream medical sub-specialty.

Shaping & Contributing to the Field
One of the most important ways is by helping to play an active role in shaping government policies that affect their livelihoods and the livelihoods of their patients.

Fellow Designation (FASAM)
ASAM's Fellow designation gives recognition to and raises awareness of ASAM members who are board certified addiction specialists.

Member Only Pricing
Recieved special pricing on ASAM's conferences, courses, online CME courses, and publications.

ASAM Career Center:
The ASAM Career Center offers job seekers free and confidential resume posting, automated weekly email notification of new job listings, and the ability to save jobs for later review.

CME - Member Exclusive Rates
ASAM has been an ACCME-accredited provider of continuing education since 1977, and is a recognized leader in the planning and presentation of educational events in the addiction field. Members recieve exclusive discounts on live and online ASAM courses and published texts.

Networking and Local Chapters
ASAM State Chapters provide networking, service, and professional learning opportunities for our members across the nation. Local events, courses, and meetings provide opportunities to network and develop lifelong professional relationships.

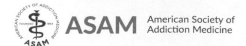 **ASAM** American Society of Addiction Medicine

www.ASAM.org/Join